PRINCIPLES OF NEURAL SCIENCE

SECOND EDITION

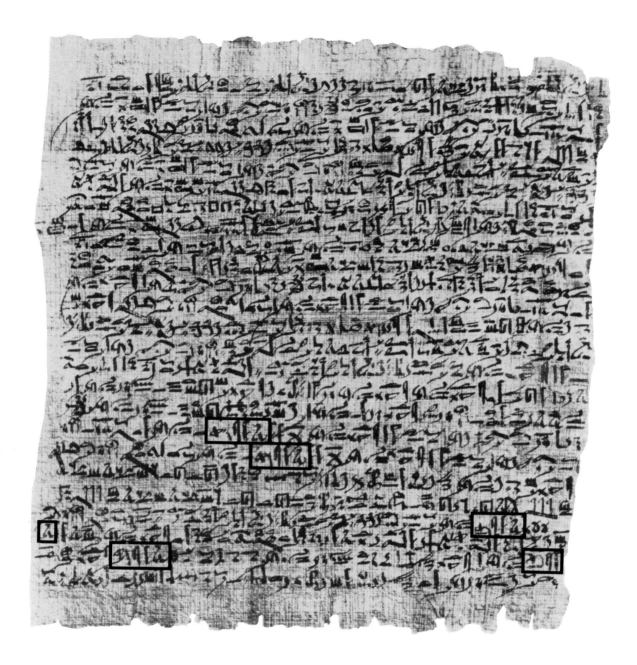

Columns II (left) and IV (right) of the Edwin Smith Surgical Papyrus

This papryus, written in the Seventeenth Century B.C., contains the earliest reference to the brain anywhere in human records. According to James Breasted, who translated and published the document in 1930, the word brain 𓄿𓏤𓇓 (ỷś) occurs only 8 times in ancient Egyptian, 6 of them on these pages of the Smith Papyrus describing the symptoms, diagnosis and prognosis of two patients, wounded in the head, who had compound fractures of the skull. The entire treatise is now in the Rare Book Room of the New York Academy of Medicine.

Reference: Breasted, James Henry. The Edwin Smith Surgical Papyrus, 2 volumes. The University of Chicago Press, Chicago. 1930.

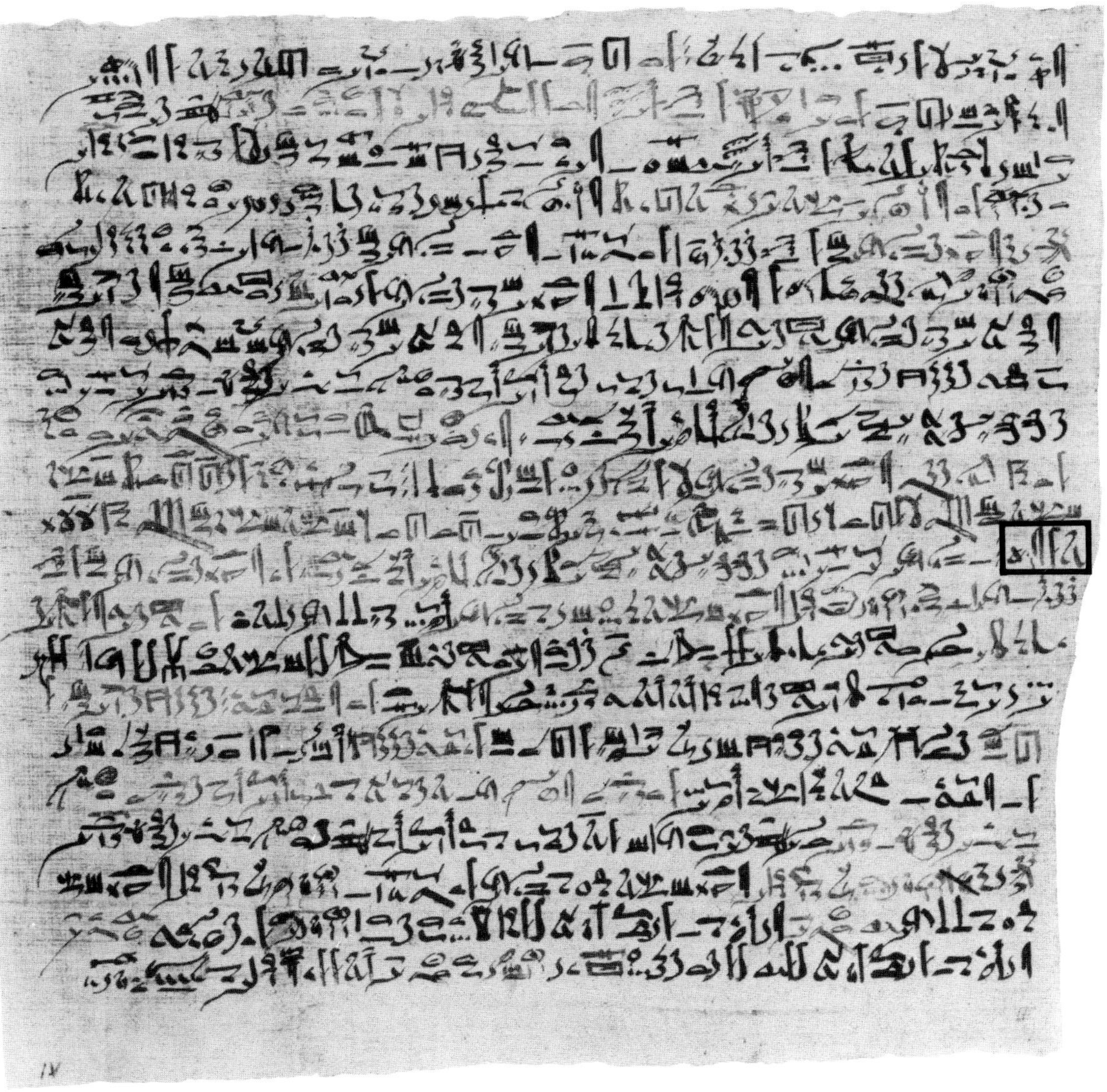

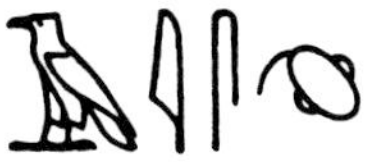

Men ought to know that from the brain, and from the brain only, arise our pleasures, joys, laughter and jests, as well as our sorrows, pains, griefs and tears. Through it, in particular, we think, see, hear, and distinguish the ugly from the beautiful, the bad from the good, the pleasant from the unpleasant . . . . It is the same thing which makes us mad or delirious, inspires us with dread and fear, whether by night or by day, brings sleeplessness, inopportune mistakes, aimless anxieties, absent-mindedness, and acts that are contrary to habit. These things that we suffer all come from the brain, when it is not healthy, but becomes abnormally hot, cold, moist, or dry, or suffers any other unnatural affection to which it was not accustomed. Madness comes from its moistness. When the brain is abnormally moist, of necessity it moves, and when it moves neither sight nor hearing are still, but we see or hear now one thing and now another, and the tongue speaks in accordance with the things seen and heard on any occasion.
But all the time the brain is still, a man can think properly.

attributed to Hippocrates,
Fifth Century, B.C.

PRINCIPLES OF NEURAL SCIENCE

SECOND EDITION

Edited by

ERIC R. KANDEL, M.D.

and

JAMES H. SCHWARTZ, M.D., PH.D.

Center for Neurobiology and Behavior
College of Physicians & Surgeons of Columbia University
and
Howard Hughes Medical Institute

Art rendered by Jonathan Dimes

ELSEVIER

New York • Amsterdam • Oxford

Elsevier Science Publishing Co., Inc.
52 Vanderbilt Avenue, New York, New York 10017

Sole distributors outside the United States and Canada:
Elsevier Science Publishers B.V.
P.O. Box 211, 1000 AE Amsterdam, The Netherlands

Library of Congress Cataloging in Publication Data

Main entry under title:

Principles of neural science.

    Bibliography: p.
    Includes index.
    1. Neurology. 2. Neurons. I. Kandel, Eric R. II. Schwartz, James H.
    [DNLM: 1. Behavior. 2. Nervous System Diseases. 3. Neurochemistry.
    4. Neurons. 5. Neurophysiology. WL 102 P9547]
QP355.2.P76   1985   599'.0188   85-4563
ISBN 0-444-00944-2

Frontispiece quotation from *Hippocrates*, Vol. 2, translated by W. H. S. Jones,
London and New York: William Heinemann and Harvard University Press, 1923,
Chapter XVII: "The Sacred Disease," p. 175.

Director of Editing Barbara A. Conover
Coordinating Editor Diane Maass
Copy Editor Ruth Melnick
Design Edmée Froment
Layout Susan Schmidler
Art Services Virginia Kudlak
Art rendered by Jonathan Dimes
                Department of Art as Applied to Medicine
                The Johns Hopkins University School of Medicine
Cover Design Paul Agule Design
Compositor The Clarinda Company
Printer and Binder Halliday Lithograph

Current printing (last digit)
10 9 8 7 6 5 4 3 2

Manufactured in the United States of America

We dedicate the second edition of this book to our many colleagues
in the neurobiology community across the country who have read earlier versions
of these chapters critically and who have offered
many useful and important suggestions for their improvement.

Contents

Preface

Four major advances have occurred since the appearance of the first edition of *Principles of Neural Science,* and they have stimulated us to undertake this revision earlier than we had planned. The *first* advance has been an application of recombinant DNA and monoclonal antibody techniques to the nervous system. These methods have made accessible the solution of many neurobiological problems; for example, it is now possible to study the genome of the nerve cell fruitfully and to determine the complete structure of several membrane proteins important for signaling. Many new neuropeptides and their precursors have also been identified. The organization of the genes that encode them is being rapidly mapped. In addition, these techniques are beginning to elucidate the molecular details that distinguish different neuronal cell types. The *second* important advance is patch clamping, which has allowed investigators to explore in intact membranes the conformational changes that occur in single ion channels. This advance is bringing our understanding of the precise molecular changes underlying synaptic transmission to a new level. It also has important implications for the future development of pharmacological agents used to treat a wide range of clinical disorders. The *third* advance, the revolution in nerve cell labeling and cell tracing methods, has clarified many previously poorly understood relationships between brain structure and behavior. *Fourth,* new, noninvasive methods of imaging have made it possible to study anatomical structures in the living human brain. Because of these last two advances, neuroanatomy can now be taught in an integrated manner with other segments of neural science.

In addition to major developments in methodology and technique, an important conceptual advance is that neural scientists have recognized that cell and molecular biology are crucial to their field. Although half a decade ago few neural scientists would have denied the importance of regarding the neuron in cell-biological terms, this approach to studying the nervous system was, until very recently, by no means central to the field, nor was it particularly useful for dealing with most day-to-day problems, either in the experimental laboratory or in the clinic. Today the view that neural science is a special—and important—part of cell biology has become commonplace. Only when neuronal function is viewed as a consequence of the activities of specific molecular components within nerve cells can the great importance of the new advances in neural science be appreciated. As the boundaries of neural science expand, and with them our understanding of the mechanisms of perception, behavior, and learning, so must the way in which neural science is taught.

The modern era in neural science began about 35 years ago. In 1953, John Eccles reviewed results based on the first intracellular recordings from single nerve and muscle cells in a book he modestly entitled *The Neurophysiological Basis of Mind.* At that time, this title seemed overly bold because so little was then known about the mechanisms of behavior. What could be learned by sticking cells with microelectrodes that could possibly help in understanding the mind? As time passed, many of us have read this marvelous book again, and each time we are more impressed with its author's prophetic insight. Eccles' book pointed the field in the right direction: its major message is the necessity to study the brain in terms of its elementary units—individual nerve cells. Only by applying analytical techniques that can resolve neural processes at a cellular level can we develop a realistic and coherent understanding of how the brain works. Studying nerve cells with analytical techniques, however, is necessary but not sufficient for understanding how the brain works (how we think, behave, feel, act, and interact with one another). It is also essential to relate cellular function to behavior.

In the years since *The Neurophysiological Basis of Mind* was published, neural science clearly has not yet fulfilled the promise implied in Eccles' title. We hope to show, however, that neural science is beginning to give insight into some of the most difficult problems of cellular differentiation on the one hand, and some of the most profound problems of behavior on the other. For example, considering that the brain is made up of a million million (10^{12}) cells, it is remarkable how much has been learned about the functioning of the nervous system as a whole by looking at nerve cells one at a time. It has become apparent from cellular studies that the building blocks of different regions of the vertebrate nervous system, and indeed of the nervous systems of all animals, are quite similar. What distinguishes one brain region from another and one brain from the next are the number of building blocks and the ways they are interconnected. Moreover, by applying a cellular approach to different sensory systems of the brain, it is possible to gain insight into how visual and other sensory stimuli are sorted out and transformed at various brain levels and how these regions contribute to perception. These cellular studies show that the brain does not simply replicate the external world or project it onto a tabula rasa, but begins at the lowest levels of the sensory system to abstract and represent reality according to its own rules by encoding it into informational signals. These developments in neural science press upon the borders of experimental psychology. We hope that the merger of neural science and experimental psychology, which we encourage in this text, will in turn lead to further advances in understanding behavior and learning.

The second edition is again designed as an introductory text for students of biology, behavior, and medicine. A major change in this edition is a more extensive treatment of neuroanatomy. The growth of functional neuroanatomy has made it possible both to describe the principles that underlie the anatomical structure of each system of the brain and to discuss each structure in terms of its physiology on the one hand, and its role in behavior and disease on the other.

Our goal in this textbook is to convey the interest and excitement surrounding the application of cell- and molecular-biological techniques to the study of the nervous system, how the brain develops, and how it controls behavior. This text also emphasizes those neurological and behavioral disorders that are both instructive scientifically and important clinically. We have again attempted to be selective and to stress the major principles that emerge from the study of the nervous system without becoming lost in detail. Toward this end we have divided the book into eleven parts, covering the following topics:

1. An overall view of the brain,
2. The cell and molecular biology of the neuron,
3. The mechanisms of synaptic transmission,
4. The anatomical organization of the nervous system,
5. The cellular basis of perception,
6. The control of movement,
7. The brain stem and reticular core,
8. Motivation and homeostasis,
9. Localization of higher cognitive functions, and the disorders of language, thought, and affect,
10. Development and the emergence of behavior, and
11. Genes, experience, and the mechanisms behavior.

In addition, we include an appendix on brain fluids, neuroophthalmology, and a discussion of current flow in neurons together with some practice problems for self study.

Our ultimate aim is to integrate information from experimental studies with practical areas of interest. For the general student, it will be important to see how basic information about the nervous system can be applied to psychology. For the student of medicine, integration with the clinical fields of neurology and psychiatry is of prime importance. Integration with neurology is relatively easy; neurology and neural science have long been interdependent. The bridge to psychiatry is more difficult. Thus far, neural science has taken only rudimentary steps toward understanding the mind. We have therefore tried to provide a systematic introduction to the biological basis of behavior and higher functions. Behavior is one of the last frontiers in biology at which we still stand in relative ignorance. We hope that this text will encourage the student to view behavior with the same combined social and biological perspective that serves so well in other areas of biology and medicine.

The past 35 years have seen splendid progress in the techniques and practice of neurology and psychiatry, but we believe that this textbook would be inadequate if it were only to summarize the information now accumulated that is directly pertinent to clinical practice. We also consider it our responsibility to impart a sense of direction for future developments by introducing students to the most important advances of our times, so that they will be able to evaluate the progress of this field in years to come. For this reason we are not content to consider only those aspects of neural science immediately relevant to neurology and psychiatry, but shall also discuss important scientific developments from current studies of animals that promise to provide a foundation for more effective understanding of normal and abnormal human behavior.

Engraved at the entrance to the Temple of Apollo at Delphi was the famous maxim "Know thyself." Central to enlightened Western culture from ancient times has been the idea that it is wise to understand oneself and one's behavior. Needed not only for clinical application, neural science is required for understanding human behavior, because all behavior is an expression of neural activity. Beyond medicine, in society at large, the problems of crowding, addiction, violence, and war are rooted in the nature of human beings. Any intelligent attempts at solving the enormous problems of human behavior, both individual and collective, must benefit from greater knowledge of neural function. Many of these problems are not yet in the domain of neural science, but progress is rapid and we can hope that neural scientists will soon be able to contribute directly to understanding them.

Eric R. Kandel
James H. Schwartz

Acknowledgments

Columbia has provided a stimulating intellectual environment that encourages interaction between basic science and clinical departments, an essential condition for writing an interdisciplinary book. It is therefore a pleasure once again to express our indebtedness to Donald F. Tapley and to the College of Physicians & Surgeons of Columbia University.

Many colleagues read portions of the manuscript critically. We are particularly indebted to John H. Martin and James P. Kelly for reading and commenting on all the anatomical chapters of the book and for helping us with the anatomical drawings. In addition, the following friends and colleagues have made constructive comments on various chapters, many of which have been incorporated into the present text: Israel Abramov, Paul Adams, Richard Aldrich, Robert Baker, Michael Bennett, Thomas Bever, Emilio Bizzi, Floyd Bloom, Robert Bowker, Dana Brooks, Michael Brownstein, Gail Burd, Paul Burgess, Robert Burke, John Byrne, Greg Clark, Bernard Cohen, David Corey, Maxwell Cowan, Joseph Coyle, John Davis, Nigel Daw, Mahlon Delong, Marc Dichter, John Dowling, Daniel Drachman, Ronald Dubner, Henry Epstein, Gerald Fischbach, Albert Fuchs, Harold Gainer, Michael Gazzaniga, Norman Geschwind, Charles Gilbert, Sid Gilman, Alexander Glassman, Mitchell Glickstein, Daniel Goldberg, Jay Goldberg, Michael Goldberg, Patricia Goldman-Rakic, Frederick Goodwin, James Gordon, Raymond Guillery, William Harris, Robert Hawkins, John Heuser, Stephen Highstein, Donald Hood, Richard Horn, James Houk, Albert Hudspeth, Jane Ellen Huttenlocher, Dorothea Jameson-Hurvich, Edward Jones, Jon Kaas, Arthur Karlin, Harvey Karten, Darcy Kelly, Donald Klein, Kenneth Knoblauch, Arnold Kriegstein, Simon LeVay, John Liebeskind, Margaret Livingstone, Rodolfo Llinás, Joseph Martin, Robert McMasters, Herbert Meltzer, Michael Merzenich, George Miller, Robert Moore, Anthony Movshon, Ralph Norgren, Sanford Palay, James Patrick, Paul Patterson, Edward Perl, Joel Pokorny, Jerome Posner, Isak Prohovnik, Edward Pugh, Dale Purves, Marcus Raichle, Pasco Rakic, Henry Ralston, Steven Rayport, Thomas Reese, Robert Rescorla, Harris Ripps, Norman Robbins, David Robinson, Paul Rozin, Kalman Rubinson, Zev Rymer, Harold Sackeim, Joseph Schildkraut, Stephen Schuetze, Carla Shatz, Gordon Shepherd, Murray Sherman, Ann-Judith Silverman, Barry Smith, Solomon Snyder, Louis Sokoloff, Nicholas Spitzer, Eliot Stellar, Peter Sterling, Charles Stevens, David Stoney, Michael Stryker, Larry Swanson, Herbert Terrace, Thomas Thach, Richard Tsien, David Van Essen, Stephen Waxman, Victor Wilson, Paul Witovsky, Kenneth Wolf, and Robert Wurtz.

We are again greatly indebted to Kathrin Hilten, who has been with the Center for Neurobiology and Behavior since its inception, for the initial preparation and final editing of the artwork. As always she took on this difficult and time-consuming task by combining expertise with judgment and good humor. We are also grateful to Sally Muir for her invaluable help. She read, edited, and improved this text, as she did its predecessor. We thank the Department of Art as Applied to Medicine, The Johns Hopkins University School of Medicine, and Terese Winslow for their work on the final figures, and Julie Ann Miller for reading and commenting on the text. We are grateful to Linda Sproviero, Barbara Sloane, and Erilyn Riley for coordinating the production of the book at Columbia, Harriet Ayers and Andrew Krawetz for typing, Ruth Melnick for copy editing the manuscript, Mildred Bobrovich for checking the bibliography, and Judy Cuddihy for preparing the index. Finally, we are grateful to Diane Maass at Elsevier for her critical assistance in producing this edition, and to Yale Altman for his enthusiastic and continued support of this book.

Contributors
College of Physicians & Surgeons of Columbia University

Craig H. Bailey, Ph.D.
Assistant Professor, Departments of Anatomy and Cell Biology
and Psychiatry; Center for Neurobiology and Behavior

John C. M. Brust, M.D.
Professor, Department of Neurology; Director of Neurology
Service, Harlem Hospital

Thomas J. Carew, Ph.D.
Professor, Departments of Psychology and Biology, Yale
University

Vincent Castellucci, Ph.D.
Associate Professor, Department of Psychiatry;
Center for Neurobiology and Behavior and the New York
State Psychiatric Institute

Shu Chien, M.D., Ph.D.
Professor, Department of Physiology; Director, Division of
Circulatory Physiology and Biophysics

Lucien Côté, M.D.
Associate Professor, Departments of Neurology and
Rehabilitation Medicine

Michael Crutcher, Ph.D.
Research Fellow, Center for Neurobiology and Behavior

Stanley Fahn, M.D.
H. Houston Merritt Professor, Department of Neurology

Michael D. Gershon, M.D.
Professor and Chairman, Department of Anatomy and Cell
Biology

Claude Ghez, M.D.
Professor, Departments of Neurology and Physiology; Center
for Neurobiology and Behavior and the New York State
Psychiatric Institute

Peter Gouras, M.D.
Professor, Department of Ophthalmology

Eric R. Kandel, M.D.
University Professor, Departments of Physiology
and Psychiatry; Center for Neurobiology and Behavior;
Senior Investigator, Howard Hughes Medical Institute

Dennis D. Kelly, Ph.D.
Associate Professor, Department of Psychiatry; New York State
Psychiatric Institute

James P. Kelly, Ph.D.
Research Scientist, Department of Anatomy and Cell Biology

John Koester, Ph.D.
Associate Professor, Department of Psychiatry; Acting Director,
Center for Neurobiology and Behavior; New York State
Psychiatric Institute

Irving Kupfermann, Ph.D.
Professor, Departments of Psychiatry and Physiology; Center
for Neurobiology and Behavior

John H. Martin, Ph.D.
Assistant Professor, Department of Psychiatry; Center for
Neurobiology and Behavior

Richard Mayeux, M.D.
Associate Professor, Department of Neurology

Lewis P. Rowland, M.D.
Henry & Lucy Moses Professor and Chairman, Department
of Neurology; Director of Neurological Service,
Presbyterian Hospital

Edward J. Sachar, M.D.
The late Lawrence C. Kolb Professor and Chairman,
Department of Psychiatry

Samuel Schacher, Ph.D.
Assistant Professor, Departments of Anatomy and Cell Biology
and Psychiatry; Center for Neurobiology and Behavior and the
New York State Psychiatric Institute

James H. Schwartz, M.D., Ph.D.
Professor, Departments of Physiology and Neurology; Center
for Neurobiology and Behavior; Investigator, Howard Hughes
Medical Institute

Steven Siegelbaum, Ph.D.
Assistant Professor, Department of Pharmacology; Center for
Neurobiology and Behavior

An Overall View

I

One of the last frontiers of science, perhaps its ultimate challenge, is to understand the biological basis of mentation: how we perceive, act, learn, and remember. What rules relate the anatomy and physiology of the brain to perception and to movement? Can these rules be discerned best by examining the brain as a whole or by studying its individual nerve cells and their important molecular constituents? How do genes contribute to behavior, and how is gene expression in nerve cells regulated by developmental and environmental processes? In Part I of this book we introduce the study of the nervous system by considering to what degree mental processes can be located to specific regions of the brain. We then go on to examine, using simple examples, how behavior can be understood in terms of the properties of specific nerve cells and their interconnections.

Eric R. Kandel

Brain and Behavior

1

The key philosophical theme of modern neural science is that all behavior is a reflection of brain function. According to this view—a view that is held by most neurobiologists and that we shall try to document in this text—the mind represents a range of functions carried out by the brain. The action of the brain underlies not only relatively simple behavior such as walking and smiling, but also elaborate functions such as feeling, learning, thinking, and writing a poem. As a corollary, the disorders of affect (emotion) and cognition (thought) that characterize neurotic and psychotic illness must result from disturbances of the brain.

The brain is made up of individual units—the nerve cells (or neurons) and the glial cells. The task of the neural sciences is to explain how the brain marshalls these units to control behavior and how, in turn, the functioning of the constituent cells in an individual's brain is influenced by the behavior of other people as well as by a host of environmental factors. In this and the next chapter we provide an introductory overall view of this task. In this chapter we shall consider the strategies used by the human brain in representing language, the most elaborate cognitive behavior. We shall examine the cerebral cortex, the part of the brain that has expanded most in recent evolution and is concerned with higher aspects of behavior. We shall illustrate how large groups of neurons are organized spatially within the nervous system and how, on the *regional level*, even the most complex behavior can be localized to a family of specific areas of the brain. In the next chapter we shall consider on the *cellular level* the relationship between nerve cells and a simple reflex behavior by examining how sensory signals are transformed into motor acts.

Two Alternative Views Have Been Advanced on the Relationship between Brain and Behavior

Current views of nerve cells, the brain, and behavior have emerged relatively recently from a fusion, at the end of the nineteenth century, of four experimental traditions: neuroanatomy, physiology, biochemical pharmacology, and the study of behavior.

The anatomical complexity of nervous tissue was not appreciated before the invention of the compound microscope. Until the eighteenth century, nervous tissue was thought to be glandular in function because of Galen's proposal that nerves are ducts conveying fluid secreted by the brain and spinal cord to the periphery of the body. Histology of the nervous system became a modern science during the nineteenth century, culminating in the investigations of Camillo Golgi and Santiago Ramón y Cajal, who shared the sixth Nobel Prize in medicine and physiology in 1906. Golgi developed the silver impregnation methods that allowed microscopic visualization of the whole neuron with all its processes: the cell body, the dendrites, and the axon. Using Golgi's staining techniques to label individual cells, Cajal showed that the nervous system is not a mass of fused cells sharing a common cytoplasm, but a highly intricate network of discrete cells. In the course of this work, Cajal developed some of the key conceptual insights and much of the empirical support for the *neuron doctrine*—the principle that the nervous system is made up of many individual signaling elements, the neurons.

Neurophysiology, the second scientific discipline fundamental to the modern view of nervous function, began in the eighteenth century when Luigi Galvani discovered that the nerve cells of animals produce electricity. During the nineteenth century the foundations of electrophysiology were laid by Emil DuBois-Reymond and Hermann von Helmholtz, who found that nerve cells use their electrical capabilities for signaling information to one another. The third discipline, biochemical pharmacology, started at the end of the nineteenth century with Claude Bernard, Paul Ehrlich, and John N. Langley, each of whom realized that drugs interact with specific receptors on the surface of cells, an insight that became the basis of the modern study of chemical synaptic transmission.

Psychology, the fourth discipline important for relating brain to behavior, has the longest history. In the West, ideas about mind and soul are derived from antiquity. Behavior, the manifestation of mind in the physical world, was not approached scientifically until the nineteenth century, when Charles Darwin's work on evolution of behavior allowed psychology to develop as a discipline independent of philosophy and to become experimental.

The merger of anatomy, physiology, and the study of behavior began with the work of the phrenologists, led by the Viennese physician and neuroanatomist Franz Joseph Gall. At the beginning of the nineteenth century, Gall had the prescience to appreciate that the functions of the mind are carried out by the brain. He postulated that the brain is not a unitary organ but a collection of at least 35 domains or centers (later others were added),

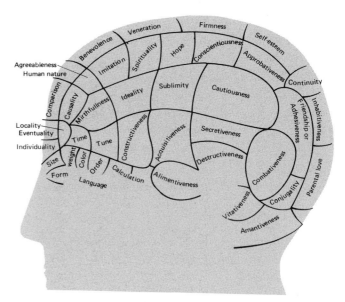

1–1 Phrenologists attempted to localize higher brain functions on the basis of bumps and ridges on the skull. This map of the skull, taken from an early nineteenth-century drawing, distinguishes more than 35 intellectual and emotional faculties and localizes them to individual and distinct areas of the cerebral cortex. (Adapted from Spurzheim, 1825.)

each corresponding to a specific mental function. Gall thought that even the most elaborate and abstract of these functions—generosity, mother love, secretiveness—were discretely localized to single areas of the cerebral cortex. Gall and the phrenologists further believed that the center for each mental function could develop and increase in size as a result of use, much as the size of a muscle is increased by exercise. As each center grew, it would give rise to specific protuberances on the surface of the head, and the location of these cranial bumps was thought to reflect the development of specific regions of the underlying brain (Figure 1–1). By correlating the personality of individuals with the bumps on their skulls, Gall sought to develop a new, objective science for describing character based on the anatomy of the brain—*anatomical personology*.

This extreme and fanciful view was an easy target for Pierre Flourens, a French neurologist working in the nineteenth century. By removing various portions of the brains of experimental animals, he attempted to determine the specific contribution of different parts of the nervous system to behavior. Flourens concluded that particular mental functions are not localized, but that the brain, and especially the cerebral cortex, acts as a whole for each mental function. He proposed that any part of the cerebral cortex is able to perform all of the cortex's functions. Injury to a specific area of the cortex would therefore affect all higher functions equally. The rapid and fairly general acceptance of this belief (subsequently called the *aggregate field* view of the brain) was based only partly on Flourens' experimental work. It also represented a philosophical reaction against the extreme localizationist view proposed by the phrenologists.

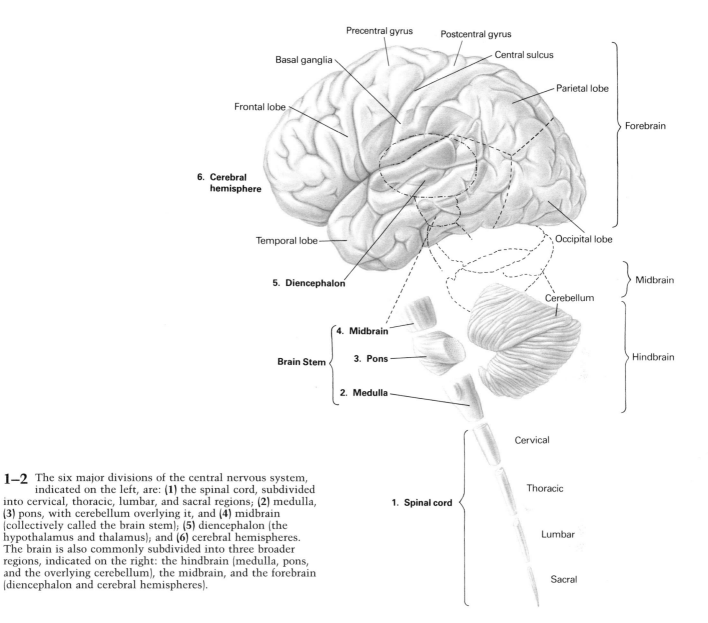

1–2 The six major divisions of the central nervous system, indicated on the left, are: **(1)** the spinal cord, subdivided into cervical, thoracic, lumbar, and sacral regions; **(2)** medulla, **(3)** pons, with cerebellum overlying it, and **(4)** midbrain (collectively called the brain stem); **(5)** diencephalon (the hypothalamus and thalamus); and **(6)** cerebral hemispheres. The brain is also commonly subdivided into three broader regions, indicated on the right: the hindbrain (medulla, pons, and the overlying cerebellum), the midbrain, and the forebrain (diencephalon and cerebral hemispheres).

In the middle of the nineteenth century J. Hughlings Jackson, a British neurologist, broke with the aggregate field view espoused by Flourens. Jackson's clinical studies of focal epilepsy (convulsions beginning in one part of the body) showed that different motor and sensory activities are localized to different parts of the brain. These studies were later elaborated systematically by the German neurologist Carl Wernicke and by Cajal into an alternative view of brain function called *cellular connectionism*. According to this view, neurons are the signaling units of the brain, and they connect to one another in precise fashion. Wernicke showed that behavior is mediated by specific regions and through discrete pathways connecting sensory and motor structures.

The history of the dispute between the proponents of the aggregate field and cellular connection views of cortical function can best be illustrated by the analysis of language, the highest and most characteristic human function. Before we consider the relevant clinical and anatomical studies concerned with the localization of language, let us briefly survey the structure of the brain.

Regions of the Brain Are Specialized for Different Functions

The central nervous system, which is bilateral and essentially symmetrical, consists of six main parts (Figure 1–2).

1. The *spinal cord*, the most caudal part of the central nervous system, receives information from the skin, joints, and muscle of the trunk and limbs, and sends out motor commands for movement, both reflex and voluntary.
2. The *medulla oblongata* is the rostral extension of the spinal cord.

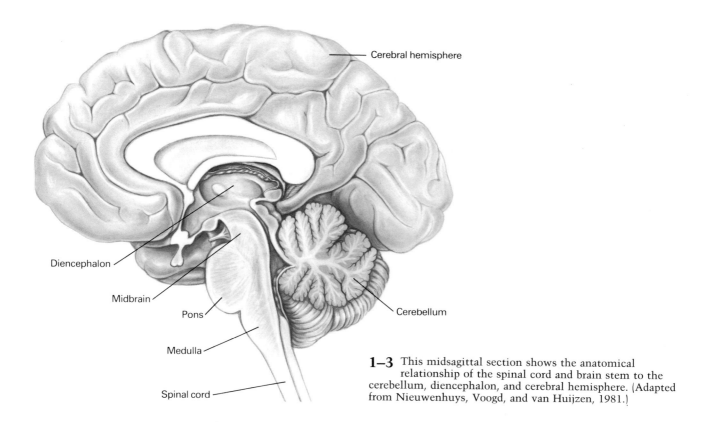

Cerebral hemisphere

Diencephalon

Midbrain

Pons

Medulla

Spinal cord

Cerebellum

1–3 This midsagittal section shows the anatomical relationship of the spinal cord and brain stem to the cerebellum, diencephalon, and cerebral hemisphere. (Adapted from Nieuwenhuys, Voogd, and van Huijzen, 1981.)

3. The *pons* and the *cerebellum* (which lies behind the pons) are rostral to the medulla. The cerebellum is concerned with modulating the force and range of movement.

4. The *midbrain* lies rostral to the pons between what is called the *hindbrain* (the medulla, pons, and cerebellum) and the *forebrain* (the diencephalon and cerebral cortex).

The medulla, pons, and midbrain—referred to collectively as the *brain stem*—mediate a wide variety of functions. The brain stem contains several collections of cell bodies, called the cranial nerve nuclei. Some of these nuclei receive information from the skin and muscles of the head and also much of the information from the special senses of hearing, balance, and taste. Other nuclei control motor output to the muscles of the face, neck, and eyes. Another key structure in the brain stem is the diffuse reticular formation, which is important in determining levels of arousal and awareness.

5. The *diencephalon* contains two key relay structures. One, the *thalamus*, processes most of the information reaching the cerebral cortex from the rest of the central nervous system. The other, the *hypothalamus*, regulates autonomic, endocrine, and visceral integration.

6. The *cerebral hemispheres* consist of the *basal ganglia* and the overlying *cerebral cortex*. Both the cortex and the basal ganglia are concerned with higher perceptual, cognitive, and motor functions.

The precise anatomical interrelationships of these several key structures are shown in Figures 1–3 and 1–4. The revolution in modern imaging techniques is making it possible to visualize these interrelationships in the living human brain (Figure 1–4B). We shall learn more about these advances in Chapter 22.

Thus, different regions of the brain are specialized for different functions. One of the reasons that this conclusion eluded Flourens and other investigators for so many years lies in another organizational principle of the nervous system known as *parallel processing*. As we shall see below, many sensory, motor, and other mental functions are subserved by more than one neural pathway. When one region or pathway is damaged, others often are able to compensate partially for the loss, thereby obscuring the behavioral evidence for localization. However, the precision with which certain higher functions are actually localized emerges clearly from a consideration of language, which we shall turn to next.

Cognitive Function Can Be Localized within the Cerebral Cortex

To understand how language is localized, we shall be concerned primarily with the cerebral cortex. The cortex of each of the brain's two hemispheres is divided into four anatomically distinct lobes: the *frontal, parietal, occipital,* and *temporal* (Figure 1–2). These lobes are specialized in function. The frontal lobe is largely concerned

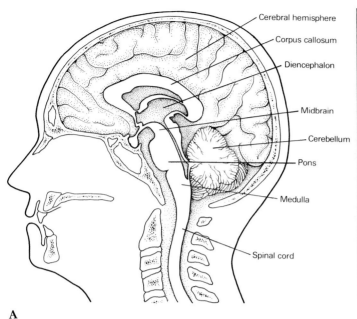

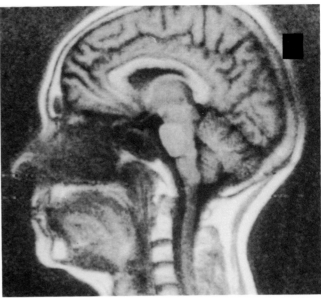

A

B

1–4 The major regions of the brain are shown here in a midsagittal view of the intact skull. **A.** The right half of the brain is shown schematically in the normal skull to indicate the position of the major brain structures in relation to external landmarks. The corpus callosum is a large fiber bundle that interconnects the left and right hemispheres. **B.** The same section as in **A** is illustrated here in the living brain by the use of magnetic resonance imaging (MRI).

with planning and with movement, the parietal with somatic sensation, the occipital with vision, and the temporal with audition as well as with learning, memory, and emotion. Each lobe has several characteristic convolutions or infoldings (an old evolutionary trick to increase surface area). The crests of the convolutions are called *gyri*. The intervening grooves are called *sulci* or *fissures*. The more prominent gyri and sulci are similar from one individual to another and therefore have specific names with respect to each other (for example, precentral gyrus, central sulcus, and postcentral gyrus).

The organization of the cerebral cortex is characterized by two important features. First, each hemisphere is concerned primarily with sensory and motor processes of the *contralateral* side of the body. Sensory information that enters the spinal cord from the left side of the body crosses over to the right side of the nervous system (either at the level of the spinal cord or later at the level of the brain stem) before being conveyed to the cerebral cortex. Similarly, the motor areas in one hemisphere exert control over the movements of the opposite half of the body. Second, the hemispheres, although quite similar, are not completely symmetrical in structure, nor are they equivalent in function.

Much of what we know about the localization of normal language has come from the study of *aphasia*, a disorder of language that is found most commonly in patients who have suffered from stroke, an occlusion of a blood vessel supplying a portion of the cerebral cortex. Many of the important discoveries in the study of aphasia occurred in rapid succession during the last half of the nineteenth century and form an exciting chapter in the history of human psychology. The first advance was made in 1861 with the publication of a paper by the French neurologist Pierre Paul Broca. Broca described the case of a patient who could understand language but who

had lost the ability to speak. The patient did not have a conventional motor deficit. He could utter isolated words and sing a melody without difficulty, but he could not speak grammatically. He could neither form fluent sentences nor express his ideas in writing. Postmortem examination of his brain showed a lesion in the posterior portion of the frontal lobe (an area now called *Broca's area*; Figure 1–5). Broca next collected eight similar cases, all of whom showed lesions that included this site. In all of these cases, the lesion was located in the left half of the brain. This discovery led Broca to announce, in 1864, one of the most famous principles of brain function: *"Nous parlons avec l'hémisphère gauche!"* ("We speak with the left hemisphere!")

Broca also noted that all those with a speech disorder from damage to the left hemisphere were right-handed individuals and all sustained a weakness or paralysis of the right hand. This observation in turn led to the generalization that there is a crossed relationship between hemispheric dominance and hand preference.

Broca's work stimulated a wider search for the cortical loci of behavioral function—a search that was soon rewarded. In 1870, nine years after Broca's initial discovery, Gustav Theodor Fritsch and Eduard Hitzig galvanized the scientific community with their discovery that characteristic movements of a limb can be produced in dogs by

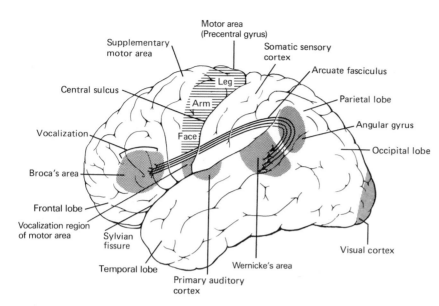

Motor area
(Precentral gyrus)

Supplementary
motor area

Somatic sensory
cortex

Central sulcus

Arcuate fasciculus

Leg

Parietal lobe

Arm

Vocalization

Angular gyrus

Face

Occipital lobe

Broca's area

Frontal lobe

Vocalization region
of motor area

Sylvian
fissure

Temporal lobe

Wernicke's area

Primary auditory
cortex

Visual cortex

1–5 This lateral view of the cerebral cortex of the left hemisphere shows some of the areas that are involved in language. The arcuate fasciculus connects Wernicke's area to Broca's area. (Adapted from Geschwind, 1979.)

electrically stimulating a certain region of the brain—the contralateral precentral gyrus in front of the central sulcus. Moreover, Fritsch and Hitzig found that there is a cortical representation for the individual muscle groups and that the small region of the cortex devoted to each group is discrete.

The next step was taken in 1876 by Carl Wernicke. At the age of 26 (having been out of medical school for only 4 years) Wernicke published a now classic paper entitled "The Symptom Complex of Aphasia: A Psychological Study on an Anatomical Basis." In this paper, he described a new type of aphasia. Wernicke's aphasia involves an impairment of comprehension rather than execution (a *receptive* as opposed to *expressive* malfunction). Whereas Broca's patients could understand but could not speak, Wernicke's patient could speak but not understand. Wernicke found that this new type of aphasia has a different locus from that described by Broca: the lesion is located in the posterior part of the temporal lobe at its junction with the parietal and occipital lobes (Figure 1–5).

In addition to this discovery, Wernicke formulated a theory of language that attempted to reconcile and extend the two existing theories of brain function. Phrenologists had argued that the cortex is a mosaic of specific functions and that even abstract mental attributes are localized to single, highly specific cortical areas. The opposing aggregate field school argued that mental functions are not at all represented topographically but distributed equally throughout the cerebral cortex. Wernicke used his discoveries and those of Broca, Fritsch, and Hitzig to propose that only basic mental functions concerned with simple perceptual and motor activities are discretely localized to single cortical areas. The elementary areas for these simple functions are interconnected in various ways, however. Therefore, according to this view, more complex mental functions (which concerned the phrenologists) arise from neural interactions among several elementary perceptual and motor areas

and are mediated by the pathways that interconnect them.

By extending the mosaic principle of the brain into a connectionist framework, Wernicke emphasized that the same function is processed serially as well as in parallel in different regions of the brain, and specific components of the function are processed at particular loci. Wernicke thus first formulated the ideas of parallel and distributed processing that are so prominent in current thinking.

Wernicke postulated that language involves separate motor and sensory regions. He proposed that Broca's area controls the *motor* program for coordinating mouth movements into coherent speech—a task for which Broca's area is suitably situated immediately in front of the motor area controlling the mouth, tongue, palate, and vocal cords (Figure 1–5). He ascribed word selection, the *sensory* component of language, to the temporal lobe area he had discovered. This area is also suitably located, being surrounded by the auditory cortex as well as by areas of cortex (called *association cortex*) that integrate aspects of audition and vision for complex perception. Thus Wernicke formulated a coherent, although somewhat simplified, model of speech that is still useful today. According to this model, auditory and visual perceptions of language are formed in their respective sensory and association areas and converge on Wernicke's area, where they are recognized as spoken or written language. Without that recognition, *comprehension* of language is lost. Once recognized, the neural representation is relayed from Wernicke's area to Broca's area, where it is transformed from auditory (or visual) representation into spoken (or written) language. Without that transformation the ability to *articulate* language is lost.

Using this powerful model, Wernicke predicted another type of aphasia, which was later discovered clinically. This form of aphasia is produced by a very different type of lesion from that in Broca's and Wernicke's aphasias: the receptive and motor speech zones are spared, but the fiber pathway that connects them, the arcuate fasciculus in the lower parietal region, is destroyed (Figure 1–5). The resulting syndrome, now called *conduction aphasia*, is characterized by the incorrect use of words (paraphasia). Patients with conduction aphasia cannot repeat simple phrases, but they can understand words that are heard and seen; they speak fluently but not correctly, omitting parts of words and substituting incorrect sounds in the words. They also are painfully aware of their own errors, but unable to correct them.

Thus, at the beginning of the twentieth century, there was compelling evidence that discrete areas of the cortex are involved in specific behaviors. Surprisingly, however, the dominant view of the brain was not the cellular connection, but the aggregate field view. During the first half of this century several major neural scientists, including the British neurologist Henry Head, the German neuropsychologist Kurt Goldstein, the Russian behavioral physiologist Ivan Pavlov, and the American psychologist Karl Lashley, continued to advocate an aggregate field view. The most influential was Lashley, Professor of Psychology at Harvard. In the tradition of his predecessor Flourens, he attempted to find the locus of learning by studying in rats the effects of various brain lesions on the complex task of learning to master a maze. Lashley could not find any specific learning center; rather, the severity of the learning defect produced by damaging the brain depended on the extent of the damage and not on its precise location. This discovery led Lashley—and, after him, many other psychologists—to conclude that learning does not have a special locus and therefore cannot be related to specific neurons. On the basis of these conclusions, Lashley reformulated the aggregate field view in a theory of brain function called *mass action*, which minimized the importance of individual neurons and of specific neuronal connections. What is important according to this mass action view is brain mass, not neuronal architecture.

Applying this logic to aphasia, Head and Goldstein argued that disorders of language cannot be attributed to specific lesions, but follow from injury to almost any cortical area. They asserted that cortical damage, regardless of site, causes the patient to regress from a higher symbolic to a simple, automatic verbal language: from an abstract to a concrete language characteristic of aphasia.

The work of Lashley and of Head has subsequently been reinterpreted. A variety of studies have demonstrated that maze learning, the task used by Lashley, is unsuitable for studying localization of function because it involves many complex motor and sensory capabilities. Deprived of one capability, an animal can still learn with another. In addition, a series of important clinical and experimental advances greatly strengthened the evidence for localization. In the late 1950s Wilder Penfield stimulated the cortex of conscious patients during brain surgery for epilepsy carried out under local anesthesia. To ensure that the surgery would not compromise the patient's communication skills, Penfield tested the cortex for areas that produced disorders of language upon stimulation. His findings, based on the verbal report of con-

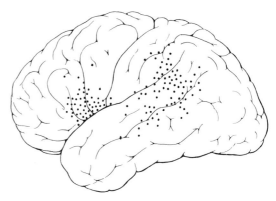

1–6 Electrical stimulation of specific points on the cerebral cortex (**black dots**) arrests speech. The anterior cluster of points overlies Broca's area; the posterior cluster overlies Wernicke's area. (Adapted from Penfield and Roberts, 1959.)

scious subjects, dramatically confirmed the localization indicated by Wernicke's studies (Figure 1–6). Moreover, extending the findings of Fritsch and Hitzig to humans, Penfield also showed that the muscles of the body are represented in the cerebral cortex in great topographical detail, which results in a map forming a motor *homunculus* (Figure 1–7). Recently, Penfield's clinical studies were extended by Norman Geschwind at Harvard, who pioneered in the modern study of functional localization in the human cerebral cortex. Experimental results from

1–7 The "homunculus" of the motor area (the precentral gyrus) of the right cerebral cortex shows the relative allotment of cortex to various muscle groups on the opposite side of the body. This map was obtained by direct electrical stimulation of the motor cortex of the human brain. The cartoon of the body surface illustrates the sequence of representation as well as the disproportionate representation given to the muscles involved in skilled movement. (Adapted from Penfield and Rasmussen, 1950.)

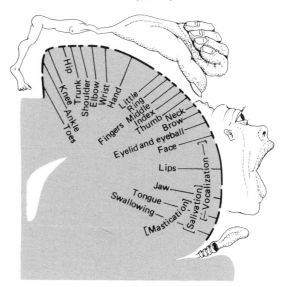

applying cellular techniques to the central nervous system, which we shall consider later in this book, have led to similar conclusions. For example, developmental and physiological studies have indicated that individual nerve cells connect to one another in a precise way. As a result, individual cells respond only to specific sensory stimuli and not to others.

Affective and Character Traits Also Are Anatomically Localizable

Even in light of the evidence for localization of cognitive functions related to language, the idea persisted that affective or emotional functions are not localizable. Emotion, it was held, must be an expression of the activity of the whole brain, a so-called emergent property. Only recently has this view been modified. Quite specific emotions can be elicited by stimulating specific parts of the brain of experimental animals. However, the three most dramatic demonstrations have come from the study of patients with certain language disorders, patients who have a particular form of epilepsy originating in the temporal lobe, and patients with acute anxiety disorders (panic attacks).

In addition to the cognitive aspects of language, represented in Wernicke's area and Broca's area in the *left* hemisphere, there is an affective component to language, consisting of the musical intonation of speech (called *prosody*), emotional gesturing, prosodic comprehension, and comprehension of emotional gesturing. Elliott Ross at the University of Texas and Kenneth Heilman at the University of Florida have found that these affective aspects of language are represented in the *right* hemisphere and that their anatomical organization mirrors that for cognitive language in the left hemisphere. Damage to the right temporal area homologous to Wernicke's area in the left hemisphere leads to disturbances in *comprehending* the emotional aspect of language, whereas damage to the right frontal area homologous to Broca's area leads to difficulty in *expressing* the emotional aspect of language. Thus, specific affective disorders of language can be localized to particular regions of the brain, and these disorders, called *aprosodias*, can be classified as sensory, motor, and conduction, in the same way that the aphasias are classified.

A second clue to the localization of affect comes from the finding that patients with chronic temporal lobe epilepsy manifest characteristic emotional changes. Some of these changes are present during the seizure itself; these are called *ictal phenomena* (Latin *ictus*, a blow or a strike). Other changes are present even in the absence of seizure; these are called *interictal phenomena*. Among the common ictal phenomena experienced by patients during temporal lobe seizures are feelings of unreality and déjà vu (the sensation of having been in a place before, or having seen a particular set of images before); transient visual or auditory hallucinations; feelings of depersonalization, fear, or anger; delusions; sexual feelings; and paranoia. However, in some ways the more impor-

tant changes are those present in patients when they are not having convulsions. These interictal changes are interesting because they represent a chronic change in personality, a true psychiatric syndrome.

A detailed personality inventory of patients with temporal lobe epilepsy has been compiled by David Bear at the National Institutes of Health. He found that many patients with temporal lobe epilepsy lose all interest in sex. This decrease in sexual interest often is paralleled by an increase in social aggressiveness. Most patients also have one or more characteristic personality traits: they can be intensely emotional, ardently religious, extremely moralistic, or lacking in humor.

Bear also found that these traits are correlated with the location of the epilepsy. Patients with right temporal lobe epilepsy display excessive emotional tendencies (hyperemotionality). In contrast, patients who have left temporal lobe epilepsy manifest ideational traits such as a sense of personal destiny, moral self-scrutinizing, and a penchant for philosophical explanation. Thus, affective functions can be localized within the temporal lobe (although they also involve other areas of the brain, as we shall see later), and hemispheric asymmetry exists for emotion as well as for cognition.

Unlike patients with temporal lobe epilepsy, patients with epileptic foci outside the temporal lobe do not generally present abnormalities in emotion and behavior. Bear has argued that the irritative lesions of epilepsy have consequences opposite to those of the destructive lesions of aphasia that Wernicke analyzed. Whereas destructive lesions bring about loss of function, often through the disconnection of specialized areas, epileptic processes may entail excessive activity in the affected regions, leading to excessive expression of emotion or an overelaboration of ideas.

Some of the symptoms seen in temporal lobe epilepsy are also seen in schizophrenia. Epileptic patients differ from those with schizophrenia, however, in that patients with temporal lobe epilepsy show a warm (rather than cold or shallow) affect, have logical thought processes, and are able to establish meaningful interpersonal relationships.

Panic attacks are a third clearly defined disorder of affect that has been localized to the temporal lobe. An acute anxiety disorder, panic attacks are recurrent, brief, spontaneous episodes of terror without clearly identifiable cause. There is a sense of impending disaster, accompanied by a racing heart and short and unsteady breathing. Using positron emission tomography (a scanning procedure that allows visualization of cerebral blood flow and metabolic changes in the brain), Eli Robins and his colleagues at Washington University in St. Louis have found a circumscribed abnormality in the right parahippocampal gyrus in patients with recurrent panic attacks. Blood flow to this area is abnormally higher than that in the corresponding area in the left hemisphere. This abnormality is present even when panic attacks are not occurring. Thus, a predisposition to this emotional disorder can be traced to a permanent and localized abnormality in the anatomy of the brain.

These clinical studies and their counterparts in experimental animals suggest that all behavior, including higher (cognitive as well as affective) mental functioning, is localizable to specific regions or constellations of regions within the brain. The role of descriptive neuroanatomy is therefore to provide us with a functional guide to localization within the three-dimensional neural space—a map for behavior. On the basis of this map we can use the patient's behavioral performance, as elicited in a clinical examination, to infer where the difficulties are located.

This discussion brings up one final point. Why has the evidence for localization, which seems so obvious and compelling in retrospect, been repeatedly rejected in the past? The reasons are both historical and scientific. As we have seen, before the work of Pierre Flourens on the aggregate function of the cerebral cortex, the phrenologists had already promulgated an extreme doctrine of localization, anatomical personology. The subsequent dialectic between the aggregate field *antilocalizationists* and the cellular connection *localizationists* thus developed as a reaction against a theory of localization that, although correct in perspective, was wrong, and indeed foolish, in detail. The concept of localization that ultimately prevailed was tempered in this controversy and emerged as much more complex than Gall would have envisioned. What is localized to discrete regions in the brain is not a set of elaborate faculties of the mind, but a large family of elementary operations often carried out in parallel. More elaborate faculties derive from the interconnections of several, even many, brain regions.

Scientifically, localization was slow to be accepted because clinicians and neural scientists were slow to appreciate which aspects of function are localized and how extensive a role parallel representations play in the processing of information by the brain. Many functions, particularly higher mental functions, are divided into subfunctions that are represented not only in series but also in parallel, so that neural processing for a given function is distributed within the brain and handled at several discrete sites. Each of these stages of processing presumably represents some distinctive elaboration of a particular subfunction. For example, we have already encountered several distinct areas for speech, each concerned with elaborating a particular component; quite probably other similar areas are still undiscovered. As a result of serial and parallel processing, damage to a single area need not lead to the disappearance of the function; or, if the function does disappear, it may partially return because the remaining parts can either assume the function or rearrange themselves to accomplish the primary task. Thus, the anatomical connections of related functions are inaccurately described as a series of functional links in a single chain, an arrangement in which all related functions would stop if the chain breaks (Figure 1–8A); rather, related functions are now seen as the product of many chains distributed in parallel (Figure 1–8B). The break of a single link will interrupt one chain, but this need not interfere permanently with the performance of the whole system.

1–8 Two models of behavioral function have been proposed within the framework of cellular connectionism. (Adapted from Uttal, 1978.) **A.** We now know that a model consisting simply of neurons connected only in series is unrealistic. This representation of brain organization is inadequate because it presupposes that all of a given function ceases when an individual neural link is broken. **B.** A somewhat more accurate model consists of chains of neurons in parallel as well as in series. When a given neural link is broken, the system typically does not fail completely because there is parallel representation of function. When part of a chain is disrupted, the system often can rearrange itself to accomplish many of the same tasks of which the original network was capable.

A corollary to this argument is that the doctrine of localization of function suffered from the lack of a mature science of behavior, a lack that, to a large degree, still persists. Various aspects of behavior are very difficult to describe and measure objectively. To study localizable brain–behavior relationships we must be able to identify in a scientifically recognizable manner the properties of the behavior we are attempting to explain.

A final and, perhaps in the long run, most important reason that it has taken so long to accept the doctrine of localization is the paucity of our knowledge of the relationship of brain anatomy to behavior. The brain is immensely complex, and the structure and the function of many of its parts are still poorly understood. The excitement in neural science today lies in the conviction that the tools are at last in hand to explore the organ of the mind, and with that excitement comes the optimism that the biological basis of mental function will prove to be understandable.

Selected Readings

Bear, D. M. 1979. The temporal lobes: An approach to the study of organic behavioral changes. In M. S. Gazzaniga (ed.), Handbook of Behavioral Neurobiology, Vol. 2. New York: Plenum Press, pp. 75–95.

Ferrier, D. 1890. The Croonian Lectures on Cerebral Localisation. London: Smith, Elder.

Geschwind, N. 1974. Selected Papers on Language and the Brain. Dordrecht, Holland: Reidel.

Geschwind, N. 1979. Specializations of the human brain. Sci. Am. 241(3):180–199.

Jackson, J. H. 1884. The Croonian Lectures on Evolution and Dissolution of the Nervous System. Br. Med. J. 1:591–593, 660–663, 703–707.

Kandel, E. R. 1976. Cellular Basis of Behavior: An Introduction to Behavioral Neurobiology. San Francisco: Freeman, chap. 1.

Lesky, E. 1976. The Vienna Medical School of the 19th Century. Baltimore: The Johns Hopkins University Press.

Penfield, W., and Rasmussen, T. 1950. The Cerebral Cortex of Man: A Clinical Study of Localization of Function. New York: Macmillan.

Ross, E. D. 1981. The aprosodias: Functional-anatomical organization of the affective components of language in the right hemisphere. Arch. Neurol. 38:561–569.

Ross, E. D. 1984. Right hemisphere's role in language, affective behavior and emotion. Trends Neurosci. 7(9):342–346.

Young, R. M. 1970. Mind, Brain and Adaptation in the Nineteenth Century. Oxford: Clarendon Press.

References

Bernard, C. 1878. Leçons sur les phénomènes de la vie communs aux animaux et aux végétaux. Paris: Baillière.

Broca, P. 1865. Sur le siége de la Faculté du langage articulé. Bull. Soc. Anthropol. 6:377–393.

Cajal, S. R. 1892. A new concept of the histology of the central nervous system. D. A. Rottenberg (trans.). (See also historical essay by S. L. Palay, preceding Cajal's paper.) In D. A. Rottenberg and F. H. Hochberg (eds.), Neurological Classics in Modern Translation. New York: Hafner, 1977, pp. 7–29.

Cajal, S. R. 1906. The structure and connexions of neurons. In: Nobel Lectures: Physiology or Medicine, 1901–1921. Amsterdam: Elsevier, 1967, pp. 220–253.

Cajal, S. R. 1908. Neuron Theory or Reticular Theory? Objective Evidence of the Anatomical Unity of Nerve Cells. M. U. Purkiss and C. A. Fox (trans.). Madrid: Consejo Superior de Investigaciones Científicas Instituto Ramón y Cajal, 1954.

Cajal, S.R. 1937. Recollections of My Life. E. Horne Craigie (trans.). Edited in 2 vols. as Memoirs of the American Philosophical Society, Philadelphia.

Darwin, C. 1860. On the Origin of Species by Means of Natural Selection. New York: Appleton.

DuBois-Reymond, E. 1848–1849. Untersuchungen über Thierische Elektricität, Vols. 1, 2. Berlin: Reimer.

Ehrlich, P. 1913. Chemotherapeutics: Scientific principles, methods, and results. Lancet 2:445–451.

Flourens, P. 1824. Recherches expérimentales sur les propriétés et les fonctions du système nerveux, dans les animaux vertébrés. Paris: Chez Crevot.

Fritsch, G., and Hitzig, E. 1870. Ueber die elektrische Erregbarkeit des Grosshirns. Arch. Anat. Physiol. Wiss. Med., pp. 300–332. G. von Bonin (trans.). In: Some Papers on the Cerebral Cortex. Springfield, Ill.: Thomas, 1960, pp. 73–96.

Gall, F. J., and Spurzheim, G. 1810. Anatomie et physiologie du système nerveux en général, et du cerveau en particulier, avec des observations sur la possibilité de reconnoître plusieurs dispositions intellectuelles et morales de l'homme et des animaux, par la configuration de leurs têtes. Paris: Schoell.

Galvani, L. 1791. Commentary on the Effect of Electricity on Muscular Motion. R. M. Green (trans.). Cambridge, Mass.: Licht, 1953.

Goldstein, K. 1948. Language and Language Disturbances. New York: Grune & Stratton.

Golgi, C. 1906. The neuron doctrine—Theory and facts. In: Nobel Lectures: Physiology or Medicine, 1901–1921. Amsterdam: Elsevier, 1967, pp. 189–217.

Head, H. 1921. Release of function in the nervous system. Proc. R. Soc. Lond. [Biol.] 92:184–209.

Head, H. 1926. Aphasia and Kindred Disorders of Speech. Cambridge, England: Cambridge University Press. Reprint, New York: Hafner, 1963.

Heilman, K. M., Scholes, R., and Watson, R. T. 1975. Auditory affective agnosia. Disturbed comprehension of affective speech. J. Neurol. Neurosurg. Psychiatry 38:69–72.

Helmholtz, H. von. 1850. On the rate of transmission of nerve impulse. Monatsber. Preuss. Akad. Wiss. Berl., pp. 14–15. Trans. in W. Dennis (ed.), Readings in the History of Psychology. New York: Appleton-Century-Crofts, 1948, pp. 197–198.

Langley, J. N. 1906. On nerve endings and on special excitable substances in cells. Proc. R. Soc. Lond. [Biol.] 78:170–194.

Lashley, K. S. 1929. Brain Mechanisms and Intelligence: A Quantitative Study of Injuries to the Brain. Chicago: University of Chicago Press.

Nieuwenhuys, R., Voogd, J., and van Huijzen, Chr. 1981. The Human Central Nervous System: A Synopsis and Atlas, 2nd rev. ed. New York: Springer-Verlag.

Pavlov, I. P. 1927. Conditioned Reflexes: An Investigation of the Physiological Activity of the Cerebral Cortex. London: Oxford University Press.

Penfield, W. 1954. Mechanisms of voluntary movement. Brain 77:1–17.

Penfield, W., and Roberts, L. 1959. Speech and Brain-Mechanisms. Princeton: Princeton University Press.

Reiman, E. M., Raichle, M. E., Butler, F. K., Herscovitch, P., and Robins, E. 1984. A focal brain abnormality in panic disorder, a severe form of anxiety. Nature 310:683–685.

Spurzheim, J. G. 1825. Phrenology, or the Doctrine of the Mind, 3rd ed. London: Knight.

Uttal, W. R. 1978. The Psychobiology of Mind. Hillsdale, N.J.: Erlbaum.

Wernicke, C. 1908. The symptom-complex of aphasia. In A. Church (ed.), Diseases of the Nervous System. New York: Appleton, pp. 265–324.

Eric R. Kandel

Nerve Cells and Behavior

2

Information coming from peripheral receptors, which sense the environment, is analyzed by the brain into components that give rise to perceptions; some of these perceptions are stored as memory. The brain also issues motor commands for the co-ordinated movements of the muscles of the body. The brain does all this with nerve cells and the connections between them. Despite the simplicity of the basic units, complexity is achieved by the enormous number of cells. The best estimate is that the human brain contains about 10^{12} nerve cells. Although these nerve cells can be classified into perhaps 1000 to 10,000 different types, they share many features in common. A key discovery in the organization of the brain is that cells with basically similar properties are able nonetheless to produce very different actions because they are connected to each other and to the periphery in different ways. Since a few principles of organization give rise to considerable complexity, it is possible to learn a great deal about how the nervous system works simply by paying attention to four general features:

1. The mechanisms by which nerve cells produce their relatively stereotypic signals.
2. The ways in which nerve cells are connected.
3. The relationship of the various patterns of interconnections to different types of behavior.
4. The means by which nerve cells and their connections are modified by experience.

In this chapter we shall introduce neuronal signaling by considering some structural and functional properties of nerve cells and their surrounding glial support cells. Next we shall examine how nerve cells are interconnected to produce a simple behavior and then briefly describe the signaling mechanisms that nerve cells use to communicate with each other.

The Nervous System Contains Two Classes of Cells

There are two distinct classes of cells in the nervous system: the nerve cells and the neuroglial cells (or glia). We shall first consider the nerve cells.

Nerve Cells

The typical neuron has four morphologically defined regions (Figure 2–1): the cell body (also called the soma or perikaryon), the dendrites, the axon, and the presynaptic terminals of the axon. Nerve cells generate active electrical signals, and each region has distinctive signaling functions. The cell body is the metabolic center of the neuron. Three organelles are characteristic of the cell body: the nucleus, which in neurons is often quite large; the endoplasmic reticulum, upon which membrane and secretory proteins are synthesized; and the Golgi apparatus, which carries out the processing of secretory and membrane components. The cell body usually gives rise to several fine arborizing extensions called *dendrites*, which serve, as we shall see later, as the chief receptive apparatus for the neuron. The cell body also gives rise to the *axon*, a tubular process that can extend considerable distances (up to 1 meter in humans). The axon constitutes the conducting unit of the neuron. Axons lack ribosomes and therefore cannot synthesize proteins. Newly synthesized macromolecules are assembled into organelles within the cell body and are moved along the axon to the presynaptic terminals by a process called axoplasmic transport, which we shall consider in Chapter 4. When severed from the cell body, the axon usually degenerates and dies (see Chapter 17). Large axons are surrounded by a fatty insulating sheath called *myelin*, which is essential for high-speed conduction of action potentials. The myelin sheath is interrupted at very regular intervals. These points of interruption are called the *nodes of Ranvier*, after the neuroanatomist Louis Antoine Ranvier, Professor at the Collège de France in Paris, who discovered them at the end of the nineteenth century.

Near its end the axon divides into many fine branches, which have specialized endings called *presynaptic terminals*. The presynaptic terminals are the transmitting elements of the neuron. By means of its terminals, one neuron contacts and transmits information about its own activity to the receptive surfaces of another neuron, a muscle, or other kinds of effector cells. The point of contact is known as the *synapse*. It is formed by the presynaptic terminal of one cell (the *presynaptic cell*), the receptive surface of the other (the *postsynaptic cell*), and the space separating them (the *synaptic cleft*). The terminals of the presynaptic neuron sometimes contact the postsynaptic neuron on its cell body, but more commonly the contacts occur on the dendrites. Less often, synapses are located on the initial or on the terminal portions of axons.

In the nineteenth century most histologists thought of the nervous system as a diffuse syncytium, a reticulated network of fused cells with interconnected cytoplasm. As we saw in Chapter 1, Santiago Ramón y Cajal, perhaps the most seminal of the modern thinkers about brain function, provided much of the evidence for the neuron doctrine, which holds instead that each neuron is a discrete cellular entity and that neurons are the basic building blocks and signaling units of the nervous system. In retrospect, it is hard to appreciate how difficult it was for Cajal and others to obtain evidence for this elementary idea. Shortly after Jacob M. Schleiden and Theodor A. Schwann put forward the cell theory in the early 1830s, it came to be accepted that cells are the structural units of all living matter, the basic elements of all tissues and organs except the nervous system. For years, most anatomists believed that the cell theory did not apply to the brain. Unlike cells of other tissues of the body, cells of the nervous system were deceptive because of their large size and complex shape, with many processes that appeared to extend endlessly. Most cells of the body are simple in shape and fit into a single field of the compound microscope, but nerve cells often do not fit into a single field or cannot easily be distinguished from the background of other nerve cells or connective tissue elements.

Only by the middle of the nineteenth century did it become clear that the axon that emerges from the cell body is continuous with it. To work out the structure of the neuron required the development of special techniques. The critical technique was discovered in 1873 by the Italian anatomist Camillo Golgi. Golgi's silver impregnation method, which is still used today, has two advantages: (1) for unknown reasons it stains only about one percent to ten percent of the total number of cells in a particular region of the brain, therefore making it possible to study a single nerve cell in relative anatomical isolation from its neighbors; and (2) the neurons that do take up the stain are delineated in their entire extent, including cell body, axon, and full dendritic tree.

By applying Golgi's method to the nervous system, and simply by looking at the structure of a nerve cell and its contacts with other cells in histological sections, Cajal gained many insights into neuronal function. Two insights proved particularly important because they form the cellular basis of the modern connectionist approach to the brain that we discussed in Chapter 1.

First, Cajal inferred the *principle of dynamic polarization*, which states that information flows in a predictable and consistent direction within each nerve cell. The flow is from the receiving sites of the neuron (the cell body and dendrites) to the impulse-initiating site in the axon, and then finally to the presynaptic sites in the axon terminal that communicate with other cells. Although, as we shall see, neurons vary dramatically in shape and function, most nerve cells adhere to this pattern of information flow. Cajal's second insight is the *principle of connectional specificity* (or cellular connectionism). According to this principle, (1) there is no cytoplasmic continuity between nerve cells, (2) nerve cells do not form random networks, and (3) each cell forms specific and precise connections, making contact only with some nerve cells but not with others.

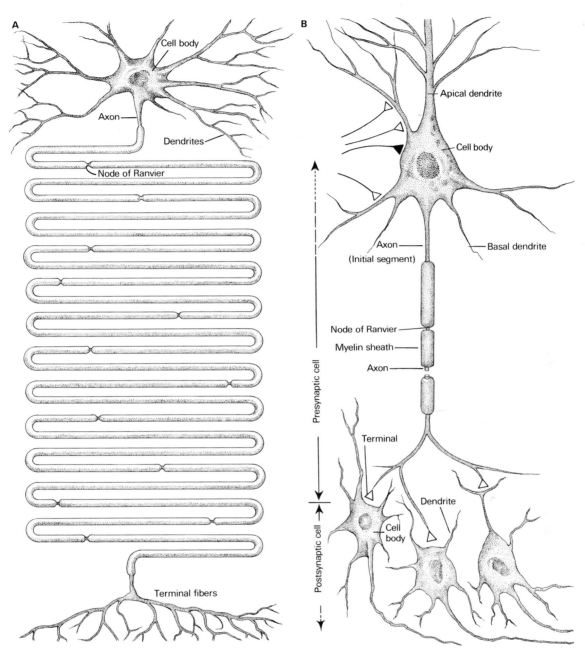

2–1 The main features of a typical neuron. **A.** A neuron
drawn to illustrate the relative extent of each region.
Axons vary greatly in length, and some extend for more than 1
meter. (The axon is folded for diagrammatic purposes. In
addition, the caliber of the axon is distorted; most axons in the
central nervous system are very thin compared with the
diameter of the cell body.) Many axons are insulated by a fatty
myelin sheath, which is interrupted at intervals by regions
known as the nodes of Ranvier. The terminal branches of the

axon form synapses with as many as 1000 other neurons. Most
synapses join the axon terminals of one neuron with the
dendrites or cell body of another neuron. Thus the dendrites
emerging from a neuron might receive incoming signals from
hundreds or even thousands of other neurons. (Adapted from
Stevens, 1979.) **B.** Typical neuron drawn to illustrate its various
regions and its points of contact with other nerve cells. By
convention, we shall indicate excitatory presynaptic terminals
as white triangles, and inhibitory terminals as black triangles.

In a long and productive career, Cajal applied Golgi's
method to almost every region of the nervous system. By
this means he described the differences between classes
of nerve cells and delineated the precise connections between many of them. Cajal and the neuroanatomists who
followed him found that the one feature that most dra-

matically distinguishes one neuron from another is
shape, and, more particularly, the number and form of a
neuron's processes. On the basis of the number of processes that arise from the cell body, neurons are classified
into three groups: unipolar, bipolar, and multipolar (Figure 2–2).

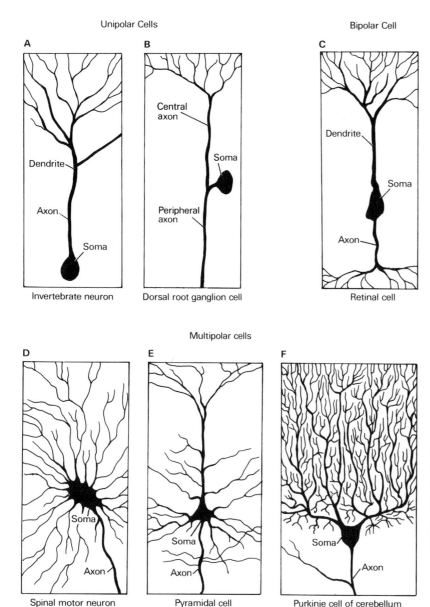

Unipolar Cells

A

Dendrite

Axon

Soma

Invertebrate neuron

B

Central axon

Soma

Peripheral axon

Dorsal root ganglion cell

Bipolar Cell

C

Dendrite

Soma

Axon

Retinal cell

Multipolar cells

D

Soma

Axon

Spinal motor neuron

E

Soma

Axon

Pyramidal cell

F

Soma

Axon

Purkinje cell of cerebellum

2–2 Neurons can be classified as unipolar, bipolar, or multipolar according to the number of processes that originate from the cell body.

A unipolar cell has a single process leaving the soma. **A.** Unipolar cells are characteristic of invertebrate nervous systems. In invertebrates, different segments of a single axonal process can serve as receptive (dendritic) surfaces or as transmitting (axonal) terminals. **B.** Neurons in the dorsal root ganglia of the spinal cord belong to a subclass of unipolar cells called pseudounipolar. In a pseudounipolar cell, the processes of the embryonic cell have apparently become fused over a short distance so that only a single process emerges from the cell body. This process then splits in a T-shaped fashion into two axons, one going peripherally to skin or muscle, the other going centrally to the spinal cord. Dorsal root ganglion cells carry information to the central nervous system from skin, muscle, and viscera.

Bipolar cells have two processes: the dendrite, which carries information toward the cell; and the axon, which transmits information away from the cell. **C.** The bipolar cell shown here is found in the retina.

The multipolar cell usually has dendrites emerging from all parts of the cell body and is common in the mammalian nervous system. **D.** This cell is a motor neuron in the spinal cord that innervates muscle fibers. **E.** A pyramidal cell is a variant of the multipolar cell. The cell body is pyramidal in shape, and dendrites emerge both from its apex (the apical dendrite) and from the base (the basilar dendrites). This pyramidal cell is from the hippocampus, a part of the brain thought to be involved in memory. Pyramidal cells are also found in the cerebral cortex. **F.** A Purkinje cell of the cerebellum, another variant of a multipolar cell, is characterized by its rich and extensive dendritic tree in one plane. (Parts B–F are adapted from Cajal, 1933.)

Unipolar cells have one primary process that may give rise to many branches. Some branches serve as dendritic receiving structures, and other branches as axons and terminal structures. Unipolar cells predominate in the nervous systems of invertebrates (Figure 2–2A) but a variant unipolar cell also occurs in vertebrates in collections of nerve cells located near the spinal cord in the sensory ganglia of the dorsal roots (Figure 2–2B).

Bipolar neurons have an ovoid soma that gives rise to one process at each end: a dendrite or peripheral process (which picks up information from the periphery), and an axon or central process (which carries information toward the central nervous system). The bipolar cells of the retina are examples of this class (Figure 2–2C).

Multipolar neurons predominate in the vertebrate nervous system. These cells have one or more dendritic branches and a single axon. In a typical multipolar cell, dendrites emerge from all parts of the cell body (Figure 2–2D); variants are the pyramidal cell (Figure 2–2E) and the Purkinje cell (Figure 2–2F). Later we shall have the opportunity to consider in detail one well-known, extensively studied class of multipolar cell—the motor cells of the spinal cord (Figure 2–2D).

Even within the category of multipolar neurons, the size and shape of different cells vary greatly. Different types of multipolar cells account for nearly all of the distinguishable neuronal types, which, as noted earlier, number between 1000 and 10,000. The morphological differences among multipolar cells are due largely to variations in two features: the number and length of the dendrites, and the length of the axon. The number and extent of dendritic processes in a given cell correlate with the number of synaptic contacts that other neurons make on that cell. A spinal motor cell, whose dendrites are moderate in both number and extent, receives roughly 10,000 contacts. The large dendritic tree of the Purkinje cell of the cerebellum receives approximately 150,000 contacts!

The length of the axon reflects the signaling function of a neuron. Neurons with long axons (sometimes called Golgi type I cells) carry information from one brain region to another; they serve as *projection* or *relay neurons*. Neurons with short axons (Golgi type II cells) primarily process information within a small, limited region of the brain. These nerve cells serve as *local interneurons* in various nuclei of the brain and in reflex pathways.

Glial Cells

There are between 10 and 50 times more glial cells than neurons in the vertebrate central nervous system. Besides being ubiquitous, glial cells are typically small and do not generate active electrical signals as neurons do. Glial cells are found between nerve cell bodies and also between axons. As a group, the various types of glial cells are thought to serve six distinct functions:

1. Glia (Greek, meaning glue) are supporting elements that provide firmness and structure for the brain, a role played by connective tissue cells in other parts of the body. They also segregate and occasionally insulate groups of neurons from each other.
2. Some glial cells are scavengers that remove debris after neuronal death or injury.
3. Certain glial cells provide myelin, the insulating sheath that covers some axons.
4. Glial cells buffer the K^+ concentration of the extracellular space and help to remove chemical transmitters released by neurons.
5. During development, certain classes of glial cells guide the migration of neurons and, possibly, direct the outgrowth of axons.
6. There is suggestive evidence that some glial cells have nutritive functions for nerve cells, although this has been difficult to demonstrate conclusively.

As we shall see below, different aspects of these functions are carried out by different types of glial cells.

Glial cells in vertebrates are generally divided into two major classes: *macroglia* (astrocytes, oligodendrocytes, and ependymal cells), and *microglia* (an assortment of phagocytic cells that are mobilized after injury, infection, or disease).

The origin of microglia is still not known. Until recently they were thought to derive from blood-borne macrophages but now are believed to derive from ectoderm, like the nervous system itself, and to proliferate as

needed from a resting population of immature glial precursor cells. Because microglia are phagocytes and belong to a physiologically distinct class of cells, unrelated to neuronal signaling, we shall not consider them further.

The two predominant types of macroglia are *astrocytes*, characterized by many processes, and *oligodendrocytes*, with few processes (Figure 2–3A and B). The *ependymal cells*, a third type, line the central canal system of the brain and spinal cord.

Astrocytes are star-shaped cells with small, irregularly shaped cell bodies and numerous extensions that ramify between the processes of nerve cells. They are commonly divided into two subclasses: fibrous and protoplasmic (Figure 2–3B). *Fibrous astrocytes* contain many filaments and are found in areas of the central nervous system containing mostly axons. These regions are called *white matter* because of the color of myelinated axons in unstained, freshly cut brain sections. The *protoplasmic astrocytes* have shorter and stouter processes that contain few filaments; these astrocytes are associated with nerve cell bodies, dendrites, and particularly synapses, which they characteristically envelop. The regions in which protoplasmic astrocytes predominate are called *gray matter* because large collections of nerve cell bodies and dendrites appear grayish in brain sections.

Astrocytes probably serve a number of functions. The processes of fibrous and protoplasmic astrocytes have end-feet that contact blood capillaries on the one hand and neurons on the other, suggesting that astrocytes have a nutritive function (Figure 2–3C). After injury, astrocytes and microglia remove neuronal debris and help seal off damaged brain tissue. Furthermore, as first shown by Stephen Kuffler, John Nicholls, and their colleagues, the resting potential of astrocytes is sensitive to small changes in K^+ concentration in the extracellular space. By taking up the excess extracellular K^+, astrocytes are thought to buffer the extracellular K^+ concentration so as to protect the membrane potential of neurons from the depolarization that might result if K^+ accumulated after repeated neuronal firing. Similarly, the protoplasmic astrocytes that surround the synaptic region have a high-affinity uptake mechanism for certain neurotransmitter substances such as γ-aminobutyric acid (GABA) and serotonin, and are thus able to remove them from the synaptic cleft.

Oligodendrocytes are small glial cells with few processes (Figure 2–3A). The one known function of oligodendrocytes is to contribute the myelin sheath to the axon, which greatly enhances the axon's conduction efficiency. They form this sheath by wrapping their membranous processes around the axon in a tight spiral. Oligodendrocytes are found in the central nervous system; their counterpart in the peripheral nervous system is the *Schwann cell*, which forms the myelin sheath around the axons of peripheral nerves. These two sheathing cells differ in that the oligodendrocyte envelops several axons in the central nervous system, whereas the Schwann cell is associated with only one axon in the periphery. Myelination will be considered in greater detail in Chapter 3.

18

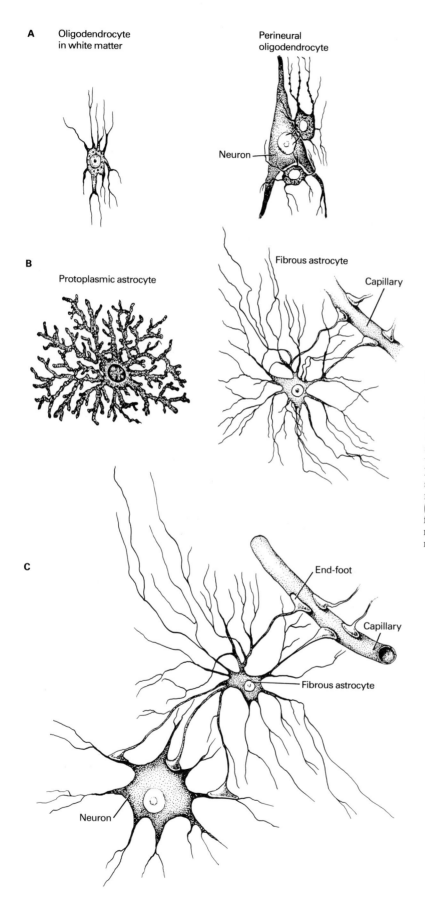

A Oligodendrocyte
in white matter

Perineural
oligodendrocyte

Neuron

B

Protoplasmic astrocyte

Fibrous astrocyte

Capillary

C

End-foot

Capillary

Fibrous astrocyte

Neuron

2–3 There are two principal types of macroglia in the nervous system, the oligodendrocytes and the astrocytes. **A.** Oligodendrocytes have few processes, which form the myelin sheath around the central axons of nerve cells. These glial cells are small and are located in gray matter, where they surround the cell bodies of neurons, as well as in white matter. (Adapted from Penfield, 1932.) **B.** Astrocytes have many processes. They are star-shaped and may either be fibrous (found in white matter) or protoplasmic (found in gray matter). (Adapted from Martinez Martinez, 1982.) **C.** The end-feet of an astrocyte contact both capillaries and neurons, and are therefore thought to have a nutritive role. (Adapted from Kuffler and Nicholls, 1976.)

Although the electrical properties of some glial cells can be altered by changes in external K^+ concentration produced by impulses in nerve cells, there is no evidence that glia are directly involved in signaling information. Signaling is the function of nerve cells.

Nerve Cells Are the Signaling Units of Behavioral Responses

To place Cajal's principle of dynamic polarization and electrical signaling by nerve cells in a behavioral context, let us examine the neuronal activity underlying a simple involuntary behavioral response—a stretch reflex, the knee jerk (Figure 2–4). The stretch reflex is the basic neural mechanism for maintaining tone (a background level of tension) in muscle. In addition to keeping otherwise relaxed muscles slightly contracted, the stretch reflex increases the tension of selected groups of muscles to provide a background of postural tone on which voluntary movements can be superimposed. For example, if the patellar tendon is tapped, the quadriceps femoris, an extensor muscle, is pulled by the tendon and briefly stretched. This initiates a reflex response that leads to a contraction of the quadriceps femoris muscle and the concomitant relaxation of the antagonist flexor muscle, the biceps femoris.

This behavior is mediated in large part by simple monosynaptic connections in the spinal cord. The reflex is called *monosynaptic* because contraction is mediated by only two types of nerve cells—here a sensory, or *afferent*, neuron[1] and a motor cell—connected to each other by only one set of synapses. The afferent neurons involved are connected to receptors in the muscle that are sensitive to stretch; these receptors are called *muscle spindles*. The afferent neurons in this reflex are a type of dorsal root ganglion cell. As we saw earlier (Figure 2–2), dorsal root ganglion cells are examples of unipolar neurons. A single axon emerges from the cell body, but then splits in two, with one branch going out to the muscle and the other running into the spinal cord, where it forms excitatory connections with the extensor motor neurons. These motor neurons in turn send axons to innervate the quadriceps muscle and control its contraction. Although only two *types* of nerve cells are involved, several hundred afferent neurons are actually activated by the stretching of a single muscle, and they excite more than 100 motor cells. (For example, in humans roughly 150,000 motor neurons innervate skeletal muscle on each side of the spinal cord, or about 5500 motor cells per segment. There are usually five to ten times more afferent neurons than motor neurons, illustrating the im-

portance of *information convergence* onto key cells, such as the motor neurons.)

The reflex mediated by these two types of neurons works as follows (Figure 2–4A): When a muscle is stretched, the afferent neuron is excited. The afferent neuron excites the motor neuron, which in turn causes the extensor muscle to contract and produce the behavior. The afferent neuron also excites many local inhibitory interneurons in the spinal cord. (An *interneuron* is a local neuron whose processes and actions are confined within a restricted area.) These interneurons inhibit the flexor motor neurons that go to the biceps, the antagonist muscle. Concurrently, the afferent neurons signal other, higher regions of the brain concerned with movement to inform them that an extensor muscle of the knee has been stretched and of what is happening in the spinal cord. Thus, the electrical signals that produce this behavior perform four functions: they convey (1) sensory information to the central nervous system, (2) reciprocal innervation to motor neurons (excitation of synergistic motor cells and inhibition of antagonistic ones), (3) motor commands from the central nervous system to muscles, the end-organs of effector behavior, and (4) information about this behavior to other parts of the central nervous system. In this example, signaling leads to a muscular reflex, a behavior that aids in maintaining posture in the presence of gravitational forces. A momentary imbalance of the body may stretch certain muscles. The sensory information that such stretching produces is conveyed to the motor cells, and motor commands to contract are sent out to the muscles so that balance will be restored.

The reflex described above activates sensory and motor projection neurons with long axons as well as local inhibitory interneurons with short axons. The signals of all these neurons depend on electrical properties of the cell membrane. Each of the nerve cells generates a resting potential and four types of electrical signals: an input membrane signal (either a receptor potential in the sensory neuron or a synaptic potential in the interneuron or motor neuron); an integrating signal; a conducting signal; and an output or secretory signal (Figure 2–4B). The resting potential and each of these four signals are briefly described below; the underlying mechanisms are treated in more detail in Part II.

Resting Membrane Potential

The neuron, like the other cells of the body, has a separation of electrical charge across its external membrane. It is positively charged on the outside and negatively charged on the inside. The separation of charge is responsible for the *resting membrane potential*. When the neuron is completely unperturbed (the quiescent state), the potential due to the separation of charge across the membrane is about 60 mV. Because the inside is negative in relation to the outside, and we arbitrarily define the outside as zero, we say that the resting potential is -60 mV. In different nerve cells the resting potential may range

---

[1]The term "afferent" (carried *toward* the nervous system) applies to all information reaching the central nervous system from the periphery, whether or not this information leads to conscious sensation. In strict usage, the term "sensory" should be reserved for that component of afferent input that ascends to the brain to generate a conscious perception.

2–4 The stretch reflex is an example of a monosynaptic reflex system.

A. The anatomical arrangement of the knee jerk. Each cell represents a population of many neurons. Information about stretch of the quadriceps femoris muscle is conveyed by afferent neurons to several loci within the central nervous system. In the spinal cord, afferent neurons act directly on the motor neurons to the quadriceps and, by means of inhibitory interneurons, indirectly on the motor neurons to the antagonistic muscle, the biceps. Both of these actions combine to produce the coordinated expression of the reflex behavior. In addition information is conveyed to higher regions of brain to update them about the information coming into the nervous system and about the behavior that is being generated. These higher centers, in turn, can act to modify the reflex behavior.

B. The sequences of signaling changes that produce the reflex action. Graded stretch of muscle produces a graded receptor potential in the muscle spindle of the afferent neuron that propagates passively to the trigger zone at the first node of Ranvier. If the potential is sufficiently large, it will trigger an action potential that will propagate actively and without fail along the axon to the terminal region. At the terminal the depolarization, the change in membrane potential, produced by the action potential gives rise to a secretory potential that leads to release of transmitter substance. The transmitter diffuses across the synaptic cleft and interacts with receptor molecules on the external membrane of the postsynaptic

motor cell to initiate a synaptic potential. The synaptic potential then propagates passively to the initial segment and in turn initiates an action potential that propagates to the terminals of the motor neuron. This action potential leads ultimately to a synaptic potential in the muscle, which initiates an action potential that produces a behavior: contraction of the muscle.

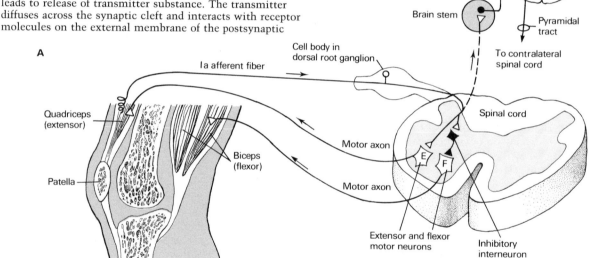

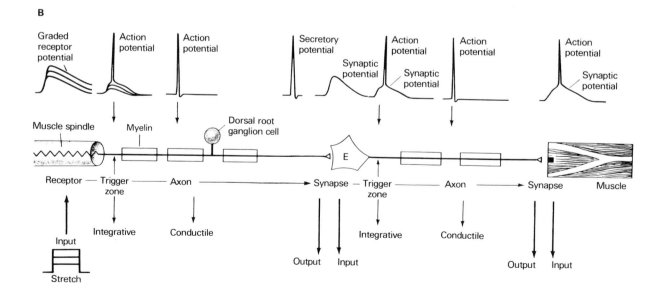

from −40 to −75 mV. In muscle cells the resting membrane potential is higher, about −90 mV. The charge across excitable membranes is of particular interest because *most signaling involves changes in the resting membrane potential* across the membrane. The resting membrane potential therefore provides the background against which signals are expressed. Signals such as the generator potential, synaptic potential, and action potential result from electrical perturbations of the membrane that cause the resting membrane potential to increase or decrease.

Because the membrane is polarized, an increase in the resting membrane potential (e.g., from −60 to −65 mV) is called *hyperpolarization*. In contrast, a reduction in membrane potential (e.g., from −60 to −45 mV) is called *depolarization*. As we shall see later, hyperpolarization decreases a cell's ability to generate an action potential and is therefore *inhibitory*; depolarization increases a cell's ability to generate an action potential and is therefore *excitatory*.

Input Signal: Receptor Potentials and Synaptic Potentials

The *receptor* (or *generator*) *potential* occurs at the receptive surface of sensory neurons and serves to transform the sensory stimulus (such as stretch, vibration, or light) into an electrical signal, the class of signal used by neurons to communicate. For example, at the receptor terminals of the sensory neuron in a stretch reflex, the mechanical energy of stretching the muscle spindle is converted into an electrical signal. This occurs because the change in spindle length releases the electrical energy stored in the resting membrane potential of the sensory nerve endings and thus produces a receptor potential. The receptor potential, like the other types of signals, is a change in the resting membrane potential of the cell membrane. However, the receptor potential of the stretch receptor has the special property of reflecting the mechanical change in the muscle in a graded, quantitative way. Thus, the larger or the longer lasting the stretch of the muscle, the larger and longer are the resulting sensory receptor potentials (see Figure 2–6).

The receptor potential in the sensory neurons is the first coded representation of stretch in the nervous system, but it alone would not cause any signals to appear in the rest of the nervous system. The receptor potential is a purely *local* signal that is restricted to the terminals of the sensory axon; because the membrane that generates this potential lacks voltage-dependent Na⁺ channels (discussed in Chapter 8), it cannot support an active signal, such as an action potential. Receptor potentials therefore propagate only passively along the neuron. Passively propagated signals (considered in greater detail in Chapters 6 and 7) decrease progressively in amplitude with distance and cannot be conveyed much farther than 1 or 2 mm. Typically, 1 mm down the axon, the amplitude of the signal will be only about one-third what it was at the site of generation.

Receptor potentials, particularly from slowly adapting or nonadapting receptors, generally last as long as the stimulus is applied. They can be either depolarizing and excitatory or hyperpolarizing and inhibitory. Depolarizing receptor potentials reduce the resting membrane potential and bring it closer to firing an action potential. Hyperpolarizing potentials increase the resting membrane potential and move it away from the firing threshold for an action potential, thereby decreasing the spontaneous generation of action potentials and the release of transmitter.

The *synaptic potentials* of central neurons (such as motor neurons) have a function comparable to that of receptor potentials. Synaptic potentials are the means by which one neuron can perturb the resting membrane potential of another cell to which it is connected and thus influence its activity. The presynaptic neuron releases a chemical transmitter that interacts with receptor molecules on the surface of the postsynaptic cell. The synaptic potential is generated in the postsynaptic cell and reflects the transformation of chemical energy into an electrical potential change. Synaptic potentials also are graded and can be either depolarizing and excitatory or hyperpolarizing and inhibitory. Synaptic potentials, like sensory receptor potentials, propagate passively from one region of the neuron to another by electrotonic mechanisms (described in Chapter 6). Synaptic potentials vary greatly in duration. They usually last several milliseconds, but some synaptic potentials last seconds or even minutes. The features of receptor and synaptic potentials are summarized in Table 2–1.

Table 2–1. Features of Receptor, Synaptic, and Action Potentials

Feature	Receptor potential	Synaptic potential	Action potential
Amplitude	Small (100 μv to 10 mV)	Small (100 μV to 10 mV)	Large (70–110 mV)
Duration	Brief (5–100 msec)	Brief to long (5 msec to 30 min)	Brief (1–10 msec)
Summation	Graded	Graded	All or none
Signal	Hyperpolarizing or depolarizing	Hyperpolarizing or depolarizing	Depolarizing
Propagation	Passive	Passive	Active

Signal Integration

As purely local signals that propagate passively, the receptor (or generator) potential and the synaptic potential cannot be faithfully transmitted because they are dissipated by the passive properties of neurons. In most neurons, the functional properties of the membrane change within 1 mm of the input component. The membrane adjacent to the input component is capable of initiating an action potential and, indeed, has the lowest threshold of any area of the cell's membrane for action potential initiation; it is thus called the *trigger zone*. The trigger zone sums the excitation and inhibition produced by the receptor potentials or synaptic potentials and determines whether or not an all-or-none action potential is discharged. Because this zone of membrane is the decision-making point, it is also called the *integrative component*. Thus if, after propagating to the trigger zone, the receptor or synaptic potentials have an integrated sum that is sufficiently excitatory, an action potential will be triggered (Figure 2–4B).

Conducting Signal: The Action Potential

Whereas input potentials propagate passively and decrease in amplitude with distance, the action potential propagates actively along the neuron without decreasing in amplitude and is therefore highly effective in signaling over a distance (Table 2–1). The action potential is a large depolarizing signal up to 100 mV in amplitude. It is often only 1 msec in duration. It differs from the graded generator and synaptic potentials in being an all-or-none signal.

Output or Secretory Signal

At the terminal region of the neuron the action potential serves as a stimulus for secretion at chemical synapses. At this type of synapse, the depolarizing effect of the action potential leads to the release of a chemical transmitter substance. As we shall see later (Chapter 11), this release is also graded because it involves a local potential, the *secretory potential*, which is triggered by the action potential and mediated by Ca^{++}. The transmitter diffuses across the synaptic cleft to the next cell, where it interacts with the input component to initiate another synaptic potential. Thus, in the monosynaptic reflex that we considered above, the secretory potential in the terminals of the dorsal root ganglion cell conveys the electrical representation of stretch to the motor cell by causing the motor cell to generate one or more synaptic potentials.

Location of Signaling Functions within Neurons

Each type of signal has a specific function; in addition, some signals are restricted to certain sites within the neuron because the neuron is regionally differentiated.

The resting membrane potential is generated by the entire surface membrane of the neuron. Different parts of the neuron usually have the same resting membrane potential, and in the absence of activity there is generally no current flow from one part of the neuron to another. In contrast, the receptor or synaptic potentials are generated only at specific input sites of the neuron. The molecular entities at the input sites responsible for receptor potentials are called *transducing receptors*; those for synaptic potentials are called the *synaptic receptors*. Both types of receptor molecules, as we shall see later, are thought to be intrinsic membrane proteins. The protein molecules of synaptic receptors are most commonly located on the plasma membrane of the dendrites and cell bodies of the neurons. Often the receptor molecules for inhibitory and for excitatory synapses are segregated from one another. For example, the inhibitory synapses are often located on the cell body of the neuron, or on the initial segment of the axon, whereas excitatory synapses are usually located on dendrites. There are typically no synapses along the main portion of the axon, but (as we shall see in Chapter 11) some axons have postsynaptic receptors on their terminals.

Integration, the algebraic summation of inhibitory and excitatory synaptic potentials (or receptor potentials), occurs in the portion of the excitable membrane that has the lowest threshold for initiating an action potential, usually the *initial segment of the axon*. In most cells the dendritic membrane cannot generate action potentials except at restricted and specialized sites, called dendritic trigger zones. Many cell bodies can generate action potentials, but they usually have a higher threshold for action potential generation than the axonal trigger zone (in the initial segment of the axon) or the dendritic trigger zones.

Similar Signaling Mechanisms Occur in All Nerve Cells

Most neurons, independent of size, shape, transmitter biochemistry, and behavioral function, can be depicted in terms of a generalized model neuron (Figure 2–5) that has four components: an input or receptive component, an integrative or summing component, a long-range signaling or conductile component, and a secretory or output component. This model neuron is thus a modern statement of the principle of dynamic polarization that Cajal inferred from examining the structure of various neural systems.

The model shown in Figure 2–5 is not accurate for all neurons, however. Some neurons do not generate action potentials (typically, neurons that have no axon or only a very short one, such as the receptor cells in the retina and certain interneurons in the brain). In cells lacking the integrative and conductile components, the input signals propagate passively to the terminal region, where they directly modulate the secretory potential and regulate transmitter release. Some cells do not have a steady resting potential and are spontaneously active. Moreover, despite many basic similarities, neurons differ in detail.

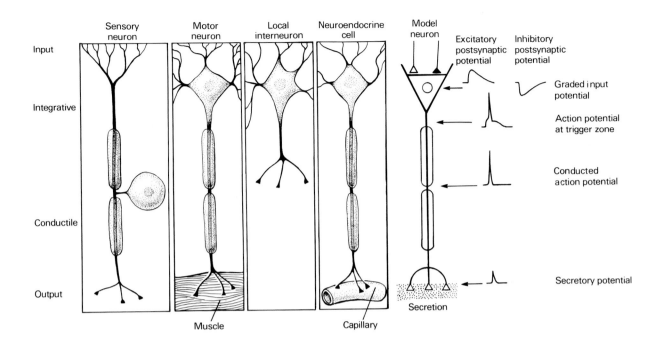

Muscle   Capillary   Secretion

Different neurons use different transmitters and have different transmitter receptors and ion channels in their membranes. Neurons are therefore biochemically quite heterogeneous. These differences account for the fact that different diseases may strike different neurons. As a result, the brain is subject to a greater number and variety of diseases, both neurological and psychiatric, than any other organ in the body. Such diseases as *amyotrophic lateral sclerosis* or *poliomyelitis* strike motor cells; other diseases, such as *tabes dorsalis*, affect sensory cells. *Diabetes insipidus* strikes only neuroendocrine cells. Within neurons, some diseases selectively affect the receptive elements, others affect the cell body, and still others affect the axon.

Nevertheless, the electrical signaling properties of all nerve cells are surprisingly similar and superficially quite stereotyped. For instance, long-range signaling varies only slightly from nerve cell to nerve cell. This feature was demonstrated by Edgar Adrian, who first approached the study of the nervous system on the cellular level in the 1920s. Adrian found that the action potential carried by a sensory axon into the nervous system is largely indistinguishable from the action potential of a motor axon carrying a command from the brain to muscles. For normal levels of excitation the firing rate of many sensory fibers and motor axons falls within the same range of 5–100 impulses per second. Different sensory fibers convey information that triggers different sensory experiences, but they do so by using the same types of action potentials. The type of signal (sensory or motor) is carried by specific sensory or motor pathways, not by different action potential mechanisms. Similarly, the intensity of the signal is conveyed by changes in the frequency of action potentials and not by changes in the magnitude or duration of the individual action potentials (Figure 2–6).

2–5 Most neurons, regardless of whether they are sensory, motor, interneuronal, or neuroendocrine, have four functional components in common: an input component, an integrative component, a conductile component, and an output component. Local interneurons often lack conductile components. On the basis of these shared features, a model neuron can be constructed that summarizes the functional organization of neurons in general.

Summarizing the results of his work on sensory fibers in 1928, Adrian wrote: ". . . all impulses are very much alike, whether the message is destined to arouse the sensation of light, of touch, or of pain; if they are crowded together the sensation is intense, if they are separated by long intervals the sensation is correspondingly feeble."

The only parameters of impulse firing in single sensory or motor neurons that are critical for signaling are the number of action potentials and the intervals between them. Given the large number of different nerve cells in the brain, it is fortunate that these two central features are shared by most neurons, because it makes the mechanism of signaling easy to understand; if we understand the mechanisms used to produce the various signals in any one kind of nerve cell, we shall be well along the way to understanding signaling in many other kinds of nerve cells.

We have now seen how individual cells produce a simple behavior and how the activation of certain movements leads to the inhibition of others so that unity of purpose is achieved. How are we to relate the functioning of individual cells to more complex behavior? No function is carried out by a single neuron; rather, behavior is generated by many cells; some perform roughly the same types of operations, others carry out related aspects of sensory analysis or motor integration. This parallel processing increases both the richness and the reliability of

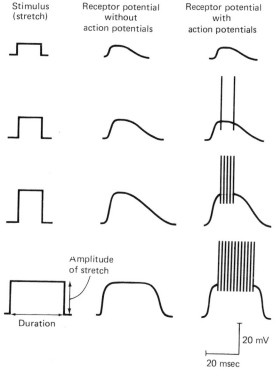

Stimulus (stretch)

Receptor potential without action potentials

Receptor potential with action potentials

Amplitude of stretch

Duration

20 mV

20 msec

2–6 Both the duration and amplitude of the receptor potential are translated into a frequency code of action potential spikes. The mechanical stimulus of stretch is transduced into an electrical signal, the receptor potential, which reflects both the amplitude and the duration of the stimulus. The receptor potential propagates passively to the initial segment of the axon, where action potentials are generated if the receptor potential is sufficiently large. The graded nature of the receptor potential is then translated into a frequency code of action potentials, or spikes. The amplitude of the receptor potential determines the frequency with which the action potentials are generated. The duration of the receptor potential determines the duration of the train of action potentials.

function within the central nervous system. Moreover, as we noted in Chapter 1 in relation to language, a key strategy used by the nervous system is spatial organization, or functional localization. Specific functions or aspects of processing are localized to particular regions or sets of regions within the brain. In addition, the brain contains distinctive regions designed to bring together neurons in various combinations that represent, in a precise topographical manner (and often repeatedly for many subfunctions), the various sensory surfaces of the body: the skin, tendons and joints, retina, basilar membrane of the cochlea, and olfactory epithelium. There is also a topographical representation for muscles and for movements, a representation that is necessary for voluntary as

well as for involuntary action. Thus, the brain contains at least two types of maps, or internal representations: one for sensory perceptions and the other for motor commands. The internal representations are interconnected in various ways.

Individual neurons within the two types of maps often do not differ greatly in their electrical properties. However, neurons with similar properties can assume different functions because they are assigned developmentally to different positions in relation to the various maps. The distinct set of input and output connections that a cell develops as a result of its position, therefore, is a key factor in determining that cell's role in behavior.

Selected Readings

Adrian, E. D. 1928. The Basis of Sensation: The Action of the Sense Organ. London: Christophers.

Cajal, S. R. 1937. Recollections of My Life. E. Horne Craigie (trans.). Edited in 2 vols. as Memoirs of the American Philosophical Society, Philadelphia.

Jones, E. G., and Cowan, W. M. 1983. The nervous tissue. In L. Weiss (ed.), Histology: Cell and Tissue Biology, 5th ed. New York: Elsevier Biomedical, pp. 282–370.

Katz, B. 1966. Nerve, Muscle, and Synapse. New York: McGraw-Hill.

Peters, A., Palay, S. L., and Webster, H. deF. 1976. The Fine Structure of the Nervous System: The Neurons and Supporting Cells. Philadelphia: Saunders.

References

Adrian, E. D. 1932. The Mechanism of Nervous Action: Electrical Studies of the Neurone. Philadelphia: University of Pennsylvania Press.

Cajal, S. R. 1933. Histology, 10th ed. Baltimore: Wood.

Jones, E. G., and Powell, T. P. S. 1973. Anatomical organization of the somatosensory cortex. In A. Iggo (ed.), Handbook of Sensory Physiology, Vol. 2: The Somatosensory System. New York: Springer, pp. 579–620.

Kandel, E. R. 1976. Cellular Basis of Behavior: An Introduction to Behavioral Neurobiology. San Francisco: Freeman, chap. 1.

Kuffler, S. W., Nicholls, J. G., and Martin, A. R. 1984. From Neuron to Brain: A Cellular Approach to the Function of the Nervous System, 2nd ed. Sunderland, Mass.: Sinauer Associates.

Martinez Martinez, P. F. A. 1982. Neuroanatomy: Development and Structure of the Central Nervous System. Philadelphia: Saunders.

Penfield, W. (ed.). 1932. Cytology and Cellular Pathology of the Nervous System, Vol. 2. New York: Hoeber.

Sears, E. S., and Franklin, G. M. 1980. Diseases of the cranial nerves. In R. N. Rosenberg (ed.), Neurology, Vol. 5: The Science and Practice of Clinical Medicine. New York: Grune & Stratton, pp. 471–494.

Stevens, C. F. 1979. The neuron. Sci. Am. 241(3):54–65.

Cell and Molecular Biology
of the Neuron

II

In this section we shall consider properties of nerve cells that are important for function. Nerve cells, the elementary signaling units of the nervous system, share many features with other cells of the body. They are distinguished from other cells by their highly developed ability to generate signals, and thus to communicate with one another and with other target cells precisely, rapidly, and over long distances. This remarkable ability derives from the presence of special membrane proteins that include channels and receptors. Some of these components are highly specific or even unique to nervous tissue. The types of channels that will primarily concern us in this part of the book are voltage-gated; they open in response to changes in the charge across the membrane in which the channel proteins are situated. Other channels are gated by the neurotransmitters released by other nerve cells. Both kinds of channels allow specific inorganic ions—Na^+, K^+, Ca^{++}, or Cl^-—to pass rapidly through the membrane.

Modern cell biology has given us considerable insights into the mechanisms by which proteins, membranes, and neurotransmitters are synthesized and processed in subcellular organelles. In these chapters, we shall therefore examine the function of neurons in the context of cell biology.

James H. Schwartz

The Cytology of Neurons

3

The Two Classes of Nerve Cells That Mediate the Stretch Reflex Differ in Morphology and Transmitter Substances
The Primary Afferent (Sensory) Neuron
The Motor Neuron

The Sensory Neuron and the Motor Neuron Differ in the Types of Receptor in Their Membranes

The Two Neurons Share Similar Na$^+$ Channels

The Two Neurons Have an Identical Na–K Exchange Mechanism

The Axons of Both Sensory and Motor Neurons Are Ensheathed in Myelin

A Major Function of the Neuron's Cell Body Is the Synthesis of Macromolecules

An Overall View

Selected Readings

References

As are other organs of the body, the brain is composed of characteristic cells that differ from the cells in other tissues. Specialization in cell type ultimately endows a tissue with its specific structure and function. Even though many brain cells are functionally similar, as we have seen in the previous chapters, the nervous system is distinctive because it contains more cell types than any other tissue. In addition to the two major types of neuroglia, there are thousands of different kinds of neurons, which are more varied in shape than any other cell type. The range of cellular diversity can be illustrated by considering the cerebellum, one part of the brain whose nerve cells have been completely catalogued. At one extreme, the cerebellum contains small granule cells, whose cell bodies are only 6–8 μm in diameter and consist of a nucleus surrounded by the thinnest shell of cytoplasm. The cerebellum also contains the Purkinje cells, which are among the largest neurons in the vertebrate nervous system; the giant cell bodies of these neurons can be 80 μm in diameter.

The cell body is only one of the four important regions of the neuron, and in most neurons it contains less than one-tenth of the cell's total volume. As we saw in Chapter 2, neurons can be classified according to the number of dendrites and axons that originate from the cell body. These processes, which usually contain more than 90% of a nerve cell's volume, differ in thickness, length, and branching pattern from neuron to neuron.

Cytological diversity is the result of the process embryologists call differentiation. Each differentiated cell synthesizes only certain macromolecules—enzymes, structural proteins, membrane constituents, and secretory products—and fails to make others. In essence, each cell *is* the macromolecules that it makes, as determined by the selection of genes it has come to express through development and differentiation. Although the particular cell type is determined by the specific classes of molecules the cell synthesizes, not all cellular constituents are specialized. Many components are found in every cell in the body; some are characteristic of all neurons, others of large classes of neurons; and still others are restricted to only a few nerve cells. Thus, each neuron consists of specific as well as general components.

In this chapter, we shall consider the cytology of the nerve cell and describe both the specific and the general components that are relevant to signaling. We shall illustrate these features with the two types of neurons that mediate the simple behavior discussed in the preceding chapter, the monosynaptic component of the stretch reflex involved in knee jerk. This component of the reflex consists only of the large sensory neurons of the dorsal root ganglion that are connected to muscle spindles, and the motor neurons in the anterior horn of the spinal cord that cause the muscle to contract. These two types of nerve cells differ in function and structure as well as in certain macromolecular components. They also display some cytological and biochemical features that are typi-cal of other neurons. In addition, they share many general components that are common to all cells of the body.

Organelles and macromolecular components are not distributed at random throughout the cell, but are situated in specific regions of the neuron. Indeed, this regional specialization of subcellular parts often determines the functions of a given cellular domain. In this chapter, we shall describe the subcellular distribution of organelles and other neuronal components. In the next chapter, we shall consider how cells synthesize macromolecules and then describe some of the mechanisms that neurons use to distribute these macromolecules to their appropriate destinations within the cell.

The Two Classes of Nerve Cells That Mediate the Stretch Reflex Differ in Morphology and Transmitter Substances

The anatomical arrangement of the neurons that mediate the stretch reflex is shown in Figure 2–4, and the role of this reflex in motor control will be discussed in Chapters 34 and 35. Essentially, the reflex consists of two cells: an afferent (or sensory) neuron and a motor neuron to which it is connected.

A Peripheral   **B** Central

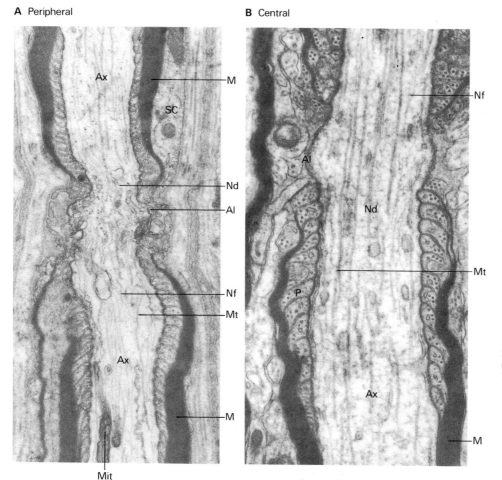

3–1 The myelin sheath of the axon is interrupted at the nodes of Ranvier. **A.** Axon from the peripheral nervous system. **B.** Axon from the central nervous system. In both **A** and **B** the axon (**Ax**) is running from the top to the bottom of the picture and is coated with many layers of myelin (**M**), which terminate at the nodes (**Nd**) in pockets of paranodal cytoplasm (**P**) of the supporting glial cell. In the peripheral nervous system this is a Schwann cell (**SC**), and in the central nervous system it is an oligodendrocyte. At the node, the axolemma (**Al**) is exposed. Within the axon, the elements of the cytoskeleton that are seen are microtubules (**Mt**) and neurofilaments (**Nf**). Mitochondria (**Mit**) are also seen. (From Peters, Palay, and Webster, 1976.)

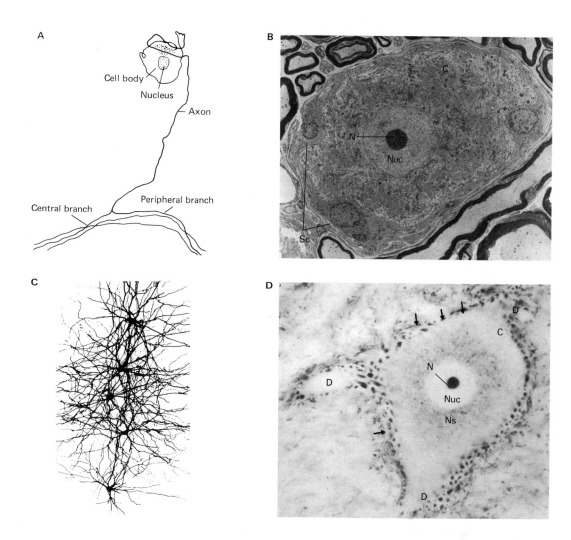

The Primary Afferent (Sensory) Neuron

The sensory ending of the primary (sensory) neuron forms a coil around a fine, specialized muscle fiber *(intrafusal fiber)* that lies within the larger stretch receptor called the *muscle spindle* (see Figures 34–9 and 34–10). In the specific instance of the knee-jerk stretch reflex, the sensory axon leaves the muscle and travels within a nerve called the sciatic nerve toward the lumbosacral region of the spinal cord. In the nerve, the diameter of the axon is 14–18 μm, and the axon is coated with a white, insulating sheath of myelin. This sheath, which is 8–10 μm thick, is regularly interrupted along the length of the axon by gaps of less than 0.5 μm that are called *nodes of Ranvier* (Figure 3–1A). In these regions, the plasma membrane of the axon, which is called the *axolemma*, is exposed to the extracellular space. Axons with smaller diameters have proportionally thinner myelin sheaths, and the distance between nodes (internodal distance) is smaller.

The round cell bodies of the primary afferent fibers are located in dorsal root ganglia at the lumbosacral portion of the spinal cord and are 60–120 μm in diameter (Figure 3–2A and B). These cells are classified as unipolar. Although they appear to give rise to only one axon, which

3–2 Two types of cells participate in the knee-jerk stretch reflex: the afferent (sensory) dorsal root ganglion cell, and the spinal motor neuron. **A.** A dorsal root ganglion cell. The cell body contains a prominent nucleus surrounded by satellite support cells. The axon of the dorsal root ganglion cell typically is quite convoluted before it bifurcates into a central and a peripheral branch. (From Dogiel, 1908.) **B.** A low-power electron micrograph showing the cell body (**C**) of a large dorsal root ganglion cell. Within the nucleus (**Nuc**) the prominent nucleolus (**N**) can be seen. The cell body of the neuron is surrounded by satellite cells (**Sc**). (Courtesy of R. E. Coggeshall and F. Mandriota.) **C.** A camera-lucida drawing of five spinal motor neuron cell bodies. These neurons have been filled with the anatomical tracer horseradish peroxidase, which reveals the many dendritic processes of the cells. (From Burke and Rudomin, 1977.) **D.** A photomicrograph of the cell body of a motor neuron. The cell membrane is contacted by an enormous number of incoming synaptic boutons (**arrows**). Three dendrites (**D**) are also shown. The nucleus with its nucleolus is surrounded by the Nissl substance (**Ns**). Synaptic input onto the cell body is prominent in this micrograph because the tissue is specially impregnated with silver. (Courtesy of G. L. Rasmussen.)

bifurcates within a few cell-body diameters into two branches, they actually derive from bipolar cells whose two processes fused during embryological development. One branch is the afferent axon (called the Ia afferent)

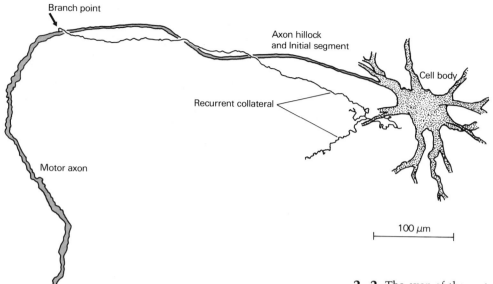

3–3 The axon of the motor neuron arises at the axon hillock, becomes myelinated after the initial segment, and gives off one to five recurrent collateral branches at branch points. This structure was demonstrated by iontophoretic staining (600 nA/min) with horseradish peroxidase. (Courtesy of R. E. Burke.)

that we have been tracing from the muscle; the other is the central branch in the dorsal root that enters the spinal cord and synapses on the motor neurons of the reflex.

The Motor Neuron

The sensory axon projects directly to motor neurons that innervate the same muscle from which the sensory axon has emerged, as well as to motor neurons of functionally synergistic muscles. These motor neurons have large cell bodies, each with a long axis up to 80 μm, and a nucleus that is distinctive because of its large size and prominent nucleolus (Figure 3–2C and D). Unlike the dorsal root ganglion cells, motor neurons have extensive dendritic trees. These cells have an average of 11 primary or first-order dendrites (with a range of 7–18), each of which ramifies 4–6 times, usually by bifurcating and occasionally by trifurcating. Because each primary dendrite ultimately gives rise to about 10 terminal branches, the total number of terminal dendritic branches per cell is over 100. The average length of a dendrite from the cell body to the termination at the end of a branch is about 10 cell-body diameters, but some branches are twice as long. Because these branches project radially, the dendritic tree of a single motor neuron can extend over an area of spinal cord with a diameter of 2–3 mm. The dendritic branching is extensive because these cells receive many inputs collected over a large area.

Although it has many dendrites, each motor neuron gives rise to only one axon, which originates from a specialized region of the cell body called the *axon hillock* (Figure 3–3). The first portion of the axon is called the

initial segment. Together, the axon hillock and initial segment extend about one cell-body diameter, at which point the axon becomes sheathed in myelin. As we saw in the last chapter, this part of the neuron functions as a *trigger zone* and is extremely important in integrating synaptic signals from other cells, which the neuron receives from synapses distributed over the dendritic tree, the soma, and the axon hillock.

In detailed morphological studies of individual motor neurons of the cat, Sebastian Conradi at the Karolinska Institute found that thousands and thousands of endings (called *synaptic boutons*) from other neurons cover about half the surface area of the axon hillock and cell body and three-quarters of the dendritic membrane. In addition to the excitatory input from the primary sensory neuron that we have been tracing, the motor neuron receives multiple excitatory and inhibitory inputs from neurons in the central nervous system that serve to modulate motor behavior. The changes in membrane potential resulting from all these synaptic inputs are tallied by mechanisms of *temporal* and *spatial summation*, and the resultant change in membrane potential is sensed at the trigger zone, whose membrane is rich in voltage-gated Na^+ channels. When these channels are activated, Na^+ ions rush in, depolarizing the membrane and initiating the propagated action potential.

Where on the motor neuron do the terminals of a primary sensory axon synapse? A. G. Brown at the University of Edinburgh, R. E. Burke at the National Institutes of Health, and their colleagues examined many individual cat motor neurons and found that the boutons from the primary sensory axons are located close to the trigger zone, either on the cell body itself (10% of boutons) or on one of its most proximal dendritic branches (Figure 3–2D). When boutons are situated on more than one dendritic branch, all of the contacts are at about the same geometric distance from the trigger zone. Each primary sensory neuron makes 2 to 6 contacts with each of 500 to 1000 motor neurons.

Communication between the primary sensory neuron and the motor neuron takes place by *synaptic transmission*. The neurotransmitter used by the primary sensory cell has not been identified with certainty, but much evidence indicates that it is a simple amino acid called *glutamate*. As we have seen, there are many synaptic boutons on the motor neuron other than the excitatory synapses from the primary sensory neuron. Among them are two classes of endings from *Renshaw interneurons* that are inhibitory in function (see below).

One striking difference between the motor neuron and the sensory cell is the localization of synaptic inputs. Both primary and modifying inputs to the motor neuron occur on the cell body and dendrites. In contrast, there are no synaptic boutons on the sensory cell bodies or on their axons within the dorsal root ganglion. The primary input to the sensory cell occurs in the muscle spindle, at the terminal coil of the peripheral axon, where a mechanical stimulus (stretch) is converted into an electrical signal by a process called *sensory transduction*. Sensory information is communicated to the central nervous system along the sensory axon by a propagated action potential. In addition to the primary input from the spindles, modifying inhibitory inputs to the sensory neuron occur within the spinal cord quite near the terminals of the central axonal branch of the dorsal root ganglion cell. These regulatory connections from neurons at higher levels of the central nervous system cause presynaptic inhibition; they will be considered in detail in Chapter 11.

Before we look at several other cytological and biochemical differences between the primary sensory neuron and the motor neuron, let us return to the description of the motor neuron by tracing its axon to its terminals in the muscle. Within the spinal cord, still close to the cell body, the motor axon gives off one to five *collateral branches* (Figure 3–3). These branches are called *recurrent* because they terminate on inhibitory interneurons called Renshaw neurons, which, in turn, synapse back on other motor neurons. (There are thought to be two types of Renshaw cells that are distinguishable on the basis of transmitter: one uses *glycine*, and the other, *γ-aminobutyric acid*. The biosynthesis of these neurotransmitters will be discussed in Chapter 13.) It has recently been discovered that a recurrent branch from the motor neuron occasionally ends directly on neighboring motor neurons without synapsing on an interneuron; sometimes the recurrent branch even ends directly on its own cell body.

The main axon, with a diameter of about 20 μm, leaves the spinal cord in the ventral root, which, in the lumbosacral region, joins the dorsal root to become the sciatic nerve. Thus, the motor axon travels along the same path as the sensory axon to the muscle that has just been stretched. When it enters the muscle, the motor axon ramifies into many branches that become thinner and thinner, reaching a diameter of only a few micrometers. Each branch then loses its myelin sheath and runs along the surface of a muscle fiber in a depression that is lined with the muscle's *basal lamina*. The basal lamina is a thin coat of connective tissue that is interposed between the presynaptic membrane of the nerve terminal and the receptors in the postsynaptic membrane of the muscle fiber. This synapse between nerve and muscle is called the *neuromuscular junction*; the site on the muscle fiber where the presynaptic terminal acts is called the *motor end-plate*. The presynaptic terminal of this synapse has a characteristic fine structure typified by a high concentration of synaptic vesicles that contain *acetylcholine* (the neurotransmitter released by the motor neuron), specialized release sites (called *active zones*), and several *mitochondria* (organelles that generate energy). The neuromuscular junction, which perhaps is the most completely characterized and best understood of all synapses, will be discussed in detail in Chapters 9 and 12.

The Sensory Neuron and the Motor Neuron Differ in the Types of Receptor in Their Membranes

As we have seen, despite similarity in signaling mechanisms, there are many cytological differences between the two cell types that mediate the knee jerk. In addition to their appearance, their place in the nervous system, and the distribution of their processes, we have also encountered two other important differences: the two neurons use different substances as neurotransmitters (although both transmitters are excitatory in function) and the two cells receive markedly different patterns of synaptic input. On one level of analysis, all of these cytological features have important consequences for the behavioral function of the neurons, which will be discussed in Part VI, in the context of the control of movement.

On another level of analysis, underlying each of these cytological features are molecular differences that ultimately stem from differential gene expression. For example, the release of acetylcholine by the motor neuron involves the formation of not only the biosynthetic enzyme choline acetyltransferase, but also several special membrane proteins that are not made in the sensory cell or in other noncholinergic neurons. Underlying the responsiveness to stretch that characterizes the transducing terminals of the sensory neuron is an ion channel that is regulated by mechanical deformation and that is not made in the motor neuron. Likewise, the motor neuron is able to respond to glutamate, γ-aminobutyric acid, and glycine because it has specific synaptic receptors, each of which is a distinct complex of integral membrane proteins. These complexes form structures that function as *chemically gated ion channels*, that is, pores in the membrane that open when a specific chemical messenger is bound to them. The molecular structure of the acetylcholine receptor at the neuromuscular junction, which is the best characterized chemically gated ion channel, will be described in Chapter 14.

The Two Neurons Share Similar Na⁺ Channels

Another class of ion channel is the voltage-gated ion channel, a pore that opens when the potential across the nerve cell membrane changes. An important member of this class is the Na⁺ channel. This ion channel is an example of a component that is expressed in almost all types of nerve cells. In both the sensory and motor neurons, the Na⁺ channel is highly concentrated in the portion of the axolemma exposed at the nodes of Ranvier; it opens to permit influx of extracellular Na⁺ ions, thereby depolarizing the axonal membrane. The Na⁺ channel functions in the propagation of the action potential. Its molecular characterization and specific arrangements along the axon will be described in Chapter 8.

Both the primary sensory neuron and the motor neuron have K⁺ channels that are concentrated in the membranes of their cell bodies and at their terminals. When the membrane in these regions is depolarized, K⁺ ions flow out of the cell through these channels. Voltage-gated K⁺ channels thus help restore the membrane potential to the resting level in these regions of the neuron. K⁺ channels have not yet been isolated or characterized. They are thought to be proteins, however, because they function according to many of the same principles as the Na⁺ channel and the acetylcholine receptor, both of which are composed of integral membrane proteins.

The synaptic endings of the primary sensory neuron and of the motor neuron contain important inward voltage-gated Ca⁺⁺ channels, another type of channel shared by all nerve cells. Ca⁺⁺ is the critical ion for the last step in the release of neurotransmitter, which occurs through the exocytosis of synaptic vesicles in which the transmitter is packaged (see Chapters 12 and 15). Therefore, this voltage-gated ion channel essentially controls the secretory function of the neuron.

The Two Neurons Have an Identical Na–K Exchange Mechanism

In the axon, maintenance of the membrane potential at the resting level is largely the result of another kind of membrane component, an enzyme called *Na–K adenosine triphosphatase* (Na–K ATPase), which acts as a pump, moving Na⁺ out of cells and K⁺ in. Pumps differ from ion channels. Channels are selective pores in the membrane that do not require metabolic energy. Pumps move ions actively using the energy produced by the hydrolysis of adenosine triphosphate (ATP) to exchange ions across the membrane. The Na–K ATPase is an example of a class of components that are universal. All cell types must maintain their membrane potential, and the use of metabolic energy for the exchange of cations is the chief mechanism by which this is accomplished. As might be expected, however, the Na–K pump is much more abundant in the membranes of excitable cells and is highly concentrated in nervous tissue.

Na–K ATPase is a multimeric complex consisting of two different polypeptides: a transmembrane catalytic subunit (with a molecular weight of 105,000) and a glycoprotein regulatory subunit (with a molecular weight of about 45,000–50,000). On its axoplasmic, or intracellular, surface the catalytic subunit has binding sites for Na⁺ and ATP, and on its extracellular surface, sites for K⁺ and for ouabain, a poison that specifically and irreversibly inhibits the pump. When ATP is split by hydrolysis, the catalytic subunit (E) forms a covalent intermediate by being phosphorylated (P) at a specific β-aspartic acid residue. This reaction depends on the presence of Na⁺:

$$E + ATP \underset{}{\overset{Na^+}{\rightleftharpoons}} \text{E-P} + ADP.$$

Protein phosphorylation changes the conformation of the complex, which leads to the removal of three Na⁺ ions from the inside of the axon to the outside in exchange for two extracellular K⁺ ions. The phosphorylated catalytic subunit (E-P) is hydrolyzed in the presence of K⁺:

$$\text{E-P} + H_2O \overset{K^+}{\rightarrow} E + P_i.$$

Although axonal membranes are an extremely rich source of Na–K ATPase, some uncertainty persists about the precise localization of the pump. There is some indication that the pump is especially concentrated in the region of the nodes of Ranvier, but the most convincing evidence suggests that it is distributed all along the axolemma, at the nodes as well as in the internodal membrane.

The Axons of Both Sensory and Motor Neurons Are Ensheathed in Myelin

Electron microscopy has revealed that the myelin sheath around axons of both types of neurons is arranged in concentric layers (Figures 3–1 and 3–4). Early microscopists were impressed with the high degree of regularity of myelin and used X-ray diffraction and polarized light (techniques appropriate for analyzing crystal structure) to investigate its structure. In 1939, F. O. Schmitt, at the Massachusetts Institute of Technology, concluded that the sheath consists of repeating layers of protein with bimolecular layers of lipids interspersed between adjacent protein layers. Biochemical analysis shows that myelin has a composition similar to that of plasma membranes, consisting of 70% lipid and 30% protein, with a high concentration of cholesterol and phospholipid.

These properties of myelin can now be explained because we understand how the sheath is formed (Figure 3–4). Before myelination, the axon in a peripheral nerve is protected by an enveloping trough formed by a series of peripheral glia called *Schwann cells*. These cells are lined up along the axon with intervals between them that will eventually become the nodes of Ranvier. The external cell membrane (plasmalemma) of each Schwann cell then surrounds the axon and forms a double-membrane struc-

A

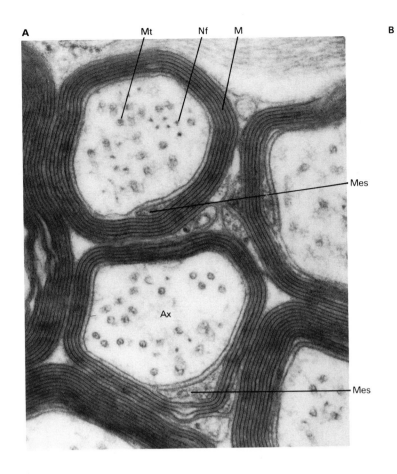

B

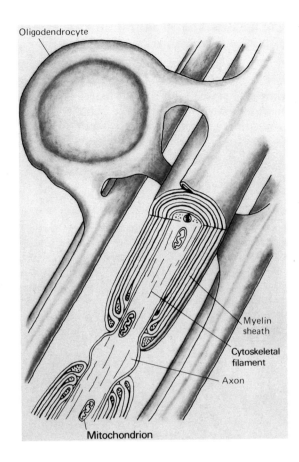

ture called the *mesaxon*, which elongates and spirals around the axon many times. The cytoplasm of the Schwann cell appears to be squeezed out as the mesaxon wraps the axonal process in concentric layers. The cytoplasmic surfaces of the Schwann cell's processes then condense into the compact lamellae of the mature myelin sheath. Because the primary sensory axon in the sciatic nerve is 1–1.5 m long, and the internodal distance is 1–1.5 mm, it can be estimated that approximately 1000 nodes of Ranvier occur along a primary afferent fiber between the leg muscle and the dorsal root ganglion, where the cell body lies. Thus, 1000 Schwann cells participate in the myelination of this sensory axon. The central axonal branch of the dorsal root ganglion cell is also myelinated. The myelin within the spinal cord differs to some degree from its peripheral counterpart because the support cell responsible for elaborating it is the oligodendrocyte rather than the Schwann cell (Figures 3–1B and 3–4A).

Although both peripheral myelin and central myelin function similarly to provide insulation, there are some specific morphological and biochemical differences between them. Peripheral myelin contains a few characteristic *glycoproteins*, which account for more than half of the total protein in the sheath. Central myelin, which lacks these glycoproteins, contains characteristic *proteo-*

3–4 Myelin ensheaths axons of both sensory and motor neurons. **A.** Transverse section through two axons (**Ax**) in the central nervous system. The spiraling lamellae of the myelin sheath (**M**) start at the internal mesaxons (**Mes**). Within the axons, microtubules (**Mt**) and neurofilaments (**Nf**) can be seen. (From Peters, Palay, and Webster, 1976.) **B.** Processes of oligodendrocyte forming myelin sheath around axons in the central nervous system. (Adapted from Bunge, 1968.)

lipids. Proteolipids are proteins soluble in organic solvents and thus differ from lipoproteins, which are soluble in water. Both central myelin and peripheral myelin contain the same predominant *basic protein*, which has a molecular weight of 18,000 and is highly antigenic. When injected into animals, this basic protein produces a cellular autoimmune response called *experimental allergic encephalomyelitis.* This laboratory disease of the central nervous system, characterized by focal areas of inflammation and demyelination, is being studied as a model for *multiple sclerosis.* A relatively common disease, multiple sclerosis primarily manifests itself as impaired sensory or motor performance because the demyelination of motor axons interferes with impulse conduction and therefore with perception and proper motor coordination (see Chapter 18).

A Major Function of the Neuron's Cell Body Is the Synthesis of Macromolecules

One of the important differences that we have already noted between the sensory neuron and the motor neuron is the role played by the motor neuron's cell body in the transmission of synaptic signals. Under normal circumstances, the action potential in the sensory neuron is transmitted directly from the peripheral axon to the central branch, although it can be detected by placing a recording microelectrode in the cell body. The invasion of the action potential into the cell body can be slowed or completely blocked if the cell body is hyperpolarized, but this blockade in no way affects the passage of the signal along the axons. What, then, is the function of the sensory neuron's cell body? The answer to this question was suggested by a critical series of experiments dating from the mid-nineteenth century in which the English physiologist Augustus Volney Waller cut the various roots and nerves of the spinal cord and studied the distribution of fibers that degenerated as a result. From the patterns of degeneration, Waller concluded that the dorsal root gan-

glion cell bodies serve to maintain the vitality of the fibers that are attached to them. In a lecture delivered to the Royal Institution of Great Britain in 1861, he said, "A nerve-cell would be to its effluent nerve-fibres what a fountain is to the rivulet which trickles from it—*a centre of nutritive energy.*"

From modern cell biology, we now know that information for the synthesis of macromolecules is encoded in the deoxyribonucleic acid (DNA) of the chromosomes within the cell's nucleus (Figure 3–5). In all cell types, there are two important ways in which this information can be processed: (1) the genetic information is passed from parent to daughter cell during cell division (heredity), or (2) a selected portion of the genetic information is *transcribed* into ribonucleic acid (RNA) and *translated* into proteins (gene expression). In most mature nerve cells, and in the two cells that we have been discussing in this chapter, cell division is no longer possible, and the chromosomes function only in gene expression.

Because mature nerve cells cannot divide, the chromosomes are not arranged in compact structures, but exist in a relatively uncoiled state. Thus, neuronal nucleo-

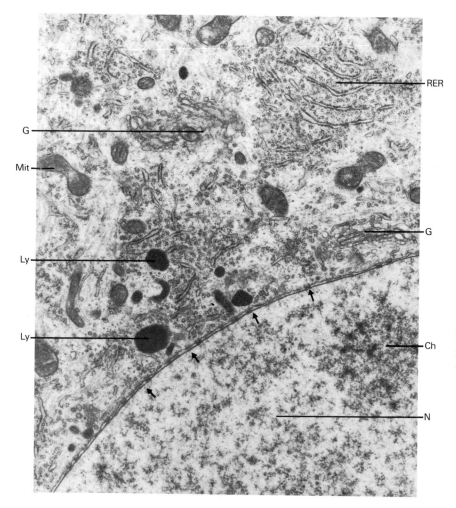

3–5 Some of the components of a spinal motor neuron that participate in gene expression for the synthesis of macromolecules. The nucleus (**N**), containing masses of chromatin (**Ch**), is bounded by a double-layered membrane, the nuclear envelope, which contains many nuclear pores (**arrows**). Messenger RNA leaves the nucleus through these pores and attaches to polyribosomes that either remain free in the cytoplasm or attach to the membranes of the endoplasmic reticulum to form the granular or rough endoplasmic reticulum (**RER**). Several parts of the Golgi apparatus are seen in various planes of section (**G**). Also present in the cytoplasm are lysosomes (**Ly**) and mitochondria (**Mit**). (From Peters, Palay, and Webster, 1976.)

plasm, even when viewed in the electron microscope, has a rather amorphous appearance, except for a prominent spherical body called the *nucleolus* (Figure 3–2B and D). The nucleolus contains the specific portion of DNA encoding the RNA (rRNA) of future *ribosomes,* complex cytoplasmic particles upon which proteins are synthesized. During development, this part of the chromosome has been reduplicated many times and is especially prominent in secretory cells, such as neurons, that make large quantities of proteins. The nucleolus can be visualized as a definite structure because it contains many repetitive sequences of DNA and RNA that cohere in a more compact organization than do the components of the rest of the chromosomes.

In addition to the ribosomal genes of the nucleus, many other genes also are actively transcribed into the precursor of messenger RNA (mRNA), called heterogeneous nuclear (hn)RNA. This is then selectively processed into mRNA. The mRNA is transported across the double-layered nuclear envelope through 65-μm pores that are arranged in rows with a center-to-center spacing of about 150 μm (Figure 3–5). Because the pores in adjacent rows are staggered, the pattern of pores appears as a roughly hexagonal array in tangential views of the nuclear membrane. The two leaflets of the nuclear envelopes are continuous only at the margin of the pores. The outer leaflet of the nuclear envelope is continuous with the highly folded membrane of the *endoplasmic reticulum,* an extensive system of sheets, sacs, and tubules that extends throughout the cytoplasm around the nucleus.

Although most of the genetic information for the synthesis of proteins is encoded in the cell's nucleus, a very small amount is contained in circular DNA molecules within mitochondria (Figure 3–5). It is in these organelles, each of which is about the size of a bacterial cell, that the energy generated by the metabolism of sugars and fats is transformed into ATP by oxidative phosphorylation. The sequence of the 16,569 nucleotides in the human mitochondrial genome has been determined; it encodes information for mitochondrial transfer RNAs (tRNAs) and rRNAs (which differ from those in the rest of the cell), and for a small fraction of the mitochondrion's proteins (cytochrome oxidase, cytochrome b, a subunit of ATP synthetase, and ten other as yet unidentified polypeptides). The rest of the mitochondrion's proteins are encoded by nuclear chromosomes, synthesized by cytoplasmic ribosomes, and then taken up into the mitochondrion, as discussed in the next chapter.

An Overall View

The word "physiology," like "physics," derives from the Greek *physis,* meaning nature; a physiologist was an inquirer into the primal elements of things. A basic tenet of neurobiology, which we considered in the first two chapters, is that the functioning of the nervous system reflects the activities of its constituent nerve cells. In this chapter, we have extended this idea by illustrating that the physiology of a cell is the expression of the macromolecules that are responsible for the particular nature of that cell. Cytology is the study of the form, location, and special composition of cells. In nervous tissue, we must also specify the target cells with which the neuron connects. Form, location, molecular composition, and specific interconnections are all reflections of the cell's developmental history and its pattern of gene expression. The variety of neuronal cell types and the resulting diversity in physiological functioning are achieved by developmental mechanisms that are only now beginning to be understood.

Like most cells, neurons contain the complex apparatus for synthesizing proteins and the genetic information in DNA to encode them. In common with other cells, they also have mitochondria and enzymes both for biosynthesis of small molecules and for intermediary metabolism—the major pathways that convert carbohydrates and other substances into usable energy. Since nerve cells are excitable, they share some membrane constituents with cells in other excitable tissues, but many components are highly specialized and are restricted to specific classes of nerve cells. Thus, only certain neurons contain one or another transmitter substance, special ion channel, membrane transport mechanism, or type of receptor molecules. Our understanding of the physiological process ultimately depends on the identification and characterization of all of these components, both general and neuron-specific. Although it is obvious that a component unique to neurons can provide insight into neuronal physiology, it is also clear that all cellular functions, from basic metabolism to neuronal signaling, are mediated by ensembles of molecular constituents, general and specific, working together.

Selected Readings

Llinás, R. R. 1984. Comparative electrobiology of mammalian central neurons. In R. Dingledine (ed.), Brain Slices. New York: Plenum Press, pp. 7–24.

Peters, A., Palay, S. L., and Webster, H. deF. 1976. The Fine Structure of the Nervous System: The Neurons and Supporting Cells. Philadelphia: Saunders.

Siegel, G. J., Albers, R. W., Agranoff, B. W., and Katzman, R. (eds.). 1981. Basic Neurochemistry, 3rd ed. Boston: Little, Brown.

Willis, W. D., and Coggeshall, R. E. 1978. Sensory Mechanisms of the Spinal Cord. New York: Plenum Press.

References

Brown, A. G., and Fyffe, R. E. W. 1981. Direct observations on the contacts made between Ia afferent fibres and α-motoneurones in the cat's lumbosacral spinal cord. J. Physiol. (Lond.) 313:121–140.

Bunge, R. P. 1968. Glial cells and the central myelin sheath. Physiol. Rev. 48:197–251.

Burke, R. E., Dum, R. P., Fleshman, J. W., Glenn, L. L., Lev-Tov, A., O'Donovan, M. J., and Pinter, M. J. 1982. An HRP study of the relation between cell size and motor unit type in cat ankle extensor motoneurons. J. Comp. Neurol. 209:17–28.

Burke, R. E., and Rudomin, P. 1977. Spinal neurons and synapses. In E. R. Kandel (ed.), Handbook of Physiology, Vol. 1: The Nervous System, Part 2. Bethesda, Md.: American Physiological Society, pp. 877–944.

Conradi, S. 1969. Ultrastructure and distribution of neuronal and glial elements on the motoneuron surface in the lumbosacral spinal cord of the adult cat. Acta Physiol. Scand. [Suppl.] 332:5–48.

Dogiel, A. S. 1908. Der Bau der Spinalganglien des Menschen und der Säugetiere. Jena: Fischer.

Fambrough, D. M., and Bayne, E. K. 1983. Multiple forms of $(Na^+ + K^+)$-ATPase in the chicken: Selective detection of the major nerve, skeletal muscle, and kidney form by a monoclonal antibody. J. Biol. Chem. 258:3926–3935.

Forgac, M., and Chin, G. 1985. Structure and mechanism of the (Na^+, K^+) and (Ca^{2+})-ATPases. In P. Harrison (ed.), Topics in Molecular and Structural Biology: Metalloproteins, Vol. 2. New York: Macmillan, pp. 123–148.

Lemke, G., and Axel, R. 1985. Isolation and sequence of a cDNA encoding the major structural protein of peripheral myelin. Cell 40:501–508.

Ochs, S. 1975. Waller's concept of the trophic dependence of the nerve fiber on the cell body in the light of early neuron theory. Clio Med. 10:253–265.

Schmitt, F. O., Worden, F. G., Adelman, G., and Dennis, S. G. (eds.). 1981. The organization of the cerebral cortex. In: Proceedings of a Neurosciences Research Program Colloquium. Cambridge, Mass.: MIT Press.

Ulfhake, B., and Kellerth, J.-O. 1981. A quantitative light microscopic study of the dendrites of cat spinal α-motoneurons after intracellular staining with horseradish peroxidase. J. Comp. Neurol. 202:571–583.

James H. Schwartz

Synthesis and Distribution of Neuronal Protein

4

The brain expresses more of the total genetic information encoded in DNA than does any other organ in the body. About 200,000 distinct messenger RNA sequences are thought to be expressed, 10–20 times more than in the kidney or liver. Some of this sequence diversity results from the greater number and variety of cell types in the brain as compared with cells in the more homogeneous body tissues; but many neurobiologists believe that each of the brain's 10^{12} nerve cells actually expresses a greater amount of its genetic information than does a liver or kidney cell. What sort of proteins are these, and where are they synthesized? With the exception of the few proteins encoded by the mitochondrial genome enumerated in Chapter 3, essentially all of the macromolecules of a neuron are made in the cell body from mRNAs that are produced in the nucleus. As in other cell types, each nerve cell makes only three classes of proteins (Figure 4–1):

1. Proteins that are cytosolic.
2. Proteins that are encoded by the cell's nucleus but that are later incorporated into mitochondria.
3. Proteins that are inserted into membranes or that become secretory products.

The mRNAs that encode the cytosolic proteins and the proteins destined to be imported into mitochondria are translated on free polyribosomes (polysomes); the mRNAs for membrane proteins and secretory products form polysomes that become associated with flattened sheets of the endoplasmic reticulum.

The three classes of proteins are common to all cell types. As in other tissues, the bulk of the protein formed in neurons is cytosolic, but because neurons are secretory cells, membrane proteins and secretory products constitute a substantial proportion of the macromolecules synthesized. Most of the macromolecules made by nerve cells appear not to differ from their counterparts in other tissues. Nevertheless, it seems axiomatic that if classes of neurons and possibly even individual nerve cells are unique, then some of the proteins synthesized by each neuron will also be unique. Indeed, cytosolic, membrane, and secretory proteins have been found that are specific to groups of neurons and even to single cells. Moreover, there is some evidence for the existence of neuron-specific mitochondria. We shall consider each of the three classes of protein in turn.

Nuclear mRNA Gives Rise to Three Classes of Proteins

Cytosolic Proteins

Cytosolic proteins constitute the two most abundant groups of proteins in the cell: (1) the fibrillar elements that make up the *cytoskeleton* (neurofilaments, tubulins, and actin, which, taken together, account for at least 20% by weight of the protein in the neuron), and (2) the numerous *enzymes* that catalyze the reactions *of intermediary metabolism.* In addition, other biosynthetic and degradative enzymes are synthesized on free ribosomes, including some that are characteristic of specific types of neurons. An example in the spinal motor neurons that we considered earlier is choline acetyltransferase, the enzyme that catalyzes the synthesis of acetylcholine.

mRNA molecules for cytosolic proteins emerge through the nuclear pores and become associated with ribosomes to form free polysomes in the neuron's cytoplasm (Figure 4–1). Typically, the proteins made on free polysomes are produced essentially in their final form. Very little modification of the polypeptide chain occurs, with the exception of small changes of functional groups in specific amino acid residues (for example, phosphorylation of serine hydroxyl groups or acetylation of N-terminal amino groups), some of which are reversible. After they are synthesized in the cell body, both the soluble components of the cytoplasm and elements of the cytoskeleton move into the dendrites and axons of the neuron by slow transport, which we shall discuss later in this chapter.

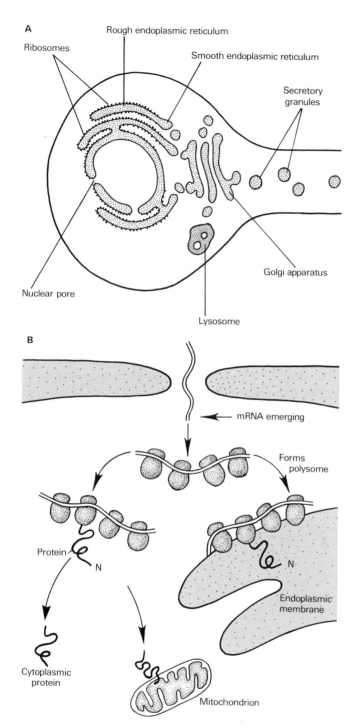

4–1 A. The organelles that are responsible for the synthesis and processing of proteins. **B.** mRNAs, transcribed from genomic DNA in the neuron's nucleus, emerge through nuclear pores to form polysomes by attaching to ribosomes. Three classes of proteins are formed. Which class of protein depends on the fate of the particular polysome and this, in turn, is determined by information encoded in the particular mRNA. Cytosolic and some mitochondrial proteins are made on polysomes that remain free in the cytosol. Proteins destined to be inserted into membranes (for example, the membranes of secretory granules or lysosomes) or proteins that ultimately will become secretory products are synthesized by polyribosomes that attach to the membrane of the endoplasmic reticulum (see Figure 4–4).

Mitochondrial Proteins

Mitochondrial proteins that are encoded by the cell's nucleus are also formed on free polysomes (Figure 4–1). Once their synthesis on polysomes is completed, these proteins attach to the outer membrane of the mitochondrion and are then imported into the organelle (Figure 4–2). Although they represent only a small fraction of the total protein produced by the neuron, mitochondrial proteins introduce an important feature of the cell biology of neurons—the mechanisms by which specific components are distributed to the organelles to which they belong. One mechanism is *posttranslational importation* of the protein *after* its synthesis has been completed on free ribosomes. The other mechanism is *cotranslational transfer*. The second mechanism is used by most membrane and secretory proteins of the neuron and will be discussed next.

Membrane Proteins and Secretory Products

mRNAs encoding proteins destined to become membrane constituents and secretory products form polysomes that become associated with flattened sheets of the endoplasmic reticulum (Figure 4–1). These membranous sheets, which are studded with ribosomes, have a granular appearance in the electron microscope and are therefore called *rough endoplasmic reticulum*. Rough endoplasmic reticulum is usually most dense in the cytoplasm nearest the nucleus but has different distributions in different neurons (Figure 4–3). In the motor neuron, for example, rough endoplasmic reticulum is densely distributed around the nucleus, where it is arranged in highly ordered parallel arrays, but it is also found in the primary dendrites, especially at their bases, where they emerge from the cell body (Figure 4–3A). In contrast, in the dorsal root sensory cell the rough endoplasmic reticulum has a more disorderly appearance (Figure 4–3B). The ribosomal RNA in the rough endoplasmic reticulum stains intensely with basic histological dyes (toluidine blue, cresyl violet, and methylene blue). In the light microscope, this basophilic complex is called Nissl substance after the Bavarian histologist who, in 1892, first described changes in the intensity and distribution of staining in neurons that occur when axons are cut. These changes, which reflect alterations in the patterns of protein synthesis in injured and regenerating neurons, will be discussed in Chapter 17. A large portion of this extensive internal membrane system lacks attached ribosomes but is continuous with the rough endoplasmic reticulum. Because of the absence of ribosomes, it is called *smooth endoplasmic reticulum.*

A polysome destined to produce a membrane protein is formed from the same population of ribosomes as that used by the free polysomes already described. As we shall see, however, the polysome for a membrane protein must eventually attach to the endoplasmic reticulum. Proteins are polypeptides, or polymers of amino acids. One end has a free amino (N-terminal) group and the other end has a carboxyl (C-terminal) group. The peptide chain begins to be synthesized at its N-terminal end. In membrane proteins, however, the N-terminus—the leading portion of the nascent polypeptide—is composed of a series of amino acid residues or *signal sequence* that does not end up in the mature protein. This region has a length of about 20 residues, many of which are hydrophobic. The signal sequence has a specific function: it causes the polysome to bind to a small ribonucleoprotein body called the *signal receptor particle*, which arrests translation of the mRNA at the end of the leader peptide sequence. This complex now attaches to the cytoplasmic surface of the endoplasmic reticulum membrane, aided

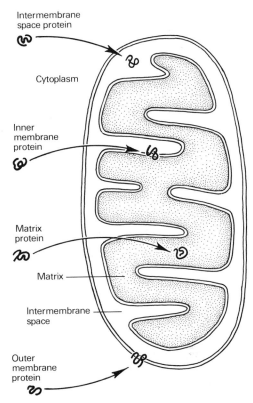

4–2 Importation of mitochondrial proteins. Many mitochondrial proteins are encoded by mRNAs synthesized in the cell's nucleus. These proteins are produced on free ribosomes in the cell's cytoplasm, and imported into the mitochondrion only after they are completed. Each kind of imported protein is destined for one of the several compartments in the organelle. The ways in which the proteins reach these compartments are shown in the diagram. All of the proteins must first bind to the outer mitochondrial membrane. This adhesion is thought to occur spontaneously. Proteins destined for the other mitochondrial compartments are then transported by energy-dependent processes through the membranes that intervene. Thus, a protein destined for the matrix must first pass through the outer membrane, traverse the intermembranous space, and then be transferred through the inner mitochondrial membrane to be released into the matrix.

by two ribosomal glycoproteins called *ribophorins*. Binding to the endoplasmic reticulum displaces the signal receptor particle, and translation begins again. In an energy-dependent process, the N-terminal end of the growing peptide threads through the lipid bilayer into the lumen of the endoplasmic reticulum, where the signal sequence peptide is removed by proteolytic cleavage. The polypeptide continues to grow in length at its C-terminal end.

There are several possible paths that the polypeptide can now take, depending on the fate of the finished protein product (Figure 4–4). An integral membrane protein with its C-terminal amino acid sequence on the cytoplasmic side and its N-terminus on the luminal side of the endoplasmic reticulum will result if transfer through

A Motor neuron

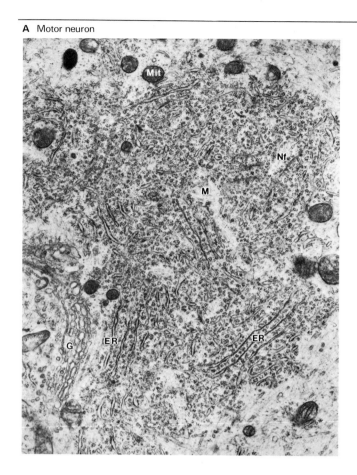

B Dorsal root ganglion cell

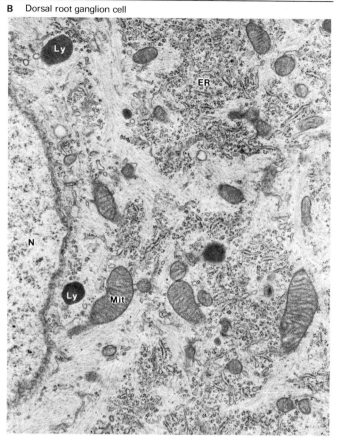

4–3 These electron micrographs show the organelles in the cell body that are chiefly responsible for synthesis and processing of proteins. **A.** The spinal motor neuron. **B.** The dorsal root ganglion. Through the double-layered nuclear envelope that surrounds the nucleus (**N**), mRNA enters the cytoplasm to form polyribosomes. Some of these polyribosomes elaborate proteins in the cytoplasm, some of which remain soluble and some of which are transported after they are synthesized into mitochondria (**Mit**). One major class of proteins is formed after the polysomes attach to the membrane of the endoplasmic reticulum (**ER**). In the light microscope, this is called Nissl substance. Both cells have similar kinds of organelles, but the particular region of the motor neuron shown in **A** also contains membranes of the Golgi apparatus (**G**), in which membrane and secretory proteins are further processed. Some of the newly synthesized proteins leave the Golgi in vesicles that move by rapid axonal transport down the axon to the synapses; other membrane proteins are incorporated into lysosomes (**Ly**). (From Peters, Palay, and Webster, 1976.)

the membrane stops before the message is fully translated (Figure 4–4A). An integral protein with several regions threaded through the membrane will result if the N-terminus doubles back through the membrane from the luminal side (Figure 4–4B). This process can be repeated several times (Figure 4–4C), as is thought to occur in the synthesis of the acetylcholine receptor (see Chapter 14). The portions of the polypeptide chain that finally remain embedded in the lipid bilayer are hydrophobic,

and therefore appropriate for the hydrophobic microenvironment in the membrane. (The endoplasmic reticulum is also a major site of lipid synthesis; thus, both constituents of membrane, protein and lipid, are produced coordinately.) A secretory protein will result if the C-terminus is completely transferred into the lumen of the endoplasmic reticulum (Figure 4–4D). Whether finally an integral membrane protein or a secretory product, these polypeptides are transferred through the membrane while the chain is being synthesized. The transfer is therefore called *cotranslational.*

Two posttranslational mechanisms distinguish membrane and secretory proteins from those made in the cytosol: (1) processing by proteolytic cleavage and (2) modification by glycosylation. The final membrane protein or secretory product is synthesized as part of a larger precursor polypeptide chain that is extensively processed by *proteolytic cleavages.* Sequential and specific tailoring of the larger precursor begins in the lumen of the endoplasmic reticulum, both rough and smooth (as we have seen for the removal of the signal peptide), and continues during the subsequent steps in the elaboration of membrane and secretory proteins in the Golgi apparatus. Indeed, processing can continue in the various finished organelles—secretory granules, lysosomes, and the plasma membrane. Production of smaller proteins from a larger polypeptide can have several physiological consequences.

One consequence is intracellular targeting. For example, the nascent precursor itself is directed to the endoplasmic reticulum. This function, common to all membrane and secretory proteins, is mediated by the N-terminal signal sequence, which is removed when it is no longer needed. Another function is the masking of a potential enzymatic activity that would be undesirable in the endoplasmic reticulum. This occurs with the precursors of proteolytic enzymes (trypsinogen, for example), which are secretory products that serve the organism best if they function extracellularly. This mode of synthesis also permits amplification or diversification of the secreted peptide products. This feature is important for hormones and neuroactive peptides (see Chapter 13). For example, in the processing of opioid peptides, more than one copy of the same peptide and several peptides with different physiological functions are cut from the same precursor. When this occurs, the polypeptide precursor is called a *polyprotein* because it contains more than one potentially active peptide.

Glycosylation, the addition of oligosaccharide chains, begins in the rough and smooth endoplasmic reticulum and is completed in the Golgi apparatus. Sugars are continuously being added; these chains are trimmed enzymatically in a specific manner both in the endoplasmic reticulum and in the Golgi apparatus. The physiological consequences of glycosylation are not yet certain, but many possible functions have been proposed. Most of the suggested functions make use of the exquisite chemical specificities of the complex sugar chains of glycoproteins. Mechanisms that require intermolecular recognition—for example, cell-to-cell recognition or adhesion that occurs during development and in the formation of synapses—could be mediated by specific binding of proteins at glycosyl residues. Moreover, since the same protein can have somewhat different oligosaccharide chains (a phenomenon called *microheterogeneity*), glycosylation could also serve to diversify the function of a given protein. For example, the same polyprotein with sugar residues at different sites along the molecule may be cleaved into different products by the same processing protease.

New membrane and secretory proteins are thought to pinch off from the smooth endoplasmic reticulum in transport vesicles that shuttle to the Golgi apparatus. The Golgi apparatus, which is found in the cell bodies of all neurons, consists of several interconnected membranous cisternae arranged in flattened stacks (Figure 4–3A). In some cells, these cisternae are quite long, extending almost concentrically around the nucleus. In other cells, the Golgi apparatus is arranged so that one of its broad aspects faces the smooth endoplasmic reticulum (*cis* or *forming* face) and the other faces the plasma membrane, axons, and dendrites (the *trans* face). The mechanisms by which new membrane is produced in the Golgi apparatus are only beginning to be understood. Components destined for assembly into several diverse organelles (secretory vesicles; synaptic vesicles; the plasma membrane, including specialized regions such as the synaptic membrane; lysosomes; and peroxisomes) all pass through the Golgi stacks, where they are biochemically tailored.

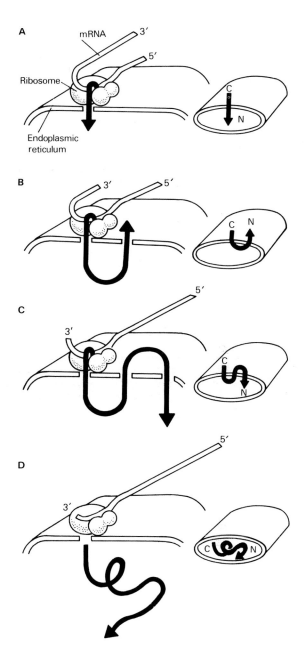

4–4 Formation of membrane and secretory proteins. This class of proteins is formed after polyribosomes attach to the membrane of the endoplasmic reticulum. Peptide chains are polymerized by translation of an mRNA from its 3' to its 5' end. Each of the many ribosomes in a polysome remains fixed to the membrane in one place while amino acid residues are being added sequentially to the C-terminal end of the nascent peptide chain. (Only one of the ribosomes in a polysome is shown in the Figure.) As the peptide elongates, the mRNA molecule moves across the ribosomes in the direction of synthesis (toward the 5' end). The N-terminus of all proteins of this class first penetrates through the membrane (**A**). The N-terminus of some polypeptides, which are destined to become integral membrane proteins, can penetrate the membrane from the luminal side of the endoplasmic reticulum (**B**), and some even repenetrate several times (**C**) as the chain grows. Proteins destined to become secretory products typically are not integrated into the membrane, but penetrate the lumen of the endoplasmic reticulum completely (**D**). A simplified diagram is shown to the right.

There they are sorted out for incorporation into the appropriate organelle by processes involving specific proteolytic cleavage, glycosylation, and the addition of other functional groups such as sulfate.

How these biochemical steps finally result in the precise and orderly segregation of membrane constituents within the neuron remains to be elucidated. These membrane components leave the Golgi apparatus in a variety of vesicles that, in electron micrographs, appear to be budding off from cisternal membrane or fusing with it. Some of the vesicles, particularly those associated with the *trans*-most cisternae, can be identified as primary lysosomes because cytochemical stains reveal that they contain acid hydrolase activity. In certain neurons, some vesicles can be identified as secretory granules because they contain some secretory product (a neuroactive peptide or a hormone) in high concentration; in other nerve cells, still other vesicles can be identified as transmitter storage granules because of their high concentration of specific neurotransmitter. These organelles from the cell body are precursors of synaptic vesicles.

Anterograde Axonal Transport Controls Intracellular Distribution of Membranes and Secretory Proteins

Neurons are secretory cells. Like gland cells, in which secretory granules are assembled in the region of the Golgi apparatus, neurons have transmitter storage granules that are the precursors of synaptic vesicles and that are formed in the internal membrane systems in the nerve cell body. In gland cells, the granules must be moved to a particular region of the plasmalemma (for example, the apical region of the gland cell that abuts the lumen of a duct), where the granule's contents are expelled by exocytosis. Although formally similar, the secretory process in neurons appears to be quite different because of the extreme regional differentiation of the nerve cell. Typically, cell bodies and nerve terminals are at considerable distances from each other. Consider, for example, the spinal motor neuron that originates in the lower back region of a 6-foot man and that innervates the muscles around the knee joint. In terms of the secretory process, this separation implies a great distance between that part of the plasmalemma specialized for exocytosis (the active zone of the presynaptic terminal membrane) and the site of origin of the synaptic or secretory vesicle (the endoplasmic reticulum and Golgi apparatus in the cell body). How do these vesicles move from the Golgi apparatus to the sites within the neuron where they must function?

Essentially all newly synthesized membranous organelles within axons and dendrites (except in the most proximal regions of primary dendrites) are exported from the cell body by fast, forward-moving *anterograde* (or *orthograde*) axonal transport. In warm-blooded animals the organelles move at a rate of about 400 mm/day. A large proportion of this material consists of synaptic ves-

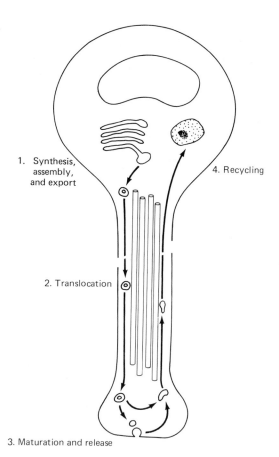

4–5 Synaptic vesicles and other membranous organelles involved in synaptic transmission are returned to the cell body for recycling after they are used at the synapse. Proteins and lipids are synthesized and incorporated into membranes within the endoplasmic reticulum and Golgi apparatus of the neuron's cell body (**1**). Organelles are then assembled from these components and exported from the cell body into the axon, where they are rapidly moved toward terminals by fast axonal transport (**2**). Some of the material is deposited along the axon to maintain the axolemma. Synaptic vesicles and their precursors reach the neuron's terminals to participate in the exocytotic release of transmitter substances (**3**). The membranes of synaptic vesicles are used many times over in the release process. At random, a small amount of the membrane becomes degraded by lysosomes, and this material is returned to the cell body by fast retrograde axonal transport. The degraded membrane is partly recycled; its residue is progressively accumulated in large, end-stage lysosomes that are characteristic of neuronal cell bodies (**4**).

icles or their precursors that must be brought to the terminals.

In the process of exocytosis at nerve terminals, the vesicle membranes are recycled many times for reuse in synaptic transmission (see Chapter 12). Membrane is constantly being renovated by new components arriving from the cell body. At a compensating rate, existing membrane components are removed from the nerve terminals and returned to the cell body for degradation or reuse (Figure 4–5).

ribosomes. *Calmodulin*, the 17,000-molecular-weight Ca^{++}-binding protein, has also been identified in this slow component. In the presence of Ca^{++}, this highly conserved protein binds reversibly to many key enyzmes and other proteins, thereby altering their function. The Ca^{++} regulation of many reactions is actually mediated by the Ca^{++}–calmodulin complex (see Chapter 14).

Fibrillar Elements Constitute the Neuronal Cytoskeleton

More recent experiments demonstrate that the proteins that constitute the cytoskeleton determine neuronal form. In addition, these proteins mediate the movements of organelles from one region of the neuron to the others. They also serve to anchor membrane constituents, such as receptors, at appropriate locations on the cell's surface. Still another important aspect of these fibrillar proteins is that they may undergo changes in diseased or aging nerve cells. The organization of the cytoskeleton in an axon is revealed in the photomicrograph of a freeze-etched preparation shown in Figure 4–10. Three types of fibrillar elements varying in thickness are the chief constituents of the cytoskeletons of neurons: microtubules, neurofilaments, and microfilaments.

Microtubules, the thickest of the neuron's cytoskeletal fibers, are long polymers of tubulin dimers composed of α, β, and two guanosine triphosphates in a tubular array with an outside diameter of 25–28 nm (Figure 4–10). They are oriented along the length of the axon. The α- and β-tubulins of neurons appear to be similar, if not identical, to the tubulins of other cell types. They are widely believed to be the tracks along which organelles move by fast transport.

Neurofilaments, 10 nm in diameter, typically are the most abundant fibers in axons and serve as the principal support system in the neuron (Figure 4–10). They were first observed by Robert Remak in 1843 at the University of Berlin. Historically, these fibers are important in the verification of the neuron theory because they are the elements impregnated with silver nitrate, the stain first applied by Golgi in 1873 and later used extensively by Cajal. Neurofilaments are related to intermediary filaments of other cell types, all of which belong to a family of proteins called the *cytokeratins*. Neurofilaments are essentially totally polymerized in the cell: like hair, to which they are also related, there is hardly any physiological condition under which these proteins can exist in solution. They also are oriented along the length of the axon. On the average, there are three to ten times more neurofilaments in an axon than microtubules, and some axons have very few microtubules. In Alzheimer's disease and other degenerative diseases, these proteins appear to be modified, forming a characteristic lesion called the neurofibrillary tangle (see Chapter 59).

Microfilaments, 5–7 nm in diameter, are the thinnest of the three types of fibers that make up the cytoskeleton (Figure 4–10). Like the thin filaments of muscle, microfilaments are polymers of globular actin monomers wound into a two-stranded helix. Actins are a

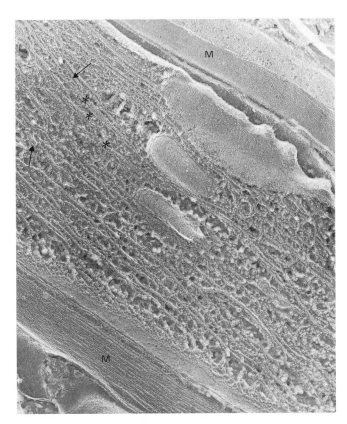

4–10 Zone near the axolemma where filamentous material contacts particles on the inner axolemmal surface. At the top of figure are two sausage-shaped organelles that probably correspond to components of the retrograde transport system. The left end of the large one is associated with a gap in the axoplasm. These organelles are in a microtubule domain of the axoplasm (bracketed by **arrows** at left) that passes obliquely through the plane of fracture and consequently has a very irregular outline. Pieces of at least five microtubules (**stars**) are evident in the vicinity of the organelles. **M**, myelin sheath. ×105,000. (Courtesy of B. Schnapp and T. Reese.)

major constituent of all cells (perhaps the most abundant single protein in nature), and are encoded by a gene family that includes, in addition to the actin of skeletal muscle (designated α), at least two other molecule forms (β and γ). Neural actin, first described by Sol Berl at Columbia University, is a mixture of the β and γ species, which differ from α-actin at a few amino acid residues. Despite these differences, most of the actin molecule is highly conserved, not only in actins from different cells of the animal, but also in actins from organisms as diverse as man and protozoa.

Microfilaments in the neuron appear to be in a state of flux. It has been estimated that about half of the total actin in neurons exists as unpolymerized monomers at any one time. Much of the actin in neurons is associated with the external membrane; in dendrites, for example, it is concentrated at spines, specialized regions upon which synapses occur. (Dendritic spines are rudimentary in the spinal motor neuron but are a prominent feature in the cerebral cortex.) Some axonal microfilaments are oriented longitudinally. In the axon and at nerve terminals, microfilaments are abundant underneath the axolemma and at the synaptic membrane. As in other cells, these filaments are attached to the external membrane by means of several structural proteins that bind actin. These structural proteins are generally tightly associated with the membrane, but they are not integral membrane proteins (proteins synthesized on rough endoplasmic reticulum whose polypeptide chains extend through the lipid bilayer of the endoplasmic reticulum and that must be treated with detergent to be extracted from the membrane). The principal anchoring protein in neurons and other cells of the body is called *fodrin*, a high-molecular-weight component that is transported along the axon with actin.

An Overall View

The flow of genetic information from the neuron's nucleus is transcribed into mRNA and carried into the cytoplasm, where it is translated into three classes of proteins: cytosolic, mitochondrial, and membrane-secretory. Each of these classes of macromolecules has distinctive physiological roles in the neuron's cell biology. Cytosolic proteins, which are distributed primarily throughout the neuron by slow axoplasmic transport, include the fibrillar elements of the cytoskeleton, which determine the shape of the cell. In addition, the cytosolic enzymes, both for intermediary metabolism and for special biosynthetic pathways, consume, use, and transfigure the many low-molecular-weight substances of the cell. Membrane-secretory proteins, which are moved along axons and dendrites by fast axonal transport, function in the interactions of the neuron with its environment—through secretion by exocytosis and maintenance of the external membrane by recycling of membrane and endocytosis. The primary function of mitochondria, which are also distributed throughout the neuron by a form of fast transport, is to generate ATP, the major molecule by which cellular energy is transferred or spent.

Which proteins are crucial to the signaling properties of nerve cells? Proteins in each of the three classes display properties and reactions that are not *directly* relevant to synaptic transmission, but some processes mediated by each class of proteins are critical. Thus, cytosolic enzymes catalyze the synthesis of the small-molecule transmitter substances; the energy of the ATP formed in mitochondria is needed in the mechanism of synaptic transmission; and one of the chief products of the membrane-secretory class of proteins in neurons is the synaptic vesicle and, in peptidergic neurons, its neurosecretory contents.

Selected Readings

Alberts, B., Bray, D., Lewis, J., Raff, M., Roberts, K., and Watson, J. D. 1983. Molecular Biology of the Cell. New York: Garland.

Fawcett, D. W. 1981. The Cell, 2nd ed. Philadelphia: Saunders.

Holtzman, E., and Novikoff, A. B. 1984. Cells and Organelles, 3rd ed. Philadelphia: Saunders College Publishing.

Schwartz, J. H. 1979. Axonal transport: Components, mechanisms, and specificity. Annu. Rev. Neurosci. 2:467–504.

References

Berl, S., Puszkin, S., and Nicklas, W. J. 1973. Actomyosin-like protein in brain. Science 179:441–446.

Brady, S.T. 1985. A novel brain ATPase with properties expected for the fast axonal transport motor. Nature 317:73–75.

Divac, I., LaVail, J. H., Rakic, P., and Winston, K. R. 1977. Heterogeneous afferents to the inferior parietal lobule of the rhesus monkey revealed by the retrograde transport method. Brain Res. 123:197–207.

Dokas, L. A. 1983. Analysis of brain and pituitary RNA metabolism: A review of recent methodologies. Brain Res. Rev. 5:177–218.

Ernster, L., and Schatz, G. 1981. Mitochondria: A historical review. J. Cell Biol. 91:227s–255s.

Gasser, S. M., Ohashi, A., Daum, G., Bohni, P. C., Gibson, J., Reid, G. A., Yonetani, T., and Schatz, G. 1982. Imported mitochondrial proteins cytochrome b_2 and cytochrome c_1 are processed in two steps. Proc. Natl. Acad. Sci. U.S.A. 79:267–271.

Glenney, J. R., Jr., and Glenney, P. 1983. Fodrin is the general spectrin-like protein found in most cells whereas spectrin and the TW protein have a restricted distribution. Cell 34:503–512.

Grafstein B., and Forman, D. S. 1980. Intracellular transport in neurons. Physiol. Rev. 60:1167–1283.

Hoffman, P. N., and Lasek, R. J. 1975. The slow component of axonal transport: Identification of major structural polypeptides of the axon and their generality among mammalian neurons. J. Cell Biol. 66:351–366.

Mori, H., Komiya, Y., and Kurokawa, M. 1979. Slowly migrating axonal polypeptides: Inequalities in their rate and amount of transport between two branches of bifurcating axons. J. Cell Biol. 82:174–184.

Oblinger, M. M., and Lasek, R. J. 1985. Selective regulation of two axonal cytoskeletal networks in dorsal root ganglion cells. In O'Lague, P. (ed.), Neurobiology: Molecular Biological Approaches to Understanding Neuronal Function and Development. The Shering Corp.: UCLA Symposium on Molecular and Cellular Biology. Vol. 24. New York: Liss.

Ochs, S. 1972. Fast transport of materials in mammalian nerve fibers. Science 176:252–260.

Peters, A., Palay, S. L., and Webster, H. deF. 1976. The Fine Structure of the Nervous System: The Neurons and Supporting Cells. Philadelphia: Saunders.

Schnapp, B. J. and Reese, T. S. 1982. Cytoplasmic structure in rapid-frozen axons. J. Cell Biol. 94:667–679.

Vale, R. D., Schnapp, B. J., Mitchison, T., Steuer, E., Reese, T. S., and Sheetz, M. P. 1985. Different axoplasmic proteins generate movement in opposite directions along microtubules in vitro. Cell 43:623–632.

Weiss, D. G., ed. 1982. Axoplasmic Transport. Berlin: Springer.

Weiss, P., and Hiscoe, H. B. 1948. Experiments on the mechanism of nerve growth. J. Exp. Zool. 107:315–395.

John Koester

Resting Membrane Potential and Action Potential

5

The modern study of the nervous system and its disorders is predicated on understanding the cellular and molecular mechanisms whereby nerve cells interact to produce behavior. This interaction, indeed the general flow of information both within and between the cells of the nervous system, is conveyed by transient electrical signals. These *transient* signals—the generator potentials, the action potentials, and the synaptic potentials—are all produced by one basic class of mechanisms: brief alterations in the electrical properties of the membrane that give rise to the *resting* membrane potential. An understanding of how the resting membrane potential is generated thus leads easily to understanding how transient signals arise; that understanding in turn explains the interactions between nerve cells that give rise to behavior.

The Membrane Potential Is Proportional to the Separation of Charge across the Cell Membrane

All neurons have an electrical charge on the membrane that results from a thin cloud of positive and negative ions spread over their intra- and extracellular surfaces. In a nerve cell at rest, there is a net excess of positive charges on the outside of the membrane and a net excess of negative charges on the inside. The membrane is able to maintain a separation of charge because it acts as a permeability barrier to the diffusion of ions. This separation of charge is responsible for the *resting membrane potential, V_R*. In most neurons, the potential difference across the resting membrane ranges from about -40 to -75 mV, with the outside taken to be zero and the inside negative with respect to the

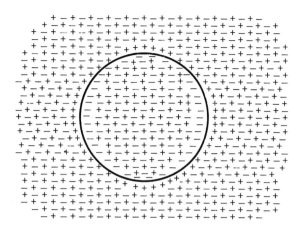

5–1 The net excess of positive charges outside and negative charges inside the membrane of a nerve cell at rest represents a small fraction of the total number of ions inside and outside the cell. (The ratio of the width of the region of charge separation to cell diameter is exaggerated here for purposes of illustration.)

outside. In these cells,

$$V_R = -40 \text{ to } -75 \text{ mV}.$$

All signaling results from changes in the resting membrane potential. Whereas the term resting membrane potential (V_R) refers to potential across the cell when it is at rest, the more general term *membrane potential* (V_m) refers to the potential across the membrane at any moment—at rest or during various types of activation—and is defined as

$$V_m = V_{in} - V_{out}$$

where V_{in} is the potential on the inside of the cell and V_{out} the potential on the outside.

The membrane potential is directly proportional to the charge separation across the membrane. To change the membrane potential by 10 mV there need only be an increase of about 600 positive charges on one side of the membrane and of 600 negative charges on the other side, per square micrometer of membrane. The relatively small number ($600 \times 6 = 3600$ charges/μm^2) of positive and negative charges that must be separated across the cell membrane to produce a resting membrane potential of -60 mV represents an insignificant fraction of the total number of positive and negative charges inside the cell (Figure 5–1). The bulk of the cytoplasm and of the extracellular fluid is electrically neutral, with an equal number of positive and negative charges. Charge separation exists only in a very narrow region, considerably less than 1 μm wide, on either side of the membrane.

To record the resting membrane potential, one electrode must be placed on each side of the membrane (Figure 5–2A). The size and shape of the extracellular electrode are not critical, but the electrode placed inside the cell must have a very fine tip in order not to damage the membrane of the cell. After amplification, the signal from the two electrodes is fed to an *oscilloscope*, which

displays the amplitude of the membrane potential as the vertical deflection of a spot of light on the face of a cathode ray tube. With both electrodes outside the cell, no electrical potential difference is recorded; but as soon as the microelectrode is inserted into the cell, the oscilloscope displays a steady deflection of about -60 mV, the resting membrane potential.

To generate an action potential, the membrane potential must be made less negative by reducing the charge separation across the membrane. Because the cell is electrically polarized at rest, the process of reducing the charge separation is called *depolarization*. A cell can be artificially depolarized in a graded fashion by using a second pair of electrodes for passing current across the membrane (Figure 5–2B). Again, one current-passing electrode is put into the surrounding fluid and a second is inserted into the cell. These two electrodes are connected to a current generator that can pass current into or out of the cell. By convention, the direction of current flow is determined by the direction of net movement of *positive* charge. By making the internal electrode positive with respect to the external electrode, the current generator delivers a pulse of current that will depolarize the cell: current (positive charge) will flow into the neuron from the intracellular microelectrode and accumulate on the inside of the cell's membrane; at the same time it will be withdrawn from the outside of the membrane by the extracellular electrode. The initial excesses of negative charge on the inside of the membrane and of positive charge on the outside are thus reduced as the cell is depolarized. The result is a progressive decrease in the normal separation of charge across the membrane, which leads to a decrease in membrane potential.

When current is injected into the cell to depolarize it, not all of the positively charged ions that pass through the intracellular electrode remain within the cell. Some of these positive ions leak out across the membrane. Thus, when positively charged ions are injected into the cell to depolarize it, there is an *outward membrane current*.

Reversing the direction of current flow—by making the intracellular electrode negative in relation to the extracellular electrode—increases the charge separation across the membrane, making the membrane potential more negative (Figure 5–2C). This increase in charge separation *hyperpolarizes* the membrane. When positive charges are withdrawn from the cell by the intracellular electrode and added to the outside by the extracellular electrode to produce a hyperpolarization, an *inward membrane current* results (Figure 5–2C). Such passive depolarizing or hyperpolarizing responses of membrane potential to current injection are called *electrotonic potentials*.

Within a certain range of membrane potential, only electrotonic potentials are evoked by current injection. A small outward current produces a small depolarization. If the outward current pulse is larger, the depolarization is proportionately larger. An active response, the all-or-none action potential, is triggered when the membrane

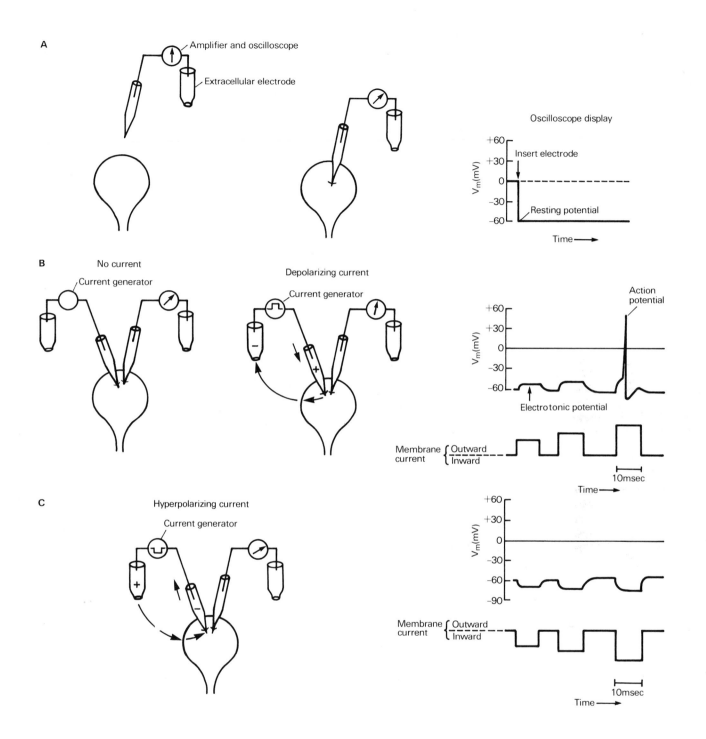

5–2 Changes in membrane potential are experimentally induced by current injection. **A.** To measure the resting potential an electrode is inserted into the nerve cell and the potential difference between the inside and the outside of the cell is recorded. The intracellular electrode is a glass pipette drawn out to a tip about 0.5 µm in diameter and filled with a concentrated solution of a salt such as KCl. The pipette acts as a "salt bridge," providing an electrical connection between the cytoplasm and a metal electrode that is connected to the electronic apparatus. A second salt bridge of the same composition is used as the extracellular electrode. Two silver wires, coated with AgCl, are inserted into the back ends of the two salt bridges. They are used to lead off the difference in transmembrane voltage to a voltage amplifier. The spot of light on the oscilloscope screen is produced by a beam of electrons which, because of its low inertia, can accurately follow the most rapid changes in V_m. Since the spot moves at a constant rate in a horizontal direction across the screen of the oscilloscope, a trace is obtained that shows how the membrane potential varies with time. **B.** Injecting positive charge into the cell through an intracellular current electrode reduces the net charge separation between the inside and outside, thereby depolarizing the cell. If the depolarization is large enough, an action potential is generated. **C.** Withdrawing positive charge from the cell (by making the electrode negative) increases the net separation of charge, thereby hyperpolarizing the cell.

potential reaches a critical level, called the *threshold* (usually about 15 mV depolarized, from -60 to -45 mV) (Figure 5–2B). The action potential differs from the electrotonic potential in magnitude, duration, and the way in which it is generated.

The mechanism by which the action potential is generated will be discussed below. First, however, we shall examine the properties of the membrane that give rise to the resting membrane potential. The mechanism of action potential generation, as well as synaptic and generator potentials, can then be understood in terms of variations in the properties of the resting membrane.

The Resting Membrane Potential Is Generated by the Differential Distribution of Ions and Selective Permeability of the Membrane

No single ion species is distributed equally on the two sides of a nerve cell membrane. Of the four major ions in cells, Na^+ and Cl^- are more concentrated outside the cell, and K^+ and organic anions (A^-) are more concentrated inside the cell. The organic anions are negatively charged amino acids and proteins. The distribution of these ions across the membrane of the squid giant axon is shown in Table 5–1. The squid giant axon, which contributes to the squid's defensive escape behavior, is widely used for experiments on neuronal function because of its large size. Similar ratios for each type of ion are found in vertebrate nerve cells, but the absolute value of the concentrations of each ion is generally three- to fourfold lower than in the squid—an animal that lives in the ocean, an environment that has a high concentration of ions.

The unequal distribution of ions raises two important questions. First, how do these ionic gradients give rise to the resting potential? Second, how are they maintained? What prevents the ionic gradients from being dissipated by passive diffusion of ions across the membrane? The answers to these questions are interrelated. We shall examine them by considering two examples of increasing complexity: the cell membrane of glial cells, which is permeable to only one species of ions, and the membrane of nerve cells, which is permeable to several species of ions.

Table 5–1. Intracellular and Extracellular Distribution of the Major Ions Across the Membrane of the Squid Giant Axon

Ion	Cytoplasm (mM)	Extracellular fluid (mM)	Nernst potential[a] (mV)
K^+	400	20	-75
Na^+	50	440	$+55$
Cl^-	52	560	-60
A^-	385	—	—

[a]The membrane potential at which there is no net flux of an ion across the cell membrane.

In Glial Cells the Membrane Is Selectively Permeable to K^+

In solutions such as the extracellular space or the cytoplasm of the cell, Na^+ and K^+ move freely. The flow of ions in response to concentration gradients such as those shown in Table 5–1 is limited only by the membrane of a cell, which acts as a physical barrier to diffusion. Most of the membrane is almost completely impermeable to ions. Ions diffuse across the membrane only at specialized intramembranous protein pores called *channels*. The various channels in the membranes are selective for the types of ions that they allow to pass. This selectivity is based on the size, charge, and hydration of the ions. The relative proportion of different types of ion-selective channels in a membrane determines its net selectivity for the permeation of various ions.

We shall first examine the membranes of glial cells, which have only K^+ channels and thus are permeable only to K^+. They differ in this respect from nerve cell membranes, which have channels for Na^+ and Cl^- as well.

A glial cell has a high concentration of K^+ and organic anions on the inside and a high concentration of Na^+ and Cl^- on the outside. Assume that initially there is no potential difference across the membrane. The glial cell membrane is selectively permeable[1] to K^+, so that K^+ diffuses out of the cell, down its concentration gradient (Figure 5–3). As the K^+ cations diffuse out, nonpermeant anions are left behind. This results in a net surplus of positively charged ions (cations) outside the cell and a net surplus of negatively charged ions (anions) inside the cell. The electrostatic attraction between the excess cations on the outside of the membrane and the excess anions on the inner surface generates a thin cloud of charge distributed over each surface of the membrane.

Although an electrostatic attraction develops between external K^+ and internal anions, there is no net movement of K^+ back into the cell because the K^+ concentration gradient is large and continues to drive K^+ out of the cell. Eventually, however, the progressive build-up of positive charge outside the cell and negative charge inside does impede the further movement of K^+ due to electrostatic repulsion. Thus, two opposing forces interact: one chemical, and the other electrical. The force of the *chemical concentration gradient* tends to push K^+ out of the cell. The force due to the charge separation results in an *electrical potential difference* that tends to push K^+ back into the cell because the outside of the cell membrane is positive in relation to the inside.

As the diffusion of K^+ continues to increase the separation of charge, the difference in electrical potential increases across the membrane. The membrane potential continues to increase until it reaches a value that has an

---

[1]The permeability of the membrane to an ion (P_i) is defined as the net flux (J_i) of that ion, divided by the product of the concentration difference of that ion across the membrane (ΔC_i) times the membrane area (A):

$$P_i = J_i/\Delta C_i A.$$

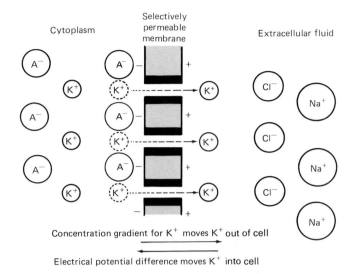

Cytoplasm

Selectively permeable membrane

Extracellular fluid

Concentration gradient for K⁺ moves K⁺ out of cell

Electrical potential difference moves K⁺ into cell

5–3 The resting potential, in a cell selectively permeable to K⁺, is generated by the efflux of K⁺ down its concentration gradient.

effect on K⁺ equal and opposite to the effect of the concentration gradient. At this value of membrane potential, which in most glial cells is about -75 mV, K⁺ is at equilibrium across the membrane. In a cell permeable only to K⁺, this K⁺ *equilibrium potential* is therefore the resting membrane potential, V_R. At the equilibrium potential, the force of the chemical concentration gradient that acts to drive K⁺ out of the cell is just equal and opposite to that of the electrical potential difference that drives K⁺ back into the cell.

In a cell that has a membrane permeable only to K⁺, no metabolic energy is required to maintain the ionic gradients shown in Table 5–1. The membrane potential automatically settles at a value where K⁺ ions are in equilibrium; that is, the efflux of K⁺ is exactly balanced by its influx. The gradients for other ions are not important, because these ions cannot pass through the membrane. Thus, once the ionic gradients are established, they will persist indefinitely with no expenditure of metabolic energy.

That the cell is truly at equilibrium under these conditions can be appreciated by examining how the membrane potential reacts to a transient deviation from its equilibrium value of -75 mV. For example, a depolarization caused by a brief current pulse has no significant effect on the *concentration* gradient for K⁺ because the net excess of positive and negative charges on opposite sides of the membrane that give rise to the membrane potential, V_m (or to changes in V_m), is only a tiny fraction of the total number of ions in the cytoplasm. The *electrical* gradient drawing K⁺ into the cell decreases, however, so that a net efflux of K⁺ develops. At the end of the current pulse, the K⁺ efflux continues until V_m has returned to -75 mV, at which point K⁺ is again in equilibrium. Conversely, a transient hyperpolarization results in an increase in the electrical gradient and therefore in a self-correcting net influx of K⁺; the influx will gradually go to zero as V_m returns to -75 mV.

The membrane potential at which K⁺ ions are in equilibrium can be calculated from an equation derived in 1888 from basic thermodynamic principles by the German physical chemist Walter Nernst. According to the Nernst equation,

$$E_K = \frac{RT}{ZF} \ln \frac{[K^+]_o}{[K^+]_i}.$$

In this equation, E_K is the value of membrane potential at which K⁺ is in equilibrium (K⁺ *Nernst potential*), R is the gas constant, T the temperature in degrees Kelvin, Z the valence of K⁺, F the Faraday constant, and $[K^+]_o$ and $[K^+]_i$ the concentrations of K⁺ on the outside and inside of the cell. To be precise, chemical activities should be used rather than concentrations.

For K⁺, $Z = +1$, and at 25°C, RT/ZF is 26 mV. The constant for converting from natural logarithms to base 10 logarithms is 2.3. Substituting the values of K⁺ concentration given in Table 5–1, we have

$$E_K = 26 \text{ mV} \times 2.3 \log_{10} \frac{20}{400} = -75 \text{ mV}.$$

The Nernst equation not only applies to K⁺ but can also be used to find the equilibrium potential of any other ion that is present on both sides of a membrane permeable to that ion. The Na⁺, K⁺, and Cl⁻ Nernst potentials for the distributions of ions across the squid axon are given in Table 5–1.

In 1902, Julius Bernstein used the Nernst equation to propose a theory of the resting potential based on the selective permeability of the membrane to K⁺. Bernstein's theory could not be tested quantitatively until the 1940s, when electronic techniques for intracellular recording were developed. It was then possible to compare the measured resting membrane potential to the value of E_K predicted from the Nernst equation (Figure 5–4). Intracellular recording showed that for most neurons, the observed values of membrane potential deviate from the theoreti-

5–4 The relationship between membrane potential and external K⁺ concentration (log scale) in nerve cells and glia. Note that the Nernst potential for K⁺ (**solid line**) predicts the glial membrane potential (**open circles**) over wide ranges of extracellular K⁺ and poorly predicts the nerve cell membrane potential, particularly at relatively low values of extracellular K⁺ (**dashed line**). (Adapted from Orkand, 1977.)

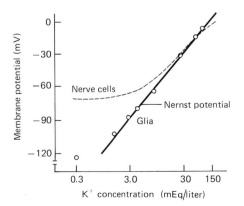

cal curve for a Nernst potential for K$^+$ at relatively low values of [K$^+$]$_o$. This suggests that neurons are permeable to one or more ions other than K$^+$. In contrast, for glial cells the fit between theoretical and observed curves is much better, with good agreement even at quite low values of [K$^+$]$_o$. Thus, glial cell membranes can be described to a first approximation as being selectively permeable to K$^+$.

In Nerve Cells the Membrane Is Permeable to Several Ionic Species

Measurements of the resting membrane potential with intracellular electrodes and flux studies using radioactive tracers indicate that nerve cells are permeable to Na$^+$ and Cl$^-$ as well as to K$^+$. Of the major ionic species present in nerve cells, only the large organic anions such as amino acids and proteins are nonpermeant. How then can concentration gradients for Na$^+$, K$^+$, and Cl$^-$ all be maintained across the cell membrane, and how do these three concentration gradients interact to determine the resting membrane potential?

To answer these questions, it will be easiest to examine first only the diffusion of K$^+$ and Na$^+$. Let us return to the simple example we considered previously of a cell permeable only to K$^+$, with unequal concentration gradients of K$^+$, Na$^+$, Cl$^-$, and A$^-$ as shown in Table 5–1. Under these conditions, the resting membrane potential is determined solely by the K$^+$ concentration gradient, so that $V_R = E_K$. Assume, then, that the membrane has a large number of K$^+$ channels, making it highly permeable to K$^+$. Now consider what happens if a few Na$^+$ channels are added to the membrane, making it slightly permeable to Na$^+$. Two forces act on Na$^+$ to propel it into the cell. First, Na$^+$ is more concentrated outside than inside and therefore tends to flow into the cell down its chemical concentration gradient. In addition, Na$^+$ is driven into the cell by the electrical gradient. The equilibrium potential for Na$^+$, calculated from the Nernst equation, is

$$E_{Na} = \frac{RT}{ZF} \ln \frac{[Na^+]_o}{[Na^+]_i}$$

$$= 26 \text{ mV} \times 2.3 \log_{10} \frac{440}{50} = +55 \text{ mV}.$$

Thus, at a resting membrane potential of -75 mV, Na$^+$ is 130 mV away from equilibrium, and a strong electrochemical force is available to drive Na$^+$ through the open Na$^+$ channels.

The influx of Na$^+$ (driven by both the concentration and electrical gradients) depolarizes the cell, tending to drive V_m toward E_{Na}. However, since the resting membrane is only slightly permeable to Na$^+$, the membrane potential actually moves only slightly away from E_K and never comes close to approaching E_{Na}. The reason for this is that once V_m begins to diverge from E_K, K$^+$ flows out of the cell, tending to counteract the Na$^+$ influx. The more V_m differs from E_K, the greater is the net electro-

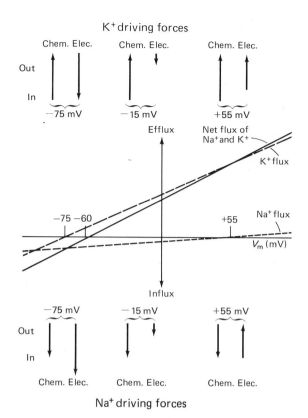

5–5 The direction and amplitude of the chemical and electrical driving forces acting on Na$^+$ and K$^+$ are shown for three different values of V_m. They result in the flux curves shown for each ion (**broken lines**) and the net flux curve for both Na$^+$ and K$^+$ (**solid line**). The change in driving force is about the same for Na$^+$ for a given change in V_m. The difference in the slopes of the Na$^+$ and K$^+$ flux curves reflects the fact that the resting membrane is more permeable to K$^+$ than to Na$^+$. The shapes of the Na$^+$ and K$^+$ flux curves as drawn here are simplified considerably. (As described in Chapter 8, these curves become quite nonlinear for values of V_m more positive than about -50 mV.)

chemical force driving K$^+$ out of the cell, and consequently the greater the K$^+$ efflux. Eventually, V_m reaches a resting potential at which the outward movement of K$^+$ just balances the inward movement of Na$^+$. As shown in Figure 5–5, this balance point (-60 mV) is more positive than E_K (-75 mV) but still far away from E_{Na} ($+55$ mV). Thus, with the resting membrane only slightly permeable to Na$^+$, V_R is shifted slightly away from E_K toward E_{Na}.

The forces acting on the cell at rest ($V_m = V_R$) are shown schematically in Figure 5–6. Because there are relatively few Na$^+$ channels, the sodium permeability, P_{Na}, is quite low. As a result, the influx of Na$^+$ is small, despite the large chemical and electrical forces driving Na$^+$ into the cell. The K$^+$ concentration gradient driving K$^+$ out of the cell is only slightly greater than the electrical force acting to hold it in the cell. Nevertheless, the small net outward electrochemical force acting on K$^+$ is enough to produce a K$^+$ efflux that balances the Na$^+$ influx because P_K, the membrane permeability to K$^+$, is relatively large.

The Passive Fluxes of Na$^+$ and K$^+$ Are Balanced by Active Ion Pumping Driven by the Na–K Pump

For the cell to have a steady resting membrane potential, the charge separation across the membrane must be constant: the net influx of charge must be balanced by the net efflux; if the fluxes of charge into or out of the cell were not balanced, they would cause the membrane potential to vary by changing the charge separation across the membrane. Therefore, in the cell at rest (Figure 5–6), the movement of K$^+$ out of the cell must be balanced by the movement of Na$^+$ into the cell. Although these steady ion leaks cancel each other, they cannot be allowed to continue unopposed for any appreciable length of time. Otherwise, [K$^+$]$_i$ would be depleted, [Na$^+$]$_i$ would increase, and the ionic gradients would run down gradually, reducing the resting membrane potential. Dissipation of ionic gradients is prevented by the ATP-dependent Na–K pump. As we saw in Chapter 3, this ion pump extrudes Na$^+$ from the cell while taking in K$^+$ (Figure 5–7). Because the pump moves Na$^+$ and K$^+$ against their net electrochemical gradients, energy must be provided to drive these actively transported fluxes. The energy that drives the pump comes from the hydrolysis of ATP.

When the cell is at rest, the active fluxes (driven by the pump) and the passive fluxes (due to diffusion) are balanced for Na$^+$ and K$^+$, so that the net flux of each of these two ions is zero. Thus, at the resting membrane potential the cell is not in equilibrium, but rather in a *steady state*: metabolic energy (derived from ATP) must be used to maintain the ionic gradients across the membrane.

In most neurons, the Na–K pump is not neutral but electrogenic; the pump produces a net flux of charge across the membrane. Typically, the pump extrudes three Na$^+$ ions for every two K$^+$ ions it brings in. In most cells, therefore, the passive Na$^+$ and K$^+$ fluxes are also not equal and opposite when the cell is at its resting potential; rather, three Na$^+$ ions diffuse into the cell for every two K$^+$ ions that diffuse out. The membrane potential at which this state occurs is a few millivolts negative to -60 mV. Because the Na–K pump is electrogenic, a slightly more negative resting membrane potential results than would be expected from a purely passive diffusion of ions.

Cl$^-$ Is Often Passively Distributed

We have not yet considered the contribution of Cl$^-$ to the generation of the resting membrane potential. How can the role of this ion be ignored in determining V_R, especially since the permeability to Cl$^-$ of most nerve cell membranes is relatively high? The answer is that V_R is ultimately determined by K$^+$ and Na$^+$ because their

Driving force (DF)		Permeability (P_i)	
Chem.	Elec.	Net DF	Net flux

5–6 The fluxes of Na$^+$, K$^+$, and Cl$^-$ across the cell membrane are a result of their chemical and electrical driving forces and the permeability of the membrane. They are shown for a cell with a membrane potential of -60 mV and the ionic gradients shown in Table 5-1. (**Horizontal arrows** signify no net driving force or no net flux.)

ionic concentrations are fixed by the Na–K pump. Cl$^-$, on the other hand, is free to diffuse into or out of the cell; in most nerve cells, Cl$^-$ is not actively pumped. Because Cl$^-$ is acted on only by passive forces (electrical and chemical gradients), the ions must be in equilibrium across the membrane. Thus, the concentration ratio of Cl$^-$ across the membrane settles at a value such that $E_{Cl} = V_R$. Because there is no net Cl$^-$ flux at E_{Cl}, Cl$^-$ has no effect on resting potential. Of the three major ions to which the membrane is permeable, only Cl$^-$ is in equilibrium at V_R. Thus, Cl$^-$ is said to be *passively* distributed across the membrane, whereas K$^+$ and Na$^+$, which are pumped, are *actively* distributed.

5–7 When the cell is at rest, the passive fluxes of Na$^+$ and K$^+$ down their electrochemical gradients through the ion channels are balanced by active transport driven in the opposite direction by the ATP-dependent Na–K pump.

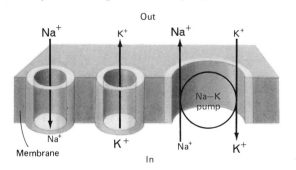

In nerve cells that do have a Cl⁻ pump, the pump is outwardly directed. As a result $[Cl^-]_o/[Cl^-]_i$ is greater than could be explained by simple passive diffusion. The Nernst potential for Cl⁻ is given by

$$E_{Cl} = \frac{RT}{ZF} \ln \frac{[Cl^-]_o}{[Cl^-]_i} = \frac{-RT}{F} \ln \frac{[Cl^-]_o}{[Cl^-]_i}$$

so that the effect of increasing the Cl⁻ gradient makes E_{Cl} more negative than V_m. This difference between E_{Cl} and V_m in the resting membrane results in a steady inward leak of Cl⁻ that is balanced by an active extrusion of Cl⁻ by the Cl⁻ pump.

The Action Potential Is Generated by a Change in the Selective Permeability of the Membrane from K⁺ to Na⁺

In the nerve cell at rest, the steady Na⁺ influx is balanced by a steady K⁺ efflux, so that the membrane potential is constant. This steady-state balance changes, however, when the cell is depolarized sufficiently to trigger an action potential. In addition to the Na⁺ channels that are open in the resting membrane, the membrane also contains a second type of Na⁺ channel that is voltage-dependent and opens only when the cell is depolarized. The more the cell is depolarized, the greater is the fraction of these gated (voltage-sensitive) Na⁺ channels that open up. A transient depolarizing potential, such as an excitatory synaptic potential, causes some voltage-gated Na⁺ channels to open, and the resultant increase in membrane Na⁺ permeability allows Na⁺ influx to outstrip the K⁺ efflux. Thus, a net influx of positive charge flows through the membrane, and positive charges accumulate inside the cell, causing further depolarization. The increase in depolarization causes more voltage-gated Na⁺ channels to open, resulting in a greater influx of positive charge, which accelerates the depolarization still further.

This regenerative, positive feedback cycle develops explosively, causing Na⁺ channels to dominate over K⁺ channels and to drive the membrane potential toward the Na⁺ equilibrium potential of +55 mV. Because net K⁺ efflux continues through the K⁺ channels, the membrane potential at the peak of the action potential reaches a value of about +50 mV, slightly below E_{Na}. In addition, there is a small diffusion of Cl⁻ into the cell at +50 mV that also counteracts the depolarizing tendency of the Na⁺ influx. Nevertheless, so many Na⁺ channels open during the rising phase of the action potential that the permeability to Na⁺ is much greater than to Cl⁻ or K⁺. To a first approximation, the membrane potential approaches E_{Na} at the peak of the action potential, just as it approaches E_K at rest, when the K⁺ permeability is predominant. The mere opening of the voltage-dependent Na⁺ channels causes the primary selectivity of the membrane permeability to change from K⁺ to Na⁺ during the rising phase of the action potential. This change in selectivity causes the potential to jump suddenly from −60 to +50 mV as a result of the passive diffusion of Na⁺ down its electrochemical gradient.

The membrane potential would remain at this large positive value indefinitely but for two somewhat slower processes that intervene to curtail the action potential by repolarizing the membrane: (1) There is an opening of voltage-dependent K⁺ channels. These K⁺ channels are gated open by depolarization, but only after a delay. Consequently, their opening lags behind that of the voltage-dependent Na⁺ channels, but once they open, these K⁺ channels increase K⁺ efflux. (2) As the depolarization continues, there is a slow turning off, or *inactivation*, of the Na⁺ channels. The increase in K⁺ efflux combines with the decrease in Na⁺ influx and results in a net efflux of positive charge from the cell, which continues until the cell has repolarized to its resting value, V_R.

The net movement of ions across the membrane during each action potential is quite small. The overall ionic concentration gradients are not altered significantly because only a relatively small number of ions must move before the charge separation across the membrane changes enough to change the membrane potential by 110 mV.

The Resting and Action Potentials Can Be Quantified by the Goldman Equation

In the example discussed above (Figures 5–5 and 5–6), the resting potential of a nerve cell with high P_K and P_{Cl} and relatively low P_{Na} was shown to be about −60 mV. As we have seen, Na⁺ and K⁺ set the value of the resting potential. V_R is equal to neither E_K nor E_{Na}, but, rather, lies between them. As a general rule, when V_m is determined by two or more ions, each ion will have an influence on V_m that is determined both by its concentrations inside and outside the cell and by the permeability of the membrane to that ion. This relationship is given quantitatively by the *Goldman equation*, which is sometimes also referred to as the Goldman-Hodgkin-Katz equation:

$$V_m = \frac{RT}{F} \ln \frac{P_K[K^+]_o + P_{Na}[Na^+]_o + P_{Cl}[Cl^-]_i}{P_K[K^+]_i + P_{Na}[Na^+]_i + P_{Cl}[Cl^-]_o}$$

The Goldman equation applies only when V_m is not changing. Its derivation is complex and will not be detailed here.[2] The equation states that the greater the concentration of a particular ionic species and the greater its membrane permeability, the greater will be its role in determining the membrane potential. In the limiting case, when permeability to one ion is exceptionally high, the Goldman equation reduces to the Nernst equation for

---

[2]There are three basic steps in the derivation of this equation as developed by Alan Hodgkin and Bernard Katz:

1. Express the flux *(J)* of each species of ion (Na⁺, K⁺, Cl⁻) across the membrane as a function of V_m, concentration, and membrane permeability: $J_i = f(V_m, conc_i, perm_i)$.
2. Convert these fluxes to membrane currents, I (e.g., an influx of Na⁺ or an efflux of Cl⁻ is an *inward* membrane current). Since V_m is constant, the charge separation across the membrane is not changing, so that $I_{Cl} + I_{Na} + I_K = 0$.
3. Substitute the equations from step 1 into the equation in step 2; rearrange terms and solve for V_m. The result is the Goldman equation.

that ion. For example, if, as in the case of glial cells, $P_K \gg P_{Cl}$, P_{Na}, the equation becomes

$$V_m \approx \frac{RT}{F} \ln \frac{[K^+]_o}{[K^+]_i}.$$

In 1949, A. L. Hodgkin and B. Katz first applied the Goldman equation systematically to the squid giant axon. They measured the variation of V_R with changing concentrations of Na^+, Cl^-, and K^+. Their results showed that if V_R is measured shortly after the concentration change, before the internal ionic concentrations are altered, $[K^+]_o$ has a strong effect on the resting potential, $[Cl^-]_o$ has some effect, and $[Na^+]_o$ has little effect. Their data could be fit accurately to the Goldman equation by assuming that, for the membrane at rest,

$$P_K : P_{Na} : P_{Cl} = 1 : 0.04 : 0.45.$$

For the membrane at the peak of the action potential, however, they calculated a quite different set of membrane permeabilities. The variation of V_m at the peak of the action potential with external ionic concentrations could be fit best by assuming the following permeability ratios:

$$P_K : P_{Na} : P_{Cl} = 1 : 20 : 0.45.$$

For this set of permeabilities (P_{Na}, P_K, P_{Cl}), the Goldman equation reduces to

$$V_m \approx \frac{RT}{F} \ln \frac{[Na^+]_o}{[Na^+]_i} = +55 \text{ mV}.$$

Thus, at the peak of the action potential, when the membrane is much more permeable to Na^+ than to any other ion, V_m approaches E_{Na}, the Na^+ Nernst potential.

An Overall View

The membrane potential is determined primarily by three ions: K^+, Cl^-, and Na^+. In general, the membrane potential is closest to the Nernst potential of the ion or ions with the greatest concentrations inside and outside the cell and the greatest membrane permeability. Because the total concentrations of K^+, Cl^-, and Na^+ are roughly equal, the relative membrane permeabilities of these three ions are most important in determining the membrane potential.

At rest, V_m is close to the Nernst potential of K^+, the ion to which the membrane is most permeable. However, because the membrane is also somewhat permeable to Na^+, there is an influx of Na^+, which drives V_m slightly positive to E_K. At this membrane potential, the electrical and chemical driving forces acting on K^+ are no longer in balance, so that a steady efflux of K^+ from the cell results. These two passive fluxes are each balanced by the active fluxes driven by the Na–K pump. In most cells, Cl^- is not actively transported and is, therefore, passively distributed so that it is at equilibrium. Under most physiological conditions, the bulk concentrations of Na^+, K^+, and Cl^- inside and outside the cell are constant. The changes in membrane potential that occur during signaling (action potentials, synaptic potentials, and receptor potentials) are caused not by changes in the concentrations of ions, which are very small, but by changes in the relative membrane permeabilities to these three ions, which are substantial.

Selected Readings

Finkelstein, A., and Mauro, A. 1977. Physical principles and formalisms of electrical excitability. In E. R. Kandel (ed.), Handbook of Physiology, Vol. 1: The Nervous System, Part 1. Bethesda, Md.: American Physiological Society, pp. 161–213.

Hille, B. 1977. Ionic basis of resting and action potentials. In E. R. Kandel (ed.), Handbook of Physiology, Vol. 1: The Nervous System, Part 1. Bethesda, Md.: American Physiological Society, pp. 99–136.

Hille, B. 1984. Ionic Channels of Excitable Membranes. Sunderland, Mass.: Sinauer.

Hubbard, J. I., Llinás, R., and Quastel, D. M. J. 1969. Electrophysiological Analysis of Synaptic Transmission. Baltimore: Williams & Wilkins, chap. 3.

Khodorov, B. I. 1974. The Problem of Excitability. New York: Plenum Press, chap. 2.

Stevens, C. F. 1979. The neuron. Sci. Am. 241(3):54–65.

References

Bernstein, J. 1902. Investigations on the thermodynamics of bioelectric currents. Translated from Pflügers Arch. 92:521–562. In G. R. Kepner (ed.), Cell Membrane Permeability and Transport. Stroudsburg, Pa.: Dowden, Hutchinson & Ross, 1979.

Goldman, D. E. 1943. Potential, impedance, and rectification in membranes. J. Gen. Physiol. 27:36–60.

Hodgkin, A. L., and Katz, B. 1949. The effect of sodium ions on the electrical activity of the giant axon of the squid. J. Physiol. (Lond.) 108:37–77.

Nernst, W. 1888. On the kinetics of substances in solution. Translated from Z. Phys. Chem. 2:613–622, 634–637. In G. R. Kepner (ed.), Cell Membrane Permeability and Transport. Stroudsburg, Pa.: Dowden, Hutchinson & Ross, 1979.

Orkand, R. K. 1977. Glial cells. In E. R. Kandel (ed.), Handbook of Physiology, Vol. 1: Cellular Biology of Neurons, Part 2. Bethesda, Md.: American Physiological Society, pp. 855–875.

John Koester

Nongated Channels and Passive Membrane Properties of the Neuron

6

Nerve cells generate electrical signals by gating—opening and closing—ion channels. The ability of nerve cells to gate their ion channels allows them to control the permeability of their membranes and thereby to regulate the diffusion of selected ions down preestablished electrochemical gradients. Although membrane permeability and ion diffusion can be measured directly with radiolabeled isotopes, these measurements lack the time resolution necessary for relating ion movement to the rapidly occurring electrical signals of the neuron. To achieve better time resolution, one usually needs to measure not the change in ionic permeability itself, but its consequences: the flow of *ionic current* and the resulting changes in *membrane potential*.

In addition to providing a remarkable time resolution (fractions of a millisecond), measuring ion fluxes as current flow rather than as permeability changes also allows us to consider the properties of the ion channels used for signaling in electrical terms. As a result, we can use a simple mathematical model derived from electrical circuits to describe the three critical features used by the nerve cell for signaling—the ion channels, the concentration gradients of relevant ions, and the ability of the membrane to store charge. In this model, called an *equivalent circuit,* all of the important functional properties of the neuron are represented by a simple electrical circuit consisting only of conductances (resistors), batteries, and capacitors. This model has two important features. First, it gives us an intuitive yet accurate sense of how current flow due to the movement of ions produces signaling in nerve cells. Second, the equations that describe this model of the neuron are very simple, much simpler than comparable equations that describe the permeability of the membrane and the diffusion of ions. An understanding of this equivalent circuit model leads to basic insights into the principles of signaling in all nerve cells and serves as an essential foundation for interpreting all clinical tests of the electrical function of nerve and muscle, including electroencephalography, electroneurography, electromyography and electrocardiography.

In this and the next chapter we shall consider the *passive electrical properties* of the neuron, the properties that *do not* change during signaling. The nerve cell has three types of passive electrical characteristics: conductance (resistance), electromotive force, and capacitance. In this chapter we shall describe the physical basis of these three properties and their role in generating the resting membrane potential. In the next chapter we shall examine how passive membrane properties function in the integration of synaptic signals and in the conduction of action potentials.

Chapters 8 through 11 deal with *active electrical properties* of the nerve cell membrane, the properties that *do* change during signaling. Among the active properties, we shall consider the voltage-gated ion channels that generate the action potential and transmitter release, and the chemically gated ion channels that generate synaptic potentials. (We shall return to this class of channels again in Chapter 23, when we consider the active ion channels in sensory nerve cells that are involved in the transduction of physical stimuli into electrical receptor potentials.)

Understanding electrical signaling requires familiarity with some principles of how current flows in an electrical circuit on the level usually taught in an introductory physics course in high school. A review of these concepts is contained in Appendix IIIA. Appendix IIIB contains a set of practice problems and their solutions, which are keyed to the material in Chapters 5–9.

A Channel Is Characterized by Its Selectivity for Ions and Its Gating Properties

The neuronal membrane is a mosaic of lipids and proteins about 8 to 10 nm thick. The continuous surface of the membrane is formed by a double layer of lipids. Embedded within this continuous sheet are various proteins.

The lipids within the membrane are very *hydrophobic;* they are immiscible with water. In contrast, the ions of the extracellular and intracellular space are *hydrophilic:* they strongly attract water molecules. Although the net charge on a water molecule is zero, there is a charge separation *within* the molecule. Consequently, water molecules have a *dipole moment.* The oxygen atom in a water molecule has slightly more electrons than protons, whereas the hydrogen atoms have slightly more protons than electrons. As a result of this charge imbalance, water creates a *polar environment.* Cations are strongly attracted electrostatically to the oxygen atoms of water molecules, and anions are attracted to hydrogen atoms. Because ions attract water they become surrounded by electrostatically bound shells of water, which are called the *waters of hydration.* For an ion to move from water into the nonpolar hydrocarbon tails of the lipid bilayer of the membrane, a large amount of energy would have to be supplied to overcome the attractive forces between the ions and the surrounding water molecules. This large difference in potential energy means that it is extremely rare for an ion to move from free solution into the lipid bilayer. Thus, the bilayer itself is almost completely *impermeable* to ions. The energy required for an ion to pass from water into another polar environment is relatively small, because the electrostatic interactions between the molecules of the new medium can substitute for the interactions of water with the ion. Such a polar environment is provided by protein pores, called ion channels, that are embedded in the membrane (Figure 6–1). To the extent that ions traverse the membrane, they do so almost exclusively by going through such channels. Not only are the channels lined with polar amino acid groups, but they have diameters large enough to accommodate water molecules, so that an ion traversing a channel need not be stripped completely of its water shell.

These ion channels, which span the membrane, fall into a class of molecules called *intrinsic membrane proteins.* Ion channels themselves can be subdivided into two categories: they are either passive or active. *Passive* channels are always open. *Active* channels have a gate

6–1 Two types of channels provide pathways for ions to permeate the membrane: passive channels are always open; active, or gated, channels have the ability to open or close in response to one of a variety of chemical, electrical, or, in some cases, physical stimuli. If this diagram were drawn to scale, inner diameters of pores would be about one-tenth of the membrane thickness, and the distances between neighboring channels would be about ten times greater than the thickness of the membrane.

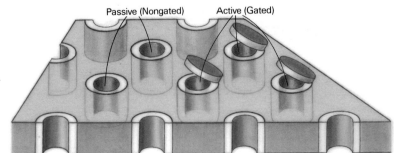

Passive (Nongated)   Active (Gated)

somewhere along their length that can be either open or closed. The gates of these active channels may be controlled by synaptic transmitters, by membrane potential, or, in the case of receptor cells, by various physical stimuli. Most active channels are closed when the membrane is at rest. Passive channels are important in determining the resting membrane potential as well as in influencing synaptic integration. Active channels generate action, synaptic, and receptor potentials.

Ion channels, whether active or passive, can also be characterized by their selectivity. Each channel behaves as if it contained a selectivity filter, or recognition site, along its length that allows only one species of ion, usually Na^+, K^+, Cl^-, or Ca^{++}, to pass through. At most, a channel will permit a select combination of ion species to move through it. In addition, there may be more than one species of channel selective for the same ion. For example, there is one class of nongated K^+ channel that is responsible for the resting K^+ flux and a second class of gated K^+ channel that contributes to the repolarization of the action potential. Most channels are not perfectly selective; K^+ channels, for instance, generally let one Na^+ ion go through for about every twelve K^+ ions that pass. For purposes of this discussion, however, it is convenient to assume that each channel is completely selective.

Electromotive Force Is Generated across the Membrane

Because ions are unequally distributed across the membrane, each open channel contributes to the generation of an *electrical potential difference* across the membrane.

6–2 A channel selectively permeable to K^+ ions gives rise to an electromotive force with a value equal to the K^+ Nernst potential; this can be represented by a battery.

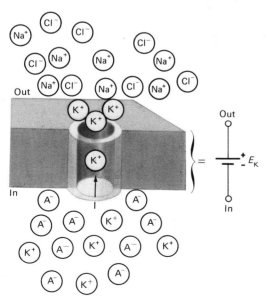

Potassium, which is present at a higher concentration inside than outside the cell, tends to diffuse out of the cell through open (nongated) K^+ channels. As we have seen, this diffusion leads to a net separation of charge across the membrane. Positive charges accumulate on the outside, leaving negative charges accumulated on the inside. The electrical potential difference that results has a value equal to the Nernst potential for K^+. The combination of a concentration gradient for K^+ and a channel selectively permeable to K^+ gives rise to a slight separation of charge across the channel that acts as a constant source of electrical potential. A source of electrical potential is called an *electromotive force* or (in this case) an *ionic battery*. The ionic battery generated in this way results from the passive diffusion of K^+ through the K^+ channel. We may therefore schematically represent the electrical potential generated across each channel with the symbol for a battery (Figure 6–2). The potential generated by this battery is equal to E_K, the K^+ Nernst potential, which, as we have seen, is typically about -75 mV.

The Membrane Has Conductive Pathways

Because ions do not dissolve well in the lipid bilayer of the membrane, it provides a poor conductance pathway for the flow of ionic current. Even a large potential difference will produce practically no current flow across a pure lipid bilayer. Consider for a moment the cell body of a typical spinal motor neuron. It has a membrane area of about 10^{-4} cm^2. If that membrane were composed solely of lipid bilayer, its electrical conductance to current flow (in the resting stage) would be only about

$$10^{-12} \text{ Siemens (S), where } 1 \text{ S} = 1 \text{ ohm}^{-1} = 1 \frac{\text{A}}{\text{V}}.$$

But because thousands of nongated ion channels are embedded in the membrane, ions constantly leak across it, so that its actual resting conductance is about 40,000 times greater, or about 4×10^{-8} S. Thus, the almost perfect insulation of the lipid bilayer is shunted by thousands of conductance pathways, the nongated ion channels.

Although an individual channel is a much better conductor of current flow than an equivalent volume of lipid bilayer, a channel still is a relatively poor conductor compared with a free solution of ions. Ion channels have diameters so narrow (at most about 0.6 nm) that only a few ions at most can carry charge through the channel at any instant in time. In addition, the narrowness of the channel, which endows the channel with selectivity, makes it much more difficult for an ion to traverse the channel than to traverse an equivalent volume of free solution. The random collisions of ions with the walls of the channel as they go through cause them to lose energy. The greater the number of collisions, the lower the conductance of the channel (the greater its resistance).

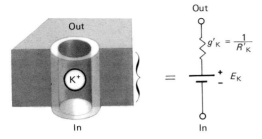

6–3 A single K^+ channel can be represented by the equivalent electrical circuit of a battery (E_K) in series with a conductance (g'_K).

As described above, each open K^+ channel generates an electromotive force by allowing diffusion of K^+ down its concentration gradient and at the same time functions as a conductance pathway with a non-zero resistance. Thus, each ion pathway can be represented by a battery in series with a conductance. The value of the battery is determined by the concentration gradient for the ion (Figure 6–3). For K^+ the value of the battery is given by the equilibrium potential for K^+ (E_K). Because the channel offers a resistance to the flow of ions, each open conductance channel can also be represented as having a resistance. We call the conductance of the K^+ channel (g'_K) the K^+ *channel conductance* and the resistance (R'_K) the K^+ *channel resistance*. The resistance of a channel is inversely proportional to its conductance:

$$R'_K = \frac{1}{g'_K}.$$

The two terms are used interchangeably for mathematical convenience when calculating current flow (see Appendix III). Of the two terms, K^+ channel conductance (g'_K) is now more commonly used because it is directly proportional to the current that flows through the open channel and therefore can be more directly related to mo-

6–4 All of the passive K^+ channels in a nerve membrane can be lumped into a single equivalent electrical structure: a series combination of a battery (E_K) and a conductance, g_K; $g_K = N_K \times g'_K$, where N is the number of passive K^+ channels and g'_K is the conductance of a single K^+ channel.

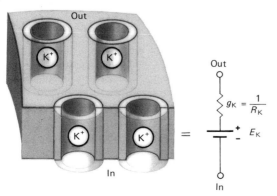

lecular structures. The conductance of a single channel (the single-channel conductance) is a measure of the ease with which K^+ moves through a single protein channel in response to an electrical potential difference.

The total K^+ conductance (g_K) of the cell membrane in its resting state is equal to the number of passive K^+ channels (N_K) multiplied by the single-channel conductance of each channel (g'_K):

$$g_K = N_K \times g'_K.$$

We may combine all the passive K^+ channels of a given area of membrane into a single equivalent structure, consisting of a conductance, g_K, in series with a battery with the value E_K (Figure 6–4).

The membrane conductance to K^+ is related to the membrane permeability to K^+, but the two terms are not interchangeable. Conductance varies with ionic concentration, whereas permeability does not. To understand this distinction, consider a limiting case in which K^+ concentration is zero on both sides of the membrane. Even if a great number of open K^+ channels were present, g_K would be zero because no K^+ ions would be available to carry current across the membrane in response to a potential difference. At the same time, K^+ permeability would be quite high, since it depends only on how many K^+ channels are open. Permeability is determined by the state of the membrane, but conductance depends on both the state of the membrane *and* the concentration of surrounding ions. Under most physiological conditions, however, a membrane with high K^+ permeability also has a large K^+ conductance.

The Resting Membrane Potential Can Be Calculated from the Equivalent Circuit of the Membrane

As we have seen, all of the passive K^+ channels can be represented by a combination of a single conductance and single battery. By analogy, all the passive Cl^- channels can be represented by a similar conductance–battery combination, as can the passive Na^+ channels (Figure 6–5). These three types of channel account for the bulk of the passive ionic pathways through the membrane.[1]

With these electrical representations of the passive Na^+, K^+, and Cl^- channels, we can calculate the resting membrane potential using a simple equivalent circuit model of the neuron. To construct this circuit, we need only connect the elements representing each type of channel at their two ends by elements that represent the extracellular fluid and the cytoplasm. These channels

---

[1]Although there is good evidence that the membrane has separate gated channels for Na^+, K^+, Cl^-, and Ca^{++}, it is not clear whether different ions have separate nongated channels or whether they all share a common (leakage) pathway. For the sake of convenience, we shall assume separate nongated channels.

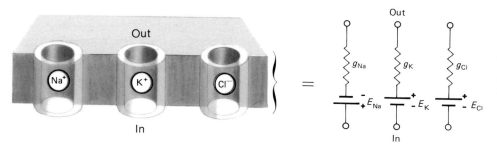

6–5 Each type of passive ion-selective channel is represented by a series combination of a battery and a conductance.

are, of course, in parallel with the conductance of the lipid bilayer. Because the conductance of the bilayer is so much lower than that of the ion channel pathways, virtually all transmembrane current flows through the channels. For this reason the negligible conductance of the bilayer can be ignored. The extracellular fluid and the cytoplasm both have relatively large cross-sectional areas with many available charge carriers, making them excellent conductors. For the purposes of this discussion, the extracellular fluid and the cytoplasm can each be approximated by a *short circuit*—a conductor with zero resistance (Figure 6–6).

To Calculate V$_m$ We Need Consider Only the Nongated K$^+$ and Na$^+$ Channels

To simplify calculation of the membrane potential, we may initially ignore the Cl$^-$ channels and begin with just two types of passive channels, K$^+$ and Na$^+$, as illustrated in Figure 6–7. Because there are more passive channels for K$^+$ than for Na$^+$, the membrane conductance for current flow carried by K$^+$ is much greater than that for Na$^+$. In Figure 6–7, g_K, which is 10×10^{-6}S, is 20 times

6–6 The neuron can be modeled by an electrical circuit that includes elements representing the ion-selective membrane channels together with the short-circuit pathways provided by the cytoplasm and the extracellular fluid.

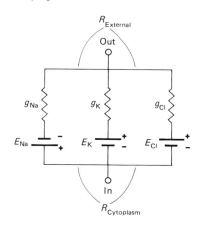

higher than g_{Na}, which is 0.5×10^{-6}S. Given these values and the values of E_K and E_{Na}, we can calculate the membrane potential as follows.

In the absence of an extrinsic current source (e.g., Figure 5–2), there can be no *net* current flow across the membrane in the resting state. If there were a net current, the separation of positive and negative charges across the membrane would change, causing V_m to change. Since V_m is constant in the resting state, the net current must be zero. I_{Na} is therefore equal and opposite to I_K:

$$I_{Na} = -I_K$$

or

$$I_{Na} + I_K = 0. \tag{6–1}$$

I_{Na} and I_K can now be easily calculated in two steps. First, we add up the separate *potential differences* across the conductance branches for Na$^+$ and K$^+$. As one goes from inside to outside across the Na$^+$ conductance branch, the total potential difference is the sum of the potential differences across E_{Na} and across g_{Na}[2]:

$$V_m = E_{Na} + I_{Na}/g_{Na}.$$

Similarly, for the K$^+$ conductance branch:

$$V_m = E_K + I_K/g_K.$$

Next, we rearrange and solve for I:

$$I_{Na} = g_{Na} \times (V_m - E_{Na}) \tag{6–2a}$$

$$I_K = g_K \times (V_m - E_K). \tag{6–2b}$$

As these equations illustrate, the ionic current through each conductance branch is equal to the conductance of that branch multiplied by the net electrical driving force. For example, the conductance for the K$^+$ branch is proportional to the number of open K$^+$ channels; and the driving force is equal to the difference between V_m and the value of the Nernst battery for K$^+$. If

---

[2]Because we have defined V_m as $V_{in} - V_{out}$, the following convention must be used for these equations: outward current (in this case I_K) is positive, inward current (I_{Na}) is negative; batteries with their positive poles toward the inside of the membrane (e.g., E_{Na}) are given positive values in the equations. The reverse is true for batteries such as the K$^+$ battery, which has its negative poles toward the inside.

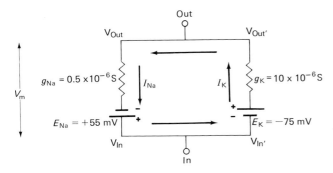

6–7 In this electrical equivalent circuit for calculating resting membrane potential, the Cl⁻ pathway has been omitted for simplicity.

V_m is more positive than E_K (-75 mV), then the driving force is positive (outward). If V_m is more negative than E_K, then the driving force is negative (inward).

In Equation 6–1 we saw that $I_{Na} + I_K = 0$. If we now substitute Equations 6–2a and 6–2b for I_{Na} and I_K in Equation 6–1, we obtain the following expression:

$$g_{Na} \times (V_m - E_{Na}) + g_K \times (V_m - E_K) = 0.$$

Multiplying through we see that:

$$(V_m \times g_{Na} - E_{Na} \times g_{Na}) + (V_m \times g_K - E_K \times g_K) = 0.$$

This can now be rearranged to yield:

$$V_m \times (g_{Na} + g_K) = (E_{Na} \times g_{Na}) + (E_K \times g_K).$$

Solving for V_m, we obtain an intuitively useful expression for the resting membrane potential:

$$V_m = \frac{(E_{Na} \times g_{Na}) + (E_K \times g_K)}{g_{Na} + g_K}. \qquad (6\text{–}3)$$

This equation allows us to calculate V_m for the equivalent circuit. Taking the circuit values of Figure 6–7, we can calculate V_m to be[3]:

$$V_m = \frac{(+55 \times 10^{-3}\text{V}) \, (0.5 \times 10^{-6}\text{S})}{0.5 \times 10^{-6}\text{S} + 10 \times 10^{-6}\text{S}}$$

$$+ \frac{(-75 \times 10^{-3}\text{V}) \, (10 \times 10^{-6}\text{S})}{0.5 \times 10^{-6}\text{S} + 10 \times 10^{-6}\text{S}}$$

$$= \frac{-722.5 \times 10^{-9}\text{V} \times \text{S}}{10.5 \times 10^{-6}\text{S}}$$

$$= -69 \text{ mV}.$$

Equation 6–3 states that V_m will approach the value of the ionic battery that is associated with the greater conductance. This principle can be illustrated with another example as we jump ahead briefly to consider what hap-

[3]An instructive alternative method for calculating the resting potential is given in Appendix IIIB, problem 1.

pens during the action potential. At the peak of the action potential, total membrane g_K is essentially unchanged from its resting value, but g_{Na} increases by as much as 500-fold! This increase in g_{Na} is caused by the opening of voltage-gated Na⁺ channels. In the example shown in Figure 6–7, a 500-fold increase would change g_{Na} from $0.5 \times 10^{-6}\text{S}$ to $250 \times 10^{-6}\text{S}$. If we substitute this new value of g_{Na} into Figure 6–7 and solve for V_m with Equation 6–3, we obtain $V_m = +50 \text{ mV}$, a value much closer to E_{Na} than to E_K. The reason V_m is closer to E_{Na} than to E_K at the peak of the action potential is that g_{Na} now is 25-fold greater than g_K, so the Na⁺ battery becomes much more important than the K⁺ battery in determining V_m.

The Equation for V_m Can Be Written in a More General Form

The resting membrane has open conductance channels not only for Na⁺ and K⁺, but also for Cl⁻. It is useful, therefore, to have a general equation to describe the resting potential as a function of all three permeable ions. If one constructs an equivalent circuit that includes a conductance pathway for Cl⁻ with its associated Nernst battery (Figure 6–8), one can derive a more general equation for V_m by following the same sequence of steps outlined above:

$$V_m = \frac{(E_K \times g_K) + (E_{Na} \times g_{Na}) + (E_{Cl} \times g_{Cl})}{g_K + g_{Na} + g_{Cl}}. \qquad (6\text{–}4)$$

This equation is similar to the Goldman equation, which we encountered in the last chapter. As in the Goldman equation, the contribution to V_m of each ionic battery is weighted in proportion to the conductance (or permeability) of the membrane to that particular ion. In the limit, if the conductance for one ion is much greater than that for the other ions, V_m will approach the value of that ion's Nernst potential.

The contribution of Cl⁻ ions to the resting potential can now be determined by comparing V_m calculated for the circuits in Figures 6–7 and 6–8. For most nerve cells, the value of g_{Cl} ranges from one-fourth to one-half of g_K. In addition, E_{Cl} is typically quite close to E_K, but slightly less negative. For the example shown in Figure 6–8, Cl⁻ ions are passively distributed across the membrane, so that E_{Cl} is equal to the value of V_m, which is determined by Na⁺ and K⁺. Note that if $E_{Cl} = V_m$ $(-69 \text{ mV}$ in this case), no net current flows through the Cl⁻ channels. If there were a net Cl⁻ current, then there would be a potential difference across g_{Cl}, and $E_{Cl} + g_{Cl}$ would not equal V_m. If one includes g_{Cl} and E_{Cl} from the Figure 6–7 in the calculation of V_m (i.e., Equation 6–4), the calculated value of V_m does not differ from that for Figure 6–6. On the other hand, if E_{Cl} were not passively distributed but actively pumped out of the cell, then E_{Cl} would be more negative than -69 mV. In that case, adding the Cl⁻ pathway to the calculation would shift V_m to a slightly more negative value.

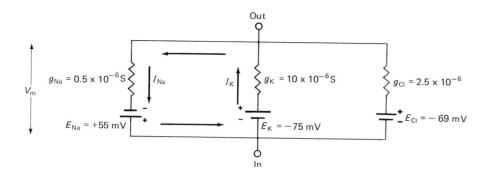

6–8 The electrical equivalent circuit of a neuron in which Cl$^-$ is passively distributed across the membrane. No current flows through the Cl$^-$ channels in this example because V_m is at the Cl$^-$ equilibrium (Nernst) potential.

The Na–K Pump Counteracts the Passive Fluxes of Na$^+$ and K$^+$

Figure 6–7 illustrates an important feature of the resting membrane: there is a steady leakage of Na$^+$ into the cell and of K$^+$ out of the cell, even when the cell is in its resting state. Referring back to the circuit in Figure 6–7, we can calculate these currents from Equations 6–2a and 6–2b:

$$I_{Na} = g_{Na} \times (V_m - E_{Na})$$

$$I_K = g_K \times (V_m - E_K).$$

Substituting the circuit values from Figure 6–7 and the value of V_m calculated above:

$$I_{Na} = (0.5 \times 10^{-6} S) \times [(-68.8 \times 10^{-3}) - (+55 \times 10^{-3})]$$

$$I_K = (10 \times 10^{-6} S) \times [(-68.8 \times 10^{-3}) - (-75 \times 10^{-3})]$$

$$I_{Na} = -62 \times 10^{-9} A.$$

$$I_K = +62 \times 10^{-9} A.$$

These steady fluxes of Na$^+$ and K$^+$ ions through the passive membrane channels are exactly counterbalanced

6–9 All major ion channels are shown in this electrical equivalent circuit of a neuron at rest. Under steady-state conditions, Na$^+$ and K$^+$ currents through membrane channels are balanced by Na$^+$ and K$^+$ fluxes (I'_{Na} and I'_K) driven by the Na–K pump.

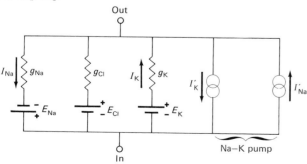

by active ion fluxes driven by the Na–K pump, as illustrated in Figure 6–9. To prevent the ionic batteries from running down, the Na–K pump continually extrudes Na$^+$ ions and pumps in K$^+$, even when the cell is at rest. The actively driven Na$^+$ current is equal and opposite to the passive Na$^+$ current, and the actively driven K$^+$ current is equal and opposite to the passive K$^+$ current.

The Membrane Has Capacitance

In addition to batteries and conductances, the third important passive electrical property of the neuron is membrane capacitance. In general, capacitance results whenever two conducting materials are separated by an insulating material. In the neuron, the conducting materials are the cytoplasm and the extracellular fluid. The insulating material is the cell membrane, especially the lipid bilayer sheet. Since the density of ion channels is low, the capacitor portion of the membrane occupies at least 100 times the area of all of the ion channels combined. A more complete equivalent circuit of the passive electrical properties of the membrane, with membrane capacitance included, is shown in Figure 6–10.

The fundamental property of a capacitor is the ability to store charges of opposite sign on its two surfaces. This maintained charge separation occurs whenever a potential difference exists between two sides of a capacitor. The net excess of positive and negative charge stored on the plates of a capacitor is given by the following equation:

$$Q = V \times C$$

where Q is the net excess of positive or negative charges on each side of the capacitor, V is the voltage difference between the two sides, and C is the capacitance.

A typical value of membrane capacitance for a nerve cell is about 10^{-6} F/cm^2 of membrane area. The net excess of positive and negative charges separated by the membrane of a cell with a resting potential of -70 mV can be calculated as follows:

$$Q = (70 \times 10^{-3} \text{ V}) \times (10^{-6} \text{ F/cm}^2)$$

$$= 7 \times 10^{-8} \text{ Coul./cm}^2.$$

We can convert charge measured in coulombs to units of

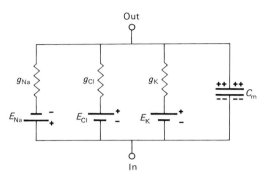

6–10 This electrical equivalent circuit of the passive electrical properties of the membrane of a neuron includes membrane capacitance (C_m).

electronic charge by using the appropriate conversion factor:

$$Q = (7 \times 10^{-8} \text{ Coul./cm}^2)$$
$$\times (6.2 \times 10^{18} \text{ charges/Coul.})$$
$$= 4.3 \times 10^{11} \text{ charges/cm}^2.$$

From this value of charge density and the membrane area, we can calculate the total amount of charge stored on the membrane capacitance. For a neuron with a cell body that is 50 μm in diameter, the soma membrane area is 7.85×10^{-5} cm^2, so that the net charge separation across the soma membrane is

$$Q = (7.85 \times 10^{-5} \text{ cm}^2)$$
$$\times (4.3 \times 10^{11} \text{ charges/cm}^2)$$
$$= 34 \times 10^{6} \text{ charges.}$$

Although this number, 34 million, may sound quite large, it represents only a tiny fraction (1/200,000) of the *total* number of positive or negative charges within the cytoplasm of the cell body.

During the action potential, the membrane potential changes from −70 to +50 mV, a total excursion of 120 mV. The number of Na$^+$ ions that must flow into the cell to change the charge on the membrane capacitance can be determined by calculating the amount of charge required to produce this change in V_m. From the calculation above, 34×10^{6} charges must be separated across the membrane to produce a 70-mV potential difference. To change the potential by 120 mV, the change in charge separation required is:

$$34 \times 10^{6} \text{ ions} \times \frac{120 \text{ mV}}{70 \text{ mV}} = 58 \times 10^{6} \text{ ions}$$

In other words, 58 million Na$^+$ ions[4] must rush into the cell to depolarize it from −70 to +50 mV.

This value of 58 million Na$^+$ ions produces only a 0.013% change in internal Na$^+$ concentration away from its typical value of 12 mM.

An Overall View

The electrical equivalent circuit of the neuron is a great aid in the study of the cellular properties of neurons. With a few of the most elementary laws of physics and some simple arithmetic, this basic model can be used to gain a fundamental understanding of the principles of electrical signaling in nerve and muscle cells. In addition, the model gives us some insights into the molecular properties of the protein channels through which the ions flow.

The equivalent circuit rests on a firm foundation of empirical data. The nerve cell actually does have conductive, capacitive, and electromotive force components that can be specifically attributed to ion channel proteins, the lipid bilayer in which they are embedded, and the ionic concentration gradient. Although they have biological reality, the three electrical properties of the membrane are functionally indistinguishable from those of a man-made electronic circuit. Moreover, these components are experimentally measurable, and only after they were measured was it possible to gain the understanding of neuronal signaling that we now have achieved.

Selected Readings

Finkelstein, A., and Mauro, A. 1977. Physical principles and formalisms of electrical excitability. In E. R. Kandel (ed.), Handbook of Physiology, Vol. 1: The Nervous System, Part 1. Bethesda, Md.: American Physiological Society, pp. 161–213.

Hubbard, J. I., Llinás, R., and Quastel, D. M. J. 1969. Electrophysiological Analysis of Synaptic Transmission. Baltimore: Williams & Wilkins, chap. 2.

---

[4]The calculated value of 58×10^{6} is a slight underestimation of the total Na$^+$ influx. A small fraction of the charge carried by Na$^+$ influx through the Na$^+$ channels does not contribute to changing the charge on C_m because it is offset by K$^+$ efflux and Cl$^-$ influx through the other ion channels.

John Koester

Functional Consequences of Passive Membrane Properties of the Neuron

7

The passive resistive and capacitive properties of the membrane have important effects on the flow of information within the nervous system. For example, the passive electrical properties of a nerve cell affect the time course of the postsynaptic potentials generated in it by other cells. The passive electrical properties of the postsynaptic cell also determine how efficiently synaptic potentials are propagated within a cell from their site of origin to the trigger zone. These features of neuronal functioning contribute to *synaptic integration*, the process by which a nerve cell adds up all incoming signals and determines whether or not it will generate an action potential. Once an action potential is generated, the speed with which it is conducted from the trigger zone to the axon terminals also depends on the passive electrical properties of the axon.

The functional aspects of passive membrane properties are best understood by considering the equivalent circuit of the neuron introduced in the previous chapter.

Membrane Capacitance Slows the Time Course of Signal Conduction

Simplified Equivalent Circuit Model

To see how membrane capacitance affects the rate of change of the membrane potential, let us refer to the simplified equivalent circuit model of the membrane shown in Figure 7–1. Since conductance and resistance are reciprocally related ($g = 1/R$), one can use either term to describe a conducting pathway in such an equivalent circuit. In the previous chapter, we used conductance because it relates directly to the number of open channels. In this chapter we shall introduce a few simple con-

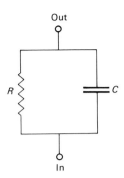

7–1 A simplified electrical equivalent circuit can be used to examine the effects of membrane capacitance on the response of a neuron to injected current. All conductance channels are lumped into a single element *(R)*, and batteries representing the electromotive forces generated by ion diffusion are ignored.

cepts that were first developed in physics and engineering. By tradition these concepts employ resistance *(R)* rather than conductance *(g)*. We shall follow that convention in the remainder of this chapter so as to be consistent with that literature from which the terms were derived.

In the diagram in Figure 7–1, the cell membrane is represented by a capacitor *(C)* in parallel with a resistor *(R)*, which represents the passive, nongated ion channels—that is, the parallel combination of the nongated R_K, R_{Na}, and R_{Cl} elements (Figure 6–10). The membrane "batteries" can be ignored for the purposes of this discussion because the batteries affect only the absolute value of V_m, not its rate of change. We can deal with only the passive membrane properties by restricting our consideration to the effects of depolarizing current pulses that are too small to open a significant number of the voltage-gated Na^+ and K^+ channels.

Rate of Change of Membrane Potential

To understand the factors that determine how long it takes for membrane potential to change in response to a current pulse passed across the membrane, let us consider a nerve cell body. Specifically, what is the response of the potential change (ΔV_m) to a pulse of current with a rectangular waveform that is passed across the membrane from an intracellular electrode to an extracellular electrode in the bathing medium (Figure 7–2)? As shown in Figure 7–3A, when current is injected into the cell to change the membrane potential, ΔV_m always lags behind the current pulse.

To account for this lag, we must first understand the two types of current that flow across the nerve cell membrane: the ionic current (I_i) and the capacitive current (I_c). The total membrane current (I_m) is the sum of these two components:

$$I_m = I_i + I_c.$$

Ionic (or resistive) membrane current represents the actual movement of ions through the ion (conductance)

channels of the membrane—for example, Na^+ ions moving through their channels from outside to inside the cell. *Capacitive* membrane current represents a change in the net charge stored on the membrane capacitance. For example, a movement of charge equivalent to an outward capacitive current is generated when positive charges are added to the inside of the membrane and an equal number of positive charges are removed from the outside of the membrane (Figure 7–3B).

An examination of the time courses of I_c and I_i reveals the reason for the delay between I_m and ΔV_m. Recall that the potential *(V)* across a capacitor is proportional to the charge *(Q)* stored on the capacitor:

$$V = \frac{Q}{C}.$$

For a change in potential (ΔV_m) to occur across the membrane, there must be a change in the charge (ΔQ) stored on the membrane capacitance:

$$\Delta V_m = \frac{\Delta Q}{C}. \qquad (7–1)$$

This ΔQ is brought about by the flow of capacitive current (I_c). Current is defined as the net movement of positive charge per unit time. The value of capacitive current is equal to the rate at which charge stored on the capacitor changes:

$$I_c = \frac{dQ}{dt}.$$

The total change in charge on the membrane capacitor (ΔQ) is the product of the average value of I_c and the duration of I_c ($\Delta t = t_2 - t_1$). If I_c has a constant value, this product is simply $I_c \times \Delta t$. If I_c varies with time, this product can be obtained by integrating I_c over the time t_1 to t_2:

$$\Delta Q = \int_{t_1}^{t_2} I_c \, dt.$$

7–2 Schematic diagram of an experimental setup (shown in detail in Figure 5–2) for measuring the rate of change of V_m in response to current injection. The equivalent circuit of the membrane is shown connected by two pairs of electrodes to the current generator and to the membrane potential monitor.

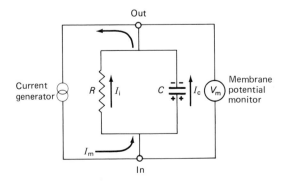

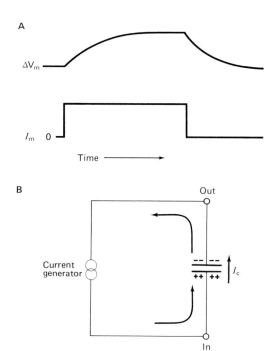

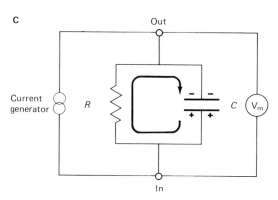

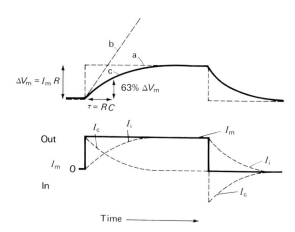

7–4 The actual shape (c) of the response of the membrane to a rectangular current pulse is intermediate between that of a pure resistive element (a) and that of a pure capacitive element (b). The product of the membrane's resistance (R) and the capacitance (C) is called the membrane time constant (τ). The total membrane current (I_m) is shown by the solid line, and the dotted lines I_i and I_c show the time course of ionic and capacitive current, respectively.

7–3 A. The time course of ΔV_m is slowed by the membrane capacitance. When V_m is changed by current injected into the cell, ΔV_m lags behind the current pulse. Outward membrane current is represented by an upward deflection, and inward current is represented by a downward deflection of the current trace. B. When capacitive current flows, positive charge builds up on one plate of the capacitor and leaves the other plate. C. At the end of the pulse, the capacitance is discharged by an inward capacitive current that drives an outward current through the membrane resistance, R.

By substituting back into Equation 7–1, we obtain

$$\Delta V_m = \frac{\int_{t_1}^{t_2} I_c \, dt}{C}.$$

The larger the value of the membrane capacitance (C), the smaller is the change in the membrane potential (ΔV_m) for a given amplitude and duration of capacitive current (I_c).

The reason for the gradual change in potential in Figure 7–3A is that the membrane capacitance and resistance are in parallel (see Figure 7–2); therefore, the potential across these two elements must be equal at all times. The potential across a capacitor cannot change until the charge stored on its plates has changed ($\Delta V_m = \Delta Q/C$). Initially, all of the membrane current flows into the capacitor to change the charge on its plates. However, as the pulse continues and ΔQ increases, more and more current must flow through the resistance, because at any instant the voltage drop across the membrane resistance ($\Delta V_m = I_i R$) must be equal to the voltage across the capacitance ($\Delta V_m = \Delta Q/C$). As a larger fraction of the membrane current flows through the resistor, less is available for charging the capacitor; thus the *rate of change* of V_m decreases with time. When ΔV_m reaches its plateau value, all of the membrane current is flowing through the resistance and $\Delta V_m = I_m R$. At the end of the current pulse, current flows around the RC loop, as the capacitor discharges and drives current through the resistor (Figure 7–3C).

The capacitance of the membrane has the effect of reducing the rate at which the membrane potential changes in response to a current pulse (Figure 7–3A). If the membrane had only resistive properties, a step pulse of outward current passed across it would change the membrane potential instantaneously (Figure 7–4, line a). On the other hand, if the membrane had only capacitive properties, the membrane potential would change slowly, in a ramplike manner, in response to the same step pulse of current (Figure 7–4, line b). Because the membrane has both capacitive and resistive properties in parallel, the actual change in membrane potential resulting from a rectangular current pulse is intermediate between the two pure responses (Figure 7–4, line c). The initial slope of V_m versus time is the same as that for a purely capacitive element, whereas the final slope and amplitude are the same as those for a purely resistive element.

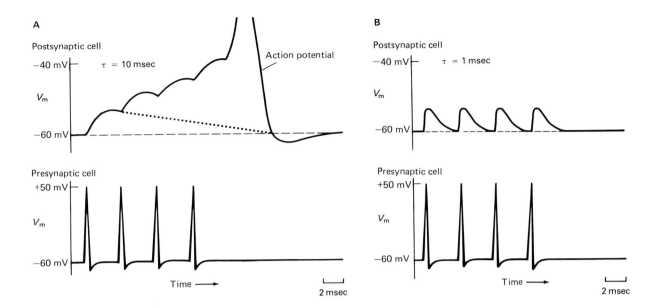

Membrane Time Constant

The waveform of the potential change shown in Figure 7–3A can be described by the following equation:

$$\Delta V_m(t) = I_m R \left(1 - e^{-t/\tau}\right).$$

In this equation, *e*, which has the value of 2.72, is the base of the system of natural logarithms, and τ equals *RC*, the product of the resistance and capacitance of the membrane. The parameter τ is called the *membrane time constant*. It can be measured experimentally. For the response of the membrane to a rectangular step of current (Figure 7–3A), τ is the time that ΔV_m takes to reach 63% of its final value.[1] The time constants of different neurons typically range from about 1 to 20 msec.

The effect of the time constant on integration of synaptic input is especially important. Most synaptic potentials are caused by brief synaptic currents triggered by neurotransmitters (see Chapter 9, Figure 9–7). The time course of the rising phase of a synaptic potential is determined by both active and passive properties of the membrane (see Chapter 9). The falling phase is purely a passive process. Its time course is a function of the membrane time constant. The longer the time constant, the longer the duration of the synaptic potential. When synaptic potentials overlap in time, they add in a process known as *temporal summation*. In this way individual excitatory postsynaptic potentials (EPSPs) that alone might be too small to trigger an action potential can sum to reach threshold. If a postsynaptic cell has a long membrane time constant, the synaptic potential is long and there is consequently more chance for temporal summa-

7–5 When the duration of the postsynaptic potential is longer than the interval between spikes in the presynaptic cell, the postsynaptic potentials overlap and their temporal summation can lead to an action potential. The larger the membrane time constant (τ) of the postsynaptic cell, the longer is the duration of the postsynaptic potential and the greater the extent of temporal summation. Here the consequences of different time constants are compared in two postsynaptic cells. In part **A,** the time constant of the postsynaptic cell is 10 msec. **Dotted line** shows the extrapolated falling phase of an individual EPSP. In part **B,** the time constant is 1 msec.

tion (Figure 7–5). In a similar fashion, temporal summation of receptor potentials also takes place in receptor cells.

Membrane and Axoplasmic Resistance Affect the Efficiency of Signal Conduction

In addition to its time constant, another electrical property of the membrane is the rate of voltage change that a signal undergoes with distance from its site of initiation. The *length constant* (also known as the *space constant*) is a measure of the distance that a potential difference can spread passively along a process of a nerve cell (an axon or dendrite). To understand this property, we must consider the three-dimensional geometry of a neuron. Consider a dendrite. Because it has a relatively small cross-sectional area, the cytoplasmic core of a dendrite exhibits a significant resistance to the longitudinal flow of current. As shown in Figure 7–6, the equivalent circuit of the dendrite may be represented as a series of identical membrane cylinders, with each adjacent cylinder connected by a short segment of cytoplasm.

The greater the length of the core, the more collisions ions experience as they carry current down the length of the dendrite. The axial resistance (r_a) therefore has units

[1] Note that 63% is equivalent to $(1 - 1/e) \times 100$.

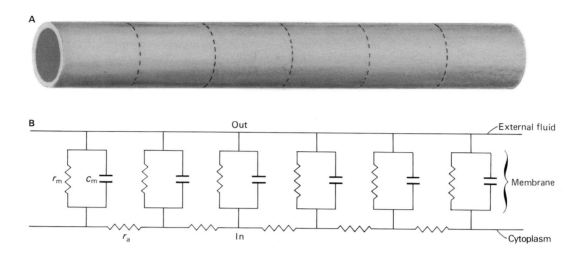

7–6 The neuronal process, either axon or dendrite, in **A** can be represented by the electrical equivalent circuit in **B**. Each unit length of the process is a circuit with its own membrane resistance, r_m, and capacitance, c_m. All the circuits are connected by resistors, r_a, which represent the axial resistance of segments of cytoplasm.

of Ω/cm. The resistance per unit length of membrane cylinder is represented as r_m. For a dendrite of a given diameter, the membrane area of a segmented membrane cylinder is proportional to the length of that cylinder; and the larger the membrane area, the lower the resis-

7–7 **A.** Current injected into a neuronal process by a microelectrode follows the path of least resistance to the return electrode in the extracellular fluid. **B.** The change in V_m produced by focal current injection decays exponentially with distance along the length of the process.

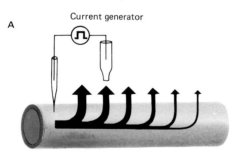

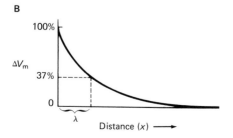

tance, because there will be a greater number of ion channels available to carry charge across the membrane. Membrane resistance (r_m) is therefore given in units of Ω-cm. The longer the segment of a dendrite, the larger r_a is and the smaller r_m. Because its volume is so great, the extracellular fluid has a negligible resistance that can be ignored for this discussion.

The capacitance per unit length of membrane cylinder is defined as c_m. Capacitance is directly proportional to membrane area. The larger the area, the greater the amount of charge that must be placed on the plates of the capacitor to produce a given voltage. For a given dendrite diameter, the membrane area of a unit length of membrane cylinder is in turn directly proportional to the length of the cylinder, so that c_m is given in units of farads per centimeter.

If a current is injected into the dendrite at one point, how will the membrane potential change with distance along the dendrite? For simplicity, let us consider the distribution of potential after the current pulse has been on for some time $(t \gg \tau)$. Under these conditions, the membrane potential has reached a steady state, so that capacitive current is zero. Because $I_c = 0$, all of the membrane current is now ionic, and $I_m = I_i$. The potential distribution is thus independent of c_m and depends solely on the relative values of r_m. The current that is injected flows out across the membrane by several possible pathways distributed along the length of the process (Figure 7–7A). Each of these pathways is made up of two components in series: a total axial resistance, R_a, and a membrane component, r_m. The total axial resistance for each current pathway is the cytoplasmic resistance between the site of current injection and any site along the dendrite. Resistors in series add, so that $R_a = r_a \cdot x$, where x is the distance along the axon from the site of current injection. The membrane component, r_m, is the same for each of these current pathways.

Because current always tends to follow the path of least resistance, more current flows across the membrane near the site of injection than at more distant regions, for which R_a is larger (Figure 7–7A). Because $V_m = I_m r_m$, the change in membrane potential produced by the current, $\Delta V_m(x)$, becomes smaller as one moves down the dendrite, away from the current electrode. This decay with distance has an exponential shape (Figure 7–7B), expressed by the following equation:

$$\Delta V_m(x) = \Delta V_0 e^{-x/\lambda}$$

where λ is the membrane length constant, x is the distance away from the site of current injection, and ΔV_0 is the change in membrane potential produced by the current flow at the site of the current electrode ($x = 0$). This equation indicates that the change in potential (ΔV_m) decays with distance along the dendrite, and the rate of decay with distance decreases as one moves away from the point $x = 0$.

The *length constant*, λ, which is the distance along the dendrite to the site where ΔV_m has decayed to $1/e$, or 37% of its value at $x = 0$, is determined by the ratio of r_m to r_a:

$$\lambda = \sqrt{\frac{r_m}{r_a}}.$$

The better the insulation of the membrane (the higher the r_m), and the better the conducting properties of the inner core (the lower the r_a), the greater is the length constant of the dendrite. The reason for this relationship is that the current is able to spread farther along the inner conductive core of the dendrite before leaking across the membrane. Typical length constant values fall in the range of about 0.1–1.0 mm.

Passive conduction of voltage changes along the neuron is called *electrotonic conduction*. The efficiency of

this process, which is measured by the length constant, has two important effects on neuronal function. First, it influences *spatial summation*. This is the process by which synaptic potentials generated in different regions of the neuron are added together at the trigger zone, the decision-making component of the neuron. For a cell with a short length constant, synaptic potentials that are initiated on the distal ends of dendrites diminish considerably as they are passively conducted to the trigger zone, so they contribute relatively little to spatial summation (Figure 7–8).

A second important feature of the length constant is its role in the propagation of the action potential. Once the membrane at any point along an axon has been depolarized beyond threshold, voltage-sensitive Na^+ channels open, causing the generation of an action potential (see Chapter 8). For conduction to continue, this local depolarization must cause the adjacent region of the membrane to reach the threshold for action potential generation (Figure 7–9). The mechanism for this spread of excitation is the passive, decremental conduction of depolarization along the axon cable. The excitation is spread by "local-circuit" current flow between the active and the inactive regions of the membrane. Once the depolarization of the inactive region of the membrane approaches threshold, this region actively contributes to its own depolarization. The voltage-gated Na^+ channels in this region of membrane open up, Na^+ rushes into the cell down its electrochemical gradient, and the depolarization becomes greater. This increase in depolarization causes more Na^+ gates to open, so that more Na^+ comes in, and so forth. Thus, as the membrane potential approaches threshold, the depolarization of this local patch of membrane changes from a passive to an active and re-

7–8 The length constant affects the efficiency of electrotonic propagation of synaptic potentials. An action potential in cell **a** elicits synaptic potentials in cells **b** and **c**. At their sites of initiation, the two synaptic potentials are equal in amplitude. Although the distance the synaptic potential must travel is the same in both cells **b** and **c**, the synaptic potential is conducted to the trigger zone much more effectively in cell **b** than in **c** because the dendrites of **b** have a much greater length constant (1 mm) than those of **c** (0.1 mm).

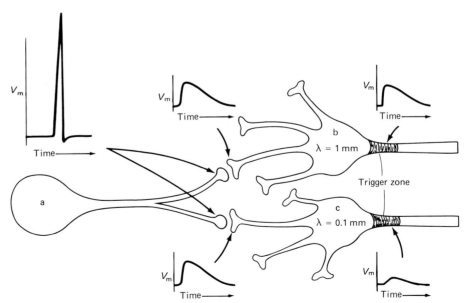

A

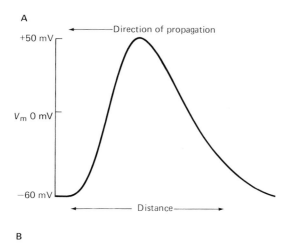

B

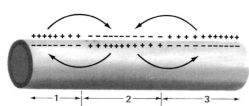

7–9 Passive conduction of depolarization along the axon contributes to action potential propagation. **A.** The waveform of an action potential propagating from right to left. **B.** The charge distribution across the membrane capacitance and the spread of depolarization from the active region (**2**) to the inactive region (**1**) ahead of the action potential results from local-circuit current flow. The spread of positive charge (current flow) along the inside of the axon from area **2** to area **3** also tends to depolarize the membrane behind the action potential. However, because g_K is increased in the wake of the action potential (see Chapter 8), this build-up of positive charge along the inside of the membrane is more than balanced by an efflux of K^+ through the membrane in area **3**.

generative process. This actively generated depolarization now spreads by passive, local-circuit flow of current to the next region of membrane, and the cycle is repeated.

Axon Diameter Affects Current Threshold

When a peripheral nerve is stimulated with a pair of extracellular electrodes, the total number of axons that generate action potentials varies with the amplitude of the current pulse. In general, the *largest axons have the lowest current threshold*. To drive the cell to threshold, the current must pass through the cell membrane. For any given axon, however, most of the stimulating current bypasses the fiber, moving instead through the low-resistance pathway provided by the other axons and by the extracellular fluid. Only a small fraction of the total stimulating current crosses the membrane of any one axon. From there it flows along the axoplasmic core, and then out again through more distant regions of axonal membrane, to the second electrode in the extracellular fluid. The larger the diameter of the axon, the smaller

the resistance of its axoplasm to longitudinal current spread because of the greater number of available intracellular charge carriers per unit length of the axon. As a result of the increase in current spread, a greater fraction of total current enters and leaves the larger axon, thereby contributing to depolarization of the membrane.[2]

Passive Membrane Properties and Axon Diameter Affect the Velocity of Action Potential Propagation

The passive spread of depolarization during conduction of the action potential is not instantaneous. In fact, it is a rate-limiting factor in the propagation of the action potential. To understand this limitation, consider the simplified equivalent circuit of the axon shown in Figure 7–10. It represents two adjacent membrane segments, connected by a segment of axoplasm, r_a. In Figure 7–10A, the two adjacent areas of membrane are both at rest. In Figure 7–10B, an action potential has been generated in the left-hand segment of membrane, and it is supplying depolarizing current to the adjacent membrane at right, causing it to depolarize gradually toward threshold.

According to Ohm's law, the larger the axoplasmic resistance, the smaller is the current flow around the loop ($I = V/R$), and thus the longer it takes to change the charge on the membrane capacitance of the adjacent segment. Recall that

$$\Delta Q = \int_{t_1}^{t_2} I_c \, dt.$$

Similarly, the larger the membrane capacitance, the more charge must be deposited on it to change the potential across the membrane. Therefore, the time it takes for depolarization to spread along the axon is determined by both the axial resistance and the capacitance per unit length of the axon (r_a and c_m); the rate of passive spread varies with the product $r_a \times c_m$. If this product is reduced, the rate of passive spread of a given depolarization increases, so that the action potential propagates faster.

Speed of action potential propagation is functionally important, and two distinct mechanisms have evolved that tend to increase it. One strategy is to increase conduction velocity by *increasing the diameter of the axon core*. Because the axial resistance (r_a) decreases in proportion to the square of axon diameter, while the capacitance per unit length of the axon (c_m) increases in direct proportion to diameter, the net effect of an increase in diameter is a decrease in $r_a c_m$. This adaptation has been

[2]Since current tends to follow the path of least resistance, a greater fraction of total current enters and leaves the larger axon, thereby contributing to depolarization of the membrane. On the other hand, the greater membrane area per length of axon in the larger diameter axon means it has a lower r_m and a larger c_m across which the current must flow to produce a depolarization. However, r_m decreases and c_m increases linearly with axon diameter, while r_a decreases with the square of the diameter. The net effect is that larger axons have lower current thresholds; gradually increasing the current strength recruits (excites) the larger axons first.

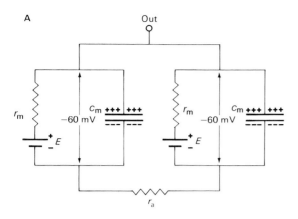

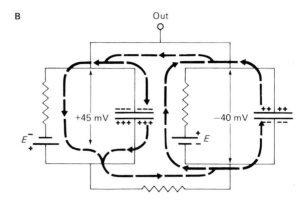

7–10 This electrical equivalent circuit represents two adjacent membrane segments of an axon, connected by a segment of axoplasm. In part **A,** both membrane segments are at rest. Part **B** shows an action potential spreading from the left-hand membrane segment to the segment on the right. **Broken lines** indicate pathways of current flow.

carried to its extreme in the giant axon of the squid, which can be as large as 1 mm in diameter. No larger axons have evolved, presumably because of the opposing need to keep neuronal size small (so that many cells can be packed into a restricted space).

A second mechanism for increasing conduction velocity and reducing $r_a c_m$ is *myelination,* the wrapping of glial cell membranes around an axon. This process is functionally equivalent to increasing the thickness of the axonal membrane by as much as 100 times. Because the

7–11 Saltatory conduction in myelinated nerves.
   A. Capacitive and ionic membrane current density are much higher at the nodes of Ranvier than in the internodal regions of the axon. Membrane current density (membrane current per unit area of membrane) is represented by the distribution of the lines depicting current flow (**arrows**).

B. Because of the low capacitance of the myelin sheath, the action potential skips rapidly from node to node. **C.** Action potential conduction is slowed down or blocked at axon regions that have lost their myelin. The local-circuit currents must charge a greater c_m, and because of the low r_m they do not spread as effectively along the length of the axon.

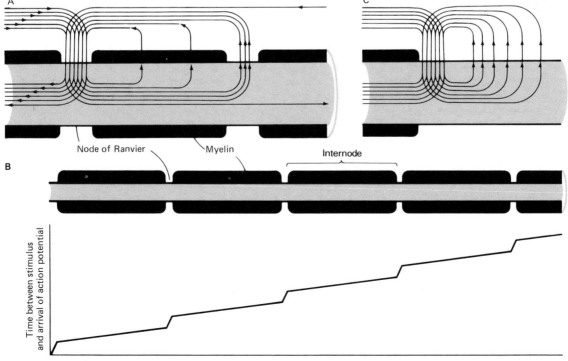

capacitance of a parallel-plate capacitor such as the membrane is inversely proportional to the thickness of the insulating material (see Appendix IIIA), myelination will decrease c_m, and thus also $r_a c_m$. The increase in *total* fiber diameter achieved by myelination causes a much larger percentage decrease in $r_a c_m$ than if the same increase in fiber diameter were achieved simply by increasing the diameter of the axon core. For this reason, conduction in myelinated axons is faster than in nonmyelinated axons of the same diameter.

Although myelin is quite effective in increasing conduction velocity, it interferes with the normal regenerative mechanism for nondecremental conduction. In a myelinated axon, the action potential is triggered at the bare axon membrane of the axon hillock. The inward current that flows through this membrane is then available to discharge the capacitance of the myelinated axon ahead of it. Even though the thickness of myelin makes the capacitance of the axon quite small, the amount of current flowing down the core of the axon from the trigger zone is limited and is not enough to discharge the capacitance along the entire length of the myelinated axon. Therefore, the action potential gradually diminishes as it spreads down the axon.

To prevent the action potential from gradually dying out, the myelin sheath is interrupted every 1–2 mm by the nodes of Ranvier. These bare patches of nodal membrane are only about 2 μm in length. Although the area of each nodal membrane is quite small, it contains a relatively high density of voltage-gated Na[+] channels and can generate an intense depolarizing inward Na[+] current in response to the passive spread of depolarization from the axon upstream. These regularly distributed nodes thus boost the amplitude of the action potential periodically, keeping it from dying out.

Because of the low capacitance of the myelin sheath, the action potential spreads quite rapidly along the internode, but slows down as it crosses the high-capacitance region of each bare node (Figure 7–11B). Consequently, if one follows the movement of the action potential down the axon, it seems to jump very quickly from node to node (Figure 7–11B). For this reason, the conduction of an action potential in a myelinated axon is called *saltatory conduction* (from the Latin *saltare*, to leap). Because ionic current flows only at the node in myelinated fibers, saltatory conduction is also favorable from a metabolic standpoint. Less energy must be expended by the Na–K

pump in restoring the Na[+] and K[+] concentration gradients, which tend to run down as a result of action potential activity.

Several diseases of the nervous system, such as multiple sclerosis and Guillain-Barré syndrome, cause demyelination. These diseases can have devastating effects on the control of behavior because they cause slowing of action potential conduction. As an action potential goes from a region where myelin is present to a bare stretch of axon (Figure 7–11C), it encounters a region of relatively high c_m and low r_m. The inward current generated at the last node before this area therefore has to flow for a longer time before it drives the adjacent membrane to threshold for generating an action potential. In addition, this local-circuit current does not spread as far as normal because it is flowing into a segment of axon that, because of its low r_m, has a short length constant. These two factors combine to slow, and in some cases actually block, the conduction of action potentials in the nerve.

Selected Readings

Barrett, J. N. 1975. Motoneuron dendrites: Role in synaptic integration. Fed. Proc. 34:1398–1407.

Graubard, K., and Calvin, W. H. 1979. Presynaptic dendrites: Implications of spikeless synaptic transmission and dendritic geometry. In F. O. Schmitt and F. G. Worden (eds.), The Neurosciences; Fourth Study Program. Cambridge, Mass.: MIT Press, pp. 317–331.

Hodgkin, A. L. 1964. The Conduction of the Nervous Impulse. Springfield, Ill.: Thomas, chap. 4.

Hubbard, J. I., Llinás, R., and Quastel, D. M. J. 1969. Electrophysiological Analysis of Synaptic Transmission. Baltimore: Williams & Wilkins, chap. 2, pp. 91–109, 257–264.

Jack, J. 1979. An introduction to linear cable theory. In F. O. Schmitt and F. G. Worden (eds.), The Neurosciences; Fourth Study Program. Cambridge, Mass.: MIT Press, pp. 423–437.

Jack, J. J. B., Noble, D., and Tsien, R. W. 1975. Electric Current Flow in Excitable Cells. Oxford: Clarendon Press, chaps. 1–5, 7, pp. 276–277.

Khodorov, B. I. 1974. The Problem of Excitability. New York: Plenum Press, chap. 3.

Rall, W. 1977. Core conductor theory and cable properties of neurons. In E. R. Kandel (ed.), Handbook of Physiology, Vol. 1: The Nervous System, Part 1. Bethesda, Md.: American Physiological Society, pp. 39–97.

John Koester

Voltage-Gated Channels and the Generation of the Action Potential

8

Because nerve cells generate and conduct action potentials, signals can be conveyed over long distances within the nervous system. The feature of action potentials crucial for long-range signaling is that the action potential does not diminish as it travels away from its site of initiation. Knowledge of the mechanisms underlying the generation and propagation of action potentials is therefore essential for an understanding of neuronal signaling.

The generation of action potentials by nerve axons and muscle fibers was first described in 1849 by the German physiologist Emil DuBois-Reymond. It was not until 100 years later, however, that it became possible to analyze the mechanism underlying action potential generation in terms of specific membrane proteins—the voltage-gated ion channels for Na$^+$ and K$^+$.

The Action Potential Is Generated by the Flow of Ions Through Voltage-Gated Na$^+$ and K$^+$ Channels

An important early clue about how action potentials are generated came from an experiment done in 1938 by K. C. Cole and Howard Curtis of the College of Physicians and Surgeons of Columbia University. Recording from the squid giant axon, they found that conductance of the membrane to ions increases during the action potential. This increase in conductance provided the first evidence that the action potential results from the movement of ions through the membrane. It also raised an important question: which ions are responsible for the action potential? A decade later, Alan Hodgkin and Bernard Katz in England found that the amplitude of the action potential is reduced when the external Na$^+$ concentration is lowered. They also found that the rate of repolarization during the falling phase of the action potential is reduced if the external K$^+$ concentration is increased.

On the basis of their own observations and those of Cole and Curtis, Hodgkin and Katz offered a specific hypothesis to explain the generation of the action potential. They proposed that the action potential is initiated by depolarization, which causes a transient change in the membrane that briefly switches its predominant permeability from K$^+$ to Na$^+$. We now know that these permeability changes occur because of voltage-sensitive channels in the membrane that allow Na$^+$ to move into the cell down its concentration gradient. These Na$^+$ channels are normally kept closed by voltage-sensitive gates. Depolarization opens these gates, allowing increased Na$^+$ influx into the cell and thereby producing the rising phase of the action potential. The falling phase of the action potential is caused by the subsequent closing of these Na$^+$ gates, which reduces Na$^+$ influx, and by the opening of gates in K$^+$ channels, which allows increased K$^+$ efflux from the cell.

To test this hypothesis, it is necessary to vary membrane potential and measure the resulting changes in the conductance through the Na$^+$ and the K$^+$ channels. This is difficult to do experimentally because there is mutual coupling between membrane potential and the Na$^+$ and K$^+$ channels. For example, if the membrane is depolarized sufficiently to open the gates of some of the active Na$^+$ conductance channels, inward Na$^+$ current flows through these channels and causes additional depolarization. This depolarization causes still more Na$^+$ channels to open and consequently induces more inward Na$^+$ current. A regenerative cycle therefore is initiated that makes it impossible to achieve a stable membrane potential. This cycle, which eventually drives V_m to the peak of the action potential, can be depicted as follows:

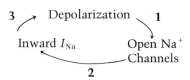

A similar technical difficulty hinders the study of the active K$^+$ conductance channels that are responsible for the falling phase of the action potential. An apparatus known as a voltage clamp was designed by Cole to overcome these problems.

Voltage-Dependent Channels Can Be Studied by Use of the Voltage Clamp

The basic function of the voltage clamp is to interrupt the interaction between the opening and closing of voltage-gated channels and membrane potential. When an axon is clamped, voltage-gated ion channels still respond to changes in membrane potential by opening or closing, but the voltage clamp prevents the resultant changes in membrane current from influencing the membrane po-

tential. The conductance of different ion channels in the membrane can therefore be measured as a function of membrane potential.

By using the voltage clamp technique on the squid giant axon in the early 1950s, Hodgkin and Andrew Huxley provided the first complete description of the ionic mechanisms underlying the action potential.

The voltage clamp is essentially a current pump connected to two electrodes, one inside and the other outside the cell. The clamp has two functions. One is to step the membrane potential rapidly to various levels of depolarization in response to "commands" from the experimenter. These commanded depolarizations, which are produced by passing current across the passive membrane resistance and capacitance, open the gates of the Na$^+$ and K$^+$ channels. The resulting movement of Na$^+$ and K$^+$ across the membrane tends to change the membrane potential to a different level. This process then calls into play the second function of the voltage clamp, which is to "clamp" the membrane potential at its commanded level.

For example, when Na$^+$ channels open in response to a depolarizing voltage step, an inward membrane current develops, mediated by Na$^+$ flowing through these channels. This Na$^+$ influx tends to depolarize the membrane by increasing the positive charge on the inside of the membrane and reducing the positive charge on the outside. The voltage clamp prevents the membrane potential from depolarizing by simultaneously pumping positive

8–1 The voltage-gated channels of the squid axon are studied by means of a voltage clamp. **A.** Basic flow diagram. **B.** Configuration of electronic components used in voltage clamping. A signal generator (**SG**) produces command potentials (**CP**) of different values. **A$_V$**, amplifier for monitoring V_m. **A$_{FB}$**, feedback amplifier for generating the current required to change V_m and to keep it clamped at the commanded level.

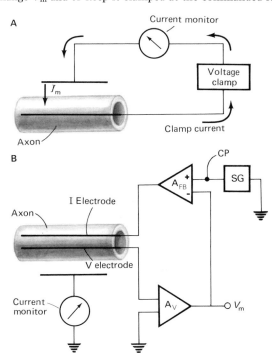

charges out of the cell into the external solution through the electronic circuitry. Thus, the flow of any membrane current that would tend to change the resting membrane potential from its commanded value is automatically counteracted by an equal and opposite current generated by the voltage clamp circuit (Figure 8–1A). Under voltage clamp conditions, the first two steps in the regenerative cycle described above are not affected directly: depolarization still causes Na^+ channels to open, which still results in an increased inward Na^+ current. The third step, however, the further depolarization caused by this extra Na^+ influx, is prevented by the clamp. By recording the current that must be generated by the voltage clamp to keep the membrane potential from changing, it is possible to measure the membrane current directly (Figure 8–1A). From the membrane current and the membrane potential, the membrane conductance can then be calculated (see below). The total membrane conductance in turn can be analyzed to obtain the relative contributions of Na^+ and K^+, and this in turn gives preliminary insight into the properties of the channels for these two ions.

The Voltage Clamp Employs Negative Feedback

The experimental apparatus used for voltage clamping a squid axon (Figure 8–1B) includes an intracellular electrode connected to an amplifier (A_V) for measuring the membrane potential. The membrane potential signal (V_m) is displayed on an oscilloscope and is also fed into one terminal of the "feedback" amplifier (A_{FB}). This amplifier has two inputs—one for the membrane potential and another for the command potential (CP). The command potential, which comes from a signal generator, is selected by the experimenter. It can be of any desired amplitude and waveform. The feedback amplifier subtracts the membrane potential from the command potential. Any difference between these two signals appears amplified several thousand times at the output of the feedback amplifier. The output of this amplifier is connected to a thin Ag–AgCl wire, the current-passing electrode that runs the length of the axon.

The voltage clamp is a negative feedback system.[1] It is designed so that the membrane potential *automatically* follows the command potential exactly. For example, if an inward Na^+ current causes the membrane potential to become more positive than the command potential, the output of the feedback amplifier becomes negative. This will make the internal current electrode negative and thereby withdraw positive charges from the cell through the voltage clamp circuit and deposit the positive charges into the external solution through the other current electrode. Since the current generated by the feedback ampli-

---

[1]A negative feedback system is one in which the value of the output of the system (V_m in this case) is "fed back" to the input of the system, where it is compared to a command signal for the desired output. Any difference between the command and the output signal activates a "controller" device (in this case A_{FB}) that automatically reduces the difference. Negative feedback is also a widely used physiological mechanism, e.g., for the control of blood pressure, blood levels of hormones, and synthesis of various metabolites and is discussed further in Chapter 47.

8–2 Records of typical squid axon voltage clamp experiments demonstrate the existence of two types of voltage-gated channels. **A.** A small depolarization is accompanied by capacitive and leakage currents (I_c and I_l, respectively). **B.** Larger depolarizing steps result in larger capacitive and leakage currents plus additional currents caused by the opening of Na^+ and K^+ channels. **C.** When the voltage step shown in **B** is repeated in the presence of tetrodotoxin (which blocks the Na^+ current) and again in the presence of tetraethylammonium (which blocks the K^+ current), records of the pure K^+ and Na^+ currents (I_K and I_{Na}, respectively) are obtained by subtraction of I_c and I_l.

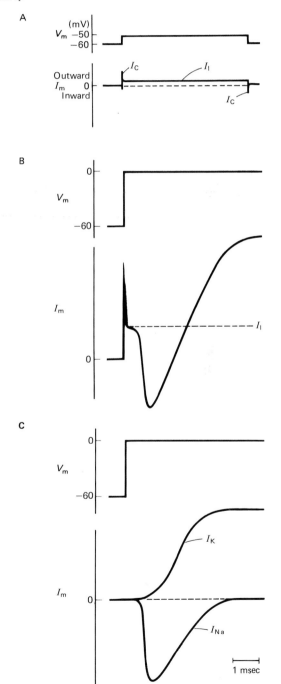

fier is exactly equal and opposite to that flowing across the membrane, two consequences follow. One, there will be no *net* change in the amount of charge separated by the membrane and therefore no significant change in V_m. Two, the current flowing through the membrane at any membrane potential can be obtained by simply setting the command to that potential.

Because the highly conductive current-passing wire short-circuits the axoplasmic resistance, reducing the axial resistance to zero, the membrane potential is the same all along the length of the axon. The presence of this low-resistance pathway along the inside of the axon makes it impossible for a potential difference to exist between different points along the axon core.

The membrane current that is recorded in a voltage clamp experiment can be separated into ionic and capacitive components. The V_m at any time is proportional to the charge on the membrane capacitance (C_m). When V_m is not changing, the charge on C_m is constant, and no capacitive current flows. Capacitive current flows *only* when V_m is changing (Chapter 7). Therefore, if the membrane potential is changed by means of a very rapid step of command potential, capacitive current flows only at the beginning and the end of the step. This capacitive current is essentially instantaneous, and it can be separated easily from the later ionic currents by inspection of the oscilloscope record.

Na$^+$ and K$^+$ Currents Move Through Two Independent Channels

Let us consider the results of a typical voltage clamp experiment (Figure 8–2). We start with the membrane potential clamped at its resting value. If a 10-mV, subthreshold depolarizing potential step is commanded, we observe that an initial, very brief outward capacitive current (I_c) instantaneously discharges the membrane capacitance by the amount required for a 10-mV depolarization (Figure 8–2A). This capacitive current is followed by a smaller, steady outward ionic current. At the end of the pulse, there is a brief inward capacitive current, and the

ionic current returns to zero. The steady ionic current is called the *leakage current*, I_l. This is the current that flows through the passive, nongated ion channels of the membrane. This population of channels is called the *leakage conductance* (g_l). As described in Chapter 6, these leakage channels, which are always open, are responsible for generating the resting potential. In a typical neuron most of the nongated leakage channels are permeable to K$^+$ ions, while somewhat smaller numbers of leakage channels are permeable to Cl$^-$ or Na$^+$ ions.

If larger depolarizing steps are commanded, the current records become more complicated (Figure 8–2B): the capacitive and leakage currents are both larger. In addition, shortly after the end of the capacitive current and the start of the leakage current, an inward current develops; it reaches a peak within a few milliseconds, declines, and gives way to an outward current. This outward current reaches a plateau that is maintained for the duration of the pulse.

A simple interpretation of these findings is that the depolarizing voltage step sequentially turns on active conductance channels for two separate ions: one type of channel for inward current and another for outward current. Because these two oppositely directed currents partially overlap in time, the most difficult part of the analysis of voltage clamp experiments is to determine their separate time courses.

Hodgkin and Huxley achieved this separation by substituting ions. By substituting a larger impermeant cation (choline) for Na$^+$ in the external bathing solution, they eliminated the inward Na$^+$ current. Recently, a simpler technique has been developed to separate inward and outward currents. This method is based on the selective pharmacological blockade of the separate voltage-sensitive conductance channels: tetrodotoxin applied to the cell membrane blocks the voltage-sensitive Na$^+$ channel, and tetraethylammonium blocks the voltage-sensitive K$^+$ channel.

To measure the current flowing through the Na$^+$ channels, I_{Na}, as a function of membrane potential, var-

8–3 Electrical equivalent circuit of a nerve cell under voltage clamp conditions.

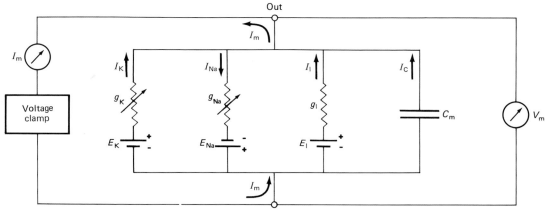

ious command pulses are given to change V_m to different levels. When tetraethylammonium is applied to the axon to block the K$^+$ channels, the total membrane current consists of I_c, I_l, and I_{Na}. The leakage conductance, g_l, is constant; it does not vary with V_m or with time. Therefore, I_l may be readily calculated and subtracted from I_m, leaving I_{Na} and I_c. Because I_c occurs only very briefly at the beginning and end of the pulse, it can be easily eliminated by inspection, leaving a pure I_{Na}. By a similar process, I_K may be measured when the Na$^+$ channels are blocked by tetrodotoxin (Figure 8–2C).

Na$^+$ and K$^+$ Conductances Are Calculated from Their Currents

Once the Na$^+$ and the K$^+$ currents have been separated (Figure 8–2C), the membrane conductances to Na$^+$ and K$^+$ can be calculated as a function of membrane potential and time. This procedure can be illustrated with a slightly more complex equivalent circuit diagram of the membrane, which includes the passive membrane capacitance (C_m) and leakage conductance (g_l), as well as the active, voltage-sensitive conductance channels for Na$^+$ (g_{Na}) and K$^+$ (g_K) (Figure 8–3). The ionic battery of the leakage channels (E_l) is equal to the resting potential. The Na$^+$ and K$^+$ conductances are shown in series with appropriate Nernst batteries.

The current through each class of active conductance channels may be calculated from Ohm's law, written in the same form used to calculate the currents through the passive channels (see Equations 6–2a and 6–2b):

$$I_K = g_K \times (V_m - E_K) \qquad (8\text{–}1a)$$

$$I_{Na} = g_{Na} \times (V_m - E_{Na}). \qquad (8\text{–}1b)$$

Rearranging and solving for g gives two equations that can be used to compute the ionic conductances for the active Na$^+$ and K$^+$ conductance channel populations[2]:

$$g_K = \frac{I_K}{(V_m - E_K)}$$

$$g_{Na} = \frac{I_{Na}}{(V_m - E_{Na})}.$$

When measured at various levels of membrane potential, the conductances through the Na$^+$ and K$^+$ channels show two basic similarities and two differences. They are alike in that both turn on in response to depolarizing

---

[2]To solve these equations for g_K and g_{Na}, one must know V_m, E_K, E_{Na}, I_K, and I_{Na}. V_m is the independent variable, set by the experimenter. E_K and E_{Na} are constants; they can be calculated from the Nernst equation or measured empirically by finding the values of V_m at which I_K and I_{Na} reverse their polarities. For example, if V_m is stepped to very positive values, I_{Na} gradually becomes less inward. At E_{Na} it goes to zero, and for values of V_m more positive than E_{Na}, I_{Na} is outward (Equation 8–1b). I_K and I_{Na} are the dependent variables and can be obtained from the current records of voltage clamp experiments by the ionic separation techniques described above (Figure 8–2C). Thus, all the data required to compute g_K and g_{Na} are available.

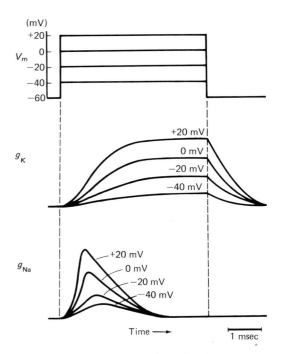

8–4 Voltage clamp experiments show that g_{Na} turns on and off more rapidly than g_K over a wide range of membrane potentials. The gradual increases and decreases in total Na$^+$ and K$^+$ conductances shown here are population phenomena that reflect shifts of thousands of voltage-gated channels between the open and closed states.

steps of membrane potential, and they both do so more rapidly and to a greater extent for larger depolarizations (Figure 8–4). They differ, however, in two respects: (1) their rate of onset and offset and (2) their inactivation. At all levels of membrane potential (Figure 8–4), g_{Na} turns on more rapidly than g_K. g_{Na} also turns off more rapidly when the depolarizing pulse is terminated (Figure 8–5,

8–5 For a brief depolarizing step (a) both g_{Na} and g_K return to their initial values when the cell repolarizes. For a longer step (b), g_{Na} inactivates even though the depolarization is maintained, while g_K reaches a plateau level that is constant for the duration of the depolarization.

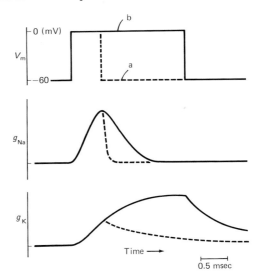

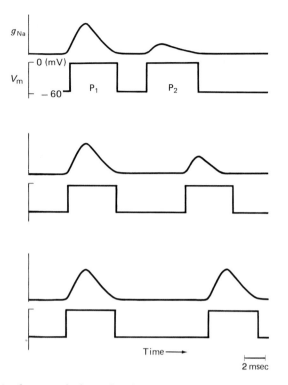

8–6 The second of two depolarizing pulses (**P₂**) produces a smaller increase in g_{Na} if the interval between the first (**P₁**) and second is brief, because Na⁺ inactivation persists for a few milliseconds after the end of the first activating pulse.

line a). In addition, with maintained depolarization, the Na⁺ channels begin to close down, or inactivate, leading to a decay of inward current (Figure 8–4 and Figure 8–5, line b). In contrast, the K⁺ channels remain open as long as the membrane is depolarized (Figure 8–5). Each Na⁺ channel can exist in three different states thought to represent three different conformations of the Na⁺ channel protein: resting, activated, or inactivated. Upon depolarization, the channel goes from the resting (closed) to the

8–7 The action potential can be reconstructed from the changes in g_{Na} and g_K that result from the opening and closing of Na⁺ and K⁺ voltage-gated channels. (Adapted from Hodgkin, 1964.)

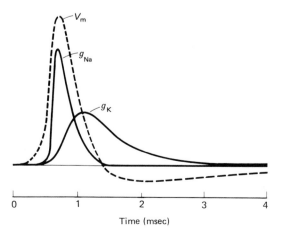

activated (open) state. If the depolarization is maintained, the channel switches to the inactivated (closed) state. Once the channel is inactivated, it is refractory: it cannot be activated (opened) by depolarization. The inactivation can be removed only by repolarizing the membrane, which allows the channel to switch from the inactivated to the resting state. This switch takes time because inactivation wanes slowly (Figure 8–6). After the channel has returned to the resting state, it again is available for activation by depolarization.

The Action Potential Can Be Reconstructed from the Individual Electrical Properties of the Neuron

By analyzing the records of depolarizing pulses of various amplitudes and durations, Hodgkin and Huxley generated a complete set of empirical equations that describe the variation of conductances through the Na⁺ and the K⁺ channels as a function of membrane potential and time. Using these equations and the values of the passive properties of the axon, they were able to compute the predicted shape and the conduction velocity of the propagated action potential. That this calculated waveform agreed almost perfectly with the action potential recorded in the unclamped axon indicates that the data accurately describe the features of the voltage-dependent conductance channels that are essential for the propagation of the action potential.

According to the Hodgkin–Huxley model, an action potential involves the following sequence of events (Figure 8–7). A depolarization of the membrane causes a rapid opening of Na⁺ channels (an increase in g_{Na}), resulting in an inward Na⁺ current. This current causes further depolarization, which results in more inward current, and the regenerative process leads to the generation of the action potential.[3] Two factors limit the duration of the action potential: (1) The depolarization of the action potential gradually inactivates the Na⁺ channels (g_{Na}). (2) The depolarization also opens, with some delay, the voltage-gated K⁺ channels, thereby increasing g_K. Consequently the Na⁺ current is followed by an outward K⁺ current that tends to repolarize the membrane (Figures 8–4 and 8–5).

In most nerve cells, action potentials are followed by a transient hyperpolarization, the hyperpolarizing afterpotential. This brief increase in the negativity of the membrane potential occurs because the K⁺ channels that open during the later phase of the action potential do not all close immediately, even after V_m has returned to its resting value. It takes a few milliseconds for all of the voltage-gated K⁺ channels to return to the closed state.

---

[3]It may at first seem paradoxical that to depolarize the cell experimentally one passes *outward* current across the membrane (see Figure 5–1), while the depolarization during the upstroke of the action potential is attributed to an *inward* Na⁺ current. Actually, in both cases *outward* current flows across the passive components, the nongated leakage channels (g_1) and the capacitance (C_m), of the membrane. This outward current across the passive membrane results because current is injected into the cell: in one case through an intracellular electrode (Figure 7–2), and in the other case by the opening of voltage-gated Na⁺ channels.

The resulting residual opening of active K$^+$ channels leads to a greater efflux of K$^+$ from the cell than occurs in the resting state. This efflux, in turn, causes V_m to hyperpolarize slightly with respect to its normal resting value (Figure 8–7).

The action potential is also followed by a brief period of refractoriness, which can be divided into two phases. The *absolute refractory period* comes immediately after the action potential; during this period, it is impossible to excite the cell no matter how large a stimulating current is applied. This phase is followed directly by the *relative refractory period*, during which it is possible to trigger an action potential, but only by applying stimuli that are stronger than normal. These periods of refractoriness, which together last just a few milliseconds, are both caused by the residual opening of K$^+$ channels and the residual inactivation of Na$^+$ channels.

Another feature of the action potential predicted by the Hodgkin–Huxley conductance data is its threshold. Action potentials are all or none in amplitude, and for depolarizations in the range of threshold an additional fraction of a millivolt may be the difference between a subthreshold stimulus and a stimulus that generates a full-blown action potential. This all-or-none behavior may seem surprising when one considers that Na$^+$ conductance (proportional to the number of Na$^+$ channels that are open) increases in a strictly graded manner as depolarization is increased (Figure 8–4). With each increment of depolarization, the number of voltage-gated Na$^+$ channels that flip from the closed to the open state increases in a gradual fashion, thereby causing a gradual increase in the Na$^+$ influx. What then gives the action potential its threshold? Although a small subthreshold depolarization increases the inward I_{Na}, it also increases two *outward* currents, I_K and I_1, by changing the driving forces that determine their values (see Equation 8–1a). In addition to increasing the driving force for I_K, the depolarization also causes a slow increase in g_K by gradually increasing the number of open K$^+$ channels (Figure 8–4). As I_K and I_1 increase with depolarization, they tend to resist the depolarizing action of the Na$^+$ influx. The steep voltage sensitivity and rapid kinetics of the Na$^+$ channel activation process ensure that, as the depolarization proceeds, it will eventually reach a point—the threshold—where the increase in inward I_{Na} outstrips the increase in outward I_K and I_1, and therefore becomes regenerative. Thus a threshold exists because there is a specific value of V_m at which the *net* ionic current ($I_{Na} + I_K + I_1$) just changes from outward to inward, depositing positive charge on the inside of the membrane capacitance.

The data reported by Hodgkin and Huxley also explain why a slowly rising stimulating current may fail to trigger an action potential when it depolarizes the cell to its usual threshold membrane potential, V_T (Figure 8–8). It fails to do so because during a slow approach to V_T the two dynamic processes that oppose the regenerative property of the membrane—inactivation of the Na$^+$ channels and the activation of the K$^+$ channels—have a chance to develop significantly before V_T is reached.

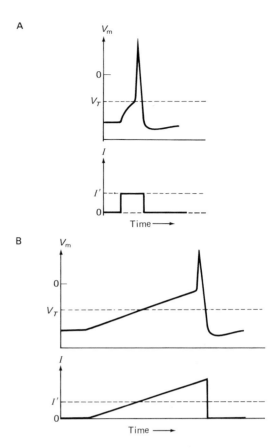

8–8 A slowly rising current pulse causes a cell's firing threshold to increase through a process called accommodation. **A.** To reach threshold (V_T) for spike generation, a rectangular (or constant-amplitude) current pulse need have an amplitude of only I'. **B.** If depolarizing current is increased gradually, accommodation occurs and the stimulating current must surpass I' before a spike is initiated.

Therefore, to activate enough Na$^+$ channels to trigger an action potential, one must depolarize the cell by a greater than normal increment. This increase in threshold resulting from the application of a slowly rising current is called *accommodation*. By decreasing the rate of rise of current even more, one can produce a depolarization so slow that, regardless of how much the cell is depolarized, an action potential is not elicited.

The Na$^+$ Channel Can Be Characterized in Molecular Terms

The empirical equations derived by Hodgkin and Huxley have been remarkably successful in describing the flow of ions through the Na$^+$ and K$^+$ channels that underlies the action potential. However, these equations describe the process of excitation only on a phenomenological level. The data of Hodgkin and Huxley tell us little about the molecular nature of the conductance channels and the mechanisms by which they are activated. Recent work on the Na$^+$ channel has been directed along these lines.

Na⁺ Channels Are Sparsely Distributed but Are Highly Efficient Pathways for Na⁺ Flux

Characterization of the Na$^+$ channel has been aided greatly by the availability of several naturally occurring neurotoxins—tetrodotoxin from the puffer fish, saxitoxin from paralytic shellfish, batrachotoxin from South American poisonous frogs, and the venom from the North African scorpion. These toxins bind tightly to the channel and therefore can be used as specific probes for localizing the channel molecules. The binding of radiolabeled tetrodotoxin molecules to axon membrane has been studied to obtain an estimate of the density of voltage-gated Na$^+$ channels per unit area of axon membrane. These studies indicate that tetrodotoxin binds to a small number of specific sites on the membrane. These specific sites are thought to represent the Na$^+$ conductance channels, because the binding constant and the kinetics of tetrodotoxin binding to these sites correspond to the values determined by physiological measurement of the tetrodotoxin blockade of Na$^+$ conductance.

Murdoch Ritchie and his colleagues at Yale estimated the number of Na$^+$ channels by measuring the total amount of tetrodotoxin that was bound when these specific binding sites were saturated. They found that the greater the density of Na$^+$ channels in the membrane of an axon, the greater the velocity at which the axon conducts action potentials (Chapter 7). This result is to be expected. A greater density of Na$^+$ channels allows more current to flow through the active membrane and along the axon core to discharge the membrane capacitance of the unexcited membrane downstream (see Figure 7–10). Depending on cell type, the values obtained for nonmyelinated axons range from 35 to 500 Na$^+$ channels per square micrometer of axon membrane.

Even at 500 channels/µm², the density of Na$^+$ channels is quite low—*about one Na$^+$ channel in 4,000 membrane molecules.* Despite this small number, quite large Na$^+$ currents can flow during the action potential. The current density through each channel must therefore be high. By dividing the total Na$^+$ current that flows during a voltage clamp pulse by the number of Na$^+$ channels in the membrane, it is possible to calculate that a single Na$^+$ channel passes up to 10^7 Na$^+$ ions/sec. Both empirical data and theoretical calculations indicate that carrier molecules cannot transport ions at this rate. The only plausible mechanism for such a high rate would be the flow of Na$^+$ ions through an aqueous channel.

Voltage-Gated Channels Open in an All-or-None Fashion

In ordinary voltage clamp experiments, the current flow through a single channel cannot be measured for two reasons: (1) the voltage clamp surveys a large extent of membrane, in which thousands of channels are opening and closing randomly; and (2) the background noise caused by current flow through passive nongated membrane channels is much larger than the current flow through any one channel. To circumvent these problems,

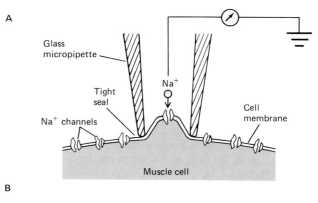

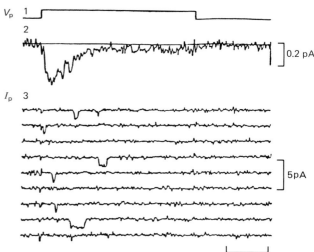

8–9 The patch clamp method is used to record current through single voltage-gated channels. **A.** A small patch of membrane containing only a single voltage-gated Na$^+$ channel is electrically isolated from the rest of the cell by the patch electrode (other non-Na$^+$ channels not shown). Na$^+$ current that enters the cell through these channels is recorded by an ultrasensitive current monitor connected to the patch electrode. **B.** Recordings of single Na$^+$ channels in cultured rat muscle cells. **1:** The time course of a 10-mV depolarizing voltage pulse applied across the patch of membrane. **2:** The computer-averaged sum of 300 trials of the inward current through the Na$^+$ channels in the patch (K$^+$ channels were blocked with tetraethylammonium and capacitive current was subtracted electronically). **3:** Nine individual trials from the set of 300, showing 6 individual Na$^+$ channel openings. These data demonstrate that the macroscopic Na$^+$ current recorded in a conventional voltage clamp record can be accounted for by the opening and closing of individual Na$^+$ channels. (From Sigworth and Neher, 1980.)

Erwin Neher and Bert Sakmann in Germany recently developed a technique called *patch clamping* for electrically isolating a tiny piece of membrane (a few µm² in area). The tip of a fire-polished glass micropipette filled with saline is brought up to the surface of an enzymatically cleaned cell membrane, and a small amount of suction is applied to the electrode. As the pipette contacts the membrane, a tight seal is formed between the membrane and the inside of the pipette. The seal has an extremely high electrical resistance. As a result, all the current produced by the opening of channels within the patch (usually about 1–3 channels/patch) flows into the pipette, where it is measured by an extremely sensitive current monitor (Figure 8–9A). This patch clamp method has made it possible to study the current flowing through individual ion channels.

These experiments have demonstrated that voltage-dependent channels generally have two conductance states, open and closed. Each channel opens in an all-or-none fashion and, when open, gives rise to a pulse of current with a variable duration but with a constant amplitude (Figure 8–9B). In the open state the conductance of a single Na^+ channel ranges from about 8 to 18 $\times$ 10^{-12} siemens, depending on the species. A single voltage-gated K^+ channel has a conductance of about 4 to 12 $\times$ 10^{-12} siemens.

Charge within the Membrane Is Rearranged When Voltage-Gated Na^+ Channels Open

In their classic series of papers on the squid axon, Hodgkin and Huxley suggested that the opening and closing of the Na^+ and K^+ channels is regulated by the movement or conformational change of a gating molecule. A gating molecule could respond to a change in membrane potential in one of three ways: (1) It could diffuse across the membrane. This would require the gating molecule to have a net charge. (2) It could rotate within the membrane. This would require the molecule to have a dipole moment (a net charge separation within the molecule) (Figure 8–10). (3) It could undergo an internal rearrangement of charge, resulting in a conformational change. Each of these three possible mechanisms requires that the gating molecule have a net charge or a dipole moment, and that in response to depolarization there be a movement within the membrane of the charged component of the gating molecule (Figure 8–10). The movement of the gating charge would, in turn, cause a small displacement of positive charge from near the inner surface of the membrane capacitance to near the outer surface (Figure 8–10B). The displacement of charge is equivalent to a reduction in the total separation of charge across the membrane capacitance. To keep the potential constant in a voltage clamp experiment, a small extra component of outward capacitive current, called *gating current*, would therefore have to be generated by the voltage clamp to maintain the constancy of the net effective charge separation across the membrane.

For technical reasons, the gating current (I_g) predicted by Hodgkin and Huxley could not be explored until the early 1970s. When the membrane current was finally examined by means of very sensitive techniques, the predicted capacitive gating current was found to flow at the beginning and at the end of a depolarizing voltage clamp pulse that opens Na^+ channels (Figure 8–10).

Analysis of the gating current has provided two critical insights into the properties of the Na^+ channel: (1) *Gating is a multistep process.* Several steps of charge movement with different kinetics occur before the channel opens in response to depolarization. (2) *Activation and inactivation are coupled processes.* For short depolarizing pulses, net movement of negative gating charge toward the inside of the membrane at the beginning of the pulse is balanced by an equal outward movement of gating charge at the end of the pulse. If the pulse lasts long enough for significant Na^+ inactivation to occur, however, the movement of gating charge back across the membrane at the end of the pulse is delayed. The gating charge is temporarily "immobilized" near the inner surface of the membrane and becomes free to move back across the membrane only as the Na^+ channels recover from inactivation. Clay Armstrong and his colleagues at the University of Pennsylvania have interpreted this charge immobilization to mean that the activation gate cannot close as long as the channel is in the inactivated state.

The Na^+ Channel Selects for Na^+ on the Basis of Size, Charge, and Energy of Hydration

After the gates of the Na^+ channel have opened, how does this protein channel discriminate between Na^+ and other ions? Bertil Hille has examined the selectivity of the Na^+ channel by measuring its relative permeability to several different types of organic and inorganic cations that differ in size and in hydrogen-bonding characteristics. He found that the channel acts as if it contains a filter or recognition site that selects partly by acting as a molecular sieve, with a pore size of 0.3 $\times$ 0.5 nm (Figure 8–10). The relative ease with which ions with good hydrogen-bonding characteristics pass through the channel led Hille to suggest that part of the inner wall of the protein channel is made up of amino acids that are rich in oxygen atoms. Ann Woodhull also found that when the pH of the fluid surrounding the cell is lowered, the conductance of the open channel is reduced gradually, and this reduction exactly parallels the titration curve for the carboxylic groups of amino acids. On the basis of these results, Hille proposed the following mechanism by which the channel selects for Na^+ ions. There are negatively charged carboxylic acid groups located at the outer mouth of the pore that perform the first step in the selection process by attracting cations and repelling anions. Cations that are larger than 0.3 $\times$ 0.5 nm in diameter are too large to pass through the pore. Cations smaller than this critical size pass through the pore, but only after losing most of the waters of hydration they normally carry in free solution. The negative carboxylic acid group, as well as the oxygen atoms that line the pore, can substitute for these waters of hydration, but the degree of effectiveness of this substitution varies for different ions. The greater the effectiveness of this substitution for a given ion species, the more readily that ion permeates the Na^+ channel.

The Major Subunit of the Na^+ Channel Is a Large Glycoprotein

To understand fully the mechanism of the selectivity filter and the gating functions, it will be necessary to determine the chemical structure of the Na^+ channel. The

84

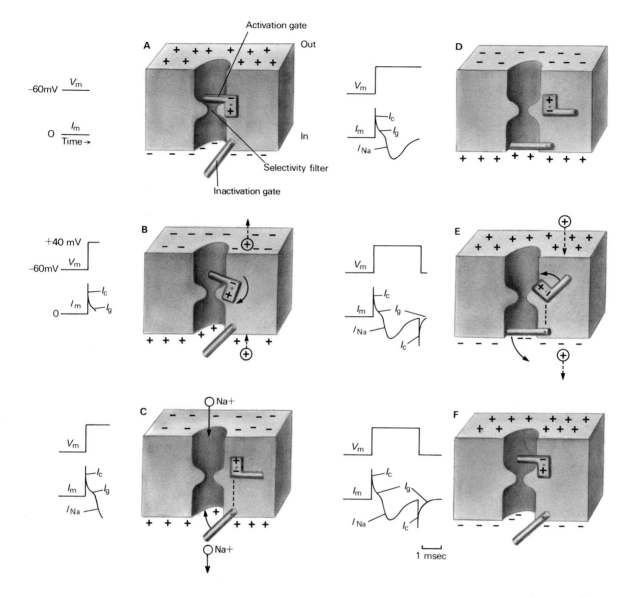

8–10 Schematic diagram of the changes in charge distribution of the Na$^+$ channel activation gate that give rise to gating current when the cell is voltage clamped. The voltage sensitivity of the activation gate may arise from (1) movement within the membrane of a molecule with a net charge, (2) a change in separation of charge within the gating molecule, or (3) as illustrated here, rotation of a gating molecule with a dipole moment in response to a change in membrane potential. **A.** The cell is in its resting state. The Na$^+$ activation gate is closed and the inactivation gate is open. **B.** The cell is stepped to a depolarized value by the voltage clamp. The standard passive capacitive current, I_c, flows only during the brief instant when V_m is changing. Once V_m has changed, the activation gates of the various channels begin to open, as the dipole moment of each gating molecule reorients itself with respect to the new electric field across the membrane. As the gate for each channel flips into the open configuration, a small outward capacitive current, the gating current (I_g), is generated by the clamp to keep the net charge separation across the membrane constant. The gates for different channels flip in a random fashion—most open right away, but some take a longer time. As a result, the capacitive

gating current is spread out in time, and does not occur instantaneously. **C.** By this time most of the Na$^+$ channels have opened, and the inward Na$^+$ current is maximal. **D.** As the depolarization is maintained, channels that have opened begin to close because the inactivation gates shut. Because no gating current is associated with the inactivation process, it is assumed that the voltage dependence of inactivation derives indirectly from some sort of coupling between the activation and inactivation processes (**dashed lines** in Parts **C** and **E** reflect this coupling). For example, the inactivation gate may have a tendency to close spontaneously, independent of voltage, but this tendency may be prevented when the activation gate is closed. **E.** Right after the membrane is repolarized, the activation gates of the Na$^+$ channels again reorient themselves, giving rise to an *inward* capacitive gating current. This "off" gating current is spread out over a longer time than the "on" gating current, perhaps because the activation gates cannot close until the inactivation gates have opened—a relatively slow process. This interpretation again is consistent with the hypothesis of coupling between the activation and inactivation processes. **F.** The channel has returned to its resting state.

first step in this direction, biochemical identification and purification of the Na$^+$ channel molecules, has been accomplished using the naturally occurring neurotoxins that bind specifically to the channel. William Catterall at the University of Washington has photoaffinity labeled the Na$^+$ channel from the rat brain by treating the rat brain membranes with a radioactively labeled azido nitrobenzoyl derivative of scorpion toxin. In the dark, this derivative binds reversibly to the same sites in the protein as does the toxin, but it can form a covalent bond with amino acid residues at the binding site when exposed to ultraviolet light. With this and related approaches, Catterall isolated three subunits that are thought to be present in the functional channel in equal proportions: one large glycoprotein with a molecular weight of 270,000 (α) and two smaller polypeptides with molecular weights of 39,000 (β_1) and 37,000 (β_2). Only the α and the β_1 subunits bind toxin; the β_2 subunit does not bind toxin but is linked to the α subunit by a disulfide bond.

Robert Barchi at the University of Pennsylvania has found that the Na$^+$ channel from muscle also has a large glycoprotein α subunit, but monoclonal antibodies raised against this subunit from muscle do not cross-react with brain Na$^+$-channel protein. It is therefore possible that Na$^+$ channels in excitable tissues other than neurons, although similar in function, may differ at the molecular level.

The electric organ of the electric eel has a Na$^+$ channel composed solely of the large α subunit. William Agnew and his associates at Yale University have been able to reconstitute the function of the purified Na$^+$ channel by inserting it into an artificial lipid bilayer. Using patch clamp techniques, they demonstrated that activity of the reconstituted channel matches that of the normal channel in the membrane. Carrying this molecular analysis a step forward, Shosaku Numa and his colleagues at Kyoto University in Japan have used gene-cloning techniques to determine the amino acid sequence for the Na$^+$ channel from electroplax. They isolated the gene from a cDNA library made by replicating the mRNA of electroplax cells. Individual cDNA molecules were then cloned and tested for their ability to code for proteins that react with antibodies to the Na$^+$ channel. (These antibodies were purified by Michael Raftery and his colleagues at the California Institute of Technology.) The nucleotide sequence of the specific cDNA clone that tested positive was then obtained by DNA sequencing techniques. Next, using the genetic code, the investigators inferred the corresponding amino acid sequences of the α subunit protein.

On the basis of the amino acid sequence, Numa and his colleagues have generated several hypotheses concerning the evolution and structure–function relationships of the Na$^+$ channel. For example, there are four similar sequences of about 150 amino acid residues each within the molecule. This homology led Numa and colleagues to suggest that the channel may have evolved from a single ancestral DNA segment that was duplicated within the gene three times. By looking at the way in which individual amino acids are distributed along the entire peptide of 1820 residues, they were also able to identify several candidate domains concerned with the various functional properties of the Na$^+$-channel molecule. In particular, several long hydrophobic stretches are postulated to pass through the membrane; other regions possess a high density of charged amino acids that could serve in the gating process, in cation selectivity, and in binding positively charged blocking drugs (tetrodotoxin). It will be possible to test these hypotheses in the future by altering the nucleotide sequence at specific sites within the clone, thereby changing one or more individual amino acids in the channel protein. With this procedure, called "site-directed mutagenesis," modified channels can be tested for functional changes: after synthesis, the modified protein can be inserted into artificial lipid bilayer membranes for voltage clamp analysis.

Membrane Channels Vary among Cell Types and among Different Regions of the Same Cell

Hodgkin and Huxley studied the axon of the squid. To what degree does their model for action potential generation apply to the other components of the cell—the cell body and the presynaptic terminals? Two general conclusions have emerged from studies designed to test the generality of the Hodgkin–Huxley model for the cell bodies of neurons. First, the cell body of almost every type of neuron examined has conductance channels similar to the Na$^+$ and K$^+$ channels in the squid axon described by Hodgkin and Huxley. Second, the cell bodies of most types of neurons have other kinds of channels as well. Many cell bodies have voltage-sensitive Ca^{++} channels and at least two additional species of K$^+$ channels. One type of K$^+$ channel, called the *Ca^{++}-activated K$^+$ channel*, is activated by depolarization, but only if the intracellular Ca^{++} concentration is greater than a certain threshold level. Another type of K$^+$ channel, the *early K$^+$ channel*, is activated about as rapidly as the Na$^+$ channel, and also inactivates rapidly with maintained depolarization. Thus, a single ion species such as K$^+$ can traverse the membrane through several distinct ion channels, each with its own characteristic time and voltage-dependent properties.

The pattern of voltage-sensitive channels found in a given neuron's cell body determines how that cell will respond to synaptic input. Some cells respond to a constant excitatory input with a decelerating train of action potentials. Others respond with an accelerating train. In some cells, small changes in the strength of synaptic inputs produce a large increase in firing rate, whereas in other cells the sensitivity of action potential frequency to input is relatively small. The marked diversity of input–output characteristics displayed by different neurons is explained by cell-to-cell variations in the combination of channel types that differ in ion selectivity, activation kinetics, and voltage sensitivity.

The properties of the presynaptic terminal have been less extensively studied, but it is clear that Ca^{++} channels are typically most dense at axon terminals, where Ca^{++} influx is involved in the release of transmitter. Thus, in addition to variations in channel distribution among cells, important differences also occur in the topographic distribution of channel types between the different regions of an individual neuron. These topographic variations of membrane conductance properties between different regions of a cell have important functional effects. For example, the membrane of the dendrites, cell body, and axon hillock has more types of conductance channels than does the axon membrane. Perhaps axons need not have as much channel complexity because they usually serve as simple relay lines between the input and output zones of a cell. The input and output zones, on the other hand, must transform the signals they receive. The input zone converts synaptic or sensory input into a temporally patterned spike train, whereas the output zone converts the spike train into a series of synaptic potentials.

An Overall View

The explanation of the mechanism for action potential generation developed by Hodgkin and Huxley is often referred to as the ionic hypothesis. According to this hypothesis, the action potential waveform is produced by ions moving passively across the membrane through voltage-gated channels. The ions can move only after the channels are opened. These fluxes change the charge distribution across the membrane capacitance. The influx of Na^+ discharges (and reverses) the resting charge distribution, after which K^+ efflux repolarizes the membrane capacitance and restores the original charge distribution.

Two major technical advances have provided an intellectually satisfying explanation of the biological functioning of voltage-gated channels. The original voltage clamp technique has been extended to patch clamp recording and gating current analysis. In addition, isolation of neurotoxins that bind selectively to different membrane channels has made it possible to estimate the density of Na^+ channels and to isolate the channel to explore its molecular structure. Studies using these two approaches are leading to an understanding of how the Na^+ channel functions on the molecular level. With more refined ultrastructural studies and recombinant DNA technology, it should be possible to gain a more complete picture of the structure of the Na^+ channel, how it is expressed, and how it functions.

Selected Readings

Armstrong, C. M. 1981. Sodium channels and gating currents. Physiol. Rev. 61:644–683.

Catterall, W. A. 1984. The molecular basis of neuronal excitability. Science 223:653–661.

Hille, B. 1984. Ionic Channels of Excitable Membranes. Sunderland, Mass.: Sinauer.

Hodgkin, A. L. 1964. The Conduction of the Nervous Impulse. Springfield, Ill.: Thomas.

Hodgkin, A. L. 1976. Chance and design in electrophysiology: An informal account of certain experiments on nerve carried out between 1934 and 1952. J. Physiol. (Lond.) 263:1–21.

Khodorov, B. I., 1974. The Problem of Excitability. New York: Plenum Press, chaps. 3–9.

Koester, J., and Byrne, J. H. (eds.). 1980. Molluscan Nerve Cells: From Biophysics to Behavior. Cold Spring Harbor, N.Y.: Cold Spring Harbor Laboratory.

Llinás, R. R. 1984. Comparative electrobiology of mammalian central neurons. In R. Dingledine (ed.), Brain Slices. New York: Plenum Press.

Noble, D. 1966. Applications of Hodgkin–Huxley equations to excitable tissues. Physiol. Rev. 46:1–50.

Ritchie, J. M., and Rogart, R. B. 1977. The binding of saxitoxin and tetrodotoxin to excitable tissue. Rev. Physiol. Biochem. Pharmacol. 79:1–50.

Sakmann, B., and Neher, E. (eds.). 1983. Single-Channel Recording. New York: Plenum Press.

Schuetze, S. M. 1983. The discovery of the action potential. Trends Neurosci. 6:164–168.

References

Cole, K. S., and Curtis, H. J. 1939. Electric impedance of the squid giant axon during activity. J. Gen. Physiol. 22:649–670.

Hodgkin, A. L., and Huxley, A. F. 1952. A quantitative description of membrane current and its application to conduction and excitation in nerve. J. Physiol. (Lond.) 117:500–544.

Hodgkin, A. L., and Katz, B. 1949. The effect of sodium ions on the electrical activity of the giant axon of the squid. J. Physiol. (Lond.) 108:37–77.

Noda, M., Shimizu, S., Tanabe, T., Takai, T., Kayano, T., Ikeda, T., Takahashi, H., Nakayama, H., Kanaoka, Y., Minamino, N., Kangawa, K., Matsuo, H., Raftery, M., Hirose, T., Inayama, S., Hayashida, H., Miyata, T., and Numa, S. 1984. Primary structure of *Electrophorus electricus* sodium channel deduced from cDNA sequence. Nature 312:121–127.

Rosenberg, R. L., Tomiko, S. A., and Agnew, W. S. 1984. Single-channel properties of the reconstituted voltage-regulated Na channel isolated from the electroplax of *Electrophorus electricus*. Proc. Natl. Acad. Sci. U.S.A. 81:5594–5598.

Sigworth, F. J., and Neher, E. 1980. Single Na^+ channel currents observed in cultured rat muscle cells. Nature 287:447–449.

Elementary Interactions between Neurons: Synaptic Transmission

III

In the last two sections, we considered nerve cells as the elementary signaling units of the nervous system. Communication between nerve cells and their targets takes place at synapses, and in this part of the book we shall focus on synapses and synaptic transmission. The brain functions by connecting individual neuronal units in highly specific ways based on their structure, biochemistry, and electrical properties. One of the key ideas that we wish to convey in this book is how this wiring gives rise to perception, motor action, behavior, and learning.

An average neuron forms about 1000 synaptic connections and receives even more. Since the human brain contains at least 10^{12} neurons, it can be estimated that 10^{15} synaptic connections are formed in the brain. Thus, there are more synapses in the human brain than there are stars in the galaxy! Fortunately, only a small number of mechanisms are responsible for producing synaptic transmission at all of these many connections.

In addition to low molecular-weight molecules, a great variety of peptides can serve as messengers at synapses. Fortunately, in the last several years, recombinant DNA techniques have helped to elucidate the structure of these peptides and to analyze how they are synthesized and processed in the presynaptic cell. The methods of molecular biology are also being used to characterize receptor molecules in postsynaptic target cells that bind and respond to the chemical messengers.

In the first seven chapters we shall consider synaptic transmission at its most elementary level, the contacts made first by one, and then by a few presynaptic neurons on a single postsynaptic cell. We shall begin by examining the physiology of synaptic function by analyzing the postsynaptic and presynaptic contributions to synaptic transmission. We shall next discuss the fine structure of synapses and then analyze the molecular machinery of synaptic actions. This background will permit us then to consider how injury and disease disrupt function by interfering with one or another component of the synapse.

Serious injury to nerve cells often leads to their death, and therefore to a reduction in the total number of nerve cells. Although most neurons do not multiply, after certain kinds of injury neurons can sometimes regenerate parts of their axons. We shall consider two aspects of the relationship between function and injury or disease. On the cell-biological level, we shall consider some of the morphological and functional consequences of injury to individual nerve cells. On the clinical level, we shall consider the role of nerve cell injury in the diagnosis of neurological disease. The diagnosis of a neurological disease usually involves two steps. First, the anatomical site of the lesion in the nervous system is determined, and second, the cause of the lesion is inferred. In this part of the text we shall be concerned primarily with the first step. Because neurons are specifically connected with other cells and mediate specific functions, lesions of a neuron produce characteristic deficits in functions. Through clinical examination, it is therefore often possible to infer the precise site of the lesion within the nervous system.

Eric R. Kandel and Steven Siegelbaum

Principles Underlying Electrical and Chemical Synaptic Transmission

9

Nerve cells differ from other cells in the body in their ability to communicate rapidly with one another, sometimes over great distances and with great precision. Axonal conduction and synaptic transmission provide the means for this rapid and precise communication. Synaptic transmission is therefore central for understanding how the nervous system works, and by extension for understanding behavior: how we perceive, move, feel, learn, and remember. Consequently, we are fortunate that aspects of synaptic transmission have now been analyzed in molecular detail.

In this chapter, we shall begin to examine synaptic transmission by considering the two major classes of synapses in the nervous system—electrical and chemical—and how their function derives from their ultrastructure. We shall then focus on the chemical excitation at the nerve–muscle synapse and use it as a model for examining the gating of transmitter-sensitive channels by a specific transmitter molecule, acetylcholine. In later chapters, we shall examine the crucial role of synaptic transmission in behavior and its abnormalities.

Synaptic Transmission Can Be Electrical or Chemical

Charles Sherrington introduced the term *synapse* (Greek *synapsis*, junction) at the turn of the century to refer to the specialized contact zone, described histologically by Ramón y Cajal, where one neuron communicates with another. In the 1930s a great debate ensued between the physiologists (led by John C. Eccles) and the pharmacologists (led by Henry Dale) about the mechanism of synaptic

A

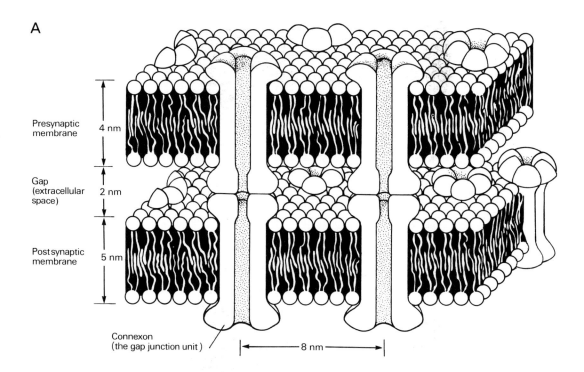

Presynaptic membrane   4 nm

Gap (extracellular space)   2 nm

Postsynaptic membrane   5 nm

Connexon (the gap junction unit)   ⟵ 8 nm ⟶

9–1 The gap junction at an electrical synapse is spanned by channels called connexons, which bridge the cytoplasm of two neighboring cells. **A.** Three-dimensional model of the connexon as revealed by X-ray diffraction studies. (Adapted from Makowski et al., 1977). **B.** Freeze-fracture of gap junctions at an electrical synapse between a presynaptic terminal and the cell body of a class of motor neuron in fish (× 20,000). Freeze-fracture cleaves the plasma membrane through its hydrophobic interior, thus exposing two complementary faces (face refers to the internal aspect of one membrane, which is revealed when it is split). The inner half of the membrane (that closest to the cytoplasm) is the protoplasmic or P leaflet and the outer membrane half adjacent to the extracellular space is referred to as the extracellular or E leaflet. The fractured and replicated surfaces of these leaflets have two distinct appearances and are called the P and E faces. The outwardly directed inner half-membrane or P face (**PF**) contains numerous, randomly distributed globular particles. The inwardly directed outer half membrane or E face (**EF**) is relatively smooth, containing many fewer particles than the P face. In the synapse illustrated here the E face of the membrane of the cell body is primarily seen. Two small *gap junctions* (**GJ**) are seen to the left, and a large junction occupies much of the central region. Each gap junction shows

transmission. Both sides assumed that synaptic transmission operates by a single, universal mechanism. The physiologists argued that synaptic transmission is electrical—that it is due to current flow from the presynaptic neuron spreading directly to the postsynaptic cell. The pharmacologists argued that it is chemical—that it is due to a chemical mediator (a transmitter substance) released by the presynaptic neuron that initiates current flow in the postsynaptic cell.

When physiological techniques improved in the 1950s and 1960s, it became clear that all synapses do not operate with one mechanism. The work of Paul Fatt and Bernard Katz, of Eccles and his colleagues, and of Edwin Furshpan and David Potter showed that both modes of transmission occur in the nervous system. Most synapses use a chemical transmitter. Some, however, operate by purely electrical means. Moreover, as it became technically possible to examine the fine structure of synapses, electron microscopists discovered that synaptic transmission does not occur at every point where neurons contact one another; rather, transmission occurs only at certain critical points in the nervous system where specialized areas of the presynaptic and the postsynaptic neurons are brought into appropriate apposition. On the basis of the morphology of the zone of apposition, it is possible to divide all synapses into two major morphological classes: those with bridges interconnecting the cytoplasms of the pre- and postsynaptic cells; and those in which the cyto-

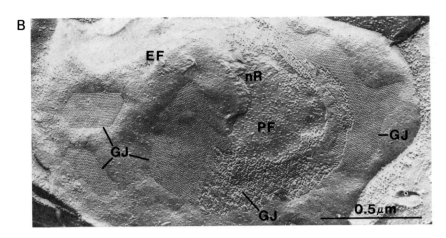

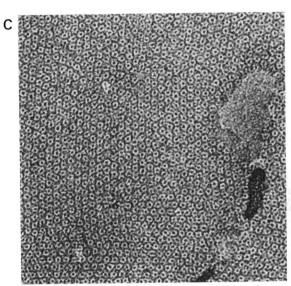

a highly ordered arrangement of pits. The P face of the axonal membrane (**nR**) is exposed near the center. It displays the particulate face of the large gap junction. (Adapted from Bennett, Sandri, and Akert, 1978.) For details on freeze-fracture, see Figure 12–3. **C.** Gap junctions isolated from rat liver that have been negatively stained (× 307,800). This technique creates a reversal or negative image of the macromolecules and reveals a regular hexagonal lattice of particles. This lattice has a periodicity of approximately 10 nm, which corresponds to the lattice observed in thin sections. Each particle is a connexon. The darkly staining central pore in each connexon represents the channel of the junction and is about 2 nm in diameter. (Courtesy of N. Gilula.)

plasms are not bridged and the neurons are separated by a cleft. These two morphological classes correspond to, and account for, the two functional classes: the electrical and the chemical synapses.

The *bridged junctions* are *gap junctions* similar to those found in many other cells in the body. At these junctions the zone of apposition is bridged by channels that run from the cytoplasm of the presynaptic neuron to that of the postsynaptic cell. These junctions mediate electrical transmission. At electrical synapses the normal extracellular space separating the pre- and postsynaptic cells is narrowed (Figure 9–1A). Between the bridges, the outer limits of the junctional plasma membranes (when cut perpendicularly), are separated by a gap of only 2 nm

(20 Å). This is about one-tenth the size of the separation between the membranes at regions where gap junctions are not present. Freeze-fracture studies show clusters of membrane particles that span the gap (Figure 9–1B). Ions and small molecules (with molecular weights up to 1000 or a diameter of up to 1.5 nm)—for example, cyclic adenosine 3′,5′-monophosphate (cyclic AMP), sucrose, or small peptides—can pass from one cell to another through the junction. Thus, the spanning structures are thought to be walls of intercellular channels that bridge two cells and allow for metabolic and electrical communication yet impose an upper limit on the size of molecules that can get through.

Because gap junctions can be isolated from homoge-

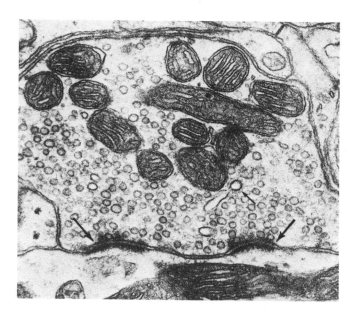

9–2 At the chemical synapse the synaptic cleft separating the presynaptic from the postsynaptic membrane is unbridged. The presynaptic terminal occupies most of this electron micrograph. The large dark structures are mitochondria. These subcellular organelles provide energy for synaptic transmission and, together with the endoplasmic reticulum, are thought to buffer the level of free Ca^{++} in the presynaptic terminal. The many round bodies are vesicles that contain the transmitter acetylcholine. The fuzzy dark thickenings (**large arrows**) along the presynaptic side of the cleft are active zones—specializations that are thought to serve as docking sites for vesicles before they release their transmitter by exocytosis. Active zones are discussed in Chapter 12. **Small arrow** points to cisternal element. (Courtesy of J. E. Heuser and T. S. Reese.)

nized nervous tissue (or from liver, where they can be obtained in even greater abundance), it is possible to characterize them. Their spanning structures are made up of six protein subunits, hexagonally arranged into assemblies called *connexons* (Figure 9–1A and C). At the cell junction, each of the two cells contributes one connexon to each bridge, and the connexons join in register to form a channel that connects the interiors of the two cells. Each of the six subunits of the connexon is composed of a protein called *connexin* with a molecular weight of approximately 25,000. Although gap junctions electrically couple adjoining cells, they do not occlude the extracellular space completely, as do tight junctions, nor do they provide adhesive coupling, as do desmosomes (similar structures in other types of cells).

In the *unbridged junction*, or chemical synapse, the pre- and postsynaptic neurons are not contiguous (Figure 9–2). There is a discrete separation, the synaptic cleft, between the presynaptic and postsynaptic elements. This separation (30–50 nm) is typically slightly wider than the adjacent extracellular space (20 nm). In addition, the pre- and postsynaptic membranes are often morphologically specialized, and the presynaptic terminals contain localized collections of vesicles (called *synaptic vesicles*).

The main functional properties of the two types of synapse are summarized in Table 9–1. Many of these differences can be illustrated by injecting the presynaptic cell with current. This current will flow outward across its membrane as shown in Figure 9–3. The current deposits positive charge on the inside of the membrane of the presynaptic cell, reducing the negative charge present on the capacitance at rest and thereby depolarizing the cell. The current flows out across the nongated conduct-

Table 9–1. Main Functional Properties of Electrical and Chemical Synapses

Electrical synapses	Chemical synapses
1. Reduced extracellular space (2 nm); cytoplasmic continuity between pre- and postsynaptic cell	1. Increased extracellular space (typically 30–50 nm); no cytoplasmic continuity between pre- and postsynaptic elements
2. Mediating agent is ionic current	2. Mediating agent is a chemical messenger (acetylcholine, norepinephrine, peptides, etc.)
3. Little synaptic delay; transmission is limited only by the speed of electrotonic transmission across the short distance separating the presynaptic and postsynaptic elements at the synapse	3. Significant synaptic delay (at least 0.3 msec, sometimes 1 to 5 msec, or even longer). Part of the delay is caused by the time required for the opening of the Ca^{++} channels and the secretory process in the presynaptic terminals. Another, small component of the delay is the time required for the transmitter to diffuse across the synaptic cleft, bind to its receptors, and initiate a synaptic potential. In some cells, further time is required for an intracellular second messenger to activate the ion channels.
4. Typically bidirectional	4. Unidirectional

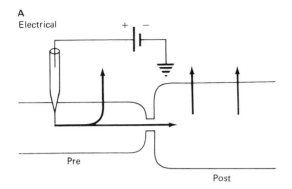

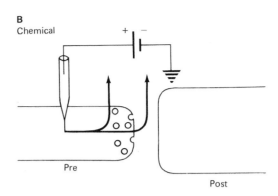

ance channels of the membrane as well. At an electrical synapse, some current also flows into the low-resistance, high-conductance channels that bridge the pre- and postsynaptic cells. The current then deposits positive charge on the inside of the membrane capacitance of the postsynaptic cell, depolarizing it, and finally flows out across the nongated conductance channels of the postsynaptic cell (Figure 9–3A). At a chemical synapse, too, the outward current injected into a presynaptic cell flows out across the presynaptic membrane. However, because current seeks the path of lowest resistance (highest conductance), it follows the low-resistance pathway offered by the extracellular fluid of the synaptic cleft. Little or no current crosses the high resistance of the external membrane of the postsynaptic cell (Figure 9–3B).

In some ways, the presynaptic terminals of chemical synapses resemble endocrine glands, and chemical transmission resembles, to a certain degree, the action of hormones. Both endocrine glands and synaptic terminals release a chemical mediating agent. The main difference between the two is the distance over which they operate. The apposition of the postsynaptic receptive membrane to the presynaptic releasing site at most chemical synapses has two advantages over endocrine signaling: it increases both the speed of action and the selectivity of the action with respect to its target. As we shall see in Chapter 12, at certain chemical synapses (nondirected synapses) the presynaptic neuron is farther away from the postsynaptic cell, and here the distinction between synaptic transmission and hormonal transmission becomes blurred. In addition, the same chemical agent can serve as a transmitter at one locus by acting directly on neighboring cells, and can be a modulator at another locus, where it produces a more diffuse action. At a third locus, it can be released into the blood stream to act as a hormone.

Transmission across electrical synapses is very rapid. In addition, electrical synapses can cause a group of interconnected neurons to fire synchronously. These synapses are usually rather limited in function, however, and not very sensitive to the activity that has occurred beforehand. Consequently, they are thought to be used for

9–3 Outward current is injected into a presynaptic cell to illustrate the difference between electrical and chemical synapses. **A.** In electrical synapses, some of the injected current flows through the channels of the gap junction, which bridges the cytoplasms of the two cells, and depolarizes the postsynaptic cell. **B.** In chemical synapses, little or none of the injected current crosses the membrane of the postsynaptic cell. Two vesicles (**semicircles**) are illustrated as having fused with the membrane and are in the process of releasing their transmitter by exocytosis (see Chapter 12).

interconnecting nerve cells that are responsible for stereotypic behavior, such as the rapid saccadic eye movements produced by the extraocular motor neurons in certain species of fish, or the release of defensive secretions by certain invertebrate animals. Chemical synapses (which are also much more numerous) are slower, but they are much more flexible, or plastic, and often reflect the history of their previous activity (as we shall see later in Chapters 11 and 62). Chemical synapses interconnect neurons for more variable and complex behavior. These distinctions are thought to be important and may account for the preponderance of chemical or electrical synapses in various regions of the brain.

In the remainder of this chapter, we shall consider chemical transmission. From a physiological point of view, chemical transmission can be divided mechanistically into two sets of processes. The *presynaptic transmitting processes* determine the release of the chemical messenger. The *postsynaptic receptive processes* determine the interaction between the transmitter and the receptor molecule in the postsynaptic cell. This interaction leads in turn to the gating of specific ion channels and gives rise to current flow that produces the various synaptic potentials.

We shall focus here on postsynaptic receptive processes. In Chapter 11, we shall consider the presynaptic mechanisms responsible for transmitter release. The best understood postsynaptic mechanism is that which mediates excitation at the synapses of the motor neuron to skeletal muscle. We shall therefore use this peripheral synapse to begin our consideration of how transmitters

9–4 The terminals of a motor neuron form synapses on a skeletal muscle fiber at the end-plate, a specialized region that contains a high density of ACh receptors. The presynaptic terminals consist of a collection of varicosities called synaptic boutons. Each bouton contains release zones, synaptic vesicles, and mitochondria. On their outside surface, synaptic boutons are covered by a thin layer of Schwann cells. The boutons are always separated from the postsynaptic cell by a cleft—the synaptic cleft—which is about 50 nm wide. Each skeletal muscle fiber is usually innervated by only one motor neuron, but each motor neuron may innervate between 1 and 1000 different muscle fibers. The bottom sketch shows the neuromuscular junction in detail. (Adapted in part from McMahan and Kuffler, 1971.)

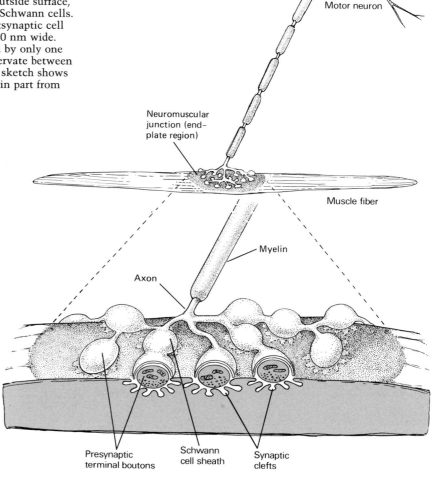

Motor neuron

Neuromuscular junction (end-plate region)

Muscle fiber

Myelin

Axon

Presynaptic terminal boutons

Schwann cell sheath

Synaptic clefts

exert their synaptic actions. In the next chapter we shall extend this treatment to transmitter actions on central nerve cells.

Synaptic Excitation of Skeletal Muscle by Motor Neurons Is Chemical and Is Now Understood in Molecular Terms

The synapse of the motor neuron on skeletal muscle provides a particularly convenient preparation for studying the synaptic actions of neurotransmitters. Because muscle cells are large, they can accommodate several micro-electrodes for electrophysiological measurements. With interference microscopy, one can visualize the region of nerve–muscle contact and precisely locate the postsynaptic membrane. Moreover, a single muscle fiber usually is innervated by only one motor axon, and the transmitter is known. These technical advantages have made the study of this synapse particularly fruitful.

Motor neurons use acetylcholine (ACh) as their transmitter. Receptors to ACh are densely inserted into a specialized region of the muscle membrane called the *end-plate*, where the terminal arborization of the motor neuron's presynaptic axon innervates the muscle (Figure

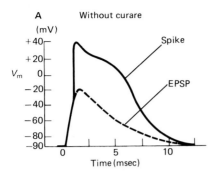

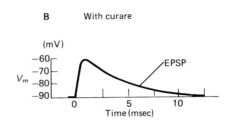

9–5 The excitatory postsynaptic potential (EPSP) produced by ACh in a skeletal muscle fiber can be reduced in amplitude by the competitive inhibitor curare. The values for the resting potential, synaptic potential, and action potential shown in these intracellular recordings are typical of vertebrate skeletal muscle. **A.** Under normal circumstances, stimulation of the motor axon produces in the muscle fiber a large excitatory synaptic potential that surpasses threshold and triggers an action potential. **B.** In the presence of curare, the synaptic potential is reduced below threshold and does not trigger an action potential. As a result, the reduced synaptic potential can be studied in isolation from action potentials.

9–4). Stimulation of the motor axon leads to the release of ACh, which then interacts with the ACh receptors in the muscle membrane to produce an excitatory synaptic action called the *end-plate potential.*

The nerve–muscle synapse is unusual. Many synaptic potentials produced by a single presynaptic neuron are small, less than 1 mV in amplitude. As a result, the postsynaptic cells are excited only when the connections of several (often many) presynaptic neurons summate to discharge the cell. At the nerve–muscle synapse, however, the synaptic potential produced by the single motor cell that innervates the fiber is very large, about 60 mV, and under normal circumstances this synaptic potential is suprathreshold and invariably triggers an action potential. Nonetheless, as we shall see in the following chapter, this synaptic potential has properties similar to those of the much smaller synaptic potentials produced on central neurons, such as those produced on the motor neuron itself by the afferent fibers from stretch receptor sensory neurons.

The synaptic (end-plate) potential at the nerve–muscle synapse was first studied with intracellular microelectrodes by Paul Fatt and Bernard Katz at University College London. To separate the synaptic action from the propagated action potential, Fatt and Katz reduced the amplitude of the synaptic potential below threshold for the action potential by exposing the muscle to curare (Figure 9–5). (Curare is a drug extracted from plants and used by South American Indians as an arrowhead poison to paralyze their quarry.) Curare reduces the sensitivity of the ACh receptors by blocking the binding of ACh to the receptor. Using curare, Fatt and Katz found that the synaptic potential produced in muscle cells by the action of the motor neuron is generated at a specific point on the muscle fiber membrane, the end-plate region. As they moved an intracellular recording electrode down the

muscle fiber, away from the end-plate region, the amplitude of the synaptic potential decreased progressively (Figure 9–6). From this analysis, Fatt and Katz concluded that the synaptic potential is due to the localized flow of a net inward synaptic current in the region of the endplate. As the synaptic potential propagates passively away from the end-plate down the muscle fiber, its amplitude is diminished because of the leakiness of the resting membrane of the muscle (see Chapter 6).

The rapid rise of the end-plate potential reflects the rapid rise in the concentration of ACh at the end-plate. The rise occurs after the transmitter is released from the presynaptic nerve terminal into the synaptic cleft and diffuses to the end-plate. Once ACh is released, however, its concentration in the synaptic cleft is not maintained but decays quickly to zero. The ACh is removed rapidly from the cleft by two processes: (1) it is hydrolyzed by the enzyme *acetylcholinesterase* localized in the basal lamina (a mesh of fibrillar proteins) that lies on the surface of the muscle at the site of the synapse (see Chapter 15); and (2) it diffuses rapidly out of the synaptic cleft. The ACh concentration diminishes so rapidly that it normally does not determine the time course of decay of the synaptic current; rather, the time course of the synaptic potential reflects both the properties of the ion channels activated by ACh and the time constant of the membrane (Figure 9–7).

The Excitatory Synaptic Potential at the End-Plate Involves the Simultaneous Movement of Na$^+$ and K$^+$

Because the end-plate potential causes a depolarization, it must result from a net inward movement of positive charge. Akira and Norika Takeuchi at the University of Kyoto first used the voltage clamp technique to study di-

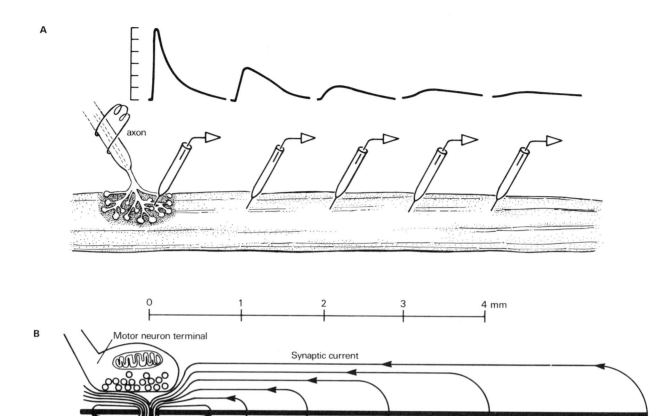

9–6 The synaptic potential is largest at its site of origin at the end-plate region and propagates from there passively. **A.** Recording from the end-plate and along the muscle fiber at various distances away from the end-plate shows that the peak amplitude of the synaptic potential decays **(top traces)** with distance away from the end-plate region. **B.** The decay illustrated in **A** results from the leakiness of the muscle fiber membrane. The inward synaptic current at the end-plate region gives rise to a return flow of outward current that leaks out across the membrane through nongated channels all along the length of the muscle membrane. (Adapted from Miles, 1969.)

rectly the time course and properties of the inward end-plate current that generates the end-plate potential.

As Figure 9–7 shows, Takeuchi and Takeuchi found that the time course of the end-plate current is faster than the resultant end-plate potential change: the end-plate current rises to its peak value more rapidly and then decays to the baseline more quickly. This is because the time course of the end-plate potential is partially determined by the passive properties of the muscle. As we saw in Chapter 7 (Figure 7–3), it takes some time both to charge and to discharge the muscle membrane capacitance.

Which ions move to produce this synaptic action? An important clue to the ions involved can be obtained by systematically changing the membrane potential and determining the reversal potential for the synaptic potential. The *reversal potential* is the potential at which the synaptic potential has zero amplitude. Does the reversal potential of the end-plate potential coincide with the

equilibrium potential for a specific ion species, such as -90 mV for K^+ or $+55$ mV for Na^+?

At the normal resting potential of the muscle, the end-plate current is inward throughout its entire course (Figure 9–7). What happens to the end-plate current at different levels of membrane potential? Just as Ohm's law was used in Chapter 8 to predict how the ionic currents flowing through voltage-gated channels vary as a function of membrane potential, it can now be used to describe the change in current flowing through transmitter-gated channels. According to Ohm's law, the current responsible for the end-plate potential, or excitatory postsynaptic potential (I_{EPSP}), is given by:

$$I_{EPSP} = g_{EPSP} \times (V_m - E_{EPSP}).$$

Here g_{EPSP} represents the conductance of the channels activated by ACh (the synaptic conductance), and the term $V_m - E_{EPSP}$ represents the electrochemical driving force

9–7 The time course of the excitatory synaptic (end-plate) *potential*, recorded with an intracellular voltage electrode, is considerably slower than the underlying inward synaptic (end-plate) *current*, recorded under voltage clamp using two intracellular electrodes, one for recording voltage and one for passing current. The synaptic potential changes slowly because synaptic current must first flow to alter the charge on the capacitance of the muscle membrane. Only when this has occurred can the potential change (see Chapter 6).

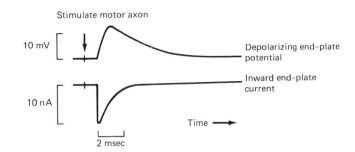

9–8 The reversal potential for the end-plate current demonstrates that *both* Na$^+$ and K$^+$ are flowing through the channels activated by ACh. **A.** Idealized traces drawn as though the end-plate current were due only to Na$^+$ moving through the Na$^+$ channels, much like the ascending limb of the action potential. Under those circumstances, the reversal potential of the end-plate current would occur at +55 mV, the equilibrium potential for Na$^+$ (E_{Na}). **B.** Actual traces showing that the end-plate current reverses not at +55 mV but at 0 mV because the channel is not specific for Na$^+$ but is permeable to both Na$^+$ and K$^+$.

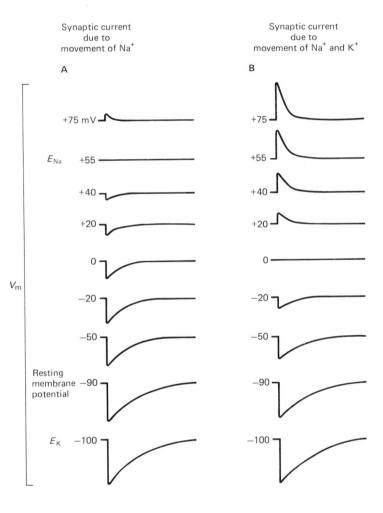

for ionic flow through the channel (where V_m is the membrane potential and E_{EPSP} is the equilibrium potential for the excitatory postsynaptic potential).

If an influx of Na$^+$ were responsible for the end-plate potential, then E_{EPSP} would be +55 mV (the equilibrium potential for Na$^+$). One would therefore predict that as the membrane potential is changed experimentally from −90 mV to +55 mV, the end-plate current would become progressively smaller because of the reduction in the electrochemical driving force on Na$^+$ (the term V_m − E_{EPSP}). At +55 mV, the inward current flow would be abolished, and at potentials more positive than +55 mV,

the end-plate current would reverse in direction and become outward (Figure 9–8A). However, this is not what investigators found! Rather, as the membrane potential was reduced, the end-plate current rapidly became smaller and was abolished at 0 mV instead of at +55 mV (Figure 9–8B). As the membrane potential was made more positive than 0 mV, the end-plate current reversed direction and became outward.

These experiments defined an unexpected reversal potential! Which ion species is in equilibrium at 0 mV? None of the major cations or anions has its equilibrium potential at this peculiar value of membrane potential.

Fatt and Katz, who first determined the reversal potential for the end-plate potential, immediately appreciated that this potential must represent a reversal potential produced by more than one type of ion. Later, Takeuchi and Takeuchi found that during the end-plate potential Na⁺ flows into the cell and K⁺ flows outward. The combined influence of these ions explains why the reversal potential is 0.

There Are Fundamental Differences between Chemically Gated and Voltage-Gated Channels

From this analysis, it would appear at first that the mechanism for generating synaptic excitation at the nerve–muscle synapse is similar to that for generating the action potential in the axon. In both the synapse and the axon, Na^+ and K^+ move down their concentration gradients through channels formed by transmembrane proteins. However, synaptic excitation differs in two important ways from the generation of an action potential, and these differences are presumed to result from differences in the structure of the respective ion channel proteins and in the mechanisms by which the channels are gated.

One difference is that the movement of Na^+ and K^+ during the action potential is sequential, whereas during the synaptic potential it is simultaneous. That the ACh-activated channel permits simultaneous movement of Na^+ into and K^+ out of the muscle seems at first somewhat unexpected. Only the increase in Na^+ influx leads to excitation (depolarization). The increase in K^+ efflux actually dampens this excitatory action. The differences in ion movement during the action and synaptic potentials are explained by differences in the molecular properties of the ion channels responsible for these two signals. During the action potential, membrane depolarization leads to the opening of two independent channels—first, one selective for Na^+, and then another selective for K^+. To produce the synaptic potential, however, the transmitter opens a special channel whose size and shape allow both Na^+ and K^+ to pass with nearly equal permeability. Indeed, the channel is so large that it allows larger cations,

such as Ca^{++}, NH_4^+, and even certain organic cations, to pass. Anions such as Cl^- are excluded, however. This cation selectivity suggests that the channel has a negative charge at its mouth that attracts a variety of cations below a certain size and repels anions because of their charge. Bertil Hille and his co-workers at the University of Washington have estimated that the channel activated by ACh is substantially larger in diameter than the Na^+ or K^+ channel. At its narrowest point in cross section, the dimensions of the channel pore are approximately 0.65 nm × 0.65 nm (0.65 nm = 6.5 Å). In contrast, the Na^+ channel is 0.31 nm × 0.51 nm and the K^+ channel is only 0.33 nm × 0.33 nm (Figure 9–9).

A second difference between synaptic potentials and action potentials is that the increase in Na^+ influx produced by the action potential is regenerative, whereas that produced by the synaptic potential is not. The Na^+ and K^+ channels responsible for the action potential are voltage-sensitive; they are opened by depolarization and closed by hyperpolarization. The opening of the channel responsible for the excitatory synaptic action is not controlled by voltage but depends on the concentration of a specific chemical transmitter—ACh. As a result, the depolarization produced by the transmitter does not lead to further increases in the number of channels that are open (and therefore does not increase the total *synaptic conductance*, g_{EPSP}). This observation explains why synaptic potentials tend to be relatively small and additive compared with the large all-or-none amplitude (+110 mV) of the action potential.

As might be expected from these two differences in molecular properties, the channels opened by the transmitter differ pharmacologically from those opened by the action potential. The influx of Na^+ produced by excitatory transmission is not blocked by tetrodotoxin, the drug that blocks the voltage-gated Na^+ channel activated by the action potential. Similarly, α-bungarotoxin, a protein that blocks the action of ACh, does not interfere with voltage-gated Na^+ or K^+ channels.

The difference between chemically gated and voltage-gated channels is summarized in Figure 9–10, and the interaction between them in the membrane of the postsyn-

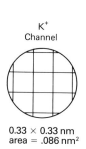

K⁺
Channel

0.33 × 0.33 nm
area = .086 nm²

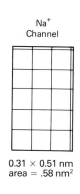

Na⁺
Channel

0.31 × 0.51 nm
area = .58 nm²

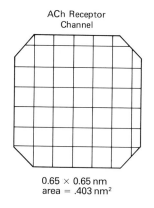

ACh Receptor
Channel

0.65 × 0.65 nm
area = .403 nm²

9–9 A comparison of the dimensions of ionic selectivity filters for the K⁺, Na⁺, and ACh receptor channels. This sketch illustrates the minimum size of the pore that will pass the known permeant ions for these three channels in the nerve and muscle of the frog. Grid marks in 0.1-nm (1-Å) steps. Sizes were evaluated from space-filling models of the permeant and impermeant ions. (From Hille, 1984.)

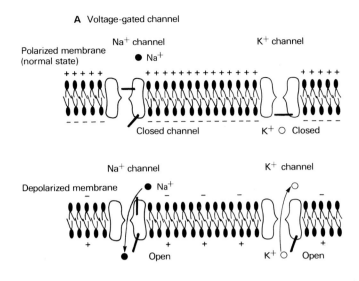

A Voltage-gated channel

B Transmitter-gated channel   **C** Concentration gradients

9–10 Voltage-gated and transmitter-gated channels operate by different mechanisms. **A.** Channels that contribute to the action potential are voltage-gated and selective for different cations. A separate channel exists for Na$^+$ (**filled circle**) and for K$^+$ (**open circle**). **B.** In contrast, the transmitter-gated channels activated by excitatory transmitters (such as ACh in skeletal muscle) are not gated by voltage and are permeable to *both* Na$^+$ and K$^+$. **C.** The ionic concentration gradients for the ions are the same for both classes of channels. (Adapted from Alberts et al., 1983.)

aptic cell is shown in Figure 9–11. The opening of the transmitter-gated channel by ACh depolarizes the muscle membrane. This depolarization activates the voltage-gated Na$^+$ channel, which in turn triggers an action potential in the muscle fibers.

Studies of Single Chemically Gated Channels Reveal Information about Conformational Changes and the Molecular Mechanisms of Transmitter Action

The ACh-activated channel is a large integral membrane protein made up of several subunits that span the membrane. As we saw in the previous chapter, Erwin Neher and Bert Sakmann have recently developed the *patch clamp* technique. This can be used to record the very small ionic currents that flow in the muscle membrane during the opening of a single ACh-gated channel. Each patch of membrane beneath the electrode is about 5 to 10 μm^2 in area. Under optimal circumstances—best found slightly away from the center of the synaptic region at the end-plate—a patch contains only a single active channel, a single protein molecule (Figure 9–12)!

Chemically Gated Channels Open in an All-or-None Fashion

Neher, Sakmann, and their colleagues found that the ACh channel opens in an all-or-none fashion giving rise to square pulses of inward current at the resting level of membrane potential. In the absence of ACh, the channels are always closed. In the presence of ACh, the channels open randomly with a mean open time of about 1 msec. When open, each channel has the same elementary conductance, about 30×10^{-12} siemens (30 pS) at the frog end-plate. At a resting potential of -90 mV, each channel contributes a rectangular current pulse of about 2 pA. During the period a single channel is open, roughly 20,000 Na$^+$ ions flow into the cell and a somewhat smaller number of K$^+$ ions flow out.

Changing the membrane potential of the patch changes the magnitude of current flow through the channel. This happens because changes in driving force ($V_m - E_{EPSP}$) have the identical effect on single channels that they have on the total current at the end-plate (Figure 9–13). Thus, whereas Ohm's law for synaptic current is

$$I_{EPSP} = g_{EPSP} \times (V_m - E_{EPSP}),$$

the equivalent expression for current flow through a single channel is simply:

$$i_{EPSP} = \gamma \times (V_m - E_{EPSP}),$$

where i_{EPSP} is the amplitude of current flow through a single open channel and γ is the single-channel conductance (which for the ACh channel is 30 pS).

Current Flow Depends on the Number of Open Channels and Transmitter Concentration

The total macroscopic synaptic conductance, g_{EPSP}, of a large population of ACh channels simply results from the summed conductance contributions of the various individual channels. It is thus given by $g_{EPSP} = n \times \gamma$, where

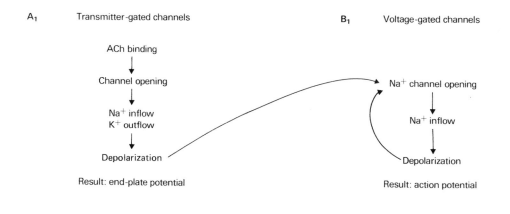

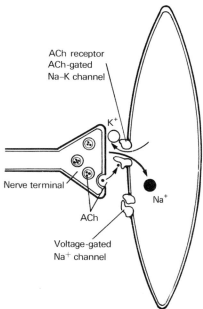

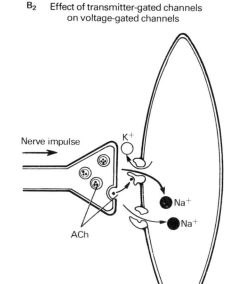

9–11 Transmitter-gated channels and voltage-gated channels interact so that the binding of ACh leads to the initiation of an action potential in the postsynaptic muscle fiber. **A₁ and B₁.** Flow chart of the steps leading from ACh binding to the initiation of the action potential in muscle showing some of the gated channels involved in the stimulation of muscle contraction by a nerve impulse. **A₂ and B₂.** Schematic diagram of the series of events illustrated in **A₁ and B₁.** (Adapted from Alberts et al., 1983.)

n is the number of open channels. The macroscopic end-plate current can therefore be written as

$$I_{EPSP} = n \times \gamma \times (V_m - E_{EPSP}).$$

This equation shows that the current for the end-plate potential is fundamentally determined by three factors: (1) the number (n) of channels gated by ACh; (2) the conductance (γ) of each channel; and (3) the driving force $(V_m - E_{EPSP})$ that acts on the ions. The number of open channels (n) depends primarily on the concentration of the transmitter and not on the value of membrane potential because the channels are opened by the transmitter and not by voltage.

In the absence of transmitter, no channels are open, so that the synaptic conductance (g_{EPSP}) is zero. Increasing concentrations of transmitter open up a larger fraction of the total number of channels, leading to a progressive increase in the number of open channels (n) and therefore increasing g_{EPSP}.

As illustrated in Figure 9–14 the waveform of the synaptic current produced by nerve stimulation results from the summed action of the opening and subsequent closing of a large number of channels. In a cell at rest, the opening of a single channel produces a depolarization of only 0.3 μV. When the presynaptic nerve terminal generates an action potential, it releases a large quantity of

9–12 The patch clamp method can be used to record single ACh channels in the postsynaptic membrane of either muscle or nerve cells. **A.** A small fire-polished glass microelectrode filled with salt solution (and a low concentration of ACh) is brought into close contact with the surface of the muscle membrane. Gentle suction is then applied to the distal end of the electrode so that the membrane forms a tight seal on the open tip of the pipette. When the seal is tight, almost all the current generated by the opening and closing of the ion channel can be collected by the recording apparatus. (Adapted from Alberts et al., 1983.) **B.** Single-channel currents recorded in the presence of 100 nM ACh from a frog muscle fiber. The resting membrane potential is −92 mV. **1:** The opening of a channel produces a rectangular pulse of inward current, which is recorded as a downward deflection. **2:** When plotted in a histogram, the amplitudes of these rectangular pulses have a distribution with a single peak. This indicates that the patch contains only a single type of active channel and that the size of the elementary current through this channel varies randomly around a mean of 2.69 pA (1 pA = 10^{-12} A). This mean is called the elementary current. It is equivalent to an elementary conductance of about 30 pS. **C.** Single-channel currents recorded in the presence of 100 nM ACh from a frog muscle fiber at a membrane potential of −130 mV. The patch contains several channels, which open independently of one another. Simultaneous channel openings cause the individual current pulses to add linearly. In this record up to three channels are open at any instant so that the individual channel currents superimpose to form amplitude levels that are multiples of −3.9 pA. (Parts **B** and **C** are courtesy of B. Sakmann.)

A

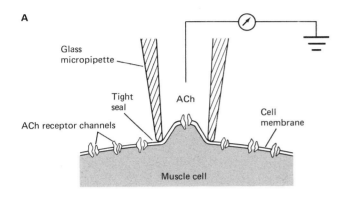

Glass micropipette

Tight seal

ACh

ACh receptor channels

Cell membrane

Muscle cell

B **1**

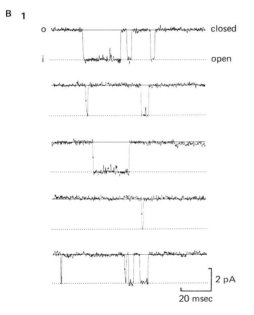

o — closed

i ..... open

2 pA

20 msec

B **2**

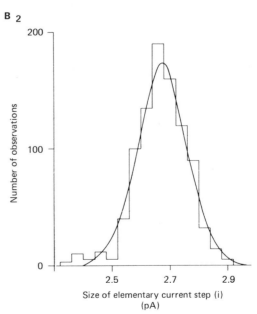

Number of observations

200

100

0

2.5   2.7   2.9

Size of elementary current step (i)
(pA)

C

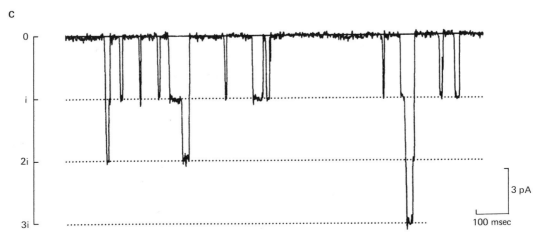

0

i

2i

3i

3 pA

100 msec

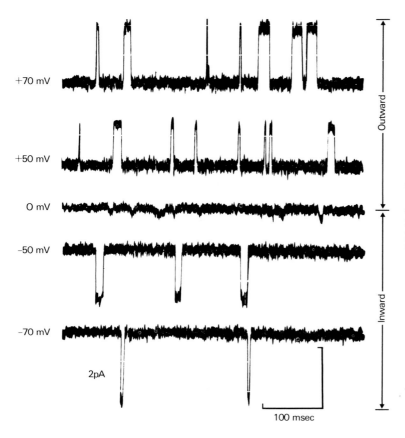

+70 mV

+50 mV

0 mV

−50 mV

−70 mV

Outward

Inward

2pA

100 msec

9–13 A single-channel current has the same reversal potential (0 mV) as does the macroscopic current (Figure 9-8B). The current is inward below 0 mV and outward above 0 mV. The voltage across the patch was systematically varied and the membrane was exposed to 2 μM ACh. (Courtesy of B. Sakmann.)

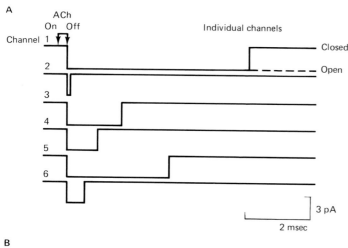

A

ACh
On Off

Channel 1

2

3

4

5

6

Individual channels

Closed

Open

3 pA

2 msec

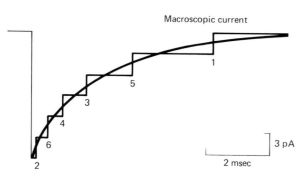

B

Macroscopic current

3 pA

2 msec

9–14 The end-plate current is the summed action of the single-channel currents. **A.** Individual ACh-activated ion channels respond to a brief pulse of ACh (**arrows**) in a manner that is similar to the effect of the brief release of ACh during the end-plate potential. Channels all open rapidly in response to ACh but remain open for variable times because of the random nature of channel closing. **B.** Summation of individual ion channels shown in **A** yields a net current with a more continuous decay (**stepped trace**). The summation of more than 200,000 such channels leads to the end-plate current seen in voltage clamp experiments. (Adapted from D. Colquhoun, 1981.)

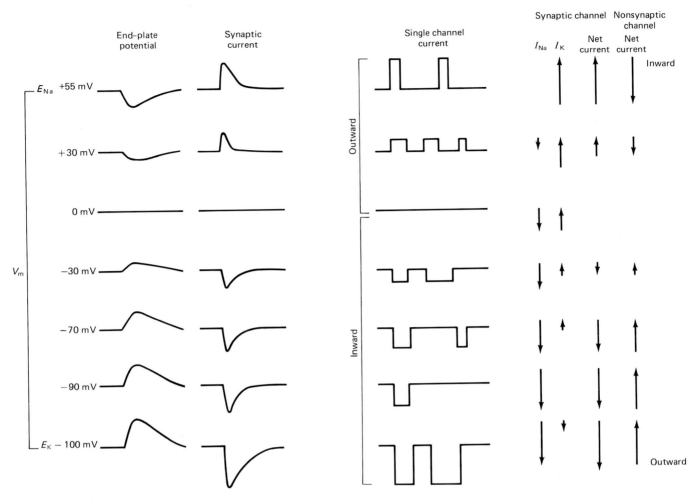

9–15 The resting membrane potential level affects single-channel currents, total synaptic current, and the end-plate potential in a similar way. At the normal muscle resting potential of −90 mV, the ACh-activated single-channel currents and total synaptic current (made up of more than 200,000 single-channel currents) are large and inward because of the large negative driving force on current flow through the synaptic channels. This large inward current produces a large depolarizing end-plate potential. As the level of membrane potential is made more positive (depolarized), the size of the single-channel currents and the magnitude of the synaptic current decrease because the inward driving force on the Na⁺ is decreased, thus reducing the size of the end-plate potential. At 0 mV, the reversal potential, there is no inward synaptic current flow and thus no change in V_m. Further depolarization to +30 mV inverts the synaptic current and direction of the end-plate potential change. On either side of the reversal potential, the synaptic current drives the membrane potential toward the reversal potential. The **arrows** on the right indicate how the individual Na⁺ and K⁺ fluxes in the channel are altered by changing V_m. The algebraic sum of the Na⁺ and K⁺ fluxes gives the *net current* that flows through the transmitter-gated (synaptic) channels. This net synaptic current is equal in size and opposite in direction to that of the net extrasynaptic current flowing in the return pathway of the nongated (nonsynaptic) channels and membrane capacitance. (The size of the **arrows** indicates the relative magnitude of the current.)

transmitter into the synaptic cleft. This leads to the rapid opening of more than two hundred thousand channels in the postsynaptic membrane and produces the fast rising phase of the synaptic current and a synaptic potential of 60 mV. The acetylcholine concentration in the synaptic cleft then rapidly decays because of diffusion and hydrolysis by acetylcholinesterase (as we shall see in Chapter 13). Once the transmitter disappears from the synaptic cleft, the channels begin to close, and each clos-

ing produces a small square step-like decrease in inward synaptic current (Figure 9–14A). The apparent smooth decay of the total synaptic current and the synaptic potential results from the sum of the closings of many thousands of channels (Figure 9–14B).

The relationships among single-channel current, total synaptic current measured under the voltage clamp, and end-plate potential over a wide range of membrane potentials are illustrated in Figure 9–15.

An Overall View

The resolution of single-channel events by means of patch clamp techniques is bringing the study of transmitter action to the level of molecular mechanisms. This in turn allows us to understand the steps that link the binding of transmitter (acetylcholine) to the receptor in order to open the ion channel. As we shall see in Chapter 14, the complete amino acid sequence of the ACh receptor has been obtained with the help of gene-cloning techniques. Thus, we should soon be in a position to answer the ultimate question: How does the molecular structure of the ACh receptor control its physiological functioning?

Acetylcholine is but one of many neurotransmitters used by the nervous system, and the end-plate potential is but one of many examples of postsynaptic transmitter actions. How similar are other transmitter actions to those produced by ACh at the nerve–muscle synapse? Do the same principles also apply to transmitter actions on neurons in the central nervous system, or are novel mechanisms involved? In the past, such questions were difficult to answer because of the small size and great complexity of nerve cells in the central nervous system. However, recent advances have opened to investigation an entirely new range of neurotransmitter actions. It is already clear that although many neurotransmitters produce their actions by a mechanism similar to that of ACh at the end-plate, other important types of transmitter actions also exist. In the next chapter we shall explore some of the rich variety of effects that neurotransmitters can exert on the neurons of the central nervous system.

Postscript: The Synaptic Current Flow during the Excitatory Postsynaptic Potential Can Be Calculated on the Basis of a Simple Equivalent Circuit

To appreciate in a more quantitative way how the opening of channels gated by ACh leads to the depolarization of muscle fiber, it is useful to examine the current that flows into and out of the muscle membrane during the excitatory postsynaptic potential. As we have seen in this chapter, the flow of current through a population of end-plate channels can be simply described by Ohm's law. To fully understand the flow of electrical current during the synaptic potential, however, we need to consider not only the chemically gated end-plate channels that are activated by ACh, but also all other nongated channels in the surrounding membrane that can serve as the return pathway for current flow. Since channels are integral proteins that span the lipid bilayer of the membrane, we must also take into consideration the capacitance properties of the membrane and the ionic batteries determined by the distribution of Na^+ and K^+ inside and outside the cell.

Such a model will allow us to examine the flow of current at the end-plate region of the muscle fiber by using rules governing the flow of current in passive electri-

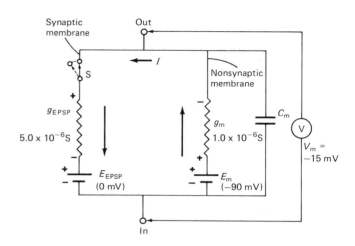

9–16 The equivalent circuit of the end-plate potential with two parallel current pathways. One consists of a synaptic battery, E_{EPSP}, in series with a single synaptic conductance channel, g_{EPSP} (the ACh channel). The other pathway consists of the battery of the resting potential (E_m) in series with the conductance of the nonsynaptic membrane (g_m). In parallel with both of these conductance pathways is the membrane capacitance (C_m). At rest, the synaptic conductance channel is closed, and no current flows through it. This is depicted as an open electrical circuit in which the synaptic conductance is not connected to the rest of the circuit. The release of ACh opens the synaptic channel. This event is equivalent electrically to throwing the switch (**S**) that connects the synaptic conductance pathway (g_{EPSP}) in parallel with the nonsynaptic membrane conductance (g_m), the conductance formed by the nongated channels. As a result, current now flows inward through the synaptic conductance channels, and outward both through the nonsynaptic membrane conductance channels and across the membrane capacitance (C_m). With the indicated values of conductances and batteries, the membrane will depolarize from -90 mV (its resting value) to -15 mV (at the peak of the synaptic potential).

cal devices that consist only of resistors, capacitors, and batteries (see Chapter 6). We can depict the end-plate region with an equivalent circuit that has three parallel branches: (1) a branch representing the flow of synaptic current through the transmitter-gated channels; (2) a branch representing the return current flow through nongated channels; and (3) a third branch representing current flow across the membrane capacitance (Figure 9–16).

Since the end-plate current is carried by both Na^+ and K^+, we could depict the synaptic branch of the equivalent circuit as two parallel branches, each representing the flow of a different ionic species. This corresponds to the treatment that was used to obtain the equivalent circuit for the axonal membrane. However, as we have seen, Na^+ and K^+ flow through the same ion channel at the end-plate. It is therefore more convenient to combine the separate synaptic ion pathways into a single conductance, in series with a battery, representing the channel gated by ACh. The exact conductance of this pathway depends on the number of channels opened, which in

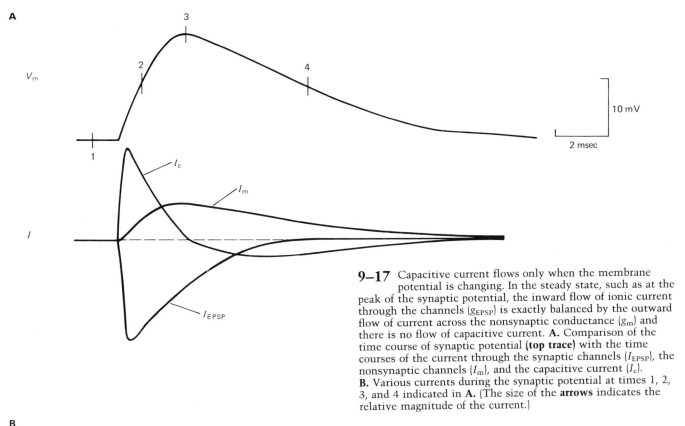

9–17 Capacitive current flows only when the membrane potential is changing. In the steady state, such as at the peak of the synaptic potential, the inward flow of ionic current through the channels (g_{EPSP}) is exactly balanced by the outward flow of current across the nonsynaptic conductance (g_m) and there is no flow of capacitive current. **A.** Comparison of the time course of synaptic potential (**top trace**) with the time courses of the current through the synaptic channels (I_{EPSP}), the nonsynaptic channels (I_m), and the capacitive current (I_c). **B.** Various currents during the synaptic potential at times 1, 2, 3, and 4 indicated in **A.** (The size of the **arrows** indicates the relative magnitude of the current.)

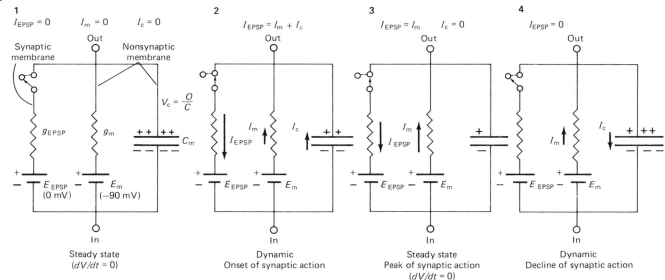

turn depends on the concentration of transmitter. In the absence of transmitter, the conductance is zero (no channels); as the transmitter concentration is increased, causing more and more channels to open, the conductance increases. When most of the end-plate channels are open, the conductance of this pathway has a value of 5

$\times$ 10^{-6} S (or a resistance of 2×10^5 Ω). This is about five times the conductance of the parallel branch (1×10^{-6} S) representing the nongated channels, or nonsynaptic membrane (G_m).

The end-plate conductance is in series with a battery (E_{EPSP}) whose value is given by the reversal potential for synaptic current flow (0 mV) (Figure 9–16). As discussed above, this value is the weighted algebraic sum of the Na$^+$ and K$^+$ batteries.

The current flowing during the excitatory postsynaptic potential (I_{EPSP}) is given by

$$I_{EPSP} = g_{EPSP} \times (V_m - E_{EPSP}).$$

Using this equation and the equivalent circuit of Figure 9–16, we can analyze the synaptic potential at the end-plate in terms of the flow of ionic current. At the onset of the excitatory synaptic action (the dynamic phase), an inward current flows through the synaptic channel because of the increased conductance to Na$^+$ and K$^+$. Since current flows in a closed loop, the inward synaptic current (I_{EPSP}) must leave the cell as outward current. From the equivalent circuit of Figure 9–16, we see that there are two parallel pathways for outward current flow: a conductance pathway due to current flow through the nonsynaptic channels (I_m), and a capacitive pathway due to current flow across the membrane capacitance (I_c). Thus,

$$I_{EPSP} = -(I_m + I_c).$$

During the earliest phase of the synaptic potential, the membrane potential, V_m, is still close to its resting value, E_m (Figure 9–17, A$_1$ and $_2$, B$_1$ and $_2$). As a result, the outward driving force on current flow through the nonsynaptic channels ($V_m - E_m$) is small. Therefore, most of the current crosses the cell membrane as capacitive current and the membrane depolarizes rapidly. As the cell depolarizes, the outward driving force on current flow through the nonsynaptic channels increases while the inward driving force on synaptic current flow decreases somewhat. Eventually, the membrane potential attains its peak level, where the flow of inward synaptic current is exactly balanced by outward current flow through the nonsynaptic channels (Figure 9–17, A$_3$, B$_3$). At this point, $I_{EPSP} = -I_m$, there is no current flow into or out of the capacitor, and the membrane potential will have reached a steady-state value ($dV/dt = 0$). As the synaptic channels close, I_{EPSP} decreases. Now I_{EPSP} and I_m are no longer in balance and the membrane potential starts to repolarize because the outward current flow due to I_m is larger than the inward synaptic current. During most of the declining phase of the synaptic action, no more current flows through the synaptic membrane (the switch is again open); current now flows only through g_m and into and out of C_m (Figure 9–17, A$_4$, B$_4$).

A convenient feature of the synaptic potential at its peak or steady-state value is that we can ignore the capacitive current (since $dV/dt = 0$). The value of the membrane potential (V_m) at the peak of the synaptic potential can then be easily calculated because in the steady state there can be no net entry of current into the muscle. As a result, the inward current flow through the synaptic channels (I_{EPSP}) must be exactly balanced by outward current flow through the nongated channels (I_m)

and we can write:

$$I_{EPSP} + I_m = 0. \tag{9–1}$$

From Ohm's law the current flowing through the active ACh channels (I_{EPSP}) and that flowing through the passive nongated membrane channels (I_m) is given by:

$$I_{EPSP} = g_{EPSP} \times (V_m - E_{EPSP}), \text{ and}$$

$$I_m = g_m \times (V_m - E_m).$$

By substituting these two expressions into Equation 9–1, we obtain

$$g_{EPSP} \times (V_m - E_{EPSP}) + g_m \times (V_m - E_m) = 0.$$

To solve for V_m, all we need do is multiply the two terms of the equation by the two conductances and rearrange so that all terms in voltage appear on one side:

$$(g_{EPSP} \times V_m) + (g_m \times V_m) = (g_{EPSP} \times E_{EPSP}) + (g_m \times E_m).$$

By factoring out V_m on the left-hand side we finally obtain:

$$V_m = \frac{(g_{EPSP} \times E_{EPSP}) + (g_m \times E_m)}{(g_{EPSP} + g_m)}. \tag{9–2}$$

As we can see, this equation is similar to that used for calculating the resting and action potentials in Chapter 6. Upon opening up the synaptic conductance channels, the membrane potential will depolarize (because of inward synaptic current flow) until it reaches a level where the inward synaptic and outward nonsynaptic ionic currents are equal and opposite. According to Equation 9–2, this voltage is a weighted average of the electromotive forces (EMFs) of the two batteries for synaptic and nonsynaptic currents. The weighting factors are given by the relative magnitudes of the two conductances. If the synaptic conductance is much less than the nonsynaptic conductance ($g_{EPSP} \ll g_m$), the term $g_{EPSP} \times E_{EPSP}$ will be negligible compared with the term $g_m \times E_m$. In this case, V_m will remain close to E_m. This situation occurs when only a very few channels are opened by ACh, as, for example, in response to a low concentration of transmitter. On the other hand, when g_{EPSP} is much larger than g_m, Equation 9–2 states that V_m approaches E_{EPSP}, the synaptic reversal potential. This situation applies when a large number of channels are opened and the concentration of ACh is very high. At intermediate ACh concentrations with a moderate number of synaptic channels open, the peak synaptic potential lies somewhere between E_m and E_{EPSP}.

We can now use this equation to calculate the peak end-plate potential for the specific case shown in Figure 9–15, where $g_{EPSP} = 5 \times 10^{-6}$ S; $g_m = 1 \times 10^{-6}$ S; $E_{EPSP} = 0$ mV; and $E_m = -90$ mV. Substituting these values into Equation 9–2 yields:

$$V_m = \frac{(5 \times 10^{-6} \text{ S})(0 \text{ mV}) + (1 \times 10^{-6} \text{ S})(-90 \text{ mV})}{(5 \times 10^{-6} \text{ S}) + (1 \times 10^{-6} \text{ S})}$$

or

$$V_m = \frac{(1 \times 10^{-6}\ S)(-90\ mV)}{(6 \times 10^{-6}\ S)}$$

$$V_m = -15\ mV.$$

The peak amplitude of the end-plate potential is then

$$\Delta V_{EPSP} = V_m - E_m$$

$$= -15\ mV - (-90\ mV)$$

$$= 75\ mV.$$

As a check for consistency, we can see whether, at the peak of the end-plate potential, the synaptic current is in fact equal and opposite to the nonsynaptic current so that the net membrane current is zero.

$$I_{EPSP} = (5 \times 10^{-6}\ S) \times (-15\ mV - 0\ mV),$$

$$I_{EPSP} = -75 \times 10^{-9}\ A.$$

and

$$I_m = (1 \times 10^{-6}\ S) \times [-15\ mV -(-90\ mV)],$$

$$I_m = 75 \times 10^{-9}\ A.$$

Here we see that solving Equation 9–2 ensures that $I_{EPSP} = -I_m$.

Selected Readings

Bennett, M. V. L. 1977. Electrical transmission: A functional analysis and comparison to chemical transmission. In E. R. Kandel (ed.), Handbook of Physiology, Vol. 1: The Nervous System, Part 1. Bethesda, Md.: American Physiological Society, pp. 357–416.

Eccles, J. C. 1964. The Physiology of Synapses. Berlin: Springer.

Eccles, J. C. 1976. From electrical to chemical transmission in the central nervous system. The closing address of the Sir Henry Dale Centennial Symposium. Notes Rec. R. Soc. Lond. 30:219–230.

Fatt, P., and Katz, B. 1951. An analysis of the end-plate potential recorded with an intra-cellular electrode. J. Physiol. (Lond.) 115:320–370.

Furshpan, E. J., and Potter, D. D. 1959. Transmission at the giant motor synapses of the crayfish. J. Physiol. (Lond.) 145:289–325.

Hertzberg, E. L., Lawrence, T. S., Gilula, N. B. 1981. Gap junctional communication. Annu. Rev. Physiol. 43:479–491.

Heuser, J. E., and Reese, T. S. 1977. Structure of the synapse. In E. R. Kandel (ed.), Handbook of Physiology, Vol. 1: The Nervous System, Part 1. Bethesda, Md.: American Physiological Society, pp. 261–294.

Katz, B., and Miledi, R. 1970. Membrane noise produced by acetylcholine. Nature 226:962–963.

Neher, E., and Sakmann, B. 1976. Single-channel currents recorded from membrane of denervated frog muscle fibres. Nature 260:799–802.

Sakmann, B., and Neher, E. (eds.). 1983. Single-Channel Recording. New York: Plenum Press.

Stevens, C. F. 1979. The neuron. Sci. Am. 241(3):54–65.

References

Alberts, B., Bray, D., Lewis, J., Raff, M., Roberts, K., and Watson, J. D. 1983. Molecular Biology of the Cell. New York: Garland.

Bennett, M. V. L., Sandri, C., and Akert, K. 1978. Neuronal gap junctions and morphologically mixed synapses in the spinal cord of a teleost, Sternarchus albifrons (gymnotoidei). Brain Res. 143:43–60.

Cajal, S. R. 1894. La fine structure des centres nerveux. Proc. R. Soc. Lond. 55:444–468.

Cajal, S. R. 1911. Histologie du Système Nerveux de l'Homme & des Vertébrés. L. Azoulay (trans.). Vol. 2. Paris: Maloine. Republished in 1955. Madrid: Instituto Ramón y Cajal.

Colquhoun, D. 1981. How fast do drugs work? Trends Pharmacol. Sci. 2:212–217.

Dale, H. 1935. Pharmacology and nerve-endings. Proc. R. Soc. Med. 28:319–332.

Dwyer, T. M., Adams, D. J., and Hille, B. 1980. The permeability of the end-plate channel to organic cations in frog muscle. J. Gen. Physiol. 75:469–492.

Furshpan, E. J., and Potter, D. D. 1957. Mechanism of nerve-impulse transmission at a crayfish synapse. Nature 180:342–343.

Hille, B. 1984. Ionic Channels of Excitable Membranes. Sunderland, Mass.: Sinauer.

Kuffler, S. W., Nicholls, J. G., and Martin, A. R. 1984. From Neuron to Brain: A Cellular Approach to the Function of the Nervous System, 2nd ed. Sunderland, Mass.: Sinauer.

Makowski, L., Caspar, D. L. D., Phillips, W. C., and Goodenough, D. A. 1977. Gap junction structures. II. Analysis of the X-ray diffraction data. J. Cell Biol. 74:629–645.

McMahan, U. J., and Kuffler, S. W. 1971. Visual identification of synaptic boutons on living ganglion cells and of varicosities in postganglionic axons in the heart of the frog. Proc. R. Soc. Lond. [Biol.] 177:485–508.

Miles, F. A. 1969. Excitable Cells. London: Heinemann.

Neher, E. 1982. Unit conductance studies in biological membranes. In P. F. Baker (ed.), Techniques in Cellular Physiology, Vol. Pl/II (P. 121). County Clare, Ireland: Elsevier/North-Holland, pp. 1–16.

Sherrington, C. 1947. The Integrative Action of the Nervous System, 2nd ed. New Haven: Yale University Press.

Takeuchi, A. 1977. Junctional transmission. I. Postsynaptic mechanisms. In E. R. Kandel (ed.), Handbook of Physiology, Vol. 1: The Nervous System, Part 1. Bethesda, Md.: American Physiological Society, pp. 295–327.

Eric R. Kandel

Chemically Gated Ion Channels at Central Synapses

10

The excitatory synapses that motor neurons make onto skeletal muscle in mammals are unusual in several ways. First, most muscle fibers receive innervation from only one motor cell. Second, all the synaptic connections that each muscle fiber receives are excitatory—there are no inhibitory synapses onto mammalian skeletal muscle. Finally, in the absence of drugs or disease, the connections are highly effective, each synaptic potential invariably producing an action potential.

Although many of the same principles govern the function of synaptic connections in the central nervous system, the details differ. A given central nerve cell, such as the motor neuron, receives not one but thousands of connections from a large variety of neurons. In addition to excitatory synaptic connections, there are also inhibitory connections. As a result, a central neuron has in its surface membrane many species of receptor proteins sensitive to various chemical transmitters, and these receptor molecules control different ion channels.

In this chapter, we shall consider synaptic transmission within the central nervous system. We shall continue to focus on the postsynaptic aspects of chemical synaptic transmission and examine three questions: (1) How do the ion channels mediating inhibitory synaptic actions differ from those mediating excitatory synaptic actions? (2) Do all synaptic actions involve the opening of ion channels, as is the case for acetylcholine at the nerve–muscle synapse, or can transmitters act on channels in other ways? (3) How does a neuron integrate the inhibitory and excitatory synaptic information coming from many different sources?

Studies of many synaptic connections have shown that transmitters produce synaptic potentials by acting on ion channels in two ways: transmitters can open ion channels that are closed at the resting potential, and thereby increase the overall conductance of the postsynaptic membrane; or transmitters can close ion channels that are open at the resting potential, thereby decreasing the overall conductance of the membrane. Synaptic actions resulting from an opening of ion channels resemble those at the nerve–muscle synapse and are therefore better understood. We shall consider them first.

Some Synaptic Actions Are Due to the Opening of Ion Channels That Are Closed at the Resting Potential

Our understanding that chemical synaptic actions in the central nervous system can lead to the opening of ion channels is based largely on the work of John Eccles and his colleagues on spinal motor cells. This work, in turn, derives from the work of Fatt and Katz on the nerve–muscle synapses of crab and frog, some of which we reviewed in the preceding chapter.

Experimental Background

The spinal motor neurons are large motor cells that lie in the ventral portion of the spinal cord (the ventral horn). These nerve cells are useful for examining synaptic mechanisms because they receive both excitatory connections (from afferent axons innervating the same or synergistic muscles) and inhibitory connections (from axons innervating antagonistic muscles). Among the first sets of synaptic connections that Eccles and his colleagues analyzed were those that mediate the stretch reflex, the simple behavior we considered in Chapters 2 and 3 (Figure 10–1).

Eccles selectively stimulated a group of the large axons of the stretch receptor neurons that innervate the stretch receptor organs (the muscle spindles) in the quadriceps muscle. (These axons, as we saw in Chapters 2 and 3, are called primary afferent fibers; they are described more fully in Chapters 34 and 35.) The same experiments can now be done by stimulating a single afferent fiber or simply by inserting a microelectrode into the cell body of one of the afferent neurons in the dorsal root ganglion. By passing stimulating current through the microelectrode, a single stretch receptor nerve cell can be excited (Figure 10–2). The firing of an action potential in a single stretch receptor neuron that innervates the quadriceps muscle produces an excitatory postsynaptic potential (EPSP), which depolarizes and excites the motor neurons to that muscle (Figure 10–2, right-hand side). This depolarization is usually less than 1 mV and clearly is insufficient to depolarize the membrane potential of the motor neuron to threshold for spike initiation. Stimulating a stretch receptor neuron that innervates the biceps, an antagonist muscle, produces an equally small but inhibitory postsynaptic potential (IPSP) that hyperpolarizes and inhibits the same motor neurons. The antagonist inhibitory pathway is disynaptic, involving an interposed inhibitory interneuron. These inhibitory neurons can also be recorded from and stimulated intracellularly (Figure 10–2, left-hand side).

Although a single excitatory postsynaptic potential is not large enough to elicit an action potential in the motor neuron, many converging excitatory synaptic connections onto a cell can summate spatially and temporally to produce a depolarization sufficient for threshold to be

10–1 Connections of neurons mediating the stretch reflex that were used by Eccles and his colleagues and by Stephen Redman in their studies of synaptic excitation and inhibition.

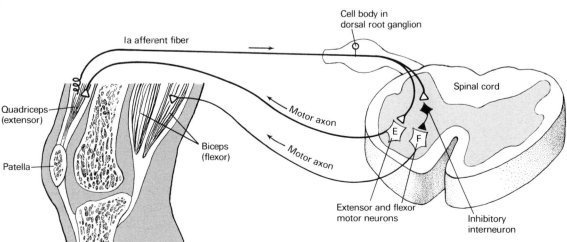

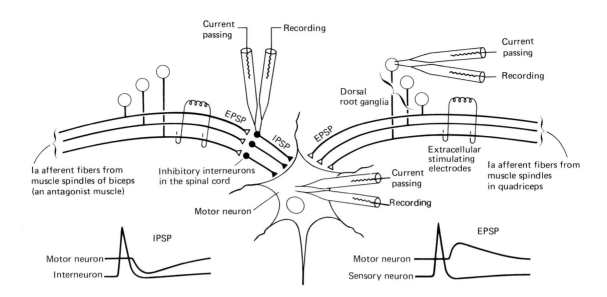

10–2 In this hypothetical, idealized experiment for studying inhibition and excitation of a motor neuron, the inhibitory interneuron in the pathway to the biceps and the receptor neuron from the quadriceps muscle are stimulated with intracellular electrodes. Alternatively, the whole muscle nerve from the biceps or the quadriceps or single axons can be stimulated electrically with gross electrodes. Typical intracellular recordings of the inhibitory and excitatory actions are shown below the experimental setup.

reached and an action potential to be initiated. The inhibitory synaptic potentials, on the other hand, have a subtractive effect that counteracts the excitatory actions. If the sum of inhibition is strong enough, these inhibitory synaptic potentials can prevent the membrane potential from reaching threshold (Figure 10–3). In addition, inhib-

10–3 Interactions of excitatory and inhibitory synaptic potentials in an otherwise silent cell. These synaptic potentials are usually produced by the synchronous activity of many presynaptic neurons.

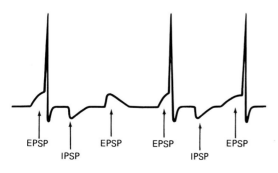

itory synaptic actions can exert powerful regulatory control over endogenously active cells. By suppressing the spontaneous generation of action potentials, inhibitory synaptic actions can determine the pattern of impulse activity. This function of inhibition is called the *sculpturing role* of inhibition (Figure 10–4).

We shall first consider excitatory synapses.

Excitatory Postsynaptic Potentials on Motor Neurons

Eccles and his colleagues discovered that the excitatory postsynaptic potential results from the opening of transmitter-gated ion channels that are permeable to both Na^+ and K^+, similar to the channels in skeletal muscle activated by ACh. As the stimulus strength is increased, more afferent fibers are recruited until the excitatory synaptic potential becomes sufficiently large to bring the membrane potential of the initial segment (the integrative component) of the neuron to threshold for spike generation.

Current That Flows during the EPSP

As we saw in Chapter 9, the best way to study the ionic basis of the EPSP is to use the voltage clamp technique. This technique has recently been successfully applied to motor neurons by Alan Finkel and Stephen Redman at the National University in Canberra, Australia (Figure 10–5). Even earlier, Eccles and his colleagues and Redman had been able to gain considerable insight into the ionic nature of the EPSP simply by measuring the size and polarity of the EPSP while varying the membrane potential (Figure 10–5). This can be done by passing cur-

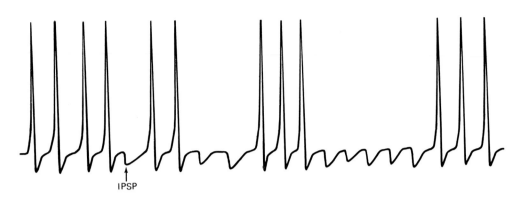

10–4 Inhibition performs a sculpturing role by producing changes in the firing pattern of a spontaneously active neuron.

IPSP

rent across the membrane with an intracellular micro-electrode. The size of the EPSP (V_{EPSP}) depends both on the magnitude of the synaptic current (I_{EPSP}) and on the cell's nonsynaptic membrane conductance (g_m), the non-gated conductance channels (see Chapter 9). To a first approximation[1] we can write

$$V_{EPSP} = \frac{I_{EPSP}}{g_m}.$$

Figure 10–5B shows how the current flows into the cell through synaptic channels and out of the cell through these nongated nonsynaptic channels. As with ACh at the nerve–muscle synapse, the channels opened by the excitatory transmitter are not voltage dependent. As a result, the number of conductance channels that are opened by the transmitter (which determines the total synaptic conductance, g_{EPSP}) depends *only* on the concentration of the transmitter; the number of channels opened does not vary when the membrane potential is changed. Thus, changes in the amplitude of the EPSP at various levels of membrane potential largely reflect changes in the I_{EPSP} produced by changes in driving force, that is, by changes in the difference between the membrane potential (V_m) and the reversal potential for the EPSP (E_{EPSP}). Thus,

$$I_{EPSP} = g_{EPSP} \times (V_m - E_{EPSP}).$$

Most nerve cells have a resting membrane potential of approximately −55 mV; this resting potential is considerably lower than that of the muscle cell (−90 mV),

which we considered in the last chapter. As the membrane potential of the nerve cell is increased from −55 to −70 mV, the EPSP increases in amplitude, much as does the synaptic potential in muscle. This occurs because more inward current flows through the synaptic channels as the driving force ($V_m - E_{EPSP}$) is increased—as the membrane potential is moved further away from the Na$^+$ equilibrium potential (E_{Na}) of +55 mV and closer to the equilibrium potential for K$^+$ (E_K), which, for central nerve cells, is about −70 mV. The resulting increase in the inward driving force on Na$^+$ and the decrease in the outward driving force on K$^+$ cause a greater Na$^+$ influx and a reduced K$^+$ efflux through the synaptic channels. If V_m is moved to a more negative potential than the K$^+$ equilibrium potential of nerve cells, the K$^+$ current through the synaptic channels actually reverses and flows inward.

As the membrane potential is progressively depolarized, however, the EPSP diminishes, until it is abolished near 0 mV, the *reversal potential* of the EPSP. Here the inward Na$^+$ current that flows through the synaptic channels is reduced because the membrane potential is now closer to E_{Na}, and the outward K$^+$ current is increased because it is further from E_K. The inward Na$^+$ current now is balanced by the outward K$^+$ current with the result that there is no net current flow through the synaptic channels. Additional depolarization produces a hyperpolarizing EPSP. Now the outward K$^+$ current is greater than the inward Na$^+$ current, resulting in a net outward ionic current because the membrane potential is closer to E_{Na} than to E_K. When Finkel and Redman used the voltage clamp to examine the synaptic current (rather than the synaptic potential) as a function of different membrane potentials, they obtained similar results. The net current was nullified at 0 mV and reversed from inward to outward as the membrane potential was depolarized further.

Because the reversal potential for excitation (E_{EPSP}) is about 0 mV, the excitatory synaptic actions tend to drive the membrane potential from its resting level (−55 mV) past threshold (−45 mV) in the direction of the reversal potential for the EPSP.

---

[1]This equation is only an approximation. First, as we saw in the last chapter, it ignores the current flow across the membrane capacitance. Unless the time course of the EPSP is very slow compared with the membrane time constant, a part of I_{EPSP} leaves the cell across the capacitance, and thus this equation overestimates the size of V_{EPSP}. Second, when the resting V_m is altered by current passing through the intracellular microelectrode, g_m does not, in general, remain constant but varies with the opening or closing of voltage-dependent ion channels in response to the changes in V_m. These problems are circumvented with the voltage clamp technique, in which V_m is held at a fixed, steady level during the I_{EPSP}.

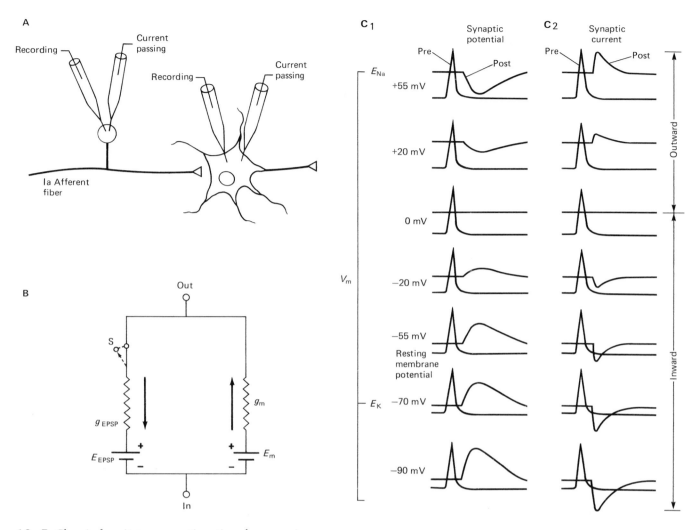

10–5 Chemical excitatory synaptic actions from opening conductance channels to both Na$^+$ and K$^+$.

A. In this experimental system, an intracellular electrode is used to stimulate the presynaptic neuron. In the postsynaptic neuron, one intracellular electrode measures membrane potential and a second passes current either to alter the level of the resting membrane potential (a method of membrane control called *current clamp*) or to keep the membrane potential fixed during the flow of synaptic current (the method of membrane control called *voltage clamp*).

B. The simplified equivalent circuit consists of a synaptic current pathway in parallel with nonsynaptic membrane. The synaptic pathway is represented by a battery, E_{EPSP}, in series with the synaptic conductance, g_{EPSP}. Na$^+$ and K$^+$ pass through the same conductance pathway (ion channel) and the battery, E_{EPSP}, is a weighted average of the two batteries for E_{Na} and E_K. The nonsynaptic membrane consists of the battery representing the resting membrane potential (E_m) in series with resting membrane conductance, g_m. The nonsynaptic conductance consists of the nongated channels of the membrane. The synaptic action is equivalent to throwing the switch (**S**), which closes the circuit by placing the pathway for synaptic conductance (g_{EPSP}) in parallel with the nonsynaptic membrane conductance (g_m). As a result, current flows inward through the synaptic channels and outward through the nonsynaptic membrane, depolarizing the membrane.

C. A unique reversal potential for the EPSP can be determined. **1:** Current clamp experiment. When the membrane potential is at its resting value (−55 mV), a presynaptic spike produces a depolarizing EPSP, which increases when the membrane potential is increased (hyperpolarized) to −90 mV. However, as the membrane potential is depolarized to −20 mV, the EPSP becomes smaller, and as the membrane potential reaches the reversal potential of 0 mV, the EPSP is nullified. Further depolarization to +20 mV inverts the synaptic potential, causing hyperpolarization. On either side of the reversal potential, the synaptic action drives the membrane potential toward the reversal potential, E_{EPSP}. **2:** Voltage clamp experiment. At the resting membrane potential and at more negative holding potentials (−70 and −90 mV), the synaptic current is large and inward because the electrochemical driving force ($V_m − E_{EPSP}$) is inward. This inward current generates the EPSP. As the membrane potential is made less negative (−20 mV), the magnitude of the inward synaptic current decreases and, at the reversal potential of 0 mV (E_{EPSP}), it becomes zero. Positive to the reversal potential, at +20 or +55 mV, the synaptic current is outward. (Adapted from Finkel and Redman, 1983.)

Chemical Transmitters for Excitation

In their basic features the synaptic channels in motor neurons are similar to those of skeletal muscle. There are, however, some important gaps in our understanding of central synaptic action. We know that motor neurons release acetylcholine to excite skeletal muscle, but we are still uncertain about the transmitter that the dorsal root ganglion neurons connected to Ia afferent fibers use to excite the motor neurons. Pharmacological evidence suggests that two simple amino acids, glutamate and aspartate, are the most likely candidates for the excitatory transmitter at this synapse.

Inhibitory Postsynaptic Potentials on Motor Neurons

Eccles and his colleagues found that inhibitory postsynaptic potentials (IPSPs) inhibit by keeping the membrane potential of the initial segment of the axon (the integrative component) from reaching threshold for spike generation. Inhibitory synaptic potentials usually do this by increasing (hyperpolarizing) the membrane potential. The IPSPs also reduce the synaptic actions produced by excitatory synapses in ways we shall consider below. Inhibitory transmitters activate either Cl^- or K^+ channels. Although they are usually activated independently, these two distinct ion channels are similar in that the reversal (or Nernst) potential for both K^+ and Cl^- is more negative than the threshold for spike initiation. In a typical nerve cell, E_K equals -70 mV and E_{Cl} equals about -60 mV, whereas the resting potential lies at -55 mV. Because the resting potential is just above these two values, the cell is hyperpolarized when either chemically gated Cl^- or K^+ channels are activated.

Chloride ions are in high concentration (150 mM) on the outside of the cell and in low concentration inside (10 mM). Opening of Cl^- channels therefore leads to the movement of Cl^- down its concentration gradient, into the cell. The inward flow of the negatively charged Cl^- is equivalent to the outward flow of the positively charged K^+. Thus, once the transmitter opens the channels for Cl^- or K^+, the net electrochemical driving force on either ion leads to a *net outward ionic current*. Movement of Cl^- into the cell therefore has consequences similar to the movement of K^+ out of the cell. With movement of either ion, there is a net increase of the negative charge on the inside of the membrane capacitance leading to hyperpolarization of the membrane. For K^+ this increase is achieved by the removal of positive charge through efflux, and for Cl^-, by the addition of negative charge through influx.

In the spinal motor neurons studied by Eccles, the inhibitory transmitter opens channels to Cl^-. Inhibitory transmitters also open Cl^- channels in many other central neurons, including those of the cerebral cortex and hippocampus. At some central synapses, inhibitory transmitters open K^+ channels. Certain cells have more than one species of inhibitory receptors. In those cells

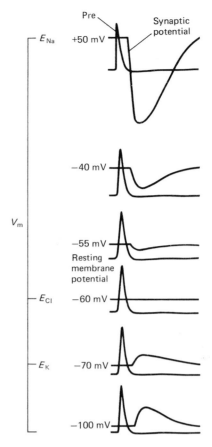

10–6 Chemical inhibitory synaptic action that results from opening ion channels to Cl^- (g_{Cl}). In this hypothetical experiment, one electrode is placed in the presynaptic cell and two are placed in the postsynaptic cell. One electrode in each cell is for passing current—in the presynaptic cell to produce an action potential, and in the postsynaptic cell to alter the membrane potential systematically (current clamp). The other electrode is for recording the membrane potential. At the resting value (-55 mV), a presynaptic spike produces a hyperpolarizing IPSP, which increases in amplitude as the membrane is artificially depolarized. However, as the membrane potential is hyperpolarized to -60 mV, the IPSP goes to zero; this is the reversal potential for the IPSP and it lies at E_{Cl}, the Nernst potential for Cl^-. With further hyperpolarization, the IPSP is inverted to a depolarizing synaptic potential (-70 and -100 mV). Even this depolarizing action is inhibitory, however, because it brings the membrane potential only toward, but not beyond, the reversal potential, which is considerably below the firing level (-45 mV).

one receptor can control a K^+ channel for inhibition and another receptor can control a Cl^- channel.

Current That Flows during the IPSP

The flow of current due to inhibitory synaptic action (I_{IPSP}) can be inferred in a way similar to that of excitation by artificially changing the membrane potential (V_m) and seeing how the changes affect the IPSP (Figure 10–6). As the membrane potential is depolarized, the IPSP be-

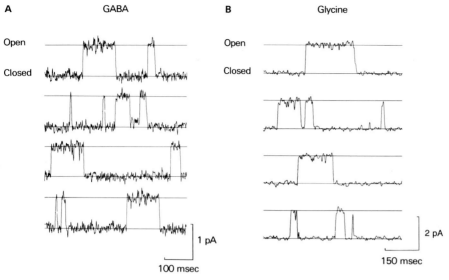

10–7 Recordings of single chemically gated Cl⁻ inhibitory channels in mouse spinal neurons at a membrane potential of 0 mV. **A.** Openings induced by GABA (10 μM). **B.** Openings induced by glycine (10 μM). Both types of inhibitory transmitters (GABA and glycine) act on different receptors that control a similar ion channel. Both channels are shown producing similar elementary pulses of outward currents, indicating the opening of similar Cl⁻ channels in response to their respective inhibitory transmitter. (Courtesy of B. Sakmann.)

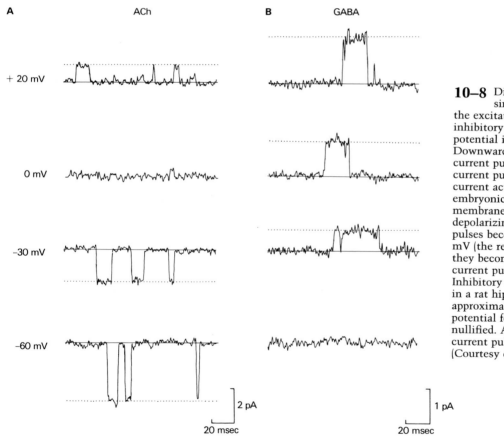

10–8 Differences in the response of the single-channel currents activated by the excitatory transmitter, ACh, and by the inhibitory transmitter, GABA, as membrane potential is systematically altered. Downward deflection indicates inward current pulses, upward deflection, outward current pulses. **A.** Elementary excitatory current activated by ACh (2 μM) in an embryonic muscle of the rat. As the membrane potential is moved in a depolarizing direction (−30 mV), the current pulses become smaller (less inward). At 0 mV (the reversal potential for the EPSP), they become nullified, and at +20 mV the current pulses invert and are outward. **B.** Inhibitory current activated by GABA (5 μM) in a rat hippocampal neuron. At approximately −60 mV (the reversal potential for the IPSP), this current is nullified. At more depolarized levels, the current pulses are always outward. (Courtesy of B. Sakmann.)

comes larger because the driving force on Cl⁻ ($V_m - E_{Cl}$) becomes larger as V_m is moved further away from E_{Cl}. The force due to the concentration gradient that promotes the movement of Cl⁻ from outside to inside the cell remains the same, but the force due to the electrical gradient that opposes the movement of Cl⁻ is reduced.

Therefore more Cl⁻ flows across the synaptic channel. If the membrane potential is now increased by moving it in the hyperpolarizing direction to −60 mV, the IPSP decreases to zero. This null point is defined as the *reversal potential* for the IPSP (E_{IPSP}). For Cl⁻, it is E_{Cl}. At the null point, V_m equals E_{Cl} and the electrical driving force acting on Cl⁻ is exactly equal to the force due to the concentration gradient. Even when g_{Cl} is increased, there is no net current through the channel. If the membrane potential is further increased to -70 mV, the electrical driving force exceeds the driving force of the concentration gradient, and Cl⁻ begins to move out of the cell. The Cl⁻ current flowing out of the cell is equivalent to current (positive charge) flowing into the cell through the synaptic channel (and outward through the nonsynaptic membrane).

The fact that the resting potential of a central neuron is so close to the Cl⁻ equilibrium potential raises some interesting questions: What happens in cells that have a resting potential of -60 mV, right at the Cl⁻ equilibrium potential? In these cells, synaptic inhibition due to an opening of conductance channels does not change the membrane potential at all; the inhibition does not hyperpolarize the cell. Does it nevertheless inhibit the cell from firing? By opening conductance channels to Cl⁻, the inhibitory transmitter increases the overall conductance of the membrane of the postsynaptic cell (g_m). As discussed earlier, the amplitude of an excitatory synaptic potential is given by

$$V_{EPSP} = \frac{I_{EPSP}}{g_m}.$$

In the presence of inhibition, the amplitude of an excitatory synaptic potential is therefore reduced because when g_m is increased an EPSP will be smaller than when, as in the absence of inhibition, g_m is normal.

Thus, synaptic inhibition due to the opening of Cl⁻ (or K⁺) conductance channels inhibits the postsynaptic cell in two ways. First, it invariably increases the membrane conductance and thereby reduces the effectiveness of an EPSP. This property is called the *short-circuiting* action of inhibition due to opening of conductance channels. Second (except in cells that have a high resting potential, where $V_m = E_{Cl}$), an IPSP due to the opening of ion channels usually hyperpolarizes the membrane potential and moves it further away from threshold.

The increase in the conductance to Cl⁻ (or to K⁺) produced by the chemical transmitter has one other interesting property. As is the case for synaptic excitation, the opening of Cl⁻ (or K⁺) channels is not influenced by membrane voltage. A change in the membrane potential does not alter the number of channels opened by the transmitter. This again reflects the fundamental difference between the channels that are chemically gated by synaptic actions and the channels that are electrically gated by the action potential.

Chemical Transmitters for Inhibition

In contrast to the paucity of information about transmitters that mediate excitation by opening channels, there is now solid evidence that gamma-aminobutyric acid (GABA) is an extremely common inhibitory transmitter in the brain and in the spinal cord, and that glycine, a less common transmitter, is used by the interneurons activated by the Ia afferent fibers from stretch receptors of antagonistic muscles.

Bert Sakmann and his colleagues have obtained single-channel recordings from spinal neurons in culture showing that both GABA and glycine give rise to outward elementary current steps due to the movement of Cl⁻ (Figure 10–7). In Figure 10–8 the reversal potential of elementary excitatory currents produced in the muscle membrane in response to ACh is compared with the reversal potential of the elementary inhibitory currents produced in neurons of the hippocampus in response to GABA.

In the transmitter-gated channels so far considered, the receptor site that recognizes the transmitter, the channel that conducts ions, and the gate that opens and closes the channel are known or thought to coexist in a single macromolecule. The binding of the transmitter to the receptor causes a simple conformational change, which acts on the gate and opens the channel (Figure 10–9A). But in addition to these channels, there is a second class (which we will consider below) in which the channel and the receptor are different proteins, and where the receptor communicates with its channel not directly but by means of an intracellular second messenger. The second messengers, in turn, activate a protein kinase that modifies the channel covalently either by phosphorylating it directly or by phosphorylating a regulatory protein that acts on the channel (Figure 10–9B).

Other Synaptic Actions Are Due to the Closing of Ion Channels That Are Open at the Resting Potential

We have thus far considered only the role of conductance increases in producing synaptic potentials. Work on the neurons of sympathetic ganglia and on neurons from various invertebrate animals has shown that it is possible to produce synaptic excitation by closing K⁺ channels that are open at rest.

In certain cells, some of the K⁺ channels that contribute to the resting membrane potential are not simply passive, or nongated, but are controlled by synaptic action. Transmitters that close these channels depolarize the cell. For example, there are two basic types of receptors to ACh: *nicotinic* and *muscarinic*. Both bind ACh, but there are agonists (substances that simulate the actions of ACh), such as nicotine or muscarine, as well as antagonists (substances that block the receptor), such as curare and hexamethonium, that bind exclusively to one type of ACh receptor or the other. The two types of receptors differ biochemically, and they serve different functions in the nervous system. The receptors located in the skeletal muscle fibers that receive synapses from motor neurons are *nicotinic*. In sympathetic neurons and in certain neurons of the hippocampus and the cerebral cortex, ACh also acts on a *muscarinic* receptor. Paul Adams and his colleagues at State University of New York at Stony Brook have found that the muscarinic action of ACh leads to the closing of a K⁺ channel, which they have called the *M* (muscarinic) *channel*, to distinguish it from other K⁺ channels, such as the one de-

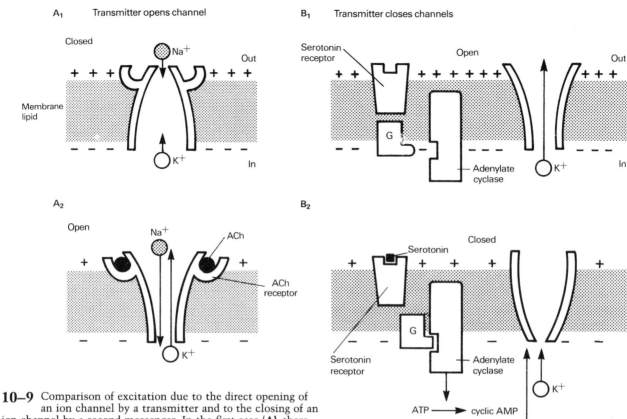

10–9 Comparison of excitation due to the direct opening of an ion channel by a transmitter and to the closing of an ion channel by a second messenger. In the first case (**A**), there is a direct coupling between the recognition site for the transmitter and the ion channel, leading to channel opening. In the other case (**B**), the receptor acts to close the channel through several coupling proteins and an intracellular messenger. **A.** A transmitter such as ACh or glutamate acts directly on the channel protein, opening a channel that is permeable to Na$^+$ and K$^+$. **B.** A transmitter such as serotonin binds to a receptor in the postsynaptic cell. When the receptor binds serotonin it causes a coupling protein (G protein) to activate an adenylate cyclase—an enzyme that synthesizes cyclic AMP from adenosine triphosphate (ATP). The cyclic

AMP in turn activates a protein kinase—an enzyme that phosphorylates proteins. The cyclic AMP-dependent kinase phosphorylates an unidentified substrate protein (perhaps the channel itself or a regulatory protein that acts on the channel), which causes the K$^+$ channel to close.

scribed by Hodgkin and Huxley that underlies the repolarization of the action potential.

At some synapses, the K$^+$ channels closed by the transmitter are not simply restricted to the membrane directly underneath the presynaptic terminals, which contains the receptors for the transmitter, but appear to be distributed more widely over the surface of the cell. In these cases, the action of the transmitter on the receptor triggers the synthesis of an intracellular second messenger that diffuses throughout the inside of the cell to act on widely distributed channels. For example, an EPSP produced by serotonin in certain sensory neurons of the marine snail *Aplysia* is caused by closure of a species of K$^+$ channel, called the *S channel* because it is modulated by serotonin. In this synaptic action, the transmitter binds to a receptor that is not itself part of an ion channel. Rather, the receptor is part of an enzymatic cascade, which is diagrammed in Figure 10–9. Once occupied by the transmitter (in the case of this example, serotonin),

the receptor causes a coupling protein (the G protein) to activate the enzyme adenylate cyclase that converts ATP to cyclic AMP. The increased level of cyclic AMP leads to the activation of another enzyme, the cyclic AMP-dependent protein kinase, which phosphorylates a substrate protein that is either the S channel itself or a regulatory protein that acts to close this species of K$^+$ channel.

Roger Nicoll and his colleagues at the University of California in San Francisco have found that a similar mechanism is involved in the actions of the transmitter norepinephrine on cortical neurons. The norepinephrine-secreting cells of the brain originate in the brain stem in a group of cell bodies called the *locus ceruleus*. Cells from this nucleus innervate the hippocampus and extend widely over the surface of the cerebral cortex. Norepinephrine acts through cyclic AMP to close a species of K$^+$ channels. (In this case, the channels that are closed represent still another class of K$^+$ channel, the Ca^{++}-activated K$^+$ channels.)

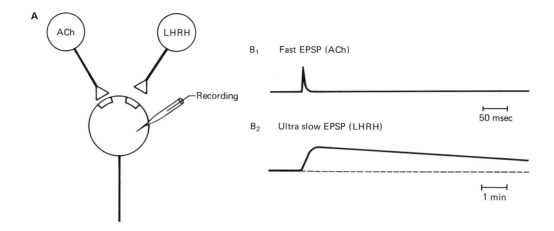

B₁ Fast EPSP (ACh)

50 msec

B₂ Ultra slow EPSP (LHRH)

1 min

The closure of K⁺ channels produces excitatory synaptic actions in two ways. First, closure of K⁺ channels that are normally open at the resting potential produces a depolarization, bringing the membrane potential closer to threshold for firing an action potential. This is because, as we saw in Chapter 5, the resting membrane is permeable to Na⁺ (and to Cl⁻), as well as to K⁺, and the resting potential is therefore a compromise among the permeabilities to the three species of ions. Closure of some K⁺ channels therefore moves V_m to a new value somewhat closer to E_{Na}. Second, because of the decrease in the number of open K⁺ conductance channels, the effective membrane conductance, g_m, is reduced. Thus, any other excitatory input that generates an EPSP now produces a greater depolarization ($V_{EPSP} = I_{EPSP} / g_m$). This is just the reverse of the situation we considered in the case of synaptic inhibition due to the opening of Cl⁻ conductance channels, in which an increase in g_m decreases the effectiveness of excitatory synaptic inputs. Decreased-conductance synaptic actions that modulate the excitability and thus the response of a postsynaptic cell are often called *modulatory*. Conventional increased conductance synaptic actions, on the other hand, are called *mediating*.

Synaptic actions due to closure of ion channels are also distinguished from synaptic potentials due to opening of ion channels by their much slower time course—in several known cases, they are 10,000 times slower.

10–10 Certain neurons in sympathetic ganglia receive independent convergent excitatory connections from two different sets of neurons. One set of neurons uses acetylcholine as its transmitter, the other uses a peptide: luteinizing hormone-releasing hormone (LHRH). ACh produces an EPSP through the opening of ion channels to Na⁺ and K⁺. LHRH produces an EPSP through the closing of channels for K⁺. **A.** This cartoon illustrates the convergent input. The neurons that use ACh make a conventional directed synaptic contact. The neurons that use LHRH make a nondirected contact. Their release site is the same distance from the target cell (this distinction is discussed further in Chapter 12). **B.** In the same neuron, the time course of the decreased-conductance EPSP is much slower than that of an increased-conductance EPSP. **B₁.** The increased-conductance EPSP induced by ACh lasts 20 msec. **B₂.** In contrast, the decreased-conductance EPSP induced by LHRH is very slow, lasting 10 min. (Adapted from Jan, Jan, and Kuffler, 1979.)

Stephen Kuffler and his colleagues Yuh Nung Jan and Lily Yeh Jan have described a decreased-conductance EPSP in a sympathetic ganglion produced by presynaptic neurons that use a peptide hormone (luteinizing hormone-releasing hormone) as a transmitter substance. This EPSP also results from the closure of the M species of the K⁺ channel and lasts 10 min. In contrast, the increased-conductance EPSP on the same neurons lasts 20 msec (Figure 10–10). Similarly, the EPSP produced when serotonin closes the K⁺ channels in the sensory neurons in *Aplysia* can last more than one-half hour. As we shall

Table 10–1. Comparison of Synaptic Excitation Produced by the Opening and Closing of Ion Channels

Properties	EPSP due to opening of channels	EPSP due to closing of channels
Ion channels involved	Cation channel for Na⁺ and K⁺	Channel for K⁺
Effect on total membrane conductance	Increase	Decrease
Contribution to action potential	None	Modulates current of action potential
Time course	Usually fast (msec)	Slow (sec or min)
Intracellular second messenger	None	Cyclic AMP (or other second messengers)
Nature of synaptic action	Mediating	Modulating

Table 10–2. Common Features of Signaling Potentials

Potentials	Channel specificity	Gating mechanism	Properties
Resting potential	Mostly nongated K^+ and Cl^- channels; some nongated Na^+ channels; occasionally, chemically gated K^+ channels	Usually nongated channels	Usually steady, ranging in different cells from -35 to -70 mV
Action potential	Independently gated Na^+ and K^+ channels	Voltage	All or none; about 100 mV in amplitude; 1–10 msec in duration
Receptor potential	Modality-specific gated Na^+ and K^+ channels	Sensory stimulus	Graded; fast, several milliseconds in duration; several millivolts in amplitude
Electrical PSP	None	None	Passive propagation of presynaptic potential change
Increased-conductance EPSP	Simultaneous gating of single class of non-voltage-gated channels for Na^+ and K^+ (channels are selective for cations)	Chemical (extracellular messenger)	Graded; fast, several milliseconds to seconds in duration; several millivolts in amplitude
Increased-conductance IPSP	Non-voltage-gated K^+ or Cl^- channels (channel is thought to be selective for small ions)	Chemical (extracellular messenger)	Graded; fast, several milliseconds to seconds in duration; several millivolts in amplitude
Decreased-conductance EPSP	Closure of leakage channels for K^+	Chemical (intracellular messenger)	Graded; slow, seconds to minutes in duration; 1 to several millivolts in amplitude; channel contributes to the action potential
Decreased-conductance IPSP	Closure of leakage channels for Na^+ or Ca^{++}	Chemical (? intracellular messenger)	Graded, slow, seconds to minutes in duration, 1 to several millivolts in amplitude

see later (Chapter 62), these slow synaptic actions are important for modulating neuronal activity over the long term (Table 10–1).

Finally, K^+ channels closed by transmitters to produce excitation differ in still one other way from channels that are opened to produce synaptic actions. The channels that are opened by transmitters characteristically are not affected by membrane potential and do not contribute to the currents of the action potential. In contrast, the various K^+ channels that generate the decreased conductance EPSP can contribute to the currents of the action potential.

Ionic Mechanisms for Signaling Have Features in Common

The resting potential, action potential, receptor (generator) potentials, IPSPs, and EPSPs all have certain common features (Table 10–2). They all result from ions moving down their concentration gradients through transmembrane protein channels. But the various types of potentials used for signaling differ in the specific ions involved, in the properties of the channels through which the ions move, in whether the channels are opened or

closed, and, if opened, in the nature of the stimulus that gates the channel (such as voltage for the Na^+ and K^+ channels of the action potential, transmitter for the channels of synaptic actions, pressure for the channels that produce the generator potential of various stretch or touch receptors, and light for retinal receptors involved in vision). The same species of ions can move through different channels and give rise to different actions. Thus, K^+ can move through a nongated channel during the resting potential, a voltage-gated channel during the action potential, and a chemically gated channel during certain inhibitory synaptic actions. Finally, when two ionic conductances are activated, different potentials are produced depending on whether ions move simultaneously or sequentially. For example, both the action potential and certain excitatory synaptic actions involve increases in Na^+ influx and K^+ efflux. During an EPSP, however, Na^+ and K^+ move simultaneously through the same channels. In the action potential, on the other hand, Na^+, which is activated first, and K^+, activated later, move through different channels. In addition, many (but not all) of the chemically activated channels are not voltage-gated and lack the regenerative link between conductance and voltage that is critical for the explosive all-or-none nature of the action potential.

Integration of Signals Determines Firing of Action Potential

To discharge an action potential, the membrane potential has to reach the threshold critical for spike generation. This usually is -45 mV. As we have seen, EPSPs excite because they drive the membrane potential toward threshold. In most cases the synaptic potentials produced by a single presynaptic neuron are small: most sensory neurons connected to a muscle spindle produce EPSPs of 0.2 mV in a motor cell, whereas a motor neuron requires a depolarization of about 15 mV to reach threshold. If the EPSPs were to sum linearly (which they do not), at least 75 afferent neurons would have to fire to discharge a motor neuron. The summing of synaptic inputs from different neurons is called *spatial summation* because each synaptic input occupies a slightly different area on the membrane of the postsynaptic cell. The degree of spatial summation is determined by the time constant and the length constant of the postsynaptic cell. We have considered the importance of these passive properties in Chapter 7. A presynaptic neuron can also increase its effect on the membrane potential of the postsynaptic neuron by firing repeatedly, giving rise to *temporal summation*. The degree of temporal summation is determined by the time constant of the postsynaptic cell.

In addition to excitatory signals, the postsynaptic cell also receives inhibitory signals that can reduce the effectiveness even of large EPSPs. As we have seen, a single cell such as a motor neuron receives 1000 or more synapses from presynaptic neurons, some capable of exciting it, some of inhibiting it. Different numbers and combinations of presynaptic neurons are active at different times. The total input determines whether the motor neuron will discharge an action potential and, if so, what the frequency and pattern of the discharge will be.

The cell bodies of some neurons cannot generate an action potential. Even in neurons whose cell bodies can trigger an action potential, the threshold for spike generation in the cell body is usually high (-30 mV), whereas that of the trigger zone in the initial segment of the axon is relatively low (-45 mV). As a result, whether an impulse is discharged is determined at the trigger zone, a point often remote from the synaptic region. The trigger zone is called the integrative component of the neuron because at this region the sum of the excitatory and inhibitory inputs onto the cell is tallied. This integrative action, in turn, reduces to the control of the membrane potential of the trigger zone. The cell will fire if, and only if, excitation exceeds inhibition at the trigger zone by a critical minimum.

As Edgar Adrian first pointed out, once a series of action potentials is initiated in a cell, such as a motor neuron, "the messages are scarcely more complex than a succession of dots in the Morse Code." The amplitude of the action potential is all or none. Therefore, the information for signaling the next cell is contained in the frequency and temporal pattern—the number of spikes in the train and the duration of the train.

Selected Readings

Adrian, E. D. 1932. The Mechanism of Nervous Action: Electrical Studies of the Neurone. Philadelphia: University of Pennsylvania Press.

Dale, H. 1935. Pharmacology and nerve-endings. Proc. R. Soc. Med. 28:319–332.

Eccles, J. C. 1964. The Physiology of Synapses. Berlin: Springer.

Nicoll, R. A. 1982. Neurotransmitters can say more than just "yes" or "no." Trends Neurosci. 5:369–374.

Takeuchi, A. 1977. Junctional transmission. I. Postsynaptic mechanisms. In E. R. Kandel (ed.), Handbook of Physiology, Vol. 1: The Nervous System, Part 1. Bethesda, Md.: American Physiological Society, pp. 295–327.

References

Adams, P. 1982. Voltage-dependent conductances of vertebrate neurones. Trends Neurosci. 5:116–119.

Cajal, S. R. 1894. La fine structure des centres nerveux. Proc. R. Soc. Lond. 55:444–468.

Cajal, S. R. 1911. Histologie du Système Nerveux de l'Homme & des Vertébrés. L. Azoulay (trans.). Vol. 2. Paris: Maloine. Republished in 1955. Madrid: Instituto Ramón y Cajal.

Coombs, J. S., Eccles, J. C., and Fatt, P. 1955. The specific ionic conductances and the ionic movements across the motoneuronal membrane that produce the inhibitory post-synaptic potential. J. Physiol. (Lond.) 130:326–373.

Eccles, J. C. 1957. The Physiology of Nerve Cells. Baltimore: Johns Hopkins Press.

Fatt, P., and Katz, B. 1952. Spontaneous subthreshold activity at motor nerve endings. J. Physiol. (Lond.) 117:109–128.

Finkel, A. S., and Redman, S. J. 1983. The synaptic current evoked in cat spinal motoneurones by impulses in single group Ia axons. J. Physiol. (Lond.) 342:615–632.

Hamill, O. P., Bormann, J., and Sakmann, B. 1983. Activation of multiple-conductance state chloride channels in spinal neurones by glycine and GABA. Nature 305:805–808.

Hodgkin, A. L., and Huxley, A. F. 1952. A quantitative description of membrane current and its application to conduction and excitation in nerve. J. Physiol. (Lond.) 117:500–544.

Jan, Y. N., Jan, L. Y., and Kuffler, S. W. 1979. A peptide as a possible transmitter in sympathetic ganglia of the frog. Proc. Natl. Acad. Sci. U.S.A. 76:1501–1505.

Redman, S. 1979. Junctional mechanisms at group Ia synapses. Prog. Neurobiol. 12:33–83.

Sherrington, C. S. 1897. The Central Nervous System. In M. Foster (ed.), A Text Book of Physiology, Part III, 7th ed. London: Macmillan.

Siegelbaum, S. A., Camardo, J. S., and Kandel, E. R. 1982. Serotonin and cyclic AMP close single K^+ channels in *Aplysia* sensory neurones. Nature 299:413–417.

Eric R. Kandel

Factors Controlling Transmitter Release

11

Current research in neurobiology indicates that some of the most remarkable activities of the brain, such as memory and learning, emerge from elementary properties of chemical synapses. The distinctive feature of chemical synapses is that the action potentials in the presynaptic terminals lead to the secretion of chemical messengers. In this chapter, we shall consider how the electrical events in the presynaptic terminals are coupled to the secretory process for the release of neurotransmitters.

Certain Ion Species Are Necessary for Transmitter Release

By examining in detail the intermediary steps between the action potential and the release of chemical transmitter, Bernard Katz and his collaborators have contributed much of what we know about transmitter release. As we have seen, the action potential results from two sequential steps. First, voltage-gated Na$^+$ channels open, allowing Na$^+$ to move into the cell. This is followed by an opening of voltage-gated K$^+$ channels and movement of K$^+$ out of the cell.

Is either of these two processes responsible for triggering the release of the transmitter substance? This question was successfully approached by studies using two agents that selectively block one, but not the other, ion channel: tetrodotoxin blocks the Na$^+$ channel, and tetraethylammonium blocks the K$^+$ channel. As we have seen in Chapters 8 and 9, these agents are amazingly selective: tetrodotoxin does not affect the K$^+$ channel nor does it affect the slight resting leak of Na$^+$ that normally occurs through the membrane. Tetrodotoxin also does not interfere with properties of the postsynaptic receptors or of the channel that it controls. Thus, at a cholinergic synapse, which uses acetylcholine as a transmitter, tetrodotoxin blocks the presynaptic Na$^+$ spike, but ACh will still produce an excitatory synaptic potential when applied directly to the postsynaptic receptors. This is not surprising since, as we saw in the last chapter, the Na$^+$ channels activated by the action potential are distinct from those activated by the synaptic potential. These drugs are thus examples of a key principle of neuropharmacology. Certain drugs are able to act selectively at specific regions of the neuron and, in those regions, on specific molecular entities.

Na$^+$ Influx Is Not Necessary

To explore the contribution of Na$^+$ and K$^+$ to transmitter release, Katz and Ricardo Miledi utilized the giant synapse of the squid because it is large enough to allow the insertion of two electrodes into the presynaptic terminal (one for stimulating and one for recording), and, at the same time, a recording electrode into the postsynaptic cell (Figures 11–1A and 11–2A).

Before treatment with tetrodotoxin, the presynaptic cell produces a full-blown action potential of 110 mV, which leads to transmitter release and the generation of a large synaptic potential in the postsynaptic cell. In the presence of tetrodotoxin, the presynaptic action potential becomes progressively smaller with time and the postsynaptic potential is reduced (Figure 11–1B). As the presynaptic spike is reduced below 25–40 mV, the synaptic potential disappears. From these results it might appear that Na$^+$ influx is essential for transmitter release. However, with the Na$^+$ channels fully blocked, Katz and Miledi next artificially depolarized the presynaptic membrane in steps of up to 150 mV by passing current out of

the terminal through a second intracellular microelectrode. By this means they found that, as the terminal is depolarized beyond a threshold of 25–40 mV, progressively greater amounts of transmitter are released (as judged by the appearance and amplitude of the postsynaptic potential). In the range of depolarization at which chemical transmitter is released (about 40–70 mV), a 10-

11–1 Experiments at the squid giant synapse in the stellate ganglion show how gradually blocking the Na$^+$ channels with tetrodotoxin (TTX) progressively affects the amplitude of the presynaptic action potential and the resulting postsynaptic potential.

A. In this experimental arrangement, recording electrodes are inserted in both the pre- and postsynaptic fibers of the giant synapse.

B. As the amplitude of the presynaptic action potential gradually decreases with time after TTX is added, the postsynaptic potential also gradually decreases. **1:** 7 min after TTX is added, the presynaptic spike still produces a suprathreshold postsynaptic potential that triggers an action potential in the postsynaptic cell. **2 and 3:** 14 and 15 min after TTX is added, the presynaptic spike gradually becomes smaller and produces smaller postsynaptic potentials. **4:** When the presynaptic spike is reduced to 40 mV or less it fails to produce a postsynaptic action.

C. The gradual blockade of the Na$^+$ channel for the action potential can be used to obtain an input–output curve for transmitter release. **1:** In this experiment, the presynaptic spike had to be 40 mV to produce a postsynaptic potential. Beyond this threshold the relationship of the amplitude of the presynaptic spike to that of the postsynaptic potential is steep. **2:** As illustrated on the semilogarithmic plot of these data, the relationship between the presynaptic spike and the PSP is logarithmic; a 10-mV increase in the presynaptic spike produces a tenfold increase in the postsynaptic potential. (Parts A–C adapted from Katz and Miledi, 1967a.)

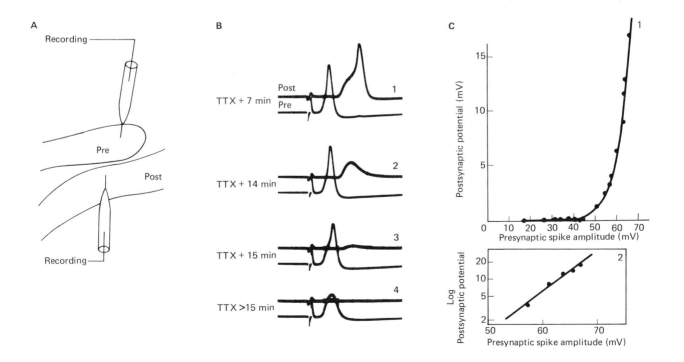

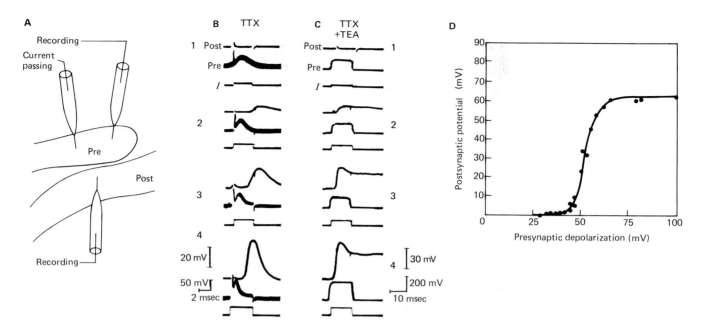

11–2 Blocking the voltage-sensitive Na$^+$ channels and K$^+$ channels in the presynaptic terminals with tetrodotoxin (TTX) and tetraethylammonium (TEA) affects the amplitude and duration of the presynaptic action potential and the resulting postsynaptic potential. It does not, however, block the capability to release transmitter, since postsynaptic potentials can still be produced by injecting depolarizing current presynaptically.

A. Experimental arrangement is the same as in Figure 11–1, except that a current-passing electrode has also been inserted into the presynaptic cell.

B. The Na$^+$ channels of the action potentials have been blocked with TTX. The three traces in each group represent (from bottom to top) the current pulse injected into the presynaptic terminal *(I)*, the resulting (electrotonic) potential in the presynaptic terminal **(Pre)**, and the postsynaptic potential generated in the postsynaptic cell **(Post)**. Progressively stronger current pulses produce correspondingly greater depolarizations of the presynaptic terminal and larger postsynaptic potentials. These depolarizations and the corresponding synaptic potentials are not maintained in amplitude throughout the duration of the depolarizing pulse because of the delayed activation of the K$^+$ current **(1–4)**.

C. After the Na$^+$ channels of the action potential were blocked with TTX, TEA was injected into the presynaptic terminal to block the K$^+$ channels (traces as in **B**). This now resulted in a maintained presynaptic depolarization and an increase in the duration of the postsynaptic potential in response to progressively stronger current pulses. Under these conditions, larger presynaptic depolarizations still produce larger postsynaptic potentials **(1–4)**.

D. A more complete input–output curve than that shown in Figure 11–1C systematically generates synaptic potentials as a function of different depolarization steps in TEA and TTX. (The initial level of the presynaptic membrane potential was about − 70 mV.) (Adapted from Katz and Miledi, 1967a.)

mV depolarization produces a tenfold increase in transmitter release (Figures 11–1C and 11–2D). Thus, in the absence of influx through voltage-sensitive Na$^+$ channels, the presynaptic terminal can still release the transmitter. A passive potential change in the terminal is just as effective in releasing transmitter and in producing a postsynaptic response in the absence as in the presence of Na$^+$. Therefore, the cause of the transmitter release is not the regenerative Na$^+$ entry that occurs during the action potential but some other event associated with the presynaptic depolarization.

K$^+$ Efflux Is Not Necessary

The opening of K$^+$ channels is unaffected by tetrodotoxin. This is demonstrated in Figure 11–2B by the decrease in presynaptic potential and in transmitter release during the current pulse. To examine the contribution of the K$^+$ efflux to transmitter release, Katz and Miledi used the same experimental setup as before but blocked both the voltage-sensitive K$^+$ and Na$^+$ channels by using tetraethylammonium and tetrodotoxin together (Figure 11–2). They then passed a depolarizing current through the presynaptic terminals and found that transmitter was released in amounts comparable to those produced by the normal action potential. Transmitter release was now maintained because the effective depolarization was maintained (Figure 11–2C); but otherwise the input–output curve of the synapse was unaltered (Figure 11–2D). Katz and Miledi therefore concluded that neither Na$^+$ nor K$^+$ is required for release. This discovery was important because it separated the ionic mechanisms responsible for the action potential from the mechanisms critical for transmitter release.

Ca⁺⁺ Influx Is Necessary

Because Ca^{++} was the major cation remaining, it became the next candidate for the ion critical to transmitter release. Indeed, even earlier, José del Castillo and Katz had found that Ca^{++} is required for transmitter release. Lowering the extracellular Ca^{++} concentration reduces and ultimately blocks synaptic transmission. Conversely, increasing the extracellular Ca^{++} concentration enhances transmitter release. The facilitating effect of Ca^{++} on synaptic transmission is blocked by Mg^{++}. Hodgkin and Baker had found that a small amount of Ca^{++} moves into the squid giant axon with each action potential through voltage-gated channels that are fairly selective for Ca^{++}. These channels, however, are sparsely distributed. Katz and Miledi therefore proposed that these Ca^{++} channels might be much more abundant at the terminal than they are in the axon and that Ca^{++} is not simply a carrier of charge (as are Na$^+$ and K$^+$), but that it serves as an intracellular messenger: Ca^{++} influx is the critical factor for coupling the action potential to transmitter secretion. Consistent with this prediction, they found that with the Na$^+$ and K$^+$ channels blocked by tetrodotoxin and tetraethylammonium, Ca^{++} influx actually produces a *secretory potential* in the terminals—a regenerative Ca^{++} action potential! This does not occur in the preterminal part of the axon because Ca^{++} channels are not sufficiently dense in the axon. Ca^{++} currents are small even in the terminal region, and consequently they are normally masked by the Na$^+$ and K$^+$ currents, which are

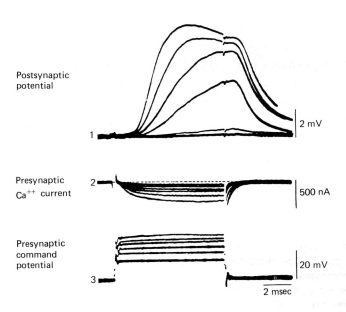

11–3 Transmitter release as a function of Ca^{++} influx into the presynaptic terminal. With the voltage-sensitive Na$^+$ and K$^+$ channels blocked by tetrodotoxin and tetraethylammonium, the amount of transmitter released (reflected by the size of the postsynaptic potentials in the top traces **[1]**) can be seen to correlate in a graded manner with the magnitude of the inward Ca^{++} current that accompanies the depolarization **(2)**. The presynaptic terminal was voltage-clamped and the membrane potential was stepped to six different command levels of depolarization **(3)**. (Adapted from Llinás, in Llinás and Heuser, 1977.)

11–4 This experiment at the nerve–muscle synapse of the frog demonstrates that Ca^{++} must be present for transmitter release. In turn, Mg^{++} can block release by antagonizing the action of Ca^{++}. **A.** The experimental chamber is devoid of Ca^{++} to block transmitter release and contains TTX to block action potentials. As a result, release from a set of terminals can be completely controlled by two external electrodes (**NaCl** for depolarizing the terminal and **CaCl₂** for injecting Ca^{++}). The consequences of transmitter release are recorded intracellularly from the muscle fiber. **B.** Electrical recordings of the postsynaptic response are shown in the **top traces**. A brief depolarizing pulse (**P**, bottom traces) is applied

through the NaCl electrode in each of three conditions: (1) alone, (2) just after a pulse of Ca^{++}, or (3) just before a pulse of Ca^{++}. Only when the Ca^{++} pulse precedes the depolarizing pulse by a critical interval is transmitter released (as indicated by the production of a postsynaptic potential). Thus, for Ca^{++} to be utilized, it must be present during the depolarization. **C.** In the presence of Ca^{++}, transmitter release is blocked by a pulse of Mg^{++}, a Ca^{++} antagonist. Transmitter release is again turned on by Ca^{++} when Mg^{++} is no longer present. The Mg^{++} is applied by a third pipette filled with MgCl, which is not shown in the diagram. (Adapted from Katz and Miledi, 1967b.)

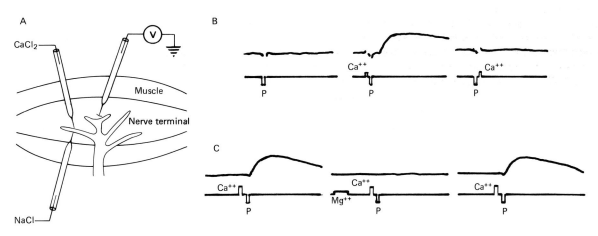

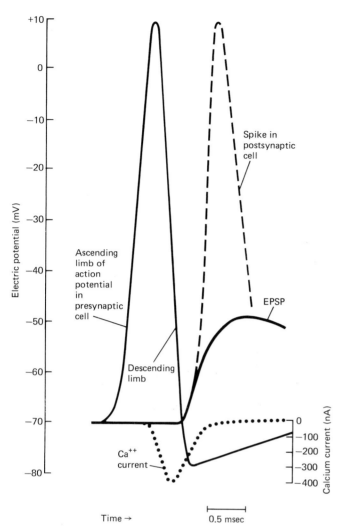

11–5 Comparison of the time course of four events related to synaptic transmission: (1) the presynaptic action potential, (2) the Ca^{++} current in the presynaptic neuron, (3) the synaptic potential (EPSP) in the postsynaptic cell, and (4) the action potential (spike) in the postsynaptic cell. An action potential in the presynaptic cell leads to the release of transmitter from the terminal by causing Ca^{++} channels to open and a Ca^{++} current to flow into the terminal. The Ca^{++} current is turned on only late during the presynaptic action potential during the falling phase. The postsynaptic response to the transmitter begins soon afterward and, if sufficiently large, will trigger an action potential in the postsynaptic cell. (Adapted from Llinás, 1982.)

10–20 times larger. Rodolfo Llinás and his colleagues have voltage-clamped the presynaptic terminals in the presence of tetrodotoxin and tetraethylammonium and shown directly that the graded depolarizations of the terminals activate an inward Ca^{++} current in a graded manner; the Ca^{++} influx that carries this current in turn leads to graded release of transmitter (Figure 11–3). Unlike the Na^{+} channels, the Ca^{++} channels do not inacti-

vate readily, but stay open as long as the presynaptic depolarization lasts.

To study the timing of the action of Ca^{++} and to find out at what stage of the presynaptic depolarization external Ca^{++} is involved, Katz and Miledi used a nerve–muscle preparation bathed in tetrodotoxin and Ca^{++}-free Ringer's solution. In addition to the normal microelectrode for recording inside the muscle fiber, they also used two external electrodes. One electrode, filled with NaCl, served as a stimulating electrode that depolarized the terminals, and the other electrode, filled with CaCl$_2$, was used to raise the local Ca^{++} concentration at a critical moment before or after the depolarizing pulse (Figure 11–4A). By this means Katz and Miledi found that Ca^{++} must be present during depolarization to produce transmitter release (Figure 11–4B). When the Ca^{++} pulse is delayed until the end of the depolarization, no release occurs. This action of Ca^{++} is once again blocked by Mg^{++} (Figure 11–4C).

These findings suggest that the depolarization produced by the action potential in the terminals opens the Ca^{++} channels. Ca^{++} can then move down its steep concentration gradient into the terminal and reach the sites from which transmitter is released. Indeed, the voltage clamp experiments of Llinás and his colleagues indicate that a large part of the synaptic delay—the time from the onset of the action potential in the presynaptic terminals to the onset of the synaptic potential in the postsynaptic cell—is due to the time that is required for the Ca^{++} channels to open in response to depolarization. Because of this delay, the Ca^{++} channels open and the Ca^{++} starts to flow only at the end of the action potential, as the membrane potential in presynaptic terminals begins to return to the resting level. Once the channels have opened, however, Ca^{++} diffuses only a short distance and acts within 0.2 msec to achieve transmitter release (Figure 11–5). As we shall see later in this chapter, the fact that the Ca^{++} channels begin to open only at the end of the action potential and do not inactivate readily makes the duration of the action potential an important determinant of the amount of Ca^{++} that flows into the terminal. If the action potential is prolonged, more Ca^{++} flows in to affect release.

Transmitter Is Released in Packets Called Quanta

How and where does Ca^{++} produce its actions? To answer that question we need to consider the quantal nature of transmitter release.

Although the release of synaptic transmitter substance appears graded, it has been shown to be quantized at all chemical synapses examined thus far. Each packet, or quantum, of transmitter gives rise to a small elementary unit of potential of fixed size (called the *unit synaptic potential* or *miniature synaptic potential*). The normal synaptic potential is made up of varying numbers of these unit potentials. The synaptic potentials and the input–output curves of Figures 11–1 and 11–2 appear to be graded because each unit potential is small and the number of units released is graded. Fatt and Katz discovered the quantal nature of transmission when they recorded at the nerve–muscle synapse of the frog in the absence of presynaptic stimulation. They observed small, spontaneously occurring potential changes of about 0.5–1.0 mV; similar results have been obtained in mammalian muscle. Because the synaptic potentials at vertebrate nerve–muscle synapses are called end-plate potentials (after the postsynaptic specialization called the end-plate region), Fatt and Katz called these small, spontaneously occurring potentials *miniature end-plate potentials.*

The time course of the miniature end-plate potentials and the effects of various drugs on them are almost indistinguishable from those seen when the end-plate potential is evoked by nerve stimulation. The nerve–muscle synapse in the frog uses ACh as its transmitter and, like the end-plate potentials, the miniature end-plate potentials are enhanced and prolonged by prostigmine, a compound that inhibits the hydrolysis of ACh by acetylcholinesterase. The miniature end-plate potentials are also abolished by agents that block the ACh receptor, such as *d*-tubocurarine. In the absence of stimulation the miniature end-plate potentials occur at random intervals. Their frequency can be increased by depolarizing the presynaptic terminal; they disappear if the presynaptic nerve degenerates and they reappear with reinnervation, indicating that they represent small amounts of ACh that are continuously being released at the presynaptic nerve terminal.

Now, how small is small? And what could account for the fixed size of the spontaneous miniature synaptic potentials? One possibility that had been suggested is that the unitary size of these potentials represents the responses of the receptor to single ACh molecules, and that the receptor response is quantized. Del Castillo and Katz tested this hypothesis by applying ACh iontophoretically to the frog muscle end-plate: a positive potential source was applied to an electrode containing acetylcholine chloride, and the positively charged transmitter molecules were moved electrophoretically out of the pipette in amounts controlled by current. Del Castillo and Katz failed, however, to find quantized receptor responses that resembled miniature end-plate potentials. The potential change produced by the interaction of the postsynaptic receptor with a single molecule of ACh could be shown to be much smaller than the 0.5-mV potential change produced by the miniature end-plate potential.

Katz and Miledi later were able to estimate the elementary ionic conductance event—the opening of a single synaptic channel caused by the interaction of two ACh molecules with a single ACh receptor. They did this by analyzing the fluctuations in membrane potential (ACh noise) produced by applying small amounts of ACh to the receptor membrane. They presumed that the small fluctuations in potential (noise) that resulted from the small amounts of ACh represent the sum of many randomly occurring channel openings and closings. Using "noise analysis," they estimated that the elementary ACh potential produced by the opening of a single conductance channel is only about 0.3 µV, or 1/1000 of the amplitude of a spontaneous miniature potential. As we saw in Chapter 9, this has been confirmed by Erwin Neher and Bert Sakmann, who, using patch clamp techniques, made direct measurements of the currents in single channels responsive to ACh.

To produce a miniature end-plate potential of 0.5 mV, the elementary depolarizations caused by the opening of about 1000 channels would have to summate. But it actually requires *more* than 1000 molecules of ACh to produce a miniature end-plate potential. For a single channel to open, two ACh molecules usually must bind to the receptor. In addition, some of the released ACh is lost by diffusion in the synaptic cleft or by hydrolysis and does not interact with receptor molecules at all. Thus, between 5000 and 10,000 molecules are necessary to produce a miniature end-plate potential. This number is similar to that estimated on the basis of direct chemical measurement of the ACh released. Thus, a miniature synaptic potential is produced not by a single molecule but by a packet containing up to 10,000 ACh molecules. As we shall see below, there is good reason to believe that these multimolecular packets of ACh are stored and released from the terminal by specialized organelles called *synaptic vesicles*, which are abundant in electron-microscopic pictures of synaptic terminals.

Amount of Ca^{++} Influx Affects the Number of Quanta Released

We can now ask some important questions: What happens during normal transmission? Are these packets the standard unit of release for ACh? Is ACh also released in quantal packets during synaptic transmission, or is it released in a continuously graded fashion? If ACh is released in quanta, one can go further and ask: How does Ca^{++} exert its action? Does Ca^{++} influence the size of each quantum by determining the number of ACh molecules packaged into each synaptic vesicle or, alternatively, does Ca^{++} influence the probability that a quantum (a synaptic vesicle) will be released?

These questions can be answered by decreasing the external concentraton of Ca^{++} and determining whether Ca^{++} acts on the size of the quantum or on the number of quanta released (Figure 11–6). Del Castillo and Katz found that when the neuromuscular junction was bathed in solutions low in Ca^{++}, the evoked end-plate potential (normally 70 mV) was reduced markedly (0.5–2.5 mV) and often failed. The minimum response above zero (the unit synaptic potential) was, however, identical in size and shape to the spontaneously occurring miniature end-plate potential, and the larger end-plate potentials were integral multiples of the unit potential. Thus, in histograms of the amplitude of the responses to a large number of stimuli, there is a peak of failures (zero responses) followed by a multimodal response distribution (Figure

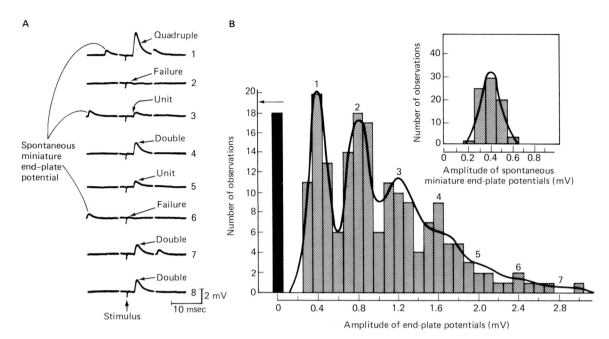

11–6 Comparison of the amplitudes of the spontaneous miniature end-plate potentials and the evoked end-plate potentials indicate that transmitter is released in quantal packages that are fixed in amplitude but variable in number.

A. Intracellular recording from a rat nerve–muscle synapse shows a few spontaneous miniature end-plate potentials and the synaptic responses (end-plate potentials) evoked by eight consecutive stimuli to the nerve. (The stimulus artifact evident in the records is produced by current flowing between the stimulating and recording electrodes in the bathing solution.) In a Ca^{++}-deficient (and Mg^{++}-rich) solution designed to reduce transmitter output, the end-plate potentials are small and show considerable fluctuations: two impulses produce complete failures (**2** and **6**), two produce a unit potential (**3** and **5**), and still others produce responses that are two to four times the amplitude of the unit potential. Comparison of the unit potential and the spontaneously occurring miniature end-plate potential illustrates that they are the same size. (Adapted from Liley, 1956.)

B. Distribution of amplitudes of the spontaneous miniature end-plate potentials and the evoked end-plate potentials. Synaptic transmission has again been reduced (this time with only a high-Mg^{++} solution). The histograms of the evoked end-plate potential illustrate peaks that occur at **1, 2, 3,** and **4** times the mean amplitude of the spontaneous potentials (0.4 mV). The distribution of the spontaneous miniature end-plate potentials shown in the **inset** is fitted with a Gaussian curve. The Gaussian distribution for the spontaneous miniature potentials is used to calculate a theoretical distribution of the evoked end-plate potential amplitudes (based on the Poisson equation) that predicts the number of failures, unit potentials, twin, triplet responses, and so on. The fit of the data to the theoretical distribution is remarkably good (**solid line**). Thus, the actual number of failures (**black bar at 0 mV**) was only slightly lower than the theoretically expected number of failures (**arrow above black bar**). (Adapted from Boyd and Martin, 1956.)

11–6B). The first response peak occurs at the voltage of the unit potential; this voltage is also identical to the amplitude of the spontaneous miniature end-plate potential. The voltage of each subsequent peak is an integral multiple of the value of the first response peak: that of the second response peak is twice that of the first, and that of the third peak is three times that of the first. The series of peaks is broad rather than sharply defined because of the statistical variation in the size of the individual miniature end-plate potentials (Figure 11–6B, inset). Thus, alterations in external Ca^{++} concentration do not affect the *number* of ACh molecules packaged into each quantum but the *probability* that a given quantum is released. As more Ca^{++} comes into the terminals, more quanta are released.

The dramatic stepwise fluctuations in the amplitude of the end-plate potentials at low levels of release and the

finding that the unit potential has the same mean amplitude as the spontaneously released miniature end-plate potentials prompted del Castillo and Katz to propose the *quantal hypothesis* for synaptic transmission. According to this hypothesis, the normal end-plate potential (60 mV) is caused by the release of more than 200 quanta. The amplitude of the end-plate potential in response to consecutive stimuli fluctuates because the exact number of quanta released varies slightly from stimulus to stimulus.

Quantal transmission has been demonstrated at all chemical synapses so far examined. However, at the vast majority of synapses each action potential releases not 200 quanta, as it does at the nerve–muscle synapse, but a much smaller number ranging typically between 1 and 10. Thus, the excitatory synapses made onto the motor neurons by the afferent fibers from a single sensory neuron, which we considered in the last chapter, release on the average only 1 quantum per presynaptic action potential.

Morphological studies indicate that in the resting state the presynaptic terminal contains accumulations of synaptic vesicles, which are thought to serve as packages for transmitter (discussed in Chapters 12 and 13). Each vesicle contains one quantum (several thousand molecules) of transmitter. The vesicles are thought to fuse to the inner surface of the presynaptic terminal at specific release sites. The fused vesicle then opens transiently and extrudes its entire contents, in an all-or-none fashion, into the extracellular space of the synaptic cleft by a process of exocytosis (reverse pinocytosis).

What is the relationship between the quantal mechanism of release and the Ca^{++} hypothesis? Katz and Miledi proposed that Ca^{++}, brought into the terminal by the action potential, interacts with specialized release sites inside the terminal, where it causes or facilitates a transient fusion of the vesicular membrane with the terminal membrane, thereby enhancing the probability that a given quantum of transmitter will be released (Figure 11–7). The fact that Ca^{++} acts so rapidly once its channels are open suggests that the Ca^{++} channels must be located near the active sites where the vesicles fuse to the membrane. It is not known whether Ca^{++} promotes fusion directly or whether it acts together with a Ca^{++}-binding protein, such as calmodulin or a related molecule, that promotes fusion. There is also some evidence from Joseph Dudel, Hannah Parnas, and Itzhak Parnas indicating that at some synapses the ease with which Ca^{++} promotes fusion may be voltage dependent.

This theoretical schema has proved very important not only for understanding synaptic transmission, but also because it helps explain the final issues that we want to consider: the special, plastic properties of chemical synapses that make them sensitive to their previous history. The plastic capabilities of chemical synapses derive from the fact that the Ca^{++} channels of the terminals, which control transmitter release, are, in turn, controlled by two factors: (1) membrane potential and (2) synaptic input, each of which is capable of exerting a long-term effect.

Amount of Transmitter Release Can Be Controlled by Altering Ca^{++} Influx

As we saw in Chapter 9, one property of chemical synapses that is lacking in electrical synapses is flexibility: chemical synapses are sensitive to their previous history. The process by which the effectiveness of chemical synapses can change as a result of their previous pattern of activity is called *synaptic plasticity*. Two classes of regulatory processes can produce short-term changes in synaptic effectiveness: (1) intrinsic processes within the neuron, such as changes in the membrane potential and activity, and (2) extrinsic processes such as the synaptic input of other neurons that produce presynaptic inhibi-

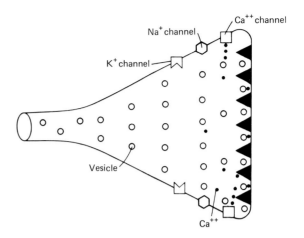

11–7 An action potential in the presynaptic terminal membrane of a neuron opens a number of Ca^{++} channels (**squares**) in parallel with the Na^{+} channels of the membrane (**hexagons**), leading to an increase in influx of Ca^{++}. In the presynaptic terminals Ca^{++} is thought to be important in allowing the vesicles to bind to release sites.

tion or facilitation. Each of these factors can modify the influx or accumulation of Ca^{++} within the presynaptic terminal.

Intrinsic Regulatory Processes (Membrane Potential and Activity) Can Alter Ca^{++} Influx and Accumulation within the Terminal

Intrinsic regulatory processes are mechanisms within the cell that affect how much transmitter will be released. In some cells there is a small steady influx of Ca^{++} across the membrane of the presynaptic terminals even at the resting level of the membrane potential. This influx is thought to occur through a class of Ca^{++} channels that is voltage dependent and inactivates very little, if at all. This resting Ca^{++} influx is enhanced by depolarization and decreased by hyperpolarization. Because of the steep dependence of transmitter release on intracellular Ca^{++} concentration, small changes in this steady-state Ca^{++} influx into terminals produce significant changes in the amount of Ca^{++} that accumulates in the terminals and therefore in the amount of transmitter released. Thus, a slight decrease in membrane potential (depolarization)—produced artificially by injected current or naturally by transmitter substances—can increase the steady-state Ca^{++} influx and enhance the amount of transmitter released by subsequent action potentials. A slight increase in membrane potential has the opposite effect (Figure 11–8). Slight changes in the resting membrane potential of the synaptic terminal can therefore alter the amount of Ca^{++} influx into the terminal and make an effective synapse inoperative or a weak synaptic connection highly effective.

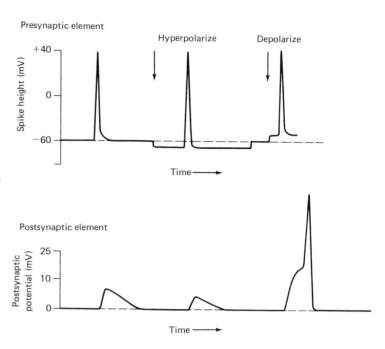

11–8 Changes in membrane potentials of the presynaptic terminal affect the amount of transmitter released as assayed by measuring the amplitude of the postsynaptic potential. When the membrane potential of the presynaptic terminal is at the normal resting potential, an action potential produces a postsynaptic potential of about 8 mV. When it is hyperpolarized by 10 mV, the steady-state (leakage) Ca^{++} influx is decreased and the presynaptic spike produces a postsynaptic potential of only 5 mV. When the presynaptic neuron is returned to the resting level and then depolarized by 10 mV, the steady-state Ca^{++} influx is increased and the resulting presynaptic action potential produces a synaptic potential of 15 mV, which triggers an action potential in the postsynaptic cell.

11–9 Intracellular recordings demonstrate posttetanic potentiation of postsynaptic potentials by a high rate of activity in the presynaptic neuron. To show events that occur over a long time, the sweep speed of this experiment has been compressed so that the amplitude of each presynaptic potential and the postsynaptic potential it produces appears as a simple line. During the control period the presynaptic neuron is stimulated at a rate of 1 per sec and a postsynaptic potential of about 1 mV is produced. The presynaptic neuron is then stimulated for several seconds at a higher rate of 5 per sec. During this tetanic stimulation, the postsynaptic potential increases in size. This increase is called facilitation. After several seconds of stimulation, the presynaptic neuron is returned to its control rate of firing of 1 per sec; however, the postsynaptic potential it produces continues to be facilitated for many minutes and, in the synapses of some cells, for several hours. This facilitation, which persists after the tetanus, is called *posttetanic potentiation*.

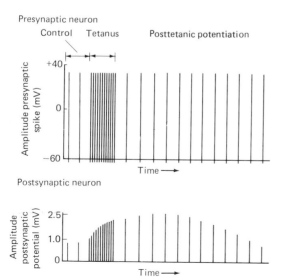

In many cells activity can affect synaptic effectiveness. In particular, a train of high-frequency action potentials will be followed by a period during which each subsequent spike will produce a larger EPSP than normal. The high rate of stimulation of the presynaptic neuron (which for some cells can reach 500–1000 action potentials/sec or even higher) is called a *tetanic stimulation*: the increase in the size of the EPSP during tetanic stimulation is called *facilitation*. The facilitation that persists after the tetanic stimulation is called *posttetanic potentiation*; this enhancement usually lasts several minutes but it can persist for 1 hr or more in some cells (Figure 11–9).

Posttetanic potentiation has been shown to result from a transient saturation of the Ca^{++} buffering systems in the terminals (the mitochondria and the endoplasmic reticulum) owing to the relatively large influx of Ca^{++} that occurs during a train of action potentials. This *residual* Ca^{++} increases the concentration of free Ca^{++} in the terminals and thereby enhances synaptic transmission for many minutes or longer.

Here then is the simplest kind of memory! This neuron remembers that it has generated a train of impulses by increasing the intracellular concentration of Ca^{++} in its terminals, and now each action potential in the presynaptic neuron, playing upon this memory, produces more transmitter release than before.

Extrinsic Regulatory Processes (Presynaptic Inhibition and Facilitation) Can Also Alter Ca^{++} Influx and Accumulation

Extrinsic regulatory processes are those that involve other cells that synapse on the presynaptic terminals of a neuron and influence transmitter release. Neurons inner-

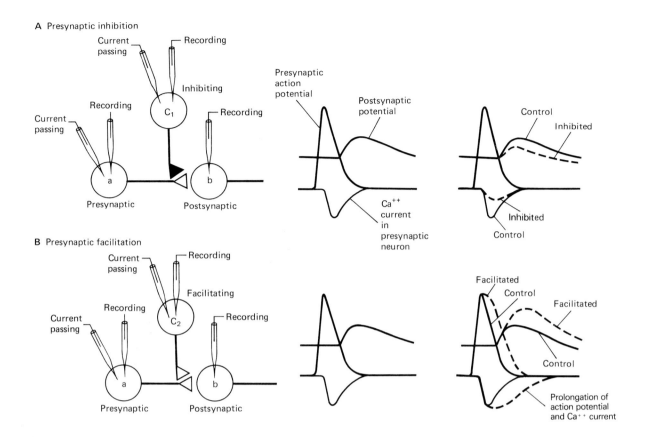

11–10 Axo-axonic synapses can inhibit or facilitate transmitter release by altering Ca^{++} influx. In each example three cells are shown: a presynaptic cell (**a**), a postsynaptic cell (**b**), and either a presynaptic inhibitory neuron (C_1), or a presynaptic facilitating neuron (C_2). **A.** Presynaptic inhibition occurs as the result of the activity of the presynaptic inhibitory neuron, which causes a depression of the Ca^{++} current accompanying the action potential of the presynaptic neuron. Because the decreased Ca^{++} influx leads to a reduction in the amount of transmitter released, the synaptic potential recorded in the postsynaptic cell is depressed. **B.** Presynaptic facilitation occurs as a result of the activity of the presynaptic facilitating neuron. This causes a depression of the K^+ current in the presynaptic neuron, leading to an increase in the duration of the action potential and therefore of the Ca^{++} current. Consequently, transmitter release is increased and, as a result, so is the amplitude of the synaptic potential recorded in the postsynaptic cell.

vate each other not only at the cell body and dendrites, where they can control impulse activity, but also at their terminals, where they can control transmitter release. The synapses that one presynaptic terminal makes with another are called *axo-axonic* or *presynaptic*. Axo-axonic synapses can exert their actions because the presynaptic terminals of certain neurons contain receptors for various transmitters *(presynaptic receptors)*. Some neurons even have receptors to their own transmitter on their terminals; these are called *autoreceptors*. Presynaptic receptors are thought to exert their action in several ways. One important way is by controlling the Ca^{++} current of the terminals.

The presynaptic actions of neurons can either depress or enhance transmitter release, processes called *presynaptic inhibition* and *presynaptic facilitation*, respectively (Figure 11–10). The best analyzed instances of presynaptic inhibition and facilitation are in the neurons of invertebrate animals and in mechanoreceptor afferent neurons (dorsal root ganglion cells) of vertebrates studied in dissociated cell tissue culture. These studies and those in the intact spinal cord of mammals indicate that there are at least two mechanisms for presynaptic inhibition. One is due to a synaptically mediated depression of the Ca^{++} current, leading to a decrease in the influx of Ca^{++} into the terminal. The other is due to an increased conductance to Cl^- that leads to a decrease (or short-circuiting) in the height of the action potential in the

presynaptic terminal. As a result, less depolarization is produced, fewer Ca^{++} channels are activated by the action potential, and, therefore, less Ca^{++} flows into the terminals.

Conversely, presynaptic facilitation is due to enhanced influx of Ca^{++}. The transmitter acts to depress a K^+ current, thereby broadening the action potential and allowing the Ca^{++} influx to persist for a longer period of time (Figure 11–10).

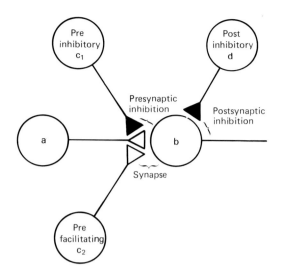

11–11 In presynaptic actions, the inhibitory neuron (**c₁**) or facilitating neuron (**c₂**) acts on the terminals of the presynaptic neuron (**a**); in postsynaptic inhibition, the inhibitory neuron (**d**) acts on the cell body or dendrite of the postsynaptic neuron (**b**).

The distinction between the pre- and postsynaptic actions of neurons is important, so let us make sure that it is clear. We shall use inhibition as an example, as illustrated in Figure 11–11. *Post*synaptic inhibition is a process in which one neuron (cell *d*) hyperpolarizes the cell body or dendrites of another (cell *b*), thereby decreasing the likelihood of cell *b* firing. In contrast, during *pre*synaptic inhibition, a neuron (cell *c₁*) may have no effect on the membrane potential of the presynaptic terminals of another cell (cell *a*), and therefore no effect on its probability of firing; however, it can reduce the amount of transmitter released by cell *a* to another cell (cell *b*). This action is presynaptic because it is exerted on the presynaptic terminals rather than at the trigger zone of cell *a*; it is inhibitory because it interferes with transmitter release.

Presynaptic actions tend to occur at points of sensory inflow. For example, presynaptic inhibition is found in the retina, spinal cord, and dorsal column nuclei. Presynaptic actions are useful because they allow selective control of the actions of individual branches of a neuron.

Thus, a variety of different mechanisms for synaptic plasticity share aspects of a common action—the regulation of the free Ca^{++} concentration in the presynaptic terminal. Whereas we now know a fair amount about short-term changes in synaptic effectiveness—changes that last minutes and hours—we know little about long-term changes that persist days, weeks, and longer. It is quite likely that these long-term changes will involve more than alterations in Ca^{++} and will also require structural changes in the machinery of the synapse.

An Overall View

In his book entitled *Ionic Channels in Excitable Membranes*, Bertil Hille summarizes the importance of Ca^{++} in the regulation of neuronal function:

Electricity is used to gate channels and channels are used to make electricity. However, the nervous system is not primarily an electrical device. Most excitable cells ultimately translate their electrical excitation into another form of activity. As a broad generalization, excitable cells translate their electricity into action by Ca^{++} fluxes modulated by voltage-sensitive Ca^{++} channels. Calcium ions are intracellular messengers capable of activating many cell functions.

. . . Ca^{++} channels . . . serve as the only link to transduce depolarization into all the nonelectrical activities controlled by excitation. Without Ca^{++} channels our nervous system would have no outputs.

What are the molecular mechanisms by which Ca^{++} leads to transmitter release? This is one of the pressing questions in neurobiology today. One possibility is that Ca^{++} simply acts to facilitate directly the physical fusion of two lipid bilayer membranes, that of the vesicle membrane and that of the external membrane. A second possibility is that Ca^{++} acts through one or more Ca^{++}-sensitive proteins such as calmodulin, a calmodulin-sensitive protein kinase, or a phospholipid kinase to accomplish vesicle fusion. The importance of calmodulin and certain Ca^{++}-dependent protein kinases in nonneuronal secretory processes makes it likely that steps such as these will be involved in at least certain central synapses. The next task for understanding transmitter release, therefore, is clear. To follow Ca^{++}, we need to move from the membrane channel to the regulatory machinery for release within the cell.

Selected Readings

Kandel, E. R. 1981. Calcium and the control of synaptic strength by learning. Nature 293:697–700.

Katz, B. 1969. The Release of Neural Transmitter Substances. Springfield, Ill.: Thomas.

Katz, B., and Miledi, R. 1967a. A study of synaptic transmission in the absence of nerve impulses. J. Physiol. (Lond.) 192:407–436.

Klein, M., Shapiro, E., and Kandel, E. R. 1980. Synaptic plasticity and the modulation of the Ca^{2+} current. J. Exp. Biol. 89:117–157.

Kretz, R., Shapiro, E., Connor, J., and Kandel, E. R. 1984. Post-tetanic potentiation, presynaptic inhibition, and the modulation of the free Ca^{++} level in the presynaptic terminals. *Exp. Brain Res.* Suppl. 9:240–256.

Llinás, R. R. 1982. Calcium in synaptic transmission. Sci. Am. 247(4):56–65.

Martin, A. R. 1977. Junctional transmission. II: Presynaptic mechanisms. In E. R. Kandel (ed.), Handbook of Physiology, Vol. 1: The Nervous System, Part 1. Bethesda, Md.: American Physiological Society, pp. 329–355.

Neher, E., and Sakmann, B. 1976. Single-channel currents recorded from membrane of denervated frog muscle fibres. Nature 260:799–802.

Reichardt, L. F., and Kelly, R. B. 1983. A molecular description of nerve terminal function. Annu. Rev. Biochem. 52:871–926.

References

Baker, P. F., Hodgkin, A. L., and Ridgway, E. B. 1971. Depolarization and calcium entry in squid giant axons. J. Physiol. (Lond.) 218:709–755.

Boyd, I. A., and Martin, A. R. 1956. The end-plate potential in mammalian muscle. J. Physiol. (Lond.) 132:74–91.

Del Castillo, J., and Katz, B. 1954. The effect of magnesium on the activity of motor nerve endings. J. Physiol. (Lond.) 124:553–559.

Erulkar, S. D., and Rahamimoff, R. 1978. The role of calcium ions in tetanic and post-tetanic increase of miniature end-plate potential frequency. J. Physiol. (Lond.) 278:501–511.

Fatt, P., and Katz, B. 1952. Spontaneous subthreshold activity at motor nerve endings. J. Physiol. (Lond.) 117:109–128.

Hille, B. 1984. Ionic Channels in Excitable Membranes. Sunderland, Mass.: Sinauer.

Katz, B., and Miledi, R. 1967b. The timing of calcium action during neuromuscular transmission. J. Physiol. (Lond.) 189:535–544.

Liley, A. W. 1956. The quantal components of the mammalian end-plate potential. J. Physiol. (Lond.) 133:571–587.

Llinás, R. R., and Heuser, J. E. 1977. Depolarization-release coupling systems in neurons. Neurosci. Res. Program Bull. 15:555–687.

Llinás, R., Steinberg, I. Z., and Walton, K. 1981. Relationship between presynaptic calcium current and postsynaptic potential in squid giant synapse. Biophys. J. 33:323–351.

Nicoll, R. A. 1982. Neurotransmitters can say more than just "yes" or "no". Trends Neurosci. 5:369–374.

Smith, S. J., Augustine, G. J., and Charlton, M. P. 1985. Transmission at voltage-clamped giant synapse of the squid: Evidence for cooperativity of presynaptic calcium action. Proc. Natl. Acad. Sci. U.S.A. 82:622–625.

Michael D. Gershon, James H. Schwartz, and Eric R. Kandel

Morphology of Chemical Synapses and Patterns of Interconnection

12

Physiology is concerned primarily with the analysis of function in *time*; in contrast, morphology is concerned with the analysis of function in *space*. Thus, morphological studies have revealed that the communication between nerve cells or between neurons and effector cells is mediated by one of two types of spatially discrete membrane specializations. The two types of synapses are unrelated ontogenetically. Electrical synapses, which correspond to the gap junctions found in many other epithelial cell types in the body, interconnect the cytoplasm of two adjacent cells and permit small molecules to flow between them. Chemical synapses, however, are regions of the neuron specialized for the release and reception of neurotransmitter. Ontogenetically, the presynaptic specializations of chemical synapses can be considered to have differentiated from subcellular components used in the universal process of secretion.

In this chapter we shall focus on the fine structure of chemical synapses. Morphological studies have shown that several subclasses of chemical synapses exist. In addition, improved techniques have recently yielded new insights into the mechanisms by which vesicles are released and vesicular membrane is recycled.

Chemical Synapses Can Be Classified into Directed and Nondirected Types

The chemical synapse includes the region of the transmitting neuron where neurotransmitter is released and the receptor region of the target cell. The transmitting region of a neuron is, in many instances, a well-differentiated structure at the end of an axonal process, but there are many variations. For example, transmitter can be released directly from cell bodies or even from dendrites. Thus, the usual histological division of a neuron into receptive and transmitter poles does not always apply. The dendritic arbor may be both receptive and transmitting. Although the geometries of axon terminals vary greatly, some subcellular features within the presynaptic element are characteristic. Essentially invariable is a high concentration of vesicles, not always uniform in size, but usually with diameters ranging from 30 to 150 nm. Mitochondria are consistently observed at synapses. Frequently seen, but not always present, are specializations at the plasma membrane that will be described later in this chapter.

Chemical synaptic transmission is a form of neurosecretion in which the area of the postsynaptic target and its distance from the presynaptic site of transmitter release vary among different types of synapses. This variability is physiologically significant and accounts for an important feature of chemical synapses—their degree of *directedness*. The most directed synapses release their transmitter onto a postsynaptic area of less than 1 μm^2 at a distance of 30 nm from the release site; these dimensions vary greatly in other types of synapses. Nondirected neurons, the neuroendocrine cells, release hormones into the blood stream that signal distant targets. Synapses of the autonomic (or visceral) nervous system are probably an intermediate form, working over a large but local area.

The synaptic cleft of directed synapses is sometimes filled with a meshwork of fibrous materials that are only now being characterized morphologically and biochemically. The *postsynaptic element* is the most difficult part of the synapse to typify. The receptor area is greatly dependent on the cell type and the region of the cell on which the connection occurs. It can be simple, showing no morphological differences from noninnervated regions of the same cell, or complex, showing many specialized membranous features not seen in surrounding noninnervated regions.

To illustrate the importance of distance and target area as physiological features, we shall first consider two well-studied peripheral synapses that have served as models for directed and relatively nondirected synapses: the neuromuscular junction (the synapse between motor neurons and skeletal muscle), and the synapse between autonomic postganglionic neurons and their targets. We shall then examine the synapses in the central nervous system, where forms resembling both extremes as well as a family of transitional types occur.

The Nerve–Skeletal Muscle Synapse Is an Example of a Directed Synapse

Chemical synapses can be conveniently divided into two components: (1) the presynaptic component, which is secretory; and (2) the postsynaptic component, which is receptive and transductive. The synaptic cleft separates them. Using primarily the nerve–muscle synapse (Figure 12–1) as a prototype, we shall examine each of these components in detail.

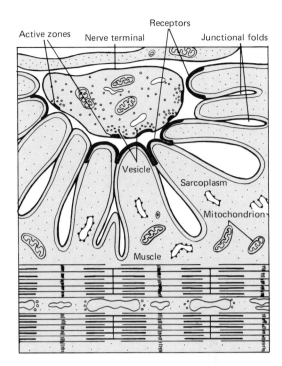

12–1 The vertebrate neuromuscular junction is a highly directed chemical synapse that contains all the elements characteristic of this type of synapse. There are specific active zones in the presynaptic terminal from which vesicles release transmitter by exocytosis. The active zones lie in appropriate apposition to specialized regions of muscle, the end-plate regions, that contain a high density of acetylcholine receptors.

The Presynaptic Terminal: Vesicles, Exocytosis, and the Active Zone

An essential feature of the presynaptic terminal is an accumulation of vesicles, membranous sacs that are thought to contain chemical transmitter. The discovery of this array of vesicles in terminals in the first electron micrographs of synapses occurred about the same time as the physiological observations of del Castillo and Katz, which indicated that transmitter release is quantal. These electron micrographs suggested to del Castillo and Katz, in 1957, that vesicles are the structural unit of quantal release. They imagined that the whole extent of presynaptic membrane contains release sites and that the vesicles mill around the nerve terminals in Brownian motion; when a vesicle strikes a release site it initiates the exocytotic release process. The idea that release sites are distributed along the whole presynaptic membrane is consistent with Sherrington's original view of the synapse as an extensive area of functional contact between cells—a region where the electrical activity of one neuron is brought to bear upon another.

Active Zones. Within several years of del Castillo and Katz's proposal, Sanford Palay at Harvard Medical School obtained high-resolution electron micrographs of central nervous system synapses. These pictures revealed that

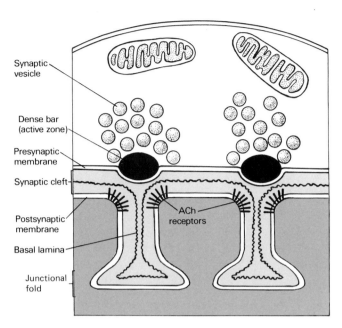

Synaptic vesicle

Dense bar (active zone)

Presynaptic membrane

Synaptic cleft

Postsynaptic membrane

Basal lamina

Junctional fold

ACh receptors

12–2   This diagram of a transmission electron micrograph shows the active zones at a neuromuscular junction. Note the clustering of small, clear synaptic vesicles (40–50 nm) around dense bars in the synaptic terminals and the clustering of ACh receptors at the apices of junctional folds. The line running through the synaptic cleft is the basal lamina. Cholinesterase attaches to the collagen of the basal lamina. Compare this view with the diagram in Figure 12–3B. (Adapted from Kuffler, Nicholls, and Martin, 1984.)

synaptic vesicles are not uniformly distributed along the entire length of the presynaptic membrane but, rather, are clustered at regions where the neighboring membranes of two neurons appear thicker and more dense than elsewhere.

Using tissue treated with phosphotungstic acid (a method first introduced to stain contractile proteins in muscle and in neurons), René Couteaux in Paris found that the presynaptic thickening is not an increased thickness of the plasma membrane itself, but a paramembranous specialization consisting of a series of dense bars attached to the internal face of the membrane (Figure 12–2). These dense bars are located directly above the postsynaptic (junctional) folds in the muscle. The synaptic vesicles collect in rows along the edges of these bars, where Couteaux occasionally found images that he interpreted to be vesicles undergoing exocytosis. He therefore called the transverse dense bars and the aligned vesicles the *active zone*, the term now used to describe the specialized and restricted regions within the presynaptic terminal where transmitter is actually released.

The discovery of the dense bars indicated that synaptic vesicles collect preferentially around specific points in the presynaptic membrane, from which they seemed destined to discharge. But are these the only sites where exocytosis occurs? This question is difficult to investigate

in conventionally fixed tissue, because the chance of finding a discharging vesicle is extremely small. For example, a thin section through a terminal at the neuromuscular junction of the frog shows only 1/4000 of the total prejunctional membrane.

Freeze-Fracture Reveals the Panoramic Interior of Synaptic Membranes. Because only relatively small areas of synaptic membrane can be examined in the ultrathin sections (50–100 nm) required for transmission electron microscopy, and because the exocytotic opening of each vesicle is less than the thickness of the section, many workers in the 1970s began to apply freeze-fracture techniques to this problem. With these techniques, frozen tissue is fractured or broken open in a high vacuum, and the freshly exposed surface is replicated by evaporating platinum and carbon on it. The advantage of this approach is that the fracture tends to split the frozen membranes through their hydrophobic interiors between the bimolecular layer of lipids. Fracture occurs there because the lipid bilayer is weakest in the middle, where the bimolecular leaflets of lipid are held together only by noncovalent interactions between the hydrophobic ends of lipid molecules. Two complementary fracture faces result: the face of the half-membrane bordering the interior of the cell is called the protoplasmic (P) face, and the face that borders the extracellular space is the external (E) face. Because freeze-fracture normally exposes not the true surface of the cell but an intramembranous view, large expanses of the presynaptic area are revealed. Consequently, deformations of the active zone membrane that occur where synaptic vesicles are attached are readily apparent and easily mapped (Figure 12–3A). The comprehensive view of the region of active zones that the freeze-fracture technique offers is best appreciated by comparing Figure 12–3B with the conventional transmission electron-microscopic image of the active zone (Figure 12–2).

Using freeze-fracture, Thomas Reese and John Heuser made four key observations: (1) The dense bars described by Couteaux are easily identified because they displace the plasmalemma slightly toward the mouth of the subadjacent transverse fold. (2) One or two rows of unusually large intramembranous particles lie along both margins of each bar (Figures 12–3B and 12–4A). These large intramembranous particles seem to be permanent specializations involved in vesicle discharge. Their function is not yet known, but they may represent the Ca^{++} channels. This idea would be consistent with the voltage clamp data obtained by Llinás (discussed in Chapter 11), which indicate that the synaptic delay between the onset of the Ca^{++} current and the release of transmitter at the squid giant synapse is short. This short latency suggests that the Ca^{++} channels and the vesicle release sites are very near one another. (3) During synaptic activity, deformations become apparent alongside the rows of intramembranous particles (Figure 12–4B), which is exactly the region of nerve terminal where electron-microscopic thin

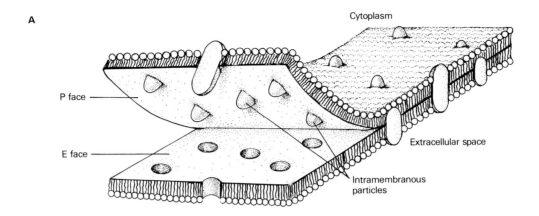

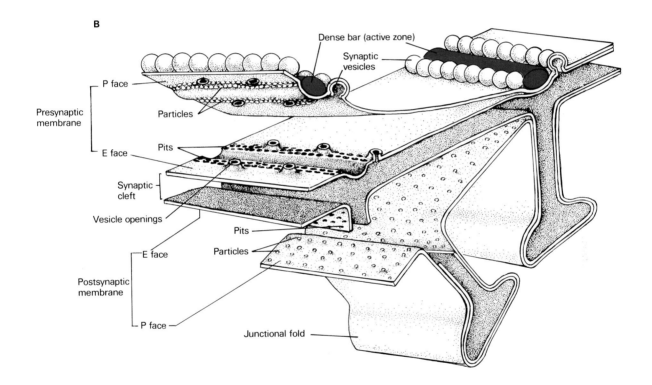

12–3 Freeze-fracture techniques reveal details of synaptic membrane structure. The cytosolic projections of integral membrane proteins are anchored to cytoskeletal elements to restrict the appropriate proteins to the active zone. **A.** In the freeze-fracture method, the lipid bilayer is split. The path of membrane cleavage is along the hydrophobic interior of the lipid bilayer, resulting in two complementary fracture faces. The inner half-membrane, or P face, faces the exterior and contains most of the projecting globular proteins (particles). The outer half-membrane, or E face, is directed toward the P face and shows pits complementary to the protein particles. (From Fawcett, 1981.) **B.** This three-dimensional view of pre- and postsynaptic membranes shows active zones and an immediately adjacent row of synaptic vesicles. The plasma membranes are split to illustrate structures observed upon freeze-fracturing. (Adapted from Kuffler, Nicholls, and Martin, 1984.)

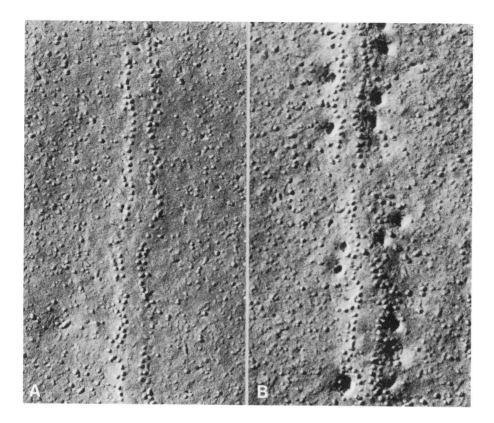

12–4 Detailed structure of the presynaptic active zone of the frog neuromuscular junction is shown by freeze-fracture replicas made after the nerve has been stimulated. **A.** After 3 msec, there is as yet no evidence of fusion of synaptic vesicles. A double row of intramembranous particles is seen extending down the P face of the presynaptic membrane. These membrane proteins may be Ca^{++} channels or structural proteins to which vesicles attach. **B.** After 5 msec the stimulation has caused synaptic vesicles to fuse with the presynaptic membrane and form pockets representing vesicles in exocytosis. (Courtesy of J. E. Heuser and T. S. Reese.)

sections show invagination of the plasmalemma. (4) These deformations do not persist after the transmitter has been released; rather, they seem to be transient distortions that occur only at the very moment of vesicle discharge.

Thus, morphological traces of the exocytotic process are visible in the presynaptic membrane when the nerves are fixed during stimulation (under conditions of enhanced quantal release) and are almost never present when the nerves are fixed at rest. Although these results are consistent with the idea that vesicles are vehicles for quantal transmission, they do not provide compelling quantitative evidence.

To catch vesicles in the act of exocytosis, a quick-freezing machine has been constructed that flings tissue onto a copper block cooled by liquid helium. This device also allows stimulation of the presynaptic axon in flight so that the tissue is frozen at precisely defined intervals after the nerve has been stimulated. The neuromuscular junction can thus be caught just as the action potential invades the terminal and exocytosis occurs. Using this device and the drug 4-aminopyridine (a tetraethylammoniumlike substance that blocks K^+ channels, broadens the action potential, and increases the number of quanta discharged with each nerve impulse), Heuser, Reese, and their colleagues have studied the morphological events accompanying exocytosis quantitatively.

Their observations of vesicles during exocytosis at the frog neuromuscular junction indicate that one vesicle un-

dergoes exocytosis for each quantum of transmitter that is discharged. Statistical analyses of the spatial distribution of synaptic vesicle discharge sites along the active zones show that individual vesicles fuse with the plasma membrane independently of one another. This result is expected from the physiological studies indicating that quanta are discharged independently. These studies therefore provide independent and direct morphological evidence that the synaptic vesicle is the transmitter storage organelle and that exocytosis is the release mechanism.

Recycling of Vesicle Membranes. If no process compensated for exocytosis, the membrane of the terminal would be enlarged as a result of nerve stimulation, because vesicle membrane would be added continuously to the plasmalemma. The expected increase does not occur, however, because the vesicle membrane added to the terminal membrane is retrieved and recycled.

Neurons stimulated extensively show a depletion of vesicles but a conservation of membrane. The total amount of membrane in vesicles, cisternae, and plasma membrane remains constant. Additional evidence for the recycling of membranes has come from studies using the enzyme horseradish peroxidase, whose reaction product can be located by electron microscopy. Some of the vesicles entering the terminal by endocytosis are also marked by coats of the protein clathrin; horseradish peroxidase probably enters the clathrin-coated endocytotic vesicles as a bulk marker. Most of the horseradish peroxidase first taken up into stimulated axons appears in coated vesicles. Tracer eventually appears in cisternae, and finally, after a period of rest, in synaptic vesicles. It is subsequently released from these vesicles when the nerve is again stimulated. The retrieval of vesicle membrane can also be shown by binding cationized ferritin to the membrane. Results from such studies indicate that this process is specific: the only membrane component retrieved is the membrane of the synaptic vesicle.

The precise ways in which recycling takes place have not yet been fully determined. One mechanism, based on the work of Miller and Heuser, is shown in Figure 12–5. According to this explanation for the retrieval of vesicle at the nerve-muscle synapse, excess membrane contributed to the plasmalemma of the terminal by vesicles that have undergone exocytosis is recycled by one of two routes.

The first pathway is believed to be the major endocytotic process for recycling membrane at normal physiological rates of stimulation. This is the slower of the two processes, peaking at 30 sec after exocytosis and lasting for more than 1 min. In this pathway, excess membrane

anywhere in the terminal except at the active zone forms a pit coated with clathrin. The clathrin coat forms a regular lattice around the pit, which finally pinches off as a small coated vesicle (Figure 12–5, pathway 1). After shedding this clathrin coat, these vesicles can serve again as synaptic (exocytotic) vesicles.

The second pathway handles only a small portion of the membrane, and the amounts recycled through it are thought to be significant only at unphysiologically high rates of stimulation. In this process, membrane is taken up directly and rapidly from the plasmalemma and reenters the terminal as large, uncoated vacuoles or cisternae (Figure 12–5, pathway 2). Most of this uptake occurs close to the release site, but some membrane can also be retrieved away from the active zone.

Some of the retrieved membrane is not recycled into functioning vesicles but is degraded. The studies with horseradish peroxidase described above have shown that, during synaptic activity, some of the tracer ultimately winds up in cell bodies within lysosomes. Therefore, synaptic vesicle membrane turnover involves retrograde axonal transport of membranes to the cell body for further processing, including lysosomal degradation. The old and

12–5 Vesicle membrane at the frog neuromuscular junction can be recycled through two pathways. In the first and physiologically most important pathway **(1)**, excess membrane is retrieved by means of coated pits. These coated pits are selective and concentrate intramembranous particles. They are not found at the active zones but only on the open area of the terminal. As the membrane enlarges with time after the beginning of the exocytotic event, more membrane invaginations have coated cytoplasmic surfaces. The path of the coated pits is shown by **solid arrows.** In the second pathway **(2)**, excess membrane reenters the terminal by budding from uncoated pits. These uncoated cisternal structures are formed in highest concentration at the active zones. Nearly all of the uncoated pits form during the first few seconds after exocytosis has occurred. However, during the normal functioning of the synapse, the second pathway may not be used at all. (Adapted from Miller and Heuser, 1984.)

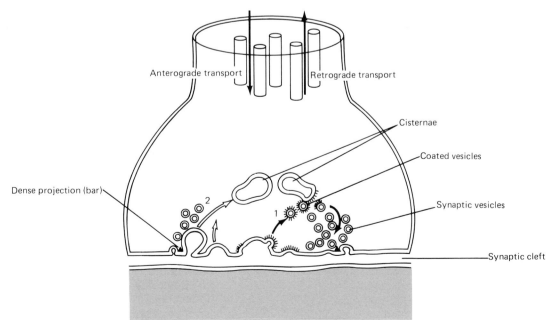

Anterograde transport   Retrograde transport

Cisternae

Coated vesicles

Dense projection (bar)

Synaptic vesicles

Synaptic cleft

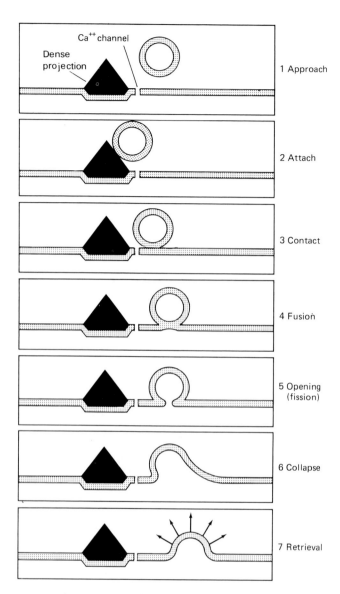

12–6 The exocytosis of synaptic vesicles and vesicle
membrane retrieval can be divided into separate stages.
Seven distinct stages can be recognized on the basis of
morphological studies. (Adapted from Llinás and Heuser, 1977.)

to the presynaptic membrane even in the absence of a
nerve impulse. The entry of Ca^{++} with each nerve impulse (perhaps through channels provided by the intramembranous particles next to the dense projections)
leads to contact (3) and fusion (4) of the vesicle membrane and the external (plasma) membrane by an as yet
unknown mechanism. Fusion is followed by a fission (5)
of all the intervening membrane components, which
opens up the synaptic vesicle. The vesicle membrane
then collapses (6) and coalesces into the external membrane, presumably as a consequence of membrane fluid-
ity. Finally, some vesicle membrane is retrieved for reuse
(7), and some leaves the terminals within lysosomes to
be degraded and returned to the cell body.

*There Is Now Electrical Evidence for Exocytosis and
for Membrane Retrieval.* The collapse of the vesicle
membrane during exocytosis and the consequent coales-
cence of this membrane with the external membrane
leads to a transient increase in surface area of the external membrane. In certain favorable circumstances, this
series of events can be detected in electrical measurements of membrane capacitance because, as we saw in
Chapter 6, the capacitance of the membrane is proportional to its surface area. This discovery was made by
Erwin Neher and his colleagues using a modified patch
clamp procedure. In adrenal medullary cells, and particularly in mast cells of the rat peritoneum, where exocytosis is massive and often involves about 1000 large vesicles (0.8 μm in size), the increase in surface area of the
external membrane is sufficiently great (several-fold) that
it can be readily detected as a change in the capacitance
of the external membrane (Figure 12–7A). Analysis of
the size distribution of these capacitative changes indicates that each fusion event represents a distinctive elementary change in capacitance. In addition, Neher and
his colleagues have detected decreases in capacitance
after massive release, which presumably reflect retrieval and recycling of the excess membrane (Figure
12–7B).

The Postsynaptic Component

A mesh of connective tissue called *basal lamina* is present in the gap between the pre- and postsynaptic membranes of the neuromuscular junction but not at other
synapses. Bound to the basal lamina is acetylcholinesterase, which functions to inactivate transmitter. (The basal
lamina may also play a role in development and in neural
regeneration by determining the site at which synapses
form on muscle cells.)

The postsynaptic receptors for ACh at the neuromuscular junction are highly localized to the plasma membrane of the junctional folds, although receptors are also
inserted into nonjunctional membrane of the muscle cell
after denervation. The receptor molecules can be localized by autoradiography after application of labeled snake
neurotoxins (α-bungarotoxin or cobra venom), which
bind to nicotinic ACh receptors (see Chapter 14).

used vesicles are replaced by new vesicles brought into
the terminals by anterograde axonal transport (considered
in Chapter 4).

According to Heuser and Reese, synaptic vesicle exocytosis and membrane retrieval can be divided into the
stages illustrated in Figure 12–6: The vesicles initially
approach the active zone (1), perhaps by some energy-
requiring process that may involve the dense projections
seen in transmission electron microscopy. These structures may consist of some contractile or cytoskeletal proteins because they are artifactually condensed by almost
all fixation procedures used. Vesicles closest to the dense
projections appear to be attached to them (2) and can be
seen in thin-section electron micrographs to hover close

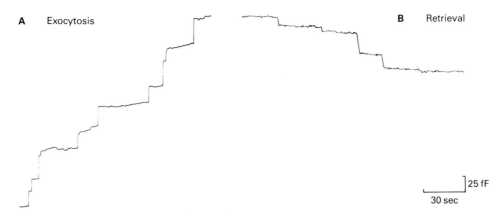

A Exocytosis   **B**   Retrieval

25 fF

30 sec

12–7 Both exocytosis of the vesicle and retrieval produce changes in surface area that can be detected electrically by measuring membrane capacitance in femtofarads (fF). **A.** Step changes in the capacitance of a rat peritoneal mast cell undergoing massive exocytotic release of its large granules. Capacitance was tracked with an 18-mV sinusoidal signal of 800 Hz. The rat mast cell was dialyzed internally with a solution rich in guanosine triphosphate (GTP), which is required for granule release. Capacitance increments associated with the release of granules occur in stepwise fashion, in agreement with the concept of vesicle fusion. The step increases ("on" steps) are not associated with measurable changes in membrane conductance and occur independently of the membrane potential. **B.** Step decreases of capacitance ("off" steps) after release of granules. The cell's capacitance now typically follows a downward trend and this also occurs in stepwise fashion. (Courtesy of Fernandez, Neher, and Gomperts, 1984).

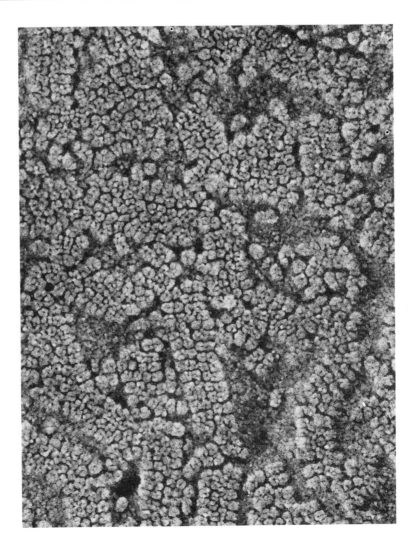

12–8 Acetylcholine receptors are densely packed in the postsynaptic membrane of a cell in the electric organ of *Torpedo californica*, a fish that can deliver an electric shock. This electron micrograph shows the platinum-plated replica of a membrane that had been frozen and etched. The size of the platinum particles limits the resolution to features larger than about 2 nm. According to recent evidence, the channel protein molecule, which measures 8.5 nm across, consists of five subunits surrounding a channel whose narrowest dimension is 0.8 nm. (Courtesy of J. E. Heuser and S. R. Salpeter.)

The structure of the postsynaptic membrane containing the receptors has been analyzed in detail by quick-freezing and freeze-fracture techniques. This analysis has been done more extensively in the electrocyte (electrical cell), a muscle cell that makes up the electric organs of certain rays, eels, and electric fish, than in the neuromuscular junction, but the organelles and molecular components of the two types of cholinergic synapse are similar. The new technique of quick-freezing tissue (the freeze-slam method, utilizing a liquid helium-cooled copper block, described above), followed by freeze-fracturing, shallow freeze-drying, and covering the dry tissue with platinum deposited in many directions simultaneously (rotary replication) permits visualization of the external surface of the membrane as well as both internal faces of the fractured membrane (Figure 12–8). The external face and the true surface of the postsynaptic membrane contain a geometrical lattice of 8.5-nm projections rising out of the membrane surface. These projections, which look like small doughnuts when properly negatively stained by shadowing with an electron-opaque material, are arranged in the membrane as dimers or tetramers in orderly rows; there are about 10,000 particles per square micrometer of membrane. Each particle is thought to represent the complex of the five protein subunits that constitute the ACh receptor (see Chapter 14).

The Autonomic Postganglionic Synapse Is an Example of a Nondirected Synapse

The presynaptic structures that constitute the active zone can be thought of as part of the directional apparatus of the synapse, which ensures that vesicles arrive at the right site for exocytosis. Many, but not all, chemical synapses function in this way. There is a major type of synapse that lacks this specialization. At such synapses, transmitter release appears not to be directed. These nondirected synapses often use a biogenic amine or a peptide as their transmitter. An example of this type of synapse occurs in the postganglionic neurons of the autonomic nervous system.

The axon terminals of these neurons arborize diffusely, and the branches resemble beads on a string (Figure 12–9). The terminal branches have this appearance because they consist of a series of swellings or varicosities connected by thin intervaricose segments (Figure 12–9, inset). Transmitter is released from the varicosities, but there are no recognizable presynaptic dense projections, and the vesicles in the varicosities show no preferred orientation toward any surface membrane. In addition, in contrast to directed synapses, where the synaptic gap is about 30 nm, the synaptic gap at nondirected synapses may be as wide as 400 nm, and the postsynaptic membrane is not modified.

The autonomic synapse appears to be specialized to ensure that the effect of the transmitter will be widespread. The extensive system of varicosities, the wide synaptic gap, and overlapping axons (called the autonomic ground plexus) contribute to this diffuse action in

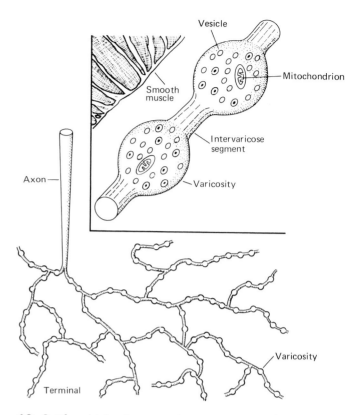

12–9 The peripheral autonomic synapse is a nondirected chemical synapse. The axon terminals are highly branched and consist of varicosities and intervaricose segments.

the peripheral autonomic nervous system. Thus, sympathetic stimulation affects large areas of blood vessels; it does not lead simply to the twitches of one smooth muscle cell in a single artery.

Synapses in the Central Nervous System Have Diverse Morphologies

Although they adhere to the general features we considered above, central synapses vary greatly in detail. Variation occurs in the extent of presynaptic specializations, in the types of vesicles that the presynaptic terminals contain, in the geometry of the zone of apposition, and in the sites where the pre- and postsynaptic cells contact one another.

Extent of Presynaptic Specialization

The nerve–muscle synapses and the synapses of autonomic postganglionic neurons represent extremes in synaptic specialization: the first type shows prominent and numerous specializations, whereas the latter shows few. The central nervous system contains both of these extremes and many intermediate forms. Like autonomic neurons of the peripheral nervous system, some neurons in the central nervous system that release monoamines have varicosities distributed over relatively widespread target areas. It was once believed that membrane specializations are rare or absent in these endings, but recent work on central adrenergic, dopaminergic, and serotonergic varicosities indicates that active zones are the rule in most monoaminergic terminals.

Transmission electron microscopy shows that most central synapses have prominent specializations—discrete dense projections—of the presynaptic plasma membrane. As in directed synapses in the peripheral nervous system, these structures are arranged in more or less triagonal arrays, each of which extends from the presynaptic membrane into the cytoplasm for some distance and is typically surrounded by synaptic vesicles (Figure 12–10). As at peripheral synapses, it is uncertain whether these discrete structures exist as such in the unfixed neuron or are formed from cytoskeletal elements during fixation. In any case, this close spatial relationship suggests that vesicles adhere to the components that form the dense projections in preparation for discharge. The dense projections appear to be interconnected by fine strands forming a "presynaptic grid." Adjacent dense projections are just far enough apart so that the synaptic vesicle can nestle between them and thus reach the presynaptic membrane. The spacing between the dense projections is narrower in synapses that contain smaller synaptic vesicles.

Examples of the more directed type of synapse are two common classes referred to as Gray type I and type II (after E. G. Gray, who described them) (Figure 12–11). In the type I synapse, the cleft is slightly widened to approximately 30 nm, the active zone is 1–2 μm^2 in area, dense projections are prominent, and the vesicles tend to be round. In addition, there is an extensive postsynaptic density, and amorphous dense material appears in the synaptic cleft. Type I synapses are often excitatory. In the type II synapse, the cleft is 20 nm across. The active zone is smaller (less than 1 μm^2), the presynaptic dense projections and the postsynaptic density are modest, and there is no material in the cleft. Characteristically, the vesicles of type II synapses tend to be oval, with a flattened appearance. Type II synapses are often inhibitory.

Varicosities of the presynaptic terminals in the central nervous system often have more than one active zone. In extreme examples, found in some specialized synapses,

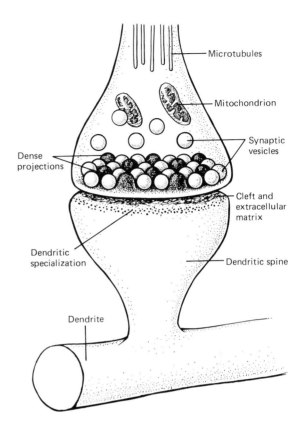

12–10 Dense projections are surrounded by vesicles at the active zone of the presynaptic membrane at a Gray type I synapse.

12–11 Gray type I and type II central synapses differ in the nature of their clefts and pre- and postsynaptic properties.

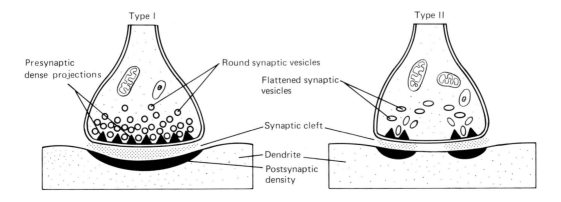

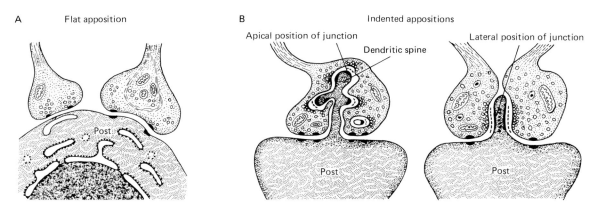

12–12 Central synapses can have flat or indented zones of apposition. **A.** In the flat apposition, the pre- and postsynaptic membranes are parallel to one another with only a slight widening at the synaptic cleft. **B.** In the indented appositions, the postsynaptic cell sends a fingerlike process into the presynaptic terminal.

they may have several hundred. This suggests that, for some unknown reason, there may be an upper limit to the size of the single active zones that any neuron can construct. As a result, a contact between neuron and target may be constrained to use multiple synaptic release sites rather than one very large active zone.

Types of Synaptic Vesicles

There are other variations in the size and electron density of the synaptic vesicles in central synapses. As a general rule, ACh and the amino acid transmitters are stored in electron-lucent and relatively small vesicles, 30–50 nm at their largest diameter. In contrast, vesicle populations appear to be heterogeneous in neurons that secrete peptides. These neurons contain many large vesicles (80–150 nm) that have electron-dense cores of varying sizes, and some smaller vesicles that vary in electron density. Axons that release biogenic amines also have both large and small vesicles at their terminals. When specialized fixation is used, noradrenergic terminals can be identified by their content of small (40–50 nm) dense-core vesicles. Fixatives containing permanganate and chromium salts reveal these endings.

Geometry of the Zone of Apposition

The zone of apposition can be flat and relatively simple (the sort that we have considered up to this point), or it can be indented and more elaborate, with the postsynaptic process typically protruding into the presynaptic one (Figure 12–12). The functional differences between these two types are not yet known. Perhaps the indented appositions (which, in some synapses, contain more vesicles per area of active zone than do flat appositions) are more effective than the flat appositions.

Site of Contact

All three regions of the nerve cell—the axon, dendrite, and soma—can be the site of synaptic contact. Among the known sites of contact are the following (by convention, the presynaptic element is named first): *axosomatic, axodendritic (axospinous), axo-axonic, dendrodendritic,* and *somasomatic.* Some of these contacts are depicted in Figure 12–13.

Does the region of a neuron where synaptic contact is made have any functional significance? The proximity of a synapse to the trigger zone of the postsynaptic cell is obviously important. Axosomatic contacts tend to be closer to the trigger zone than remote axodendritic contacts. As a result, a given synaptic current generated by an axosomatic input has a greater effect on the trigger zone than distant inputs on the dendrites. Axo-axonic synapses have no direct effect on the trigger zone of the postsynaptic cell that they innervate. As we have seen in Chapter 11, they produce their actions not by affecting the threshold of the neuron but by controlling the amount of transmitter released by the presynaptic terminal.

Inputs onto a Neuron Can Be Highly Segregated

We have previously considered synapses as individual entities. Neurons typically have many synaptic inputs. The motor neuron, for example, may have as many as 100,000. Some of these inputs are excitatory, others are inhibitory; some are strong, others weak. Clearly, in cells with many inputs, no one synapse is likely to be capable of exciting the cell above its threshold for firing. Function depends not only on the existence of excitatory and inhibitory synapses, but also on their strategic location, size, shape, terminal diameter, relationship to glial insulation, and the proximity of other synapses. Certain principles bear on these relationships between cells.

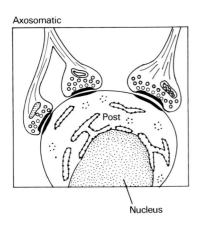

Axosomatic

Post

Nucleus

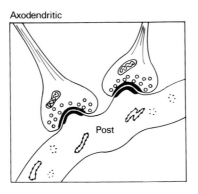

Axodendritic

Post

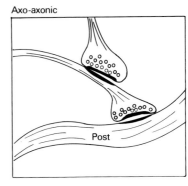

Axo-axonic

Post

12–13 Various sites of contact at synapses. (Presynaptic neurons are shown on top of postsynaptic neurons.)

For a given cell type, the synapses made by different afferents have characteristic positions and structures. For example, the pyramidal cells of the hippocampus, which have a consistent dendritic structure, receive seven major categories of inputs. Each input comes from a different afferent source. Six of these inputs are rigidly segregated: their synapses are restricted to different zones of the dendritic tree (Figure 12–14). Thus, there is not only cell–cell specificity in connections, but a specific set of axons of one cell ends on a *specific region* of the target cell. The seventh input, from neurons with short axons, innervates the dendritic tree throughout its extent and presumably serves a diffuse modulatory function. The various inputs also have different synaptic specializations.

Another example is the cerebellar Purkinje cell (Figure 12–15). These cells receive input from four principal sources:

1. Weak excitation comes from as many as 800,000 granule cell axons (known as parallel fibers) that end on dendritic spines. These spines resemble little thorns that project from the shaft of the dendrites. (Synaptic endings on spines are often excitatory.)
2. Weak inhibition comes from stellate cells that contact primary and secondary dendrites.
3. Strong inhibition comes from the combined terminals of 10–20 basket cell axons that form a basket-shaped cluster around the axon hillock.
4. Finally, very strong excitation, overriding everything else, is exerted by a single climbing fiber that runs over the soma and the entire dendritic tree, and synapses repeatedly over much of that huge area of contact.

The importance of this segregation is that the position of a synaptic input along a dendritic arbor determines its interaction with other synaptic inputs and its effect on the firing pattern of the cell. Although there are important exceptions, dendrites of many cells do not generate propagated action potentials; rather, synaptic potentials are conducted passively to the cell body, where integration occurs and the *net* effect is read out at the axon hil-

12–14 Synapses on a single cell can vary in source, location, and type. Inputs to a single hippocampal pyramidal cell are segregated on the dendritic tree according to their afferent source; only the input from short-axon neurons is distributed throughout.

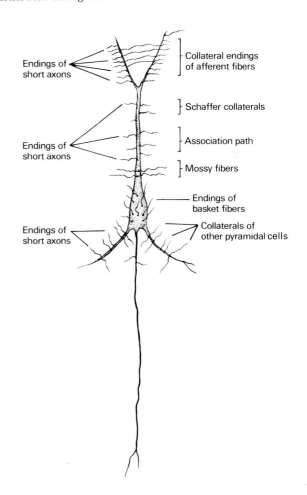

Endings of short axons

Collateral endings of afferent fibers

Schaffer collaterals

Association path

Mossy fibers

Endings of short axons

Endings of basket fibers

Collaterals of other pyramidal cells

Endings of short axons

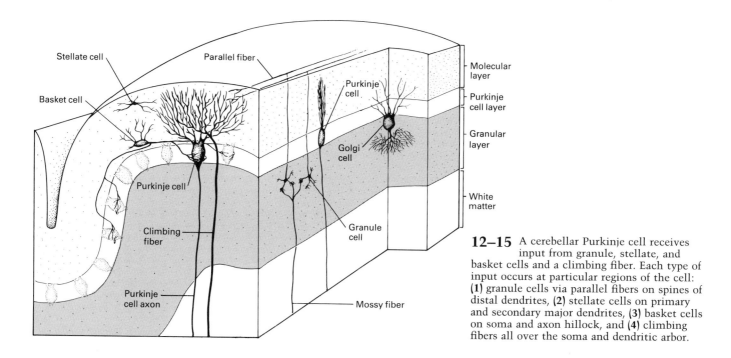

12–15 A cerebellar Purkinje cell receives input from granule, stellate, and basket cells and a climbing fiber. Each type of input occurs at particular regions of the cell: **(1)** granule cells via parallel fibers on spines of distal dendrites, **(2)** stellate cells on primary and secondary major dendrites, **(3)** basket cells on soma and axon hillock, and **(4)** climbing fibers all over the soma and dendritic arbor.

lock. Therefore, a synaptic input that opens a given number of ion channels near the soma will be more effective than a more distant input opening the same number of channels. Similarly, synapses relegated to the branches of apical dendrites are less effective than those placed on the dendrite itself. Inhibitory endings, which generally open channels to K^+ or Cl^-, are more effective when they make contact near the site where the action potential is generated. Their short-circuiting action far out on dendrites affects only nearby excitatory synapses on the same dendrite. Perhaps for this reason, many inhibitory inputs end on the cell soma, the axon hillock, or the most proximal parts of the dendritic arbor.

Interconnections Give Rise to Local Processing of Information

Most of the discussion in this chapter has focused on the polarized model of the neuron first outlined by Cajal and considered in Chapter 2. The dendritic arbor constitutes the receptive pole in this model; the axon, the conducting portion; and the axon terminal (which can be long, varicose, and branched, as in the autonomic nervous system, or can be a more compact terminal bouton), the transmitting pole. With this model in mind, we naturally think of the nervous system as being composed of information-transforming relays (or nuclei) made up of cell bodies and dendritic arbors receiving information, and tracts of axons acting as pathways connecting the relays. Some brain nuclei or relays, however, process and integrate information locally in addition to relaying information from place to place. These nuclei are character-

ized by neurons with short axons that do not project out of the region. As we saw in Chapter 2, these short-axon cells are classified as local interneurons or Golgi type II neurons. (The long-axon *principal*, or projection, *cells* whose axons project out of the local area, such as the Purkinje cell, are classified as Golgi type I cells.)

The processing of information is also accomplished in some regions by dendrodendritic interactions among the dendritic arbors themselves. The existence of dendrodendritic synapses indicates that (1) the dendritic arbor is not always strictly receptive but can have active release zones, and (2) impulse activity is not always necessary for transmitter release because many dendrites release transmitters without generating action potentials. Large excitatory postsynaptic potentials generated near active release zones in dendrites can activate sufficient Ca^{++} influx to initiate transmitter release.

An example of a region where dendrodendritic connections are important in processing is the olfactory bulb (Figure 12–16). There, the input and output are separate. The input comes to the bulb from olfactory receptors. The output is directed to the olfactory cortex. Cells in the bulb are located in discrete layers. The principal cell in the bulb is the *mitral cell*. This Golgi type I cell receives an input from olfactory receptors in complex synaptic structures called *glomeruli* and sends its axons to the cortex. Other types of neuron are interneurons (Golgi type II) and are confined within the olfactory bulb. One of these types is the *periglomerular cell*, which sends a small dendritic tuft into a glomerulus and has a short axon that terminates nearby. Another interneuron is the granule cell, which has two long vertical dendrites covered with spines, but *this cell has no axon at all*.

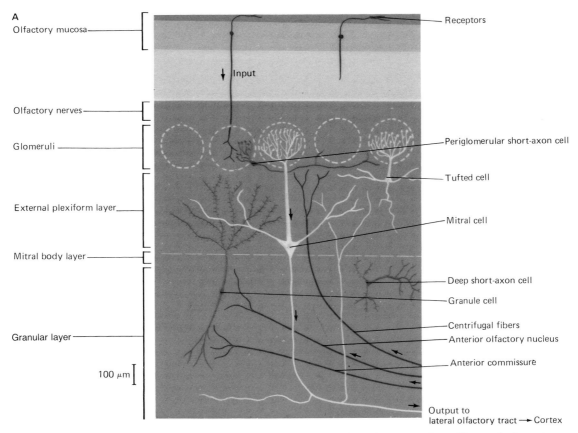

A

Olfactory mucosa

Olfactory nerves

Glomeruli

External plexiform layer

Mitral body layer

Granular layer

100 μm

Input

Receptors

Periglomerular short-axon cell

Tufted cell

Mitral cell

Deep short-axon cell

Granule cell

Centrifugal fibers

Anterior olfactory nucleus

Anterior commissure

Output to
lateral olfactory tract → Cortex

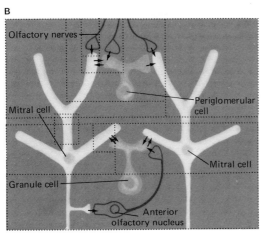

B

Olfactory nerves

Mitral cell

Granule cell

Periglomerular cell

Mitral cell

Anterior olfactory nucleus

12–16 In the mammalian olfactory bulb various types of connections process messages among the different neuronal elements. **A.** Neuronal elements. The principal neurons are the mitral cell and the tufted cell. Input comes from afferent fibers (from above) from olfactory receptors, and central fibers (from below) from three sources: centrifugal fibers from the nucleus of the horizontal limb of the diagonal band, ipsilateral fibers from the anterior olfactory nucleus, and contralateral fibers from the anterior commissure. The deep short-axon cell, periglomerular short-axon cell, and granule cell are interneurons within the bulb. (Adapted from Shepherd, 1974.) **B.** Organization of functional units. **Dotted lines** enclose *functional units*, each defined as the morphological substrate for a specific function. The units differ in size and complexity: the single synapse with its pre- and postsynaptic terminals; reciprocal synapses and other patterns involving dendritic terminals and axonal inputs; parts of dendritic trees with their associated input–output ensembles of processes; and long-distance "loop units" through neighboring structures (anterior olfactory nucleus). **Arrows** indicate functional polarity of synapses. (Adapted from Rakic, 1975.)

When the axon of the mitral cell is experimentally stimulated to fire an action potential, the mitral cell undergoes long-lasting recurrent inhibition. This is due to retrograde invasion of the mitral cell body by the spike generated in the axon, which, in turn, leads to electrotonic invasion of the dendritic arbor. The mitral dendritic arbor then excites granule cells, which, reciprocally and in an anterograde manner, now inhibit the mitral cell (as well as neighboring mitral cells). All of this is made possible by dendrodendritic synapses. The periglomerular

cells contact the mitral cell's dendrites inside the glomerulus, and these two cell types also make reciprocal dendrodendritic inhibitory synapses with one another.

These dendrodendritic connections are a logical and economical way to organize synaptic interactions in a minimal space. The reciprocal dendrodendritic circuit is as compact a synaptic circuit as any that exists. It has therefore been called a *microcircuit* (or local circuit). Such circuits have been found in parts of the brain other than the olfactory bulb. These include structures that we shall consider later, such as the retina, basal ganglia, cerebral cortex, thalamus, fifth nerve nucleus, and suprachiasmatic nucleus.

An Overall View

Synaptic contacts between cells range in complexity from the most simple, the electrical synapse, to more complex directed chemical synapses. Electrical synapses are ideal for synchronizing cellular events but allow little flexibility and integration. Chemical synapses are flexible and serve integration. The simplest chemical synapse is the autonomic postganglionic terminal axon, a long-branched chain of vesicle-filled varicosities. These structures disperse transmitter by means of exocytosis over a wide area and are not suited for discrete control. For discrete, directed release of transmitter, a more complex chemical synapse has evolved. This synapse has a well-defined active surface with pre- and postsynaptic membrane specializations. The synaptic vesicles are directed to the active zone, where exocytosis occurs. The vesicle membrane is then either recycled locally in terminals or, in a process that involves retrograde axonal transport, it is retrieved from the presynaptic terminals, packaged in lysosomes, and degraded in the cell body. The directed synapse produces highly localized excitatory or inhibitory responses, which makes a great deal of integration possible through the spatial distribution of synapses on receptive cells. Directed synapses can be segregated and meaningfully arranged on a single postsynaptic neuron. In much of the nervous system, the dendritic arbor is specialized as the receptive pole of the neuron, and the axon terminal as the transmitting pole; however, in certain instances, microcircuits use dendrodendritic synapses.

Selected Readings

Bennett, M. V. L., and Goodenough, D. A. 1978. Gap junctions, electrotonic coupling, and intercellular communication. Neurosci. Res. Program Bull. 16:371–486.

Burnstock, G., Hökfelt, T., Gershon, M. D., Iversen, L. L., Kosterlitz, H. W., and Szurszewski, J. H. 1979. Non-adrenergic, non-cholinergic autonomic neurotransmission mechanisms. Neurosci. Res. Program Bull. 17:377–519.

Fernandez, J. M., Neher, E., and Gomperts, B. D. 1984. Capacitance measurements reveal stepwise fusion events in deregulating mast cells. Nature 312:453–455.

Heuser, J. E., and Reese, T. S. 1977. Structure of the synapse. In E. R. Kandel (ed.), Handbook of Physiology, Vol. 1: The Nervous System, Part 1. Bethesda, Md.: American Physiological Society, pp. 261–294.

Heuser, J. E., and Reese, T. S. 1981. Structural changes after transmitter release at the frog neuromuscular juncture. J. Cell Biol. 88:564–580.

Llinás, R. R., and Heuser, J. E. 1977. Depolarization-release coupling systems in neurons. Neurosci. Res. Program Bull. 15:555–687.

Molliver, M. E., Grzanna, R., Lidov, H. G. W., Morrison, J. H., and Olschowka, J. A. 1982. Monoamine systems in the cerebral cortex. In V. Chan-Palay and S. L. Palay (eds.), Neurology and Neurobiology, Vol. 1: Cytochemical Methods in Neuroanatomy. New York: Liss, pp. 255–277.

Neher, E., and Marty, A. 1982. Discrete changes of cell membrane capacitance observed under conditions of enhanced secretion in bovine adrenal chromaffin cells. Proc. Natl. Acad. Sci. U.S.A. 79:6712–6716.

Palay, S. L., and Chan-Palay, V. 1977. General morphology of neurons and neuroglia. In E. R. Kandel (ed.), Handbook of Physiology, Vol. 1: The Nervous System, Part 1. Bethesda, Md.: American Physiological Society, pp. 5–37.

Peters, A., Palay, S. L., and Webster, H. deF. 1976. The Fine Structure of the Nervous System: The Neurons and Supporting Cells. Philadelphia: Saunders.

Shepherd, G. M. 1978. Microcircuits in the nervous system. Sci. Am. 238(2):92–103.

Tremblay, J. P., Laurie, R. E., and Colonnier, M. 1983. Is the MEPP due to the release of one vesicle or to the simultaneous release of several vesicles at one active zone? Brain Res. Rev. 6:299–314.

References

Buckley, K. M., Schweitzer, E. S., Miljanich, G. P., Clift-O'Grady, L., Kushner, P. D., Reichardt, L. F., and Kelly, R. B. 1983. A synaptic vesicle antigen is restricted to the junctional region of the presynaptic plasma membrane. Proc. Natl. Acad. Sci. U.S.A. 80:7342–7346.

Cajal, S. R. 1911. Histologie du Système Nerveux de l'Homme & des Vertébrés. L. Azoulay (trans.). Vol. 2. Paris: Maloine. Republished in 1955. Madrid: Instituto Ramón y Cajal.

Ceccarelli, B., Hurlbut, W. P., and Mauro, A. 1973. Turnover of transmitter and synaptic vesicles at the frog neuromuscular junction. J. Cell Biol. 57:499–524.

Couteaux, R. 1974. Remarks on the organization of axon terminals in relation to secretory processes at synapses. Adv. Cytopharmacol. 2:369–379.

Couteaux, R., Akert, K., Heuser, J. E., and Reese, T. S. 1977. Ultrastructural evidence for vesicle exocytosis. Neurosci. Res. Program Bull. 15:603–607.

Couteaux, R., and Pécot-Dechavassine, M. 1970. Vésicules synaptiques et poches au niveau des "zones actives" de la jonction neuromusculaire. C. R. Hebd. Séances Acad. Sci. Sér. D. Sci. Nat. 271:2346–2349.

Del Castillo, J., and Katz, B. 1957. La base "quantale" de la transmission neuro-musculaire. In Microphysiologie comparée des éléments excitables. Colloq. Int. Cent. Natl. Rech. Sci. 67:245–258.

Fawcett, D. W. 1981. The Cell, 2nd ed. Philadelphia: Saunders.

Geffen, L. B., and Livett, B. G. 1971. Synaptic vesicles in sympathetic neurons. Physiol. Rev. 51:98–157.

Gray, E. G. 1963. Electron microscopy of presynaptic organelles of the spinal cord. J. Anat. 97:101–106.

Heuser, J. E., Reese, T. S., Dennis, M. J., Jan, Y., Jan, L., and Evans, L. 1979. Synaptic vesicle exocytosis captured by quick freezing and correlated with quantal transmitter release. J. Cell Biol. 81:275–300.

Holtzman, E. 1977. The origin and fate of secretory packages, especially synaptic vesicles. Neuroscience 2:327–355.

Ko, C.-P. 1984. Regeneration of the active zone at the frog neuromuscular junction. J. Cell Biol. 98:1685–1695.

Kuffler, S. W., Nicholls, J. G., and Martin, A. R. 1984. From Neuron to Brain: A Cellular Approach to the Function of the Nervous System, 2nd ed. Sunderland, Mass.: Sinauer.

Llinás, R. R. 1982. Calcium in synaptic transmission. Sci. Am. 247(4):56–65.

Makowski, L., Caspar, D. L. D., Phillips, W. C., Baker, T. S., and Goodenough, D. A. 1984. Gap junction structures. VI. Variation and conservation in connexion conformation and packing. Biophys. J. 45:208–218.

Miller, T. M., and Heuser, J. E. 1984. Endocytosis of synaptic vesicle membrane at the frog neuromuscular junction. J. Cell Biol. 98:685–698.

Palay, S. L. 1958. The morphology of synapses in the central nervous system. Exp. Cell. Res. Suppl. 5:275–293.

Pappas, G. D., and Waxman, S. G. 1972. Synaptic fine structure—morphological correlates of chemical and electrotonic transmission. In G. D. Pappas and D. P. Purpura (eds.), Structure and Function of Synapses. New York: Raven Press, pp. 1–43.

Pfenninger, K., Sandri, C., Akert, K., and Eugster, C. H. 1969. Contribution to the problem of structural organization of the presynaptic area. Brain Res. 12:10–18.

Rakic, P. 1975. Local circuit neurons. Neurosci. Res. Program Bull. 13:289–446.

Shepherd, G. M. 1979. The Synaptic Organization of the Brain, 2nd ed. New York: Oxford University Press.

Sherrington, C. S. 1897. The Central Nervous System. Part III of M. Foster, A Text Book of Physiology, 7th ed. London: Macmillan.

Thesleff, S., and Molgó, J. 1983. Commentary. A new type of transmitter release at the neuromuscular junction. Neuroscience 9:1–8.

Vrensen, G., Nunes Cardozo, J., Müller, L., and Van Der Want, J. 1980. The presynaptic grid: A new approach. Brain Res. 184:23–40.

James H. Schwartz

Chemical Messengers:
Small Molecules and Peptides

13

What is the chemical basis of synaptic transmission? To what degree can synaptic transmission be explained in terms of specific molecules? As a class, neurons are distinguished from other cells of the body by certain molecular properties. Many of these characteristic properties are responsible for the signaling activities of neurons considered in previous chapters. These activities include (1) conducting electrical impulses, (2) communicating with other cells by synaptic transmission, and (3) responding to the chemical messengers released by other cells by altering channels for common ions (Na^+, Cl^-, K^+, Ca^{++}). Underlying each of these three physiological functions are biochemical processes and cellular components that are currently being characterized and understood at the molecular level. Some of these components are characteristic of specific neurons, whereas others occur in other cell types as well.

In this and the next two chapters we shall consider synaptic transmission in molecular terms. In this chapter we shall focus on the characterization and synthesis of chemical messengers. In the next chapter, we shall concentrate on the structure and function of receptors. Finally, in Chapter 15 we shall consider the molecular steps involved in the storage, release, and removal of transmitters from the synaptic cleft, as well as the long-term regulation of transmitter biosynthesis.

The Nature of Chemical Messengers

Before we consider in detail the biochemical processes involved in synaptic transmission, it is important to make clear what is meant by a *chemical transmitter*. The concept had become familiar by the early 1930s, after Otto Loewi demonstrated the release of ACh from vagus terminals in frog heart and Henry Dale reported his work on cholinergic and adrenergic transmission. It has been continually modified since that time to accommodate new information about the cell biology of neurons and the pharmacology of receptors.

As a first approximation we can define a *transmitter* as a substance that is released synaptically by one neuron and that affects another cell (neuron or effector organ) in a specific manner. As with many other operational concepts that emerge in biology, the concept of a transmitter is quite clear at the center but can be somewhat fuzzy at the edges. Thus, most neural scientists would agree that eight low-molecular-weight substances can indisputably function as transmitters, but many other transmitter candidates exist about which there are varying degrees of uncertainty. Moreover, it is often difficult to prove in all instances that one of the accepted substances is a transmitter at any given synapse. Because of these (often, but not always, scholastic) difficulties, a set of experimental criteria has been developed. Strictly speaking, a substance will not be accepted as the transmitter at a particular synapse of a neuron unless the following four criteria are met:

1. It is synthesized in the neuron.
2. It is present in the presynaptic terminal and is released in amounts sufficient to exert its supposed action on the postsynaptic neuron or effector organ.
3. When applied exogenously (as a drug) in reasonable concentrations, it mimics exactly the action of the endogenously released transmitter (for example, it activates the same ion channels in the postsynaptic cell).
4. A specific mechanism exists for removing it from its site of action (the synaptic cleft).

Needless to say, it is often impossible experimentally to demonstrate *all* of these features at a given synapse; this has resulted in the very cautious use of the word *transmitter*.

Despite these words of caution, a great many nerve cells have been characterized with respect to their transmitter biochemistry, and an important generalization has emerged: *a mature neuron makes use of the same transmitter substance at all of its synapses*. This generalization, attributed to the great British pharmacologist Henry Dale, was actually formulated as a principle in 1957 by John Eccles. Eccles had been studying the motor neuron of the spinal cord, which has a cholinergic peripheral synapse at the neuromuscular junction. He correctly predicted—on the basis of Dale's discussions of work on cholinergic and adrenergic neurons in the autonomic nervous system, dating from the early 1930s—that the synapse from the recurrent central branch (onto the Renshaw cells of the cord) would also be cholinergic. During the intervening years, much more information on the chemistry and cell biology of synaptic transmission has been obtained, and the number of accepted transmitter substances has increased from the two that had been recognized in the 1930s, ACh and norepinephrine. Since most neurons examined were found to use only one transmitter substance, Dale's principle became a doctrine of neuronal specificity.

It is certain that the spirit of Dale's law is *not obeyed in some developing neurons*, which have been shown to synthesize, and to release, more than one transmitter substance. In recent years, many mature neurons have also been described that contain more than one potential chemical messenger. This situation, called *coexistence*, usually involves a low-molecular-weight transmitter and a neuroactive peptide. Several different neuroactive peptides can also be released together because peptides typically are processed from larger polyprotein precursors (discussed below). As a consequence, to conserve Dale and Eccles' important cell-biological insight, this principle of neuronal specificity may now have to be reformulated to state that *a neuron makes use of the same combination of chemical messengers at all of its synapses*. Most adult neurons, however, are differentiated so that only the biochemical apparatus specific to one transmitter is present; consequently, a mature neuron contains an exclusive set of biochemical processes that endows that cell with its differentiated character. Neuronal differentiation, in this respect, is thought to resemble the specialization of cells in other body tissues (e.g., liver cells

Table 13–1. Small-Molecule Transmitter Substances and Their Key Biosynthetic Enzymes

Transmitter	Enzymes
Acetylcholine	Choline acetyltransferase (specific)
Biogenic amines	
Dopamine	Tyrosine hydroxylase (specific)
Norepinephrine	Tyrosine hydroxylase and dopamine β-hydroxylase (specific)
Serotonin	Tryptophan hydroxylase (specific)
Histamine	Histidine decarboxylase (specificity uncertain)
Amino acids	
γ-Aminobutyric acid	Glutamic acid decarboxylase (probably specific)
Glycine	General metabolism (specific pathway undetermined)
Glutamate	General metabolism (specific pathway undetermined)

Table 13–2. Neuroactive Peptides: Mammalian Brain Peptides Categorized According to Principal Tissue Localization

Hypothalamic-releasing hormones	Gastrointestinal peptides
Thyrotropin-releasing hormone	Vasoactive intestinal polypeptide
Gonadotropin-releasing hormone	Cholecystokinin
Somatostatin	Gastrin
Corticotropin-releasing hormone	Substance P
Growth hormone–releasing hormone	Neurotensin
	Methionine-enkephalin
Neurohypophyseal hormones	Leucine-enkephalin
Vasopressin	Insulin
Oxytocin	Glucagon
Neurophysin(s)	Bombesin
	Secretin
Pituitary peptides	Somatostatin
Adrenocorticotropin	Thyrotropin-releasing hormone
β-Endorphin	Motilin
α-Melanocyte-stimulating hormone	
Prolactin	Others
Luteinizing hormone	Angiotensin II
Growth hormone	Bradykinin
Thyrotropin	Sleep peptide(s)
	Calcitonin
Invertebrate peptides	CGRP (calcitonin gene-related peptide)
FMRF amide[a]	Neuropeptide Yy
Hydra head activator	

Source: From Krieger, 1983.   [a]Phe-Met-Arg-Phe-NH$_2$

differentiate to make albumin, but not insulin; fibroblasts make collagen, but not albumin; and red blood cells make hemoglobin, but not immunoglobulin).

The nervous system makes use of two main classes of chemical substances for signaling: (1) small-molecule transmitters (Table 13–1), and (2) neuroactive peptides, which are short chains of amino acids (Table 13–2). The biochemical distinctions between these two classes are fundamental, so we shall consider each in turn.

Small-Molecule Transmitter Substances

All of the eight accepted low-molecular-weight transmitter substances are amines; seven of them are amino acids or their derivatives. These chemical messengers therefore share many structural similarities. All of them are charged small molecules that are formed in relatively short biosynthetic pathways, and all are synthesized from precursors that ultimately derive from the major carbohydrate substrates of intermediary metabolism. Like other pathways of intermediary metabolism, synthesis of these neurotransmitters is catalyzed by enzymes that almost without exception are cytosolic. (One exception is dopamine β-hydroxylase.)

The particular transmitter used by a neuron is determined by a specific set of biosynthetic enzymes. A specific set of enzymes is a necessary but not a sufficient determinant of transmitter specificity, however, because other biochemical processes intervene between synthesis of the transmitter and its release at synapses, for example, packaging of the transmitter into synaptic vesicles that mediate synaptic release (described in Chapter 15).

In any biosynthetic pathway, there is some controlling element. Thus, in *all* transmitter pathways there is an enzymatic step at which the overall synthesis of the transmitter is regulated; the controlling enzyme ordinarily is characteristic of (or specific to) the neuron and endows the cell with the property of being cholinergic, norepinephrinergic (noradrenergic), dopaminergic, serotonergic, etc.

Acetylcholine

Acetylcholine is the only accepted low-molecular-weight transmitter substance that is not derived directly from an amino acid. The biosynthetic pathway for ACh has only one enzymatic reaction, that of choline acetyltransferase (step **1** in the reaction below); this enzyme is the determining and characteristic enzyme in ACh biosynthesis. The biosynthesis of the cosubstrate acetyl coenzyme A (acetyl CoA) is not specific to cholinergic neurons, since it participates in many metabolic pathways. Nervous tissue cannot synthesize choline, which is ultimately derived from the diet and delivered to neurons through the blood stream.

$$\text{Acetyl CoA + choline}$$
$$(1) \Big\Downarrow$$
$$\overset{O}{\underset{\text{Acetylcholine}}{CH_3-C-O-CH_2-CH_2-\overset{+}{N}-(CH_3)_3 + CoA}}$$

Acetylcholine is the transmitter used by the motor neurons of the spinal cord and, therefore, at all nerve–skeletal muscle junctions in vertebrates. In the autonomic nervous system, it is the transmitter for all preganglionic neurons and for the parasympathetic postganglionic neurons as well. Centrally, ACh is used at many synapses throughout the brain, but cell bodies synthesizing ACh are highly concentrated in the nucleus basalis with widespread projections to the cerebral cortex. The large Betz cells of the motor cortex that send their axons into the pyramidal tract in the spinal cord are also cholinergic.

Biogenic Amine Transmitters

Catecholamines are substances that have a catechol nucleus—a 3,4-dihydroxylated (adjacent) benzene ring. The catecholamine transmitters—dopamine, norepinephrine, and epinephrine—are all synthesized from tyrosine in a common biosynthetic pathway that contains five enzymes: tyrosine hydroxylase; aromatic amino acid decarboxylase; dopamine β-hydroxylase; pteridine reductase; and phenylethanolamine-*N*-methyltransferase.

The first enzyme, tyrosine hydroxylase (1), is an oxidase that converts the amino acid tyrosine to L-dihydroxyphenylalanine (L-DOPA). This enzyme is rate limiting for both dopamine and norepinephrine synthesis. It is present in all cells producing catecholamines and requires a reduced pteridine (Pt) cofactor, which is reoxidized by another enzyme, pteridine reductase (4). This reductase is not specific to neurons.

L-DOPA is next decarboxylated by a decarboxylase (2) to give dopamine and CO_2.

The third enzyme, dopamine β-hydroxylase (3), converts dopamine to norepinephrine.

In the central nervous system, norepinephrine-containing nerve cell bodies are prominent in the locus ceruleus, a nucleus of the brain stem. These cells are unusual: although few in number, they project diffusely throughout the cortex, cerebellum, and spinal cord. In the peripheral nervous system, norepinephrine is the transmitter in the postganglionic neurons of the sympathetic nervous system.

In the adrenal medulla, in addition to these four adrenergic biosynthetic enzymes, another enzyme, phenylethanolamine-*N*-methyltransferase (5), methylates norepinephrine to form epinephrine. This reaction requires *S*-adenosylmethionine as methyl donor.

Not all cells that release catecholamines express all five of these biosynthetic enzymes, although cells that release epinephrine do. Neurons that make norepinephrine do not express the methyltransferase, and neurons releasing dopamine do not express either the transferase or dopamine β-hydroxylase. Thus, during development the expression of the genes encoding the catecholamine-synthesizing enzymes can be differentially turned on. This insight prompted Tong Joh and his colleagues at Cornell University Medical Center to examine the genetic organization of these enzymes. Using recombinant DNA technology, Joh found a high degree of similarity in amino acid sequences and also considerable homology in the nucleic acid sequences encoding for three of the biosynthetic enzymes: tyrosine hydroxylase, dopamine β-hydroxylase, and phenylethanolamine-*N*-methyltransferase, which appear to be linked together on the same chromosome. As we shall see in Chapter 15, the gene expression of these three enzymes can be regulated coordinately: physiological conditions that alter the synthesis of one of them also change the synthesis of the others. Joh has therefore suggested that the genes for these enzymes, which behave as if they are situated together on the chromosome, have evolved from a common ancestral gene by reduplication and divergence.

Several other naturally occurring amines derived from catecholamines may also be transmitters: tyramine and octopamine have both been found to be active in invertebrate nervous systems.

Serotonin belongs to a group of aromatic compounds called indoles with a five-membered ring containing nitrogen joined to a benzene ring. The synthesis of serotonin (5-hydroxytryptamine) involves two enzymes: tryptophan hydroxylase (1), an oxidase similar to tyrosine hydroxylase, which puts a hydroxyl group in the 5 position on the indole ring of the amino acid tryptophan; and 5-hydroxytryptophan decarboxylase (2), which forms serotonin.

The controlling step is tryptophan hydroxylase, the first enzyme in the pathway. Interestingly, L-DOPA decarboxylase and 5-hydroxytryptophan decarboxylase seem to be identical. An enzyme with similar activity,

L-aromatic amino acid decarboxylase, is present in many tissues, including organs outside the nervous system, but it is not yet certain whether these enzymes are identical in structure or whether different molecular forms of the enzyme (specific isozymes) exist in the different tissues.

Serotonergic cell bodies are found in the midline raphe nucleus of the brain stem; the fibers of these cells (like those of the noradrenergic cells in the locus ceruleus) have a widespread distribution throughout the brain and spinal cord.

Histamine is an imidazole because it contains a characteristic five-membered ring with two nitrogen atoms. It has been convincingly shown to be a transmitter in invertebrates, and binding sites for certain kinds of antihistaminic drugs have been localized to neurons in the vertebrate brain. This putative vertebrate transmitter substance is concentrated in the hypothalamus. It is synthesized from the amino acid histidine by decarboxylation. Although not extensively analyzed, the decarboxylase (1) catalyzing this step appears to be characteristic of histaminergic neurons.

$$\text{Histidine} \xrightarrow{\text{(1)}} \underset{\underset{\text{Histamine}}{HN \diagdown N}}{\boxed{}} CH_2{-}CH_2{-}NH_2 + CO_2$$

Histidine is also the precursor of two dipeptides that are found in nervous tissue. A synthetase catalyzes the formation of carnosine (β-alanyl histidine) with the amino acid β-alanine and ATP. The same enzyme forms homocarnosine (β-aminobutyrylhistidine) with GABA. Although the role of homocarnosine is not known, there is some evidence that carnosine, which is highly concentrated in olfactory areas of the brain, acts as a neurotransmitter there.

The biochemical similarity between the synthetic pathways of the catecholamines and the indolamines suggests that the two classes of neurons that use these transmitters are closely related, and that the genes encoding their biosynthetic enzymes may have evolved from common ancestors. This kind of suspected relationship may have predictive clinical value: disorders that now appear predominantly to involve neurons of one transmitter type (for example, dopamine in Parkinson's disease and in schizophrenia, and norepinephrine and serotonin in depression) may also affect homologous components in the other cell type. Thus, although the disorder may present primarily as a disturbance in the metabolism of one transmitter, a complete understanding of a disease and appropriate therapy would depend on the identification of all the cell types affected. Histamine is an imidazole, and its biochemistry is remote from the catecholamines and the indolamines. Nevertheless, all of these substances are frequently referred to as biogenic amines.

Amino Acid Transmitters

Acetylcholine and the biogenic amines are substances that are not intermediates in general biochemical pathways. Consequently, their production occurs only in certain neurons. In contrast, there is a group of amino acids that are released as neurotransmitters and that also are universal cellular constituents. Glycine, glutamate, and aspartate are 3 of the 20 common amino acids that are incorporated into the proteins of all cells; GABA, like glutamate, can serve as a substrate in intermediary metabolism.

Glutamate and aspartate are synthesized in familiar metabolic pathways that we shall not review here. The case for glutamate as a transmitter in the cerebellum and the spinal cord is fairly strong; aspartate's role is more controversial.

Glycine, which is probably synthesized from serine, is thought to be one of the inhibitory transmitters in spinal cord interneurons. Its specific biosynthesis in neurons has not been studied, but its pathways in other tissues are well known.

γ-Aminobutyric acid is synthesized from glutamate in a reaction catalyzed by glutamic acid decarboxylase (1).

$$\underset{\text{Glutamate}}{\begin{array}{c} COOH \\ | \\ CH_2 \\ | \\ CH_2 \\ | \\ H_2N{-}CH \\ | \\ COOH \end{array}} \xrightarrow{\text{(1)}} \underset{\text{GABA}}{\begin{array}{c} COOH \\ | \\ CH_2 \\ | \\ CH_2 \\ | \\ H_2N{-}CH_2 \end{array}} + CO_2$$

Although detectable in other tissues (especially pancreas and adrenal gland), GABA is present in much higher concentrations in the central nervous system, where it is widely distributed. An important class of inhibitory interneurons in the spinal cord is gabaminergic. In the brain, GABA is highly concentrated and is thought to serve as a transmitter in granule cells of the olfactory bulb, in amacrine cells of the retina, in Purkinje cells of the cerebellum, and in basket cells of both the cerebellum and the hippocampus. In the basal ganglia, there is an important inhibitory tract with endings on dopaminergic cells of the substantia nigra.

It might at first seem puzzling how common amino acids can act as transmitters in some neurons but not in others. This phenomenon can be taken as an indication that the presence of a substance, even in substantial amounts, is insufficient evidence that the substance is used as a transmitter. To illustrate this point, let us consider the following example. GABA is the inhibitory transmitter at the neuromuscular junction of the lobster (and of other crustacea as well as insects) and glutamate is the excitatory transmitter. Edward Kravitz and his coworkers at Harvard University showed that the concentration of GABA in inhibitory cells is about 20 times greater than that in excitatory cells, which supports the idea that GABA is the inhibitory transmitter. On the other hand, the concentration of glutamate (the excitatory transmitter) was found to be the same in both the excitatory and inhibitory cells. Glutamate must be compartmentalized within these neurons: *transmitter* glutamate is somehow kept separate from *metabolic* glutamate. What mediates the compartmentalization of the amino acid transmitters is not yet certain. With ACh and the biogenic amines it has been convincingly demonstrated that the transmitter substances are packaged in specific and characteristic membranous vesicles. Vesicles with a similar appearance are present in the terminals of neurons that use the amino acid transmitters, and, although it has not yet been proved, it is likely that these vesicles constitute the transmitter compartment (see Chapter 15).

Neuroactive Peptides

With rare exceptions (for example, dopamine β-hydroxylase), the enzymes that catalyze the steps in the synthesis of the low-molecular-weight neurotransmitters that we considered above are cytoplasmic. Although these enzymes are synthesized on free polysomes in the cell body, they become distributed throughout the neuron by slow axoplasmic transport (see Chapter 4). Because these biosynthetic enzymes are distributed throughout the cell, the small-molecule transmitter substances whose synthesis they catalyze can be formed in all parts of the neuron; most important, they can be synthesized at the nerve terminal where the transmitter is released. In contrast to the small-molecule transmitter substances, whose biosynthesis is catalyzed by cytosolic enzymes, the neuroactive peptides derive from the processing of secretory proteins that are formed in the cell body on polyribosomes that attach to the cytoplasmic surface of the endoplasmic reticulum (discussed in Chapter 4). Like other secretory proteins, neuroactive peptides or their precursors leave the Golgi apparatus within secretory granules and are moved to terminals by fast axonal transport.

In recent years, over 30 short peptides that are pharmacologically very active have been found in neurons (Table 13–2). These peptides cause inhibition, excitation, or both when applied iontophoretically to target neurons. Some of these peptides were previously identified as hormones, with known targets outside the brain (for example, angiotensin and gastrin), or as products of neuroendocrine secretion (for example, oxytocin, vasopressin, somatostatin, luteinizing hormone, and thyrotropin-releasing hormone). Neuronal or regional localization in the brain on the one hand, and specific target action on the other, have spurred the idea that, in addition to being hormones in some tissues (i.e., substances released at a considerable distance from their intended sites of action), these peptides act in other tissues as chemical messengers that are released essentially directly onto the site of intended action. The study of neuroactive peptides is important because certain peptides have been implicated in modulating sensibility and emotions. For example, some peptides (substance P and enkephalins) are preferentially localized in brain regions thought to be involved in the perception of pain and pleasure; and others in brain regions regulating responses to stress (γ-melanocyte-stimulating hormone, adrenocorticotropin, and β-endorphin).

The diversity of neuroactive peptides is enormous. Nevertheless, with the information now at hand, we can attempt to outline the main features of the cell biology of this class of chemical messengers, even if only in a preliminary manner.

The first important feature of these peptides is that they all are produced only in a restricted group of cells: neurons and gland cells that are known to derive from embryological precursors of nervous tissue (for example, chromaffin cells of the adrenal medulla, pancreatic islet cells, and secretory enterochromaffin cells in the gut). Thus, although every cell in the body elaborates membrane proteins that are processed in their endoplasmic reticulum and Golgi apparatus, only a small group of cells, which can be presumed to be closely related developmentally, expresses genes for neuroactive peptides.

A second striking generality about neuroactive peptides is that they are grouped in families. At least seven families have already been recognized (Table 13–3). Members of each family are structurally related: they contain stretches of similar amino acid residues. Where extensive sequence homology is lacking, family members often reveal their relatedness through similarities in molecular conformation: a sufficient degree of homology exists so that the polypeptides fold in the same way. Individual members of a family may be expressed both in the nervous system and in nonneural tissues (most often gut and pancreas), or only in one tissue or the other.

How is relatedness between peptides determined? Ultimately, the most direct way to show relatedness is to compare either the actual amino acid sequences of the peptides or the nucleotide base sequences in their genomic DNA. Similarity in function is the first clue to structural similarity; relatedness is suspected if two peptides mediate the same or similar physiological processes. Because the types of physiological processes that we have been discussing are mediated by the interaction of a chemical messenger with specific receptors, functional similarity indicates that the peptides are recognized by the same or similar receptors (see Chapter 14). Receptors are presumed to recognize a peptide because of its structure. Therefore, receptor recognition is one index

Table 13–3. Families of Neuroactive Peptides

Opioid: opiocortins, enkephalins, dynorphin, FMRF amide

Neurohypophyseal: vasopressin, oxytocin, neurophysins

Tachykinins: substance P, physalaemin, kassinin, uperolein, eledoisin

Secretins: secretin, glucagon, vasoactive intestinal peptide, gastric inhibitory peptide, growth hormone releasing factor, peptide histidine isoleucineamide

Insulins: insulin, somatomedins, relaxin, nerve growth factor

Somatostatins: somatostatins, pancreatic polypeptide

Gastrins: gastrin, cholecytokinins

of structural similarity between peptides, primary (amino acid sequence) or conformational. Conformation of a polypeptide ultimately is determined by its primary structure, and therefore receptor binding can be thought of as a highly specific bioassay for a particular amino acid sequence. Family members may not have similar biological activities, however, or may be only poor analogues of each other. Thus, family members glucagon and secretin are functionally divergent, but secretin and vasoactive intestinal peptide can recognize each other's receptor, although each binds to its own receptor with much greater affinity.

Immunoreactivity is a less restricted biological assay for amino acid sequences. Unlike the receptor, which is constrained to bind only with quite specific regions of the polypeptide, resulting in the physiological response, many different stretches of amino acids can serve as antigenic determinants. (Consequently, an antibody can recognize regions of the peptide that may or may not be directly involved in the physiological function.) Receptor binding and immunological cross-reactivity both may sometimes be artifactual—receptors can be tricked by unrelated analogues and immunoreactivity may lack specificity.

The determination of amino acid sequences with modern techniques of protein chemistry proceeds slowly (about one residue per day), and a relatively large amount of the purified peptide is needed. Sequencing is much more rapid through recombinant DNA technology (more than 100 residues per day). The mRNA encoding the polypeptide contains the precise information for its amino acid sequence. Because RNA is unstable and therefore inconvenient to work with, it is copied by the enzyme reverse transcriptase into copy (c) DNA. The cDNA is stable and carries exactly the same information in the form of the nucleotide code as the mRNA that has been copied. Moreover, the nucleotides in cDNA can be rapidly sequenced by one of two convenient and widely used techniques—one developed by Allan Maxam and Walter Gilbert at Harvard University, and the other by Frederick Sanger at Cambridge University. The amino acid sequence of the polypeptide is then inferred from the nucleotide code.

Structural analyses of neuroactive peptides, especially in those studies in which recombinant DNA technology has been used, have demonstrated a third key feature of this class of chemical messengers. In most instances, several different neuroactive peptides are encoded by a single continuous mRNA, which is translated into one large polyfunctional protein precursor or *polyprotein* (Figure 13–1). Production from a large precursor can sometimes serve as a mechanism for amplification, since more than one copy of the *same* peptide can be produced from one polyprotein. Examples can be found in the opioid family: 18 distinct peptides with opioid activity all contain the sequence Tyr-Gly-Gly-Phe; these peptides arise from three different polyprotein precursors, each of which is the product of a distinct gene (see Chapter 26). Another example is the precursor of glucagon, which contains two copies of the hormone. In other instances, the biological purposes served are more complicated, since peptides with either *related* or *antagonistic* functional capacities can be generated from the same precursor. Processing of more than one functional peptide from a single polyprotein is a mechanism by no means unique to peptide chemical messengers, but was first described by David

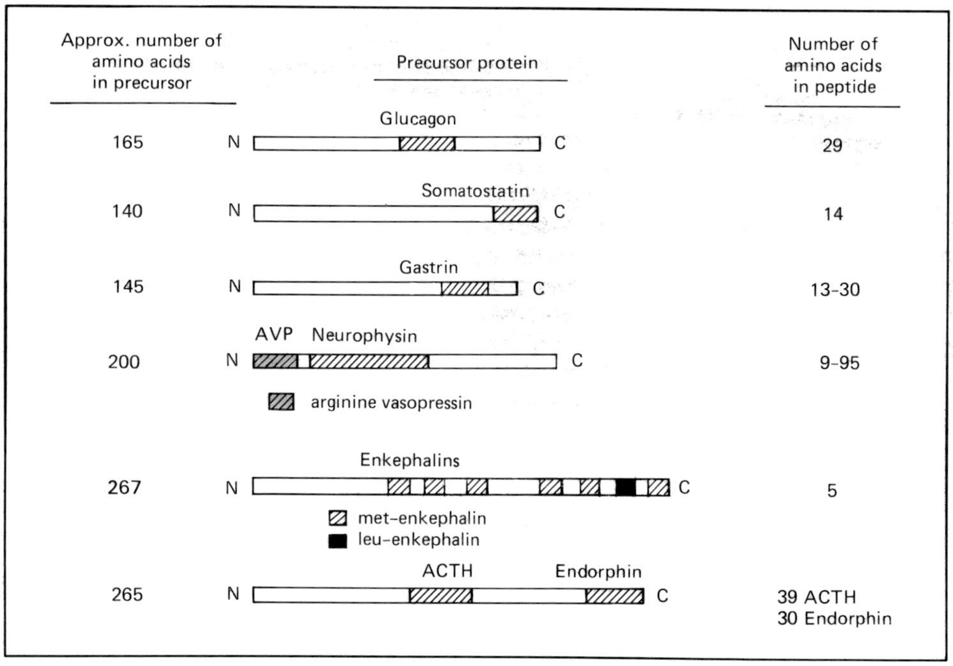

13–1 Small neuroactive peptides are derived from large precursor proteins. (From Herbert et al., 1983.)

Baltimore at the Massachusetts Institute of Technology for proteins encoded by small RNA viruses. Since there are several viral polypeptides produced and all contribute to the generation of new virus particles, it seems evident that, at least in this case, the polyprotein mechanism serves a concerted biological purpose.

Processing of neuroactive peptide precursors takes place within vesicles, as discussed below and in Chapter 4. Multiple peptides are produced from a single polyprotein by limited and specific proteolytic cleavages that are catalyzed by proteases present within these internal membrane systems. As yet, little information is available about these proteases, because so few examples have been studied. Some of these enzymes are serine proteases, a class that also includes trypsin and chymotrypsin. They are called serine proteases because they all have a serine residue at their active site that catalyzes the cleavage reaction. As with trypsin, the peptide bond cleaved is determined by the presence of dibasic amino acid residues (lysine and arginine); in neuroactive peptides, this bond often is between the carboxyl of a residue N-terminal to a *pair* of dibasic residues (Lys-Lys, Lys-Arg, Arg-Lys, or Arg-Arg). The *kallikreins* are a group of serine proteases that are present in gland tissue. Some members of this group can remain tightly bound to the processed peptide after a cleavage has taken place, thereby becoming part of the peptide complex released. Presumably, the binding of the protease to the polyprotein contributes to the specificity of the cleavage. Although cleavage at dibasic residues is quite common, polyproteins can also be cleaved at bonds between other amino acids.

Processing is a critical step in determining which peptides a peptidergic neuron releases. Of course, the types of peptides that can be produced depend first on the particular gene expressed by the neuron; the genetic information also specifies the positions within the polyprotein of those amino acid residues that can determine sites of possible proteolytic cleavage, for example, the dibasic amino acids lysine and arginine. The polyprotein is then subject to specific processing. One polyprotein can give rise to several sets of chemical messengers, because the same protein precursor can be processed differently in different neurons. An example is proopiomelanocortin (POMC), one of the three branches of the opioid family. The mRNA for POMC is found in the anterior and intermediate lobes of the pituitary in the hypothalamus and in several other regions of the brain, as well as in the placenta and the gut, but different peptides are produced and released in these different tissues. It is not yet known how differential processing occurs. Information about the biochemistry of membrane proteins and secretory products discussed in Chapter 4 suggests two plausible mechanisms: two neurons might process the same polyprotein differently because each cell contains proteases with different specificities within the luminal spaces of their internal membrane systems and vesicles. Alternatively, the two neurons might contain the same processing proteases, but each cell might glycosylate the common polyprotein at different sites and thereby protect different regions of the polypeptide from cleavage.

The production of the same or similar peptides from a single polyprotein could explain why some neuroactive peptides are related. The mRNA, which is the template for several copies of the same or of partly homologous peptides, is transcribed from genomic DNA that might have evolved by a series of duplications of a simpler DNA ancestor. Amplification of products by reduplication appears to have been a common occurrence during evolution. In the genes for polyproteins that contain neuroactive chemical messengers, reduplication followed by divergence could result in the production of related but diversified sets of peptides. This is called *divergent* evolution. Another possibility is *convergent* evolution. By this mechanism, a nucleotide sequence with the potential to code for a physiologically active peptide might originally have occurred at a variety of sites in the ancestral chromosome. During evolution these sequences could become organized together in a similar way in all of the genes that code for the polyproteins of a given gene family. Whether the result of divergent or convergent evolution, the similarities in the genetic structure of the various members of a gene family can be presumed to have a selective advantage—at the level of transcription into mRNA, at the level of translation into the polyproteins, or at the posttranslational level of protein processing.

Peptides and Small-Molecule Transmitters Differ in Several Presynaptic Features

Many of the established criteria for classical neurotransmitters have been met by some neuroactive peptides, but no peptide has met all of them. Moreover, certain features of the metabolism and action of peptides differ from those of the accepted (small-molecule) transmitters. Although these neuroactive peptides have been shown to be present in some neurons in relatively high concentrations, they are formed only in the cell body because their synthesis requires peptide bond formation on ribosomes, whereas the small-molecule transmitters can be synthesized locally at terminals.[1] Furthermore, although the Ca^{++}-dependent synaptic release of some neuroactive peptide messengers has been demonstrated, release patterns can be expected to be quite different between peptides and classical small-molecule substances. Because vesicles can be refilled rapidly with the classical transmitters that are resynthesized at terminals, release can be both rapid and sustained. It is not yet clear how the dif-

---

[1]Distinguishing between the two classes of chemical messengers by mode of synthesis can present some semantic difficulty because the peptide bond can also be catalyzed by cytosolic enzymes. Synthesis of peptides from amino acids without the participation of mRNA, however, usually results in short polymers, many of which involve the carboxyl group in the gamma position rather than the alpha, for example, carnosine, homocarnosine, and glutathione, as well as in other γ-glutamyl peptides.

Table 13–4. Neuroactive Peptides That Coexist with a Small-Molecule Transmitter Substance

Transmitter	Peptide
Acetylcholine	Vasoactive intestinal peptide
Norepinephrine	Somatostatin
	Enkephalin
	Neurotensin
Dopamine	Cholecystokinin
	Enkephalin
Adrenalin	Enkephalin
Serotonin	Substance P
	Thyrotropin-releasing hormone

Evidence for the coexistence of a classical transmitter substance with a neuroactive peptide has been reported for these combinations; with the information thus far available, it is not yet possible to determine the specificity of the pairs and their physiological significance.

ferences in the biosynthesis of neuroactive peptides affect the kinetics of signaling. In addition, as we shall see in the next chapter, there are important differences between the postsynaptic receptors for peptides and for the small-molecule transmitters, as well as differences in mode of inactivation after release.

Peptides and classical transmitters can coexist in the same neuron (Table 13–4), as first demonstrated by Tomas Hökfelt at the Karolinska Institute and by Victoria Chan-Palay at Harvard University. Hökfelt, Jan Lundberg, and their collaborators have shown that ACh and vasoactive intestinal peptide can be released together during synaptic transmission and work synergistically on the same target cells. Moreover, neurons releasing peptides processed from polyproteins can release several neuroactive components with potentially different postsynaptic actions. The coordinated release of several substances with potentially different postsynaptic activities suggests many new possibilities about how neurons can signal their targets (see discussion of the reticular core in Chapter 41).

Chemical Messengers Can Be Localized within Neurons

A major problem in studying the functioning of neurons is to identify the chemical messengers they might use. There now are powerful cytological techniques for localizing both small-molecule transmitter substances and neuroactive peptides. Specific histochemical and autoradiographic methods can be used to localize the biogenic amines and to show that vesicles contain transmitter. Catecholamines and serotonin, when reacted with formaldehyde vapor, form fluorescent derivatives. The Swedish neuroanatomists Falck and Hillarp found that under properly controlled conditions the reaction can be used to locate transmitters on histological sections under the fluorescence (light) microscope. Because individual vesicles are too small to be resolved by the light microscope,

histofluorescence can localize transmitters only to particular regions of nerve cells. Vesicular position can be inferred by comparing the distribution of fluorescence under the light microscope with the position of vesicles under the electron microscope. Histochemical analysis can be extended to the ultrastructural level: fixation of nervous tissue under special conditions intensifies the electron density of vesicles containing biogenic amines. Thus, fixation in the presence of potassium permanganate, chromate, or silver salts brings out dense-core vesicles that are characteristic of aminergic neurons.

It is now also possible to identify histochemically neurons in which the gene for a particular transmitter enzyme or peptide precursor is active. Many methods for detecting specific mRNAs depend on the phenomenon of nucleic acid *hybridization*. One particularly elegant method is in situ hybridization, applied to the nervous system by James Roberts at Columbia University (Figure 13–2). Two single strands of a nucleic acid polymer will pair if the sequence of bases is complementary or homologous. (The degree of homology required for pairing depends on the conditions used for annealing the two strands; under stringent experimental conditions, hybridization occurs only between two strands whose homology is 80% or greater.) In in situ hybridization, radiolabeled cDNA encoding the peptide is applied to tissue sections under conditions suitable for hybridizing with endogenous mRNA. Autoradiography reveals the location of neurons that contain the complex formed between the labeled cDNA and the homologous mRNA.

Transmitter substances can also be localized directly to vesicles by electron-microscopic autoradiography and by immunocytochemistry. A necessary condition for autoradiography is that the labeled transmitter should not have been washed out of the tissue during preparation for microscopy. Amino acid transmitters and biogenic amines can be successfully localized by autoradiography because they have a primary amino group that permits their covalent fixation in place within the neuron; this group becomes cross-linked to proteins by glutaraldehyde or formaldehyde, the usual fixatives used in microscopy. For immunohistochemical localization, specific antibodies to the transmitter substance are necessary. Specific antibodies have been raised that combine with serotonin and with many of the neuroactive peptides. When these antibodies are labeled with fluorescein (a fluorescent tag) they can be used under the light microscope to localize antigens to regions of individual neurons (e.g., cell bodies, axons, and sometimes terminals). Ultrastructural localization can be achieved by immunohistochemical techniques, usually involving a peroxidase–antiperoxidase system developed by the American immunologist Ludwig Sternberger.

An Overall View

An important functional aspect of neuronal diversity is the type or types of chemical messengers that a nerve cell uses. For the most part, each mature neuron is restricted in the types of messengers it uses in much the same way

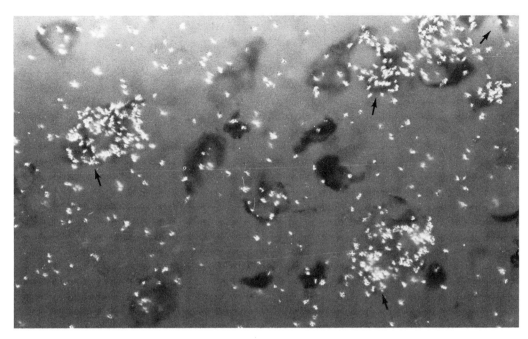

13—2 Photomicrograph made after in situ hybridization reveals that some hypothalamic neurons express proopiomelanocortin (POMC). The periarcuate region of the rat hypothalamus at the level of the median eminence has been probed with a tritium-labeled cDNA that encodes POMC sequences; periarcuate nerve cell bodies that are heavily labeled **(arrowheads)** contain POMC mRNA. When adjacent serial tissue sections are processed with an antibody to ACTH (one of the peptides contained in the POMC polyprotein), these same neurons also stain immunocytochemically. This shows that the POMC mRNA detected by the cDNA probe is translated into protein. For this experiment, 10-μm cryostat sections were exposed to the cDNA that had been radioactively labeled by nick-translation to permit hybridization. At the end of the hybridization step the sections were washed to remove the unhybridized cDNA probe, dehydrated, and coated with photographic emulsion. After development the tissue was counterstained with the dyes hematoxylin and eosin. The micrograph was taken using a combination of bright field and polarized light epiluminescence illumination so that the silver grains developed in the autoradiographic emulsion appear white and the counterstained cells dark. Not all neurons in the arcuate nucleus are labeled (unlabeled neurons appear the same as background). × 500. (Courtesy of J. N. Wilcox and J. L. Roberts.)

that other secretory cells selectively release specific secretory products. With the small-molecule transmitters this differentiation involves not only biosynthetic enzymes but also, as we shall discuss in Chapter 15, specific membrane components—vesicles with special properties appropriate to the specific messengers used, and specific pump mechanisms (proteins in the neuron's membrane for recapturing transmitter from the extracellular space after it has been released).

The two major types of chemical messengers differ in their modes of synthesis. Small-molecule transmitters all are positively charged ions that are synthesized in the cytoplasm in short enzymatic pathways from precursors that stem from the major cycles of intermediary metabolism. Their synthesis is catalyzed by enzymes that are distributed throughout the neuron, so that a small-molecule transmitter can be formed at nerve endings as well as in other neuronal regions. In contrast, neuroactive peptides are processed from secretory proteins that can be formed only in the cell body.

Are these two classes the only types of chemical messengers? Some evidence now indicates still a third class. All secretory granules and synaptic vesicles thus far examined biochemically contain substantial amounts of ATP (see Chapter 15). Therefore all neurons probably release purines, and some postsynaptic cells have receptors for them. For these cells, the released purine may be a chemical transmitter. The metabolism of ATP, synthesized in the mitochondria, is quite different from that of either the small-molecule transmitters or the neuroactive peptides.

Selected Readings

Chan-Palay, V. 1982. Immunocytochemical and autoradiographic methods to demonstrate the coexistence of neuroactive substances: Cerebellar Purkinje cells have glutamic acid decarboxylase and motilin immunoreactivity, and raphe neurons have serotonin and substance P immunoreactivity. In V. Chan-Palay and S. L. Palay (eds.), Neurology and Neurobiology, Vol. 1: Cytochemical Methods in Neuroanatomy. New York: Liss, pp. 93–118.

Chan-Palay, V., and Palay, S. L. (eds.). 1984. Coexistence of Neuroactive Substances in Neurons. New York: Wiley.

Cooper, J. R., Bloom, F. E., and Roth, R. H. 1982. The Biochemical Basis of Neuropharmacology, 4th ed. New York: Oxford University Press.

Hökfelt, T., Johansson, O., Ljungdahl, Å., Lundberg, J. M., and Schultzberg, M. 1980. Peptidergic neurones. Nature 284:515–521.

Krieger, D. T., Brownstein, M. J., and Martin, J. D. (eds.). 1983. Brain Peptides. New York: Wiley.

Loh, Y. P., Brownstein, M. J., and Gainer, H. 1984. Proteolysis in neuropeptide processing and other neural functions. Annu. Rev. Neurosci. 7:189–222.

McGeer, P. L., Eccles, J. C., and McGeer, E. G. 1978. Molecular Neurobiology of the Mammalian Brain. New York: Plenum Press.

References

Dale, H. 1935. Pharmacology and nerve-endings. Proc. R. Soc. Med. 28:319–332.

Eccles, J. C. 1957. The Physiology of Nerve Cells. Baltimore: Johns Hopkins University Press.

Falck, B. 1962. Observations on the possibilities of the cellular localization of monoamines by a fluorescence method. Acta Physiol. Scand. Vol. 56 [Suppl.] 197:6–25.

Falck, B., Hillarp, N. Å., Thieme, G., and Torp, A. 1962. Fluorescence of catechol amines and related compounds condensed with formaldehyde. J. Histochem. Cytochem. 10:348–354.

Geffen, L. B., and Jarrott, B. 1977. Cellular aspects of catecholaminergic neurons. In E. R. Kandel (ed.), Handbook of Physiology, Vol. 1: The Nervous System, Part 1. Bethesda, Md.: American Physiological Society, pp. 521–571.

Gershon, M. D. 1977. Biochemistry and physiology of serotonergic transmission. In E. R. Kandel (ed.), Handbook of Physiology, Vol. 1: The Nervous System, Part 1. Bethesda, Md.: American Physiological Society, pp. 573–623.

Herbert, E., Oates, E., Martens, G., Comb, M., Rosen, H., and Uhler, M. 1983. Generation of diversity and evolution of opioid peptides. Cold Spring Harbor Symp. Quant. Biol. 48:375–384.

Hökfelt, T., and Bjorklund, A. 1985. Handbook of Chemical Neuroanatomy, Vol. 3: Classical Transmitters and the Transmitter Receptors in the CNS, Part 2. Amsterdam: Elsevier.

Joh, T. H., Baetge, E. E., Ross, M. E., and Reis, D. J. 1983. Evidence for the existence of homologous gene coding regions for the catecholamine biosynthetic enzymes. Cold Spring Harbor Symp. Quant. Biol. 48:327–335.

Kravitz, E. A. 1967. Acetylcholine, γ-aminobutyric acid, and glutamic acid: Physiological and chemical studies related to their roles as neurotransmitter agents. In G. C. Quarton, T. Melnechuk, and F. O. Schmitt (eds.), The Neurosciences: A Study Program. New York: Rockefeller University Press, pp. 433–444.

Krieger, D. T. 1983. Brain peptides: What, where, and why? Science 222:975–985.

Loewi, O. 1960. An autobiographic sketch. Perspect. Biol. Med. 4:3–25.

Maxam, A. M., and Gilbert, W. 1980. Sequencing end-labeled DNA with base-specific chemical cleavages. Meth. Enzymol. 65:499–560.

Mayeux, R., Stern, Y., Côté, L., and Williams, J. B. W. 1984. Altered serotonin metabolism in depressed patients with Parkinson's disease. Neurology 34:642–646.

Otsuka, M., Kravitz, E. A., and Potter, D. D. 1967. Physiological and chemical architecture of a lobster ganglion with particular reference to gamma-aminobutyrate and glutamate. J. Neurophysiol. 30:725–752.

Pearse, A. G. E. 1969. The cytochemistry and ultrastructure of polypeptide hormone-producing cells of the APUD series and the embryologic, physiologic and pathologic implications of the concept. J. Histochem. Cytochem. 17:303–313.

Pearse, A. G. E., Polak, J. M., and Bloom, S. R. 1977. The newer gut hormones: Cellular sources, physiology, pathology, and clinical aspects. Gastroenterology 72:746–761.

Sanger, F., and Coulson, A. R. 1975. A rapid method for determining sequences in DNA by primed synthesis with DNA polymerase. J. Mol. Biol. 94:441–448.

Scatton, B., Javoy-Agid, F., Rouquier, L., Dubois, B., and Agid, Y. 1983. Reduction of cortical dopamine, noradrenaline, serotonin and their metabolites in Parkinson's disease. Brain Res. 275:321–328.

Shine, J., Manson, A. J., Evans, B. A., and Richards, R. I. 1983. The kallikrein multigene family: specific processing of biologically active peptides. Cold Spring Harbor Symp. Quant. Biol. 48:419–426.

Sternberger, L. A. 1974. Immunocytochemistry. Englewood Cliffs, N. J.: Prentice-Hall.

Teitelman, G., Joh, T. H., and Reis, D. J. 1981. Linkage of the brain–skin–gut axis: Islet cells originate from dopaminergic precursors. Peptides 2 [Suppl.] 2:157–168.

Tuček, S. 1978. Acetycholine Synthesis in Neurons. London: Chapman and Hall.

Watson, J. D., Tooze, J., and Kurtz, D. T. (eds.). 1983. Recombinant DNA: A Short Course. San Francisco: Freeman.

James H. Schwartz

Molecular Aspects
of Postsynaptic Receptors

14

Release of chemical messengers enables neurons to communicate with other neurons or with target cells. None of the substances described in the preceding chapter, whether small-molecule or peptide, reacts effectively with any of the *universal* constituents of cell membranes, even if these substances are administered in concentrations much higher than those achieved in the synaptic cleft during synaptic transmission. Thus, as a class of chemicals, these messenger molecules have no direct action on the lipid bilayer of the postsynaptic membrane, as would detergents, for example. They also do not act directly on integral membrane proteins in general, as would denaturants such as urea, phenols, strong acids, or bases. Rather, to be effective, transmitters must interact with receptors—special protein complexes that are present in the membranes of some cells but not others. Although transmission at each type of synapse is highly individualized—because of the specific chemical messengers released and the great specificities of the receptor molecules present—the postsynaptic events at all synapses have important features in common.

In this chapter, we shall describe how all instances of synaptic transmission thus far analyzed result from one of two types of transmembrane transductions in the postsynaptic cell, caused by the transient binding of a specific messenger to a receptor. Depending on the receptor, there is either a rapid change in the conductance of ions through channels of the postsynaptic membrane, or a direct change in biochemical activity within the postsynaptic cell.

Structure and Function of Receptors

The postsynaptic effects of a chemical messenger are not specifically characteristic of the transmitter as a chemical but result from its interactions with specific receptors. For example, ACh can excite at some synapses, inhibit at others, and do both simultaneously at others. Catecholamines (e.g., norepinephrine) may inhibit at some synapses, while at others they bring about changes in excitability by increasing the synthesis of cyclic AMP; at still others, they may do both.

It is the receptor that determines whether a synapse is excitatory or inhibitory. Within a group of closely related animals (for example, vertebrates) a given transmitter substance binds to similar receptors and is associated with specific physiological functions. For example, ACh is the transmitter at the vertebrate neuromuscular junction, where it is associated with synaptic transmission; ACh slows the vertebrate heart (excitatory transmission to the heart is adrenergic). As we shall see in later chapters (especially Chapters 53 and 54), emotional state is related to central biogenic amines. This close association between transmitters and physiological functioning should not be surprising. From the standpoint of evolution, muscle, heart, and even mind are each quite similar in all vertebrates. It is therefore understandable that organs in similar species share common modes of innervation. In contrast, heart and muscle of phylogenetically distant animals are not necessarily excited or inhibited by the same transmitter substances.

At first the notion of a receptor was a mental construct or operational model proposed to account for the site on a membrane that is sensitive to a drug. The great German biological chemist Paul Ehrlich introduced the idea of receptors to explain the selective action of toxins and other pharmacological agents and the specificity of immunological reactions. In his Croonian lecture of 1900, Ehrlich said that "chemical substances are only able to exercise an action on the tissue elements with which they are able to establish an intimate chemical relationship. . . . [This relationship] must be specific. The [chemical] groups must be adapted to one another . . . as lock and key." A receptive substance in skeletal muscle sensitive to curare and nicotine was postulated in 1906 by John N. Langley, Professor of Physiology at Cambridge University. As discussed below, this receptive substance has now been isolated and characterized as the ACh receptor of the neuromuscular junction. Receptor theory was subsequently developed by Langley's students—in particular, Eliot Smith and Henry Dale—and was greatly influenced by the study of both enzyme kinetics and cooperative interactions between small molecules (ligands) and proteins (a historically important example of which is the binding of O_2 to hemoglobin).

Receptors for chemical messengers have two common biochemical features:

1. Their location is in the membrane facing outward; this is important for their interaction with the transmitter arriving from across the synaptic cleft.

2. They are proteins with active sites that bind the messenger.

In a few instances, progress has been made in isolating receptor molecules. Some receptors can be localized in tissues autoradiographically or assayed in isolated preparations of membranes by radiochemical binding studies using radiolabeled ligands. Most often, specific pharmacological antagonists are used because of their high affinity for the receptor. Neurotoxins have turned out to be most useful because they bind specifically with great avidity, but radioactive transmitter analogues have also been used. Especially useful are derivatives of transmitters that are modified with special chemical groups that are sensitive to ultraviolet radiation. When irradiated, these photoaffinity reagents form covalent linkages to the receptor at the transmitter binding site. The labeled receptor protein can then be isolated and characterized biochemically.

There Are Two Classes of Receptors, One That Mediates Changes in Membrane Conductance and Another That Mediates Changes in the Metabolic Machinery of the Postsynaptic Cell

The Nicotinic Acetylcholine Receptor Is a Multimeric Intrinsic Membrane Protein

Because of the pioneering work of David Nachmansohn at Columbia University and of his students Arthur Karlin and Jean-Pierre Changeux, as well as many other investigators, the most completely characterized receptor is the nicotinic ACh receptor from the electric organ of electric fish. Electric organs are a rich source of the receptor because they contain densely innervated cells that are derived embryologically from striated muscle. This chemically gated ion channel is a multimeric, intrinsic membrane glycoprotein that traverses the postsynaptic membrane. The native receptor has a molecular weight of about 275,000, and can be seen in shadowed preparations of membrane from the electric organ (Figure 12–8). It can be isolated from electric tissue by extraction in solutions containing relatively mild (non-ionic) detergents and is purified by affinity chromatography on columns containing gels substituted with quaternary ammonium groups (for example, immobilized choline carboxymethyl groups). Biochemical and biophysical studies reveal that the receptor is formed from five subunits, with the stoichiometry $\alpha_2\beta\gamma\delta$ (Figure 14–1). Two molecules of the transmitter can bind to this multimeric complex: each ACh molecule binds to a site on one of the two α subunits of the receptor.

When sulfhydryl groups are reduced and the complex is dispersed in the strong ionic detergent sodium dodecyl sulfate, the four types of subunits can be separated from each other by polyacrylamide gel electrophoresis. These four polypeptide chains have apparent molecular weights of 40,000 (α), 48,000 (β), 58,000 (γ), and 64,000 (δ).

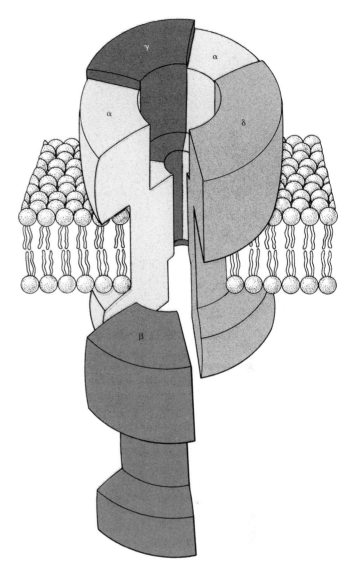

14–1 A three-dimensional model of the nicotinic acetylcholine receptor consistent with current biophysical and biochemical information. The biophysical data are of two kinds. Electron microscopy of isolated, negatively stained receptor complexes reveals its doughnut-like shape in face-on views. The relative positions of the different subunits in this doughnut, the overall length of the receptor, and its extension above the plane of the postsynaptic membrane are also indicated by electron microscopy. The overall dimensions of the receptor have been obtained by X-ray scattering as well. Finally, the radius of gyration of the receptor has been obtained by neutron scattering. The model also makes use of biochemical information such as the amino acid sequences of the four types of subunits of the receptor, their molecular weights, and their stoichiometries. The presence of hydrophobic stretches in the sequences suggests that each subunit traverses the membrane four or five times. In addition, chemical modification with impermeant affinity labels and partial proteolytic digestion of receptor while still in the membrane also have indicated that a large N-terminal portion of each of the subunits is extracellular. (The model is drawn from two-dimensional views in Karlin, 1983).

A snake venom, α-bungarotoxin, binds specifically and essentially irreversibly to the receptor, also on the α subunits. This toxin has been used extensively as a probe for the isolation and characterization of ACh receptors in a variety of tissues because it can be labeled with radioactive iodine or made fluorescent when tagged with rhodamine or fluorescein (Figure 14–2).

In the past five years, dramatic insights have been obtained into the molecular biology of the ACh receptor. Shosaku Numa and his colleagues in Kyoto have shown that each of the four subunits is translated from its own mRNA, and each mRNA is transcribed from its own gene. Both α subunits are encoded by the same gene. The cDNAs corresponding to all four mRNAs have been sequenced, and much of the structure of the genomic DNA has been analyzed. The true molecular weight of the α subunits derived from these sequence data is 50,000. A comparison of the nucleotide sequences encoding the four receptor subunits shows a high degree of homology among them. As in some of the instances of sequence homology mentioned in Chapter 13, the gene structure of the ACh receptor is thought to have arisen by divergent evolution, that is, by gene duplication and subsequent divergence; all four of the modern genes are thought to have derived from a single ancestor.

Amino acid homologies among the subunits may also be important for the orientation of the receptor proteins within the membrane. The subunits are arranged as barrel staves around a central pore (Figure 14–1). There is evidence that each subunit threads through the membrane several times, with its N-terminal portion on the extracellular face of the membrane. Homologous domains of both hydrophilic and hydrophobic amino acids permit all of the subunits to be arranged *in register*. The

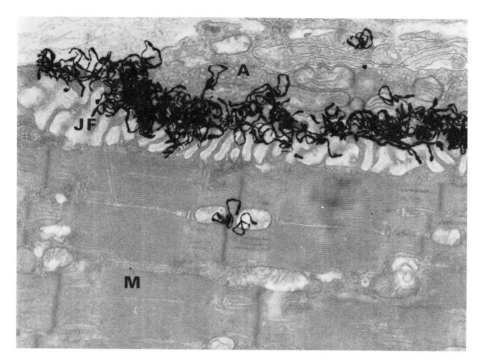

14-2 The ACh receptors in an end-plate from mouse sternomastoid muscle have been labeled with radioactive α-bungarotoxin. The muscle tissue was incubated with ^{125}I-labeled α-bungarotoxin until all neurally evoked muscle contractions were blocked. **A.** This electron-microscopic autoradiograph is overexposed (i.e., the emulsion is saturated with developed grains) to show that the label is not uniformly distributed throughout the postjunctional membrane but is concentrated near the axonal interface. **JF**, junctional folds. **A**, axon. **M**, muscle. × 21,000.

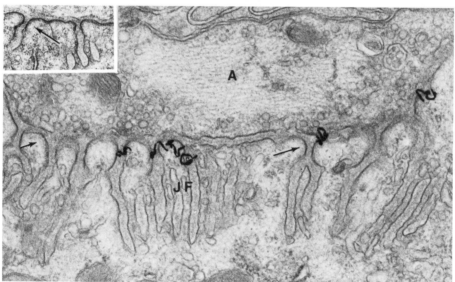

B. This autoradiograph (not overexposed) shows the subneural location of the developed grains, which are again concentrated at the postjunctional membrane nearest the primary cleft, and not distributed throughout the folds. × 37,500. **Inset:** Section after lead citrate staining (the autoradiographs are not lead stained) emphasizes that postsynaptic membrane densities are concentrated near the muscle surface and dip partly down into the folds **(arrows)**. These densities may be related to the receptor specializations. × 21,000. (Adapted from Fertuck and Salpeter, 1974.)

homologous hydrophobic regions are embedded in the lipid bilayer. The hydrophilic N-terminal portions of all five subunits, which are glycosylated, are exposed on the extracellular surface of the membrane and appear in electron micrographs as petals around a central pit (Figure 12–8). The exposed regions of the two α subunits contain the transmitter binding sites.

The subunits are thought to be inserted through the membrane by the mechanisms described for membrane proteins in Chapter 4. How the separate subunits are brought together and assembled into the completed receptor complex within the postsynaptic membrane is not yet understood, but it involves processing and glycosylation within the internal membrane systems of the cell (discussed in Chapter 4). Once inserted into the membrane at the neuromuscular junction, the receptor has a half-life of about a week. Accelerated degradation or turnover of ACh receptors in the presence of autoantibodies is believed to cause the neurological disorder myasthenia gravis (see Chapter 16).

Current ideas about mechanism suggest that the receptor complex mediates two functions: (1) binding of the transmitter (receptor function) and (2) forming a channel in the membrane through which ions flow (ionophore) (Figure 14–3). Increased permeability to ions is postulated to be the result of a cooperative rearrangement of the subunits brought about by interaction of the binding portion with the transmitter molecules. This in turn widens the channel through the membrane, thereby permitting the influx of ions (Figure 14–3). As we have seen in Chapter 9, the channel formed by the ACh receptor is not very selective: in addition to Na^+ and K^+, it permits some divalent ions, including Ca^{++}, to enter the muscle cell.

Partial Characterization of Other Ionophoric Receptors Indicates That They Also Are Large Membrane Protein Complexes

Other receptors that change membrane permeability are thought to operate like the ACh receptor. They are categorized by the chemical messenger to which they respond and by their reaction to specific drugs (activated by agonists or inhibited by blocking agents). This type of receptor is not restricted to small-molecule transmitter substances; peptides also mediate changes in membrane ion conductances. Further characterization of these receptors should include a determination of whether specific ion species are involved; some channels are quite specific and carry only K^+ or Cl^-, whereas some are permissive and allow any cation or anion to pass. This type of characterization is most conveniently done with isolated nervous tissue because the ionic environment can be manipulated experimentally (see Chapter 9).

Receptors that mediate changes in membrane conductance are considered *chemically gated* ion channels. The molecular structures of few ion channels other than the ACh receptor have been characterized, and none nearly as thoroughly. But information about the ACh receptor and the Na^+ channel (Chapters 3 and 5) suggests that all ion channels are large integral membrane protein complexes that form a tubular structure that traverses the lipid bilayer. This accounts in part for the large size of the receptor. Moreover, as we saw for the ACh receptor, in addition to the channel region within the membrane, which is hydrophobic, a ligand-gated ion channel requires a more hydrophilic domain on the outer face of the postsynaptic membrane to form the binding sites for the transmitter. In the receptor for γ-aminobutyric acid (GABA), there is evidence for still other functional regions. In addition to the domain that binds the transmitter and a domain that serves as a channel selective for Cl^-, there seem to be regulatory subunits that can modulate the activity of the receptor. Suggestive evidence for this type of subunit in the receptor for GABA has been obtained by studying the binding to nervous tissue of a group of tranquilizing drugs, the benzodiazepines, such as diazepam (Valium) and chlordiazepoxide (Librium), and the barbiturates (hypnotic drugs that include phenobarbitol and secobarbitol).

Consistent with the idea that the GABA receptor might be composed of several subunits is its large size. This receptor, which is widely distributed in the brain

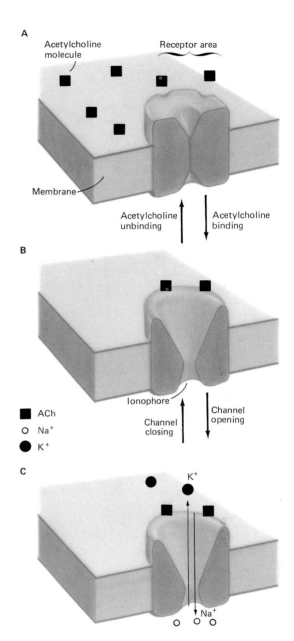

14–3 The nicotinic ACh receptor in the postsynaptic membrane changes conformation when it binds ACh to allow the passage of ions through the membrane. **A.** The receptor at rest does not pass ions. **B.** Two molecules of ACh bind rapidly to the portions of the α subunits exposed on the external surface of the muscle cells to form a receptor–ACh complex. The complex then changes its conformation, and this change results in the opening of a channel in the portions of the five subunits that are embedded in the lipid bilayer of the membrane. **C.** The channel now allows Na^+ and other ions to rush into the cell, causing the postsynaptic changes in membrane potential. Because the concentration of K^+ is greater in the muscle, this ion can leave the cell. (Adapted from Stevens, 1979.)

and spinal cord, has not been successfully purified from membranes. Therefore its size has not yet been measured directly, but it appears to be similar in size to the ACh receptor. The mass of the crude GABA receptor solubilized by treating membranes with detergent can be assessed at 200,000–300,000 daltons by centrifugation on sucrose gradients, by filtration through sizing gels, and by radiation target size analysis. It can be shown that any one of the three types of ligands (GABA, benzodiazepine, or barbiturate) influences the binding of the other two. For example, when GABA is bound to the receptor, a benzodiazepine (or a barbiturate) will bind more tightly. Another indication for a physical interaction between the three bindings sites is that the binding of any one of the ligands to the receptor complex can protect the binding sites for the other two from being inactivated when the membranes are heated.

The binding site for the transmitter is distinct from the sites for the two drugs, which, in turn, are distinct from each other, despite the evidence that all three sites can interact with each other. This can be explained if the GABA receptor complex, in addition to the transmitter-binding site and the Cl^- channel, consists of two other types of subunits that are regulatory in function. The two groups of drugs bind to and block the inhibitory action of the regulatory components in the receptor, thereby permitting GABA to interact with its binding site more effectively. Their binding results in the enhanced influx of Cl^- when the transmitter is present. These biochemical results are consistent with the pharmacology of both the benzodiazepines and the barbiturates, which, like GABA, are physiologically inhibitory. The use of radiolabeled photoaffinity benzodiazepine reagents is beginning to yield information about the actual polypeptides constituting the GABA receptor complex.

An Important Class of Receptors Mediates Changes in the Metabolic Machinery of the Postsynaptic Cell

Not all receptors mediate changes in ionic conductances directly. An important class of receptors responds to the binding of the chemical transmitter by changing the metabolic machinery of the postsynaptic cell through a mechanism involving the formation of intracellular second messengers—cyclic AMP or certain lipids. Cyclic AMP activates cyclic AMP-dependent protein kinases that phosphorylate proteins within the cell. Lipid second messengers, such as diacylglycerol, activate lipid-dependent protein kinases called *protein kinase C.*

The introduction of the charged phosphoryl group can alter the conformation of a protein and thereby modify the function of an enzyme, a regulatory protein, or an ion channel subunit. For example, by decreasing an enzyme's affinity for its substrate or by changing its localization within the cell, phosphorylation can diminish the activity of that enzyme. Conversely, enhanced activity can result if phosphorylation increases the affinity for substrate, positions the enzyme in a more efficient subcellular locale, or prevents the association of the enzyme with an inhibitor. As we have seen in Chapter 10, in

some neurons protein phosphorylation can lead to the closure or the opening of ion channels and thereby modulate the signaling properties of those cells. In neurons these changes, which depend on the presence of elevated concentrations of the second messenger in the postsynaptic cell, usually are of only moderate duration. Even though they are much more prolonged than the electrophysiological changes produced by the receptors that open ion channels in the membrane, these biochemical changes last only minutes because there are intracellular enzymes that rapidly inactivate the second messengers and there are protein phosphatases that remove the phosphoryl group from the proteins.

The mechanism described for the ACh receptor explains the activity of the class of receptors that causes changes in membrane permeability. Receptor molecules that alter intracellular metabolism are thought in principle to behave in an analogous manner—by altering their conformation in the membrane. Receptors that alter the cell's biochemistry, however, initiate a more complex chain of events because they participate in a cascade of reactions involving several distinct proteins. At the present time, the mechanism is known in any molecular detail only for receptors that provoke increased synthesis of cyclic AMP; one example is the β-adrenergic receptor that is present in cardiac and other muscle cells as well as in uninnervated cells such as the erythrocyte, where it has been extensively studied.

Like the ACh receptor, the β-adrenergic receptor binds the transmitter on the external surface of the postsynaptic cell. Instead of forming a channel through the membrane, however, the transmitter–receptor complex interacts with a coupling protein. The receptor and the cyclase do not interact directly, but are coupled by transducer proteins that shuttle through the membrane. There are several kinds of G-proteins: one is known to be stimulatory (G_s) and another is inhibitory (G_i). These proteins bind GTP or GDP. When the transmitter is bound to the receptor and the complex is associated with G_s, GTP displaces GDP at the nucleotide site on the transducer. The G-protein now associates with the catalytic subunit of adenylate cyclase, stimulating it to catalyze the conversion of ATP to cyclic AMP. The GTP-G-protein and the catalytic subunit of the cyclase together constitute the active form of cyclase. (When GTP is bound to G_i, the complex inhibits cyclase activity.) The duration of cyclic AMP synthesis is regulated by the GTPase activity of G_s. Its potency as an activator of the cyclase is again restored by interacting with the transmitter–receptor complex at the external surface of the cell.

Unlike the intramembranous portion of the ACh receptor, which forms the transmembrane ion channel, transducer proteins are not a part of the β-adrenergic receptor molecule. Cells without the receptor contain G-protein, which is not an integral membrane component, but only a loosely associated (peripheral) membrane protein. Moreover, in cells with the receptor, the G-protein exists in amounts far greater than the receptor itself. In

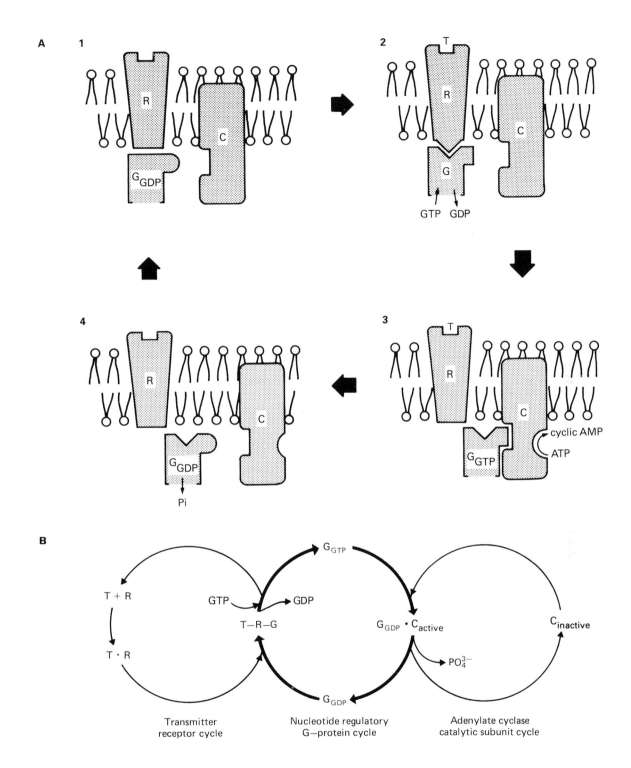

14–4 The synthesis of cyclic AMP that results when transmitter (**T**) binds to the β-adrenergic receptor (**R**) is mediated through a transducer, or G-protein (**G**). **A.** The GDP at the nucleotide site of the G-protein (**1**) is replaced by GTP when the transmitter–receptor complex interacts with the G-protein (**2**). The G-protein associates with the catalytic subunit of adenylate cyclase (**C**), which then catalyzes the conversion of ATP to cyclic AMP (**3**). This association of the G-protein with the catalytic subunit of the cyclase also results in the hydrolysis of GTP to GDP; the G-protein therefore dissociates from the catalytic subunit (**4**), and cyclic AMP synthesis stops. (Adapted from Schramm et al., 1983.) **B.** This process can also be conceived of as three interrelated cycles in which each component returns to its original state. (Adapted from Lefkowitz, Stadel, and Caron, 1983.)

fact, the molecular stoichiometry indicates that transducer proteins act to amplify the small synaptic signal (represented by the few receptor molecules) into the larger number of activated cyclase complexes needed to catalyze the synthesis of an effective concentration of cyclic AMP within the cell.

Further amplification occurs at the protein kinase reaction, the next step in the cyclic AMP cascade. The cyclic AMP activates the cyclic AMP-dependent protein kinase by causing the dissociation of its two regulatory subunits (R) from the catalytic subunits (C) according to the reaction

$$R_2C_2 + 4 \text{ cyclic AMP} \rightleftharpoons 2 R (2 \text{ cyclic AMP}) + 2 C.$$

(When combined, the tetrameric kinase complex $[R_2C_2]$ is enzymatically inactive.) When activated, the catalytic subunits function catalytically, that is, many times over, to phosphorylate protein substrates at serine or threonine residues according to the reaction

$$\text{Protein} + \text{ATP} \xrightarrow{C} \text{Phosphoprotein} + \text{ADP}.$$

In most cells, there are large numbers of protein substrates that can be phosphorylated by the kinase. Thus, the initial binding of a relatively small amount of chemical messenger to the receptor results in the subsequent incorporation of a much larger number of phosphoryl groups into a great variety of protein substrates within the cell.

Several important receptors, including muscarinic ACh receptors, α-adrenergic receptors, and receptors for some peptides, neither alter membrane conductances nor stimulate synthesis of cyclic AMP. These receptors have been found to stimulate the enzymatic hydrolysis of phosphatidylinositol, a lipid, in the postsynaptic membrane, to produce diacylglycerol and inositol tris phosphate. Diacylglycerol activates protein kinase C, and increasing evidence indicates that the lipid acts as a second messenger for these receptors.

Another important second messenger is Ca^{++}. This ion also brings about protein phosphorylation through Ca^{++}-dependent protein kinases. In addition, as the complex Ca^{++}–calmodulin (which is thought to mediate most if not all of the effects of Ca^{++} on enzymatic processes), Ca^{++} activates various enzymes: the form of adenylate cyclase that predominates in brain, one of the two major types of cyclic nucleotide phosphodiesterases (the enzymes that inactivate cyclic AMP by converting it to AMP), and a protein phosphatase, calcineurin, which is enriched at synapses, as well as several other enzymes. One of those enzymes is phosphorylase kinase, which is also phosphorylated (at two sites) by a cyclic AMP-dependent protein kinase. Moreover, Ca^{++} is also necessary for the activation of certain forms of the lipid-dependent protein kinase C. Further interaction between the lipid second messenger system and regulation by Ca^{++} is strongly indicated by the increasing evidence that inositol tris phosphate (one of the products of the hydrolysis of phosphatidylinositol that was already mentioned) can mobilize Ca^{++} from internal stores (for example, the en-

doplasmic reticulum), and thereby raise the concentration of free Ca^{++} within the cell.

The difference between receptors like the ACh receptor and the class that mediates changes in the metabolic machinery of the postsynaptic cell is important but not fundamental. Remember that some Ca^{++} enters the muscle cell along with Na^+ through the ACh receptor channel and that more Ca^{++} is released from the sarcoplasmic reticulum within muscle cells as a direct consequence of the depolarization of the muscle membrane caused by cholinergic synaptic transmission. To be sure, the intracellular Ca^{++} triggers the contraction of the actomyosin filaments (through troponin-C, a Ca^{++}-binding protein distantly related to calmodulin). But, as mentioned above, Ca^{++} also activates phosphorylase kinase, thereby enhancing breakdown of glycogen in order to supply ATP for the contractile process. Therefore, in muscle, the nicotinic ACh receptor is not only ionophoric, changing membrane permeability, but also operates through the release of Ca^{++} as a second messenger to change the metabolism of the postsynaptic cell.

The three second-messenger systems do not achieve their regulatory effects independently of each other. All three systems—cyclic AMP, Ca^{++}, and lipid—already have been shown to interact and influence each other at several key reactions, and many other points of intersection between these pathways undoubtedly remain to be discovered. Protein phosphorylation, used by all these systems, has complex regulatory effects because metabolic transformations consist of many reaction sequences that interlock and interact. These reactions are catalyzed by enzymes, many of whose activities are regulated by phosphorylation. In addition to the complexity of the pathways themselves, regulation by phosphorylation is also complicated because individual enzymes can be modified at more than one site in the molecule. Furthermore, the different phosphorylation reactions often are mediated by protein kinases that are dependent on several different second messengers. For example, as we shall see in the next chapter, phosphorylation of tyrosine hydroxylase can result in the augmented production of norepinephrine when adrenergic neurons are stimulated briefly. This rate-limiting enzyme of the catecholamine biosynthetic pathway can be activated in different ways by a cyclic AMP-*dependent* phosphorylation or a cyclic AMP-*independent* phosphorylation, or by both types of phosphorylation together.

Characterization of Receptors by Speed of Onset and by Duration of Action

Physiologists often classify receptors as fast or slow. This distinction refers to the speed of onset of the postsynaptic effect. The opening of ion channels, which is an intramolecular change in conformation, is usually a rapid process. Therefore, ionophoric receptors usually act rapidly—on the order of tens of milliseconds. Not all receptors of this sort are fast, however. The effects of some receptors for small molecules and for most peptides typically are slow in onset (hundreds of milliseconds to seconds), even though the action mediated is a conductance change in the postsynaptic cell. In contrast, receptors that bring about biochemical changes in the postsynaptic cell are typically slow, as might be expected because the several molecular steps involved each take time.

Duration of action depends on several molecular features. As discussed above, metabolic changes initiated by second messengers can persist long after the chemical messenger has been removed from the synaptic cleft. Receptor activity is largely determined by the lifetime of the chemical messenger and its effective concentration. A substance that is active at a low concentration and is removed slowly from the synaptic cleft will continue to act for a longer period than a substance that is active at relatively high concentrations and is rapidly destroyed. As a rule, peptides are effective at very low concentrations (10^{-9} M or lower), whereas the effective concentrations of small-molecule transmitters are much higher (10^{-7} M or greater). As we shall see in the next chapter, peptides are only slowly removed from the synaptic cleft. The difference in effective concentration is a postsynaptic feature that distinguishes peptidergic signaling from synaptic transmission with small-molecule transmitters.

An Overall View

Two of the three receptor mechanisms that have been described for other cells have now been shown to be used for neuronal signaling. The first of these mechanisms brings about direct changes in membrane excitability and is mediated by chemically gated ion channels. The second is mediated by receptors through transmembrane transduction that uses second messengers. This kind of mechanism also alters the excitability of the membrane, but only as a consequence of extensive and coordinated changes in the metabolism of the postsynaptic cell. The third receptor mechanism has not yet been shown to be used in synaptic signaling. This mechanism brings about changes in gene expression within the target cell either through surface membrane receptors that are internalized (like those for insulin) or by receptors already present within the cytoplasm of the target cell (like those for steroid hormones). When activated, this type of receptor alters the functioning of the genome by entering the cell's nucleus. The molecular basis of each of the three receptor mechanisms generally approximates and conforms to the speed of the actions they mediate: thus, chemically gated ion channels operate most rapidly, and underlie physiological processes that require speed. The physiological paradigm used to illustrate neuronal signaling in Chapters 2 and 3, the simple knee-jerk reflex, is but one example. Similar fast processes also include synaptic connections that produce much of the animal's motor behavior.

In recent years it has become increasingly clear that neurons also mediate longer lasting activities in target cells. Indeed, even in muscle contraction, sustained activity requires regulation of the muscle cell's metabolism. This regulation is mediated by receptor mechanisms that are slower in onset and that persist for longer periods of time. Furthermore, activities of neurons in the integrating centers of the brain involve both rapid and longer-lasting forms of synaptic transmission, and both ionophoric and transmembrane-transducing receptors have been found in neurons within these regions of the central nervous system.

As we shall see in the next chapter—where we consider the long-term changes in the catecholamine biosynthetic pathway that occur in noradrenergic neurons—changes in gene expression take hours and even days to be reflected in alterations of activity at nerve terminals. It therefore has not been thought useful to include the third receptor mechanism as a type of synaptic transmission. Nevertheless, from the logic of cell biology, it is now attractive to consider this mechanism also. Because it is the slowest and most persistent receptor mechanism known, it is appropriate for the persistent changes that are believed to underlie long-term memory. Moreover, its inclusion would serve to unify our view of the molecular basis of synaptic transmission.

Selected Readings

Cooper, J. R., Bloom, F. E., and Roth, R. H. 1982. The Biochemical Basis of Neuropharmacology, 4th ed. New York: Oxford University Press.

Kennedy, M. B. 1983. Experimental approaches to understanding the role of protein phosphorylation in the regulation of neuronal function. Annu. Rev. Neurosci. 6:493–525.

Nestler, E. J., and Greengard, P. 1984. Protein Phosphorylation in the Nervous System. New York: Wiley.

Reichardt, L. F., and Kelly, R. B. 1983. A molecular description of nerve terminal function. Annu. Rev. Biochem. 52:871–926.

Snyder, S. H. 1984. Drug and neurotransmitter receptors in the brain. Science 224:22–31.

References

Anderson, D. J., and Blobel, G. 1981. In vitro synthesis, glycosylation, and membrane insertion of the four subunits of Torpedo acetylcholine receptor. Proc. Natl. Acad. Sci. U.S.A. 78:5598–5602.

Changeux, J.-P. 1981. The acetylcholine receptor: An "allosteric" membrane protein. Harvey Lect. 75:85–254.

Claudio, T., Ballivet, M., Patrick, J., and Heinemann, S. 1983. Nucleotide and deduced amino acid sequences of Torpedo californica acetylcholine receptor γ subunit. Proc. Natl. Acad. Sci. U.S.A. 80:1111–1115.

Cohen, P. 1983. Control of Enzyme Activity, 2nd ed. London: Chapman and Hall.

Ehrlich, P. 1900. On immunity with special reference to cell life. Croonian Lecture. Proc. R. Soc. Lond. 66:424–448.

Fertuck, H. C., and Salpeter, M. M. 1974. Localization of acetylcholine receptor by ^{125}I-labeled α-bungarotoxin binding at mouse motor endplates. Proc. Natl. Acad. Sci. U.S.A. 71:1376–1378.

Gilman, A. G. 1984. G proteins and dual control of adenylate cyclase. Cell 36:577–579.

Harden, T. K. 1983. Agonist-induced desensitization of the β-adrenergic receptor-linked adenylate cyclase. Pharmacol. Rev. 35:5–32.

Hesketh, R. 1983. Inositol trisphosphate: Link or liability? Nature 306:16–17.

Karlin, A. 1983. The anatomy of a receptor. Neuroscience Comment. 1:111–123.

Karlin, A., Holtzman, E., Yodh, N., Lobel, P., Wall, J., and Hainfeld, J. 1983. The arrangement of the subunits of the acetylcholine receptor of Torpedo californica. J. Biol. Chem. 258:6678–6681.

Langley, J. N. 1906. On nerve endings and on special excitable substances in cells. Proc. R. Soc. Lond. [Biol.] 78:170–194.

Lefkowitz, R. J., Stadel, J. M., and Caron, M. G. 1983. Adenylate cyclase-coupled beta-adrenergic receptors: Structure and mechanisms of activation and desensitization. Annu. Rev. Biochem. 52:159–186.

Noda, M., Furutani, Y., Takahashi, H., Toyosato, M., Tanabe, T., Shimizu, S., Kikyotani, S., Kayano, T., Hirose, T., Inayama, S., and Numa, S. 1983. Cloning and sequence analysis of calf cDNA and human genomic DNA encoding α-subunit precursor of muscle acetylcholine receptor. Nature 305:818–823.

Noda, M., Takahashi, H., Tanabe, T., Toyosato, M., Kikyotani, S., Furutani, Y., Hirose, T., Takashima, H., Inayama, S., Miyata, T., and Numa, S. 1983. Structural homology of Torpedo californica acetylcholine receptor subunits. Nature 302:528–532.

Olsen, R. W. 1982. Drug interactions at the GABA receptor–ionophore complex. Annu. Rev. Pharmacol. Toxicol. 22:245–277.

Raftery, M. A., Hunkapiller, M. W., Strader, C. D., and Hood, L. E. 1980. Acetylcholine receptor: Complex of homologous subunits. Science 208:1454–1457.

Schramm, M., Korner, M., Neufeld, G., and Nedivi, E. 1983. The molecular mechanism of action of the β-adrenergic receptor. Cold Spring Harbor Symp. Quant. Biol. 48:187–191.

Schworer, C. M. and Soderling, T. R. 1983. Substrate specificity of liver calmodulin-dependent glycogen synthase kinase. Biochem. Biophys. Res. Comm. 116:412–416.

Sigel, E., Stephenson, F. A., Mamalaki, C., and Barnard, E. A. 1983. A γ-aminobutyric acid/benzodiazepine receptor complex of bovine cerebral cortex. J. Biol. Chem. 258:6965–6971.

Stevens, C. F. 1979. The neuron. Sci. Am. 241(3):54–65.

James H. Schwartz

Molecular Steps
in Synaptic Transmission

15

The metabolism of neurotransmitter substances is complex, reflecting many aspects of neuronal cell biology. For simplicity, a general scheme can be used to describe chemical transmission in terms of four steps—two presynaptic and two postsynaptic. These steps are: (1) synthesis of transmitter substance, (2) storage and release of transmitter, (3) interaction of transmitter with receptor in the postsynaptic membrane, and (4) removal of the transmitter from the synaptic cleft (Figure 15–1). Even though most of the transmitter molecules actually released are synthesized locally at nerve endings, other parts of a neuron contribute significantly to the process. As described in Chapters 3 and 4, the terminal is dependent on the cell body for all of the macromolecular components needed for transmission—biosynthetic and degradative enzymes, proteins of synaptic vesicles (both those in membranes and those that may be contained within the vesicle in soluble form), and most (but not all) of the lipid. While much of a neuron's small-molecule transmitter is synthesized locally at nerve terminals, the cell bodies of neurons that use peptides as chemical messengers must supply synapses with the peptide itself as well as with the vesicles in which peptides are processed and packaged, and by which they are ultimately released. After being synthesized in the cell body, these macromolecular components are rapidly moved along the axon to nerve terminals by fast axonal transport.

In this chapter we shall consider, from a biochemical point of view, the intracellular vesicle membrane system that is used by neurons to store and release chemical messengers. We shall also discuss the three known mechanisms for removing chemical messengers from the synapse and their pharmacological manipulation. Because the binding

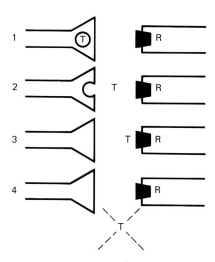

15–1 There are four biochemical steps in synaptic transmission: **1**, synthesis of the neurotransmitter substance (**T**); **2**, release of transmitter into the synaptic cleft; **3**, binding of the transmitter to the postsynaptic receptor (**R**); and **4**, removal or destruction of the transmitter substance.

of a transmitter to the postsynaptic receptor is a reversible process, and because removal of the transmitter from the synaptic cleft stops synaptic transmission, these removal mechanisms can be considered the molecular basis of punctuating the synaptic message. Finally, the concentration of transmitter substance available for release at synapses is maintained by biosynthetic pathways in the neuron's cytoplasm. We shall examine several kinds of metabolic control mechanisms by which neurons control the synthesis of neurotransmitters.

Vesicles Store and Release Chemical Messengers

The storage and release of a chemical messenger are mediated by vesicles that accumulate the transmitter and release it at the synapse by the process of exocytosis. In the nerve terminal, these vesicles are called *synaptic vesicles*. Nerve cells viewed by electron microscopy reveal characteristic vesicular profiles that are greatly concentrated at nerve endings (see, for example, Figure 9–2). The morphological appearance of these vesicles varies in different neurons, but the diameters of all of them range between 30 and 150 nm. In the other regions of the neuron, the vesicles that store transmitter are called *transmitter storage granules*. At present, it is uncertain whether all types of storage granules eventually develop into synaptic vesicles, but it is likely that some of the granule's membrane is used to form the vesicles.

Storage in Vesicles Protects the Transmitter from Degradation

There is abundant experimental evidence for vesicular localization of small-molecule transmitters. If free in the cytoplasm, these transmitters would be subject to intracellular degradative enzymes. For example, the *monoamine oxidases*, which are situated in the outer mem-

brane of mitochondria, degrade biogenic amines. There are at least two types of monoamine oxidases, A and B, which can be distinguished on the basis of their substrate specificity. Vesicular stores constitute a large reserve of transmitter that is protected from these intracellular enzymes.

Several neuroactive peptides have also been shown to be localized within vesicles (for example, substance P in terminals of neurons in the substantia nigra, and enkephalins in chromaffin granules), and it is expected that all types of peptides used as messengers will ultimately be found to be contained in vesicles. Because of the manner in which neuroactive peptides are synthesized, it can be assumed that essentially all of the peptide within a neuron is packaged in vesicles. Unlike the small-molecule transmitters, none of the peptide is synthesized in the cytosol, and therefore no mechanism for regulating the *cytoplasmic* level of peptide need exist. The absence of specific enzymes for controlling the intracellular store of these messengers is another point of difference between classical transmitters and neuroactive peptides.

Subcellular Fractionation Allows Biochemical Study of Vesicles

Additional biochemical information about transmitter vesicles has been obtained by means of *subcellular fractionation*. This is usually accomplished by differential centrifugation. Transmitter vesicles can be separated from other subcellular organelles because they differ in size, density, or shape. Isolation of synaptic vesicles is facilitated by an artifact of homogenization of nervous tissue: when neurons are ground gently in an isotonic solution, entire synaptic terminals can be pinched off. These artifactual sacs were named *synaptosomes* by Victor Whittaker, the British neurochemist who first described them and who has subsequently developed techniques for their preparation. They are fairly stable and much larger (about 1 μm across) than most subcellular membrane structures. They therefore can be isolated by differential centrifugation using either step- or continuous density-gradients created by layering or mixing viscous solutions of inert, impermeable substances such as sucrose or polysaccharide polymers. Centrifugation is carried out at high speeds in the ultracentrifuge; this method has been used for over two decades for separating subcellular organelles and viruses. Once separated from the smaller cellular components, the isolated synaptosomes can be broken by osmotic shock when diluted into water. This process releases synaptic vesicles, which in turn can be separated from all the other constituents of synaptosomes by another differential centrifugation step because the vesicles are considerably smaller.

After the vesicles are isolated, they can be characterized biochemically. Biochemical measurements of the amount of ACh in a single vesicle (2000 molecules) are somewhat lower than those estimated from neurophysiological experiments (about 5000 molecules per quantum). This quantitative discrepancy is probably small enough to disregard. Neurophysiological evidence for packaging of transmitters in vesicles has been described in Chapter 11, where the quantal hypothesis was considered.

Studies of vesicles isolated from adrenergic neurons show a heterogeneous population of vesicles; these vesicles can be classified into at least two types, large and small. Less extensive work suggests that serotonergic and histaminergic neurons similarly have more than one type of transmitter vesicle. The large aminergic vesicle contains both a higher concentration and more transmitter than does the smaller vesicle. Nevertheless, the small vesicle, which is similar in size to the cholinergic vesicle, is believed to be the one that mediates synaptic release of biogenic amine transmitters at active zones in aminergic nerve endings. In aminergic neurons precise measurements of quantal size by electrophysiological methods are more difficult to make than in cholinergic neurons.

Isolated synaptic vesicles contain other substances in addition to neurotransmitter. Both cholinergic and aminergic vesicles contain ATP. The large adrenergic vesicles contain at least two soluble proteins, called *chromogranins*. Large and small adrenergic vesicles also contain the enzyme dopamine β-hydroxylase, partly in a soluble state within the vesicle and partly bound to the membrane of the vesicle. Within vesicles, ATP and the chromogranins may serve to form complexes with transmitter. Because osmotic pressure depends on the *number* of molecules in a solution and not on their size, formation of complexes within the vesicle could serve to decrease the osmotic activity that would otherwise result from the high intravesicular concentration of free transmitter.

At some synapses, ATP and its degradation products—for example, adenosine—may act as chemical messengers. Adenine and guanine and their derivatives are called *purines*; the evidence for *purinergic* transmission is especially strong for purines released from sympathetic neurons on muscle fibers of the heart, from nerve plexuses on smooth muscle in the gut, and from dorsal root ganglion cells that synapse with some neurons in the dorsal horn of the spinal cord. The amount of ATP at some of these synapses appears to be considerably greater than at other nerve endings. At other synapses, even though ATP has been shown to be released, purines have no effect on postsynaptic targets. Presumably whether these common metabolites can act in synaptic transmission depends on the presence of a postsynaptic receptor that is sufficiently sensitive to purines.

Transmitter Is Actively Taken up into Vesicles

How do the vesicles concentrate small-molecule transmitters? What is the driving force? Catecholamines have been shown to move across the membrane of aminergic vesicles because of a pH gradient. This chemiosmotic mechanism was first proposed by Peter Mitchell in 1961 to explain oxidative phosphorylation (pH gradients also underlie the formation of ATP in mitochondria). Vesicle membrane contains a transport mechanism that is activated by the hydrolysis of ATP; this mechanism both brings in protons—making the inside of the vesicle more acid than the cytoplasm—and also generates a positive electrical potential. The pH of the vesicle is 5.5; that of the cytoplasm is 7.

There are several plausible models for explaining the detailed molecular steps by which the energy generated by the proton gradient is coupled to transport of the transmitter. One explanation presumes that only uncharged biogenic amine molecules are transported. (Biogenic amine transmitters exist as charged and uncharged species.) The pK of the primary amine group in catecholamines is about 9; therefore, at the neutral pH of cytoplasm, only about 0.5% of the amine exists in uncharged form. The cytoplasmic surface of the vesicle membrane contains specific receptor sites at which the biogenic amine binds in its charged (cationic) form. Once bound, the amine becomes uncharged by dissociating a proton. The neutral transmitter molecule is then translocated into the vesicle by carrier-mediated transport. Because the pH of the inside of the vesicle is 5.5, the proportion of uncharged amine inside is about 70-fold lower than in the cytoplasm. Consequently, when a molecule of uncharged amine comes into the vesicle, it is protonated and does not escape. According to this view, the transmitter is actively translocated into the vesicle and is concentrated there both by ion trapping and by the formation of complexes with ATP and internal proteins.

Vesicles Are Involved in Transmitter Release

Although there is still some debate, the vesicle hypothesis has been generally accepted, and there is little doubt that synaptic vesicles are directly involved at the site in the synaptic membrane at which transmitter molecules are released from the neuron (see Chapter 12).

The best biochemical evidence that exocytosis is involved in transmitter release comes from experiments of W. W. Douglas in which the cells of the adrenal medulla (which embryologically can be thought of as postganglionic adrenergic neurons of the sympathetic nervous system) were stimulated to release their content of biogenic amine (norepinephrine and epinephrine) into the circulation. When the materials released with the catecholamines were assayed, it was found that ATP, the chromogranins, and dopamine β-hydroxylase were released into the blood, in addition to the amines; furthermore, these constituents were present in the same molar ratios in which they occurred in isolated chromaffin granules. Only the soluble fraction of dopamine β-hydroxylase was released: no membrane proteins were lost from the gland. Historically, these experiments have been quite persuasive and are often cited as proof of exocytosis.

More recent morphological and biochemical observations suggest that synaptic transmission, although an exocytotic process, differs in certain respects from glandular release and neurosecretion. Release by the adrenal medulla involves large vesicles that contain high concentrations of amine complexed to chromogranins; these large vesicles interact slowly with the external membrane of the *gland* cell. Synaptic transmission, on the other hand, is mediated by smaller vesicles. These have been isolated by subcellular fractionation of tissue rich in true aminergic nerve endings; they have been found to contain less transmitter and few if any core proteins. It is therefore likely that synaptic transmission mediated by small vesicles at active zones in the terminals of neurons is a specialized form of neurosecretion.

Vesicle Membranes Differ with Type of Neuron

The biochemical make-up of storage granules and synaptic vesicles differs in neurons of different transmitter type. In addition to a specific biosynthetic pathway, each type of neuron has a characteristic system of membranes involved in packaging its particular transmitter substance. This vesicular apparatus is also the vehicle by which transmitter is released into the synaptic cleft by exocytosis. It is generally believed that a potential transmitter cannot be used unless it is packaged; thus, in addition to the specificity built into the biosynthetic enzymatic pathway, there is a *specificity to the packaging apparatus* in these cells. These various specificities are interesting not only theoretically, but also practically, because whenever a biological system has a specificity, it can be interfered with pharmacologically.

Any specificity recognition system within neurons can easily discriminate between naturally occurring transmitters, such as ACh and serotonin, because they are chemically quite dissimilar. There are drugs that are sufficiently similar to the normal transmitter substance that they can act as *false transmitters*, however; after they have been taken up by the cell, they are packaged in the vesicles and released as if they were true transmitters. They often have less potency in interacting with the receptor than the true transmitter. Therefore, their release decreases the efficacy of transmission at specific synapses. It has been suggested, for example, that several β-hydroxylated phenylethylamines and drugs that can be hydroxylated after being taken up into adrenergic vesicles owe some of their effects on adrenergic systems to their ability to replace norepinephrine in synaptic vesicles. When released, these drugs are not as potent as norepinephrine at postsynaptic adrenergic receptors.

Transmitter Is Removed from the Synaptic Cleft to Terminate Synaptic Transmission

The way in which a neuron disposes of transmitter to end the signal is critical to synaptic transmission, because if a released transmitter substance persisted for a very long time, a new signal could not get through. There are three mechanisms by which nervous tissue disposes of soluble or unbound transmitter substance: (1) diffusion, (2) enzymatic degradation, and (3) reuptake. Diffusion will remove some fraction of *all* chemical messengers; it can be an important means by which the synaptic cleft is cleared of transmitter.

Enzymatic degradation of transmitter substance is used primarily by the cholinergic system, and the extracellular enzyme involved is acetylcholinesterase. Although this enzyme is important in shortening synaptic transmission, its chief role is probably to make possible the recapture of choline, which, unlike ACh, is readily taken up by the neuron from the extracellular space (see below and Chapter 13).

There are many enzymatic pathways that degrade transmitter substances within the neuron and in nonneural tissues of the body. These enzymes can be important for controlling the concentrations of the transmitter *within* the neuron or in detoxifying transmitters that have escaped, but they are not involved specifically in terminating synaptic transmission. Many of these pathways are nevertheless important clinically: they provide sites for drug action and opportunity for diagnosis. Monoamine oxidase inhibitors, for example, which block degradation of amine transmitters within the cell, are currently used in medicine for the control of hypertension and in psychiatry for treating depression. Another example is the intracellular enzyme catechol-*O*-methyltransferase, which is important in degrading biogenic amines. It is found in the cytoplasm of most cells, including neurons, but is most prominent in liver and kidney. Concentrations of this enzyme's metabolites in body fluids serve as an indirect or diagnostic indication of the efficacy of drugs that affect the synthesis or degradation of the biogenic amines in nervous tissue.

The slow rate of removal is another postsynaptic feature that distinguishes neuroactive peptides from classical transmitters. Little is currently known about the way neuroactive peptides are removed, if indeed there are any mechanisms other than diffusion and slow proteolysis by extracellular peptidases. The slow removal contributes to the long duration of the action of the peptides and makes their metabolism seem more akin to that of hormones.

Reuptake of the transmitter substance from the synaptic cleft is probably the most common mechanism used for inactivation. At nerve endings there are high-affinity uptake mechanisms for the released transmitter or its metabolites. Choline, for example, is taken up specifically. Biogenic amines are also taken up into the presynaptic terminal by specific concentrating mechanisms. Some psychotropic drugs are effective because they block these uptake processes (for example, cocaine and imipramine). In the central nervous system, amino acid transmitters are taken up from the synaptic cleft by glial cells as well as by neurons. The application of appropriate drugs to block uptake prolongs and enhances the action of the biogenic amines and GABA. No uptake mechanism for peptides has yet been described.

A Late Consequence of Transmitter Action: Control of Transmitter Biosynthesis in the Postsynaptic Cell

We have seen that synaptic transmission operates by changing ion conductances and by activating second messengers. Transmitters also have other actions on the postsynaptic cell. One important metabolic process in a postsynaptic neuron that might be expected to be influenced by presynaptic input is the production of transmitter substance. In the absence of any regulatory mechanisms, the consequence of prolonged synaptic excitation would be depletion of transmitter in the postsynaptic cell. Conversely, uncontrolled synthesis of transmitter by an inactive neuron might result in overproduction. What are the ways by which a neuron can control biosynthesis of its transmitters?

There are three possible mechanisms by which the rate of an enzymatic pathway can be modulated:

1. Altering the availability of substrates or cofactors to the pathway.
2. Inhibiting or stimulating the activity of enzymes (usually the rate-limiting ones) in the pathway. Often the end-product of the pathway is the governing element; this is called feedback or end-product inhibition.
3. Increasing the synthesis of enzymes (usually the rate-limiting ones); this is called induction and is the consequence of a change in gene expression.

As we saw from the discussion on the regional differentiation of the neuron in Chapter 4, any *rapid* changes in transmitter concentration at synapses cannot involve the synthesis of new enzyme. Because the synapses are separated from the cell body and materials must be moved over relatively great distances, changes in protein synthesis are effective only after considerable delay. In a warm-blooded animal, for example, it takes about 18 hr to move an organelle 1 ft by fast transport, and most transmitter biosynthetic enzymes move by slow transport, which is at least 100 times slower.

To illustrate our current understanding of how neurons modulate their content of neurotransmitter substances, we shall examine two pathways: one in the adrenergic neuron, and the other in the cholinergic neuron.

Catecholamine Biosynthesis

The formation of norepinephrine is extraordinarily plastic. Under normal conditions, the amount of norepinephrine available for release remains constant in noradrenergic terminals despite moderate variation in functional activity. This steady level of transmitter is regulated by *short-term* mechanisms. *Long-term* processes come into play, however, under stressful conditions that result in intense sympathetic activity (for example, exposure to cold, forceful immobilization of the animal, and administration of the drug reserpine). Both types of regulatory mechanisms have been studied in greatest detail in the autonomic nervous system (in adrenergic neurons of sympathetic ganglia and in the adrenal medulla), but most of the processes have also been shown to take place in adrenergic cells in the central nervous system (principally in neurons whose cell bodies are situated in the locus ceruleus).

Short-term regulatory mechanisms involve modulation of the first enzyme in the synthetic pathway, tyrosine hydroxylase. This modulation occurs primarily at nerve terminals. The activity (V_{max}) of the hydroxylase in extracts has been shown to be about 50 times lower than that of aromatic amino acid decarboxylase and 1000 times lower than that of dopamine β-hydroxylase (see Chapter 13 for the biosynthetic pathway). What mechanisms can influence this enzyme's activity or production? In addition to being dependent on the concentration of the substrate, tyrosine, the enzyme also requires a pteridine cofactor—for example, tetrahydrobiopterin. In the adrenal medulla, the concentration of tetrahydrobiopterin is about one-half that of the enzyme's Michaelis constant ($K_m = 20$ μM); consequently, hydroxylase activity there should normally be limited by the availability of the cofactor. Indeed, addition of a pteridine to isolated sympathetic tissue has been found to increase the enzyme's activity. At normal plasma concentrations of tyrosine, tyrosine hydroxylase is saturated, indicating that availability of the substrate is not a critical factor under physiological conditions. Enzyme activity is reversibly inhibited by norepinephrine and dopamine, the end-products of the pathway; these feedback inhibitors act by competing with the binding of the oxidized form of the pteridine cofactor.

Phosphorylation of tyrosine hydroxylase by a cyclic AMP-dependent protein kinase increases the enzyme's affinity for both tyrosine and the pteridine cofactor and diminishes the effects of end-product inhibition. Cyclic AMP-dependent phosphorylation thus can enhance the enzyme's activity. A *further* increase can be achieved by another protein phosphorylation that is not dependent on cyclic AMP or on Ca^{++}. In the hydroxylase from adrenal medulla, this second phosphorylation results in an increase in the activity of the enzyme when substrate is saturating (V_{max}) without changing the affinity (K_m) of the enzyme for either substrate or cofactor. Dependence of the second phosphorylation on Ca^{++} and calmodulin has been reported for the hydroxylase from the striatum, and it is possible that phosphorylation might be lipid-dependent.

Finally, the activity of tyrosine hydroxylase can be influenced by the enzyme's subcellular localization. If free in the cytoplasm, it is less active than when bound to subcellular organelles. Fractionation studies have revealed that most of the enzyme is soluble, but in vitro some is recovered in a particulate form bound to membrane or cytoskeleton, and transient association may also occur within nerve terminals in vivo. It is still uncertain how this compartmentalization of the enzyme might be related to its state of phosphorylation.

We have discussed the rather large number of possible mechanisms that *could* account for the observed short-term regulation of catecholamine biosynthesis. All of the mechanisms described might influence the activity of tyrosine hydroxylase in the animal, presumably controlling synthesis of transmitter under different physiological circumstances. It is also important to appreciate that the data on the regulation of tyrosine hydroxylase come from experiments with the enzyme from several tissues (the peripheral and central nervous system and the adrenal medulla). Although a cyclic AMP-dependent phosphorylation regulates the hydroxylase from all adrenergic tissues, the types of protein kinases that carry out the other phosphorylations of the molecule and their effects on enzyme activity can vary from tissue to tissue. This complexity should not be surprising when viewed from the vantage of cell biology, since the principal molecular process at work is the post-translational modification of the hydroxylase, which could differ in detailed mechanism in the different tissues. As with other proteins, the same gene product can be processed differently in different cells.

Short-term increase in production of norepinephrine occurs within minutes and is rapidly reversible. Severe stress to the animal results in *long-term* changes whose effects can take days to be perceived. Increases in norepinephrine are observed within hours in cell bodies (in the autonomic nervous system, in sympathetic ganglia and adrenal medulla; in the central nervous system, in the locus ceruleus). Only much later (several days to 1 week) are they seen in terminals. Increased production of transmitter in this instance has been shown to result from the induction of new enzyme protein. The long-term change is not restricted to the first enzyme in the biosynthetic pathway. As discussed in Chapter 13, the genes for tyrosine hydroxylase, dopamine β-hydroxylase, and phenylethanolamine *N*-methyltransferase, which show sequence homology and appear to be related structurally, can show coordinate changes in gene expression. (In noradrenergic neurons, where the transferase gene is unexpressed, stimulation results only in the increased synthesis of the two hydroxylases; in the adrenal medulla and in the recently discovered class of neurons that synthesize epinephrine, however, the synthesis of all three enzymes is increased.) The change in gene expression is specific: the formation of other proteins, including aromatic amino acid decarboxylase and monoamine oxidase, is not affected.

These enzymes, like all proteins, are synthesized only in the cell body. The delay between the inducing environmental stimulus and the manifestation of the effects at synaptic terminals is a reflection of the time it takes for the newly synthesized enzyme to reach nerve terminals by slow axonal transport.

Acetylcholine Biosynthesis

In contrast to the plastic mechanisms regulating the enzymes concerned with the synthesis of norepinephrine, choline acetyltransferase is controlled only through the availability of its substrate, choline. As we have seen, the concentration of choline within nerve terminals depends on a high-affinity uptake process that accumulates choline from the extracellular space; sufficient choline to restore normal levels of the transmitter within the terminal after the neuron is fired becomes available when ACh is broken down after being released into the synaptic cleft (see the biosynthetic pathway in Chapter 13). This specific uptake mechanism is present only in cholinergic axons and terminals; it is absent in cholinergic cell bodies and in *all* parts of neurons that are not cholinergic.

Recent evidence indicates that high-affinity uptake of choline—which depends on the presence of Na^+ (as do many other carrier-mediated transport processes)—is also voltage-dependent: it is enhanced when cholinergic terminals are depolarized. Coupling of choline uptake and depolarization, perhaps through an effect on the conductance of Na^+, would serve to bring more substrate into the neuron when it is most needed, since depolarization triggers the synaptic release of the transmitter. Unlike the situation in the catecholamine pathway, no changes in amount of enzyme protein have been described in response to increased function of cholinergic neurons, and there is no indication of any long-term adaptive process.

An Overall View

Communication at synapses depends upon two classes of molecules: (1) chemical messengers and (2) chemically gated receptors. In the last two chapters, we considered the variety of small-molecule transmitters and neuroactive peptides, and we described both ionophoric and biochemical receptors; we also considered how the molecular properties of the messengers and receptors might contribute to the character of the synaptic transmission that they mediate. In this chapter, we examined the vesicles that package the chemical messengers within the neuron. These vesicles play a different role in the metabolism of the two major classes of chemical messengers—small-molecule transmitters and neuroactive peptides. After synthesis in the cytoplasm, small-molecule transmitters are concentrated in the vesicles, where they are protected from intracellular degradative enzymes that serve to maintain a constant cytoplasmic level of the transmitter substance. Because nerve endings contain so high a concentration of synaptic vesicles into which the locally synthesized transmitter is concentrated, and because the contents of the vesicular compartment are being continuously depleted by synaptic release, it is to be expected, from dynamic considerations, that much of the transmitter in the neuron must be synthesized at terminals. In contrast, the polypeptide precursors of neuroactive peptides are introduced during protein synthesis into the internal membrane systems that ultimately become the secretory granules and synaptic vesicles that are transported from the cell body to terminals. Unlike the vesicles that contain the small-molecule classical transmitters, these vesicles cannot be refilled at the terminal.

While certain aspects of vesicle function are quite different in different neurons, one role is shared by all neurons—those that use small-molecule transmitter substances and those that use peptides. Vesicles mediate the release of the chemical messenger through exocytosis. It seems axiomatic that the understanding of the molecular strategy of chemical transmission begins with the identification of the *contents* of the synaptic vesicle: only if a molecule can be released, does it have the potential of activating a receptor. Not all of the molecules released function as chemical messengers, however—only if the appropriate receptor is within the range of the substance released can that substance serve as a transmitter.

Synaptic transmission depends on the sustained availability of the transmitter molecules. Although complex, regulation of metabolism is a well studied aspect of cell biology. When viewed against a background of the information available about the control of biosynthetic processes in other cell types, the mechanisms by which a neuron can regulate its level of low-molecular-weight transmitter substance fall into place: short-term mechanisms all involve brief changes in the flow of small molecules through enzymatic pathways; these changes are mediated by *transient* alterations in the functioning of the macromolecular constituents of those pathways (enzymes and membrane proteins that serve as carrier or uptake molecules). Memory at the molecular level is quite short, however: there are no known mechanisms for maintaining altered functioning of existing macromolecules for periods longer than minutes once the stimulus has ceased. It is therefore to be expected that synthesis of new macromolecules is implicated in those changes in metabolism that persist for longer periods of time. Thus, long-term alterations in the production of transmitters depend on changes in gene expression.

Selected Readings

Blusztajn, J. K., and Wurtman, R. J. 1983. Choline and cholinergic neurons. Science 221:614–620.

Cooper, J. R., Bloom, F. E., and Roth, R. H. 1982. The Biochemical Basis of Neuropharmacology, 4th ed. New York: Oxford University Press.

Kelly, R. B., Deutsch, J. W., Carlson, S. S., and Wagner, J. A. 1979. Biochemistry of neurotransmitter release. Annu. Rev. Neurosci. 2:399–446.

Zigmond, R. E. 1980. The long-term regulation of ganglionic tyrosine hydroxylase by preganglionic nerve activity. Fed. Proc. 39:3003–3008.

Zigmond, R. E., and Bowers, C. W. 1981. Influence of nerve activity on the macromolecular content of neurons and their effector organs. Annu. Rev. Physiol. 43:673–687.

References

Andrews, D. W., Langan, T. A., and Weiner, N. 1983. Evidence for the involvement of a cyclic AMP-independent protein kinase in the activation of soluble tyrosine hydroxylase from rat striatum. Proc. Natl. Acad. Sci. U.S.A. 80:2097–2101.

Burnstock, G. 1976. Purinergic receptors. J. Theor. Biol. 62:491–503.

Dodd, J., Jahr, C. E., Hamilton, P. N., Heath, M. J. S., Matthew, W. D., and Jessell, T. M. 1983. Cytochemical and physiological properties of sensory and dorsal horn neurons that transmit cutaneous sensation. Cold Spring Harbor Symp. Quant. Biol. 48:685–695.

Douglas, W. W. 1968. Stimulus-secretion coupling: The concept and clues from chromaffin and other cells. Br. J. Pharmacol. 34:451–474.

El Mestikawy, S., Glowinski, J., and Hamon, M. 1983. Tyrosine hydroxylase activation in depolarized dopaminergic terminals—involvement of Ca^{2+}-dependent phosphorylation. Nature 302:830–832.

Gilman, A. G., Goodman, L. S., and Gilman, A. (eds.). 1980. The Pharmacological Basis of Therapeutics, 6th ed. New York: Macmillan.

Holtzman, E. 1977. The origin and fate of secretory packages, especially synaptic vesicles. Neuroscience 2:327–355.

Johnson, R. G., Carty, S., and Scarpa, A. 1982. A model of biogenic amine accumulation into chromaffin granules and ghosts based on coupling to the electrochemical proton gradient. Fed. Proc. 41:2746–2754.

Johnson, R. G., and Scarpa, A. 1979. Protonmotive force and catecholamine transport in isolated chromaffin granules. J. Biol. Chem. 254:3750–3760.

Kuhar, M. J., and Murrin, L. C. 1978. Sodium-dependent, high affinity choline uptake. J. Neurochem. 30:15–21.

Lisman, J. E. 1985. A mechanism for memory storage sensitive to molecular turnover: A bistable autophosphorylating kinase. Proc. Natl. Acad. Sci. U.S.A. 82:3055–3057.

Mitchell, P. 1961. Coupling of phosphorylation to electron and hydrogen transfer by a chemi-osmotic type of mechanism. Nature 191:144–148.

Saitoh, T., and Schwartz, J. H. 1985. Phosphorylation-dependent subcellular translocation of a Ca^{++}/calmodulin-dependent protein kinase produces an autonomous enzyme in *Aplysia* neurons. J. Cell Biol. 100:835–842.

Shkolnik, L. J., and Schwartz, J. H. 1980. Genesis and maturation of serotonergic vesicles in identified giant cerebral neuron of *Aplysia*. J. Neurophysiol. 43:945–967.

Schworer, C. M., and Soderling, T. R. 1983. Substrate specificity of liver calmodulin-dependent glycogen synthase kinase. Biochem. Biophys. Res. Comm. 116:412–416.

Usdin, E., Kopin, I. J., and Barchas, J. (eds.). 1979. Catecholamines: Basic and Clinical Frontiers. New York: Pergamon Press.

Whittaker, V. P., Michaelson, I. A., and Kirkland, R. J. A. 1964. The separation of synaptic vesicles from nerve-ending particles ('synaptosomes'). Biochem. J. 90:293–303.

Youdim, M. B. H., Banerjee, D. K., and Pollard, H. B. 1984. Isolated chromaffin cells from adrenal medulla contain primarily monoamine oxidase B. Science 224:619–621.

Lewis P. Rowland

Diseases of Chemical Transmission at the Nerve–Muscle Synapse: Myasthenia Gravis

16

In previous chapters we have examined the morphological structures that mediate chemical transmission and analyzed the electrical and molecular events that occur in the presynaptic nerve terminal and at the receptor in the postsynaptic membrane of the target cells. In this chapter we shall discuss a disease that illustrates a disorder in a specific synaptic function. Several human diseases are caused by impaired function of chemical synapses; the best understood of these is *myasthenia gravis* (Latin, severe muscle weakness), a disorder of function at the synapses between cholinergic motor neurons and skeletal muscle. Studies of myasthenia gravis illustrate how analysis of a human disease can illuminate our understanding of the normal physiology of the synapse.

Myasthenia Gravis Is Defined by Means of Clinical, Physiological, and Immunological Criteria

Myasthenia gravis provides a good illustration of how a disease can be delineated clinically and defined in rigorous terms. To be useful, the definition of a disease should include a statement about the cause (etiology) and the disordered process (pathogenesis and pathophysiology); it should also account for the clinical and laboratory abnormalities that appear in every patient affected by the disorder. The definition may be extended to include manifestations that occur frequently but not invariably.

Myasthenia gravis is an autoimmune syndrome that is caused by antibodies to the nicotinic ACh receptor. The antibodies reduce the number of functional receptors or impede the interaction of ACh with the receptors. As a result, there is weakness of skeletal muscle, which has four special characteristics:

1. The weakness is especially likely to affect cranial muscles (eyelids, eye muscles, and oropharyngeal muscles) as well as limb muscles (Figure 16–1A).
2. Unlike any other disease of muscle or nerve, there is a tendency for the severity of the weakness to vary within the course of a single day, from day to day, or over longer periods (remissions and exacerbations).
3. There are no conventional clinical signs of denervation that characterize disorders of the motor unit, such as fasciculation, loss of tendon reflexes, or atrophy of muscle, and there are no electromyographic signs of denervation. (Signs of denervation are described in Chapter 18.)
4. The weakness is reversed by the administration of drugs that inhibit acetylcholinesterase, the enzyme that degrades ACh at the neuromuscular junction (Figure 16–1B).

This clinical definition does not include the word "fatigue." Traditional definitions often consider myasthenia as a state of "abnormal fatigability," said to be brought on or increased by exercise and relieved by rest. That view is faulty, however; fatigue is not a reliable diagnostic criterion for several reasons. First, "fatigue" in this clinical sense implies diminishing strength after exercise, but the properties of fatigue in normal muscle have not been characterized and must vary according to occupational history, athletic experience, or age of the individual. Second, muscles weakened from any disease or injury might be expected to fatigue more rapidly than normal. Third, in myasthenia the eye muscles may be completely paralyzed but show no signs of fatigue at all. Fourth, when patients actually complain of fatigue, they usually describe a sense of exhaustion, a need to lie down and rest, but they do not describe the specific limitation of physical acts that follows true weakness of limb muscles as is found in myasthenia. Patients with a primary complaint of fatigue usually have emotional problems, or *psychasthenia* rather than *myasthenia*. The emphasis on fatigue has led many physicians to misdiagnose depression as myasthenia, and to treat the muscles rather than the psychiatric disorder that really causes the symptoms.

Emphasis on fatigue has even muddied the history of myasthenia. The first recorded case is usually attributed to Sir Thomas Willis, famed discoverer of the arterial circle at the base of the brain. In 1672 he wrote,

At this time I have under my charge a prudent and honest woman, who for many years hath been obnoxious to this sort of spurious Palsie, not only in her members, but also in her tongue; she for some time can speak freely and readily enough, but after she has spoke long, or hastily, or eagerly, she is not able to speak a word, but becomes mute as a Fish, nor can she recover the use of her voice under an hour or two.

This quaint description fulfills the expectations of abnormal fatigue; muscle function disappears after exercise and reappears after rest. It is true that slurred speech

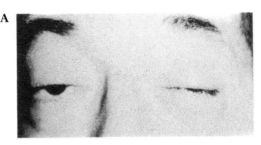

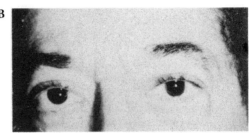

16–1 **A.** Severe drooping of the eyelids, or ptosis, is characteristic of myasthenia gravis. In addition, this patient could also not move his eyes to look to either side. **B.** One minute after he received an intravenous injection of 10 mg edrophonium, an inhibitor of cholinesterase, both his eyes were open and he could move them freely. (From Rowland, Hoefer, and Aranow, 1958.)

(dysarthria) is common in myasthenia, and it may become worse after prolonged speaking. However, *anarthria,* to become "mute as a Fish," never occurs in myasthenia and it is remarkable that myastheniologists have accepted Willis's case, despite their own daily experience to the contrary. Anarthria, like fatigue, is more apt to be psychogenic.

The modern history of our understanding of myasthenia gravis can be divided into two periods. The first period extends from the delineation of the syndrome, in the nineteenth century, to about 1970. The second, characterized by the revolutionary development of new ideas about the etiology of the disease, extends from 1973 to the present. Throughout our discussion of these two periods it is important to follow two intertwined themes, which offer a framework for describing the disease. One is a physiological approach, concerned with the abnormality of cholinergic transmission between the motor nerve terminal and skeletal muscle; the other is an immunological approach, concerned with the production of antibodies to the patient's own ACh receptors.

The Essential Characteristics of the Disease Were Defined between 1877 and 1970

The first well-documented example of myasthenia gravis was reported in 1877 by Samuel Wilks of Guy's Hospital in London. By 1900, neurologists had described the important clinical characteristics of the disease. In 1900, however, diseases were still defined primarily in terms of morphological lesions found at postmortem examination rather than in terms of physiological or etiological criteria. In myasthenia, the brain, spinal cord, peripheral nerves, and muscles all appeared normal at postmortem, and the disease was therefore considered a disorder of function.

Physiological Studies Showed a Disorder of Neuromuscular Transmission

By the mid-1930s, two discoveries provided the information essential to identify myasthenia as a disease of neuromuscular transmission. First, Henry Dale, Wilhelm Feldberg, and Marthe Vogt, working in England, demonstrated that the neuromuscular junction operates by means of chemical transmission, and they identified ACh as the transmitter. Second, Mary Walker, in England, found that physostigmine and neostigmine are effective in treating the symptoms of myasthenia gravis. These drugs are inhibitors of acetylcholinesterase, the enzyme that hydrolyzes ACh and thereby terminates its action.

In the years between 1940 and 1960, A. M. Harvey and his colleagues at the Johns Hopkins Hospital described the physiological basis of the disorder. When a motor nerve is stimulated electrically, the summed electrical activity of a population of muscle fibers can be measured with surface electrodes. At stimulation rates of 2–5/sec, the amplitude of the compound action potential evoked in normal human muscle remains constant. In myasthenia, the amplitude of evoked action potentials decreases rapidly. This abnormality resembles the abnormality induced in normal muscle by d-tubocurarine (curare). Curare (an arrow poison once used by South American Indians) antagonizes the action of ACh at the neuromuscular junction by blocking ACh receptors. In fact, patients with myasthenia show a heightened sensitivity to curare. Neostigmine, which increases the duration of action of ACh at the neuromuscular junction, reverses the decrease in amplitude of evoked action potentials in myasthenic patients (Figure 16–2).

Mary Walker's findings and those of A. M. Harvey raised an important question: What accounts for the disordered physiological response? Any of three possible mechanisms might cause this abnormality: (1) the cholinesterase activity in myasthenia is excessively high, (2) the motor nerve terminals release inadequate amounts of ACh, or (3) the postjunctional receptor is reduced in its response or blocked by an endogenous curarelike factor.

For several reasons, a receptor defect seemed most likely. However, in 1964, Dan Elmqvist, in the laboratory of Steven Thesleff in Sweden, reported what seemed to be the definitive microelectrode study of human intercostal muscle. They found that the amplitude of miniature end-plate potentials was greatly reduced in myasthenia. Prolonged washing failed to remove any curarelike substance. Depolarization of the terminal (by application of K^+) caused the release of a normal amount of ACh, indicating that there was no abnormality in the mechanisms of release. Similarly, the store of ACh in nerve terminals was normal. Depolarization of the end-

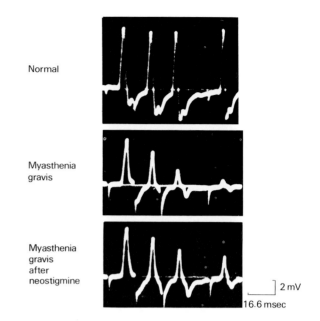

16–2 Electrical recordings of action potentials evoked by a train of four stimuli at 16.6-msec intervals demonstrate the effect of neostigmine in a patient with myasthenia. **A.** In the normal person, stimulation evokes action potentials of consistent amplitude. **B.** In the myasthenic patient, there is a rapid decrease in amplitude with repeated stimulation. **C.** After 2 mg neostigmine was injected into the brachial artery of the myasthenic patient, the decrease in amplitude was partially reversed. Calibration: 2.0 mV. (From Harvey, Lilienthal, and Talbot, 1941.)

plate by the ACh agonists carbachol or decamethonium produced a normal end-plate potential, implying that the postjunctional responses were normal. Because these tests did not indicate that the response of the postsynaptic receptor was reduced, the investigators concluded that the defect in myasthenia gravis was presynaptic: they suggested that synaptic vesicles released subnormal amounts of ACh in each quantum. The abnormally low amount of ACh might be due either to a defective binding of ACh in the vesicles or to the presence in the vesicles of a false transmitter. These papers are still admired as model applications of neurobiological methods and thinking to a human disease. Nevertheless, the conclusions of those skilled and careful investigators later proved to be wrong, as we shall see.

Immunological Studies Indicated That Myasthenia Is an Autoimmune Disease

Soon after the clinical syndrome had been identified, it was recognized that benign tumors of the thymus occur in about 15% of adult patients with myasthenia. In 1939, Alfred Blalock first reported improvement in a myasthenic patient after removal of a thymoma. After World War II, he and A. M. Harvey systematically performed thymectomy on patients with the disease and initiated what has now become standard therapy. There has never been a controlled trial of thymectomy, but it is now generally agreed that more than 75% of patients improve after surgery and that patients with a thymoma do not do as well as those without a tumor.

Why these tumors are associated with myasthenia and why thymectomy is beneficial remained mysteries because the immunological role of the thymus was not established until 1960. At that time, John Simpson, a neurologist in Scotland, suggested that myasthenia is an immunological disorder because it frequently occurs in patients who also have other diseases that are thought to be autoimmune, such as rheumatoid arthritis. The strongest experimental evidence indicating that an antibody might be involved was provided at Columbia University College of Physicians and Surgeons by Arthur Strauss and William Nastuk. They found antibodies to muscle striations in the serum of about one-third of all patients with myasthenia and in almost all patients with both myasthenia and a thymoma. Serum that reacted with muscle also reacted with thymus, presumably with *myoid* (striated muscle-like) cells in the gland.

It was soon evident, however, that the muscle antibodies of Strauss and Nastuk could not be the immediate cause of symptoms. The antibodies were not present in all patients, and, when present, there was no correlation between titer of antibodies and severity of symptoms. There was also no correlation between the presence or absence of antibodies and the occurrence of neonatal myasthenia in infants born to myasthenic mothers. Moreover, some patients with thymomas had the antibodies but no symptoms of myasthenia and no evidence of latent myasthenia (no abnormal response to repetitive stimulation and no abnormal sensitivity to neuromuscular blocking agents such as *d*-tubocurarine). Most important, antibodies that bind to striations in muscle could not explain the abnormality of junctional transmission. It still is not known what components of skeletal muscle are recognized by those antibodies.

Therefore, in 1969, myasthenia seemed an ill-defined autoimmune disease. The best evidence suggested that the physiological disorder was presynaptic, despite the lingering impression that there was a curarelike postsynaptic abnormality. This confused state of affairs was to be dramatically reversed in the next few years.

Identification of Antibodies to ACh Receptor Initiated the Modern Period of Research

The Antibodies Make Animals Myasthenic

With the isolation and characterization of the nicotinic ACh receptor, the modern concept of myasthenia emerged. Dale, in England, and David Nachmansohn, at Columbia University, had proposed that ACh exerts postsynaptic effects by interacting with a specific protein receptor, but numerous early attempts failed to isolate the receptor. In 1966, two chemists, C. C. Chang and C.-Y. Lee, were concerned with a local public health problem in Taiwan—poisonous snakebite. One of the

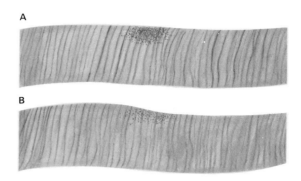

16–3 The ACh receptors in human muscle fiber are marked with ^{125}I-labeled α-bungarotoxin and detected in autoradiograms (drawn here). **A.** Normal fibers show a dense accumulation of silver grains over a limited junctional area, the end-plate, and a paucity of grains outside this region. **B.** In myasthenic fibers the grains are still mostly localized over the end-plate region, but their number per unit area is markedly reduced, indicating a reduced density of functional reactive sites. (Adapted from Fambrough, Drachman, and Satyamurti, 1973.)

toxins they isolated from snake venom, α-bungarotoxin, was found to cause paralysis by binding (essentially irreversibly) to the motor end-plate. By 1971, Ricardo Miledi and David Potter, in England, and Lee and Jean-Pierre Changeux, in France, had used the toxin to isolate and purify ACh receptors from the electric organ of the electric eel and *Torpedo* (see Chapter 14).

In 1973, Douglas Fambrough and Daniel Drachman at the Carnegie Institute and at Johns Hopkins used radioactive α-bungarotoxin to label the ACh receptors in human end-plates. They found that in myasthenia there are fewer binding sites than in controls (Figure 16–3). In the same year, James Patrick and Jon Lindstrom of the Salk Institute injected ACh receptors purified from eel electroplax into rabbits, intending to use antibodies to study the properties of eel ACh receptors. When the expected antibodies appeared, the rabbits became "myasthenic." The rabbits became weak, and the weakness was reversed by edrophonium or neostigmine. The animals were sensitive to neuromuscular blocking agents such as *d*-tubocurarine, and the response of the summated action potentials in muscle decreased with repetitive stimulation, as it does in humans with myasthenia gravis. A similar syndrome can be induced in mice (Figure 16–4).

Between 1973 and 1975, workers in several laboratories demonstrated that all the essential characteristics of human myasthenia gravis are reproduced in experimental autoimmune myasthenia gravis. In addition to the observations of Patrick and Lindstrom described above, these characteristics included reduced amplitude of the miniature end-plate potentials, simplification of postjunctional folds, loss of ACh receptors from the tips of postjunctional folds, and deposition at postjunctional sites of antibody and complement (a serum protein that participates in an immunological attack on antigens). The ACh receptors from *Torpedo* induced experimental autoimmune

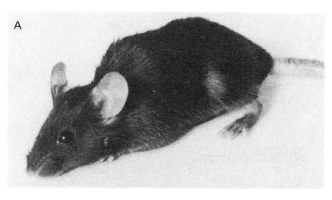

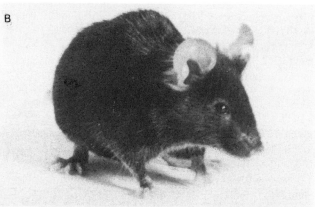

16–4 Posture of a myasthenic mouse before and after treatment with neostigmine. To produce the syndrome, the mouse was immunized with 15 μg ACh receptors from *Torpedo californica* and boosted 45 days later with another 15 μg of the receptor. **A.** Before treatment, the mouse is inactive. **B.** Twelve minutes after receiving an intraperitoneal injection of 37.5 μg/kg neostigmine bromide, the mouse is standing. (From Berman and Patrick, 1980.)

myasthenia gravis in several experimental animals, including mice, rats, and monkeys, suggesting that the nicotinic receptors to ACh are sufficiently similar in vertebrates that antibodies to the receptor of one species are also effective against the receptors of others. Moreover, experiments with inbred rats demonstrated that the disease could be transferred by thymus-derived (T) lymphocytes (which modulate the response of the B lymphocytes that secrete antibody). Thymectomy in early life prevented induction of experimental autoimmune myasthenia gravis in these rats.

The Antibodies Lead to Symptoms in Humans

After experimental autoimmune myasthenia gravis was characterized, antibodies to ACh receptors were shown in human myasthenia. In addition, when B cells from patients were cultured, antibodies to ACh receptors were produced in the culture. The idea that the human antibodies actually cause the symptoms of myasthenia was also supported by additional observations. First, Drachman and K. V. Toyka at Johns Hopkins found that re-

peated injection of mice with human myasthenic serum reproduced the electrophysiological abnormalities and reduced the number of α-bungarotoxin–binding sites in skeletal muscle. Similar results were obtained by Isao Kamo and colleagues in Japan when they injected mice with monoclonal antibodies to ACh receptors. These antibodies had been produced in culture by a permanent B lymphocyte line established from myasthenic patients.

More supporting evidence was that antibodies were found in infants with neonatal myasthenia; as the clinical syndrome abated, the level of antibodies declined. In adults, draining lymph from the thoracic lymph duct improved symptoms; the symptoms recurred when the lymph fluid was returned to the patient, but not when lymphocytes were replaced. Furthermore, symptoms improved and antibody levels declined when patients were subjected to *plasmapheresis*, a procedure in which blood is removed from a patient, cells are separated from plasma, and then the cells are returned to the patient but the plasma (which contains the antibodies) is discarded. Finally, clinically typical myasthenia seems to be inordinately frequent in patients taking the drug penicillamine (usually to treat rheumatoid arthritis); these patients also have antibodies to ACh receptors. When penicillamine therapy is discontinued, the myasthenic symptoms remit and the antibodies disappear. Penicillamine has been found to cross-link the sulfhydryl groups of ACh receptors, presumably altering the antigenicity of the receptors and provoking autoantibodies.

In 1976, Edson Albuquerque and his associates at the University of Maryland repeated the electrophysiological experiments of Elmqvist and Thesleff and found that the responsiveness of myasthenic muscle to ACh was decreased. Albuquerque's approach was similar to that of Elmqvist and Thesleff; technical refinements in the intervening decade accounted for the difference. Better microelectrodes had become available, and it was now possible to deliver ACh iontophoretically rather than applying it in the bathing medium.

The Immunological Changes Cause the Physiological Abnormality

As we have seen, A. M. Harvey and associates found that the physiological basis of myasthenia is an abnormal decrease in the amplitude of the summed action potentials when affected muscle fibers are stimulated repeatedly. How do the immunological observations that we have just considered account for the characteristic decrease in the response of myasthenic muscle to repetitive stimulation?

Normally, an action potential in the motor axon releases enough ACh from vesicles to induce an excitatory end-plate potential that is about 70–80 mV in amplitude (Chapter 10). Since the normal resting potential is −90 mV and the threshold for spike generation is about −45 mV, the normal end-plate potential far exceeds the threshold needed to initiate an action potential. Thus, in normal muscle the difference between the threshold and

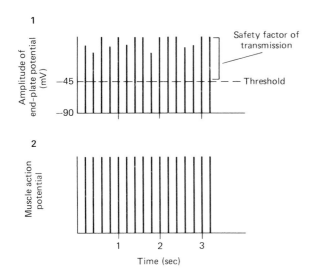

A   Normal junction

B   Myasthenic junction

16–5 The normal safety factor of transmission is greatly
reduced in myasthenia. **A.** In the normal
neuromuscular junction the amplitude of the end-plate
potential is so large that all fluctuations in the efficiency of
transmitter release occur well above the minimal level required
to elicit a muscle action potential (**1**). Therefore, surface
recording of a compound muscle action potential during
repetitive stimulation reveals a constant and unvarying
response amplitude (**2**). **B.** In the myasthenic neuromuscular
junction, postsynaptic changes have reduced the amplitude of
the end-plate potential in response to a given amount of ACh,
so that under optimal circumstances the end-plate potential

may be just sufficient to produce a muscle action potential.
Fluctuations in the efficiency of transmitter release that
normally accompany repeated stimulation now cause the end-
plate potential to drop below this threshold, leading to
conduction failure at that junction (**1**). When the action
potential is recorded from the surface of a myasthenic muscle,
the total amplitude—a measure of contributions from all fibers
in which synaptic transmission is successful—shows a
progressive decline and only a small variable recovery (**2**). This
sequence is characteristic of the myasthenic response. (From
Lisak and Barchi, 1982.)

the actual end-plate potential—called the *safety factor*—
is quite large (Figure 16–5A). The amount of ACh released can be reduced to 25% of normal before transmission fails to initiate an action potential in the muscle.

Most of the ACh released into the synaptic cleft by an
action potential is rapidly hydrolyzed by acetylcholinesterase, and the rest diffuses away. When the density of
ACh receptors is reduced, as it is in myasthenia, it is less
probable that a molecule of ACh will find a receptor before it is removed from the synaptic cleft. Moreover, the

geometry of the end-plate is also disturbed in myasthenia. The normal infolding is lost (including the tips of
the folds that usually have the highest density of receptors), and the synaptic cleft is enlarged (Figure 16–6).
These morphological changes further reduce the ability
of transmitter to find the few remaining functional receptors. As a result, the amplitude of the end-plate potential
is reduced and approaches threshold. Thus, transmission
is blocked readily even though the vesicles in the presynaptic terminals contain a normal amount of ACh and the

16–6 The morphological changes in the
myasthenic neuromuscular junction
reduce the likelihood of synaptic transmission.
The myasthenic junction has a normal nerve
terminal but shows reduced numbers of ACh
receptors, sparse, shallow postsynaptic folds, and
a widened synaptic space. (Adapted from
Drachman, 1983.)

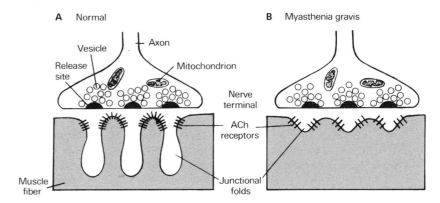

A Neurotransmitter binds receptor

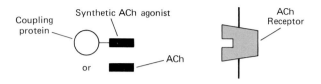

B Generate antibody to synthetic neurotransmitter (agonist)

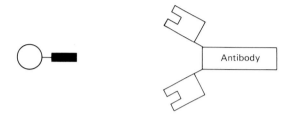

C Generate antibody (anti-idiotype) for antibody to transmitter

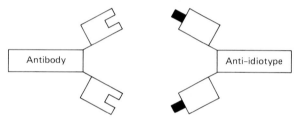

D Anti-idiotypic antibody will now bind to ACh receptor

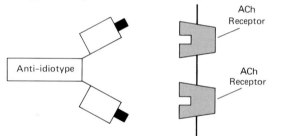

16–7 Antibodies to a receptor can be produced without using isolated receptors or transmitter. **A.** The neurotransmitter and a synthetic agonist of the neurotransmitter both bind to the receptor for the transmitter. **B.** The synthetic agonist, an analogue of the transmitter, is used to raise an antibody that has binding characteristics of the receptor. **C.** This antibody against the synthetic agonist can be used, in turn, as an immunogen to generate a new antibody. The new (anti-idiotypic) antibody has the property of reacting with the combining site of the first antibody. **D.** This anti-idiotypic antibody also has the property of reacting with the original receptor. Another way to express this concept is that the antineurotransmitter is equivalent to the receptor; therefore, the anti-antineurotransmitter is equivalent to an antireceptor antibody.

mechanisms of exocytosis and release are intact (Figure 16–5B). The loss of transmission at muscle fibers causes the clinical symptoms due to weakness and gives rise to the decremental response recorded with surface electrodes. Both the physiological abnormality (the decremental re-

sponse) and the clinical symptoms (muscle weakness) are partially reversed by drugs that inhibit cholinesterase because the ACh molecules remain intact for a longer time and are therefore more likely to reach a receptor.

The uncertainty of neuromuscular transmission in myasthenia is also assessed by the clinical technique of single-fiber electromyography, which measures the intervals between discharges of different muscle fibers of the same motor unit. The normal variation in intervals is called *jitter.* The normal time limits of jitter have been defined and include the sum of several effects: velocity of conduction in nerve terminals, transmitter release, and activation of the postsynaptic membrane. Jitter therefore may increase in different neurogenic diseases, but increased jitter is especially characteristic of myasthenia. When the intervals are very long, expected action potentials fail to appear. This phenomenon is called *blocking.* The number of blockings increases in myasthenia because of the reduced safety factor.

Antireceptor Antibodies Can Now Be Produced without Receptor

Still another observation indicates the power of the combined immunological–neurobiological approach. When an antibody is prepared to react with a small molecule that is an agonist of ACh receptors, the binding sites of antibody and receptor should be similar; the antiligand should be functionally equivalent to the receptor. Indeed, Bernard F. Erlanger and his colleagues at Columbia University made antibodies to a synthetic agonist of ACh, and the antibodies had binding properties similar to those of ACh receptors. Moreover, if antibodies can be made against the binding sites of the antiligand antibodies, the new (anti-idiotypic) antibodies should have antireceptor activity (Figure 16–7). This was also found by Erlanger and his co-workers. The anti-idiotypic antibodies did have antireceptor activity and actually induced manifestations of experimental autoimmune myasthenia gravis in the immunized animals. Thus, it is possible to produce antibodies to a receptor—such as ACh receptor—without actually isolating the receptor. This approach has since been used to make monoclonal antibodies to receptors for neurotransmitters when receptors were difficult to purify.

Important Problems Remain to Be Solved

Even though the central role of antibodies to ACh receptors in the pathogenesis of myasthenia seems to be established—so much so that myasthenia is now the prototype of human autoimmune disease—important problems still remain. We still do not know what initiates the production of antibodies to the ACh receptor. One possibility is that a persistent viral infection could alter surface membrane properties, rendering them immunogenic; but this has not been shown.

How do the antibodies cause symptoms? The antibodies do not simply act by blocking the binding site of

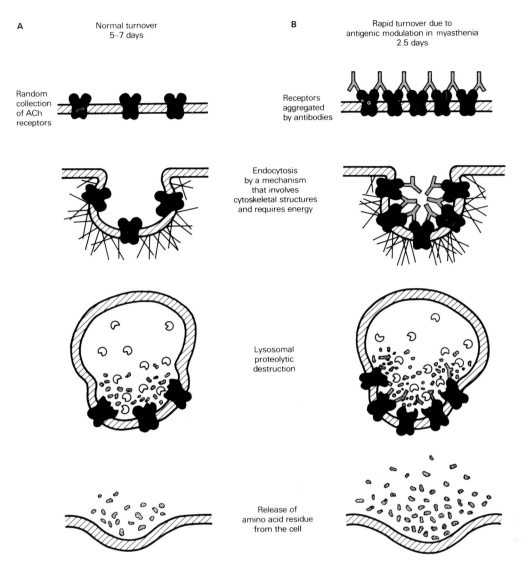

A Normal turnover 5–7 days

B Rapid turnover due to antigenic modulation in myasthenia 2.5 days

Random collection of ACh receptors

Receptors aggregated by antibodies

Endocytosis by a mechanism that involves cytoskeletal structures and requires energy

Lysosomal proteolytic destruction

Release of amino acid residue from the cell

16–8 The normal rate of destruction of ACh receptors is increased in myasthenia. The degradation of the receptor is schematically illustrated as occurring in consecutive steps. **A.** Normal turnover of randomly spaced ACh receptors takes place every 5–7 days.
B. In myasthenia gravis and in experimental autoimmune myasthenia gravis the primary mechanisms of ACh receptor loss are antigenic modulation and complement-mediated focal lysis of the postsynaptic membrane. The cross-linking of ACh receptors by the antireceptor antibody facilitates the normal endocytosis and phagocytic destruction of the receptors, which leads to a two- to threefold increase in the rate of receptor turnover. Binding of antireceptor antibody activates complement, which is involved in focal lysis of the postsynaptic membrane. This focal lysis is probably primarily responsible for the alterations of postsynaptic membrane morphology (Figure 16–6) that characterize myasthenia. (Adapted from Lindstrom, 1981, and Drachman, 1983.)

the receptor for ACh because the antibodies must react with determinants on the receptor molecule other than the α-bungarotoxin–binding site (and therefore the ACh-binding site). This property of the antibody—that it reacts with a site other than the ACh recognition site—is actually the basis of the conventional assay for the antibodies. To serve as test antigen, ACh receptors are labeled by ^{125}I-α-bungarotoxin, which then occupies the ACh-binding site. Nevertheless, the antibody recognizes and combines with other antigenic determinants in the receptor molecule. Thus, one effect of the antibodies might be steric hindrance of the interaction of ACh and

the receptor. However, the loss of functional receptors is attributed primarily to increased turnover and degradation of ACh receptors. This, in turn, is attributed to the ability of myasthenic antibodies to cross-link many molecules of ACh receptors (Figure 16–8). Some antibodies to ACh receptors bind complement and may induce lysis of the postsynaptic membrane.

Not all patients have demonstrable circulating antibodies, however, and there is no consistent relationship between the titer of antibodies to ACh receptors and the severity of symptoms. A dramatic example of this was seen in a woman who completely recovered from myasthenia and was in remission when she became pregnant. The woman had very high levels of antibodies although she was asymptomatic; the infant had both high antibody levels and severe symptoms. A similar situation can be produced in experimental animals. Experimental autoimmune myasthenia gravis is produced by immunizing animals with the native receptor. Immunization with *denatured* ACh receptors, however, results in the formation of high titers of antibody but no symptoms of experimental autoimmune myasthenia.

The antibodies found in the serum of myasthenic patients or in animals with experimental autoimmune myasthenia gravis are polyclonal; they are produced by different B cells in response to different antigenic determinants and are therefore heterogeneous in specificity. This kind of heterogeneity has been demonstrated by the study of monoclonal antibodies (produced by clones from a single B cell) that differ in capacity to interact with purified ACh receptors. Some monoclonal antibodies to the ACh receptors induce manifestations of experimental autoimmune myasthenia gravis in mice, but others have no effect, presumably because they do not react with or cross-link the receptors effectively or because they fail to bind complement. Therefore, some people with high titers of antibodies to the receptor but few or no clinical symptoms might have a type of antibody that is limited in ability to interfere with synaptic transmission. In contrast, other patients with severe myasthenia might have low titers of antibodies that are very effective in interfering with the functioning of the receptor.

The role of the thymus in myasthenia is also open to question. It is not clear why, when improvement occurs after thymectomy, it is usually delayed for months or years. It also is not clear whether thymectomy removes the cells that produce antibody, the antigenic stimulus, both, or neither.

Several other important questions remain unanswered: If the disease is due to circulating antibodies, why are some muscles affected and others spared? What is responsible for the remissions and exacerbations? Abnormal lymphocyte responses to ACh receptors have also been identified in human myasthenia; what is the role of altered cell-mediated immunity? Finally, what is the relationship between the antibodies to ACh receptors and the striation-binding antibodies of Nastuk and Strauss?

Myasthenia Gravis May Be a Heterogeneous Syndrome

One result of the modern analysis of myasthenia has been the increased support for the idea that myasthenia gravis may be a heterogeneous syndrome. This had been suspected earlier but was difficult to prove. For instance, it had long been recognized that congenital myasthenia (symptoms present from birth in children whose mothers do not themselves have myasthenia) is often familial. Now it seems that patients with congenital myasthenia do not have antibodies to ACh receptors. Therefore, there may be two distinct major categories of myas-

thenia: an acquired autoimmune form in older children and adults (with ACh receptor antibodies), and a nonimmune hereditable congenital myasthenia (without ACh receptor antibodies).

Further heterogeneity among the congenital cases has been suggested by the biophysical and immunocytochemical studies of Andrew Engel, Edward Lambert, and their colleagues at the Mayo Clinic, and of Angela Vincent, John Newsom-Davis, Stuart Cull-Candy, and their colleagues in London. Some cases seem to be due to a presynaptic abnormality, with impaired release of ACh from nerve terminals. Others are apparently due to postsynaptic disorders, including congenital lack of acetylcholinesterase, altered capacity of ACh receptors to react with ACh, or abnormally low numbers of ACh receptors. On the basis of the clinical picture alone, these differences could not have been imagined.

Current Therapy Is Effective but Not Ideal

Despite the revolutionary impact of immunological advances, treatment of myasthenia is still a problem—although progress has been considerable. Twenty-five years ago, the mortality rate of the disease was about 33%. Now, few patients die of myasthenia itself; normal life expectancy is probably reduced very little, and other complicating diseases are much more likely to cause death. Years ago, the respiratory-care units of hospitals were usually populated by patients with myasthenia who suffered respiratory crisis; the number of patients in crisis seems to have decreased dramatically. The cause of these changes is not clear. Some investigators attribute the improvement to widespread use of thymectomy and steroid therapy; skeptics point to improved respiratory care, so that the disease is not fatal and a new type of natural history emerges.

There are two general types of therapy: anticholinesterase medication, and measures that are designed to alter the course of the disease by immunological manipulation. Drugs that inhibit cholinesterase provide symptomatic relief but do not alter the course of the disease; moreover, they rarely relieve symptoms completely. For more prolonged treatment, the clinician must choose among thymectomy, steroids, immunosuppressive drugs (azathioprine and cyclophosphamide are most popular), and plasmapheresis. The best sequence and combination of these choices are still being debated.

Other Disorders of Neuromuscular Transmission: Presynaptic (Facilitating) Neuromuscular Block

In some patients with carcinoma, weakness is associated with a neuromuscular disorder that is the opposite of myasthenia. Instead of a myasthenic response that declines with repetitive stimulation, these patients show an incremental response of "facilitating neuromuscular block." The first response to stimulation is abnormally small. Subsequent responses increase with repetition, so that the final summated action potential (in a population of muscle fibers) produced by a train at 5/sec is two to four times the amplitude of the first potential. This syndrome is called the *Eaton-Lambert syndrome*, after the investigators at the Mayo Clinic who identified it. This disorder may also be an autoimmune disease that results from antibodies directed against an as yet unidentified molecular component of the presynaptic motor terminals. A similar presynaptic physiological abnormality is seen in human botulism, and experimental studies have indicated that botulinum block is due to impaired release of ACh. Both Eaton-Lambert syndrome and botulism are treated with calcium gluconate and with guanidine, agents that promote the release of ACh.

An Overall View

Myasthenia gravis, a disease in which the number of ACh receptors is reduced, is improved by drugs that inhibit cholinesterase and thereby prolong the action of the transmitter. Facilitating neuromuscular block, in which the number of transmitter quanta is reduced, is improved by calcium gluconate, which presumably is effective because Ca^{++} enhances release. In principle, these findings suggest an insight into the strategy for treatment of diseases of synaptic function. Ideally, one should determine whether the cause of a disorder of transmission is presynaptic (a disease of transmitter release) or postsynaptic (a disease of the receptor). Once the cause is identified, the treatment most likely to give symptomatic relief is one that either corrects the affected step in transmission or eliminates the pathogenic agent. This insight emphasizes the importance of a theoretical understanding of synaptic transmission for analyzing and treating human diseases.

In practice, however, the history of work on myasthenia gravis illustrates that progress in our understanding of neurological diseases often depends on a complex interplay of insights from both clinical and basic research. For example, the clinical observation that thymectomy is therapeutically valuable became meaningful when the immunological role of the thymus was discovered and when clinical evidence identified the disease as autoimmune. Similarly, the clinical observation that neostigmine is an effective treatment established myasthenia as a disease of neuromuscular transmission because the drug is an inhibitor of acetylcholinesterase. Clinical insights have consistently proved important in weaving together the various strands of evidence that contribute to our understanding of neurological diseases.

Selected Readings

Drachman, D. B. 1981. The biology of myasthenia gravis. Annu. Rev. Neurosci. 4:195–225.

Grob, D. (ed). 1981. Myasthenia gravis: pathophysiology and management. Ann. N.Y. Acad. Sci. 377:1–902.

Lindstrom, J. 1979. Autoimmune response to acetylcholine receptors in myasthenia gravis and its animal model. Adv. Immunol. 27:1–50.

Lindstrom, J. 1983. Using monoclonal antibodies to study acetylcholine receptors and myasthenia gravis. Neurosci. Comment. 1:139–156.

Lindstrom, J. M., and Lambert, E. H. 1978. Content of acetylcholine receptor and antibodies bound to receptor in myasthenia gravis, experimental autoimmune myasthenia gravis, and Eaton-Lambert syndrome. Neurology 28:130–138.

Lisak, R. P., and Barchi, R. L. 1982. Myasthenia Gravis. Philadelphia: Saunders.

Rowland, L. P. 1977. Myasthenia gravis. In E. S. Goldensohn and S. H. Appel (eds.), Scientific Approaches to Clinical Neurology, Vol. 2. Philadelphia: Lea & Febiger, pp. 1518–1554.

Rowland, L. P. 1980. Controversies about the treatment of myasthenia gravis. J. Neurol. Neurosurg. Psychiatry 43:644–659.

Swift, T. R. 1981. Disorders of neuromuscular transmission other than myasthenia gravis. Muscle Nerve 4:334–353.

Vincent, A. 1980. Immunology of acetylcholine receptors in relation to myasthenia gravis. Physiol. Rev. 60:756–824.

Wilks, S. 1883. Lectures on Diseases of the Nervous System Delivered at Guy's Hospital, 2nd ed. Philadelphia: P. Blakiston, Son and Co.

References

Albuquerque, E. X., Rash, J. E., Mayer, R. F., and Satterfield, J. R. 1976. An electrophysiological and morphological study of the neuromuscular junction in patients with myasthenia gravis. Exp. Neurol. 51:536–563.

Berman, P. W., and Patrick, J. 1980. Experimental myasthenia gravis: A murine system. J. Exp. Med. 151:204–223.

Berman, P. W., Patrick, J., Heinemann, S., Klier, F. G., and Steinbach, J. H. 1981. Factors affecting susceptibility of different strains of mice to experimental myasthenia gravis. Ann. N.Y. Acad. Sci. 377:237–257.

Berrih, S., Morel, E., Gaud, C., Raimond, F., Le Brigand H., and Bach, J. F. 1984. Anti-AChR antibodies, thymic histology, and T cell subsets in myasthenia gravis. Neurology 34:66–71.

Bever, C. T., Jr., Dretchen, K. L., Blake, G. J., Chang, H. W., Penn, A. S., and Asofsky, R. 1984. Augmented anti-acetylcholine receptor response following long-term penicillamine administration. Ann. Neurol. 16:9–13.

Blalock, A., Mason, M. F., Morgan, H. J., and Riven, S. S. 1939. Myasthenia gravis and tumors of the thymic region. Report of a case in which the tumor was removed. Ann. Surg. 110:544–561.

Changeux, J.-P., Kasai, M., and Lee, C.-Y. 1970. Use of a snake venom toxin to characterize the cholinergic receptor protein. Proc. Natl. Acad. Sci. U.S.A. 67:1241–1247.

Dale, H. H., Feldberg, W., and Vogt, M. 1936. Release of acetylcholine at voluntary motor nerve endings. J. Physiol. (Lond.) 86:353–380.

Drachman, D. B. 1983. Myasthenia gravis: Immunobiology of a receptor disorder. Trends Neurosci. 6:446–451.

Eaton, L. M., and Lambert, E. H. 1957. Electromyography and electric stimulation of nerves in diseases of motor unit. Observations on myasthenic syndrome associated with malignant tumors. J.A.M.A. 163:1117–1124.

Elmqvist, D., Hofmann, W. W., Kugelberg, J., and Quastel, D. M. J. 1964. An electrophysiological investigation of neuromuscular transmission in myasthenia gravis. J. Physiol. (Lond.) 174:417–434.

Engel, A. G. 1980. Morphologic and immunopathologic findings in myasthenia gravis and in congenital myasthenic syndromes. J. Neurol. Neurosurg. Psychiatry 43:577–589.

Erlanger, B. F., Wassermann, N. H., Cleveland, W. L., Penn, A. S., Hill, B. L., and Sarangarajan, R. 1984. Anti-idiotypic route to antibodies to the acetylcholine receptor and experimental myasthenia gravis. In J. C. Venter, C. M. Fraser, and J. Lindstrom (eds.), Receptor Biochemistry and Methodology, Vol. 4: Monoclonal and Anti-idiotypic Antibodies: Probes for Receptor Structure and Function. New York: Liss, pp. 163–176.

Fambrough, D. M., Drachman, D. B., and Satyamurti, S. 1973. Neuromuscular junction in myasthenia gravis: Decreased acetylcholine receptors. Science 182:293–295.

Harvey, A. M., Lilienthal, J. L., Jr., and Talbot, S. A. 1941. Observations on the nature of myasthenia gravis: The phenomena of facilitation and depression of neuromuscular transmission. Bull. Johns Hopkins Hosp. 69:547–565.

Harvey, A. M., and Masland, R. L. 1941. The electromyogram in myasthenia gravis. Bull. Johns Hopkins Hosp. 69:1–13.

Kamo, I., Furukawa, S., Tada, A., Mano, Y., Iwasaki, Y., Furuse, T., Ito, N., Hayashi, K., and Satoyoshi, E. 1982. Monoclonal antibody to acetylcholine receptor: Cell line established from thymus of patient with myasthenia gravis. Science 215:995–997.

Lang. B., Newsom-Davis, J., Wray, D., Vincent, A., and Murray, N. 1981. Autoimmune aetiology for myasthenic (Eaton-Lambert) syndrome. Lancet 2:224–226.

Lee, C.-Y., 1972. Chemistry and pharmacology of polypeptide toxins in snake venoms. Annu. Rev. Pharmacol. 12:265–286.

Lee, C.-Y., and Chang, C. C. 1966. Modes of actions of purified toxins from elapid venoms on neuromuscular transmission. Mem. Inst. Butantan Simp. Internac. 33:555–572.

Lindstrom, J. 1981. Acetylcholine receptors: structure, function, synthesis, destruction and antigenicity. In A. Engel and B. Banker (eds.), Clinical Myology. New York: McGraw-Hill, Chapter 27.

Lindstrom, J. 1986. Function and molecular structure of the acetylcholine receptor. In A. Engel and B. Q. Banker (eds.), Clinical Myology. New York: McGraw-Hill, chap. 27, in press.

Miledi, R., Molinoff, P., and Potter, L. T. 1971. Isolation of the cholinergic receptor protein of *Torpedo* electric tissue. Nature 229:554–557.

Nachmansohn, D. 1959. Chemical and Molecular Basis of Nerve Activity. New York: Academic Press.

Patrick, J., and Lindstrom, J. 1973. Autoimmune response to acetylcholine receptor. Science 180:871–872.

Rowland, L. P., Hoefer, P. F. A., and Aranow, H., Jr. 1960. Myasthenic syndromes. Res. Publ. Assoc. Nerv. Ment. Dis. 38:548–600.

Simpson, J. A. 1960. Myasthenia gravis: A new hypothesis. Scott. Med. J. 5:419–436.

Smit, L. M. E., Jennekens, F. G. I., Veldman, H., and Barth, P. G. 1984. Paucity of secondary synaptic clefts in a case of congenital myasthenia with multiple contractures: Ultrastructural morphology of a developmental disorder. J. Neurol. Neurosurg. Psychiatry 47:1091–1097.

Strauss, A. J. L., Seegal, B. C., Hsu, K. C., Burkholder, P. M., Nastuk, W. L., and Osserman, K. E. 1960. Immunofluorescence demonstration of a muscle binding, complement-fixing serum globulin fraction in myasthenia gravis. Proc. Soc. Exp. Biol. Med. 105:184–191.

Toyka, K. V., Drachman, D. B., Pestronk, A., and Kao, I. 1975. Myasthenia gravis: Passive transfer from man to mouse. Science 190:397–399.

Tzartos, S. J. 1984. Monoclonal antibodies as probes of the acetylcholine receptor and myasthenia gravis. Trends Neurosci. 9:63–67.

Vincent, A., Newson-Davis, J., Newton, P., and Beck, N. 1983. Acetylcholine receptor antibody and clinical response to thymectomy in myasthenia gravis. Neurology 33:1276–1282.

Walker, M. B. 1934. Treatment of myasthenia gravis with physostigmine. Lancet 1:1200–1201.

Walker, M. B. 1935. Case showing the effect of prostigmin on myasthenia gravis. Proc. R. Soc. Med. 28:759–761.

James P. Kelly

Reactions of Neurons to Injury

17

In this chapter we shall consider the responses of neurons to physical trauma. To simplify matters, we shall again use the motor neuron of the spinal cord and the afferent (sensory) neurons of the associated dorsal root ganglia as models for analyzing the consequences of cutting the axon *(axotomy).* Damage to nervous tissue is particularly serious because most neurons in the adult mammalian central nervous system have withdrawn from the mitotic cycle and are no longer capable of cell division. Consequently, any physical injury that causes neurons to die will not be followed by regeneration of cells, as would happen to cells in the liver, but will bring about a permanent change in the structure of the nervous system. This structural change is usually accompanied by long-lasting alterations in the functions of the affected areas.

Cutting an axon interrupts both rapid axonal transport and the slower axoplasmic flow, the two mechanisms that carry materials synthesized in the cell body to the axon terminals (see Chapter 4). Therefore, the axon and synaptic terminals degenerate when deprived of their normal metabolic interaction with the cell body. Because axonal transport also occurs in the retrograde direction along the axon, it would be logical to predict that changes might also occur in the cell body after axotomy: *retrograde* changes indeed are found quite frequently after axotomy; in some instances they are severe and can result in death of the neuron.

In previous chapters we have seen that sensory information is first encoded by receptors and other afferent neurons, and that the series of synaptic interactions that follows eventually leads to the generation of the motor output, which constitutes a behavioral act. To understand the consequences of nerve injury, it is important to know that synapses mediate not only electrical signals but also nutritive, or *trophic,* interactions between neurons. Although the mechanisms underlying trophic interactions between neurons are not as well understood as those underlying synaptic interactions, trophic factors are crucial for the normal maintenance of these cells. Like synaptic interactions, trophic interactions are thought to occur via a neuron's synaptic contacts. Deprived of its synaptic terminals, a neuron may shrink, atrophy, or degenerate. Therefore, if a bundle of axons in the central nervous system is severed, degenerative changes may be found not only in the damaged neurons but also in neurons that *receive* synapses from the damaged neurons. In some injuries the presynaptic neurons that synapse on the damaged cells are also affected. Such reactions are called *transsynaptic* or *transneuronal* because they cross from one neuron to the next via the synapse. These influences can be mild, or they can be drastic and cause degeneration of the affected neurons. Transneuronal changes of various kinds are important in explaining why a lesion at one site in the central nervous system can have effects on sites distant to the lesion, sites that are distributed according to the connections that the lesion interrupts.

Degenerative reactions after injury have been studied in detail by neurologists over the past century. As a result, anatomical methods have been devised that utilize these reactions to trace synaptic connections within the brain. These anatomical methods are useful adjuncts to the modern cell-labeling techniques—rapid anterograde and retrograde transport of electron-dense and radiolabeled markers—that we considered in Chapter 4. We shall consider some of the applications of these tracing procedures later in this chapter.

In addition to neurons, nervous tissue contains glial cells (oligodendrocytes, astrocytes, ependymal cells, Schwann cells, and microglia). Some of these cells play an important role in healing. Certain types of supporting cells absorb the cellular debris that results from neuronal injury by taking up and destroying (phagocytosing) toxic products of degeneration. On the other hand, supporting cells can sometimes interfere with healing if their proliferation blocks the restoration of severed synaptic connections within the brain and spinal cord. Therefore, the healing processes that are activated in the central nervous system by neuronal injury can be both helpful (phagocytosis) and troublesome (blocked regeneration)—a rule that holds true for many of the restorative processes employed by the body.

Cutting the Axon Causes Changes in the Neuron and in Glial Cells

If a bundle of axons is cut, either by sectioning of a tract within the brain or by sectioning of a peripheral nerve, the site where the lesion is located is termed the *zone of trauma.* The part of the axon still connected to the cell body is the *proximal segment,* and the part isolated from the rest of the cell is the *distal segment.* The cut ends of both parts of the axon lose axoplasm immediately after injury, but the ends soon become sealed off by fusion of the axon membrane, retract from one another, and begin

to swell. The swollen *retraction bulbs* that result are formed largely by materials carried along the axon by axonal transport and axoplasmic flow. Mitochondria, vesicles, multivesicular bodies, and much unidentified membranous material pile up in the sealed end of each axon segment. Both the proximal and the distal segments swell because fast axonal transport occurs in two directions. The proximal end swells more, however, because newly synthesized neurofilaments, microtubules, and microfilaments, traveling by slow axoplasmic flow, come from the cell body only.

At a zone of trauma in the central nervous system, the axon and myelin sheath undergo rapid local degeneration. Because blood vessels are usually interrupted by a lesion, macrophages from the general circulation can enter the area and phagocytose axonal debris. Glial cells (astrocytes and microglia) also proliferate and act as phagocytes. In the central nervous system, however, the proliferation of fibrous astrocytes *leads to the formation of a glial scar* around the zone of trauma. Scarring can block the course taken by regenerating axons and establish an effective barrier against the reformation of central connections.

Degeneration spreads in both directions along the axon from the zone of trauma, but only for a short distance in the proximal segment, usually up to the point of origin of the first axon collateral. After 2–3 days, a retrograde reaction is seen in the cell body. If the entire cell body dies, then degeneration spreads from the axon hillock down along the remainder of the proximal segment. In the distal segment, outside the zone of trauma, degeneration first appears in the axon terminal about 1 day after the occurrence of the lesion. In approximately 2 weeks, the synapses formed by the distal segment degenerate completely; this process is called *terminal degeneration.* Degeneration of the distal axon itself takes place over a period of 1–2 months. This is termed *Wallerian degeneration* because it was first described by the English physician Augustus Waller in the nineteenth century. Eventually, cells that are either pre- or postsynaptic to the injured neuron may also be affected. This transneuronal degeneration may be anterograde or retrograde: it is anterograde if the affected cell receives synapses from the injured neuron and retrograde if the affected cell makes synapses on the injured neuron. The various types of reaction to a severed axon are depicted in Figure 17–1. We shall consider each of them in turn.

Terminal Degeneration Leads to the Rapid Loss of the Presynaptic Terminal

The axon terminal is very sensitive to interruption of contact with the parent cell body. If the axon of a motor neuron to a skeletal muscle is severed by cutting a peripheral nerve, within a matter of hours degenerative changes begin to occur at the presynaptic terminals of the motor axon because the maintenance of its integrity is critically dependent on fast axonal transport. Intracellular recordings from muscle fibers after the motor axons that innervate them are severed have shown that synaptic transmission fails soon after the axon is cut, even be-

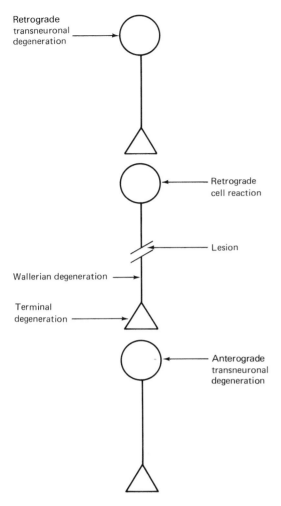

17–1 Axotomy can result in degeneration not only in the injured cell, but also in those cells with which it shares synapses.

fore the first morphological signs of degeneration become evident in the synaptic terminal. The onset of transmission failure is very rapid if the axon is cut close to the synaptic terminal region, and slower if the axon is cut close to the cell body. This indicates that axonal transport continues for some time in the distal segment until the entire axon is depleted of metabolic products required for synaptic transmission.

The degenerative changes that occur in the synaptic terminal itself are similar to the changes that take place in degenerating synapses in the central nervous system. Within 1 day after axotomy, the terminal and its mitochondria begin to swell. In some cases the terminal becomes filled with swirls of neurofilaments surrounding a central packet of disrupted mitochondria. Alternatively, the terminal may become filled with more homogeneous electron-dense products of degeneration (Figure 17–2). After 6 or 7 days the terminal is pushed away from its contacts with postsynaptic neurons by invading glial cells. At the neuromuscular synapse, eventually the Schwann

cells around the synaptic terminal of the motor axon de-differentiate and proliferate to form phagocytes that absorb the degenerating terminal. Soon afterward, the whole distal axon breaks up into short, beaded segments that are then phagocytosed by Schwann cells.

Wallerian Degeneration Leads to the Slow Loss of the Distal Axon Segment

About 1 week after the initial degenerative changes appear in the axon terminal, degeneration begins in the entire distal axon. The myelin sheath draws away from the axon and breaks apart (Figure 17–3B). The axon swells and then becomes beaded. Neurofilaments and neurotubules (collectively termed *neurofibrils* by light microscopists) soon fill the axon. Fragments of the axon and the myelin sheath are absorbed by *local* phagocytes derived from the glial cell population in the central nervous system or from Schwann cells in the peripheral nervous system. In the central nervous system, macrophages from the general circulation do not absorb the debris produced by Wallerian degeneration, as they do in the zone of trauma.

The sequence of axonal degeneration in the peripheral nervous system differs from the sequence that occurs in the central nervous system. If the *peripherally* directed process of a dorsal root ganglion cell is cut, or if a motor axon is cut, then the distal segment of the severed axon will degenerate as described earlier. However, the connective tissue sheath that surrounds the nerve in which the severed axon ran originally may remain intact. In many instances, depending upon the nature of the injury, the proximal segment of a severed axon can regenerate and reconnect to its previous synaptic sites as long as its cell body remains alive. The regenerating axons run along the connective tissue sheath, which acts as a conduit leading the growing axons back to the peripheral target (Figure 17–3C). On the other hand, if the *centrally* directed branches of dorsal root ganglion cells are cut, the glial scar that forms around the degenerating axons in the dorsal aspect of the spinal cord prevents any axons that might regenerate from reaching their central targets.

The disappearance of myelin from degenerating fibers in the central nervous system provides a means of tracing neural pathways. Normal myelin can be stained a dark blue with the *Weigert method* using a combination of chromium salts and hematoxylin. When a tract in the brain is cut, the myelin wrapping the distal portions of the fibers disappears. These degenerating fibers are not stained by the Weigert method, and thus provide a negative image of the route taken by the interrupted pathway. Because the loss of myelin persists indefinitely after a lesion, revealing fiber loss with the Weigert stain is often the only method available for tracing pathways in human pathological material. The Weigert method was one of the first techniques used to study the central connections of dorsal root ganglion cells, and much of what is known about the anatomical organization of afferent pathways in the human spinal cord has come from observations made with this technique.

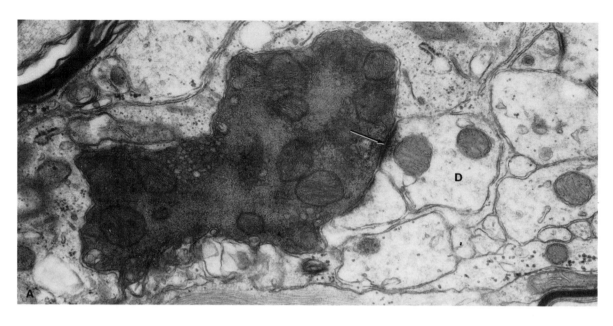

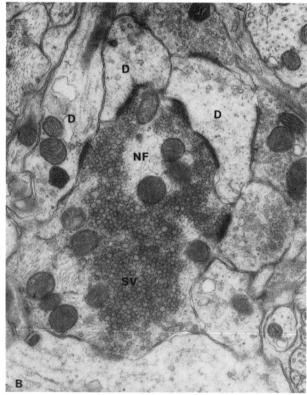

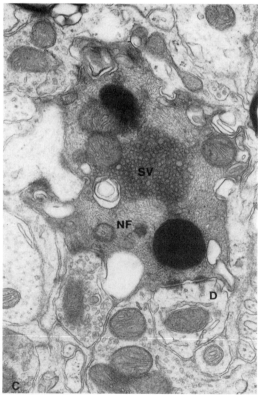

17-2 Synaptic terminals in the spinal cord dorsal horn of the monkey exhibit degeneration following lesions of the dorsal roots. **A.** Advanced degeneration resulting in a very electron-dense appearance of the synaptic profile. The degenerating profile forms a synapse (**arrow**) with a dendrite (**D**). **B.** Early degeneration in which neurofilaments (**NF**) appear among clumps of synaptic vesicles (**SV**). The altered profile forms synaptic contacts on several adjacent dendrites (**D**). **C.** Advanced degeneration in which neurofilaments (**NF**) form a dense matrix adjacent to a clump of synaptic vesicles (**SV**). The degenerating profile contacts a dendrite (**D**). Approximately × 40,000. (Courtesy of H. J. Ralston, III.)

The hypertrophy of neurofilaments or of electron-dense products of degeneration in damaged axons also provides a means of tracing connections. For example, neurofilaments found in the axons and cell bodies of normal neurons bind silver selectively. If the staining of normal fibers is suppressed with an oxidizing agent, the degenerating fibers can still be stained intensely because of their increased content of argyrophilic neurofibrils. Degenerating axons appear as black, beaded profiles against a pale background. This is, in part, the basis of the *Nauta*

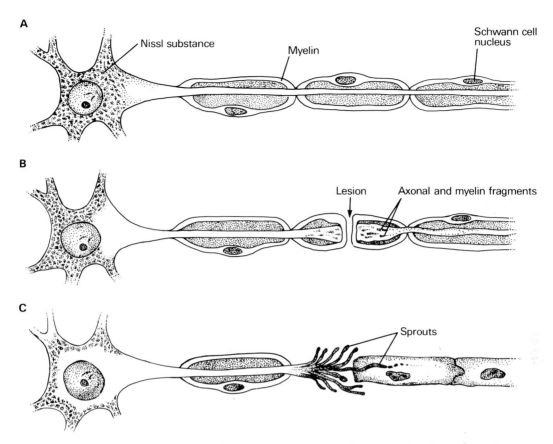

17–3 When an axon is severed, there are changes in the distal axon segment and in the parent neuron after the terminal has degenerated. **A.** Normal cell body and portion of axon. (The axon terminal and its changes are omitted.) **B.** Retrograde cell reaction and Wallerian degeneration. About 2–3 days after the axon is severed, the cell body begins to swell, and the nucleus swells and migrates. About 1 week after axotomy, the myelin sheath withdraws from the axon and fragments; the axon swells and beads, and then fragments. **C.** Retrograde cell reaction and axon regeneration. The cell body and nucleus continue to swell, and finally, the Nissl substance undergoes chromatolysis in preparation for regeneration of the proximal axon segment.

method, a procedure for tracing fiber degeneration that is widely used today in experimental studies of the anatomy of the brain because it stains both unmyelinated and myelinated degenerating axons.

The Neuronal Cell Body Also Reacts to Axotomy

There are two major ways in which the cell bodies of different classes of neurons respond to axotomy. After an axon is severed, some neurons undergo distinctive regenerative changes as they prepare metabolically for the regrowth of a new axon. For example, cutting the peripheral axon of a dorsal root ganglion cell or a spinal motor neuron causes characteristic changes in the parent neuron within 2–3 days (Figure 17–3B). The cell body first begins to swell; it may double in size. The nucleus moves to an eccentric position, usually opposite the axon hillock, and also begins to swell. Finally, the rough endoplasmic reticulum breaks apart and moves to the periphery of the swollen cell body (Figure 17–3C). Rough endoplasmic reticulum in the cell bodies of normal neurons can be stained a bright blue with basic dyes, such as

thionin, that bind to the acidic proteins in ribosomes. Clumps of endoplasmic reticulum stained in this way are termed *Nissl substance. Chromatolysis*, or the dissolution of Nissl substance, can therefore serve as a histological indication that the axon of a neuron has been severed.

Chromatolysis commonly lasts for 1–3 weeks. During this period the number of free polysomes in the cell body increases, as does the total amount of protein; RNA synthesis in the nucleus increases as well. These changes suggest that chromatolysis involves massive synthesis of proteins necessary for regenerating the severed parts of the axon. If proper connections are restored after regeneration of the axon, chromatolysis ceases and the cell body usually regains its normal appearance. If proper connections are not restored, the cell will atrophy or degenerate totally.

In experimental animals or in human nervous tissue, chromatolysis can therefore be used to identify which cells in the central nervous system give rise to peripheral nerves. In fact, observations of the distribution of chromatolytic neurons in the anterior horn of the spinal cord after motor nerve lesions provided the first anatomical maps of the motor neuron pools that innervate particular muscle groups.

Many cells do not undergo chromatolytic or regenerative changes after axon section. Thalamic neurons, for example, degenerate rapidly after their axons are cut, and they may either degenerate completely or remain shrunken indefinitely. Purkinje cells of the cerebellum do not undergo chromatolytic changes after axotomy. Furthermore, section of the centrally directed processes of the dorsal root ganglion cells or of the cells in the sensory ganglia of the cranial nerves produces no change in the cell bodies of these neurons.

Two generalizations can be made about chromatolysis: (1) Chromatolysis is more pronounced in young animals. Axotomized neurons commonly undergo chromatolysis but then degenerate, failing to regenerate their axons. A similar population of adult neurons may undergo chromatolysis after axotomy, regenerate, and return to its former state. (2) Chromatolysis is more profound if the lesion is close to the cell body. Consequently, the age of the animal, the site of the lesion, and the nature of the injury are important considerations in judging the potential for functional recovery after nerve section.

Neurons with processes confined to the central nervous system may undergo chromatolysis after axotomy, but they then either degenerate or remain in a state of severe atrophy. This is presumably because they cannot restore appropriate synaptic connections. Whatever the mechanism, the prognosis for the recovery of axotomized neurons within the brain is very poor. One of the key questions in experimental neurology is why damaged neurons are prevented from regrowing their central axons and reinnervating their target cells. Answers to this question might eventually lead to relief from the disabling and often tragic effects of stroke or trauma of the nervous system.

Central Axons Can Regenerate under Certain Favorable Circumstances

Why is it that central axons cannot regenerate but peripheral axons can? Is the deformation produced by the glial scar the only barrier to the regrowth of central neurons, or are these neurons simply incapable of regenerating an axon? Alternatively, perhaps the Schwann cell sheaths of peripheral nerves facilitate the outgrowth of axons after damage by releasing a factor that promotes regeneration. To test whether the environment created by the sheaths of peripheral Schwann cells can induce regeneration of central axons, Alberto Aguayo and his coworkers at the Montreal Neurological Institute inserted a piece of sciatic nerve between the cut ends of the spinal cord in a mouse. The peripheral axons in the nerve graft degenerated, but central axons from the spinal cord grew into the graft readily and traversed the gap between the cut ends of the spinal cord. In contrast, when regenerating peripheral axons were exposed to central glial cells

(astrocytes and oligodendrocytes), their normal regenerating outgrowth was inhibited. Thus, peripheral Schwann cells seem to release a factor that encourages the outgrowth of axons, whereas central glial cells lack this growth-promoting factor.

Does regeneration stimulate protein synthesis within the outgrowing axon? Mark Willard and his colleagues at Washington University have addressed this question and discovered that growth-associated proteins (GAPs) are indeed increased in regenerating nerves and may be essential for the reformation of the axon. Several of them are also transported in large amounts in the developing nervous system. If GAPs are required for axonal growth, then gene expression must be altered in damaged neurons to cause the synthesis of GAPs. The lack of regenerative capacity characteristic of most mature neurons in the brain and spinal cord may therefore reflect the absence of one or more steps necessary to induce GAP production.

It is not yet known whether regenerating central axons establish functional synaptic connections, but the study of nerve grafts and growth-associated proteins offers strong promise that the outgrowth of axons will be understood and that a reliable means for promoting the regeneration of damaged central axons will eventually be developed.

Glial Cells Absorb the Debris Caused by Injury

It is important to recognize the role played by glial cells in normal function as well as in response to disease or damage of the central nervous system. Two types of glial cells—astrocytes and oligodendrocytes—vastly outnumber neurons. Astrocytes predominate in gray matter. They have small (3–5 μm) cell bodies that are packed with fascicles of glial filaments about 100 nm in diameter (Figure 17–4). Numerous processes radiate from the cell body in various directions, and many of these come into close contact with blood vessels. The physiological importance of astrocytes is not known. In electron micrographs they are often found wrapping individual presynaptic terminals, and this has led to the idea that they may insulate synaptic terminals from their neighbors. In the damaged brain, however, it is known that astrocytes phagocytose neuronal debris. The term sclerosis (Latin sclera, scale) is often used to describe disease states, such as multiple sclerosis, that affect populations of axons in the brain. The term refers to the palpably hard scar of astrocytes that replaces phagocytosed debris resulting from the disease process.

Oligodendrocytes, which form myelin in the central nervous system, predominate in white matter. They have smaller cell bodies (1–3 μm in diameter) and give off fewer processes than astrocytes; each process appears to participate in forming myelin for a single axon (see Figure 3–4B). In the central nervous system, each oligodendrocyte contributes to the myelin sheath of several (as many as 20) axons by means of its different processes.

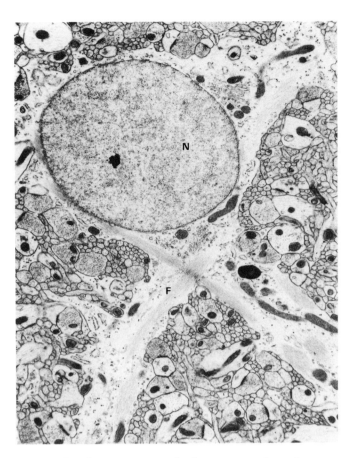

17–4 This electron micrograph of an astrocyte from the cerebral cortex of a cat shows the nucleus (**N**) and fascicles of glial filaments (**F**). (Courtesy of Dr. E. G. Jones.)

Glial cells proliferate around chromatolytic neurons and assume the appearance of phagocytes. Glial cells have been observed displacing presynaptic terminals along the proximal dendrites and cell bodies of axotomized motor neurons. The pre- and postsynaptic elements of the synapse appear to be pushed apart by the invading glial cells. This stripping of synapses has been confirmed by intracellular recording from cell bodies of chromatolysing motor neurons. Damaged neurons receive reduced synaptic inputs, and the evoked excitatory postsynaptic potentials are smaller in amplitude, as if synapses on the cell body and proximal dendrites were removed by encroachment of glial cells. Even though somatic synapses are displaced, chromatolysing motor neurons can still be activated because remote synapses on their dendritic tree that are normally ineffective begin to excite the cell. After the normal input to the soma is removed, new trigger zones develop on the cell body and along the axon. A reorganization of this type may enable the cell to maintain normal activity in the absence of a normal number of synapses. If appropriate connections with muscles are established by the regenerating motor axons, then the normal input to the cell body of the motor neuron returns. The reason synapses are shed in the first place, however, is still unknown.

What is the signal for chromatolysis? Most likely, axotomy interrupts the flow of some trophic substance moving back along the axon from the terminal to the cell body, and deprivation of this substance elicits chromatolysis.

Transneuronal Degeneration Leads to Changes in Cells to Which the Damaged Neuron Connects

As noted earlier, transneuronal degeneration is one facet of a broad class of trophic interactions known to occur between neurons that are in synaptic contact as well as between neurons and their peripheral target organs. Transneuronal degeneration was first observed in the visual system of the brain. The axons of the retinal ganglion cells join together to form the optic nerve, which terminates in an area of the thalamus called the lateral geniculate nucleus. The postsynaptic neurons in this nucleus send their axons to the visual cortex of the occipital lobe. When the optic nerve is cut, the retinal terminals in the lateral geniculate nucleus degenerate rapidly. After several months, the postsynaptic neurons in the nucleus undergo severe atrophy (Figure 17–5). This type of reaction to injury is called *anterograde transneuronal degeneration* (Figure 17–1). It does not occur in all brain pathways. When transneuronal degeneration does occur, the degree of atrophy is related to the percentage of total input removed from a population of neurons by a lesion. Other sources of input can reduce the severity of transneuronal degeneration.

Two speculative mechanisms have been proposed to explain transneuronal degeneration. The first is that neurons require a certain amount of stimulation to survive. Cutting the axons that provide input to a population of cells could reduce activity below a critical level, and the deafferented cells might atrophy as a consequence of this reduced activity. However, activity may not be the sole factor (see Chapter 56). The second is that some trophic substance necessary for the normal survival of neurons is released by synaptic terminals. Degeneration of the terminals removes this substance and leads eventually to the atrophy of the postsynaptic cell. Of course, the two mechanisms could be related if the release of the trophic factor is tied to the level of activity in the presynaptic fiber.

Transneuronal degeneration may cross more than one synapse. For example, some changes are seen in the neurons of the visual cortex after the optic nerve has been sectioned. Cutting the optic nerve causes neurons in the lateral geniculate nucleus to atrophy, and they subsequently induce degeneration in cortical cells receiving input from the thalamus. Transneuronal degeneration can also move along a neural pathway in a retrograde direction. Lesions in the visual cortex cause neurons in the lateral geniculate nucleus to undergo severe retrograde degeneration. The retinal ganglion cells that synapse upon the affected neurons in the lateral geniculate nucleus may then atrophy after a few months. Evidence of this kind reveals the degree to which neurons are depen-

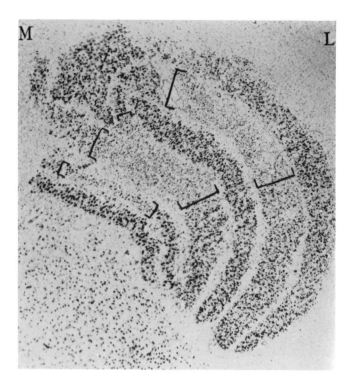

17–5 This photomicrograph of a Nissl preparation of monkey tissue shows transneuronal degeneration of the nerve cells in three of the laminae of the lateral geniculate body of the thalamus after a retinal lesion. **M,** medial. **L,** lateral. (Adapted from Le Gros Clark and Penman, 1934.)

dent on one another for survival, and illustrates the widespread changes brought about by damage confined to a small part of the brain.

The Prognosis for Recovery from Damage to the Cells of the Brain May Soon Be Improved

The use of peripheral nerve grafts to stimulate the regeneration of damaged central axons is one of several recently developed techniques designed to improve prognosis for recovery from damage to the central nervous system. A second line of research that may alleviate the effects of damage is the transplantation of the cells from fetal or neonatal animals into the brains of adults. Anders Björklund and his co-workers in Sweden have used this approach in experiments with rats lacking a dopaminergic pathway to the basal ganglia. These animals have a characteristic movement disorder that is corrected by the transplantation of embryonic dopaminergic neurons into appropriate sites within the brain. As a result of this procedure, axons grow out from the graft and form synapses with neurons in the host brain; but dopamine may also be released diffusely by the transplanted cells to act as a neuromodulator of host synapses. Transplantation research of this kind may provide a means of reversing damage to particular neurotransmitter systems in the brain, such as the damage that occurs in Parkinson's disease.

Finally, although most neurons in the adult mammalian brain are postmitotic and are no longer capable of dividing, Fernando Nottebohm and his colleagues at Rockefeller University have shown that some populations of neurons in the brains of adult songbirds can increase in number. Using [3H]thymidine autoradiography, Nottebohm found that certain central neurons in adult songbirds are capable of synthesizing DNA and of dividing. These new nerve cells generate action potentials and display normal synaptic potentials, suggesting that they can be integrated into circuits with normal physiological functions.

An Overall View

The analysis of both accidental and experimental lesions has provided much useful information about the contribution of particular neurons and groups of neurons to behavior. Moreover, the information gained in this way reinforces the principle that the behavioral role of a nerve cell is determined by its location in the brain and by its connections, its input–output relationships. A similar injury has very different behavioral consequences depending on which neuron it strikes. For example, severance of the axons of motor neurons that innervate skeletal muscle (lower motor neurons) results in the paralysis of individual muscles on the side of the lesion. These muscles undergo a reduction in mass (atrophy), tone, and reflex activity. In contrast, a lesion produces a different disorder of behavior when it severs axons of cortical motor cells (upper motor neurons) as they run in the white matter soon after they leave the cerebral cortex. In this case, groups of muscles rather than individual muscles are disturbed and the disturbance is on the side opposite the lesion (since the axons of the upper motor neurons cross to the other side of the brain at the level of the brain stem during their descent). Muscle mass diminishes because of inactivity, but muscle tone and reflex activity are increased. Thus, the effects of lesions in different parts of the nervous system demonstrate clearly that the importance of specific nerve cells for behavior is determined largely by their location in the brain and their pattern of interconnection.

Selected Readings

Brodal, A. 1981. Neurological Anatomy in Relation to Clinical Medicine, 3rd ed. New York: Oxford University Press, pp. 3–45.

David, S., and Aguayo, A. J. 1981. Axonal elongation into peripheral nervous system "bridges" after central nervous system injury in adult rats. Science 214:931–933.

Lieberman, A. R. 1971. The axon reaction: A review of the principal features of perikaryal responses to axon injury. Int. Rev. Neurobiol. 14:49–124.

Mendell, L. M., Munson, J. B., and Scott, J. G. 1976. Alterations of synapses on axotomized motoneurones. J. Physiol. (Lond.) 255:67–79.

Paton, J. A., and Nottebohm, F. N. 1984. Neurons generated in the adult brain are recruited into functional circuits. Science 225:1046–1048.

Vaughn, J. E., Hinds, P. L., and Skoff, R. P. 1970. Electron microscopic studies of Wallerian degeneration in rat optic nerves. 1. The multipotential glia. J. Comp. Neurol. 140:175–205.

References

Baitinger, C., Cheney, R., Clements, D., Glicksman, M., Hirokawa, N., Levine, J., Meiri, K., Simon, C., Skene, P., and Willard, M. 1983. Axonally transported proteins in axon development, maintenance, and regeneration. Cold Spring Harbor Symp. Quant. Biol. 48:791–802.

Björklund, A., and Stenevi, U. 1979. Regeneration of monoaminergic and cholinergic neurons in the mammalian central nervous system. Physiol. Rev. 59:62–100.

Björklund, A., Dunnett, S. B., Stenevi, U., Lewis, M. E., and Iversen, S. D. 1980. Reinnervation of the denervated striatum by substantia nigra transplants: Functional consequences as revealed by pharmacological and sensorimotor testing. Brain Res. 199:307–333.

Jones, E. G., and Cowan, W. M. 1977. Nervous tissue. In L. Weiss and R. O. Greep (eds.), Histology, 4th ed. New York: McGraw-Hill.

Le Gros Clark, W. E., and Penman, G. G. 1934. The projection of the retina in the lateral geniculate body. Proc. R. Soc. Lond. [Biol.] 114:291–313.

Schmidt, R. H., Björklund, A., and Stenevi, U. 1981. Intracerebral grafting of dissociated CNS tissue suspensions: A new approach for neuronal transplantation to deep brain sites. Brain Res. 218:347–356.

Lewis P. Rowland

Diseases of the Motor Unit: The Motor Neuron, Peripheral Nerve, and Muscle

18

Information about the response of nerve cells to injury and about other aspects of neurobiology enables clinicians to diagnose and understand the manifestations of neurological disease. In a reciprocal manner, the manifestations of particular human diseases help us understand how the nervous system functions. Nowhere is this mutual benefit of clinical and basic science more evident than in diseases of the motor unit. As a group, diseases of the motor unit illustrate a key principle of modern neurobiology: the most useful insights come from combining clinical observations with experimental findings from a variety of basic disciplines—morphology, physiology, biochemistry, immunology and genetics. To analyze the consequences of these diseases, we need to be familiar with the cell biology of neurons, the organization of the motor unit, the conduction of the nerve impulse, the factors that control the excitability of the muscle membrane, and the trophic effects of nerve on muscle that are lost by denervation. Diseases of the motor unit raise questions that are central for clinical neurology and also compel interest from the view of cell biology.

The Motor Unit Is the Functional Element of the Motor System

Although each mature mammalian skeletal muscle fiber is innervated by only one motor neuron, each motor neuron innervates more than one muscle fiber. As we have seen, synaptic transmission at the nerve–muscle synapse normally is so effective that every action potential in the motor neuron leads without fail to the contraction of every muscle fiber innervated by that neuron. Charles Sherrington

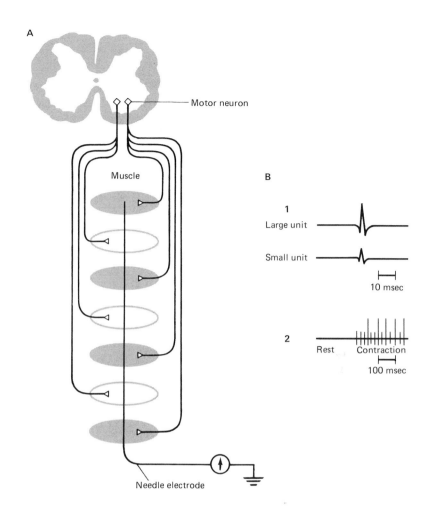

18–1 The motor unit consists of a single motor neuron and the population of muscle fibers it innervates.

A. The experimental arrangement for recording the electrical activity of two motor units shows that the muscle fibers innervated by a single motor neuron do not usually lie adjacent to one another. A needle electrode inserted into the muscle records an all-or-none unit potential when a unit fires because the highly effective transmission at the neuromuscular junction ensures that each action potential in the motor neuron produces a contraction in every fiber that it innervates.

B. Electrical recordings of the unit potentials vary in size in proportion to the number of muscle fibers that contribute to them. The small motor unit that innervates three muscle fibers produces a small spike; the larger motor unit produces a large spike. Muscular contraction usually recruits smaller units first and then the larger ones. The action potentials from the separate units are shown on a fast time base (**1**). The two units are displayed together on a slow time base during a contraction (**2**).

introduced the term *motor unit* to refer to the motor neuron in the spinal cord and the population of muscle fibers that it innervates (Figure 18–1). The motor unit has four functional components: (1) the cell body of the motor neuron, (2) the axon of the motor neuron that runs in the peripheral nerve, (3) the neuromuscular junctions, and (4) the muscle fibers innervated by that neuron. We have considered diseases of junctional transmission separately because of their special manifestations (see Chapter 16). Therefore, in this chapter we shall consider only disorders that affect the cell body, axon, or muscle.

The number of muscle fibers innervated by a single motor neuron varies greatly according to the function served by particular muscles. Motor units that control fine movements—for example, those of the ocular muscles or the small muscles of the hand—consist of only three to six muscle fibers. In contrast, there are about 2000 muscle fibers in each motor unit of the gastrocnemius, the ankle extensor that is involved in gross movements of the leg; large numbers of muscle fibers are also found in motor units of other muscles, such as the trapezius of the back, used in postural control.

Contraction of muscle is the final expression or readout of the motor system. Variations in the range, force, or type of movement are determined by the pattern of recruitment and the frequency of firing of different motor units. The motor unit can therefore be considered the elementary unit of behavior in the motor system.

Neurogenic and Myopathic Diseases Are Defined by the Component of the Motor Unit That Is Affected

Most diseases of the motor unit cause weakness and wasting of skeletal muscles. These diseases may differ in other features, however, depending upon which of the four components of the motor unit is primarily affected. Distinctions among diseases were originally established at postmortem examination. When pathologists of the nineteenth century studied patients who had died from diseases characterized by progressive weakness and wasting of limb muscles, they found different morphological changes in patients with different symptoms or signs. Some patients had pronounced changes in the nerve cell bodies or peripheral nerves but only minor changes in

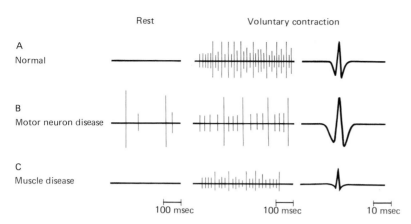

18–2 Some characteristic electromyogram features in three populations: **A.** Normal subjects. **B.** Patients with neurogenic diseases. **C.** Patients with myogenic diseases. Spontaneous activity is seen at rest in denervated muscle, but not in normal muscles and only under special conditions in myopathy. In chronic denervation, muscle action potentials become larger in amplitude and longer in duration (see Figure 18–3). In myopathies, the action potentials become smaller (see Figure 18–4).

muscle fibers. These diseases were called *neurogenic* and were subdivided into those that primarily affected the cell bodies *(motor neuron diseases)* and those that primarily affected the peripheral axons *(peripheral neuropathies).* Other patients had advanced degeneration of muscles, with little change in motor neurons or axons; these diseases were called *myopathic* diseases.

These pathological findings demonstrate two important features of neurological disease. First, disease can be functionally selective; some diseases affect only sensory systems, others only motor systems. Second, a disease may be regionally selective, affecting only one component of the neuron (for example, the axon rather than the cell body). Thus the distinctions among the different components of the neuron (considered in Chapter 2) have important clinical implications; reciprocally, clinical observations can provide valuable insights into the functional significance of these components.

The clinical consequences of neurogenic disease are most obvious when a peripheral nerve is cut. The muscles innervated by that nerve are immediately paralyzed and then waste progressively. Tendon reflexes are lost immediately, as is sensation in the area innervated by the nerve because the nerve carries sensory as well as motor fibers. In neurogenic diseases similar effects of denervation appear more slowly; the muscles gradually become weak and wasted.[1]

In the myopathies there is dysfunction of muscle without evidence of denervation. The main symptoms are due to weakness of skeletal muscle and often include difficulty in walking or lifting. Less commonly, other muscle symptoms occur, such as inability to relax *(myotonia)*, cramps, pain *(myalgia)*, or the appearance in the urine of the protein that colors the muscle red *(myo-*

globinuria). The *muscular dystrophies* are a group of myopathies with special characteristics: they are hereditary; all symptoms are due to weakness; the weakness becomes progressively more severe; and, histologically, there is evidence of degeneration and regeneration, with no storage of abnormal metabolites.

Neurogenic and Myopathic Diseases Are Distinguished by Clinical and Laboratory Criteria

Because both neurogenic and myopathic diseases are characterized by weakness of muscle, differential diagnosis may be difficult. Classification and diagnosis of these diseases involve both clinical and laboratory criteria.

Clinical Evidence

Neurogenic disorders tend to cause distal limb weakness, and myopathic disorders tend to cause proximal limb weakness. But, because there are many exceptions to this generalization, location of weakness cannot be regarded as a reliable differential sign. Some signs, however, are restricted to neurogenic diseases. Denervated muscle fibers tend to fire spontaneous motor unit potentials that give rise to spontaneous twitches of muscle called fasciculations and fibrillations.

Fasciculations are visible twitches of muscle that can be seen as ripples under the skin. They result from the synchronous and involuntary contractions of the muscle fibers innervated by the same motor neuron (a motor unit).

Fibrillations, on the other hand, arise from spontaneous activity within single denervated muscle fibers. They are not clinically visible but can be recognized only by electromyography. For reasons that are not clear, clinically visible fasciculations are characteristic of slowly progressive diseases of the motor neuron and are uncommon in peripheral neuropathies.

Another unequivocal sign of neurogenic disease is the

---

[1]*Atrophy* (literally, lack of nourishment) means wasting away of a once-normal muscle. By historical accident, "atrophy" appears in the names of several diseases that are all thought to be neurogenic. Therefore, in describing the appearance of a patient's muscles, it is best to use the word *wasting* unless the condition is known to be neurogenic.

combination of overactive reflexes (evidence of disease of upper motor neurons) in a weak, wasted, and twitching limb (evidence of disease of the lower motor neuron); this combination of apparently incongruous signs is virtually diagnostic of amyotrophic lateral sclerosis, a condition that involves both the upper and the lower motor neurons.

When the sole manifestation of a disease is limb weakness, as often happens, clinical criteria alone rarely suffice to distinguish between neurogenic and myopathic diseases. To assist in this differentiation, clinicians rely upon several laboratory tests.

Laboratory Evidence

The sarcoplasm of muscle is rich in soluble enzymes that are also found in the serum in low concentrations. In many muscle diseases, the serum level of these sarcoplasmic enzymes is increased, presumably because changes occur in the properties of muscle surface membranes that ordinarily retain soluble enzymes within the

sarcoplasm. Slight increases are also found in some denervating diseases, but the increases are usually much less than in a myopathy. The enzyme activity most commonly measured for diagnosing myopathy is that of creatine kinase (CK), an enzyme that phosphorylates creatine and is important in the energy metabolism of muscle; assays for serum glutamic oxaloacetic transaminase (SGOT) and lactate dehydrogenase (LDH) are also used.

Some abnormalities can be diagnosed by *electromyography,* a routine clinical procedure in which a small needle is inserted into a muscle to record the electrical activity of several neighboring motor units (Figure 18–2). Attention is given to three measurements: spontaneous activity at rest, the number of motor units under voluntary control, and the duration and amplitude of each motor unit potential. Because each motor unit fires in an all-or-none fashion, it gives rise to an all-or-none motor unit potential. Normally, there is no activity in a resting muscle (Figure 18–2A). During a weak voluntary contraction, a series of motor unit potentials is recorded as different motor units are recruited. Normal values have been es-

18–3 In motor neuron disease, fewer units are under voluntary control, but sprouting and reinnervation can lead to increased individual unit potentials. **A.** The motor neuron on the left is undergoing degeneration. Muscle fibers formerly supplied by this anterior horn cell have become denervated and atrophic; there is no longer a motor unit potential. However, the surviving neuron on the right has sprouted an axonal branch that has reinnervated one of the denervated muscle fibers. **B.** Because of the additional innervation, the surviving motor neuron produces a unit potential that is larger than normal. In addition, axons of the surviving motor unit fire spontaneously even at rest, giving rise to fasciculations, another characteristic of motor neuron disease. The unit potential is shown on a fast (**1**) and a slow (**2**) time base.

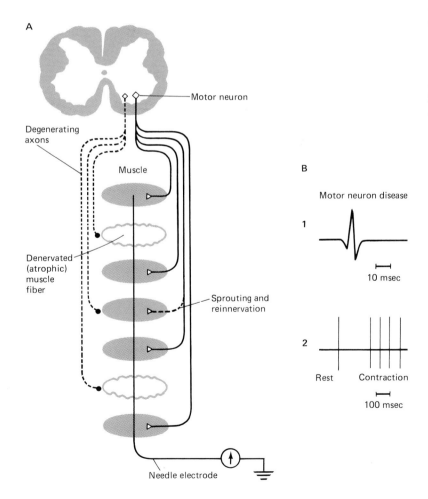

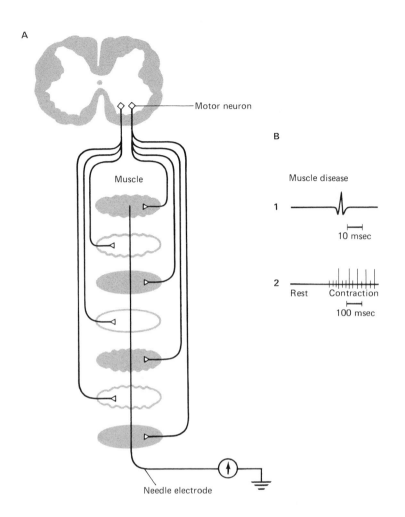

18–4 In muscle disease, the fewer the muscle fibers in each unit, the smaller the individual unit potentials. **A.** Some muscle fibers innervated by each of the two motor neurons have shrunk and become nonfunctional. **B.** The unit potentials have not decreased in number, but they are smaller than normal in amplitude and shorter in duration. The unit potential is shown on a fast **(1)** and a slow **(2)** time base.

tablished for the amplitude and duration of these unit potentials. The amplitude of the unit potential is determined by the number of muscle fibers within the motor unit.

In denervated muscle (Figure 18–2B), there is spontaneous activity even at rest (fibrillation and fasciculation). On volitional movement few motor units contract because the motor axons have been lost and there are fewer units under voluntary control. The amplitude and duration of individual potentials may be increased, presumably because remaining nerve fibers sprout and reinnervate denervated fibers, so that surviving units contain more than the normal number of muscle fibers (Figure 18–3). In myopathic diseases (Figure 18–2C), there is no activity at rest and no change in the number of units firing during a contraction, but because there are fewer surviving muscle fibers in each motor unit, individual motor unit potentials are smaller in amplitude and of shorter duration (Figure 18–4).

Electrical stimulation and recording can also be used to measure the *conduction velocities* of peripheral motor axons. Motor conduction velocity is slowed in *demyelinating neuropathies*, as we shall see later. In neuropathies without demyelination *(axonal neuropathies)*, conduction velocity is normal.

Finally, muscle can be biopsied and the muscle fibers examined histologically. As we shall see again in Chapter 34, two types of muscle fibers can be distinguished histochemically. One histochemical type corresponds to the fast-twitch or pale fibers. The predominant metabolic enzymes present in these muscle fibers are those of glycolytic metabolism. The other type corresponds to the red slow-twitch fibers, which rely primarily on oxidative metabolism. Although this distinction is probably an oversimplification and there may be subtypes within the major classes, the biochemical differences can be demonstrated vividly by histochemical stains for specific enzymes of either class. By stimulating a single axon in

18–5 **A.** Gastrocnemius muscle from a normal adult. Pale (type I) muscle fibers and dark (type II) fibers are roughly equal in incidence and seem to be distributed in a random fashion. Myofibrillar (myosin) ATPase, preincubation at pH 9.4, ×100.

B. Gastrocnemius muscle from a patient with a chronic sensorimotor polyneuropathy. Muscle fibers of the same histochemical fiber type form distinct groups. This phenomenon of fiber-type grouping is thought to result from repeated episodes of denervation and reinnervation by axon sprouts from surviving motor units. Eventually, a single motor neuron innervates several contiguous muscle fibers, which acquire uniform histochemical and physiological properties specified by that neuron. Myofibrillar ATPase, preincubation at pH 9.4, ×100.

C. Gastrocnemius muscle from another patient with a chronic sensorimotor polyneuropathy. A large group of atrophic muscle fibers is surrounded by fibers that are normal in size or hypertrophied. This large group atrophy of fibers is pathognomonic of disorders of the lower motor neuron. Modified Gomori trichrome, ×60.

D. Vastus lateralis muscle from a 4-year-old boy with Duchenne muscular dystrophy. The section demonstrates the focal character of the damage to muscle fibers, manifested as hypercontracted (hyaline) fibers **(large arrows)** and necrotic fibers **(small arrows)**. The **arrowheads** indicate muscle fibers with cytological signs of regeneration. Modified Gomori trichrome, ×60. (All four figures courtesy of A. P. Hays.)

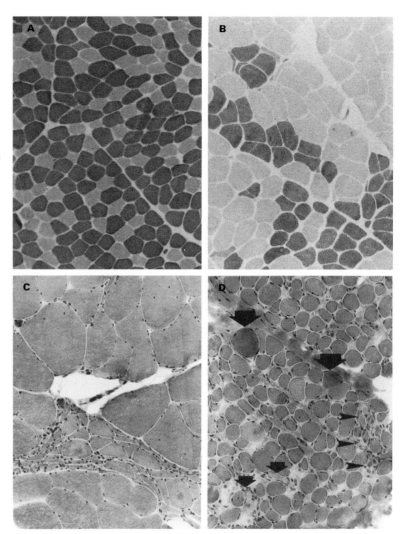

a ventral root for a prolonged period, it is possible to deplete the enzyme stores of the muscle fibers in only that one motor unit; this can be demonstrated by appropriate histochemical stains. Experiments of this kind indicate that all of the muscle fibers innervated by a single motor neuron are of the same histochemical type. However, these muscle fibers do not lie side by side; instead, they are interspersed among the muscle fibers of other motor units. Therefore, in normal muscle, when an enzyme stain is used that is selective for only one type, a cross section of the muscle has the appearance of a checkerboard, with the stained and unstained fiber types alternating in an irregular pattern (Figure 18–5A).

In chronic neurogenic diseases of the denervating type, muscle fibers innervated by a dying neuron become atrophic and some of them disappear; axons of surviving neurons tend to sprout and innervate some of the muscle fibers left by the dying neurons. Because the neuron determines histochemical type, these reinnervated fibers become histochemically homogeneous. As a result, instead of a normal checkerboard pattern, the fibers become clustered by type *(fiber-type grouping)* because the surviving motor unit is larger than normal (see Figures 18–3B and 18–5). When the neurons in these motor units are ultimately affected, atrophy occurs in groups of muscle fibers all belonging to the same histochemical type *(group atrophy)* (Figure 18–5C).

In myopathic diseases, muscle fibers are affected in a more or less random fashion by signs of cell death (necrosis) and regeneration, sometimes with an inflammatory cellular response and sometimes with prominent infiltration of the muscle by fat and connective tissue (Figure 18–5D).

The main clinical and laboratory features that serve in the differential diagnosis of diseases of the motor unit are listed in Table 18–1. Some of the major diseases that affect the motor neuron, axons, or muscle are listed in Table 18–2. We shall consider each of them in turn.

Table 18–1. Differential Diagnosis of Neurogenic and Myopathic Diseases

Finding	Neurogenic	Myopathic
Weakness	+	+
Wasting	+	+
Loss of reflexes	+	+
Fasciculations	+ (ALS)	0
Sensory loss	+ (PN)	0
Hyperreflexia, Babinski	+ (ALS)	0
Cerebrospinal fluid protein increased	+ (PN)	0
Slow nerve conduction velocity	+ (PN)	0
Electromyography		
Duration and amplitude of potentials	Increased	Decreased
Fibrillation, fasciculation	+	0
Number of potentials	Decreased	Normal
Serum enzymes increased	±	+ + + +
Muscle biopsy	Group atrophy, fiber-type grouping	Necrosis and regeneration

Abbreviations: ALS, amyotrophic lateral sclerosis; PN, peripheral neuropathy.

Diseases of the Motor Neuron

It is useful to distinguish *lower motor neurons* in the spinal cord and in the brain stem that innervate skeletal muscles directly from *upper motor neurons* that originate in higher regions of the brain and act on the lower motor neurons to convey descending commands for movement; axons of upper motor neurons make up the corticospinal (pyramidal) tract. Disorders of lower motor neurons result in atrophy, fasciculations and fibrillations, decreased muscle tone, and loss of tendon reflexes. Disorders of upper motor neurons and their axons result in spasticity, overactive tendon reflexes, and abnormal extensor reflexes (Babinski signs).

Chronic and Acute Diseases

The best-known disorder of motor neurons is amyotrophic lateral sclerosis. *Amyotrophy* is another word for neurogenic atrophy of muscle. *Lateral sclerosis* refers to the sense of hardness when the spinal cord is palpated at autopsy. This hardness is due to the proliferation of astrocytes and scarring of the lateral columns of the spinal cord. Scarring is caused by disease of the corticospinal tracts that carry the axons of upper motor neurons from

cell bodies that lie in the cortex and brain stem to the spinal cord. There is progressive degeneration of upper motor neurons in the cortex and of lower motor neurons in the brain stem and spinal cord. Remarkably, some motor neurons are spared, notably those supplying ocular muscles and those involved in voluntary control of bladder sphincters. The cause of amyotrophic lateral sclerosis is not known.

Symptoms usually start with painless weakness of the arms or legs. Typically, the patient, most often a man in his 60s, discovers that he has become awkward in executing fine movements of the hands (typing, playing the piano, fingering coins, or working with tools). This weakness is associated with wasting of the small muscles of the hands and feet and fasciculations of the muscles of the forearm and upper arm. These signs of lower motor neuron disease are often paradoxically associated with *hyperreflexia*, the increase in tendon reflexes that is characteristic of upper motor neuron disease. The condition is inexorably progressive and may affect muscles of respiration. Sensation is always normal. There is no effective treatment for this uniformly fatal condition.

Other variants of motor neuron disease are recognized. Sometimes the first symptoms are restricted to muscles innervated by cranial nerves, with resulting *dysarthria* (difficulty speaking) and *dysphagia* (difficulty swallow-

Table 18–2. Examples of Neurogenic and Myopathic Diseases

Neurogenic		Myopathic	
Motor neuron	Peripheral nerve	Inherited	Acquired
Amyotrophic lateral sclerosis	Guillain-Barré syndrome	Duchenne dystrophy	Dermatomyositis
		Facioscapulohumeral dystrophy	Polymyositis syndrome
	Chronic peripheral neuropathy	Limb-girdle dystrophy	Endocrine myopathies
		Myotonic dystrophy	Myoglobinurias

ing). When cranial symptoms occur alone, the syndrome is called *progressive bulbar palsy*. (The term "bulb" is synonymous with "medulla.") If only lower motor neurons are involved, the syndrome is called *spinal muscular atrophy*. Spinal muscular atrophy is characterized by weakness, wasting, loss of reflexes, and fasciculation, but hyperreflexia and other signs of disease of the upper motor neuron are lacking. Spinal atrophy in adults is probably the same disease as amyotrophic lateral sclerosis because autopsy usually reveals some demyelination in the corticospinal tracts even though upper motor neuron signs were not clinically evident in life. Presumably, the more advanced degeneration of the lower motor neurons in spinal muscular atrophy prevents clinical expression of upper motor neuron signs.

Amyotrophic lateral sclerosis and its variants are restricted to motor neurons of skeletal muscle. The disease does not affect sensory neurons or autonomic neurons to viscera, and therefore illustrates dramatically the individuality of nerve cells and the principle of *selective vulnerability*. For instance, the motor neuron is also selectively vulnerable to poliomyelitis virus, which causes a disease that is restricted to motor neurons but is acute (lasting days) rather than chronic (progressing for years) like amyotrophic lateral sclerosis. Although the basis of this selectivity is not yet understood, it might be explained in both acute disease (polio) and chronic (amyotrophic lateral sclerosis) by characteristic biochemical components in the membrane of motor neurons that act as receptors for specific *neurotropic viruses* (viruses that attack the nervous system). Another possibility suggested by Mark Gurney at the University of Chicago is that antibodies are directed against motor neurons themselves or against nerve growth factors that are necessary for the health (or sustenance) of motor neurons.

Pathophysiology

Aspects of motor neuron disease can be understood in terms of the physiology of the motor neuron and the influences that the motor neuron exerts on the muscles it innervates. The weakness characteristic of motor neuron disease results from loss of motor neurons and consequent denervation.

At first, the surviving motor neurons may send sprouts to neighboring muscle fibers that have been stripped of normal innervation (see Figure 18–3). Ultimately, so many motor nerve cells are affected that the number of innervated and functioning muscle fibers declines progressively. The motor axons of surviving motor neurons seem to function normally, whereas those that are seriously compromised do not function. As a result, the conduction velocity of peripheral nerves from surviving anterior horn cells is normal or only slightly slow. Tendon reflexes are lost because motor efferents are affected, and the denervated muscles waste away or become atrophic in the absence of presynaptic trophic in-

fluences that are essential for survival, as we shall see in Chapter 56. The muscles also become inactive, and lack of activity is an additional cause of wasting *(disuse atrophy)*.

As we have seen, motor neuron disease also leads to two types of spontaneous activity in the motor axon and in the muscle: fasciculation and fibrillation. The cause of fasciculation is not known. The electromyographic counterpart of a visible twitch is a compound motor unit potential, and these electrical changes may also be seen in disorders of nerve roots or peripheral nerves. In all of these conditions the electrical activity may persist after nerve block (by injection of a local anesthetic) or even after section of the nerve. Nerve block eliminates all activity central to the site of injection (the spinal cord, dorsal and ventral roots, and proximal nerve). Under these circumstances, if spontaneous muscle activity persists, it must arise distal to the block—in the remote axon just before it branches, in the terminals, or at the neuromuscular junction. Acetylcholine seems to be involved because the fasciculations of motor neuron disease can be abolished by *d*-tubocurarine and because neostigmine (an inhibitor of cholinesterase) can induce fasciculation in a normal mammalian nerve–muscle preparation. However, it is uncertain precisely where and how acetylcholine acts.

Fasciculations involve activation of one or more whole motor units and therefore produce visible twitching of the skin, but fibrillation results from the discharge of a single muscle fiber and is too small to be seen through the skin; nevertheless, it can be detected electromyographically. In some circumstances, fibrillations are thought to be due to the insertion of new voltage-dependent Na^+ and Ca^{++} channels into the external membranes of denervated muscle fibers. These new channels make the fiber spontaneously active, much like the pacemaker cells of the heart. This cannot be the entire explanation, however, because fibrillations are increased by intra-arterial injection of acetylcholine or epinephrine, suggesting that there may be more than one mechanism.

Diseases of Peripheral Nerves (Peripheral Neuropathies)

Because motor and sensory axons run in the same nerves, disorders of peripheral nerves usually cause symptoms of both motor and sensory dysfunction. Some patients with peripheral neuropathy often report abnormal sensory experiences, frequently unpleasant. Similar sensations are recognized by normal individuals after local anesthesia is used for dental work; these sensations are variously called "numbness," "pins-and-needles," or "tingling." When these sensations occur spontaneously without a proximate sensory stimulus, they are called *paresthesias*. Patients may be unable to discriminate between hot and cold. Lack of pain perception may lead to painless injuries. Examination of patients with paresthesias usually reveals impaired perception of cutaneous modalities of sensation (pain and temperature) due to selective loss of the small myelinated fibers that carry these sensations; the sense of touch may or may not be involved. Proprioceptive sensations (position and vibration) may be lost without loss of cutaneous sensation. The sensory disorders are always more prominent distally (the *glove-and-stocking* pattern), presumably because the distal portions of the nerves are most remote from the cell body and therefore more susceptible to disorders that interfere with axonal transport of essential metabolites and proteins. This concept of *dying-back* is invoked to explain why both weakness and sensory loss are usually more severe in distal parts of the arms and legs.

The motor disorder of peripheral neuropathy is first manifested by weakness, which may be predominantly proximal in acute cases and is usually distal in chronic cases. Tendon reflexes are usually depressed or lost. Fasciculation is only rarely seen, and atrophy does not ensue unless the weakness has been present for many weeks. Protein content in the cerebrospinal fluid is often increased, presumably because of altered permeability of the nerve roots within the subarachnoid space of the spinal cord.

Neuropathies may be either acute or chronic. The best known acute neuropathy is the Guillain-Barré syndrome, which achieved notoriety in 1976 when many cases seemed to follow vaccination against the swine influenza virus. Most cases, however, follow a more banal respiratory infection or occur without preceding illness. This condition may be mild, or so severe that mechanical ventilation is required. Cranial nerves may also be affected, leading to paralysis of ocular, facial, and oropharyngeal muscles. Although the condition may be life-threatening, some improvement occurs in every survivor, and return to normal function is possible no matter how severe the original state. Many patients are left with some disability, however. The disorder is believed to be due to an autoimmune cellular attack on peripheral nerves. It is therefore often treated with corticosteroids, although the efficacy of this treatment has not been proved.

The chronic neuropathies also vary from the mildest manifestations to incapacitating or even fatal conditions, and the list of possible causes seems almost endless, including genetic diseases (acute intermittent porphyria, Charcot-Marie-Tooth disease), metabolic disorders (diabetes, B_{12} deficiency), intoxications (lead), nutritional disorders (alcoholism, thiamine deficiency), carcinomas (especially carcinoma of the lung), and immunological disorders (plasma cell diseases, amyloidosis). Some are amenable to therapy, such as the neuropathy of B_{12} deficiency in pernicious anemia. The variety of conditions associated with neuropathy implies a variety of different pathogenetic mechanisms.

In addition to being acute or chronic, neuropathies may be categorized as demyelinating or axonal. Demyelinating neuropathies are probably more common. As might be expected from the role of the myelin sheath in saltatory conduction, the velocity of conduction is slow in axons that have lost myelin. In axonal neuropathies, the myelin sheath is not affected, and conduction velocity is normal. The clinical manifestations may be due in part to disorders of axonal transport.

Positive and Negative Symptoms

Both axonal and demyelinating neuropathy may lead to two kinds of symptoms, positive or negative. The *positive symptoms* of peripheral neuropathies consist of paresthesias that are attributed to abnormal impulse activity in sensory fibers. These paresthesias may arise from spontaneous activity of injured nerve fibers or from electrical cross-talk interactions between abnormal axons (a process called *ephaptic transmission* to distinguish it from normal *synaptic transmission*). Electrical cross-talk does not normally occur between healthy nerve fibers but has been shown in experimentally damaged nerves. For reasons that are not known, damaged nerves also become *hyperexcitable.* This is evident in the Tinel sign, named after a French neurologist who studied the effects of nerve injuries in World War I. He found that tapping the site of injury evoked a burst of unpleasant sensations in the distribution of the nerve. This sign is useful both for showing that there is actually peripheral nerve damage and for pinpointing the site of the lesion.

The *negative symptoms* consist of weakness or paralysis, loss of tendon reflexes, and impaired sensation. Weakness and loss of tendon reflexes result from damage to motor axons. The specific loss of sensation depends on the category of sensory fibers affected. Early in many neuropathies there is loss of position sense or in the perception of low-frequency vibration, indicating damage to large-diameter fibers. Disordered pain and temperature perception indicates that small-diameter fibers are also affected.

Pathophysiology of Demyelinating Neuropathies

These negative symptoms have been studied most thoroughly in demyelinating neuropathy and can be attributed to three basic mechanisms: conduction block, slowed conduction, and impaired ability to conduct impulses at higher frequencies.

Conduction block was first recognized in 1876 by the German neurologist Wilhelm Erb, one of the first clinicians to study human nerves with electrical methods. He found that in patients with some peripheral nerve injuries, he could still evoke muscular contraction by stimulating the nerve below the site of injury. In contrast, there was no response when he stimulated above the site of injury. Erb argued that even though the nerve distal to the lesion still functions, impulses of central origin cannot pass through the blockade imposed by the lesion. Later experimental studies illustrated that diphtheria and other toxins produce conduction block by causing demyelination at the site of application.

Why does demyelination cause nerve block? And how does it lead to slowing of conduction velocity? As we have seen in Chapters 3 and 7, conduction velocity is much more rapid in myelinated fibers than in unmyelinated axons for two reasons. First, the axons of myelinated fibers tend to be larger in diameter, and there is a direct relationship between conduction velocity and diameter. Second, in the myelinated axon, the action potential propagates discontinuously, in saltatory jumps from one node of Ranvier to the next (Figure 18–6A), which is a more rapid process than the continuous propagation that occurs in unmyelinated axons. The axon membrane in the region of the nodes of Ranvier differs from that at the internode (Figure 18–6A). At the node the membrane has a high density of voltage-sensitive Na^+ channels, about 10,000 channels/μm^2. In contrast, the membrane at the internode contains fewer than 25 Na^+ channels/μm^2. The voltage-sensitive K^+ channels are distributed in a complementary manner. Most K^+ channels are in the internodal membrane and do not normally play an important role in repolarizing the action potential (Figure 18–7).

In an axon that has become demyelinated, as in diabetic neuropathy or an inherited neuropathy, the high-resistance, low-capacitance insulation of the myelin sheath is damaged or lost completely. The current at the leading front of the action potential is now short-circuited by the abnormally low resistance and high capacitance of the internode, so that less current is available to depolarize the next node (Figure 18–6B). This shunting of current in the local circuit is enhanced because demyelination unmasks the voltage-gated K^+ channels of the internode (Figure 18–7). These channels are opened by depolarization, and they therefore provide additional pathways for outward current to escape from the axon. The net result of this shunting process is a decrease in the amount of depolarizing current at the next node. Consequently, it takes longer than usual to discharge the capacitance of the nodes and to reach the voltage threshold for action potential.

Reflecting the different degrees of demyelination along the axon, the action potentials in the axons of a nerve begin to conduct at slightly different velocities, with the result that the nerve loses the normal synchrony of conduction. This slowing and the temporal dispersion are thought to account for some of the early clinical signs of neuropathy. For example, functions that normally depend upon the arrival of synchronous bursts of neural activity, such as tendon reflexes and vibratory sensation, are lost soon after onset of a chronic neuropathy. Although at this early point the average conduction velocity may be reduced only slightly, the very fact that the individual axons no longer fire synchronously leads to clinical symptoms. As demyelination becomes more severe, conduction becomes blocked. This block may be either *intermittent*, occurring only at high frequencies of activity, or *complete*. Block of conduction in the largest and fastest fibers of a nerve could also contribute to *overall*

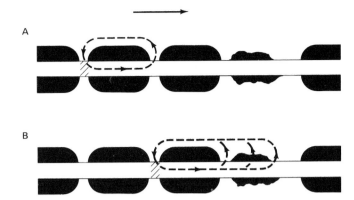

18–6 The demyelinated region of a nerve fiber does not conduct an impulse as well as the normal, myelinated region. The **solid arrow** indicates the direction of impulse conduction; the **hatched area** indicates the region occupied by the impulse. Current flow is indicated by the **broken arrows**. **A.** In normally myelinated regions the high-resistance, low-capacitance myelin shunts the majority of current to the next node of Ranvier. **B.** In contrast, in the demyelinated region current is lost through the damaged myelin sheath or denuded regions of the axon. (From Waxman, 1982.)

18–7 The concentrations of Na^+ channels and K^+ channels differ in the myelinated and unmyelinated regions of the axon. **A.** At a node of Ranvier, Na^+ channels (g_{Na}) are clustered in a high concentration, but they are sparse or absent in the internodal axon membrane. The K^+ channels (g_K) are located beneath the myelin sheath in internodal regions. The nodal regions of the axon membrane (**broken lines**) therefore have different conduction properties than the internodal regions (**solid lines**). **B.** The properties of the internodal axon membrane are not important for conduction in normally myelinated internodes (e.g., between nodes N_1 and N_2) but are highly relevant to the function of demyelinated axons (e.g., between N_2 and N_3). (From Waxman, 1982.)

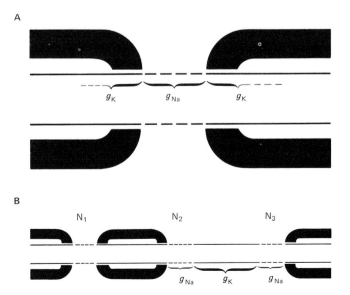

slowing of the average conduction velocity in mixed sensory and motor nerves that contain axons with a variety of diameters.

Diseases of Muscle (Myopathies) Can Lead to Weakness or Myotonia

Muscle diseases are conveniently divided into those that are inherited and those that seem to be acquired.

Inherited Myopathies

The best known inherited diseases are the *muscular dystrophies*, which are separated on the basis of clinical and genetic patterns into four major types (Table 18–3). Two types can be distinguished that are characterized by weakness alone: the Duchenne and facioscapulohumeral dystrophies. The *Duchenne* type starts in the legs, affects boys only (because it is transmitted as an X-linked recessive trait), and progresses relatively rapidly, so that the boys are in wheelchairs by age 12 and usually die in the third decade. In Duchenne dystrophy the concentration of sarcoplasmic enzymes in serum is markedly increased. The *facioscapulohumeral* type differs in genetic pattern (autosomal dominant), affects the two sexes equally, starts later (usually in adolescence), affects the shoulder, girdle, and face early, and may be much milder, compatible with an almost normal life span. These clinical and genetic differences imply different biochemical abnormalities, which have not been identified. Increasing evidence suggests that Duchenne dystrophy is due to a genetic fault of the muscle surface membrane.

A third type of inherited muscular dystrophy, called *myotonic muscular dystrophy*, also causes weakness but has an additional and characteristic feature—myotonia. Myotonia is a delayed relaxation of muscle after vigorous voluntary contraction, percussion, or electrical stimulation (Figure 18–8). The delayed relaxation is caused by repetitive firing of the muscle action potentials and is independent of nerve supply because it persists after nerve block or curarization. The molecular fault is not known but may involve an abnormality of the Cl^- channels of the muscle membrane, as described later. In addition to myotonia, the dystrophy has other special characteristics: it involves cranial muscles, and the limb weakness is primarily distal rather than proximal. The symptoms are not confined to muscles; for instance, cataracts are found in all patients, and testicular atrophy and baldness are common in affected men. Like most autosomal dominant diseases, myotonic dystrophy may be so mild that the patient is literally asymptomatic, or so severe that disability occurs at an early age.

Forms of inherited muscular dystrophy that do not fit these three major types are lumped into a fourth group termed *limb-girdle dystrophy*. This category probably includes more than one type, because affected families differ in distribution of weakness, age at onset, and genetic patterns.

Acquired Myopathies

The prototype of an acquired myopathy is *dermatomyositis*, defined by two clinical features: rash and myopathy. The rash has a predilection for the face, chest, and extensor surfaces of joints, including the fingers. The myopathic weakness primarily affects proximal limb muscles. Both rash and weakness usually appear simultaneously and become worse in a matter of weeks. The weakness may be mild or life-threatening, and the disorder affects children and adults. The cause is not known, but about 10% of the adult cases are associated with malignant tumors. Although the pathogenesis is also not known, the prominence of lymphocytic infiltration of muscle suggests a cell-mediated autoimmune disorder. Corticosteroid therapy is therefore used routinely, but its efficacy has not been proved because the disease may remit spontaneously and muscle function may return partly or completely.

Of the several possible manifestations of myopathy, we shall consider the pathophysiology of only two: weakness and myotonia.

Degeneration of Muscle Fibers May Not Be the Only Cause of Weakness in Muscle Disease

The weakness seen in any myopathy is conventionally ascribed to degeneration of muscle fibers. At first, the missing fibers are replaced by regeneration, but ulti-

Table 18–3. Major Forms of Muscular Dystrophy

Features	Duchenne	Facioscapulohumeral	Limb-girdle	Myotonic
Sex	Male	Both	Both	Both
Onset	Before age 5	Adolescence	Adolescence	Infancy or adolescence
Initial symptoms	Pelvic	Shoulder-girdle	Either	Hands or feet
Face involved	No	Always	No	Often
Pseudohypertrophy	80%	No	Rare	No
Progression	Rapid	Slow	Slow	Slow
Inheritance	X-linked recessive	Autosomal dominant	Autosomal recessive	Autosomal dominant
Serum enzymes	Very high	Normal	Slight increase	Normal
Myotonia	No	No	No	Yes

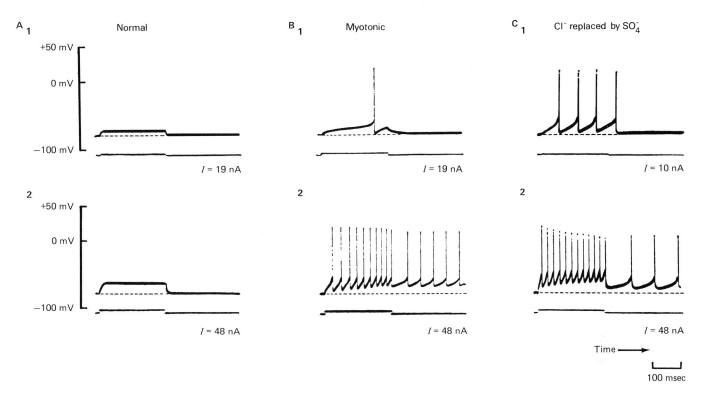

18-8 The delayed muscle relaxation in myotonia is demonstrated by responses to injection of depolarizing current pulses in three types of goat intercostal muscle fibers: **A.** Normal fiber. **B.** Myotonic fiber. **C.** Normal fiber with a reduced Cl⁻ conductance (achieved by substituting SO_4^-, an impermeant anion, for Cl⁻), which mimics the myotonic condition. The **bottom trace** in each section is proportional to the amplitude and duration of the current pulse; the amplitude of the current pulse is given numerically below each voltage trace. Because the myotonic fiber has higher membrane resistance than normal, less current is required to reach action potential threshold (**B₁**). Moreover, a slow depolarizing afterpotential builds up during the spike train. For high-frequency trains, the afterpotential results in extra spikes that outlast the period of current injection (**B₂**). (Adapted from Adrian and Bryant, 1974).

mately renewal cannot keep pace and fibers are lost progressively. As we have seen in discussing electromyography, this leads to compound motor unit potentials of brief duration and reduced amplitude. The decreased number of functioning muscle fibers would then account for the diminished strength. This interpretation may be correct. However, the reverse need not be true. In another form of inherited myopathy, the *glycogen storage diseases*, which are due to a lack of phosphorylase or phosphofructokinase, large amounts of glycogen accumulate within the cells because there is a block of glycogen breakdown. The glycogen accumulations disrupt the normal architecture of many muscle fibers, as seen by light microscopy; at the ultrastructural level there is major distortion of the myofilaments. Despite these severe physical changes, however, the patient may have no symptoms of weakness. Thus, muscle damage does not invariably lead to weakness. Conversely, it is also possible that muscle weakness in some myopathies may be due to a biochemical or physiological abnormality instead of, or in addition to, loss of muscle fibers.

Some Forms of Myotonia May Be Due to Decreased Numbers of Cl⁻ Leakage Channels

Myotonia, impaired relaxation after a forceful contraction, is a manifestation of several inherited disorders. *Myotonic muscular dystrophy* is characterized by weakness as well as myotonia. On the other hand, in another form of myopathy, *myotonia congenita*, myotonia occurs without weakness. Myotonia can also be induced in humans and in experimental animals—for example, by administering diazacholesterol, a drug used clinically to lower blood lipids in efforts to prevent atherosclerosis. Other drugs and chemicals, especially aromatic monocarboxylic acids or clofibrate, induce myotonia in experimental animals.

In all of these conditions, the myotonia seems to arise from an abnormality of the plasma membrane of the muscle that causes the muscle to fire repetitively. The myotonia is thought to arise in muscle because it persists after curarization and because treatment with diazacholesterol leads to the accumulation of an abnormal sterol in surface membranes. All forms of myotonia are ameliorated by treatment with drugs that stabilize membrane excitability, such as phenytoin or quinine.

In three forms of myotonia (myotonia congenita, an inherited form of myotonia found in goats, and the experimental myotonia produced by carboxylic acids)—but not in myotonic muscular dystrophy—the resistance of the muscle membrane is increased. This resistance is attributed to a specific reduction of membrane conductance to Cl^- ions, possibly because of a reduction in Cl^- leakage channels. Unlike nerve membranes, in which the leakage channels are permeable primarily to K^+ at rest, normal muscle membranes at rest have about the same leakage conductance for both Cl^- and K^+. Normally, a train of action potentials in muscle leads to an accumulation of K^+ in the T-tubules of the muscle. This local increase in extracellular K^+ causes the K^+ Nernst potential to shift in a depolarizing direction, resulting in a depolarizing afterpotential.

In normal muscle, this afterpotential is attenuated by the high resting Cl^- leakage conductance, which tends to resist any shift of membrane potential beyond the Cl^- equilibrium potential (about -80 mV). In myotonic muscle, the number of functional Cl^- leakage channels is reduced. As a result, the braking effect of Cl^- is attenuated, and the depolarizing afterpotential due to accumulation of K^+ may persist long enough to trigger an extra spike, once the refractory period has waned. This extra spike will, in turn, generate its own depolarizing afterpotential, and in this way a self-sustaining train of spikes can be evoked that substantially outlasts the neurally evoked train (Figure 18–8).

A different mechanism must be responsible for myotonic muscular dystrophy (the most common dystrophy), however, because Cl^- conductance is normal. The basis of this disease, still unknown, may be an abnormal Na^+ channel.

An Overall View

At the moment there is no treatment for most diseases of motor neuron or muscle. Nevertheless, muscle is a target of nerve cell action and is accessible for biochemical study or for cell biological study in tissue culture. Moreover, many of these diseases are heritable; we can hope that the new techniques of molecular genetics will soon lead to identification of the elusive gene products that are affected in these diseases. If that can be achieved, rational therapy should follow.

Selected Readings

Adrian, R. H., and Bryant, S. H. 1974. On the repetitive discharge in myotonic muscle fibres. J. Physiol. (Lond.) 240:505–515.

Barchi, R. L. 1982. A mechanistic approach to the myotonic syndromes. Muscle & Nerve 5:S60–S63.

Brooke, M. H. 1977. A Clinician's View of Neuromuscular Diseases. Baltimore: Williams & Wilkins.

Culp, W. J., and Ochoa, J. (eds.). 1982. Abnormal Nerves and Muscles as Impulse Generators. New York: Oxford University Press.

Dyck, P. J. 1982. Diseases of the peripheral nervous system. In J. B. Wyngaarden and L. H. Smith, Jr. (eds.), Cecil Textbook of Medicine, 16th ed. Philadelphia: Saunders, pp. 2153–2165.

Dyck, P. J., Thomas, P. K., Lambert, E. H., and Bunge, R. (eds.). 1984. Peripheral Neuropathy, 2nd ed. Philadelphia: Saunders.

Eliasson, S. G., Prensky, A. L., and Hardin, W. B., Jr. (eds.). 1978. Neurological Pathophysiology, 2nd ed. New York: Oxford University Press.

Erb, W. 1883. Handbook of Electro-therapeutics. L. Putzel (trans.). New York: Wood.

Gurney, M. E. 1984. Suppression of sprouting at the neuromuscular junction by immune sera. Nature 307:546–548.

Roth, G. 1984. Fasciculations and their F-response: Localisation of their axonal origin. J. Neurol. Sci. 63:299–306.

Rowland, L. P., and Layzer, R. B. 1977. Muscular dystrophies, atrophies, and related diseases. In A. B. Baker (ed.), Clinical Neurology, Vol. 3. New York: Harper & Row, pp. 1–109.

Rowland, L. P. (ed.). 1982. Human Motor Neuron Diseases. New York: Raven Press.

Rowland, L. P. 1985. Diseases of muscle and neuromuscular junction. In J. B. Wyngaarden and L. H. Smith, Jr. (eds.), Cecil Textbook of Medicine, 17th ed. Philadelphia: Saunders, pp. 2198–2216.

Serratrice, G., Cros, D., Desnuelle, C., Gastaut, J.-L., Pellissier, J.-F., Pouget, J., and Schiano, A. 1984. Neuromuscular Diseases. New York: Raven Press.

Sumner, A. J. (ed.). 1980. The Physiology of Peripheral Nerve Disease. Philadelphia: Saunders.

Walton, J. (ed.). 1981. Disorders of Voluntary Muscle, 4th ed. Edinburgh: Churchill Livingstone.

Waxman, S. G. 1982. Membranes, myelin, and the pathophysiology of multiple sclerosis. N. Engl. J. Med. 306:1529–1533.

Functional Anatomy
of the
Central Nervous System

IV

In 1948, Alf Brodal, the great Norwegian anatomist, published *Neurological Anatomy in Relation to Clinical Medicine.* Widely regarded as the most readable, coherent, and influential textbook in neuroanatomy, this remarkable book asks the questions we first have to consider here: Why do we need to know anatomy? Can it help us to understand behavior? Is it useful in the diagnosis and treatment of disorders of the nervous system? Stated more boldly: Is the need for anatomical knowledge greater in neurology (and psychiatry) than in other fields of medicine? Brodal points out that, from a clinical perspective, the purpose of anatomical knowledge is not simply to acquaint the student with the common sites of disturbance produced by the major illnesses that affect the brain. If that were all, a smattering of anatomical knowledge would be sufficient. The student of neural science, however, wants to comprehend how the brain works: how we think, feel, act, and remember. From a clinical perspective this means understanding the symptomatology of *each individual patient* and determining for each person the exact site and the nature of the lesion as accurately as possible. For this goal, knowledge of the principles of neuroanatomy is indispensable. Only with this knowledge will the student be able to understand normal mental function and the deviations produced by diseases.

Brodal ends his book by summarizing three principles that form the basis of current anatomical knowledge, which we shall consider in this and subsequent sections of our book. First, there is a high degree of order in the anatomical organization of the nervous system. This is true down to the most minute structural feature. For example, the fiber projections to and from the cerebral cortex are topographically organized. There is also a strict topographical organization in the connections between many nuclei and between a given nucleus and the cerebral cortex. Even regions once considered to be diffusely organized, such as the reticular formation of the brain stem or the association cortices, are now known to be specific in their anatomical organization. Moreover, this topographical organization is carried to the level of individual cells. Different afferent fibers establish synaptic contacts at different sites on the dendrites or on the cell body of a given category of nerve cells, and great complexity is achieved because these afferent fibers originate from different parts of the nervous system.

Second, the brain is composed of many small units, or modules, each with its particular structural organization, as well as its characteristic connections with other units. It therefore follows that there must be in the nervous system as many minor functional units as there are structural ones.

Third, the investigation of the structure of the nervous system is a prerequisite for progress in studies of its function. The two are inseparable both conceptually and clinically.

Our aim in this section, much influenced by Brodal, is to convey a modern approach to neuroanatomy, an approach in which structure and function are inseparable. We do not attempt to cover comprehensively all known facts or topographical relationships. We have focused, rather, on the principles of neuroanatomical structure as they relate to normal function and to disease. In the four chapters of this section we introduce the subject and pro-

vide an overall view of the structural and functional organization of the brain and spinal cord. In our functional approach to the anatomy of the brain, the emphasis will be on topics that are significant, interesting scientifically, and important for clinical medicine.

In the first chapter we shall examine the functional systems that operate during the execution of a simple behavioral act and discuss the principles that underlie the anatomical organization of these systems. In the next chapter, we shall take a closer look at the structural organization of each level of the central nervous system by following the course of sensory information from the periphery as it flows into the spinal cord and brain, is transformed into an appropriate motor command, and descends back through the spinal cord to produce a motor response.

For clinical neurology and psychiatry it is also important to grasp the three-dimensional structure of the brain. As an initial and simplifying approach to this task, we examine, in Chapter 21, the principles of development responsible for the three-dimensional architecture of the brain. The final chapter in this section is designed to illustrate how modern imaging techniques have revolutionized our understanding of both the three-dimensional architecture of the brain and its relationship to function by allowing the exploration of three-dimensional structure and function together in the living brain. In subsequent sections we shall explore each of the systems of the brain in turn and examine how their structure contributes to their characteristic function.

James P. Kelly

Principles of the Functional and Anatomical Organization of the Nervous System

19

To understand normal and abnormal behavior, it is necessary to appreciate how the nervous system is organized in space. Although complex, the architecture of the nervous system is governed by a relatively simple set of functional, organizational, and developmental principles. Taken together, these principles provide a foundation that brings order to the myriad details of brain anatomy. In this chapter, we shall first briefly review the parts of the central nervous system and then consider the functional systems related to perception, motor coordination, and motivation that are called into play during the execution of a simple behavioral act. We shall then discuss four general principles that underlie the anatomical organization of these systems.

The Central Nervous System Has an Axial Organization

To begin, it is necessary to become familiar with the language of neuroanatomy. Since many of the terms used to designate particular structures are derived from Greek or Latin or from the names of scientists who first described them, the task of learning neuroanatomy actually resembles learning a new language. The root words of neuroanatomical terms sometimes convey important structural information, so the English translation of these terms will be given as each is introduced.

The brain and spinal cord are organized along two major axes. To understand these axes, it is convenient first to consider the case of a simpler vertebrate such as an amphibian. In these animals, there is a rostral–caudal axis and a dorsal–ventral axis. Here, *rostral* means toward the nose (Latin, *rostrum*, beak), *caudal* toward the tail (Latin,

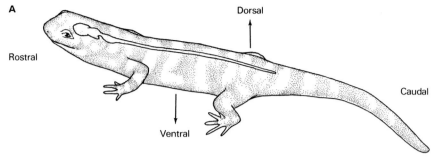

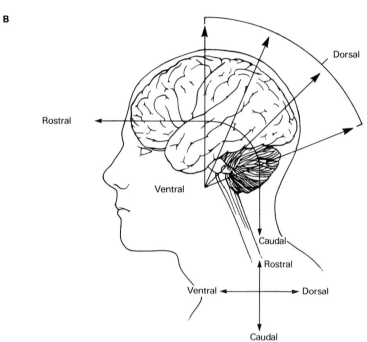

19–1 The axes of the nervous system. **A.** The nervous system of lower vertebrates develops along a straight line, and consequently the orientation of its axes is invariant. **B.** In humans, because of the cephalic flexure at the juncture between the midbrain and the diencephalon, the direction indicated by the terms rostral, caudal, dorsal, and ventral changes systematically at higher levels of the brain. Thus, above the diencephalon rostral means toward the nose, caudal toward the back of the head, ventral toward the jaw, and dorsal toward the top of the skull. The neuraxis is the longitudinal axis of the brain and spinal cord. A coronal section is roughly perpendicular to the neuraxis at levels of the nervous system above the brain stem.

cauda, tail), *dorsal* toward the back (Latin, *dorsum,* back), and *ventral* toward the abdomen (Latin, *venter,* belly)—a straightforward terminology that is accurate for all parts of the nervous system (Figure 19–1A).

However, during human development the long axis of the nervous system bends, or flexes, at the juncture between the brain stem and the region just above it, the diencephalon. As a consequence, the terms used to describe the positions of neural structures in the human nervous system vary in their meaning as a function of the position of these structures relative to the flexure. In the spinal cord, the terminology used in simpler vertebrates is maintained: rostral means toward the neck, caudal toward the coccyx, ventral toward the belly, and dorsal toward the back. Above the flexure, however, rostral means directly toward the nose, caudal toward the back of the head, ventral toward the jaw, and dorsal toward the top of the head (Figure 19–1B). At any level of the brain or spinal cord, a transverse section is one that is cut perpendicular to the nervous system's longitudinal axis, whether it is vertical or bent.

The Central Nervous System Is Subdivided into Six Main Regions

As we saw in Chapter 1, the central nervous system consists of six main regions (Figure 19–2):

1. The *spinal cord,* the most caudal part of the central nervous system, receives information from the skin, joints, and muscles in the trunk and limbs, and it is the final way station for issuing commands for movement. In the spinal cord there is an orderly arrangement of motor and sensory nuclei controlling the limbs and trunk. In addition to nuclei, the spinal cord contains afferent pathways for sensory information to flow to the brain and efferent pathways for commands necessary for motor control to descend from the brain to motor neurons. *Afferent pathways* carry information to the central nervous system; *efferent pathways* carry commands out of the central nervous system. The spinal cord also receives sensory information from the internal organs and controls many autonomic functions.

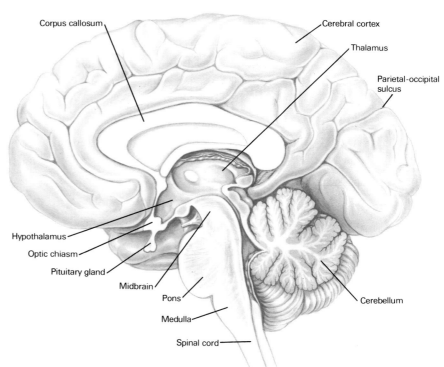

19–2 The major parts of the central nervous system and important landmarks shown in midsagittal section.

The spinal cord continues rostrally as the *brain stem*, which comprises the next three main divisions of the central nervous system:

2. The *medulla*
3. The *pons*
4. The *midbrain*

The *medulla* is the most direct rostral extension of the spinal cord and resembles the spinal cord in aspects of its organization.

The *pons*, which lies rostral to the medulla, contains a massive set of neurons that relay information from the cerebral hemispheres to the cerebellum. The *cerebellum* is not part of the brain stem, but because of its position dorsal to the pons, it is commonly grouped together with the pons. The cerebellum is important for determining the timing sequence and the pattern of muscles activated during movement. Recent evidence suggests that it may also play a role in reflex modification and motor learning.

The *midbrain* lies rostral to the pons and is important in the control of eye movement. The midbrain also contains an essential relay in the auditory pathway and several structures critically involved in motor control of skeletal muscles.

Like the spinal cord, the three divisions of the brain stem contain motor and sensory nuclei, but most of these are related to structures in the head and neck, rather than in the limbs or trunk. In addition to the afferent and efferent systems that innervate skin and skeletal muscles, the brain stem contains systems that innervate blood vessels and glands in the head and neck, and the viscera of the body. Neural structures unique to the brain stem mediate some of the special senses, for example, hearing and taste. Each level of the brain stem also contains fiber tracts that descend from the higher levels of the brain to regulate activity in the brain stem and spinal cord, and tracts that relay sensory input from the spinal cord to the cerebral cortex.

Many of the neurons in the brain stem are grouped into orderly clusters with specific afferent and efferent fiber systems and reasonably well-delineated functions. The brain stem also contains clusters of neurons lying among the bundles (fascicles) of crossing fibers and outside the more discrete nuclear groups. These neurons constitute the *reticular formation* (Latin, *reticulum*, little net). Many reticular neurons have axons that spread widely in both directions, up and down the brain stem. As we shall see in later chapters, they also have a unique functional role in the regulation of overall levels of brain activity and the modification of spinal reflexes. Other reticular neurons have a more conventional pattern of either ascending or descending projections.

5. The *diencephalon* contains two key subdivisions, the thalamus and the hypothalamus. The *thalamus* (Greek, inner chamber) processes and relays most of the information coming from the lower regions of the central nervous system en route to the cerebral cortex. We shall consider the organization of the thalamus in greater detail in the next chapter. The *hypothalamus* (lying below the thalamus) is important for integration in the autonomic nervous system and for regulating hormonal secretion by the pituitary gland.

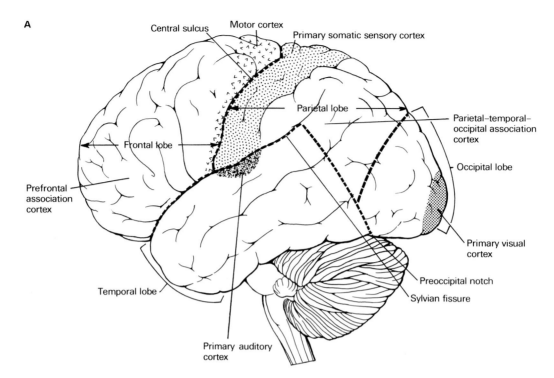

19–3 The major divisions of the human cerebral cortex.
A. Lateral view of the hemisphere. In this view, it is easier to appreciate both the primary cortical areas and the association areas. The primary auditory cortex lies near the junction of the temporal and parietal lobes. Two large association areas are visible: the prefrontal association cortex and the parietal–temporal–occipital association cortex. The Sylvian fissure is the most prominent cleft visible in a lateral view of the brain. **B.** Dorsal view, with anterior toward the left. The sagittal fissure separates the two hemispheres. The frontal

6. The *cerebral hemispheres* consist of the *cerebral cortex* and the *basal ganglia*. Collectively termed the *cerebrum*, these structures are concerned with perceptual, cognitive, and higher motor functions. Some of these complex functions and other specific behavioral functions have now been localized to specific regions of the cerebral cortex.

The Cerebral Cortex Is Further Subdivided into Four Lobes

The cerebral cortex is thrown into infoldings called fissures and sulci. In the sixteenth and seventeenth centuries, Vesalius, Sylvius, and other Renaissance anatomists found that some of the most prominent infoldings are invariant from one human brain to the next. Using these invariant features as landmarks, they separated the brain into distinct regions. These anatomists recognized that the most prominent fissure, which they called the *sagittal fissure*, separated the brain along the midline into two hemispheres (Figure 19–3B). These hemispheres are fairly symmetrical. Each hemisphere, in turn, can be divided into four *lobes*, which are named for the overlying bones of the skull: *frontal, parietal, temporal,* and *occipital* (Figure 19–3A). A cleft called the *central sulcus* separates the frontal lobe (by far the largest lobe) anteriorly from the parietal lobe, which lies caudal to it. The parietal lobe is also separated from the occipital lobe by

the *parietal-occipital sulcus*, which is present only on the medial aspect of the hemisphere. The temporal lobe lies ventral to another consistent cleft within each hemisphere, the *Sylvian fissure* or lateral fissure.

Not surprisingly, large regions of the cerebral cortex are committed to movement and sensation (Figure 19–3A). Areas that are directly committed are called *primary, secondary,* and *tertiary* sensory or motor areas. For example, the *primary motor cortex*, which lies within the precentral gyrus, contains neurons that project directly to the spinal cord. The *primary sensory areas* (the visual, auditory, somatic sensory, and gustatory areas) receive information from peripheral receptors with only a few synapses interposed. The *primary visual cortex* is located at the back of the occipital lobe on its medial aspect. The *primary auditory cortex* lies in the temporal lobe, where it makes up a portion of the lower bank of the lateral sulcus. The *primary somatic sensory cortex* lies on the postcentral gyrus.

Surrounding the primary areas are higher order (secondary and tertiary) sensory and motor areas. These areas process more complex aspects of a single sensory modality or motor function than the primary areas. The purpose of the higher order sensory areas is to achieve greater analysis and integration of information coming *from* the primary sensory areas. In contrast, the flow of information from the motor areas is in the opposite direction. Higher order motor areas distill complex infor-

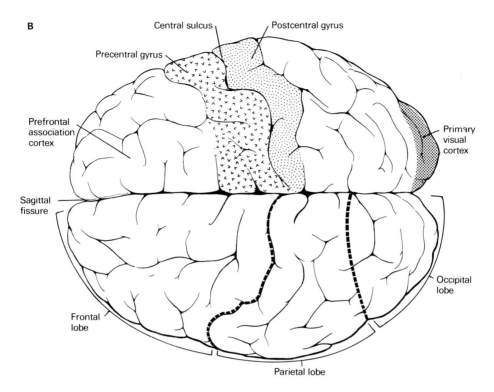

lobe is rostral to the central sulcus. The precentral gyrus of the frontal lobe contains the motor cortex. The postcentral gyrus, which contains the somatic sensory cortex, lies posterior to the central sulcus and is a part of the parietal lobe. The occipital lobe lies at the caudal margin of the hemisphere and contains the visual cortex. The temporal lobe, which lies ventrally, is not visible in this view of the brain.

mation about a potential motor act and relay it *to* the primary motor cortex, which is the site from which voluntary movement is initiated.

Also classified with the higher order areas is a portion of the posterior parietal lobe called the *posterior parietal cortex*. This region is somewhat transitional between sensory and motor functions. Not only does it serve as a higher order sensory area for both somatic sensation and vision but, in addition, it interrelates aspects of sensation and movement.

Three other large regions of cortex, called *association areas*, lie outside the primary, secondary, and tertiary areas and function mainly to integrate diverse information for purposeful action. These three regions—the parietal–temporal–occipital association cortex, the prefrontal association cortex, and the limbic association cortex—are involved to different degrees in the control of the three major functional systems of the brain: sensory reception, motor control, and motivation. The *parietal–temporal–occipital association cortex* occupies the interface between the three lobes for which it is named (Figure 19–3B). It is concerned chiefly with higher perceptual functions related to the primary sensory inputs to these lobes: somatic sensation, hearing, and vision. In this association cortex, information from different sensory modalities is combined and complex perceptions are formed. The *prefrontal association cortex* occupies most of the rostral part of the frontal lobe. One important function of

this area is the planning of voluntary movement. The *limbic association cortex* is located on the medial and inferior surfaces of the cerebral hemispheres, in portions of the parietal, frontal, and temporal lobes, and is devoted mainly to motivation, emotion, and memory. We shall consider the organization of the association areas of the cortex in greater detail in Chapter 51.

To summarize, the primary sensory areas of the cerebral cortex are devoted to the reception and initial cortical processing of sensory information. The primary areas project to higher sensory areas that further elaborate and process sensory input. The higher order areas connect to the association areas; these provide the link between sensation and action and make connections with the higher order motor areas. The higher order motor areas, in turn, constitute the final pathway to the primary motor cortex, which exerts direct control over motor neurons. (See Table 51–1 for an overview of these cortical areas.)

The Central Nervous System Surrounds an Interconnected System of Four Cavities Called Ventricles

The ventricular system consists of two lateral ventricles, a third ventricle, and a fourth ventricle (Figure 19–4). Circulating within this ventricular system is cerebrospinal fluid. The composition of this fluid is chemically similar

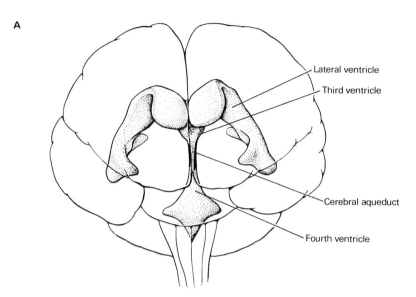

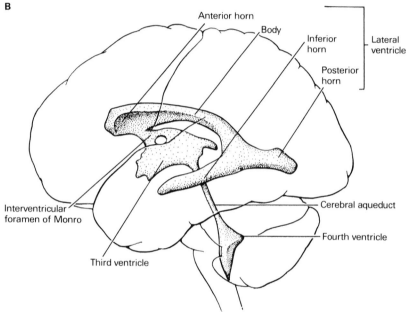

19–4 The ventricular system of the brain. **A.** Frontal view. **B.** Lateral view. (Adapted from Noback and Demarest, 1981.)

to the extracellular fluid surrounding the cells of the brain. The two lateral ventricles, one within each cerebral hemisphere, communicate with the third ventricle in the diencephalon, which leads, through a narrow aqueduct in the midbrain (the cerebral aqueduct of Sylvius), to the fourth ventricle in the medulla. Cerebrospinal fluid also bathes and cushions the outside of the brain and spinal cord by flowing through a space that covers the surface of the entire central nervous system. The ventricular system is described in greater detail in Chapter 21.

Even Simple Behavior Recruits the Activity of Three Major Sets of Functional Systems

Consider the systems called into action during even an apparently simple behavior—for example, catching a ball.

For this task, the brain must have *sensory systems* to provide at least three types of information: visual information about the motion of the ball, tactile information about the impact of the ball in the hand, and proprioceptive information about the position of the arms (and legs) in space (even though the catcher may not be looking at them).

These sensory inputs must be fed to the *motor systems* of the brain, which issue commands on the basis of integrated information about the sensory periphery. Motor commands must *select* the exact muscles in the back, shoulder, arm, and hand required for catching the ball; the commands must also *time* the coordinated contraction and relaxation of appropriate muscle groups and regulate body posture as a whole. Moreover, the motor systems must be continually *updated* about the performance of a motor command with information

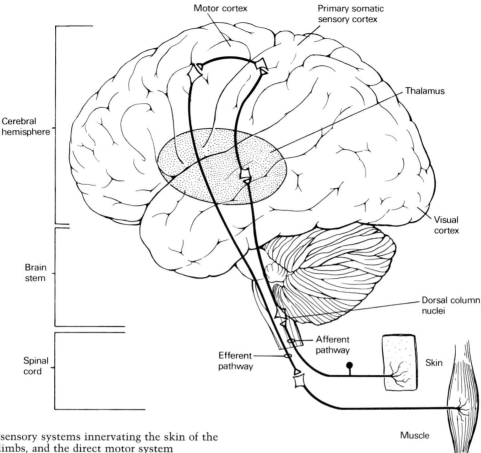

19–5 The major sensory systems innervating the skin of the trunk and limbs, and the direct motor system governing the activity of muscles in these body regions must cooperate to carry out a behavioral act. Ascending sensory input runs through the spinal cord and brain stem. It eventually reaches the somatic sensory cortex after a synaptic relay in the lower medulla and in the thalamus. The direct descending pathway runs from the motor cortex through the brain stem to the motor neurons of the spinal cord.

about the variations in muscular tension that accompany a motor act.

Finally, there must be *motivational systems* to stimulate interest in initiating and completing the behavioral sequence. The motivational systems must regulate the motor output to skeletal muscles as a reflection of the catcher's interest. How fast and accurately the ball is caught may depend on whether the catcher is excited or bored. Furthermore, the motivational systems coordinate the activity of the skeletal, or somatic, motor system with the activity of the autonomic nervous system, which regulates the endocrine glands, the viscera of the body, and the cardiovascular system. The physiological signs of excitement—such as sweating and an increase in heart rate—are therefore controlled by the same motivational systems that modulate the activity of the skeletal muscles. In this way, the motivational systems are able to orchestrate an integrated behavioral response.

The locations of the major motor and sensory systems in the brain and spinal cord are indicated in Figure 19–5; the interactions of these systems together with the motivational systems are schematized in Figure 19–6. The various sensory inputs necessary for catching a ball reach the cerebral cortex and eventually converge on the motor areas. The motor output of the cortex is modulated by the motivational systems and is conveyed to the motor neurons of the spinal cord through both direct and indirect pathways. In any behavioral act, there is constant interplay between the various components of the motor, sensory, and motivational systems so that motor output can be varied if any change is detected in the sensory periphery.

In later chapters, we shall see that these three major sets of brain systems are localized in separate neural pathways that work together to produce appropriate motor responses to sensory stimuli.

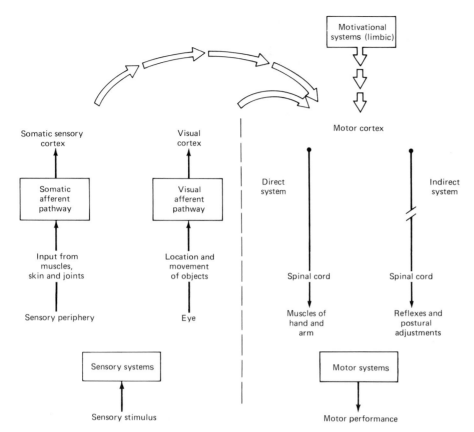

19–6 The three major brain systems—the sensory systems, the motor systems, and the motivational systems—must interact in a behavioral act such as catching a ball. Information about the movement of the ball and its eventual impact in the hand is relayed to the sensory areas of the cerebral cortex. These areas provide input to the motor cortex. The motivational systems, which include a portion of the limbic system of the brain, also send input to the motor cortex. A gap in an arrow signifies that a particular interaction may involve many synaptic relays, not simply a direct connection between two areas or systems. From the motor cortex, direct and indirect descending systems emerge. The direct system regulates the activity of motor neurons that innervate the muscles of the hand and arm, muscles involved in the fine control of movement. The indirect system plays an important role in the overall regulation of body posture.

The Motivational Systems Act Through Two Independent Motor Systems: The Autonomic and Somatic

As we saw above, the skeletal muscles involved in voluntary movements are innervated and controlled by the *somatic motor system*. The motivational systems act through the somatic motor system. But, in addition, they also act through a separate motor system, the *autonomic motor system* (also called the autonomic *nervous* system, although it controls only motor output), which provides the innervation for the endocrine and exocrine glands, for the viscera, and for smooth muscles in all organs of the body. The autonomic nervous system has two major divisions: the *sympathetic* and *parasympathetic*.[1] Both divisions are important in mediating motivational and emotional states as well as in monitoring the body's basic physiology.

The sympathetic and parasympathetic divisions sometimes act synergistically and at other times oppose one another in their actions. The *sympathetic* system often mediates the response of the body to stress: it speeds up heart rate, increases blood pressure, mobilizes the body's energy stores for emergency, and prepares for action. In contrast, the *parasympathetic* system acts to conserve the body's resources and restore homeostasis: it slows the heart, reduces blood pressure, and prepares the body for relaxation or rest.

The two divisions are segregated anatomically. The cell bodies that give rise to the sympathetic division lie in the *thoracic* and *lumbar* regions of the spinal cord (Figure 19–7). The neurons that give rise to the parasympathetic division lie above this region of the spinal cord in several brain stem nuclei associated with cranial nerves, and below it in the sacral region of the spinal cord. The autonomic nuclei in the brain stem and spinal cord contain neurons, called *preganglionic cells*, that send their axons to synapse on a second set of neurons, called *postganglionic cells*, that lie in peripheral collections of nerve cell bodies called *autonomic ganglia*. The postganglionic cells in turn innervate viscera, glands, and smooth muscle.

---

[1]In addition to the two major divisions, the autonomic nervous system has a third branch, the *enteric nervous system*. This is remarkable both anatomically and physiologically because it is virtually independent from central nervous system control. Its neurons are located in two ganglionated plexuses within the bowel, the submucosal and the myenteric, and function as an *intrinsic* nervous system of the gut. As a result, the gut, alone among the organs of the body, can manifest reflex activity in the complete absence of input from the central nervous system.

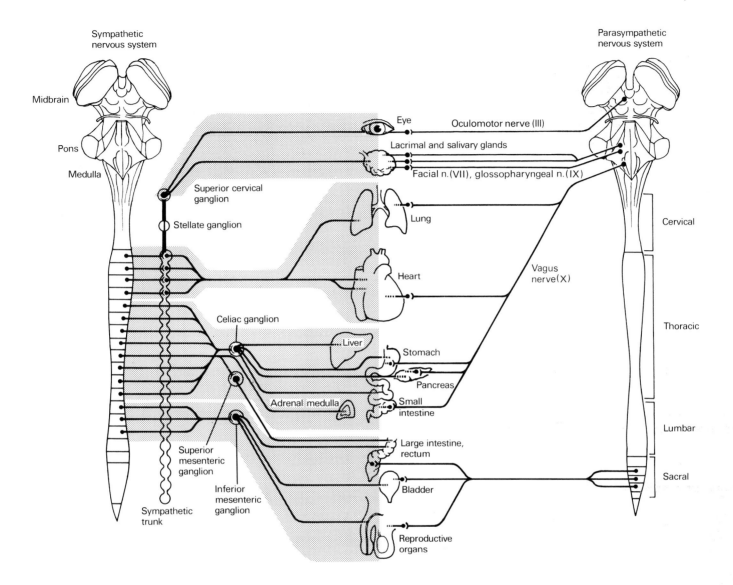

19–7 The autonomic motor system consists of the sympathetic and parasympathetic divisions. The connections of both systems with the hypothalamus and higher brain centers have been omitted in this figure. **Solid lines,** preganglionic axons. **Broken lines,** terminals of postganglionic axons. (The sympathetic innervation of blood vessels, sweat glands and piloerector muscles is not shown.) **Shading** indicates the distribution of the sympathetic nervous system.

The ganglia of the sympathetic division are located in bilateral chains called the *sympathetic trunks.* The sympathetic trunks lie close to the spinal cord, along the anterolateral surfaces of the vertebral column, and extend from the base of the skull to the coccyx. The axons of preganglionic sympathetic neurons tend to be short because they go to a nearby structure, whereas the axons of the postganglionic neurons are long. This situation is reversed in the parasympathetic division. Parasympathetic preganglionic axons must often travel considerable distances to reach their terminal ganglia, which are situated within or very close to the organs innervated.

This anatomical difference has an important functional consequence in the specificity with which each system acts on the body. Because the ganglia of the sympathetic division lie close to the spinal cord, the axons from an individual ganglion are able to spread out to innervate many organs. In contrast, the location of parasympathetic ganglia allows the innervation from this division to be more specifically directed to an individual organ. Consequently, sympathetic reactions tend to be widespread, affecting the response of the organism as a whole, whereas parasympathetic reactions can be restricted to particular organs or glands. Some sympathetic preganglionic axons do not terminate in the sympathetic trunk, but run through it to form splanchnic nerves. The fibers in these nerves synapse in several collateral ganglia (the celiac and mesenteric) containing postganglionic cells that innervate the viscera. The cranial outflow of the parasympathetic nervous system terminates in the parasympathetic ganglia of the head and neck. Postganglionic axons derived from neurons in these ganglia innervate the salivary and lacrimal glands, glands in the nasal and oral mucosa, and the smooth muscles associated with the eye. (From Schmidt and Thews, 1983.)

The main control center for the autonomic motor system is the hypothalamus, which is also critically involved in the regulation of feeding and drinking. The hypothalamus sends out descending fibers that regulate sympathetic and parasympathetic nuclei in the spinal cord and brain stem, axons that control the release of hormones by the anterior pituitary gland, and axons that release hormones directly into the posterior pituitary gland. The hypothalamus receives information from many other structures, including higher levels of the motivational systems: the cerebral cortex and the reticular formation. The activity of the hypothalamus is also influenced by the concentrations of insulin and glucose circulating in the blood. Thus, in its role as central governor of the autonomic motor system, the hypothalamus directly regulates autonomic output and endocrine function, and also is responsive to a broad spectrum of behaviorally important stimuli.

Four Principles Govern the Organization of the Functional Systems of the Brain

Each Major System in the Brain Is Composed of Several Distinct Pathways in Parallel

The sensory, motor, and motivational systems have subdivisions that perform subtasks. Thus, the sensory systems have separate divisions for each of the senses, and each of these divisions has components. The visual system, for example, enables us not only to perceive stationary objects but also to track their motion. These functions are performed by separate visual pathways that work together to coordinate perceptual abilities with the control of eye and limb movement. Similarly, anatomically separate somatic sensory pathways, such as those for touch and for pain, relay information to the cerebral cortex from receptors in the skin that are sensitive to these different stimuli. The motor systems also consist of several pathways that run from the highest centers of the brain to the spinal cord. The pyramidal tract, a pathway that descends from the cerebral cortex to the spinal cord, mediates the performance of accurate voluntary movements of the hand. Other motor pathways control overall body posture and regulate spinal reflexes. Thus, multiple pathways are required to mediate complex sensations and motor acts; multiple pathways are also thought to be involved in motivation.

Each Pathway Contains Synaptic Relays

Each of these multiple sensory, motor, and motivational pathways of the central nervous system is interrupted, usually at several points, by synaptic relays. These relays are not simply one-to-one connections between presynaptic and postsynaptic neurons, but a complex convergence of neurons. At these sites the sensory input, motor output, or motivational component is modified by processing that occurs within the relay nucleus itself as well as by inputs from other parts of the brain that converge on the relay nucleus. Relay nuclei commonly contain several types of neurons. Two of these types are particularly important: (1) *Projection* (or *principal*) *cells* have long axons that constitute the output from that nucleus. These axons leave the nucleus to synapse upon other nuclei or the cortex. (2) *Local interneurons* have axons that remain confined to the area around the cell body. We shall encounter many synaptic relays or nuclei in both the spinal cord and the brain, but perhaps the most important relay structure is the thalamus because it is a collection of many separate nuclei that relay information to the cerebral cortex. Indeed, almost all of the sensory information that reaches the cerebral cortex does so after first having been processed by a relay nucleus in the thalamus.

Each Pathway Is Topographically Organized

The most striking feature of sensory pathways is that the peripheral receptor surface, be it the retina or the skin, is represented in an organized way within a particular pathway. For example, functionally related neighboring groups of cells in the retina connect with similar neighboring groups in the thalamus, which in turn connect with corresponding neighboring regions of the visual cortex. Adjacent parts of the visual field are therefore represented in adjacent regions of the cerebral cortex, so that an orderly map of the visual field is found at each successive level, from lowest to highest in the brain. This visuotopic map does not represent each part of the visual field equally, but distorts it: the central region, which has the capacity for high-acuity vision, is represented by a disproportionately large cortical area. Similarly, there is a somatotopic map, a map of the body surface, in the cerebral cortex. This map is also highly distorted in favor of regions that are particularly important for somatic sensibility, such as the finger tips and the lips, whose representation occupies a relatively large cortical area. At each level of the auditory pathway, distinct regions of the relay nuclei are selectively responsive to particular frequencies of sound, thereby generating a tonotopic map of the sound spectrum to which the ear is sensitive.

Somatotopic, visuotopic, and tonotopic maps are found throughout the somatic sensory, visual, and auditory pathways and show the orderly organization of synaptic connections in the brain. In the secondary sensory areas of the cerebral cortex, several additional maps of the sensory periphery are usually found, implying that these areas may be further subdivided on a functional basis. In the motor pathways, the neurons that regulate the activity of particular muscle groups also are clustered together to form a motor map, which, as we saw in Chapter 1, is particularly clear in the motor cortex. The motor map, like the sensory maps, is distorted, and reflects the fineness of control of individual muscles. These central sensory and motor maps are clinically important; knowledge of them permits the neurologist to localize lesions in the central nervous system with precision because damage to a particular subdivision of a pathway will produce specific deficits in restricted aspects of motor or sensory function.

Most Pathways Are Crossed

An important but as yet unexplained aspect of the organization of the brain is that many of the bilaterally symmetrical neural pathways cross the midline. Because the information crosses, sensory and motor events on one side of the body are interpreted and controlled by the cerebral hemisphere on the opposite side. Furthermore, the pathways cross at different anatomical levels in different systems. In the somatic sensory system, crossing usually occurs soon after the *first* synapse is established by a primary afferent fiber. As a result, somatic sensation is processed on the contralateral side of the brain. The direct cortical motor pathway to the spinal cord crosses at the level of the medulla, and consequently the cerebral hemisphere on each side regulates the activity of muscles on the opposite side of the body. Crossings of this kind within the brain stem and spinal cord are usually called *decussations* (Latin, *decussare*, to cross in the shape of an X).

Crossing in the visual system is slightly more complicated. Only half of the visual field of each eye is represented in the opposite half of the brain; the other half is represented in the ipsilateral half of the brain. This arrangement is made possible by a different type of crossing, which occurs in the *optic chiasm* (Greek, from the letter *chi*, X), where the left and right optic nerves join. In the optic chiasm, axons from both eyes are segregated so that all the fibers that relay information about the same half of the visual field are brought together in the optic tract on one side. Therefore, only half of the fibers from each eye cross to the contralateral side of the brain. Other types of crossing fibers are found in the major brain *commissures* (Latin, joining together). The fibers in these commissures join functionally similar areas from each half of the brain, across the midline. By far the largest commissure, and indeed the largest fiber bundle in the brain, is the *corpus callosum* (Latin, hard body), which connects the two cerebral hemispheres (see Figure 19–2).

An Overall View

Knowledge of how motor, sensory, and motivational systems are organized anatomically is essential for understanding how the brain executes motor commands and generates perceptions of the world. Thus, neuroanatomy is basic to modern neurology and psychiatry. As we shall see in the next chapter, the anatomical details of the functional systems of the brain are quite complex. However, this complexity has a logic, as is revealed in a study of the organizational principles of the brain.

Selected Readings

Barr, M. L., and Kiernan, J. A. 1983. The Human Nervous System: An Anatomical Viewpoint, 4th ed. Philadelphia: Harper & Row.

Brodal, A. 1981. Neurological Anatomy in Relation to Clinical Medicine, 3rd ed. New York: Oxford University Press.

Gilman, S., and Winans, S. S. 1982. Manter & Gatz's Essentials of Clinical Neuroanatomy and Neurophysiology, 6th ed. Philadelphia: Davis.

Heimer, L. 1983. The Human Brain and Spinal Cord: Functional Neuroanatomy and Dissection Guide. New York: Springer.

Nieuwenhuys, R., Voogd, J., and van Huijzen, Chr. 1981. The Human Central Nervous System: A Synopsis and Atlas, 2nd rev. ed. Berlin: Springer.

References

Appenzeller, O. 1982. The Autonomic Nervous System: An Introduction to Basic and Clinical Concepts, 3rd rev. ed. New York: Elsevier Biomedical Press.

Gershon, M. D. 1981. The enteric nervous system. Annu. Rev. Neurosci. 4:227–272.

Noback, C. R., and Demarest, R. J. 1981. The Human Nervous System: Basic Principles of Neurobiology, 3rd ed. New York: McGraw-Hill.

Schmidt, R. F., and Thews, G. (eds.). 1983. Human Physiology. Berlin: Springer.

James P. Kelly

Anatomical Basis of Sensory Perception and Motor Coordination

20

The central nervous system is made up of an extremely large number of cells—about 10^{12} neurons—that are wired together in a highly precise manner. The cerebral cortex alone has at least 50 billion (5×10^{10}) nerve cells! Despite the large number of cells, however, the task of studying the nervous system is greatly simplified for two reasons. First, the neurons of the central nervous system are not randomly distributed but are clustered into discrete cellular groups called *nuclei*, which are connected to one another to form sensory, motor, or motivational systems. To understand the anatomy of the human central nervous system, one needs only to know the major nuclear groups within individual sensory and motor systems and their relationships—to each other, to the motivational systems, and to the gross topographical features of the brain. Second, because we now have a clearer idea of the functional importance of many of the key nuclear groups, brain anatomy can be studied in a more interesting and behaviorally relevant way than was possible in the past.

In this chapter we shall examine the central nervous system and consider in detail each of its six major structures. To simplify this survey, we shall focus primarily on how information from the body surface ascends through the nervous system, is processed and transformed into a motor command, and descends again to produce a motor response. Because our emphasis here is on functional relationships, this survey will not include a systematic three-dimensional description of the brain; rather, the aim is to convey a general idea of the relays and interconnections that work together to translate afferent information into appropriate behavioral responses.

In the Somatic Sensory Systems, Axons Travel Along the Spinal Cord to the Brain

Dorsal Root Ganglion Cells Provide Input to the Spinal Cord

The skin, muscles, and joints of the body contain a variety of receptors that transduce stimuli into electrical activity. The skin has tactile receptors as well as receptors for pain and temperature. These receptors are innervated by afferent axons that carry information from the receptors to the central nervous system. The cell bodies of these afferent axons lie in clusters called the *dorsal root ganglia,* located between the vertebrae and adjacent to the spinal cord.

As we saw in Chapters 2 and 3, the cells of the dorsal root ganglia have an interesting structure (Figure 20–1). Their rounded cell bodies give off a single process that bifurcates into two separate branches. One branch is directed peripherally, running in a spinal nerve with other sensory and motor axons until it reaches the receptor. The other branch runs centrally into the spinal cord through the dorsal root. The anatomical relationship of the dorsal roots to the spinal cord is illustrated in Figure 20–2.

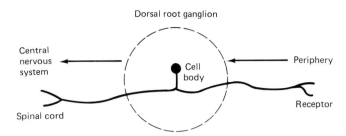

20–1 A single process emerges from the body of a dorsal root ganglion cell and divides into a branch that innervates a receptor in the periphery, and a central branch that relays input to the spinal cord.

Efferent fibers from the *ventral root* join the fibers of the dorsal root to form a mixed *spinal nerve.* The spinal nerve that enters the vertebral column therefore contains both afferent and efferent fibers, the axons of sensory as well as motor nerve cells.

The centrally directed branches of all dorsal root ganglion cells branch extensively when they enter the spinal cord, and the information they carry is forwarded to specific sites in the central nervous system that process somatic sensory modalities, such as temperature and touch. However, not all fibers branch in the same way. Different functional classes of neurons have highly specific branching patterns and, as a result, neurons mediating different sensory modalities have different patterns of central connections.

20–2 The dorsal and ventral spinal roots join to form a mixed spinal nerve before their fibers leave the vertebral column. The dorsal root breaks up into a series of fine rootlets as it enters the cord. Similarly, motor axons run in rootlets as they emerge from the cord, and these rootlets join to form the ventral root.

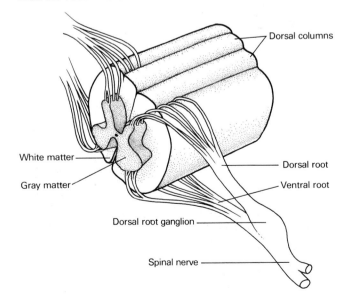

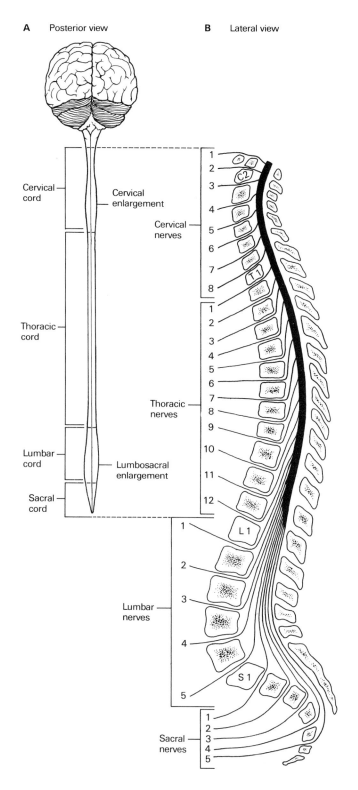

A Posterior view   **B** Lateral view

20–3 Spinal nerves are named for their site of emergence from the vertebral column.

A. Posterior view of the brain and spinal cord. The spinal cord is divided into four regions: cervical, thoracic, lumbar, and sacral. The *cervical cord* lies closest to the junction with the brain and contains the cervical enlargement. The *thoracic cord* is the longest division and is continuous with the *lumbar cord.* The lumbar cord shares the lumbosacral enlargement with the *sacral cord,* which is most caudal.

B. Lateral view. The spinal roots emerge between the individual vertebrae. There are 7 cervical vertebrae, 12 thoracic vertebrae, 5 lumbar vertebrae, and 5 sacral vertebrae. The adult spinal cord does not run the whole length of the vertebral column but terminates at about the level of the L1 vertebra. The dorsal and ventral roots that exit between the lumbar and sacral vertebrae must therefore take a long course before exiting from the vertebral column. These rootlets are collectively termed the *cauda equina.*

Despite differences in details, each class of dorsal root ganglion cell conveys three types of information by means of three types of connections:

1. Information for reflex activity through connections with the interneurons and motor neurons of the spinal cord.

2. Information for conscious perception, such as perception of touch or pain, through connections with neurons that ascend to the cerebral cortex.

3. Information for behavioral arousal (for controlling levels of awareness and attention) through connections with neurons of the reticular formation in the brain stem.

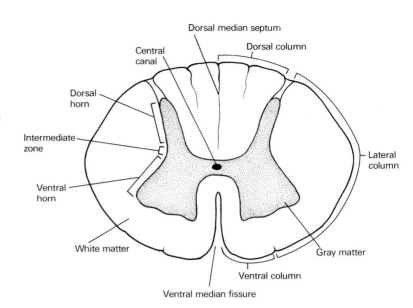

20–4 This cross-sectional view of the spinal cord shows the bilaterally symmetrical divisions of white matter and gray matter. The central gray matter is surrounded by white matter that is organized into three columns (dorsal, lateral, and ventral) running parallel to the long axis of the cord. The gray matter is divided into the dorsal and ventral horns, which are concerned, respectively, with receiving afferent input and generating the motor output of the cord.

In this chapter, we shall be concerned primarily with connections made between dorsal root ganglion cells and other neurons that lead to conscious perception of tactile information. We shall return to a consideration of the reflex function of the various types of dorsal root fibers when we discuss the motor systems (Chapter 33), and we shall examine arousal in the context of the brain stem (Chapter 41).

The Spinal Cord Is Composed of Both Gray and White Matter

The spinal cord is connected to the skeletal muscles of the limbs and trunk and to the sensory receptors in skin and muscle by the spinal nerves that emerge from the vertebral column between the individual vertebrae (Figure 20–3). A schematic section through the spinal cord is shown in Figure 20–4. At the center of the cord is the *central canal*, a remnant of the space within the primitive neural tube, which we shall consider in detail in the next chapter. The spinal cord is bilaterally symmetrical. As is true for other parts of the central nervous system, the spinal cord is divided into *gray matter*, which contains the cell bodies of neurons, and *white matter*, which contains fiber tracts (see Chapter 24). Also like the brain, the spinal cord is encased by three layers of membranes or meninges: the *pia mater*, *arachnoid mater*, and *dura mater* (see Chapter 21).

The gray matter of the spinal cord is located centrally. It surrounds the central canal and, in transverse section, is shaped like a butterfly. The wings of this butterfly contain most of the gray matter and are divided into the *dorsal* and *ventral horns*. The neurons of the dorsal and ventral horns of the gray matter are clustered into groups called *nuclei*, consisting of nerve cells that share similar functional properties—an anatomical arrangement that allows particular inputs to be focused on discrete clusters of neurons. Each dorsal horn extends toward the entering

dorsal root and contains sensory nuclei that are relay stations for somatic sensory information coming into the spinal cord. Each ventral horn contains clusters of motor neurons and interneurons. The motor neurons give rise to the axons that innervate skeletal muscles. The interneurons channel information from the dorsal horn (or from higher centers) to motor neurons or from one group of motor neurons to another. The zone between the dorsal horn and the ventral horn is called the *intermediate zone*. This zone contains neurons whose axons go to autonomic ganglia as well as neurons that connect axons from the dorsal root afferents to the cerebellum.

The white matter of the spinal cord is located peripherally and envelops the gray matter. It contains large numbers of myelinated fibers, which appear white because of their lipid-rich sheaths. Each symmetrical half of the white matter is divided into three large groups of axons arranged as longitudinally running bundles or columns—the *dorsal, lateral,* and *ventral columns*. The dorsal columns contain afferent axons carrying somatic sensory information to the brain stem. The lateral and ventral columns contain axons that ascend to higher levels as well as axons that descend from the brain to synapse upon neurons in the gray matter of the spinal cord.

The Internal Structure of the Spinal Cord Varies at Different Cross-Sectional Levels

The individual spinal nerves are related to particular levels of the cord (the *cervical, thoracic, lumbar,* and *sacral*), and each level has a distinctive structure (Figure 20–3). There are 8 cervical spinal nerves, even though there are only 7 cervical vertebrae, because the first cervical spinal nerve emerges rostral to the first cervical vertebra. The spinal nerves in the other spinal segments are named for the vertebra caudal to which they exit. There are 12 thoracic nerves, 5 lumbar nerves, and 5 sacral nerves.

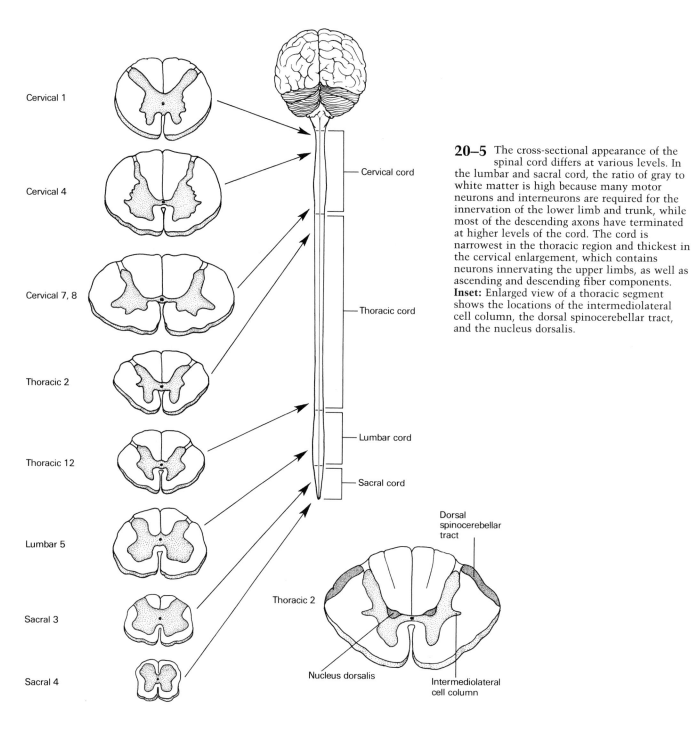

Cervical 1

Cervical 4

Cervical 7, 8

Thoracic 2

Thoracic 12

Lumbar 5

Sacral 3

Sacral 4

Cervical cord

Thoracic cord

Lumbar cord

Sacral cord

20–5 The cross-sectional appearance of the spinal cord differs at various levels. In the lumbar and sacral cord, the ratio of gray to white matter is high because many motor neurons and interneurons are required for the innervation of the lower limb and trunk, while most of the descending axons have terminated at higher levels of the cord. The cord is narrowest in the thoracic region and thickest in the cervical enlargement, which contains neurons innervating the upper limbs, as well as ascending and descending fiber components. **Inset:** Enlarged view of a thoracic segment shows the locations of the intermediolateral cell column, the dorsal spinocerebellar tract, and the nucleus dorsalis.

Thoracic 2

Dorsal spinocerebellar tract

Nucleus dorsalis

Intermediolateral cell column

The organization of the spinal cord is determined in predictable ways by two important features. First, from the lower sacral region to progressively higher lumbar, thoracic, and cervical levels, there is a sequential addition of afferent axons to the spinal cord. Because of this organization, the portion of the spinal white matter consisting of *afferent* fibers gets larger at each successively higher level. Similarly, the long descending axons originating in the brain terminate at various levels of the cord, so that fewer are left at each succeeding lower level,

with only a small number remaining in the sacral spinal cord. Thus, there is very little white matter relative to gray matter in the sacral cord (Figure 20–5, sacral 3 and 4). In contrast, there is more white matter than gray matter in the high cervical region of the cord, where there are many ascending and descending axons (Figure 20–5, cervical 1). Second, the size of the ventral and dorsal horns is greater in the regions of the spinal cord that innervate the limbs (known as the lumbosacral and cervical enlargements, respectively) than in the thoracic region, which innervates only the trunk. This is because more motor neurons and interneurons are required to innervate the arms and legs.

In addition to variations in the ventral horn, certain nuclei are present in the gray matter at some levels but not at others. For example, two important nuclei are present in the thoracic and upper lumbar segments but not elsewhere. They are the *intermediolateral cell column* and the cells of the *nucleus dorsalis* (Figure 20–5, inset). The intermediolateral cell column contains the preganglionic sympathetic neurons of the autonomic motor system. These neurons project out the ventral root to synapse on neurons in the sympathetic trunks or in prevertebral ganglia (see Figure 19–6). The cells of the nucleus dorsalis receive direct input from joint receptors and muscle spindles and send their axons into the lateral column on the same side of the cord. The axons from the cells of the nucleus dorsalis ascend to the cerebellum as the *dorsal spinocerebellar tract*, which relays information about the position and movement of the lower trunk and leg.

Axons of Dorsal Root Ganglion Cells Are Somatotopically Arranged

Some dorsal root ganglion cells terminate in the dorsal horn and in the intermediate zone to participate in local spinal activity. Other cells have branches that allow them to participate in local spinal activity and also to mediate conscious sensations by sending long ascending branches that run in the dorsal column to the brain (Figure 20–6). In the dorsal column the axons are arranged in a highly ordered manner that results from the way fibers are added to the columns. When the sacral axons enter they are packed near the midline. The axons that are added at higher levels are packed at successively more lateral positions. As a result, in the cervical cord, sensory information from the sacrum is represented medially, the leg and trunk are represented more laterally, then the skin of the arm and shoulder, and, finally, most laterally, the neck. Thus, the dorsal columns contain a representation of body receptors. This orderly representation of the body receptors is termed the *somatotopic representation. Once established at the level of the dorsal columns, somatotopic order is maintained throughout the entire ascending somatic sensory pathway.*

Axons of the Dorsal Root Ganglion Cells That Course in the Dorsal Columns Synapse in the Medulla

The axons that ascend in the dorsal columns run up the spinal cord to its rostral continuation, the *medulla*, which is the lowest portion of the *brain stem*—the part of the central nervous system that is interposed between the spinal cord and the thalamus. Like the spinal cord, the caudal part of the medulla has centrally located nuclei surrounded by fiber tracts that convey afferent information to higher levels of the brain and motor com-

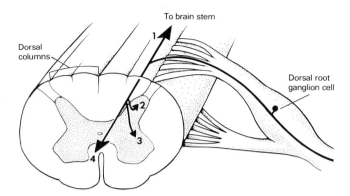

20–6 An individual dorsal root may have several types of central branches. The principal branch ascends in the dorsal column to the brain stem (**1**). Other branches terminate locally in the spinal cord (**2, 3**) or descend for a few segments (**4**). Branches **2, 3,** and **4** participate in the mediation of spinal reflexes or are involved in sensory processing within the dorsal horn.

mands to the spinal cord. The nuclei of the medulla process input from the cranial nerves that innervate the head and neck and generate the motor output of these nerves, just as the spinal cord mediates the functions of spinal nerves. The medulla is also a way station for ascending sensory input from the spinal cord. The axons of the dorsal root ganglion cells that run in the dorsal columns synapse on two important nuclei, the *dorsal column nuclei*, called the *gracile nucleus*, and the *cuneate nucleus* (Figure 20–7A and B, 3). In addition to relaying sensory information, the dorsal column nuclei receive afferents from sensory areas in the cerebral cortex. The nuclei also contain interneurons. The cortical feedback and the additional synaptic interactions within the nucleus provided by the interneurons modify the flow of sensory information along the somatic afferent pathway.

Up to this point, information about tactile input has been relayed by dorsal column axons that have entered on one side of the cord and remained on that side throughout their ascent to the dorsal column nuclei. In the medulla, however, an important crossing occurs. As the postsynaptic axons of the cells in the dorsal column nuclei emerge, they take an arc-shaped route and cross to the other side of the brain as the *internal arcuate fibers* (Figure 20–7B, 3). They continue their ascent to higher centers of the brain in a fiber bundle called the *medial lemniscus* (Latin, band or ribbon), the brain stem pathway that is most important for the mediation of sensation from the limbs and trunk. As is true of the dorsal columns and their nuclei, the medial lemniscus contains a somatotopic representation, but now of the opposite side of the body surface. The outcome of the orderly crossing of the fibers from the dorsal column nuclei to form the medial lemniscus is that the right side of the brain receives input from the sensory periphery of the limbs and trunk on the left side of the body, and vice versa.

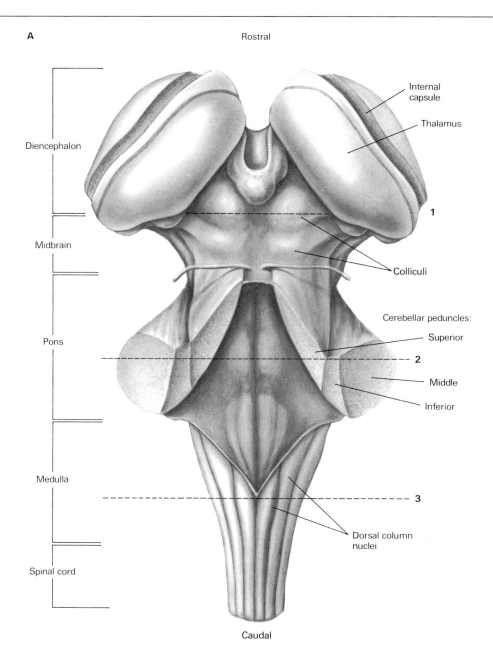

20–7 The path of the medial lemniscus serves as a landmark for locating various structures at different levels of the brain stem. **A.** Dorsal view of the brain stem with the cerebellum and cerebral hemispheres removed.

The Medial Lemniscus Ascends Through the Brain Stem

The medial lemniscus is a prominent structure through the entire brain stem, and therefore serves as a useful landmark in this region. Indeed, we can now consider the locations of the various cranial nerve and other nuclei in the brain stem in relation to the medial lemniscus. Some

of the nuclei found in the lower medulla are shown in Figure 20–7B, 3.

Whereas the dorsal columns are the prominent landmarks on the dorsal surface, the most prominent landmarks on the ventral aspect of the medulla are pyramid-shaped clusters of axons called the medullary pyramids. They contain the axons of the *corticospinal tracts*, which run from the cerebral cortex to the spinal cord and

B

1

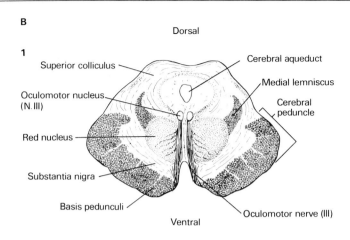

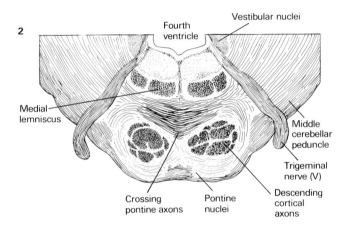

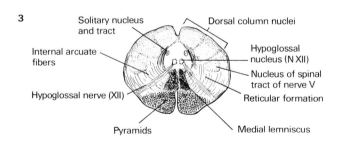

20–7 B. Cross sections made through the brain stem at the levels indicated in **A.**

1: Section through the midbrain. The dorsal portion of the midbrain at this level consists of the superior colliculus. The cerebral aqueduct, which connects the ventricular system in the diencephalon with the fourth ventricle in the pons and medulla, lies in the midline and is surrounded by the periaqueductal gray matter. Close to the midline, ventral to the aqueduct, lie the oculomotor (cranial nerve III) nuclei. The red nucleus is also a significant component of the midbrain. It gives rise to the rubrospinal tract, which descends to the spinal cord and regulates motor function. The medial lemniscus lies dorsolateral to the red nucleus in the midbrain. The most ventral portion of the midbrain is the cerebral peduncle, which has two principal components, the substantia nigra and the basis pedunculi.

2: Section through the pons. At this level axons are running to the cerebellar cortex in the middle cerebellar peduncle. Many of these axons arise from the nuclei that lie between the crossing fibers of the pons. These nuclei receive information from the cerebral cortex and pass it on to the cerebellum. The medial lemniscus lies in a mediolateral orientation in the pons. Cranial nerve V (trigeminal) is also evident here. The vestibular nuclei lie in the pons and medulla.

3: Section through the lower medulla. The dorsal column nuclei and the crossing internal arcuate fibers that form the medial lemniscus are evident at this level. The nucleus of cranial nerve XII (hypoglossal) lies medial to the solitary nucleus and tract, an important landmark for identifying sections through the medulla. A portion of the nucleus of cranial nerve V lies near the lateral margin of the medulla. The pyramids make up the ventral surface of the medulla. The medial lemniscus, shaped roughly like a triangle, lies dorsal to the pyramid and adjacent to the midline. Many neurons of the reticular formation lie between the major nuclear groups and fiber tracts of the medulla.

constitute a major motor system for the control of fine voluntary movements. We shall describe this system in detail at the end of this chapter.

As we follow the medial lemniscus up the medulla through the brain stem, the next region we encounter is the pons. The pons contains clusters of neurons (the *pontine nuclei*) that give rise to fibers that cross the midline and run to the cerebellar hemisphere on the opposite side. These axons are important for the cerebellar control of movement and posture. Within the pons, the crossing fibers are located ventral to the medial lemniscus (Figure 20–7B, 2). The pons also contains the more rostral continuation of the corticospinal tracts.

Continuing its ascent, the medial lemniscus next passes through the midbrain. The dorsal surface of the midbrain (Figure 20–7A) is composed of four swellings,

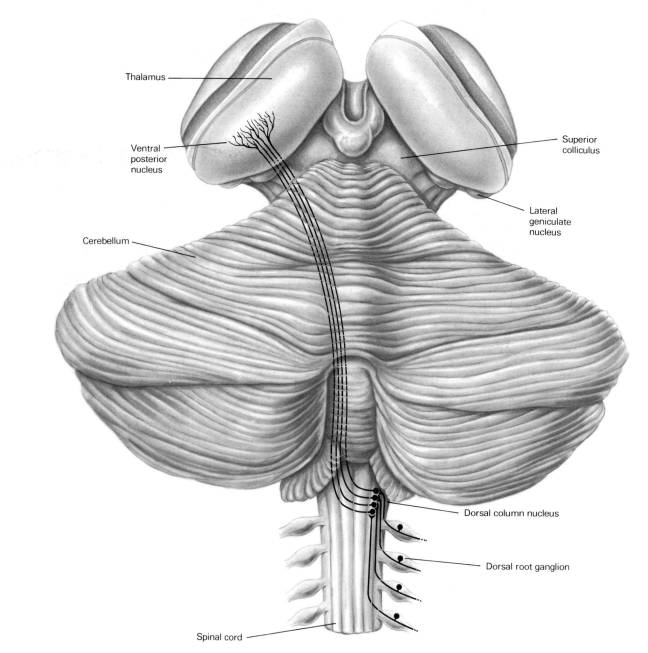

Thalamus

Ventral posterior nucleus

Cerebellum

Superior colliculus

Lateral geniculate nucleus

Dorsal column nucleus

Dorsal root ganglion

Spinal cord

20–8 In this drawing the cerebral hemispheres have been removed to show the course of the medial lemniscus from the medulla to the thalamus. The cerebellum covers the brain stem. The medial lemniscus arises from the cells of the dorsal column nuclei, which cross the midline and ascend the brain stem dorsal to the pyramids and adjacent to the midline. As the fibers ascend in the medial lemniscus, they move progressively more laterally to terminate in the ventral posterior portion of the thalamus. (Adapted from Niewenhuys, Voogd, and van Huijzen, 1981.)

two on each side, called the colliculi (Latin, little hills). The *superior colliculi* are important for involuntary visual tracking reflexes and receive direct input from the retina. This portion of the visual pathway concerned with visual reflex function is separated from the percep-

tual pathway that involves relays in the thalamus and ultimately in the visual cortex. The separation of perceptual and reflex visual pathways provides a good illustration of multiple channels within a single sensory modality. The perceptual and tracking subsystems are interrelated by axons that run from the visual cortex to the superior colliculus, as well as axons that run from the superior colliculus to the pulvinar (a portion of the thalamus, which in turn sends axons to the cerebral cortex). The *inferior colliculi* of the midbrain are functionally distinct from the superior colliculi. As we shall see, they relay auditory information from the brain stem to the thalamus and are an integral part of the pathway underlying hearing.

The base of the midbrain is formed by the cerebral peduncles (Latin, stalk). The bottom of each peduncle, the *basis pedunculi* (Figure 20–7B, 1), is a massive fiber bundle that contains axons of the corticopontine, corticobulbar, and corticospinal tracts that run from the cerebral cortex to lower centers in the pons, medulla, and spinal cord. Lying dorsal to the basis pedunculi is the *substantia nigra*, so named because some of its cells contain a dark pigment. The substantia nigra is a motor center, many of whose cells send their axons to motor nuclei in the thalamus and to higher motor regions of the brain that are a part of the basal ganglia; the organization of these structures will be described later in this chapter.

The medulla, the pons, and the midbrain also contain most of the twelve cranial nerve nuclei. These nuclei give rise to nerves that innervate structures in the head and neck (Table 41–1). Some of the cranial nerves are sensory, some are motor, and some are mixed. For example, the olfactory nerve (cranial nerve I), the optic nerve (cranial nerve II), and the vestibulocochlear nerve (cranial nerve VIII) are purely sensory and are associated with sensory relay structures in the brain. Other cranial nerves are purely motor; these nerves are found exclusively in the brain stem, where they originate from motor nuclei. Examples of pure motor nerves are the three cranial nerves that innervate the extraocular muscles, which move the eyes (cranial nerves III, IV, and VI), and the hypoglossal nerve, which innervates the muscles of the tongue (cranial nerve XII). Some cranial nerves have mixed functions. They contain both motor and sensory fibers, and are related to both motor and sensory nuclei in the brain stem. For example, the motor division of the trigeminal nerve (cranial nerve V) innervates muscles used in mastication, and the sensory division innervates the skin of the face.

The entire course of the medial lemniscus from the dorsal column nuclei through the brain stem to the thalamus is summarized in Figure 20–8. The medial lemniscus terminates in the ventral region of the thalamus near its posterior border.

The Thalamus Is Composed of Six Functionally Distinct Nuclear Groups

The importance of the thalamus cannot be overstated: It is the key structure that provides sensory input to the primary sensory areas of the cerebral cortex, and input about ongoing movement to the motor areas of the cortex. Because of its pivotal role in sensation and motor

control, we shall consider the thalamus in more detail than the other neural structures described so far. The thalamus is surrounded by a family of important structures (Figure 20–9). Ventral to the thalamus lies the hypothalamus, the endocrine and autonomic control center mentioned in Chapter 19. The boundary between the thalamus and the hypothalamus is indicated by the *hypothalamic sulcus*. Caudal and dorsal to the thalamus is the *pineal gland*, which secretes the hormone melatonin. The *subthalamic nucleus*, a motor control region, lies ventral to the thalamus and lateral to the hypothalamus. Collectively, the thalamus and these related structures form the diencephalon (Latin, between-brain), which lies between the cerebral hemispheres and the brain stem.

The thalamic nuclei establish connections with the cerebral cortex through the *internal capsule*, a massive fiber bundle that carries the vast majority of axons running *to* and *from* the cerebral hemisphere. Thus the internal capsule contains the rostral continuation of the somatic afferent pathway as well as of the corticopontine, corticobulbar, and corticospinal axons. A common, but cumbersome, terminology has been devised by anatomists to classify the various thalamic nuclei. Because this terminology is used throughout this book to distinguish the cell groups of the thalamus, we shall first explain it here. We shall then consider a functional classification of the nuclei that relates them to behavior.

The thalamus is divided into six nuclear groups:

Lateral (ventral tier and dorsal tier)	Intralaminar
	Midline
Medial	Reticular
Anterior	

The lateral, medial, and anterior groups are named according to their positions relative to a collection of axons called the *internal medullary lamina*.

The lateral group is subdivided into two tiers: ventral and dorsal (Figure 20–10). *The nuclei of the ventral tier of the lateral group are specific relay nuclei: each receives restricted sensory or motor input and projects to and receives input from a specific sensory or motor cortical region* (Table 20–1). The six nuclei of the ventral tier are named according to their position within the tier: The ventral anterior and the ventral lateral nuclei are important for motor control, the ventral posterior nucleus is important for somatic sensation. The medial and lateral geniculate nuclei (Latin *genu*, knee; *geniculus*, little knee), which are located at the posterior margin of the thalamus, are often included with the nuclei of the ventral tier. They mediate information about hearing and vision, respectively. *The nuclei of the dorsal tier of the lateral group are association nuclei; they project to association cortices* (Table 20–1). The three nuclei of this tier are called the lateral dorsal, the lateral posterior, and the pulvinar (Latin, cushion, because of its shape), which occupies most of the posterior aspect of the thalamus (Figure 20–10).

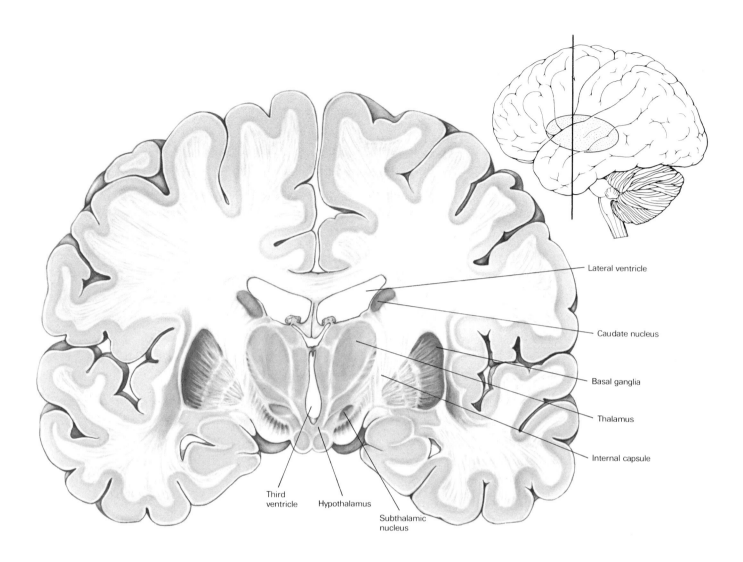

Lateral ventricle

Caudate nucleus

Basal ganglia

Thalamus

Internal capsule

Third ventricle   Hypothalamus

Subthalamic nucleus

20–9   This coronal section through the diencephalon shows that the thalamus lies dorsal to the hypothalamus and makes up the walls of the third ventricle. **Inset:** The line indicates the plane of the coronal section. (Adapted from Nieuwenhuys, Voogd, and van Huijzen, 1981.)

The nuclei of the medial group are also association nuclei. The largest component of the medial group is the medial dorsal nucleus.

The anterior nuclei are specific relay nuclei, but they participate in the regulation of emotion by relaying information from the hypothalamus to the cingulate gyrus, a portion of the cerebral cortex.

The intralaminar, reticular, and midline nuclei are nonspecific thalamic nuclei (Table 20–1). The intralaminar group consists of clusters of neurons that lie within the internal medullary lamina (Figure 20–10). The reticular nucleus caps the lateral aspect of the thalamus. The midline nuclei are located in the dorsal half of the wall of the third ventricle and are probably involved in visceral function.

Each Nuclear Group Belongs to One of Three Functional Classes

More important than the anatomical divisions just described is the fact that each of these nuclei belongs to one of three functional classes: specific relay nuclei, association nuclei, or nonspecific nuclei. Let us consider these classes in greater detail.

Specific Relay Nuclei. These nuclei (the anterior nuclei and the ventral tier of the lateral group) are characterized by three features (Table 20–1): (1) They receive discrete inputs either from a single sensory modality or a particular motor function. (2) They project upon a localized region of the cerebral cortex. The zones in the cerebral cortex where specific sensory or motor nuclei terminate are usually primary motor and sensory areas. In a primary sensory area, the first stage of intracortical processing occurs, eventually leading to the generation of a sensory perception. Each primary sensory area receives a direct input from a specific thalamic nucleus devoted to a single sensory modality. The primary motor area of the

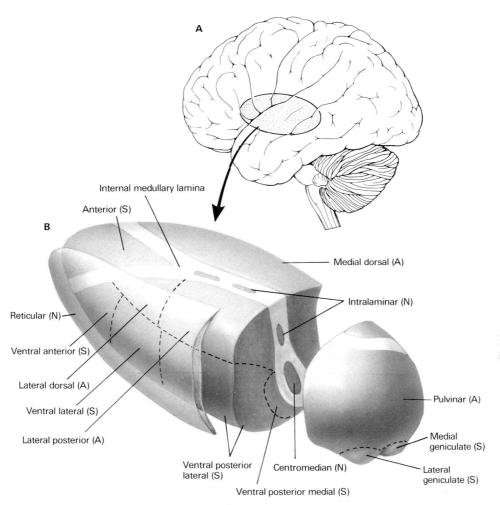

20–10 This view of the thalamus on the left side of the brain shows the location of the major thalamic nuclei. The internal medullary lamina divides the thalamus into the anterior, lateral, and medial groups of nuclei. The lateral group is divided into a dorsal and ventral tier. The ventral tier is composed of the ventral anterior, ventral lateral, and ventral posterior nuclei. The lateral geniculate nucleus, which is concerned with vision, and the medial geniculate nucleus, which is concerned with hearing, are often classed as components of the ventral tier. The nuclei of the dorsal tier are the lateral dorsal, lateral posterior, and the pulvinar. The medial dorsal nucleus is the largest of the medial group. The ventral tier nuclei are specific nuclei, while the dorsal tier and the medial group project to the association cortex. The intralaminar nuclei lie within the internal medullary lamina, while the reticular nucleus caps the lateral aspect of the thalamus. The functional class of each nucleus is indicated parenthetically: Specific relay **(S)**, association **(A)**, and nonspecific **(N)**.

cortex contains neurons that project to motor neurons and interneurons of the spinal cord. (3) Each specific relay nucleus in turn receives a recurrent connection from the region of the cerebral cortex upon which it projects. This connection presumably functions to allow the cortex to modulate its own input based on its ongoing activity.

These three points can be illustrated by considering as an example the ventral posterior nucleus, which is the major somatic sensory relay nucleus of the thalamus. It is the site of termination for the medial lemniscus. The projection cells of the ventral posterior nucleus send their axons (through the internal capsule) to the somatic sensory cortex of the postcentral gyrus. The ventral posterior nucleus also contains inhibitory interneurons that regulate the flow of sensory input and motor feedback to the cerebral cortex. The synaptic interactions between projection cells and interneurons are the basis for the integrative role that this nucleus has in sensation. Like all the specific relay nuclei, the ventral posterior nucleus receives a recurrent set of connections from the cortical area to which it projects, which allows the cerebral cortex to regulate its own thalamic input. The medial and lateral geniculate bodies are other examples of specific sensory relay nuclei that deal, respectively, with hearing and vision.

The ventral lateral and ventral anterior nuclei are specific nuclei related to the motor system. The ventral lateral nucleus receives input from the cerebellum and projects to the motor cortex of the precentral gyrus. The ventral anterior nucleus receives input from the globus pallidus (one of the large motor centers in the basal ganglia that we shall consider later) and projects that infor-

Table 20–1. Connections and Functions of Thalamic Nuclei

Nuclei	Principal afferent inputs	Major projection sites	Function
Specific relay nuclei			
Anterior nuclear group	Mamillary body of hypothalamus	Cingulate gyrus	Limbic
Ventral anterior	Globus pallidus	Premotor cortex (area 6)[a]	Motor
Ventral lateral	Dentate nucleus of cerebellum through brachium conjunctivum (superior cerebellar peduncle)	Motor and premotor cortices	Motor
Ventral posterior			
Lateral portion	Dorsal column–medial lemniscal pathway and spinothalamic pathways	Somatic sensory cortex of parietal lobe	Somatic sensation (body)
Medial portion	Sensory nuclei of trigeminal nerve (V)	Somatic sensory cortex of parietal lobe	Somatic sensation (face)
Medial geniculate	Inferior colliculus through brachium of inferior colliculus	Auditory cortex of temporal lobe (areas 41 and 42)[a]	Hearing
Lateral geniculate	Retinal ganglion cells through optic nerve and optic tract	Visual cortex of occipital lobe (area 17)[a]	Vision
Association nuclei			
Lateral dorsal	Cingulate gyrus	Cingulate gyrus	Emotional expression
Lateral posterior	Parietal lobe	Parietal lobe	Integration of sensory information
Pulvinar	Superior colliculus, temporal, parietal, and occipital lobes, and primary visual cortex	Temporal, parietal, and occipital lobes	Integration of sensory information
Medial dorsal	Amygdaloid nuclear complex, olfactory, and hypothalamus	Prefrontal cortex	Limbic
Nonspecific nuclei			
Midline nuclei	Reticular formation and hypothalamus	Basal forebrain	Limbic
Intralaminar nuclei Centromedian and centrolateral	Reticular formation, spinothalamic tract, globus pallidus, and cortical areas	Basal ganglia (striatum)	—
Reticular nucleus	Cerebral cortex and thalamic nuclei	Thalamic nuclei	Modulation of thalamic activity

[a]See Figure 20–12 for map of Brodmann's areas.

mation to the premotor cortex of the frontal lobe, which lies rostral to the primary motor area. The anterior nuclear group is related to visceral function and emotion. It receives input from the hypothalamus, and it projects to the cingulate gyrus, which is visible on the medial aspect of the cerebral hemispheres.

Association Nuclei. These nuclei (the pulvinar and the dorsal tier of the lateral group) receive input from several areas and each projects to one of the three association cortices (Table 20–1): the *parietal–temporal–occipital association cortex*, the *prefrontal association cortex*, or the *limbic association cortex*.

The pulvinar projects to the parietal–temporal–occipital association cortex, which includes Wernicke's speech

area (described in Chapter 1). The pulvinar occupies the posterior aspect of the thalamus (Figure 20–10) and makes connections quite unlike those of the specific thalamic nuclei. It receives inputs from many areas: from the superior colliculus of the midbrain, from the parietal–temporal–occipital association cortex upon which it projects, and from the primary visual cortex. Such a pattern of connections suggests that the pulvinar, the largest of the thalamic nuclei, integrates several sensory modalities (in contrast to the specific sensory nuclei of the thalamus, which are devoted to several aspects of a single modality).

The medial dorsal nucleus projects to the prefrontal association cortex. This nucleus receives connections from a cluster of nuclei called the *amygdaloid body*

(Greek, almond-shaped), which lies deep within the temporal lobe, and from the portion of the cerebral cortex that subserves olfaction. The amygdaloid nucleus is part of the limbic system and is thought to be involved in the control of emotional behavior.

The other components of the dorsal tier of the lateral group—the lateral dorsal and lateral posterior nuclei—are also association nuclei but their inputs are less well understood. The lateral dorsal nucleus, which lies close to the anterior nuclear group (Figure 20–10), projects to the limbic association cortex and specifically to the cingulate gyrus, the projection site of the anterior nuclear group. The lateral posterior nucleus projects upon the parietal–temporal–occipital association cortex.

Nonspecific Nuclei. These nuclei (the midline, intralaminar, and reticular nuclei) have patterns of connections that are much more widespread than those of either the relay or the association nuclei of the thalamus (Table 20–1). These widespread connections influence the activity of cells throughout the thalamus and the cerebral cortex. As we shall see in Chapter 46, these nuclei are part of an intrinsic system believed to govern the level of arousal of the brain.

The most significant nonspecific nuclei are the intralaminar nuclei—clusters of cells that are found within the confines of the internal medullary lamina. The largest of these cell groups is the centromedian nucleus (Figure 20–10). Cells in this nucleus receive inputs from the globus pallidus and have axons that terminate diffusely in several cortical areas and in the corpus striatum, a component of the basal ganglia. Another nonspecific nucleus, the reticular nucleus, lies over the lateral aspect of the thalamus (Figure 20–10). It receives input from most cortical areas and all thalamic nuclei, and projects upon other thalamic nuclei. The cells of the reticular nucleus have abundant collateral branches that spread widely and inhibit many thalamic neurons. The reticular nucleus is the only thalamic nucleus whose output is inhibitory. Its cells do not project to the cerebral cortex.

Relation of the Thalamic Nuclei to Cortical Function

The major functional subdivisions of the thalamus match those we considered in Chapter 19 for the cortex: sensory, motor, associative, and motivational. Each subdivision has a distinctive pattern of connections that reflects its particular role in information processing and the generation of behavior (Table 20–1). For example, each of the sensory systems forwards information about a single sensory modality to restricted regions of the cerebral cortex via specific thalamic relay nuclei. This information serves as the initial step in generating a sensory perception of the world. In the association areas of the cortex, these perceptions from several sensory systems are integrated and related to higher motor behaviors such as speech—behaviors that again involve not only specific motor nuclei, but also the association nuclei of the thalamus. The motor nuclei provide information to

the motor cortex about other regions of the brain, such as the cerebellum, that are involved in the control of motor output. Finally, the nonspecific systems are thought to regulate the overall level of brain activity and to reflect the general state of arousal and motivation.

All Other Major Sensory Systems Relay Through the Thalamus on the Way to the Cortex

As we have seen while following the ascent of information from the somatic sensory system, other sensory systems also relay through the thalamus. Let us now briefly consider these systems.

Vision. The ganglion cells of the retina receive information about form and color from the photoreceptors (already processed through two sets of synapses) and send their axons into the optic nerve. The two optic nerves join at the optic chiasm, where an important crossing of fibers occurs to form the optic tracts. The optic tracts terminate in the lateral geniculate nuclei of the thalamus, which projects upon the visual cortex in each occipital lobe.

Hearing and Balance. The eighth cranial nerve (the vestibulocochlear nerve) is composed of the centrally directed processes of ganglion cells that innervate receptors in the inner ear. These fibers terminate in two pairs of nuclei found at the level of the medulla and pons: the *cochlear nuclei* and the *vestibular nuclei.* The auditory portion of the eighth nerve relays information about sound to the brain stem. The cochlear nucleus, which receives the auditory input, lies on the lateral aspect of the inferior cerebellar peduncle. The vestibular portion of the nerve relays input from the semicircular canals, the utricle, and the saccule; these components of the inner ear detect the motion and position of the head in space. This input is critical for the coordination of head and eye movements and for the maintenance of body posture. The vestibular axons terminate in the vestibular nuclei—several groups of neurons in the dorsolateral aspect of the pons (Figure 20–7B, 2). Most of this input is used for vestibular reflexes. The eighth nerve also has auditory input that carries the primary information for the perception of sound. Ascending axons from the cochlear nucleus synapse in the inferior colliculus. Neurons in the inferior colliculus, in turn, send their axons to the medial geniculate nucleus of the thalamus, which projects upon the primary auditory cortex of the temporal lobe.

Taste. As described earlier, information about taste enters the brain stem through three cranial nerves: the facial, the glossopharyngeal, and the vagus. Fibers in each of these nerves innervate taste buds and have their cell bodies in sensory ganglia outside the brain stem. The central branches of these cells terminate in the *solitary nucleus* (Figure 20–7B, 3) of the brain stem. Cells in this nucleus send axons through the brain stem to the medial portion of the ventral posterior nucleus of the thalamus. Fibers from this nucleus project to the insular region of the cerebral cortex.

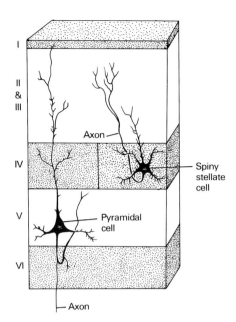

20–11 Cortical neurons are generally classified as pyramidal or stellate. Pyramidal cells are the major output neurons, but they also have axonal branches that terminate in the local area. The axons of most stellate cells terminate locally. Each layer of the cerebral cortex, with the exception of layer I, contains both stellate and pyramidal cells, but the proportions of these cells vary from layer to layer.

Smell. Primary sensory neurons in the olfactory mucosa send their axons to the olfactory bulb, which projects directly to the olfactory region of the entorhinal cortex. This phylogenetically older part of the cortex projects to the mediodorsal nucleus of the thalamus, which, in turn, projects upon the frontal lobe.

The Cerebral Cortex Consists of Layers of Neurons

The cerebral cortex is a sheet of cells that ranges from 2 to 4 mm in thickness and is folded into gyri and sulci. This folding is necessary to accommodate the large surface area of the cortex within the confines of the skull. If the cortex were not folded but spread out and flattened, it would occupy approximately 2.5 ft^2, an area about the size of a chess board.

The cortex that is visible when the brain is viewed from the outside is called *neocortex* because it is the brain's most recent evolutionary addition. The neocortex is by far the largest component of the cerebral hemispheres in the human brain and includes the four lobes described in Chapter 19. In addition to the neocortex, there are other, more primitive regions of the cortex, called the *allocortex* (Greek, *allos*, other), which arose early during vertebrate evolution. These areas lie deep within the temporal lobe near the zone where olfactory input first reaches the cerebral cortex.

The cerebral cortex is important for sensation, motor coordination, and higher cognitive functions, and many chapters in this book describe various aspects of this role. We shall limit our discussion here to the cellular anatomy of the cortex because, as we shall see in later chapters, great strides have been made in relating the cellular architecture of this region to behavior. The most striking morphological feature of the neocortex is that its cells are arranged in several well-defined layers. These layers are oriented in sheets that run parallel to the surface of the brain.

The Two Main Varieties of Cortical Neurons Are Pyramidal and Stellate Cells

The cell bodies of cortical neurons have a variety of shapes, but in general they can be distinguished as conforming to two main classes: *pyramidal cells* and *stellate cells* (Figure 20–11), each of which can be subclassified into several varieties on the basis of the dendritic branching pattern alone. However, the distinctions based solely on the configurations of cell bodies and dendrites are not rigid, and the differences between cell types are occasionally very subtle.

Pyramidal cells have a conical body, and the apex of the cone usually points toward the pial surface of the brain (Figure 20–11). A dendrite, which may be 500 μm or more in length, arises from the apex of the cell body and runs toward the pial surface, intersecting the overlying layers at roughly right angles. From the base of the pyramid, which may be 30 μm across, a number of basal dendrites branch off and course laterally within the layer containing the cell body. Stellate cells have round bodies that are smaller than those of pyramidal cells, seldom measuring more than 10 μm in diameter; dendrites arise from all aspects of the cell body, giving it a star-shaped appearance (Figure 20–11).

These two cell types can be usually distinguished on the basis of one significant feature: the distribution of their axonal branches. The axon of the pyramidal cell does not stay confined to the local cortical region; rather, it gives off several collateral branches that terminate nearby and then enters the white matter, running for some distance to terminate in another cortical area or in a more distant site in the central nervous system. In contrast, axons of stellate cells branch profusely in the cortical layers near the cell body and, with rare exception, do not leave the local cortical region. On these structural grounds, pyramidal cells seem designed to influence local processing through collateral branches and to carry the output of a cortical area, whereas stellate cells seem to be primarily involved in local intracortical processing of afferent inputs. Individual layers of the cortex do not contain equal ratios of stellate and pyramidal cells, and the predominant cell type in a layer provides an important clue about the functional role of that layer. For example, layers rich in pyramidal cells are predominantly output layers, and those rich in stellate cells are the principal sites of termination for thalamic and other afferent inputs.

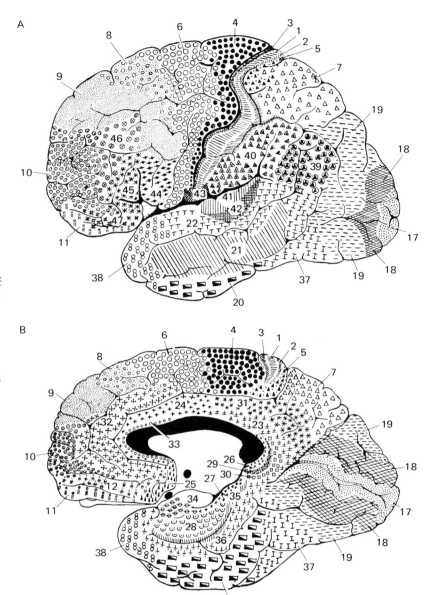

20–12 Brodmann divided the human cerebral cortex into discrete cytoarchitectonic areas. **A.** Lateral view. **B.** Medial view. Each symbol represents a distinct area, numbered as shown. Area 4, the motor cortex, occupies most of the precentral gyrus. The postcentral gyrus, where the primary somatic sensory cortex is found, is divided into areas 3, 1, and 2, each of which is organized differently. The primary visual cortex is area 17, and the primary auditory cortex is composed of areas 41 and 42. The prefrontal association cortex and the parietal–temporal–occipital association cortex are also composed of a number of distinct cytoarchitectonic areas.

The Pattern of Layering Varies in Different Cortical Areas

In the neocortex, it is usually possible to recognize six layers, numbered successively from the pial surface to the underlying white matter (Figure 20–11). Layer I, the most superficial layer, contains only a few neuronal cell bodies. It is made up largely of glial cells (similar to those found in all cortical layers) and of axonal processes running parallel to the pial surface that synapse on apical dendrites of cells lying in deeper layers and presumably interconnecting local cortical areas. In contrast, layer II is densely cellular, containing mostly small pyramidal cells. Layer III is composed primarily of somewhat larger pyramidal cells. Layers II and III provide the output that goes to other cortical regions. Layer IV is rich in stellate cells and is the layer that receives most of the afferent input from the thalamus. Layer V has the largest pyra-

midal cells; they give rise to the long descending pathways that leave the cortex and run to the corpus striatum, the brain stem, and the spinal cord. Layer VI is composed of neurons that project back to the thalamus. Just below layer VI is the white matter that carries axons to and from the cortex.

Each cortical region has a characteristic layering pattern that usually results from subdivisions and expansions of one or more of these layers and thinning of others. Nevertheless, two simple rules prevail: First, in primary sensory areas there is a large thalamic input; consequently, layer IV is usually expanded in these areas because it contains the stellate cells that are important for the initial stages of input processing. For example, in the primary visual cortex, layer IV is so thick that it can readily be subdivided into three distinct sublayers: IVa, IVb, and IVc. Second, in motor areas that give rise to long descending pathways, layer V, with its large pyramidal cells, is prominent and layer IV is much reduced in size. The association cortex has a layering pattern that is somewhat intermediate between that of the sensory and motor cortices.

Although these general principles apply to all areas of the cortex, each area has a slightly different layering pattern. This diversity was shown most clearly at the turn of the century by Korbinian Brodmann, who examined the organization of the cells and fibers in the cortex using the Nissl stain to recognize cell bodies and myelin stains for axons. On the basis of these studies, Brodmann divided the human cerebral cortex into 52 unique cytoarchitectonic areas according to the sizes of cells, their packing density, the number of layers in each region, and the density of myelinated axons. Figure 20–12 is a map of Brodmann's subdivisions that shows the relative contribution of the major cortical areas to the total cortical surface. Brodmann assigned a number to each structural area, but most of these numbers are not related to one another in a systematic way. He correctly identified the boundaries of the primary motor and sensory areas. For example, the primary visual cortex, the area that receives direct input from the lateral geniculate nucleus, corresponds exactly to Brodmann's area 17. He also suggested that there are many separate functional zones within the association areas. Recent research has shown that there are, in fact, more functional zones in the association cortex than even Brodmann anticipated.

The Descending Motor Systems Interconnect the Cortex, Basal Ganglia, and Thalamus

Now that we have examined the general organization of the brain stem, diencephalon, and cerebral hemispheres, it will be easier to understand the organization of the motor systems and pathways associated with them. The motor cortex of the frontal lobe is precisely organized so that particular regions influence the activity of specific muscle groups in the periphery, just as each region of the somatic sensory cortex is related to specific portions of the sensory periphery (Chapter 1). The activity of the motor cortex is influenced by input from sensory systems as well as by information about ongoing movement from other areas of the brain, such as the cerebellum and the basal ganglia; this information is important for the smooth performance of coordinated motor acts. Many motor acts also require tactile information about the position of an object in one's hand, visual cues, and proprioceptive information about the body's posture. Small wonder, then, that voluntary acts require many components of the motor systems, including reflex components, to work as a unit.

The anatomical connections underlying motor behavior involve both direct and indirect pathways from the motor cortex to the motor neurons of the ventral horn of the spinal cord. The motor cortex gives rise to a pathway that directly influences the motor neurons controlling muscles of the distal extremities. The red nucleus, a prominent structure in the midbrain (Figure 20–7B, 1), also gives rise to a pathway that controls the distal extremities, but this pathway is probably indirect. Also indirect is the pathway from the reticular formation that controls proximal and axial muscles.

In the sections that follow, we shall consider the pathways taken by a motor command from the cortex to the spinal cord and illustrate the various additional brain regions involved in a voluntary movement. Of these regions, the cerebellum and the basal ganglia are especially interesting. Unlike the motor cortex, the cerebellum and the basal ganglia do not project directly to the spinal cord, but exert their control over movement through the thalamic pathway to the motor cortex. Thus, the cerebellum and basal ganglia do not participate directly in the mediation of movement, but modulate movement initiated by other structures of the motor system.

The Cerebellum Is Important in Regulating the Automatic Control of Movement

As we have seen, even a simple motor act requires sensory inputs from the somatic sensory and visual systems, as well as feedback from both the spinal cord and the periphery. The cerebellum is critical for coordinating this sensory and motor information. To accomplish this coordination, the cerebellum and the cerebral hemispheres work in constant collaboration during motor acts through massive reciprocal pathways. Lesions of the cerebellum disrupt the ability to measure the precise trajectory of movements, a class of disorders called *dysmetrias*. In animal studies it has been shown that cerebellar lesions can disrupt simple learned motor actions.

The cerebellum, like the cerebral hemisphere, has an outer cortex, underlying white matter, and deep nuclei. Afferent and efferent fibers run to and from the cerebellar cortex by coursing through one of three large fiber bundles, the *cerebellar peduncles*. These peduncles, named the inferior, middle, and superior, are visible in the dorsolateral aspect of the brain stem on each side (Figure 20–7A). Most of the afferent fibers to the cerebellum run in the inferior and middle peduncles; most of the efferent fibers leave the cerebellum through the superior peduncle.

The *inferior peduncle* conveys the dorsal spinocerebellar tract to the cerebellar cortex. This pathway carries afferent input about ongoing movement. The *middle cerebellar peduncle* conveys axons from the pontine nuclei to the cerebellar cortex. The connections from the pons provide the cerebellar cortex with information from a wide variety of peripheral receptors, including visual receptors, as well as inputs from the motor and premotor areas of the cerebral cortex.

Some branches of the afferent fibers that enter the cerebellum excite neurons in the deep cerebellar nuclei—clusters of cell bodies lying within the white matter of the cerebellum. The deep cerebellar nuclei are the principal output centers of the cerebellum as a whole. Other branches of the afferent fibers terminate on cells in the cerebellar cortex. Afferent excitation in the cerebellar cortex travels through several local synaptic relays and eventually excites the major output neurons of the cor-

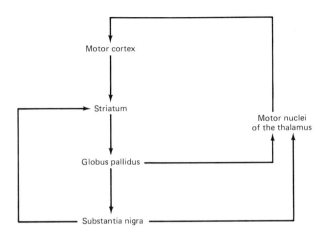

20–13 Pathways interconnect the motor components of the basal ganglia, the thalamus, and the cerebral cortex. The connections of the subthalamic nucleus, individual thalamic motor nuclei, and descending connections of the substantia nigra are discussed in Chapter 40.

tex, the Purkinje cells. The Purkinje cells send their axons to the deep cerebellar nuclei and exert an inhibitory action on these output centers. As a result, an initial burst of excitation in the deep cerebellar nuclei is followed by inhibition delivered by the Purkinje cells—an arrangement that endows the cerebellum with its ability to serve as a precise timing device.

The *superior cerebellar peduncle* is the major output pathway from the cerebellum. Through it the deep cerebellar nuclei establish connections with relays in the thalamus and the brain stem. In the thalamus, axons from the deep cerebellar nuclei terminate in the ventral lateral nucleus. This relay allows for cerebellar control of the activity of cells in the motor cortex, since the principal cells of the ventral lateral nucleus run through the internal capsule to terminate in the precentral gyrus and other motor areas. The most important projection of the

cerebellum to the brain stem runs to the red nucleus in the midbrain. The axons of the cells of the red nucleus give rise to the rubrospinal tract, which crosses the midline and descends to the spinal cord, serving as a relatively direct link between the cerebellum and the cord. By means of its output projections to the thalamus and motor cortex and to the red nucleus, the cerebellum regulates the timing necessary to generate the complex patterns of muscle activation required by any behavioral act. Moreover, it does so not through direct links with the motor neurons, but rather by acting on pathways from the motor cortex and the red nucleus (as well as pathways from the premotor cortex and from the reticular formation) that in turn project to the motor neurons. As we shall see below, the cerebellar control of motor function is in many ways analogous to the control of motor function exerted by the basal ganglia, the large masses of gray matter within the cerebral hemispheres.

The Basal Ganglia Project to the Motor Cortex via the Thalamus

The basal ganglia influence the activity of the motor cortex through connections mediated by the motor areas of the thalamus. The major components of the basal ganglia are three large subcortical nuclei: the *caudate nucleus* (Latin, tail-shaped, because it arcs into the temporal lobe), the *putamen* (Latin, shell), and the *globus pallidus* (Latin, pale body). The caudate nucleus and putamen are collectively called the *striatum* and constitute the input components of the basal ganglia. They receive input from the entire neocortex, including the association areas and the primary sensory areas, as well as from the substantia nigra in the midbrain (Figure 20–7B, 1). The cells of the caudate and putamen send their axons to the globus pallidus, the output component of the basal ganglia, *which projects back to the motor and premotor cortex by way of the ventral anterior nucleus of the*

20–14 The motor cortex receives input from many sources both directly and indirectly via the premotor cortex and thalamus. The association cortices (the prefrontal association cortex and the parietal–temporal–occipital association cortex) feed into the premotor cortex (Brodmann's area 6), which in turn projects to the primary motor cortex. The thalamus projects directly to the motor cortex as well as to the premotor cortex. The primary somatic sensory cortex also has direct connections with the motor cortex.

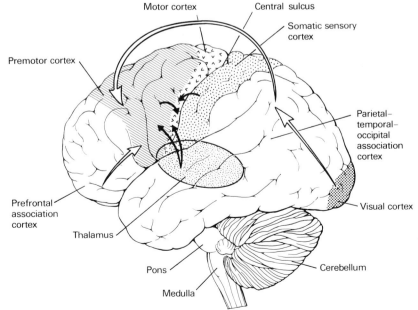

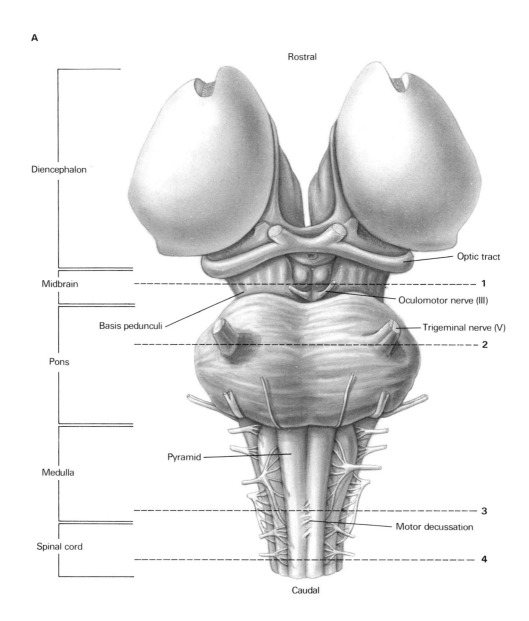

A

Rostral

Diencephalon

Optic tract

Midbrain

Oculomotor nerve (III)

1

Basis pedunculi

Trigeminal nerve (V)

2

Pons

Medulla

Pyramid

3

Motor decussation

Spinal cord

4

Caudal

thalamus (Figure 20–13). These recurrent inputs to the motor cortex, mediated by inputs from the basal ganglia to the ventral anterior nucleus, keep the motor cortex constantly updated about the performance of motor commands.

The basal ganglia are also thought to have a role in the initial generation of commands for movement. One of the characteristics of Parkinson's disease, a disorder of the basal ganglia, is difficulty in beginning movements *(akinesia)*. The basal ganglia are also functionally related to the subthalamic nucleus, but the role of this connection is not as clearly understood as other aspects of basal ganglia function. Lesions in the subthalamus cause sudden erratic movements of the limbs, termed *ballism*. The anatomical relationships between the basal ganglia, the

thalamus, and the cerebral hemispheres will be discussed in the next chapter.

Various Inputs Converge on the Motor Cortex

Three factors contribute to the central role played by the motor cortex in the execution of voluntary movement: (1) The cascade of sensory information, from primary cortical areas through association and premotor areas, provides a pathway to the motor cortex that integrates sensation with action (Figure 20–14). Both the parietal–temporal–occipital cortex and the prefrontal cortex connect to the premotor cortex (Brodmann's area 6), which lies anterior to the primary motor area. The premotor area, in turn, projects largely to the primary motor cor-

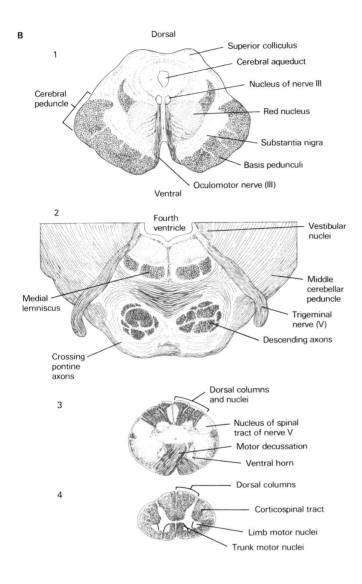

B

1

Dorsal

Superior colliculus

Cerebral aqueduct

Nucleus of nerve III

Cerebral peduncle

Red nucleus

Substantia nigra

Basis pedunculi

Oculomotor nerve (III)

Ventral

2

Fourth ventricle

Vestibular nuclei

Medial lemniscus

Middle cerebellar peduncle

Trigeminal nerve (V)

Descending axons

Crossing pontine axons

3

Dorsal columns and nuclei

Nucleus of spinal tract of nerve V

Motor decussation

Ventral horn

4

Dorsal columns

Corticospinal tract

Limb motor nuclei

Trunk motor nuclei

20–15 The course of cortical fibers descending through the brain stem to form the corticospinal tract is shown in relation to various other structures at four levels. **A.** View of the ventral surface of the brain stem. Descending cortical fibers run through the basis pedunculi at the level of the midbrain, through the pons, and into the pyramids of the medulla. The fibers that form the corticospinal tract cross the midline in the motor decussation. **B.** Transverse sections through the brain stem and spinal cord at the levels indicated in **A**. **1:** Section through the midbrain. Descending corticospinal axons run into the basis pedunculi from the internal capsule. **2:** Section through the pons. The corticopontine axons terminate in the pontine nuclei upon neurons that send their axons to the cerebellar cortex. Other descending axons continue through the pons to the medulla. Corticobulbar axons leave the group of descending axons and terminate on the motor nuclei of the cranial nerves in the brain stem. These axons mediate voluntary control of muscles in the head and neck. **3:** Section through the lower medulla. Descending axons that make up the lateral corticospinal tract cross at this level. **4:** Section through the spinal cord. These axons run in the lateral columns of the white matter and terminate upon the motor neurons of the ventral horn.

tex, thereby connecting the motor cortex with areas of the brain concerned with perception and decision making. (2) Input from the cerebellum and basal ganglia, the brain regions that ensure effective and smooth motor performance, influences the motor cortex through thalamic relays. (3) Many neurons in the motor cortex project directly upon motor neurons.

The Corticospinal Tract Is a Direct Pathway from the Cortex to the Spinal Cord

The efferent fibers that mediate motor commands leave the motor cortex and take several pathways. These separate pathways arise from neurons with cell bodies in different cortical layers—another reflection of the principle

that *cortical layers segregate cells with different patterns of connectivity.* The cells of layer VI send axons to the motor nuclei of the thalamus; the information they carry presumably regulates the flow of input to the motor cortex, in a manner similar to the recurrent control of input by the sensory cortical areas. Neurons in layer V give rise to long axons that descend to the spinal cord as the corticospinal tract. This tract is a direct pathway to the spinal cord, and we shall follow its entire course.

The corticospinal tract contains axons from several cortical areas, but the fibers that concern us come from the motor cortex of the precentral gyrus and synapse directly on the motor neurons of the spinal cord. These axons leave the local cortical area, enter the white matter, and run into the internal capsule (Figure 20–15).

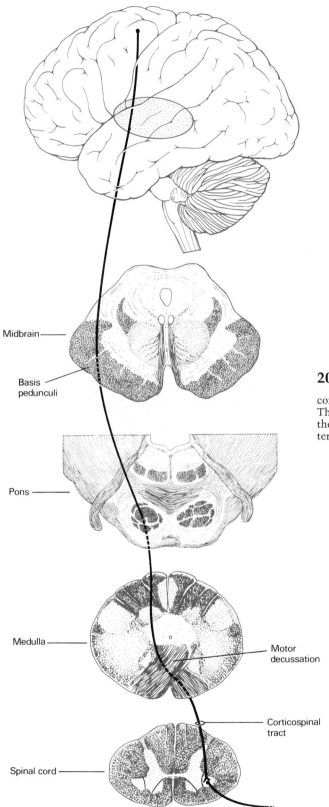

Midbrain

Basis
pedunculi

Pons

Medulla

Motor
decussation

Corticospinal
tract

Spinal cord

20–16 Summary of the origin and course of corticobulbar axons and the corticospinal tract. Only the component that takes origin from the motor cortex is shown. The tract descends through the basis pedunculi and crosses at the base of the medulla to reach the spinal cord, where it terminates directly upon motor neurons.

The descending corticospinal fibers run through the internal capsule and join the cerebral peduncle, the fiber bundle that forms the inferior portion of the midbrain (Figure 20–15B, 1). Cortical fibers that are destined for the red nucleus exit from the cerebral peduncle at this point. In addition to receiving an input from the motor cortex, the red nucleus receives a strong connection from the cerebellum directly, as described earlier. The corticospinal tract, which accounts for about 5% of the fibers in the cerebral peduncle, is surrounded on either side by *corticopontine* and *corticobulbar fibers*. The corticopontine fibers terminate in the pons. The remaining fibers from the cerebral peduncle descend into the medullary pyramids (Figure 20–15A). As the pyramid runs along the ventral aspect of the medulla, the corticobulbar fibers (so named because the bulb was an archaic term for the medulla) leave it and synapse with cranial nerve nuclei that innervate the muscles of the head and neck. Other axons leave the pyramids and terminate in the reticular formation on medullary nuclei that make descending connections in the spinal cord. These connections influence the activity of the spinal neurons concerned with the control of body posture. Unlike the corticobulbar and corticoreticular fibers, the corticospinal fibers continue directly into the spinal cord.

In our discussion of the ascending sensory system, we found that each hemisphere is concerned with sensory events on the opposite side of the body. Similarly, the corticospinal tract from each hemisphere is concerned with motor events on the opposite side of the body. Thus, at some point the corticospinal tract must cross the midline so that its fibers can contact motor neurons innervating muscles on the opposite side of the body. The corticospinal tract decussates just after it passes below the dorsal column nuclei in the medulla (Figures 20–15A and B, 3). In the decussation, about 90% of the corticospinal axons (900,000 fibers) cross the midline to reach the lateral column of the spinal cord, where they descend to the appropriate level. The remaining 10% continue on the same side until they reach the appropriate levels of spinal cord, where they too eventually cross (Figure 20–15B, 3).

The corticospinal tract is primarily concerned with regulating distal muscles that are important for precise movements, such as those of the hand. Corticospinal axons do not terminate diffusely; they end in an organized manner on groups of motor neurons or motor nuclei that innervate specific muscles. The entire course of the corticospinal tract is summarized in Figure 20–16. Other motor pathways are concerned with gross postural adjustments that occur during a behavioral act, as well as with the modification of local spinal reflexes. One of these is the *reticulospinal pathway*, which terminates upon motor neurons and interneurons that regulate the activity of trunk musculature. For an effective motor act, all the components of the motor system must work in harmony from the highest levels of the cerebrum (the cerebral cortex and the basal ganglia) to the final output at the level of the motor neurons innervating proximal and distal muscles.

The Motivational Systems Include Connections between the Limbic System and the Hypothalamus

How do emotional factors affect sensation or the performance of a motor act? The exact pathways that control the emotional quality of sensation or motor behavior are not understood completely, but one important set of connections is thought to involve the limbic system and the autonomic nervous system.

The term *limbic system* (Latin, girdle or belt) was originally used to designate several structures that encircle or border the corpus callosum and the brain stem and were thought to function as a unit to control emotion. The hippocampus of the temporal lobe, and the cingulate gyrus, which overlies the corpus callosum, are components of the limbic system; this anatomy will be described in the next chapter. Some authorities also include the hypothalamus and part of the prefrontal association cortex in the limbic system because of the extensive interconnections between these structures. By means of direct connection with the hypothalamus, the limbic system is involved in the control of the autonomic nervous system of the brain and spinal cord, which mediates the interaction between emotion and visceral function and allows for the coordination of visceral responses (such as blood pressure, heart rate, and pupillary size) with motivational state. In addition to its involvement in motivation, the limbic system influences all of the endocrine systems of the body by controlling the release of hypothalamic hormones. Finally, the hippocampal formation is important in the retention of memory.

An Overall View

While tracing the major brain pathways described in this chapter, we have seen how each pathway is wired with great specificity throughout the major structures of the spinal cord and brain. In the chapters that follow, the various regions of the nervous system encountered here will be considered again in greater detail and in the context of the behavioral functions in which they participate. Even at this early point, however, it is easy to appreciate that the brain is a marvelously complex machine, an evolutionary biological achievement that has as its foundation the specificity of connections between neurons.

Selected Readings

Brodal, A. 1981. Neurological Anatomy In Relation to Clinical Medicine, 3rd ed. New York: Oxford University Press.

References

Brodmann, K. 1909. Vergleichende Lokalisationslehre der Grosshirnrinde in ihren Prinzipien dargestellt auf Grund des Zellenbaues. Leipzig: Barth.

Nieuwenhuys, R., Voogd, J., and van Huijzen, Chr. 1981. The Human Central Nervous System, A Synopsis and Atlas. Berlin: Springer.

John H. Martin

Development as a Guide to the Regional Anatomy of the Brain

21

The central nervous system is organized into different functional systems that course through the major divisions of the brain, and even an apparently simple motor task, such as catching a ball, requires the combined effort of several systems. Because of rearrangements that have occurred throughout evolution and others that occur during development, structures belonging to unrelated systems often come to lie next to one another. As a result, insults to the nervous system that cause regional damage (trauma, a tumor, or a vascular disturbance) affect all the functional systems within a given area indiscriminately. The behavioral consequences of regional insults are therefore usually not restricted to any one functional system. To understand the consequences of this kind of damage to the nervous system, we need to learn the spatial relationships that exist between neighboring structures. Fortunately, this task has been greatly facilitated by modern imaging techniques that allow regional anatomy to be visualized in the living brain (Chapter 22).

As we saw in the previous two chapters, the functional systems of the brain are organized according to a precise logic. In contrast, the brain's regional anatomy and its subdivision into six regions—the spinal cord, medulla, pons and cerebellum, midbrain, diencephalon, and cerebral hemispheres—may seem arbitrary and forbiddingly complicated in their details. There is, however, also a logic to this aspect of brain anatomy, a logic that becomes clearer when we understand how the brain develops. In this chapter, therefore, we shall consider aspects of the development of the brain that aid in clarifying its regional anatomy. In Chapter 55 we shall return to the principles underlying the development of the nervous system on the cellular level.

The Neural Tube and Its Vesicles Are the Embryonic Precursors of the Various Brain Regions

There are three principal layers of cells in the human embryo: *endoderm*, the innermost layer; *mesoderm*, the middle layer; and *ectoderm*, the outermost layer. Nerve and glial cells of the central nervous system derive from a specialized region of the ectoderm, the *neural plate*, which lies along the dorsal midline of the embryo (Figure 21–1A). This region of ectoderm becomes committed to the formation of the nervous system by a process called *neural induction*. As we shall see in Chapter 55, the molecular mechanisms responsible for neural induction remain elusive but involve the action of molecules (inducing or triggering substances) on the ectoderm that are released from a specific part of the mesoderm, the *notochord*. The notochord survives in the adult vertebral column as the intervertebral disks.

Early in development the neural plate undergoes an indentation that deepens gradually and closes to form a hollow structure called the *neural tube* (Figure 21–1B through D). The mechanism by which the lips of the neural groove close is thought to involve cell-to-cell recognition by means of specific membrane glycoproteins located on the surface of the developing cells of the neural plate at the edge of each lip. Occasionally the neural plate fails to close completely during development. When the caudal portion of the neural tube fails to close, a crippling developmental abnormality known as *spina bifida* (Latin, cleft spine) results. In this condition the functions subserved by the lumbar and sacral spinal cord are disrupted. When closure fails at rostral levels, a condition known as *anencephaly* occurs, in which the overall structure of the brain is grossly disturbed.

The cavity of the neural tube gives rise to the ventricular system of the central nervous system. The epithelial cells that line the walls of the neural tube generate virtually all the neurons and glial cells of the central nervous system. The epithelial cells lining the neural tube are therefore called the *neuroepithelium*. The axons of the spinal and cranial motor neurons and of the preganglionic autonomic neurons spin out from the cell body and grow into the periphery. Despite the peripheral course of their axons, these neurons also arise from the cells of the neural tube. Only the nerve cells of the peripheral nervous system, whose *cell bodies* actually lie outside of the spinal cord (the dorsal root ganglion cells and the postganglionic neurons of the autonomic nervous system), originate from the *neural crest*, a population of cells originally located at the lateral margins of the neural plate.

The cells of the neuroepithelium divide repeatedly and, following a strictly programmed sequence, differentiate into both the neurons and the glial cells of the central nervous system. However, the precursors of nerve cells, called *neuroblasts*, do not proliferate uniformly along the length of the neural tube; rather, different regions within the neuroepithelium enlarge differentially

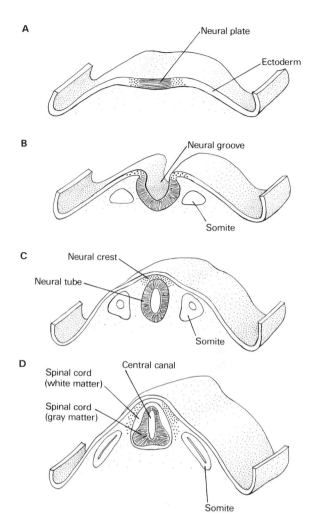

21–1 The neural tube is formed from the ectoderm of the embryo during the third and fourth weeks following conception; its development is shown in sections through the dorsal surface of the embryo. **A.** Neural plate is activated by neural induction. **B.** Neural groove forms. **C.** Opposing lips of neural groove close to form neural tube and neural crest develops. **D.** The spinal cord (and other structures of the central nervous system) begins to develop in the neural tube. (Adapted from Cowan, 1979.)

to give rise to the six functionally distinct parts of the adult central nervous system.

In the *caudal part* of the neural tube the cells proliferate to form the spinal cord (Figure 21–2A), which contains the motor neurons and many of the second-order neurons that receive somatic sensory information from the legs, arms, and trunk. In the *rostral part* of the neural tube the proliferation of cells is more complex and ultimately affects the orientation of the *neuraxis*, the longitudinal axis of the central nervous system. Initially, the rostral neural tube forms three vesicles called the *forebrain*, the *midbrain*, and the *hindbrain* (Figure 21–2A).

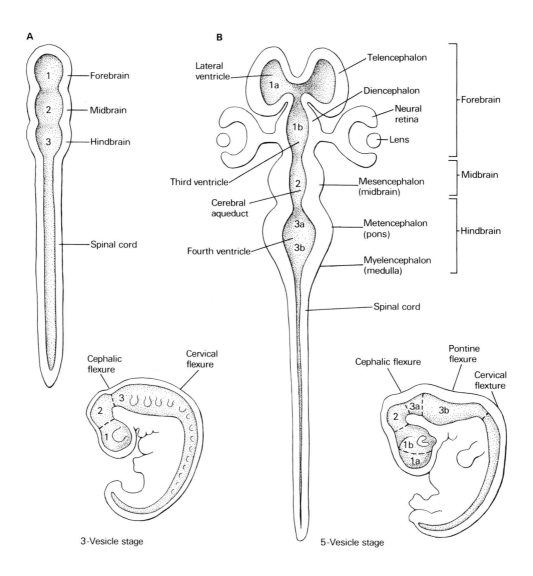

21–2 The neural tube forms the spinal cord and the brain vesicles. In early development, there are only three vesicles; later, two additional vesicles form. The vesicles at these two stages are illustrated in a dorsal straightened-out view of the neural tube, and the flexures are illustrated in a side view. **A.** Three-vesicle stage. **B.** Five-vesicle stage.

At this early stage in development (the three-vesicle stage) the brain undergoes two prominent flexures: the *cervical flexure* occurs at the junction of the spinal cord and hindbrain; the *cephalic flexure* occurs at the junction of the hindbrain and midbrain. A third flexure, called the *pontine flexure,* forms somewhat later in development (Figure 21–2B). Both the cervical and pontine flexures become much less pronounced later in development and tend to straighten out. The cephalic flexure remains prominent and thereby causes the adult forebrain to have a different longitudinal axis from the brain stem and spinal cord. Because of this bend in the neuraxis, an anatomical slice through the cerebral hemispheres that is perpendicular to the neuraxis, called a *transverse* or *cross section,* becomes a *longitudinal section* through the brain stem and spinal cord. (Figure 19–1 in Chapter 19 shows how this change of axis affects the terminology used to describe the spatial relationships in the adult human brain.)

Next, two of the three primary embryonic vesicles, the forebrain and hindbrain, each give rise to an additional subdivision (Figure 21–2B), creating the five basic regions of the brain that, together with the spinal cord, make up the six regions of the adult central nervous system. Two structures emerge from the primitive forebrain: (1) the *telencephalon* (or end-brain), which gives rise to the cerebral cortex and the basal ganglia, the two major constituents of the cerebral hemispheres; and (2) the *diencephalon* (or between-brain), lying between the hemispheres and composed principally of the thalamus and hypothalamus. (3) The *mesencephalon* (or midbrain) remains undivided. The hindbrain gives rise to (4) the *metencephalon* (or afterbrain), consisting of the *pons* and *cerebellum*; and (5) the *myelencephalon* or *medulla*. The caudal part of the neural tube remains undivided and becomes (6) the *spinal cord*. The diencephalon, basal ganglia, and cerebral cortex eventually develop more extensively than the more caudal portions of the central nervous system. The cerebral hemispheres proliferate and ultimately grow to cover most of the diencephalon and midbrain. A second region of growth occurs in the dorsal aspect of the metencephalon (the rostral part of the hindbrain); this becomes the cerebellum (Table 21–1).

Early in development the brain and spinal cord become covered by three distinct membranes collectively called the *meninges* (Greek, *meninx*, covering). The meninges consist of the dura mater, the arachnoid mater, and the pia mater (Figure 21–3). The *dura mater* (Latin, hard mother, implying a protective function) is the thickest and most external of these membranes. The *arachnoid mater* (Greek, *arachne*, spider) adjoins but is not tightly bound to the dura mater, thus allowing a potential space to exist between them. This potential space, called the *subdural space*, is important clinically. The dura mater is vascularized; breakage of one of its vessels can lead to subdural bleeding and to the formation of a blood clot (a *subdural hematoma*). In this condition the blood clot pushes the arachnoid away from the dura mater, fills the subdural space, and compresses the underlying neural tissue. Running through the *subarachnoid space*, an actual space, are filaments of arachnoid mater that give this space the appearance of a spider's web. These filaments connect to the innermost meningeal layer, the *pia mater* (Latin, soft mother), which is very

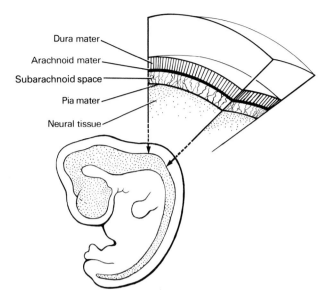

21–3 The central nervous system is covered by three meningeal layers. The dura mater is the thickest and most external. Because it is so tough it is thought to function to protect the central nervous system. The arachnoid mater is internal to the dura. The most internal layer is the pia mater, which tightly adheres to the surface of the brain and spinal cord.

fine and adheres to the surface of the brain and spinal cord. As we shall see later, the subarachnoid space is filled with cerebrospinal fluid. Much of this fluid is produced by an intraventricular structure called the *choroid plexus*; cerebrospinal fluid is derived from blood plasma but differs from plasma in its ionic composition.

Table 21–1. The Main Subdivisions of the Embryonic Central Nervous System and Their Adult Forms

Early three-vesicle stage	Later five-vesicle stage	Major adult derivatives	Related cavity
	1a. End-brain (telencephalon)	1. Cerebral cortex, basal ganglia, olfactory bulb	Lateral ventricles
1. Forebrain (prosencephalon)	1b. Between-brain (diencephalon)	2. Thalamus, hypothalamus, subthalamus, epithalamus, retinae, optic nerves and tracts	Third ventricle
2. Midbrain (mesencephalon)	2. Midbrain (mesencephalon)	3. Midbrain	Cerebral aqueduct
3. Hindbrain (rhombencephalon)	3a. Afterbrain (metencephalon)	4. Pons and cerebellum	Fourth ventricle
	3b. Medullary brain (myelencephalon)	5. Medulla oblongata	
4. Caudal part of neural tube (spinal cord)	4. Caudal part of neural tube (spinal cord)	6. Spinal cord	Central canal

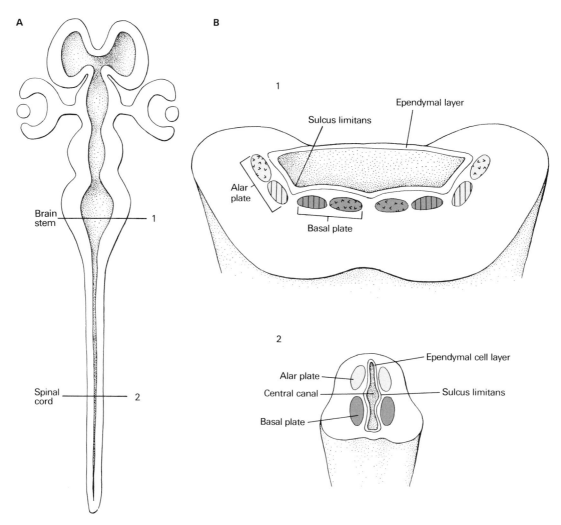

21–4 The spinal cord and brain stem share a similar developmental plan. During the development of each, there is a region that serves sensory functions (termed the alar plate) and a motor region (the basal plate). In the spinal cord the alar plate is dorsal to the basal plate. In the brain stem the alar plate is lateral to the basal plate. **A.** Dorsal view of neural tube. **B.** Schematic transverse sections of brain stem (**1**) and spinal cord (**2**) located at corresponding numbers in **A.**

The Spinal Cord and Brain Stem Have a Similar Developmental Plan

Even at an early stage of development, the primitive spinal cord is similar in organization to the adult form and is easy to understand. In the developing spinal cord there are two zones of proliferating cells in the dorsal and ventral portions of the wall of the neural tube, called the *alar plate* (Latin, *ala*, wing) and the *basal plate* (Figure 21–4A and B, 2). These plates are organized as longitudinally oriented columns of cells and are separated by a shallow groove, the *sulcus limitans*. Neuroblasts from the alar plate become projection neurons and interneurons of the dorsal horn that mediate body sensations such as touch and pain. Some neuroblasts from the basal plate differentiate into the motor neurons and interneurons of the ventral horn. Others differentiate into preganglionic autonomic neurons. Autonomic neurons that derive from

precursor cells of the developing thoracic and lumbar spinal segments become the *sympathetic division*, whereas those from the sacral spinal cord (and brain stem) become part of the *parasympathetic division*.

During development, there is surprisingly little change in the internal organization of the spinal cord. The spinal cord remains divided into a dorsal sensory region and a ventral motor region. Neurons mediating sensation or motor control become organized into cell columns (or thin sheets for some sensory neurons) that run in the rostrocaudal direction of the spinal cord. The major change in the morphology of the spinal cord is reflected in its length in relation to the length of the vertebral canal, the space within the vertebral column. Early in development the spinal cord fills the vertebral canal (Figure 21–5A). As development progresses, the vertebral column lengthens more than the spinal cord so that an increasingly smaller portion of the vertebral canal is oc-

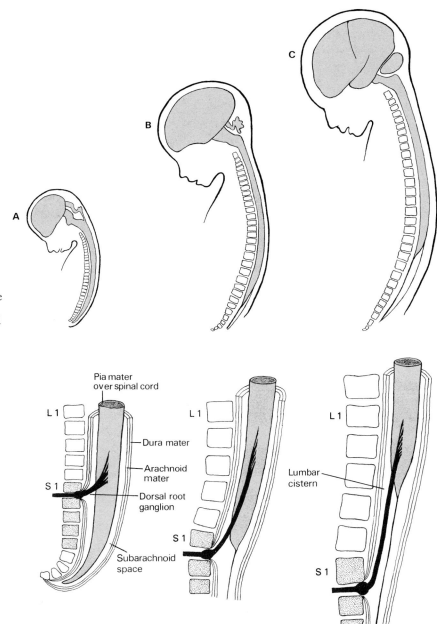

21–5 The lumbar cistern forms because the vertebral column grows in length more than the spinal cord. A side view and the detailed organization of the lumbosacral spinal cord and vertebral column are shown at three stages of development: **A.** Fetus at 3 months. **B.** Fetus at the end of 5 months. **C.** Newborn. (Adapted from Pansky, 1982.)

cupied by the spinal cord (Figure 21–5B). At birth the caudal end of the spinal cord lies at the level of the third lumbar vertebra (Figure 21–5C), and in the adult, the spinal cord extends only to the caudal margin of the first lumbar vertebra. The dorsal (or sensory) and ventral (or motor) spinal rootlets related to the lumbar and sacral segments must therefore travel a long way within the vertebral canal before they join the spinal cord (or after they leave it). These spinal rootlets are collectively called the *cauda equina* (Latin, horse's tail) and, together with the spinal cord, are wrapped in meningeal coverings.

The space around the cauda equina is part of the subarachnoid space, which surrounds the entire central nervous system. Cerebrospinal fluid accumulates here in the region called the *lumbar cistern* and can be sampled for clinical examination without risk of damaging the spinal cord. In this examination, cerebrospinal fluid is drawn by *spinal tap* or *lumbar puncture* from the space between the third and fourth lumbar vertebrae (Figure 21–6). The constituents of the cerebrospinal fluid are a sensitive indicator of some functions of the central nervous system. Infections of the central nervous system, neoplasm, or bleeding produce characteristic changes in the composition of the cerebrospinal fluid. For example, bleeding in the brain causes red blood cells to appear in the cerebrospinal fluid. Bacterial infections of the brain or the meninges cause white blood cells to appear in the cerebro-

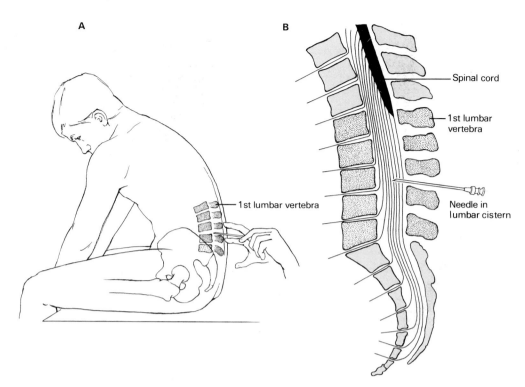

21–6 Cerebrospinal fluid is drawn from the lumbar cistern in a spinal tap. **A.** The needle is inserted into the subarachnoid space of the lumbar cistern. **B.** Schematic drawing of the caudal portion of the vertebral column and spinal cord.

The meninges have been omitted to better show the spinal rootlets in the lumbar cistern. Because the spinal cord ends rostral to the injection site, it remains undamaged during the spinal tap. (Adapted from House, Pansky, and Siegel, 1979.)

spinal fluid. Bacterial cultures of the cerebrospinal fluid may lead to isolation and identification of the offending organisms.

The brain stem is concerned with certain special senses, such as audition and taste, with control of muscles of the head and neck, and with aspects of the neural substrates of arousal and awareness. In addition, nuclei in the brain stem play a critical role in the regulation of the cardiovascular, gastrointestinal, and respiratory systems. The *caudal brain stem* follows a developmental plan that is much like that of the spinal cord (Figure 21–4A and B, 1). It too has an alar and basal plate separated by the sulcus limitans. Neuroblasts of the alar plate in the brain stem differentiate into sensory neurons that mediate taste, hearing, balance, visceral sensations, and somatic sensations from the face. Some neuroblasts of the basal plate differentiate to become the motor neurons for the muscles of the eyes, head, and neck; others become parasympathetic preganglionic neurons that give rise to the cranial autonomic outflow.

In the brain stem, as in the spinal cord, the sensory neurons in the alar plate and the motor neurons in the basal plate are organized into longitudinal cell columns (Figure 21–4B, 1). Here, neurons mediating sensation and motor control of the viscera are arranged in columns that are clearly separated from those for somatic sensation and innervation of somatic muscles. This further subdivision of the alar and basal plates in the brain stem into separate somatic and visceral cell columns is incomplete

in the spinal cord. In addition, the alar and basal plates of the brain stem, unlike their counterparts in the spinal cord, also give rise to some additional structures that are not strictly sensory or motor. For example, some neuroblasts of the basal plate differentiate into the cells of the reticular formation, important for arousal and attention.

The Cavities of the Brain Vesicles Are the Embryonic Precursors of the Ventricles

The tubular nature of the developing nervous system persists as the embryonic brain matures (Figure 21–7). The large cavities within the cerebral vesicles develop into the ventricular system of the brain, and the remaining caudal cavity becomes the central canal of the spinal cord. As the five vesicles develop, the cavity in the forebrain differentiates into the two *lateral ventricles* (formerly called the first and second ventricles) and the *third ventricle*. The rostral wall of the third ventricle is formed by the *lamina terminalis*, which, at an earlier developmental stage, represented the rostral end of the neural tube. An *interventricular foramen* (of Monro) interconnects each lateral ventricle and the third ventricle. The ventricles contain cerebrospinal fluid, which is produced by the choroid plexus present in each of them. Because the entire central nervous system is bathed by cerebrospinal fluid, the ventricles provide an important route for chemical communication between different brain regions.

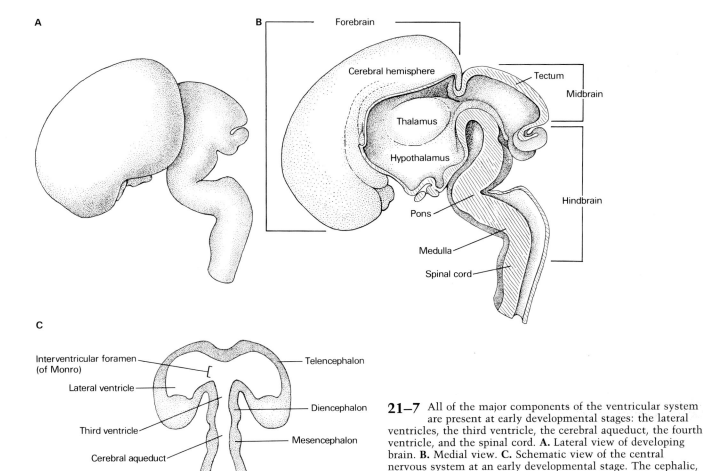

21—7 All of the major components of the ventricular system are present at early developmental stages: the lateral ventricles, the third ventricle, the cerebral aqueduct, the fourth ventricle, and the spinal cord. **A.** Lateral view of developing brain. **B.** Medial view. **C.** Schematic view of the central nervous system at an early developmental stage. The cephalic, pontine, and cervical flexures have been straightened to show the five major divisions in rostral-to-caudal sequence.

The cavity within the midbrain, somewhat dilated in the embryo, narrows to become the *cerebral aqueduct* (of Sylvius) as the dorsal region (or tectum) of the midbrain develops (Figure 21–7C). The cerebral aqueduct is a narrow conduit for the flow of cerebrospinal fluid to the *fourth ventricle,* which is located dorsal to the pons and medulla. During development a small amount of cerebrospinal fluid produced in the fourth ventricle as well as that produced in the lateral and third ventricles flows into the spinal cord through the central canal. Late in fetal life, however, the central canal closes. Thus, all cerebrospinal fluid passes through three apertures in the roof of the fourth ventricle (the two foramina of Lushka and the foramen of Magendie) to the subarachnoid space, from which it bathes the surface of the entire central nervous system. As with the subarachnoid space overlying the spinal cord, cerebrospinal fluid accumulates in cisterns in the subarachnoid space overlying the brain. The cerebral cisterns will be discussed in the next chapter because their locations can be mapped precisely using modern brain imaging techniques. The hydrostatic pressure within the subarachnoid space is maintained at a low level because cerebrospinal fluid is passively reabsorbed into the blood through small unidirectional valves, called *arachnoid granulations,* located along the major venous sinus, the superior sagittal sinus, and other sites.

Obstruction of the cerebral aqueduct during development results in *hydrocephalus.* In this condition, cerebrospinal fluid produced by the choroid plexuses of the lateral and third ventricles cannot pass freely to more caudal parts of the ventricular system and subarachnoid space. As a consequence, pressure increases within the lateral and third ventricles, eventually compressing the cerebral hemispheres and enlarging the cranium, which in the infant is still free to enlarge, since the bones of the skull have not yet fused. Left untreated, this disorder can result in mental retardation. Recently an in utero surgical technique has been developed to insert a tube that bypasses the obstruction and prevents damage to the developing forebrain.

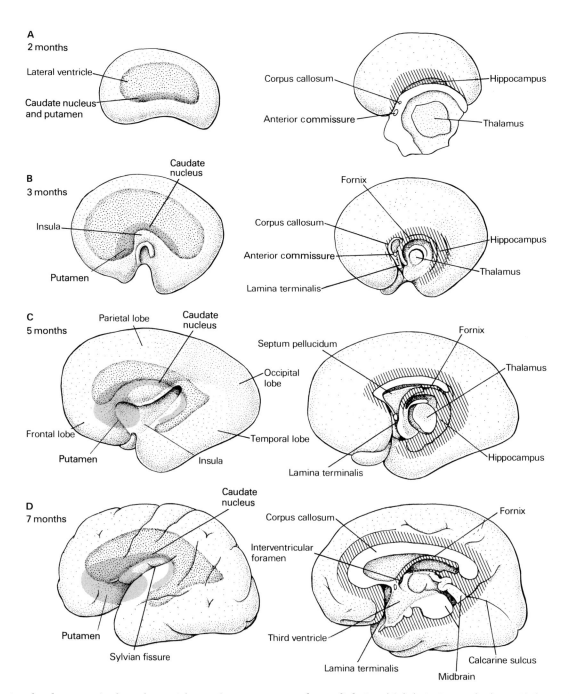

21–8 During development the lateral ventricle, caudate nucleus, and cortical limbic areas become C-shaped. The lateral ventricle (**stippled**) and the caudate nucleus (**shaded**) are best shown on the lateral view of the developing brain (**left**), whereas the cortical limbic areas (**hatched**) are seen on the medial view (**right**). At 2 months (part **A**) the caudate nucleus and putamen form a swelling on the floor of the lateral ventricle. As development of the brain proceeds (parts **B, C,** and **D**) only the caudate nucleus and lateral ventricles become C-shaped. (Adapted from Keibel and Mall, 1910–1912.)

The Ventricular System Provides a Framework for Understanding the Regional Anatomy of the Diencephalon and Cerebral Hemispheres

When the five-vesicle stage is first achieved early in development, the cerebral hemispheres and lateral ventricles are spherical and lie lateral to the diencephalon and third ventricle (Figures 21–7 and 21–8). The cells of the cerebral hemispheres undergo an enormous proliferation. As they proliferate, the cerebral cortex expands first rostrally to form the frontal lobes, then dorsally to form the parietal lobes, and finally posteriorly and inferiorly to form the occipital and temporal lobes (Figure 21–8). *As a result of this inferior and posterior expansion, the cortex loses its simple spherical shape, and the underlying structures in the hemisphere are forced into a C-shaped*

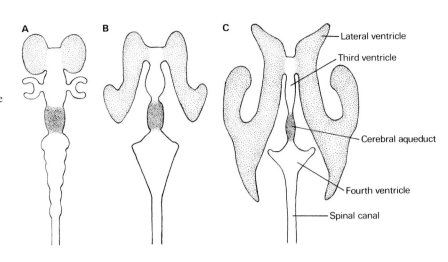

21–9 Early in development the lateral ventricles are spherical in shape and lie close to the midline (part **A,** 2 months). As the cerebral hemisphere enlarges later in development, the lateral ventricles grow with them (parts **B,** 5 months; and **C,** newborn). At these later developmental stages, portions of the lateral ventricles remain close to the midline, but others have expanded laterally.

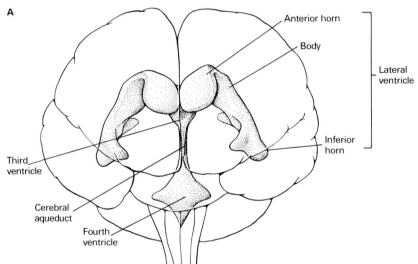

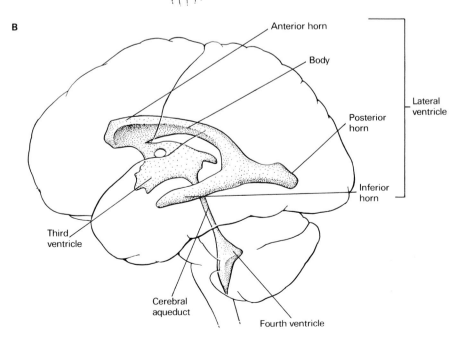

21–10 The position of the ventricles in the adult is shown in two views: **A.** Front view. **B.** Side view.

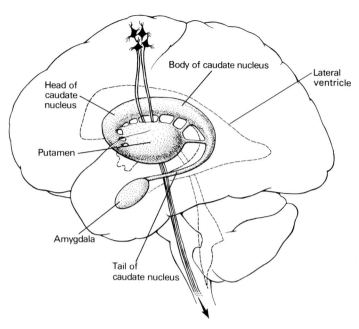

21–11 The shape of the caudate nucleus parallels that of the lateral ventricle. There are three parts to the caudate nucleus: the head, the body, and the tail. The head of the caudate lies parallel to the anterior horn of the lateral ventricle; the body of the caudate lies parallel to the body of the ventricle; and the tail of the caudate lies parallel to the inferior horn. In the adult, fibers of the internal capsule pass between the caudate nucleus and putamen. Axons of corticospinal neurons are schematically illustrated to show their path through the internal capsule en route to the spinal cord.

configuration (Figure 21–8). As the cerebral hemispheres develop, a part of the cortex becomes buried. This region is called the insula (Latin, island). The insular cortex is covered by the opercular regions (Latin, *operculum*, lid) of the frontal, parietal, and temporal lobes. Broca's area, the cortical site important in the motor mechanisms of speech, is located in the frontal operculum.

The lateral ventricles serve as useful landmarks in understanding the regional anatomy of the cerebral hemispheres. For this reason, we shall first follow their development into the adult form and then consider three anatomically related structures that also have a characteristic C-shaped configuration: the caudate nucleus of the basal ganglia, the hippocampus of the limbic system,

and the neocortical gyri of the limbic system (cingulate and parahippocampal gyri).

The development of the lateral ventricles, viewed from the lateral surface of the cerebral hemisphere, is stippled in the left half of Figure 21–8. As can be seen in Figure 21–8C, it is not until later developmental stages that the four parts of the lateral ventricle become distinct: the *anterior* (or frontal) horn, the *body*, the *posterior* (or occipital) horn, and the *inferior* (or temporal) horn. Now we also see the septum pellucidum (Latin, clear membrane), which separates the anterior horn and body of the lateral ventricles of the two hemispheres. In addition to developing inferiorly and posteriorly, the lateral ventricles assume a more lateral position (Figure

21–12 The hippocampus of the right and left hemispheres is shown below the corpus callosum.

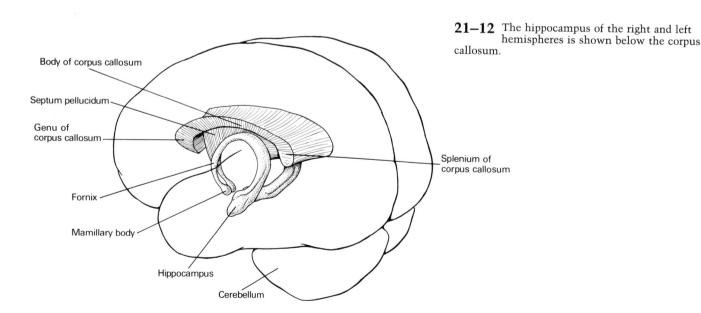

21–13 The cingulate gyrus and the parahippocampal gyrus (**stippled area**) are two components of the limbic system present on the medial surface of the cerebral hemisphere. The brain stem and a portion of the diencephalon have been removed to expose the parahippocampal gyrus.

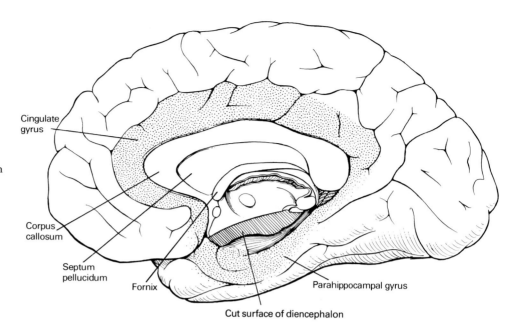

Cingulate gyrus

Corpus callosum

Septum pellucidum

Fornix

Parahippocampal gyrus

Cut surface of diencephalon

21–9). The lateral ventricles, the third ventricle, the cerebral aqueduct, and the fourth ventricle of the adult brain are shown in Figure 21–10.

The Caudate Nucleus Is C-Shaped and Parallels the Lateral Ventricles

As we saw in the last chapter, the basal ganglia are important structures in the planning and execution of movement. The three main parts of the basal ganglia are the caudate nucleus and the putamen (collectively termed the *striatum*), and the globus pallidus. Only the caudate nucleus is C-shaped. It roughly parallels the shape of the lateral ventricles. The approximate location of the caudate nucleus (and putamen) during development is shown in Figure 21–8 and in the adult in Figure 21–11.

The caudate nucleus is only incompletely separated from the putamen by fiber tracts, which are made up of axons of thalamic neurons that project to the cerebral cortex and axons that descend from the cortex. These ascending and descending fibers form the *internal capsule*. The adult caudate nucleus is composed of three parts. The *head*, or most rostral portion of the caudate nucleus, is adjacent to the anterior horn of the lateral ventricle in the frontal lobe. The *body* of the caudate nucleus runs along the lateral wall of the lateral ventricle; this structure then curves around as the *tail* of the caudate nucleus in the roof of the inferior horn of the lateral ventricle. This entire course describes a C-shaped arc. At the tip of the inferior horn of the ventricle, near the end of the tail of the caudate nucleus, lies the amygdala or amygdaloid nuclear complex (Figure 21–11), a part of the limbic system.

The head of the caudate nucleus is a critical anatomical landmark in studying both the normal brain and certain neurological disorders. For example, in Huntington's

disease—a hereditary neurological disease caused by a mutation in a single gene—the caudate nucleus during adulthood undergoes extensive cell loss and consequently diminishes in size. Normally the head of the caudate nucleus bulges into the anterior horn of the lateral ventricle, and thus it can be easily visualized with computerized X-ray tomography scans and other imaging techniques. In Huntington's disease, the shrinkage in the head of the caudate nucleus is reflected dramatically as a change in the contour of the lateral ventricle.

The Major Components of the Limbic System Are Also C-Shaped

The two other C-shaped structures comprise four major components of the limbic system. The *hippocampus* and the *fornix* form one C-shaped structure, and the *cingulate* and *parahippocampal gyri* and their connections collectively form the second. Early in development, the hippocampus and cingulate gyrus are adjacent to one another. As development proceeds, however, the hippocampus and the cingulate gyrus are pushed farther apart by a substantial increase in the number of axons that course through the large commissure, the corpus callosum that interconnects the cerebral cortices of the two hemispheres (Figure 21–8A, B). Given the early developmental proximity of the hippocampus, the cingulate gyrus, and the parahippocampal gyrus, it is easy to understand why these structures, the principal constituents of the limbic system, are so closely interconnected (Figures 21–12 and 21–13).

The limbic system has a role in both affective and cognitive functioning. On the one hand, it is concerned with emotions and with the regulation of the autonomic nervous system. As a result, the limbic system is often called the *visceral brain*. On the other hand, as we saw in Chapter 20, the limbic system is also involved in me-

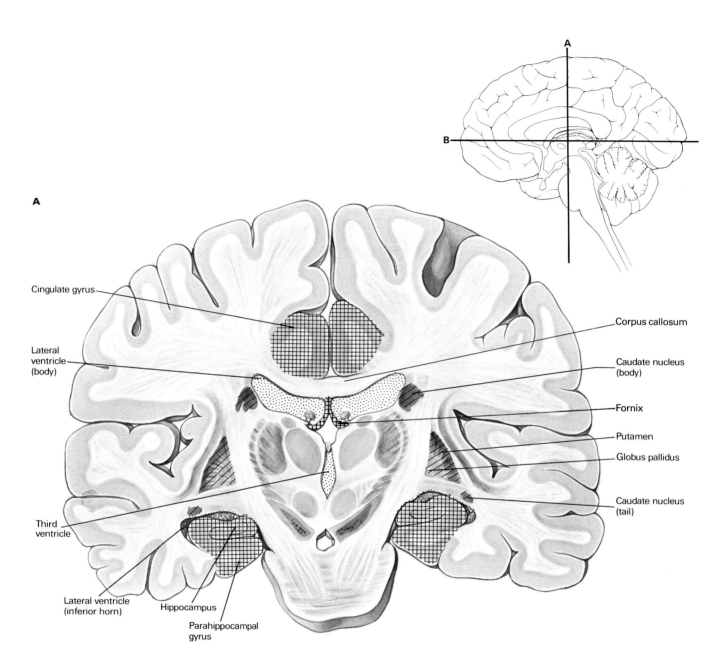

A

Cingulate gyrus

Lateral ventricle (body)

Third ventricle

Lateral ventricle (inferior horn)

Hippocampus

Parahippocampal gyrus

Corpus callosum

Caudate nucleus (body)

Fornix

Putamen

Globus pallidus

Caudate nucleus (tail)

21–14 Two-dimensional slices through the brain in the coronal and horizontal planes cut through C-shaped structures twice. The inset, a midsagittal slice, shows the planes of section in parts **A** and **B. A.** Coronal section. The C-shaped structures are seen in duplicate: first, dorsal and medial; and second, ventral and lateral. The body of the caudate nucleus forms the lateral wall of the body of the lateral ventricle, and the corpus callosum forms its roof. The cingulate gyrus and underlying cingulum bundle are located dorsal to the corpus callosum. The output pathway of the hippocampus, the fornix, hangs from the ventral surface of the corpus callosum between the lateral ventricles. In the temporal lobe, the roof of the inferior horn of the lateral ventricle is formed by the tail of the caudate nucleus and axons of the

diating learning and memory. Indeed, James Papez, a neuroanatomist at Cornell University, suggested that higher cognitive functions influence emotions and their visceral consequences via a complex pathway now called *Papez' circuit* that interconnects the association areas of the cerebral cortex with the hypothalamus. The pathway works as follows: the parietal–temporal–occipital association and prefrontal association areas first project to the cingulate gyrus. The information is then relayed from the cingulate gyrus to the parahippocampal gyrus

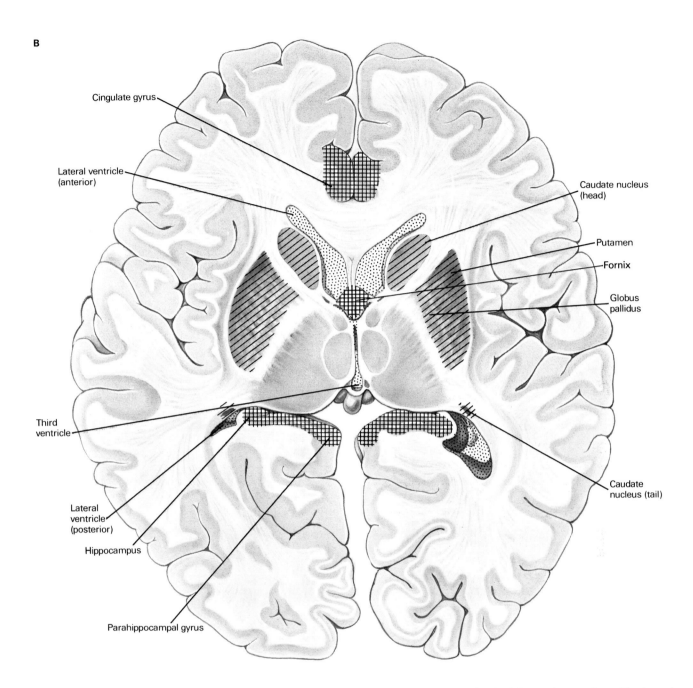

B

Cinculate gyrus

Lateral ventricle (anterior)

Caudate nucleus (head)

Putamen

Fornix

Globus pallidus

Third ventricle

Caudate nucleus (tail)

Lateral ventricle (posterior)

Hippocampus

Parahippocampal gyrus

white matter. The floor of the ventricle is formed by the hippocampus. The parahippocampal gyrus is medial and inferior to the hippocampus. **B.** Horizontal section. The C-shaped structures are seen both rostrally and caudally. The cingulate gyrus and cingulum bundle are rostral to the corpus callosum. Next we encounter the anterior horn of the lateral

ventricle, fornix, and head of the caudate nucleus. The lateral ventricle is seen caudally as the posterior horn. In this region we also see the tail of the caudate nucleus and the hippocampus, and, along the medial surface, the parahippocampal gyrus. (Adapted from Nieuwenhuys, Voogd, and van Huijzen, 1981.)

and to the hippocampus by means of a pathway called the *cingulum bundle,* which is also C-shaped. From the parahippocampal gyrus, information is relayed to the hippocampus. The hippocampus in turn projects through the fornix to the mammillary bodies of the hypothala-

mus (Figure 21–12) and from there to the anterior nuclei of the thalamus. Finally, information is relayed from the thalamus back to the cingulate gyrus. Interruption of Papez' circuit at any one of several points produces profound behavioral deficits.

An Understanding of the C-Shaped Gyri Is Necessary for Interpreting Sections Through the Brain

Most often the brain is viewed in two-dimensional sections. With such sections, it becomes particularly important to appreciate the relationships of the ventricles to the three C-shaped structures: the caudate nucleus, the hippocampus, and the cingulate and parahippocampal gyri. For example, a section may be cut through a three-dimensional structure in such a way that different portions of the structure, such as the head and tail of the caudate, will appear in two separate places (Figure 21–14). An understanding of the three-dimensional anatomy of the brain therefore greatly clarifies the interpretation of these two-dimensional images.

An Overall View

The regional anatomy of the central nervous system is a consequence of its developmental plan. The anatomy of the brain stem and spinal cord is simple in contrast to the complex anatomy of the cerebral hemispheres. Indeed, the extraordinary proliferation of neurons in the cerebral hemispheres provides the foundation for human cognitive capabilities. A precise understanding of the regional anatomy of the central nervous system can now be achieved because modern imaging techniques, de-

scribed in Chapter 22, map the complex spatial relations of the living brain. By means of imaging, the exploration of human neuroanatomy has moved from the visual examination of the fixed brain to the analysis of the dynamic actions of the brain during behavior.

Selected Readings

Cowan, W. M. 1979. The development of the brain. Sci. Am. 241(3):112–133.

Heimer, L. 1983. The Human Brain and Spinal Cord: Functional Neuroanatomy and Dissection Guide. New York: Springer.

Jacobson, M. 1978. Developmental Neurobiology, 2nd ed. New York: Plenum Press.

Nieuwenhuys, R. Voogd, J., and van Huijzen, Chr. 1981. The Human Central Nervous System: A Synopsis and Atlas, 2nd rev. ed. Berlin: Springer.

References

House, E. L., Pansky, B., and Siegel, A. 1979. A Systematic Approach to Neuroscience, 3rd ed. New York: McGraw-Hill.

Keibel, F., and Mall, F. P. (eds.). 1910–1912. Manual of Human Embryology. 2 vol. Philadelphia: Lippincott.

Pansky, B. 1982. Review of Medical Embryology. New York: Macmillan.

Papez, J. W. 1937. A proposed mechanism of emotion. Arch. Neurol. Psychiatry 38:725–743.

John H. Martin and John C. M. Brust

Imaging the Living Brain

22

Study of the regional anatomy of the living brain has been revolutionized by the development of three imaging techniques: computerized tomography, positron emission tomography, and magnetic resonance imaging (MRI) (formerly designated as nuclear magnetic resonance [NMR] imaging). Each of these methods allows the structure of the human brain to be visualized in detail. As a result, neural scientists can examine the brain while people think, perceive, and initiate voluntary actions, and clinicians can now localize lesions of the brain with remarkable accuracy, without invasive procedures that interfere with normal function and even endanger life. Because these imaging methods have so much promise, neural scientists should soon be able to apply cell-biological techniques to the study of human behavior. To utilize these advances, both the clinician and neural scientist must be familiar with the functional and regional anatomy of the human brain that we considered in the preceding chapters.

In this chapter we shall discuss the three major types of imaging techniques and how they allow a completely new approach to the study of regional anatomy. Toward that end, we shall reexamine the regions of the brain we explored in the last three chapters, but now we shall look at them in the living brain and from a functional point of view. We shall also consider how these methods of imaging can be used to identify the location of neurons that contain particular receptors on their cell membranes, to define the pattern of activity associated with different functional states, and to examine other aspects of the dynamic operation of different regions of the brain. The objective is to emphasize structural aspects of the functioning brain that are behaviorally and clinically interesting.

Computerized Tomography (CT) Scanning Has Improved the Resolution of Images of Brain Structures

Computerized tomography (CT) allows us to explore the regional anatomy of the brain in living patients suffering from neurological disease. The CT scan is an image of a single plane, or "slice," of tissue. The image produced is a computerized reconstruction of the degree to which different tissues absorb transmitted X-rays. Before we consider the principle by which CT scans are generated, we need to understand something about X-rays in general.

A conventional radiograph of the head represents a static picture of the skull and its contents. To produce a radiograph, a broad beam of X-ray photons is passed through the skull toward an X-ray film. The film reveals the lucency of different tissues in inverse proportion to their absorption of X-rays. The resolution of a conventional radiograph of the brain is limited. For example, the gray matter and white matter of the brain cannot be distinguished from one another because they differ so little in their absorption of X-rays. The bones of the skull, on the other hand, absorb a good deal of radiation and therefore appear light on radiographs (Figure 22–1A). In addition, certain brain tissues that accumulate calcium with age, such as the pineal gland (an unpaired structure in the diencephalon), also absorb radiation and can often be recognized in plain radiographs of the skull. The pineal gland is normally located in the midline and is therefore a reliable landmark for brain symmetry. Lesions of the brain that occupy space, such as a hemorrhage or a tumor, displace the pineal gland and other midline structures.

In contrast to bone and other calcified tissue, air absorbs very little radiation and appears dark in radiographs. This fact has been exploited by neuroradiologists to provide an image of the ventricular system of the brain called a *pneumoencephalogram* (Figure 22–1B). To construct such an image, a small amount of cerebrospinal fluid is removed from the subarachnoid space by spinal tap and the fluid is replaced with air. Studying the path by which air enters the ventricles enables one to review the organization of the ventricular system. When the patient assumes an erect posture, the air travels up the subarachnoid space surrounding the spinal cord and brain. Some air enters the fourth ventricle, which is located in the medulla and pons, through apertures in the roof of the ventricle. Air then travels through the cerebral aqueduct in the midbrain to the third ventricle, and then to the lateral ventricles through the interventricular foramina. However, pneumoencephalography is painful and

22–1 A. Skull radiograph. Bones and calcium-accumulating tissues absorb X-rays and appear light on the X-ray film. **B.** Pneumoencephalogram. Air replacing cerebrospinal fluid in the ventricles appears dark on the X-ray films. **Vertical arrows** indicate air in basal subarachnoid cisterns; **arrows with asterisks** indicate air in Sylvian fissures. (Courtesy of Dr. Robert McMasters, Lenox Hill Hospital.)

A

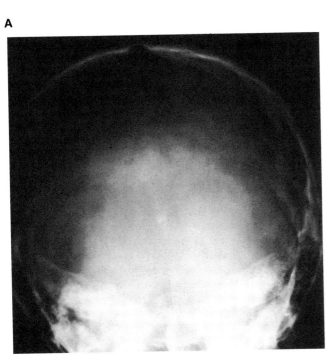

B

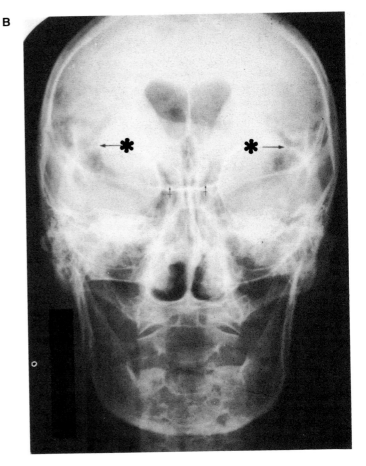

sometimes dangerous. It is therefore rarely used at present, having been superseded by CT.

Similar limitations beset *cerebral angiography*, in which a radiopaque dye is injected intra-arterially (or intravenously, using recently developed digital imaging techniques) and a radiographic image of brain vasculature is displayed. Except for vessels, angiography does not reveal the normal intracranial structures. Abnormalities are inferred from distortions in the appearance of the vasculature. For example, normal vessels may be displaced by an avascular neoplasm or a blood clot. The presence of abnormal extra vasculature could indicate either a vascular neoplasm ("neovascularization") or a congenital vascular malformation.

To overcome limitations in spatial resolution and the inability to distinguish gray matter from white matter, CT was developed. This advance was so significant that its inventors, Godfrey Hounsfield and Allan Cormack, were awarded the Nobel Prize for Physiology and Medicine in 1979. In CT, the X-ray tube gives off a series of narrow, highly collimated beams of radiation (Figure 22–2) and standard X-ray film is replaced by scintillation crystals, which are more sensitive. Even though gray and white matter, blood, and cerebrospinal fluid all differ from one another in radiodensity by less than 2%, computer-analyzed X-ray transmission profiles permit their resolution. Currently available CT equipment can produce scans that have resolution in soft tissue of less than 1 mm. To increase further the contrast between tissue constituents, radiopaque contrast material can be injected intravenously, allowing "enhancement" of regions that have either increased vasculature or impaired blood–brain barrier functions. By this means, blood vessels, tumors, or abscesses can be more effectively visualized. In fact, many features can be seen only when contrast material is used.

Ten computerized tomographic transverse slices through the normal brain are shown in Figures 22–3A through J. In Figures 22–3A and B, the most inferior (or caudal) slices pass through the orbits of the eyes and the base of the skull, displaying the eyes, optic nerves, and temporal lobes of the cerebrum and the two divisions of the cerebellum, the midline *vermis* (Latin, worm) and lateral *hemispheres*. These scans also pass through the *posterior fossa*, the intracranial region in which the cerebellum and brain stem are located. Numerous nonneural structures whose boundaries are formed by bone can also be seen (for example, the paranasal and mastoid sinuses, and the carotid canal, which is the space through which the internal carotid artery passes). In these figures radiographic artifact from adjacent bone obscures detail in the medulla and pons, a common problem with CT of the posterior fossa. Therefore, the individual lower brain stem structures that were discussed in Chapter 20 are not distinguishable. (These structures include the dorsal column nuclei, the motor nuclei to cranial muscles, the medial lemniscus, and the spinothalamic and corticospinal tracts.) The relationship of the medulla and pons to the cerebellum and fourth ventricle, however, is shown clearly.

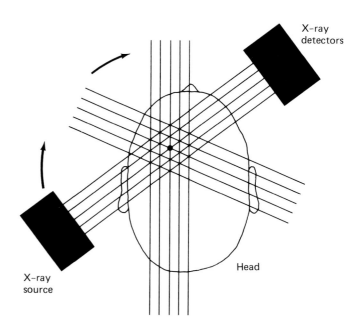

22–2 In CT scanning the transmission of X-rays through tissue is read at each point of beam intersection. Multiple narrow beams of X-rays are rotated 180° around one side of the skull while the X-ray detectors are rotated around the opposite side in an identical path. At each degree of rotation, tube and detectors, now moving linearly, make a series of transmission readings (up to several hundred, depending on the model). The transmission characteristics, or radiodensity, of a single region of tissue are calculated by summing the transmission readings of all beams passing through that region. The spatial resolution of CT scans is limited to the distance between these intersection points. The result for each "slice" of brain is a matrix computed from thousands of intersecting radiation intensity measurements, translated into numbers (*attenuation coefficients*) and visually displayed as areas that are relatively dark or light.

In Figures 22–3C and D the upper brain stem is above the bony base of the skull and therefore better delineated. The midbrain is clearly seen in cross section. The dorsal midbrain, often called the tectum, contains the inferior and superior colliculi. In the ventral midbrain the cerebral peduncles can be seen. The corticospinal tracts occupy the center of the peduncles ventrally and are flanked by descending corticopontine fibers. These corticopontine fibers synapse in the pontine nuclei, which in turn project to the cerebellum. In between the colliculi and the corticospinal tracts, however, there are a number of structures that are not observed on CT slices: the medial lemnisci, the spinothalamic tracts, the red nuclei, the oculomotor nuclei, the ascending fibers from the cerebellum, and the reticular formation. Two important parts of the dura mater are seen on these CT scans. The *falx cerebri* (Latin, *falx*, sickle) is the flap of dura in the interhemispheric fissure that separates the two cerebral hemispheres. The *tentorium cerebelli* (Latin, *tentorium*, tent) forms the roof of the posterior fossa and therefore separates the cerebellum from the cerebral hemispheres.

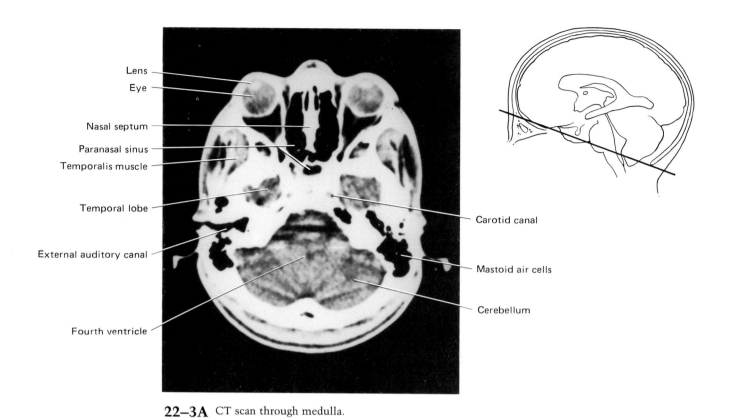

22–3A CT scan through medulla.

22–3 Detailed images of transverse slices of normal brain are obtained by CT scanning.
Insets: Plane of section ("slice") shown in each scan. (CT scans courtesy
of Dr. Sadek Hilal, Columbia University College of Physicians and Surgeons.)

22–3B CT scan through pons.

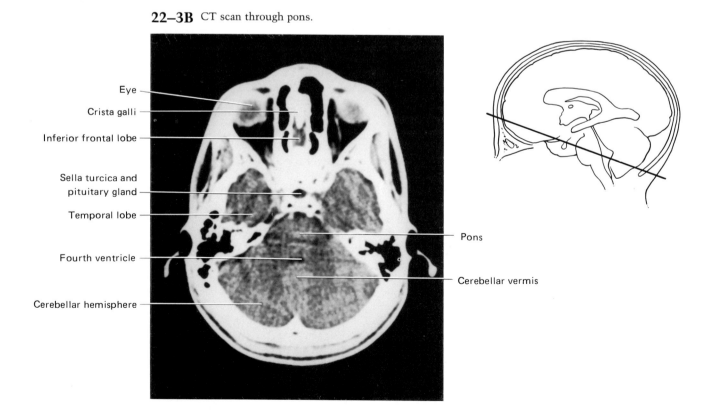

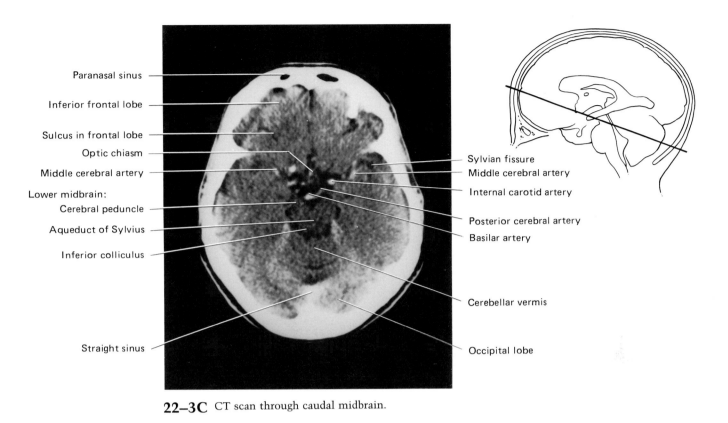

Paranasal sinus

Inferior frontal lobe

Sulcus in frontal lobe

Optic chiasm

Middle cerebral artery

Lower midbrain:

Cerebral peduncle

Aqueduct of Sylvius

Inferior colliculus

Straight sinus

Sylvian fissure
Middle cerebral artery

Internal carotid artery

Posterior cerebral artery

Basilar artery

Cerebellar vermis

Occipital lobe

22–3C CT scan through caudal midbrain.

22–3 (continued)

22–3D CT scan through upper midbrain.

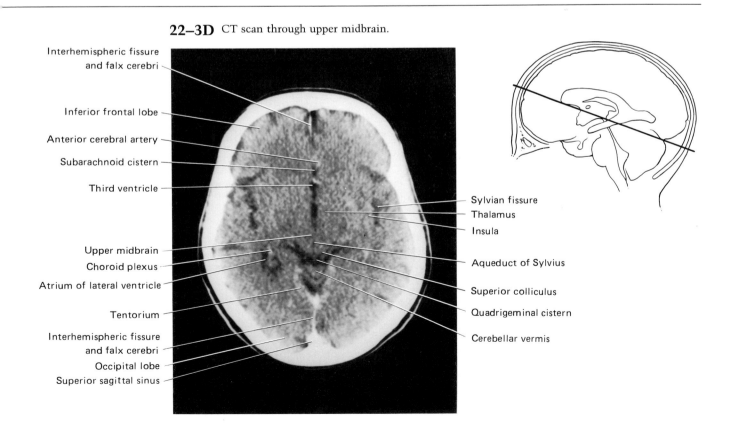

Interhemispheric fissure
and falx cerebri

Inferior frontal lobe

Anterior cerebral artery

Subarachnoid cistern

Third ventricle

Upper midbrain

Choroid plexus

Atrium of lateral ventricle

Tentorium

Interhemispheric fissure
and falx cerebri

Occipital lobe

Superior sagittal sinus

Sylvian fissure

Thalamus

Insula

Aqueduct of Sylvius

Superior colliculus

Quadrigeminal cistern

Cerebellar vermis

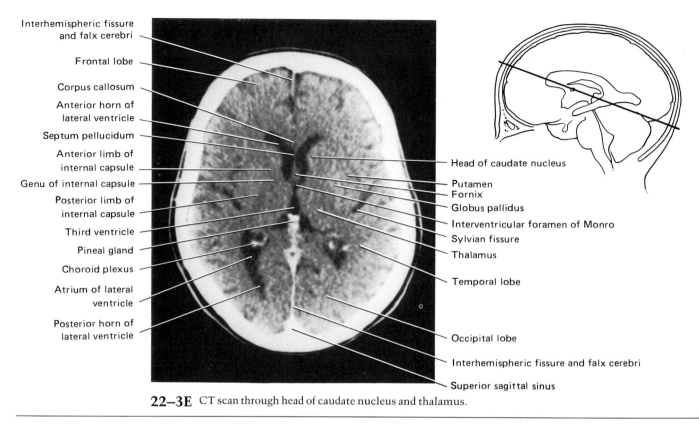

Interhemispheric fissure and falx cerebri

Frontal lobe

Corpus callosum

Anterior horn of lateral ventricle

Septum pellucidum

Anterior limb of internal capsule

Genu of internal capsule

Posterior limb of internal capsule

Third ventricle

Pineal gland

Choroid plexus

Atrium of lateral ventricle

Posterior horn of lateral ventricle

Head of caudate nucleus

Putamen

Fornix

Globus pallidus

Interventricular foramen of Monro

Sylvian fissure

Thalamus

Temporal lobe

Occipital lobe

Interhemispheric fissure and falx cerebri

Superior sagittal sinus

22–3E CT scan through head of caudate nucleus and thalamus.

22–3 *(continued)*

22–3F CT scan through dorsal diencephalon.

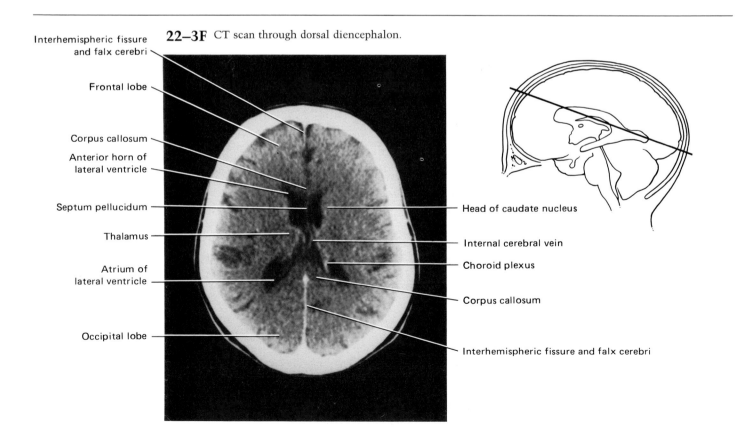

Interhemispheric fissure and falx cerebri

Frontal lobe

Corpus callosum

Anterior horn of lateral ventricle

Septum pellucidum

Thalamus

Atrium of lateral ventricle

Occipital lobe

Head of caudate nucleus

Internal cerebral vein

Choroid plexus

Corpus callosum

Interhemispheric fissure and falx cerebri

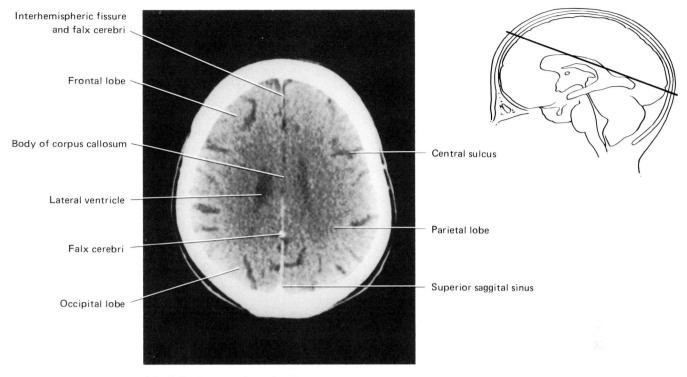

Interhemispheric fissure
and falx cerebri

Frontal lobe

Body of corpus callosum

Lateral ventricle

Falx cerebri

Occipital lobe

Central sulcus

Parietal lobe

Superior saggital sinus

22–3G CT scan through white matter of cerebral cortex.

22–3 *(continued)*

22–3H CT scan through white matter of cerebral cortex.

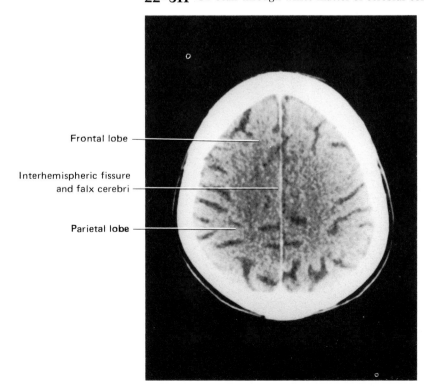
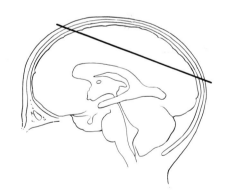

Frontal lobe

Interhemispheric fissure
and falx cerebri

Parietal lobe

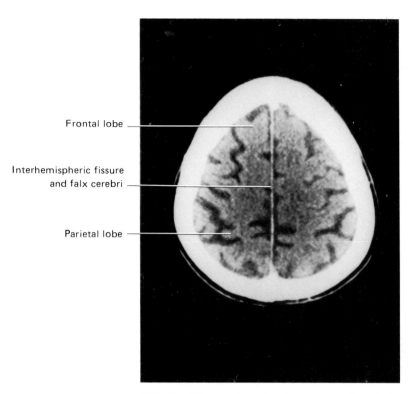
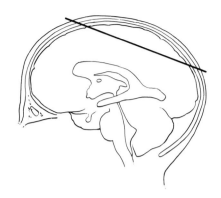

Frontal lobe

Interhemispheric fissure
and falx cerebri

Parietal lobe

22–3I CT scan through white matter of cerebral cortex.

22–3 *(continued)*

22–3J CT scan through white matter of cerebral cortex.

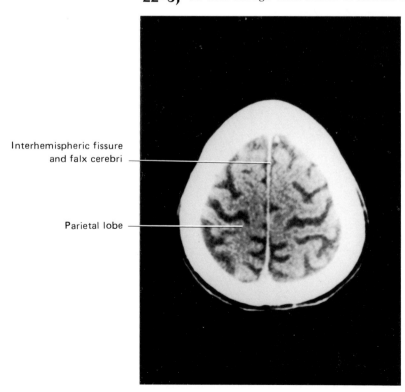
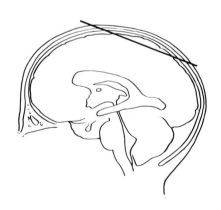

Interhemispheric fissure
and falx cerebri

Parietal lobe

The scan in Figure 22–3D illustrates how the rostral portion of the midbrain merges into the caudal parts of the thalamus. This figure also "slices" the frontal, temporal, and occipital lobes, as well as the most dorsal (superior) part of the cerebellum.

In Figures 22–3E and F aspects of the ventricular system are displayed: the third and lateral ventricles as well as their connection at the interventricular foramen of Monro. The choroid plexus in the lateral ventricles is radiopaque both because it contains calcium and because the patient received a radiopaque contrast agent intravenously. As we shall see in other figures, this technique also reveals major blood vessels. The spatial relationships of the internal capsule (the genu and posterior limb, which contains the corticospinal tract), the basal ganglia (caudate nucleus, putamen, and globus pallidus), and the thalamus are seen in Figures 22–3E and F.

The scans in Figures 22–3G through J illustrate the white matter and the cerebral cortex of the frontal, parietal, and occipital lobes. In this patient, the sulci are very prominent and clearly seen, indicating a moderate degree of cortical atrophy not uncommon in elderly patients.

Positron Emission Tomography (PET) Scanning Yields a Dynamic Picture of Brain Function

CT scanning provides a view of the living brain, but this view is *static*. It allows one to view structure but it does not explore function. *Positron emission tomography* (PET) scanning combines CT with radioisotope imaging

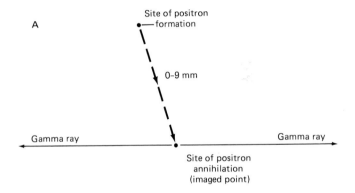

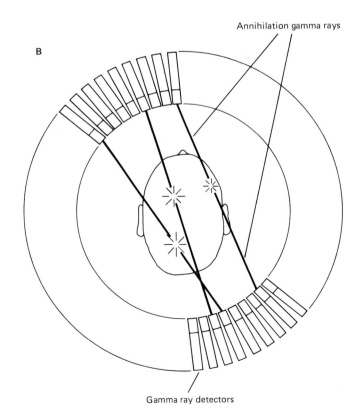

22–4 In PET scanning the emission of positrons from labeled structures is used for imaging. Nuclear imaging of neurophysiological processes requires isotopes of light elements (e.g., hydrogen, carbon, nitrogen, and oxygen) that make up biologically important compounds. Gamma emitters of such elements are few, however, and their very short half-lives (seconds) make them clinically impractical. More useful are isotopes of elements that decay after longer half-lives (minutes to hours), with the emission of positrons (positively charged electrons). Useful positron-emitting isotopes can be made by accelerating protons in a cyclotron at extraordinarily high rates into the stable nuclei of nitrogen, oxygen, carbon, and fluorine. Normally, these nuclei contain protons and neutrons in equal numbers. Incorporation of an extra proton into a nucleus produces an unstable isotope. For stability to be regained, the proton is broken down into two particles: (1) a neutron, which remains within the nucleus because a stable nucleus can manage extra neutrons; and (2) a *positron*, an unstable particle, which travels away from the site of generation, dissipating energy as it goes. Soon the positron collides with an electron. The reaction between one positron and one electron leads to their mutual annihilation and the *emission of two gamma rays* at precisely 180° from one another. **A.** In PET scanning the site of positron annihilation that is imaged may be several millimeters from the site of origin. For example, the distance between sites of origin and annihilation is 2 mm for ^{18}F and 8 mm for ^{15}O. Because of this difference, ^{18}F scans can ultimately have greater resolution than those that use ^{15}O. **B.** Gamma rays are detected by crystal photomultipliers that surround the head. The two gamma rays ultimately reach a pair of detectors that record an event when, and only when, two simultaneous detections are made. This method of coincident detection permits precise localization of the site of gamma emission and it is the method by which positron scanning produces images of the brain. (Adapted from Oldendorf, 1980.)

and makes it possible to probe function as well as structure. CT depends on *transmission tomography*, the relative absorption of X-rays passing through tissues. The X-ray source and detector are rotated around the head and radiodensities of a slice of tissue are used to generate the image. *Emission tomography* utilizes similar principles to reconstruct images of sections, but formation of the image depends on the distribution in the tissue of an injected or inhaled isotope that emits radiation. By binding positron-emitting isotopes, such as ^{11}C, ^{13}N, ^{15}O, or ^{18}F, to compounds of biological interest, such as water, glucose, or transmitter molecules, it is possible to map the distribution of these various compounds within the brain (Figure 22–4).

Therefore, unlike conventional radiographs and CT scans, which simply yield structural information, PET scanning provides images of brain function. A powerful application of PET scanning is the mapping of the sugar metabolism of neurons, an ingenious tracing method that reveals active nerve cells. Activity in a nerve cell is directly related to utilization of glucose. *2-Deoxyglucose*, an analogue of glucose, is taken up by neurons and phosphorylated by hexokinase in the same manner as glucose. Unlike glucose, however, phosphorylated deoxyglucose cannot be further metabolized, nor can it exit across the cell membrane. Therefore, it accumulates within active brain cells. By covalently bonding the positron-emitting isotope of fluorine (^{18}F) to deoxyglucose to make ^{18}F-deoxyglucose it is possible to measure glucose utilization in small regions of the brain. Because uptake of ^{18}F-deoxyglucose into neurons is proportional to the activity of the cells, active areas of the brain are more heavily labeled than inactive ones after intravenous injection of ^{18}F-deoxyglucose.

In Figure 22–5, PET scans of 14 slices are shown, each 8 mm apart and parallel to the line between the eye and the ear canal (canthomeatal line). In this scan ^{18}F-deoxyglucose was used to measure glucose metabolism in vivo in different brain regions, in this case in a normal person at rest. At the spatial resolution of these scans we can observe the contours of various cortical gyri and sulci. Among the subcortical nuclei, we can see activity within the thalamus, caudate nucleus, and the lenticular nucleus, the region that comprises the putamen and globus pallidus. The posterior and anterior limbs of the internal capsule can also be observed, and so can the brain stem, cerebellar hemispheres, and vermis.

In Figure 22–6 ^{18}F-deoxyglucose PET scans are shown that measure glucose metabolism in a normal person during visual stimulation. Transverse slices are shown with the eyes closed, open, and looking at a complex scene. With the eyes open, glucose metabolism increases in the primary visual cortex. When the subject views a complex scene, it increases further, and the visual association cortex becomes active as well.

PET scans before and during auditory stimulation (which consisted of listening to a Sherlock Holmes adventure) are shown in Figure 22–7. The subject was instructed to remember key phrases of the story. This led

to increased metabolic rate of brain tissue in primary auditory cortex (Heschl's gyri). It is presumed that activation of the hippocampus is a consequence of the verbal memory task. With this technique, we can visualize the regions of the brain that are active in response to natural sensory experience.

Although these images illustrate structure, they really are reflections of function. The scan is an index of glucose utilization, or the degree of activity, in the neurons surveyed in the particular slice of brain. Since the images confirm previous observations derived from fixed specimens, they provide a vehicle for correlating structure with function and thus pave the way for a new approach to the anatomy of the brain based on physiological function.

In addition to analogues of glucose, transmitters or their precursors can be labeled, and so can receptor ligand molecules. Recently, ^{11}C-N-methylspiperone, a ligand that preferentially binds to dopamine receptors, was used to map receptor location in living human brain (Figure 22–8). Many dopamine receptors labeled in this manner are located in the anterior part of the striatum, in the head and body of the caudate nucleus, and in the putamen.

22–8 Dopamine receptors in living brain are imaged in this PET scan in the horizontal plane. The ligand ^{11}C-N-methylspiperone, which preferentially binds to dopamine receptors, was injected intravenously 70–130 min before the scan was made. Note the accumulation of the isotope in the caudate and putamen of the basal ganglia. (Courtesy of Dr. H. N. Wagner, Johns Hopkins Medical Institutions.)

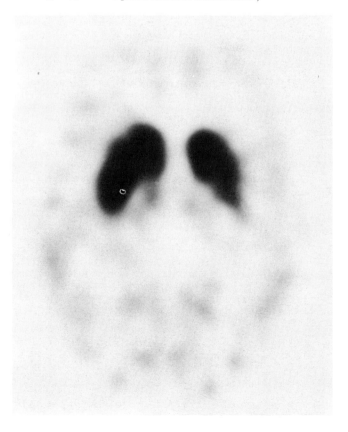

Normal resting pattern

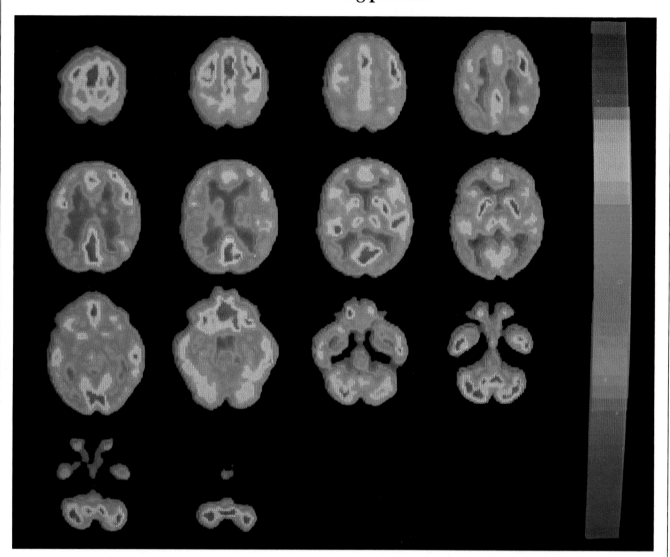

22–5 The local utilization of glucose by the normal resting brain can be seen in this series of PET scans using ^{18}F-deoxyglucose . Red represents the highest metabolic rate. These scans were made through 14 consecutive sections of the brain, from dorsal (**top**) to ventral (**bottom**) levels. Gray matter, which contains the cell bodies and dendrites of neurons as well as the regions of synaptic contact, is metabolically more active than white matter, which contains the myelinated axons. The areas of gray matter that are especially active are in the cerebral cortex, cerebellum, basal ganglia, and thalamus. (Courtesy of Drs. Michael E. Phelps and John C. Mazziotta, UCLA School of Medicine.)

Visual stimulation

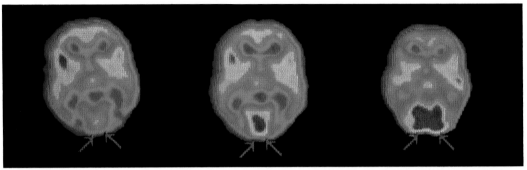

Eyes closed   White light   Complex scene

22–6 PET scans reveal neuronal regions that are active in response to visual stimulation. The scans illustrated here show that different brain regions become active in response to stimuli of differing complexity. Even simple white-light illumination (**center**) causes the primary visual cortex (area 17) to be active. This can be seen by comparing the activity in this area when the eyes are open with that when they are closed (**left**). However, higher order visual cortices (such as area 18) become active only when the subject views a complex scene (**right**). **Arrows** point to the occipital lobes. (Courtesy of Drs. Michael E. Phelps and John C. Mazziotta, UCLA School of Medicine.)

Auditory stimulation

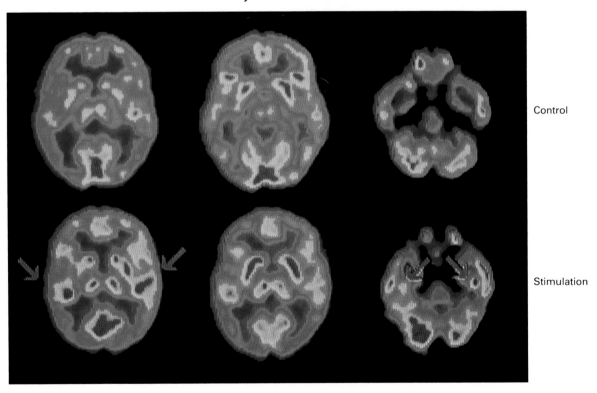

Control

Stimulation

22–7 Auditory stimulation alters the pattern of activity at three different levels of the brain. An experimental subject (**bottom**) is listening to a Sherlock Holmes story and is told to remember specific phrases. A control subject (**top**) is not exposed to auditory stimuli. Listening to the story increases metabolic activity in the experimental subject's primary and higher order auditory cortices (**arrows, bottom left scan**), as well as in the hippocampus (**arrows, bottom right scan**), a structure important for memory. (Courtesy of Drs. Michael E. Phelps and John C. Mazziotta, UCLA School of Medicine.)

Most of the dopamine in these structures comes from the nigrostriatal pathway, which originates in the substantia nigra and terminates in the striatum.

The ability of PET to reveal the distribution of specific neurotransmitters as well as metabolic substrates may permit a cell-biological approach to the human brain and lead to revisions in our present view of neuroanatomy and physiology. The major disadvantage of PET is that, because isotopes with short half-lives are involved, an on-site cyclotron is needed for generating them; this requirement makes the procedure extremely costly. Although currently the resolution of PET is relatively poor—about 4–8 mm—it is nonetheless better than that of electroencephalographic recording, the only other method available until recently for probing the dynamics of human brain activity.

Magnetic Resonance Imaging (MRI) Creates Brain Images without Using X-Rays

Magnetic resonance imaging (MRI) explores function, as does PET, but it has better resolution. MRI was first developed in the early 1950s to measure the atomic constituents of chemical samples. In recent years MRI has been combined with CT for spatial localization of atomic nuclei. This combination has resulted in a powerful imaging technique, one that can distinguish different body tissues because of their individual chemical compositions. For example, gray matter can be strikingly differentiated from white matter—more so, in fact, than by CT.

The physics of MRI is complex and thus will not be discussed in great detail (Figure 22–9). Briefly, certain atomic nuclei, when placed in suitable magnetic fields, resonate and consequently emit a radiofrequency signal. A particularly strong resonator is ordinary hydrogen, with a single proton for its nucleus. This is very fortunate for probing the chemical composition of body tissue, because 75% of the body is water, and each molecule of water has two hydrogen nuclei. Tissues, of course, vary in their water content. Gray matter contains more water than white matter, and therefore by manipulating the radiofrequency signal to which the tissue is exposed, the relaxation time of protons in water can be enhanced to produce striking gray and white matter differentiations by MRI. Dense bone contains little free water and so does not produce an image at all; this is an advantage when one is concentrating on adjacent soft tissues. In addition, disease states that produce swelling or cell death can alter the distribution of water in a given region of the brain.

At its best, the resolution of MRI is almost comparable to that seen in fixed and sectioned anatomical material because of the ability of MRI to distinguish between gray and white matter. A dramatic demonstration is shown in Figure 22–10. This midsagittal section of the living human brain clearly illustrates the six regions of the nervous system that we considered in the preceding three chapters. MRI images have suitable resolution for reviewing key aspects of the regional neuroanatomy of the human brain. We shall focus not on details, but rather on the principles important for effective clinical and scientific understanding.

MRI Images Can Provide an Atlas of Key Sections Through the Living Brain

Let us use representative two-dimensional MRI scans to reconsider the key structures discussed in this and previous chapters. We shall consider eight critical sections: (1) a midsagittal section through the medial aspect of the brain and spinal cord; (2) a parasagittal section through the brain and lateral ventricles; three transverse sections through the brain stem at the levels of (3) the medulla, (4) the pons, and (5) the midbrain; (6) a horizontal section through the thalamus and basal ganglia; (7) a horizontal section through the caudate nucleus and putamen; and (8) a coronal section through the basal ganglia.

We shall examine MRI sections together with drawings of comparable anatomical sections. In addition to locating key structures, we shall follow several systems that have been the focus of these four chapters: (1) the dorsal column–medial lemniscal system, which is important in tactile sensation and limb position sense; (2) the corticospinal tract, which is important in voluntary movement; and (3) the ventricular system and subarachnoid space, the conduits for the flow of cerebrospinal fluid.

Midsagittal Section Reveals C-Shaped Structures

To begin this survey, let us examine a view of the medial aspect of the brain, focusing on C-shaped structures (Figure 22–10). This and subsequent MRI images are based on the concentration of hydrogen ions in the living brain.

This medial brain section reveals the spinal cord and brain stem cut longitudinally, the cerebellum, the diencephalon, and the cerebral hemispheres. Like the lateral surface of the cerebral hemispheres, the medial aspect of the hemisphere is composed of *gyri* and *sulci*. The most prominent gyrus on the medial surface is the *cingulate gyrus*, which overlies the *corpus callosum*. The corpus callosum contains three major divisions, the genu, the body, and the splenium. These three divisions interconnect different portions of the cerebral hemisphere. The genu interconnects the rostral part of the frontal cortex, which is important in cognitive behavior and motor planning. The body interconnects the remaining parts of the frontal lobe and the parietal lobe. The occipital and temporal lobes, important in vision and audition, respectively, are connected through the splenium. Below the corpus callosum we see the fornix, the outflow pathway from the hippocampus, as it curves dorsally around the thalamus. The hypothalamus can be seen ventral to the thalamus.

We also see many of the components of the ventricular system: the third ventricle, the cerebral aqueduct, and the fourth ventricle. Cerebrospinal fluid produced in the

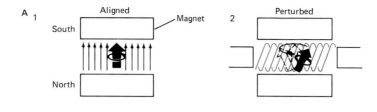

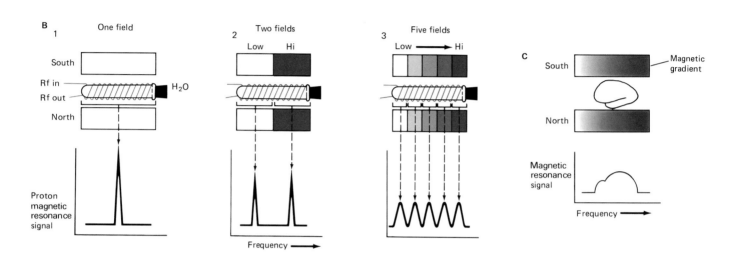

22–9 In MRI scanning an image is obtained of radiofrequency signals emitted by nuclei resonating in response to exposure to a magnetic field. **A.** Behavior of atomic nuclei in a magnetic field. When exposed to a *strong static homogeneous magnetic field,* the nuclei of odd atomic weight atoms such as hydrogen behave as tiny spinning magnets and develop a net alignment of their spin axes along the direction of the applied field (**1, large arrow**). The MRI signal is obtained from these atomic nuclei as follows. The alignment of the spin axes can be perturbed by a brief pulse of radio waves, which serves to tip the spinning nuclei away from their parallel orientation with the strong magnetic field and provides energy for their subsequent gyroscopelike motions, called *precession* (**2, large arrow**). By varying the strength of this radiofrequency pulse at a specific frequency, it is possible to produce precession of only one type of atomic nucleus at a time. When the radiofrequency pulse is turned off, the nuclei tend to return to their original orientation, and in doing so release energy in the form of radio waves. The frequencies given off are distinct for different atomic species as well as for a given atomic nucleus in different chemical or physical environments. The nuclei thus become radiofrequency transmitters, resonating at characteristic frequencies (hence magnetic *resonance* imaging) and revealing their presence by their signals. The strength of the radio wave at each frequency is proportional to the number of atomic nuclei of each kind in the sample. The rate at which a collection of nuclei return from an excited to a lower energy state is called *relaxation* and is usually described by its time constant (T). There are two types of relaxation of importance in MRI at present: spin–lattice relaxation (T_1) and spin–spin relaxation (T_2). Since relaxation times are influenced by local tissue conditions, images emphasizing one or the other relaxation time can either discriminate between normal tissues of various compositions or define pathological processes. For example, the difference between gray and white matter is best appreciated on images emphasizing T_1, whereas cerebrospinal fluid is greatly enhanced on images emphasizing T_2. **B.** For a particular nucleus, the radiofrequency of the signal depends directly upon the strength of the magnetic field to which it is exposed. For a homogeneous sample in a homogeneous magnetic field, the resultant signal is at a single frequency (**1**). For the same sample exposed to two different strength fields simultaneously, the signal is split; the nuclei positioned in the weaker magnetic field emit a signal at a lower frequency than those positioned in the higher field (**2**). If the strength of the applied magnetic field is made to change more often across the sample, each point on the frequency axis corresponds to a different spatial location within the sample, and the profile of the MRI signal as a function of frequency becomes a one-dimensional projection of the distribution of the constituent nuclei (**3**). **C.** Using this principle, one can translate signals coming from the brain into images by adding a small magnetic gradient onto the static homogeneous magnetic field. The nuclei in the higher end of the field transmit a radiofrequency signal with a higher frequency than those in the lower end. The frequency of a given signal is therefore the indicator of the spatial location. By changing the orientation of the applied magnetic gradient, one can obtain a larger series of profiles of the brain (or any other part of the body) from which sufficient information is generated to reconstruct an entire cross section using computer techniques similar to those applied to CT and PET.

ventricles (including the lateral ventricle, shown in Figure 22–11) flows through apertures in the roof of the fourth ventricle into the subarachnoid space that overlies the surface of the brain. Three major subarachnoid cisterns, which contain cerebrospinal fluid, are also visible: the *quadrigeminal cistern*, which overlies the colliculi; the *interpeduncular cistern*, which lies ventral to the hypothalamus and between the cerebral peduncles; and the *cisterna magna*, which lies below the cerebellum.

Parasagittal Section Shows Shape of the Lateral Ventricle

Each lateral ventricle consists of four parts: the anterior (frontal) horn, the body, the posterior (occipital) horn, and the inferior (temporal) horn. The structure of the posterior (occipital) and the inferior (temporal) horn and their confluence (called the atrium) with the body of the lateral ventricle can be seen in the parasagittal slice shown in Figure 22-11.

The Corticospinal Tract Is Located on the Ventral Surface of the Medulla

The resolution of MRI is still not sufficient to distinguish nuclei in the gray matter of the medulla, especially nuclei in the central region that forms part of the reticular formation. However, the fourth ventricle and the corticospinal tracts (on the ventral surface of the medulla) can be identified (Figure 22–12). The surface characteristics of the cerebellum are particularly prominent, especially the cerebellar tonsils and the vermis. Note that the contents of the posterior fossa, which are partially obscured by bone-related artifact in comparable CT slices (Figures 22–3A and B), are clearly seen here because bone is invisible in MRI proton images.

The Dorsal Surface of the Pons Forms Part of the Floor of the Fourth Ventricle

At the pontine level (Figure 22–13), regions containing the medial lemnisci and corticospinal tracts can be distinguished from the surrounding tissue, as can the fourth ventricle. The descending cortical fibers, which at this level include the corticospinal fibers as well as fibers that terminate in the pons (corticopontine) and medulla (corticobulbar), are embedded within the pontine nuclei. The cerebral cortex influences the activity of cerebellar neurons via a relay in these nuclei.

The Superior and Inferior Colliculi Form the Dorsal Surface of the Midbrain

On the dorsal surface of the midbrain we can locate the superior colliculi (Figure 22–14), ventral to which is the midbrain tegmentum. Among its many structures, the midbrain tegmentum contains the medial lemnisci, the red nuclei, the substantia nigra, the crossing outflow of

the cerebellum, the oculomotor nuclei, and the reticular formation. It also contains the spinothalamic tracts, which relay information about pain to the thalamus. Ventral to the tegmentum are the basis pedunculi, which contain the corticospinal tracts as well as descending corticopontine and corticobulbar fibers. Together, the tegmentum and the basis pedunculi comprise the cerebral peduncles. The cerebral aqueduct can be seen, as can the interpeduncular and quadrigeminal cisterns. On this slice, the medial and inferior parts of the temporal lobes are seen, as are the orbital gyri of the frontal lobes. Because of the cephalic flexure, a transverse section through the midbrain cuts through the cerebral hemispheres longitudinally.

Horizontal Section Through the Cerebral Hemispheres Allows Both Cortical and Subcortical Structures to Be Visualized

Figure 22–15 is similar to the X-ray CT of Figures 22–3E and F and the third and fourth PET scans in the second row of Figure 22–5. The *insular cortex*, which becomes buried beneath the parietal, temporal, and frontal lobes during development (see Figure 21–8), subserves many functions, including perception of taste. In the temporal lobe, lateral to the insular cortex, is the *auditory cortex*. The *visual cortex* is located on the medial surface of the occipital lobe, in the banks of the calcarine fissure.

Deep structures can also be identified in this MRI scan. The walls of the third ventricle are formed by the thalamus and hypothalamus, which are separated from the caudate nucleus, putamen, and globus pallidus by the fibers of the *internal capsule*. The internal capsule is shaped like a fan and in horizontal section it appears as an arrowhead, with its point, the genu, flanked by the anterior and posterior limbs. The anterior limb of the internal capsule separates the head of the caudate nucleus, which bulges into the anterior horn of the lateral ventricle, from the putamen and the globus pallidus. The genu and the posterior limb of the internal capsule separate the thalamus from the more lateral components of the basal ganglia. Because axons of the ascending sensory and descending motor systems form a relatively compact bundle of fibers in this area, damage to this region is often devastating. Occlusion of the vascular supply for the internal capsule can result in motor deficits on the opposite side of the body because the descending motor axons cross the midline in the caudal medulla. This slice is similar to the one shown in Figure 21-14B, 2, where we saw that the tail of the caudate nucleus is just posterior to the thalamus. The tail of the caudate nucleus forms part of the roof of the inferior horn of the lateral ventricle. This section therefore cuts the caudate nucleus and lateral ventricle twice. The anterior portion of the lateral ventricle is not well visualized in this slice. Because cerebrospinal fluid appears dark on this scan, the subarachnoid space delimits the gyral and sulcal folds of the cortex.

272

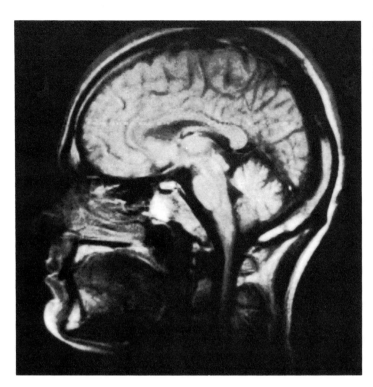

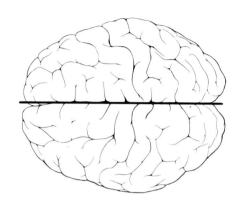

22–10 MRI scan of a midsagittal slice through the cerebral hemispheres, corpus callosum, brain stem, and spinal cord reveals C-shaped structures. Whereas dense bone is not seen on MRI, marrow is. (Courtesy of Phillips Medical Systems, Inc.)

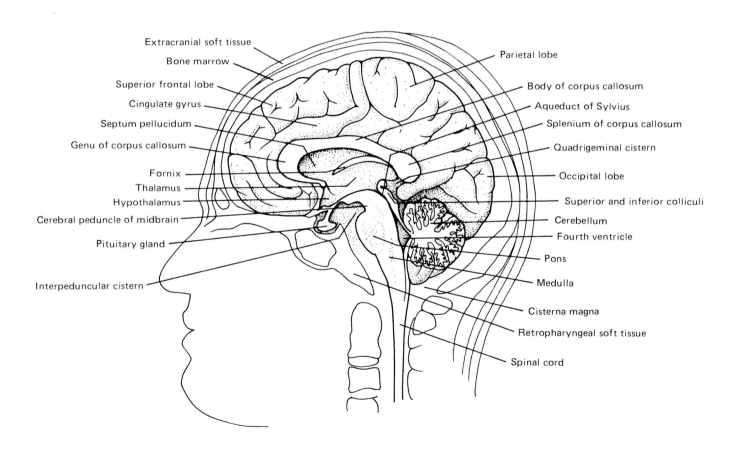

Extracranial soft tissue

Bone marrow

Superior frontal lobe

Cingulate gyrus

Septum pellucidum

Genu of corpus callosum

Fornix

Thalamus

Hypothalamus

Cerebral peduncle of midbrain

Pituitary gland

Interpeduncular cistern

Parietal lobe

Body of corpus callosum

Aqueduct of Sylvius

Splenium of corpus callosum

Quadrigeminal cistern

Occipital lobe

Superior and inferior colliculi

Cerebellum

Fourth ventricle

Pons

Medulla

Cisterna magna

Retropharyngeal soft tissue

Spinal cord

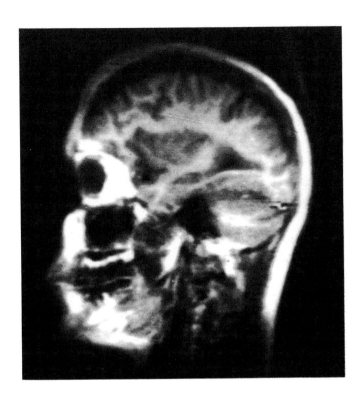

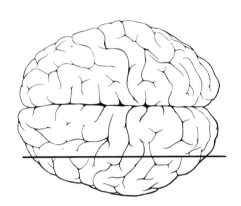

22–11 MRI scan of a parasagittal slice through the cerebral hemispheres and cerebellum shows the shape of the lateral ventricle. (Courtesy of Phillips Medical Systems, Inc.)

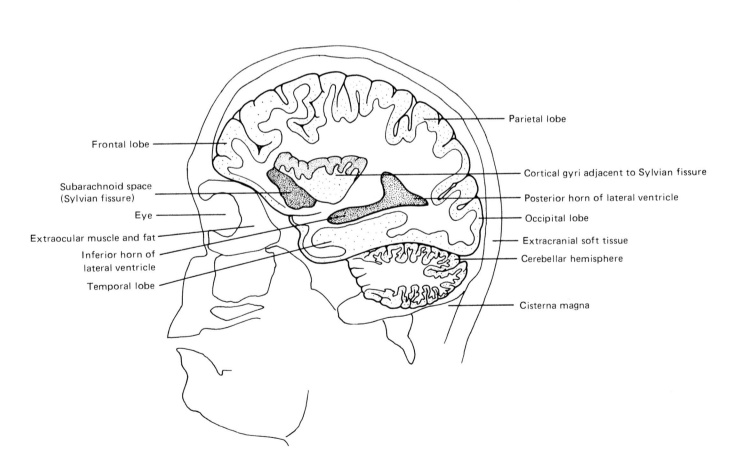

Frontal lobe

Subarachnoid space
(Sylvian fissure)

Eye

Extraocular muscle and fat

Inferior horn of
lateral ventricle

Temporal lobe

Parietal lobe

Cortical gyri adjacent to Sylvian fissure

Posterior horn of lateral ventricle

Occipital lobe

Extracranial soft tissue

Cerebellar hemisphere

Cisterna magna

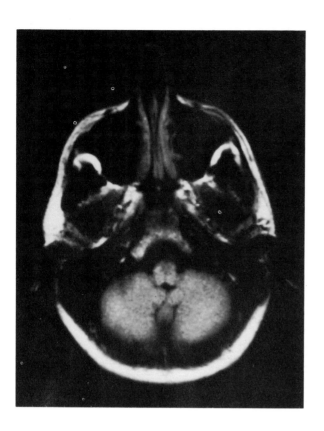

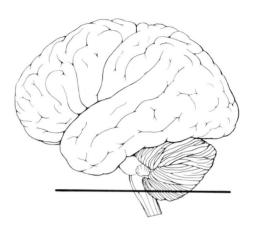

22–12 MRI scan of a transverse slice through the medulla and cerebellum shows that the corticospinal tracts are located on the ventral surface of the medulla. The tonsilar (Latin, tonsil) portion of the cerebellum is also clearly seen. (Courtesy of Phillips Medical Systems, Inc.)

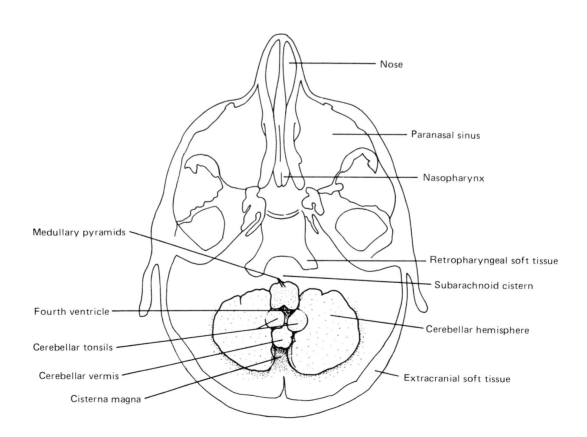

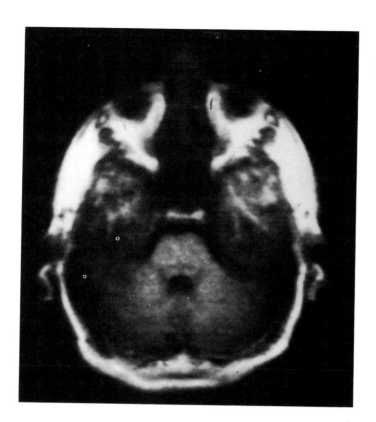

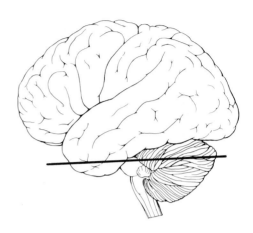

22–13 MRI scan of a transverse slice through the pons and cerebellum shows that the dorsal surface of the pons forms part of the floor of the fourth ventricle. (Courtesy of Phillips Medical Systems, Inc.)

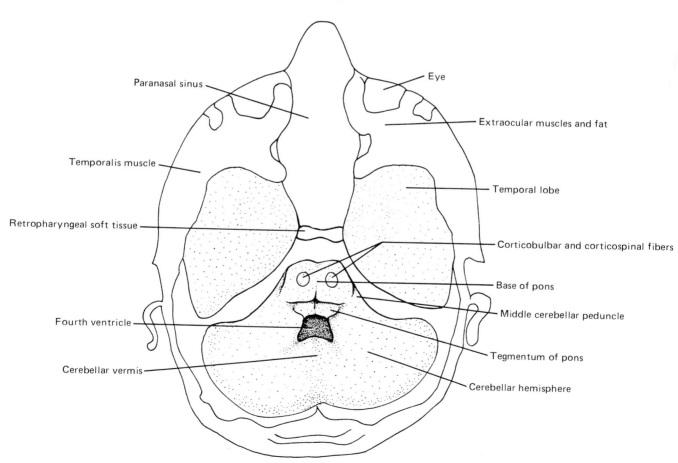

Paranasal sinus

Eye

Extraocular muscles and fat

Temporalis muscle

Temporal lobe

Retropharyngeal soft tissue

Corticobulbar and corticospinal fibers

Base of pons

Middle cerebellar peduncle

Fourth ventricle

Tegmentum of pons

Cerebellar vermis

Cerebellar hemisphere

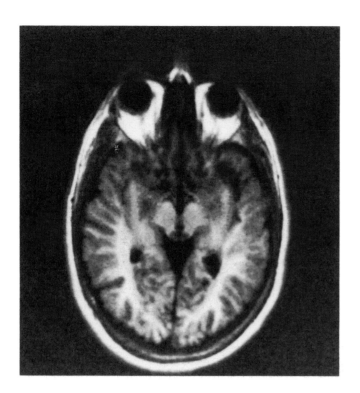

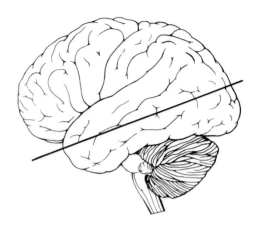

22–14 MRI scan of a horizontal slice through the hemispheres (horizontal plane) and midbrain (transverse plane) shows that the superior and inferior colliculi form the dorsal surface of the midbrain. (Courtesy of Phillips Medical Systems, Inc.)

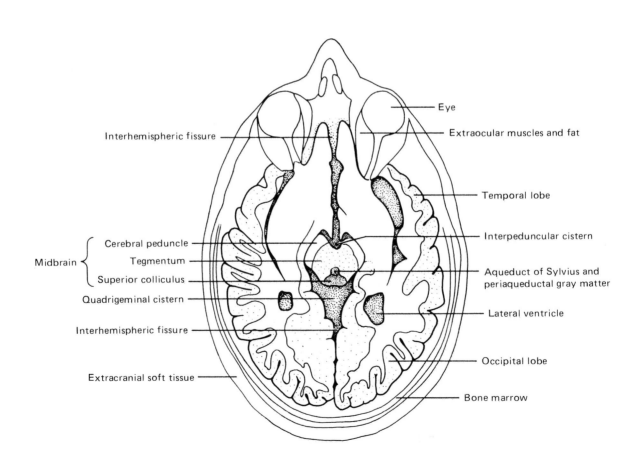

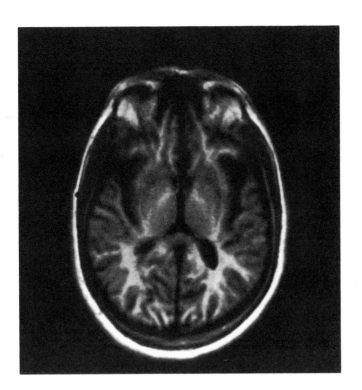

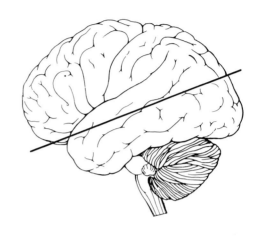

22–15 MRI scan of a horizontal section through the cerebral hemispheres and diencephalon allows both cortical and subcortical structures to be visualized. A series of alternating gray matter and white matter structures can be seen. From lateral to medial, these are (1) the insular cortex, (2) the extreme capsule, (3) the claustrum, (4) the external capsule, and (5) the lenticular nucleus. (Courtesy of Phillips Medical Systems, Inc.)

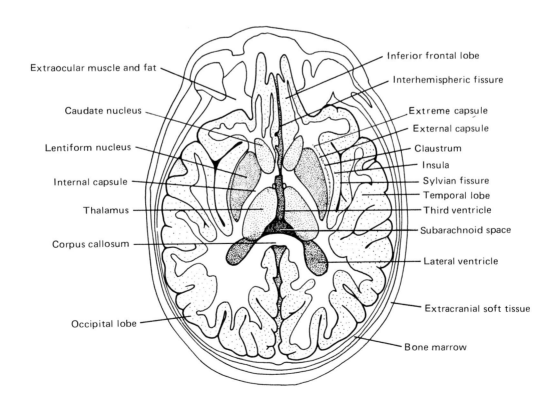

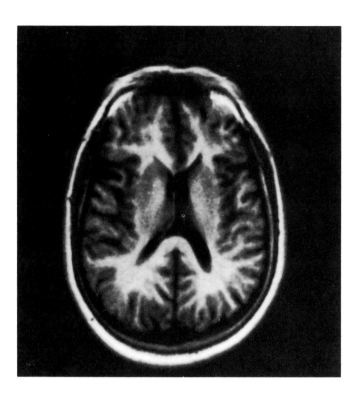

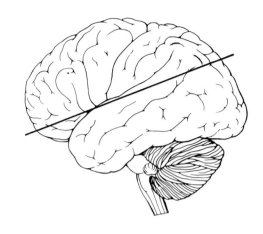

22–16 MRI scan of a horizontal slice through the cerebral hemispheres and basal ganglia shows that the caudate nucleus forms the wall of the anterior horn and body of the lateral ventricle. (Courtesy of Phillips Medical Systems, Inc.)

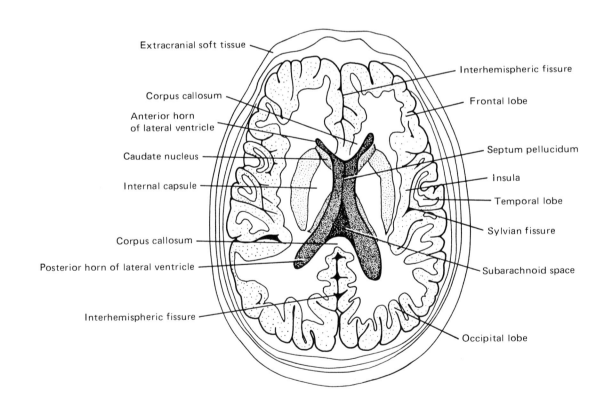

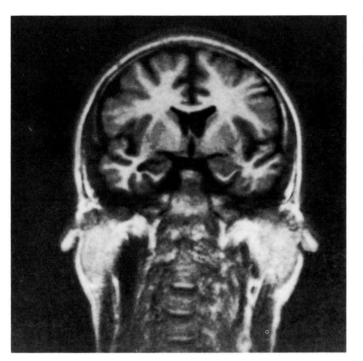

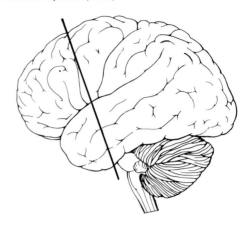

22–17 MRI scan of a coronal section through the cerebral hemispheres and basal ganglia shows that the anterior limb of the internal capsule separates the caudate nucleus from the globus pallidus and putamen. (Courtesy of Phillips Medical Systems, Inc.)

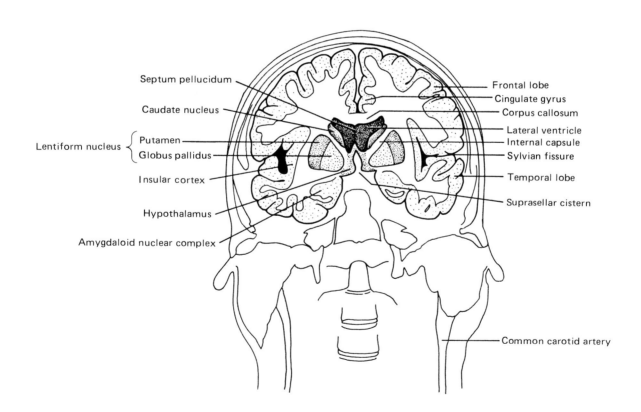

Septum pellucidum

Caudate nucleus

Lentiform nucleus { Putamen

Globus pallidus

Insular cortex

Hypothalamus

Amygdaloid nuclear complex

Frontal lobe

Cingulate gyrus

Corpus callosum

Lateral ventricle

Internal capsule

Sylvian fissure

Temporal lobe

Suprasellar cistern

Common carotid artery

*The Caudate Nucleus Forms the Wall of the
Anterior Horn and Body of the Lateral Ventricle*

The head of the caudate nucleus bulges into the anterior
horn of the lateral ventricle (Figure 22–16). The body of
the caudate nucleus forms the wall of the body of the
lateral ventricle. The putamen is located lateral to the
caudate nucleus. Collectively, the caudate nucleus and
putamen receive information from wide areas of the cerebral cortex and project via the globus pallidus to the
thalamus and then to cortical motor regions.

*The Anterior Limb of the Internal Capsule
Separates the Caudate Nucleus from the Globus
Pallidus and Putamen*

Figure 22–17 is a scan of a coronal section through the
basal ganglia, orthogonal to the horizontal section shown
in Figure 22–16. This plane of section is particularly useful for understanding the three-dimensional organization
of the brain. From lateral to medial we see the frontal
and temporal lobes, insular cortex, putamen, and globus
pallidus. The head of the caudate nucleus, which is separated from the putamen and globus pallidus by the anterior limb of the internal capsule, bulges into the lateral
ventricle.

The gray matter inferior to the globus pallidus and putamen is called the *substantia innominata* (Latin, un-
named substance). The different nuclei within this region
cannot be distinguished with current MRI scanning.
Most important among them is the *basal nucleus*, a collection of cholinergic neurons that project widely to dif-

ferent regions of cortex. In patients with Alzheimer's disease, a degenerative neurological disease characterized by
dementia, the cholinergic cells of the basal nuclei die.

Lateral and inferior to the substantia innominata are
the amygdaloid nuclear complex and the overlying cerebral cortex. Structures of the temporal lobe include the
hippocampus, a common site of epileptic seizures. As we
saw in Chapter 1, seizures originating here are often accompanied by bizarre behavior. Unlike motor seizures of the
frontal lobe, behaviors evoked by temporal lobe seizures
are influenced by psychological factors and by the environmental context in which the seizures occur. Because
part of the olfactory tract terminates in this region, olfactory hallucinations often accompany certain types of
temporal lobe seizures.

MRI Facilitates Clinical Diagnosis

The technique of MRI is based on the resonance of
atomic nuclei when placed in a strong magnetic field.
After such exposure, the time that it takes for a nucleus
to return to its previous state is called its "relaxation"
time (see Figure 22–9A). Relaxation times are variable
and depend on local tissue conditions. Figure 22–18 is an
MRI scan that incorporates particular relaxation time information into the image, increasing the contrast beyond
that obtained by mapping proton density alone. As a result, cerebrospinal fluid in the ventricles and the subarachnoid space appears white against the dark brain tissue.

Water content often varies during disease states. The
analysis of relaxation times provides a means of discriminating between normal brain tissue and that of patients
suffering from such pathological processes as small infarctions, small tumors, or the plaques of multiple sclerosis. In Figure 22–19, the diagnostic values of CT and
MRI are contrasted. In this horizontal section through
the cerebral cortex and underlying white matter of a

22–18 MRI scan of T_2 relaxation time (see Figure 22–9A
legend) produces a sharp image of cerebrospinal fluid
outlining cerebral ventricles and sulci. (Courtesy of Phillips
Medical Systems, Inc.)

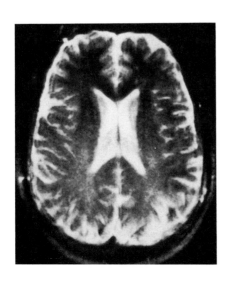

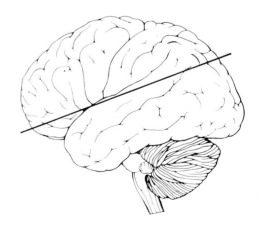

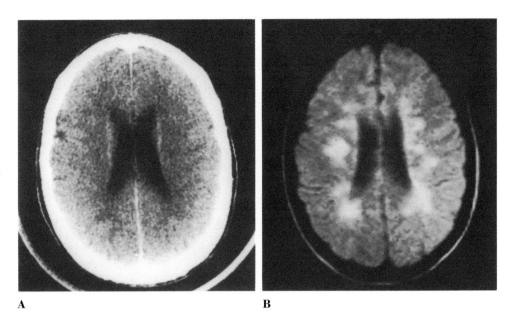

22–19 The diagnostic superiority of MRI to CT is shown in horizontal sections through the cerebral cortex and underlying white matter of a patient with multiple sclerosis. **A.** CT scan. **B.** MRI scan. Demyelination of white matter is visualized in this scan. (Courtesy of Dr. Michael Aminoff, University of California School of Medicine, San Francisco.)

A   B

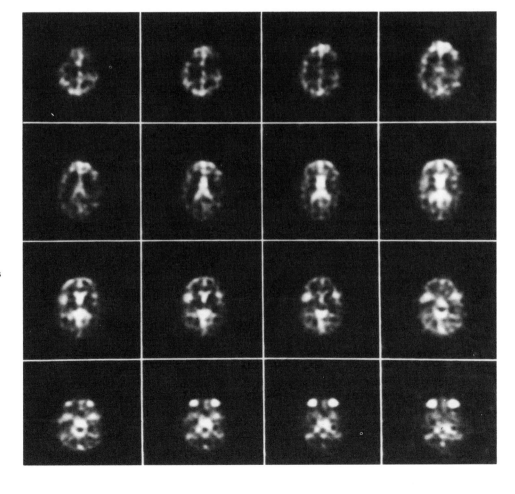

22–20 MRI scan in a normal person shows distribution of Na⁺. Slices from **top left** to **lower right** pass through successively more inferior levels of the cerebral hemispheres and brain stem. Note the prominent Na⁺ signal from cerebrospinal fluid in the lateral ventricles (**second and third rows**) and the subarachnoid space (**third row**) and from vitreous fluid of the eyes (**lower row**). (Courtesy of Dr. Sadek Hilal, Columbia University College of Physicians and Surgeons.)

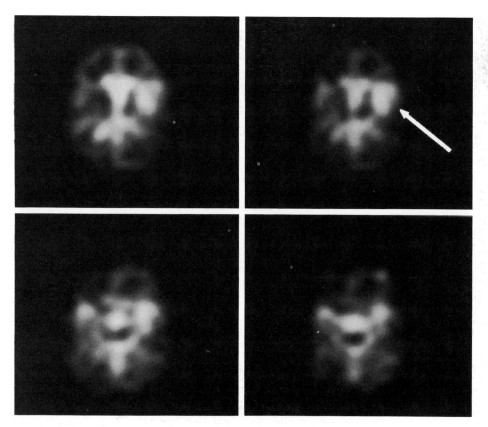

22–21 MRI scan in a patient with a recent cerebral infarction shows increased Na$^+$, indicating tissue death, at an infarction in the right frontal lobe **(arrow).** Slices are through cerebral hemispheres; most inferior **lower right,** most superior **upper left.** (Courtesy of Dr. Sadek Hilal, Columbia University College of Physicians and Surgeons.)

multiple sclerosis patient, local regions of demyelination in the white matter underlying the cerebral cortex are more clearly observed in the MRI scan.

MRI scanners are currently being developed that determine the presence of other atomic nuclei and biologically important compounds. Of particular interest are scans for Na$^+$, which is a sensitive probe for tissue death such as that which follows occlusion of a blood vessel in the brain. In dying tissue, the concentration of Na$^+$ rises more rapidly than that of water; Na$^+$ imaging may therefore reveal pathology earlier than proton imaging can. In Figure 22–20, 16 slices of a normal scan for Na$^+$ show little or no Na$^+$ signal arising from the brain parenchyma and a large Na$^+$ signal arising from the ventricles, the subarachnoid space, and the vitreous fluid of the eye; this is consistent with the fact that Na$^+$ is present primarily in the extracellular compartment. Four slices of a scan for Na$^+$ from a patient with a cerebral infarct are shown in Figure 22–21. A remarkable increase in Na$^+$ is observed at the site of the lesion (arrow).

Na$^+$ imaging requires a very strong magnetic field. So does phosphorus imaging, by which it is possible to display separately the various compounds of phosphorus involved in energy production, including organic phosphates, phosphocreatine, and ATP. Although MRI imaging is in an early stage of development, the technique is superior to CT for obtaining static images because it probes the body with non-ionizing energy that does not disrupt the molecules of living tissue. Moreover, with MRI it is possible to perform detailed chemical analysis of selected regions of body tissue in vivo.

An Overall View

High-resolution techniques are now available to provide images of the living brain—images based not only on X-ray transmission but on the biochemical activity of the tissue as well. The availability of in vivo biochemical analyses that are noninvasive allow the physician and neural scientist to probe cell-biological processes of neurons in health and disease. As our understanding of the anatomy of the living brain becomes greater, we will be able to localize disease processes and traumatic lesions in the brain more precisely, and to develop therapies to deal with them.

Selected Readings

Ascherl, G. F., Ganti, S. R., and Hilal, S. K. 1980. Neuroradiology for the clinician. In R. N. Rosenberg (ed.), The Science and Practice of Clinical Medicine, Vol. 5: Neurology. New York: Grune & Stratton, pp. 634–718.

Bradbury, E. M., Radda, G. K., and Allen, P. S. 1983. Nuclear magnetic resonance techniques in medicine. Ann. Intern. Med. 98:514–529.

Brownell, G. L., Budinger, T. F., Lauterbur, P. C., and McGeer, P. L. 1982. Positron tomography and nuclear magnetic resonance imaging. Science 215:619–626.

Oldendorf, W. H. 1980. The Quest for an Image of Brain. New York: Raven Press.

Pykett, I. L. 1982. NMR imaging in medicine. Sci. Am. 246(5):78–88.

References

Cormack, A. M. 1973. Reconstruction of densities from their projections, with applications in radiological physics. Phys. Med. Biol. 18:195–207.

Hounsfield, G. N. 1973. Computerized transverse axial scanning (tomography): Part 1. Description of system. Br. J. Radiol. 46:1016–1022.

Lauterbur, P. C. 1973. Image formation by induced local interactions. Examples employing nuclear magnetic resonance. Nature 242:190–191.

Lukes, S. A., Crooks, L. E., Aminoff, M. J., Kaufman, L., Panitch, H. S., Mills, C., and Norman, D. 1983. Nuclear magnetic resonance imaging in multiple sclerosis. Ann. Neurol. 13:592–601.

Phelps, M. E., Mazziotta, J. C., and Huang, S-C. 1982. Study of cerebral function with positron computed tomography. J. Cerebral Blood Flow Metab. 2:113–162.

Sokoloff, L. 1984. Modeling metabolic processes in the brain in vivo. Ann. Neurol. [Suppl] 15:S1–S11.

Wagner, H. N., Jr., Burns, H. D., Dannals, R. F., Wong, D. F., Langström, B., Duelfer, T., Frost, J. J., Ravert, H. T., Links, J. M., Rosenbloom, S. B., Lukas, S. E., Kramer, A. V., and Kuhar, M. J. 1984. Assessment of dopamine receptor densities in the human brain with carbon-11-labeled N-methylspiperone. Ann. Neurol. [Suppl] 15:S79–S84.

Sensory Systems of the Brain: Sensation and Perception

V

The brain functions both to perceive and to translate sensation into action. These two aspects of the nervous system are considered in the next two sections: Part V on Sensory Systems and Part VI on Motor Systems.

Familiar to all of us are the perceptions of sight, sound, smell, taste, touch, the sensation of our bodily movements (position sense and kinesthesia), and the awareness of pain. All of these perceptions originate in our sensory systems.

The modern study of these sensory systems begins with *psychophysics*, the establishment of quantitative correlations between specific aspects of physical stimuli and the sensations that they evoke. Important information can be obtained about the various classes of receptors, their specificity, the stimuli to which they respond, and the major sensory pathways that carry information from these receptors to the cerebral cortex. Thus, physiological events can be related to stimulus events, and both can be correlated with quantitative assessments of discriminative sensory behavior. As a result, we can begin to understand how the various sensory events that impinge upon us alter the activity of the brain and generate specific perceptions.

Sensory neurons—both peripheral receptors and central cells—often show remarkable specificity for a stimulus. This specificity is related to the location of the stimulus and its quality, dynamic properties, and configuration. Specificity is important for encoding within the nervous system some of the critical attributes of sensations. For encoding other attributes of sensation, however, the pattern of activity of sensory neurons also seems to be important.

A major task of current research in sensory physiology is to determine, for each sensory pathway, the extent to which codes for either specificity or pattern are used. We know, for example, that receptor specificity for sweet, sour, bitter, or salty is important in coding for different tastes. In contrast, the pitch of an auditory stimulus depends, in large part, on pattern coding. Many other sensory systems are more complicated and involve combinations of sensory neuron specificity and response pattern.

Sensory systems consist of serial chains of neurons that link the periphery with the spinal cord, brain stem, thalamus, and cerebral cortex. It is therefore important to learn which aspects of a given sensation are analyzed by structures at the different levels of the brain devoted to that sensibility. The most striking aspect of the orga- nization of sensory systems is that the peripheral recep- tor sheet (the body surface or the retina) is systematically mapped onto structures of the brain. These maps are not strictly isomorphic with the size and shape of the periph- ery but reflect the relative importance of the various re- gions of the receptive sheet.

Finally, the brain makes extensive use of parallel pro- cessing. Aspects of perception—of a visual object, a tac- tile sensation, or a melody—are carried and processed in parallel by different components of the specific sensory system committed to processing that perception. Each sensory system first decomposes the sensory information and then reconstructs the perception by using the differ- ent components that selectively process one or another aspect of the sensory experience.

John H. Martin

Receptor Physiology and Submodality Coding in the Somatic Sensory System

23

We all feel that our perceptions are precise and direct. However, as we shall see in these 10 chapters on sensory systems, this belief is an illusion—a perceptual illusion. We confront the world neither directly nor precisely, but, as Vernon Mountcastle has pointed out,

> . . . from a brain linked to what is "out there" by a few million fragile sensory nerve fibers, our only information channels, our lifelines to reality. They also provide what is essential for life itself: an afferent excitation that maintains the conscious state, the awareness of self.
>
> Sensations are set by the encoding functions of sensory nerve endings, and by the integrated neural mechanics of the central nervous system. Afferent nerve fibers are not high-fidelity recorders, for they accentuate certain stimulus features, neglect others. The central neuron is a story-teller with regard to the nerve fibers, and it is never completely trustworthy, allowing distortions of quality and measure. . . . *Sensation is an abstraction, not a replication, of the real world.*[1]

Contact with the external world occurs through specialized neural structures called *sensory receptors*. At these receptor organs, various natural stimuli that impinge upon our bodies are transformed into neurally relevant signals. We receive sensory information not only from the environment but also from within our bodies: from blood vessels, the viscera, and the actions of skeletal muscles on joints. To distinguish the systems that convey signals from these different sources the sensory systems are divided into three categories: exteroceptive, proprioceptive, and interoceptive.

---

[1]Mountcastle, V. B. 1975. The view from within: Pathways to the study of perception. Johns Hopkins Med. J. 136:109.

Exteroceptive systems are sensitive to external stimuli and include vision, audition, skin sensation, and some chemical senses. *Proprioceptive systems* provide information about the relative position of body segments to one another and about the position of the body in space. *Interoceptive systems* are concerned with internal bodily events such as blood pressure and the concentration of glucose in the blood. Unlike exteroceptive and proprioceptive stimuli, of which we are typically aware, interoceptive signals often do not reach consciousness.

The somatic sensory system, which is the subject of this and the next three chapters, receives and processes stimuli that impinge on the body surface or originate from within the deeper tissues and viscera. Thus, unlike the visual system, which is entirely exteroceptive, the somatic sensory system serves all three classes of stimulus reception. We may view the somatic sensory system as comprising several different perceptual *modalities*, or subclasses, each related to different stimuli. There are four major modalities:

1. *Tactile sensations*, elicited by mechanical stimulation applied to the body surface.
2. *Proprioceptive sensations*, elicited by mechanical displacements of the muscles and joints.
3. *Thermal sensations*, including separate cold and warm senses.
4. *Pain sensations*, elicited by noxious stimuli.

Each of the major modalities is mediated by a particular class of receptors. In this chapter we shall first consider how sensory systems are organized. Next we shall see how behavioral studies have made it possible to evaluate sensation quantitatively. These studies have therefore provided major insights into receptor function and central neural processing. After discussing how stimulus energy is encoded into neural signals, we shall examine the nature of receptor specificity and survey the types of known somatic receptors and their general physiological properties. In Chapters 24–26 we shall consider how the sensory modalities, which are initially processed by separate afferent information channels, converge in the spinal cord, then project to the thalamus, and finally reach the somatic sensory cortex.

Sensory Systems Are Organized in a Hierarchical and Parallel Fashion

Sensory systems are organized to receive, process, and relay stimulus information from the periphery to higher neural levels. Because in many ways the somatic sensory system is the most simply organized, it serves as a good introduction to the sensory systems as a whole.

The organization of a pathway for perception of somatic stimuli is schematically illustrated in Figure 23–1. The first neuron in the chain of events leading from the periphery to the central nervous system is the receptor neuron, which, in this example, is a dorsal root ganglion

cell. Receptor neurons convert or encode natural stimuli into neural events. Only the distal portion of the peripheral axonal branch of the dorsal root ganglion cell is specialized to encode stimulus energy. The remaining portion of the axon is specialized to conduct information, encoded in the form of action potentials, to the central nervous system. (In the visual and auditory systems stimulus encoding and information transmission are carried out by separate neurons.) A receptor neuron encodes stimulus information from a restricted region of the receptive surface. This region, called the neuron's *receptive field*, is the area of skin within which a stimulus excites the receptor.

Sensory systems are serially or *hierarchically organized*. Receptor neurons in the somatic sensory system converge onto second-order neurons in the central nervous system. The second-order neurons also have a receptive field because they receive input from receptor neurons. The second-order neurons, which may be located in the spinal cord or the medulla, project to third-order neurons in the thalamus. Neurons in the thalamus in turn project to the parietal lobe of the cerebral cortex. (In addition to this pathway for conscious perception, information about the stimulus is conveyed to motor neurons directly, or indirectly by interneurons, to mediate reflex functions. Movement is further controlled and modulated by afferent projections to supraspinal structures such as the cerebellum.)

Most modalities are subserved by more than one serially organized pathway (Figure 23–1). Indeed, as we shall see in Chapters 24 and 25, two important pathways mediate perception of somatic stimuli: the dorsal column–medial lemniscal pathway and the anterolateral pathway. These are examples of *parallel sensory pathways*, each serving somewhat different but overlapping functions. The parallel organization of sensory systems is important clinically because when one pathway is damaged the remaining pathway can mediate residual sensory capabilities.

Sensory Psychophysical Studies Correlate Behavior with the Physiology of Neurons

Before we consider the physiological properties of sensory neurons, let us briefly consider aspects of sensory experience that these neurons mediate. Sensory capacity reflects both the stimulus intensity necessary to elicit a perception and the precision with which the site of stimulation can be recognized. Different parts of the body vary greatly from one another in their sensory capacities. For example, the finger tips are very sensitive. When they move over a surface, their afferent fibers convey detailed sensory information about that surface to the central nervous system. In contrast, the skin over the elbow is limited to only the crudest discriminations. The need to quantify sensory experiences for scientific studies and clinical evaluation has led to the development of an

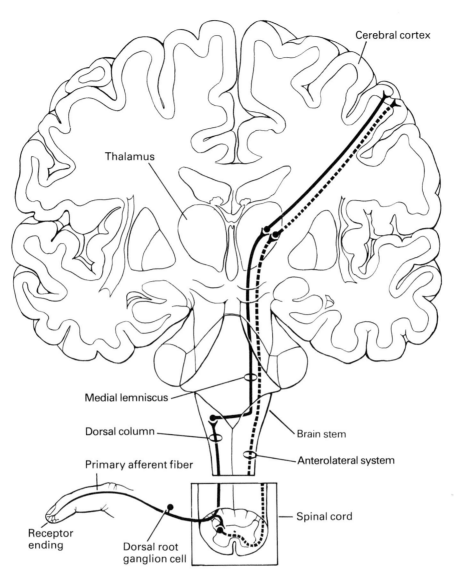

23–1 The hierarchical and parallel organization of sensory systems is demonstrated by two ascending parallel pathways: the main pathway for tactile sensations is termed the dorsal column–medial lemniscal system (**solid line**); and a circuit whose main function is to mediate pain and, to a much lesser extent, tactile sensations is termed the anterolateral system (**broken line**). Only when the dorsal column–medial lemniscal pathway becomes damaged, as in certain degenerative neurological disorders, does the anterolateral pathway assume an important role in mediating tactile sensations.

area of experimental psychology termed *sensory psychophysics.*

Psychophysical investigation allows us to explore the performance of the neural machinery that constitutes a sensory system. In addition, the quantitative methods used in psychophysics for investigating sensory phenomena provide effective tools for correlating behavior with the response properties of neurons. To illustrate this correlation we shall consider three psychophysical observations that can be explained by the properties of afferent fibers: sensory threshold, evaluation of stimulus intensity, and two-point discrimination.

Sensory Thresholds for Perception and for Afferent Fibers May Be Equal

The *absolute sensory threshold* is the lowest stimulus intensity a subject can detect. Threshold is determined statistically. If a subject is given several series of stimuli of different intensities, the intensity at which the stimulus is first detected in each series (i.e., the threshold) will differ slightly. Moreover, if a subject receives a series of stimuli whose intensity is close to the average threshold, the subject typically fails to detect a certain proportion of stimuli. It is therefore convenient to define

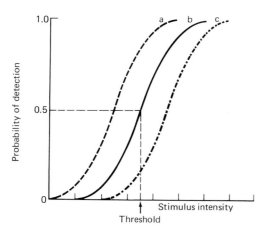

23–2 Absolute sensory threshold (**curve b**) is an idealized representation of the relationship between stimulus intensity and the probability of stimulus detection. **Curve a** would be observed if either the detectability of the sensory system increased or response criterion decreased; **curve c** illustrates the converse.

threshold as that stimulus intensity detected in 50% of the trials (Figure 23–2, curve b).

In addition to measuring a subject's threshold for detecting a stimulus, we can also measure the threshold of a particular class of afferent fibers to the same stimulus. Usually the psychophysical observations are obtained from human subjects and the afferent fiber recordings from experimental animals. Recently, however, Å. B. Vallbo and colleagues at the University of Umea, Sweden, recorded from afferent fibers in alert (unanesthetized) humans and were able to combine the psychophysical and physiological experiments. They were thus able to compare directly the subject's appraisal of a stimulus with the afferent fiber response patterns elicited by the stimulus. By this means, Vallbo and his colleagues found that the absolute sensory threshold sometimes also coincides with the threshold of the afferent fiber. In this situation, detection of a mechanical stimulus corresponds to the activity in a single afferent fiber! Although the afferent fiber threshold can represent the minimum psychophysical threshold, generally the psychophysical threshold is higher.

Why is this so? Why is the psychophysical threshold not invariably linked to the activity of a single afferent fiber? Detailed studies have shown that sensory thresholds are not fixed, but can be modified by the context of expectation in which the stimulus is detected. For example, in experiments testing sensory threshold, subjects frequently report a *false alarm*—a sensory experience (i.e., detection) when no stimulus is actually presented. The occurrence of false alarms can be reconciled with the sensory threshold by means of the theory of *signal detection* developed by W. P. Tanner and J. A. Swets. According to this theory a subject's stimulus-detecting capabil-

ities can be divided into two components, each of which can be measured separately: (1) the absolute *detectability* of the sensory system under examination, and (2) the *criterion* the subject uses to evaluate the presence (or absence) of a stimulus. In some contexts it may be advantageous never to miss the occurrence of a stimulus; in these circumstances an individual is more likely to report the presence of a stimulus when the stimulus is absent. Consider the soldier in a foxhole who might duck at the mere mention of gunfire. His anxiety, caused by danger, would manifest itself as a decrease in the observed threshold (Figure 23–2, curve a). Similarly, thresholds can increase; for example, the threshold for pain is often heightened during competitive sporting events (Figure 23–2, curve c). These changes in sensory threshold do not result from changes in receptor threshold in the periphery, but rather from changes in the threshold of neurons within the central nervous system.

Stimulus Intensity Evaluation Is Correlated with the Discharge Rate of Afferent Fibers

Not only is the somatic sensory system remarkably sensitive in detecting when stimuli occur, but it also provides information about the magnitude of the stimulus. This is important for our ability to discriminate between stimuli and to estimate stimulus intensity.

The capacity to distinguish stimuli that differ only in magnitude depends on how large the stimuli are. Consider the discrimination of two weights. One can perceive a 1-kg weight as different from a 2-kg weight; but it is very difficult to distinguish between a 50- and a 51-kg weight. Yet both sets differ by only 1 kg! This phenomenon was examined in 1834 by Ernst Weber, who developed a quantitative relationship between stimulus intensity and discrimination, now known as Weber's law. This law states that

$$\Delta S = K \times S$$

where ΔS is the minimal intensity difference that can be perceived relative to a reference stimulus S (i.e., background), and K is a constant. Thus, as the intensity of the reference stimulus increases, the difference in magnitude necessary to perceive a second stimulus as different from the reference stimulus also increases.

In 1860, Gustav Fechner modified Weber's law and described the mathematical relationship between stimulus intensity and the intensity of the sensation experienced by a subject,

$$I = K \log \frac{S}{S_0}$$

where I is the subjectively experienced intensity, S_0 is the threshold, S is the suprathreshold stimulus used in the estimation of stimulus magnitude, and K is a constant.

In 1953, S. S. Stevens at Harvard University noted that subjective experience is proportional not to the logarithm, as Fechner described, but to the nth power of the intensity of the suprathreshold stimulus. Over an extended range of stimulus intensity, subjective experience is best described by a power rather than by a logarithmic relationship:

$$I = K \times (S - S_0)^n$$

This is important because natural stimuli vary greatly in intensity. Consider the range of sounds that we experience, from a whisper to a shout.

As we shall see in our discussion of the physiological properties of peripheral receptors, an increase in discharge rate of primary afferent fibers parallels the increase in stimulus intensity. This relationship between receptor physiology and sensory experience is an important mechanism for encoding stimulus intensity.

Spatial Discrimination Is Explained by Receptor Innervation Density

Weber's early work on somatic sensation highlighted two attributes of the awareness of the spatial aspects of sensory experience: (1) the ability to localize the site of stimulation, and (2) the ability to distinguish two closely spaced stimuli. The capacity to resolve two stimuli is quantified by measuring the distance between the stimuli, a measurement that Weber called the *two-point threshold*. The two-point threshold is 1 mm at the finger tip and increases markedly for more proximal parts of the body. The palm, for instance, has a two-point threshold of 10 mm; the arm, 20 mm. As the two-point threshold increases from the finger tip to the arm, there is a corresponding decrease in the accuracy with which we are able to localize the site of stimulation. Insight into the neural mechanisms for fine spatial discriminations on the finger tips have come from the work of Vallbo and his colleagues, who have systematically evaluated the receptive fields of mechanoreceptors that innervate the glabrous, or hairless, skin of the human hand. Vallbo found that the density of receptor innervation is four times greater on the finger tips than on the palm. The greater detail in the fine-grain resolution of the receptive sheet is reflected in a greater spatial sensory capacity.

Stimulus Features Are Electrically Encoded by Receptors

Sensory Transduction Is the First Step in the Extraction of Stimulus Features

In the periphery, the unmyelinated ending of a single afferent fiber forms one kind of receptor. Here we shall consider the process by which the receptive portion of an afferent fiber converts natural stimulus energy into neural activity. This is the process of *stimulus transduction*. To activate a receptor, a stimulus must be of suitable intensity (greater than threshold) as well as of suitable quality. The dimensions of the receptive field

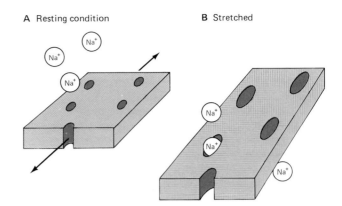

23–3 Mechanoelectric transduction changes the mechanical energy of the stimulus into electrical energy that results in the receptor potential. **A.** In the resting condition the mechanoreceptive membrane allows few Na$^+$ ions to pass because the effective channel size is small. **B.** Stretching the membrane increases the effective channel size, thereby allowing more Na$^+$ to flow across the membrane into the cell while K$^+$ can simultaneously flow out.

typically exceed the regions of tissue directly innervated, since stimulus energy can be transmitted through body tissue.

The key to understanding sensory transduction lies in the analysis of the *receptor* (or *generator*) *potential*, which is a local depolarizing potential that propagates only by electrotonic means and is therefore restricted to the receptive membrane. The potential is produced by an opening of cation channels selective for Na$^+$ and K$^+$, similar to those that produce the excitatory postsynaptic potential (see Chapter 10). The transductive process is shown schematically in Figure 23–3 for a receptor sensitive to mechanical energy (mechanoreceptor). In the resting condition few channels in the receptive membrane are open. Mechanical stimulation deforms the membrane, causing its physical characteristics to change. In this stimulated condition more channels open and more Na$^+$ and K$^+$ ions flow through the membrane.

The physiological properties of different parts of the primary afferent fiber are illustrated in Figure 23–4. Stretching the skin of the receptive field results in a receptor potential in the receptive membrane. When the amplitude of the receptor potential reaches the threshold of the trigger zone, an action potential is generated (see Chapter 10). The trigger zone is located on the myelinated portion of the axon. Because the trigger zone is close to the receptive membrane, the potential across this region reflects the sum of the receptor potential and action potentials. Farther from the receptive membrane and trigger zone, only action potentials are recorded. Suprathreshold stimuli lead to receptor potentials with faster rates of rise and greater amplitude. These receptor potentials evoke trains of action potentials at progressively higher frequencies.

A

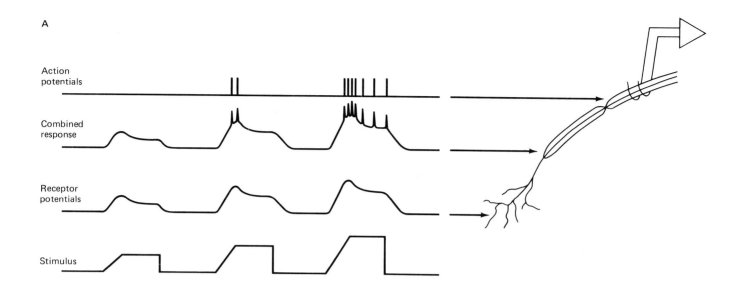

Action
potentials

Combined
response

Receptor
potentials

Stimulus

B

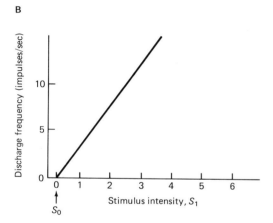

23–4 Recordings from different parts of a primary afferent fiber sensitive to skin stretch show that they differ in their physiological characteristics. **A.** Afferent fiber (**right**) and associated physiological responses of its three different portions (**left**): the receptor potential in the receptive membrane, the interaction of the receptor potential with the spike-generating membrane at the trigger zone, and the propagated impulse at the first node of Ranvier. **B.** Graph illustrates discharge frequency (recorded from myelinated portion of axon a few millimeters away from ending) as a function of stimulus intensity. Afferent fibers begin discharging action potentials when the stimulus amplitude reaches S_0 (the absolute physiological threshold). At lesser amplitudes only nonpropagated receptor potentials are generated. The absolute physiological threshold is important because stimulus information reaches the central nervous system only when action potentials are generated.

Stimulus Intensity Is Encoded by Frequency and Population Codes

Edgar Adrian first noted in the 1920s that the discharge frequency of any given afferent fiber increases with increasing stimulus intensity. This function is known as the *frequency code* for stimulus intensity. Stronger stimuli evoke larger receptor potentials, which cause not only a greater number of action potentials but also action potentials at higher frequencies (Figure 23–4B). The relationship between discharge frequency and stimulus intensity resembles the relationship between a subject's estimate of the magnitude of a stimulus and its intensity.

Stronger stimuli also activate a correspondingly greater number of receptors, so that stimulus intensity is also encoded in the size of the responding population. The term *population code* is therefore used to describe the activity of the ensemble of responding receptors. Thus, as the stimulus intensity becomes greater, it is en-

coded in two ways: (1) each afferent fiber conducts a greater number of action potentials and (2) more fibers are activated. (As we shall see in Part VI, these principles also apply to the motor systems, where an increase in both the size of the population of active neurons and their frequency of firing determine the strength of muscle contraction.)

Rapid Receptor Adaptation Is a Form of Feature Extraction

An important feature of all somatic receptors is that they adapt. The receptor potential invariably decreases in amplitude in response to a maintained and constant stimulus, but it may do so either slowly or rapidly. An example of a *slowly adapting receptor* is the muscle spindle receptor, which is located within muscle and is sensitive to stretch. An example of a *rapidly adapting receptor* is the Pacinian corpuscle, which is located in subcutaneous tissue and is sensitive to vibration. The Pacinian corpuscle responds only transiently at stimulus onset and sometimes also at the end of a step change in stimulus position.

Adaptation often results from characteristic properties of the excitable membrane of the sensory neuron. However, in the case of the Pacinian corpuscle, adaptation depends on the *nonneural accessory structure that surrounds the central unmyelinated axon.* This accessory structure consists of concentric layers of connective tissue, resembling the layers of an onion, surrounding an afferent nerve fiber terminal (Figure 23–5A). A steady stimulus applied to the outermost layer deforms the inner unmyelinated axon, but there is transverse slippage between the layers of the accessory structure so that, with time, the effective stimulus reaching the axon decreases. As a result, the accessory structure filters steady or slow components of mechanical stimuli and the receptor responds only to rapid changes in pressure (Figure 23–5B). As W. R. Lowenstein and M. Mendelson showed in 1965, removal of the connective tissue accessory structure transforms the Pacinian corpuscle from a rapidly adapting receptor into a slowly adapting one (Figure 23–5C).

Rapid adaptation in the Pacinian corpuscle is an example of a simple form of *feature extraction*—the selective detection by sensory neurons of only certain features of a stimulus. With a steady and maintained stimulus, the duration is uniquely defined by stimulus onset and offset. Any intervening neural discharges are redundant and carry no additional information.

Different Classes of Afferent Fibers Conduct Action Potentials at Different Rates

The speed at which an afferent fiber conducts action potentials is related to the diameter of the fiber (see Chapter 7). In large myelinated fibers, the conduction velocity (in meters per second) is approximately equal to six times the diameter (in micrometers). The ratio is smaller for smaller myelinated fibers and smaller still for unmyelinated fibers.

To investigate the composition of afferent fibers in peripheral nerves it is essential that efferent fibers be eliminated. The simplest way to accomplish this is to remove the efferent fibers from peripheral nerve in experimental animals by cutting both the ventral roots (which contain the axons of the somatic motor neurons) and the nerve trunks that contain the postganglionic motor supply (the gray rami). To ensure that the motor fibers distal to the transection degenerate, the animals are then allowed to recover for about 4 months before the nerves, now thought to contain *only* afferent fibers, are examined histologically.[2] The afferent fibers in the nerve then are counted, their diameters are measured, and a frequency

---

[2]Richard Coggeshall and his colleagues at the University of Texas at Galveston have shown that the ventral roots, once thought to carry only motor axons, also carry some afferent fibers. However, there are relatively few ventral root afferents, and we shall not consider them here.

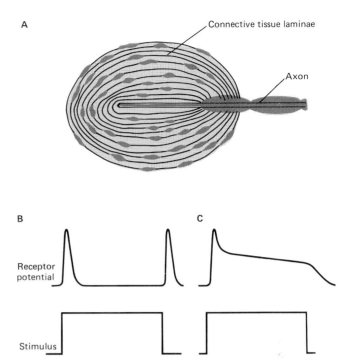

23–5 The Pacinian corpuscle is a rapidly adapting receptor in the skin that is sensitive to vibration. **A.** A cross section of this receptor reveals concentrically arranged layers of connective tissue surrounding the sensory nerve terminal. **B.** An intact Pacinian corpuscle responds with a receptor potential only to the onset and offset of a mechanical stimulus. **C.** If the connective tissue laminae are removed, the receptor responds to the same mechanical stimulus in a slowly adapting manner. (Adapted from Lowenstein and Mendelson, 1965).

distribution histogram of fiber diameter is constructed. These histograms show that afferent fibers innervating muscle differ from those innervating the skin (Figure 23–6). The histogram for an afferent nerve from muscle has four peaks, corresponding to large myelinated (I), small myelinated (II), smaller myelinated (III), and unmyelinated (IV) fibers (Figure 23–6A). Rather than adhere to this numerical classification, which is used for muscle afferents, physiologists studying cutaneous nerves chose another nomenclature: Aα, Aβ, Aδ, and C. The histogram for cutaneous nerves has only three peaks because the group I (or Aα) afferents are absent in cutaneous nerves. The physiological properties of these group I afferents will be considered in detail in Chapter 34. In Table 23–1 the numerical and the alphabetical schemes are compared, and the fiber diameters and conduction velocities are given for each group.

The conduction velocity of a fiber has important functional significance. The faster a fiber conducts action potentials, the quicker the central nervous system receives the information. Consider that in an average adult a stimulus delivered to a finger tip activates receptors that are located about 1 m from the spinal cord. An Aβ fiber,

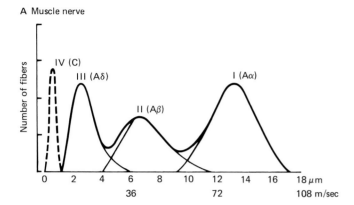

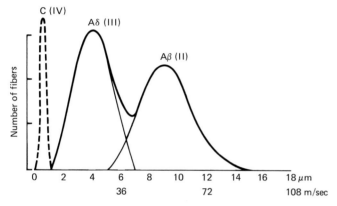

23-6 The distribution of axonal diameters (in micrometers) and conduction velocities (in meters per second) differs in different types of afferent fibers. **A.** Muscle fibers. **B.** Cutaneous fibers. (Adapted from Boyd and Davey, 1968).

conducting at 50 m/sec, conveys its information to the central nervous system in 0.02 sec. In contrast, a C fiber, conducting at the rate of 0.5 m/sec, takes 2 sec or more to convey the information it carries to the central nervous system. If the stimulus is noxious and carried only by the C fibers, damage to the finger tip can begin long before the central nervous system receives the information. Time delays also occur in the central processing of a stimulus, which further increase the possibility of damage.

Table 23-1. Afferent Fiber Groups

Muscle nerve	Cutaneous nerve	Fiber diameter (μm)	Conduction velocity (m/sec)
I		13–20	80–120
II	Aβ	6–12	35–75
III	Aδ	1–5	5–30
IV[a]	C[a]	0.2–1.5	0.5–2

[a]Unmyelinated.

Different Classes of Somatic Receptors Are Sensitive to Different Stimuli

Stimulus Quality Is Encoded by a Labeled Line Code

How do afferent fibers encode stimulus quality? Does perception of stimulus quality depend on *receptor specificity* (so that only a particular receptor responds selectively to one type of stimulus), or does quality depend on the *temporal pattern of activity* in a single class of relatively nonspecific receptors? Modern electrophysiological techniques have made it possible to distinguish between these two possibilities by demonstrating that single receptors and the afferent fibers to which they connect exhibit specificity of response. The same sensation will always be elicited whether a receptor is activated by a natural (or *adequate*) stimulus or its afferent fiber is activated artificially (by electrical stimulation). An excellent illustration of this principle is that electrical stimulation of the optic nerve produces a sensation of light. Specificity resulting from specialized or committed neural pathways was first proposed by Johannes Müller in 1826 and forms the basis for what we now call a *labeled line code*, in contrast to a *pattern code*, in which an uncommitted pathway can signal different sensations by using different patterns of firing. Pattern codes do not seem to be important for coding stimulus quality by afferent fibers in the somatic sensory system. Almost all the coding is done by labeled lines.

On the basis of their selective response to stimuli, three major classes of somatic receptors can be distinguished: nociceptors, thermoreceptors, and mechanoreceptors.

Pain Is Mediated by Nociceptors

The receptors that respond selectively to damaging stimuli are called *nociceptors* (Latin *nocere*, to injure). They are connected to axons belonging to two fiber classes: Aδ and C. There are three main types of nociceptors: (1) *Mechanical nociceptors* are activated only by strong mechanical stimulation and most effectively by sharp objects. No response is evoked in this type of nociceptor when a blunt probe is pressed firmly into the skin, but a pinprick or pinch causes a brisk response (Figure 23-7). (2) *Heat nociceptors* respond when the receptive field is heated to temperatures greater than 45°C, the heat pain threshold in humans. (3) *Polymodal nociceptors* respond equally to all kinds of noxious stimuli—mechanical, heat, and chemical. Morphologically, nociceptors are bare nerve endings. It is not known, however, whether nociceptors respond directly to the noxious stimulus or indirectly by means of one or more chemical intermediaries released from the traumatized tissue.

We recognize two different types of pain: fast and slow. *Fast pain* is an abrupt and sharp sensation that is carried by Aδ fibers. *Slow pain*, carried by C fibers, is a

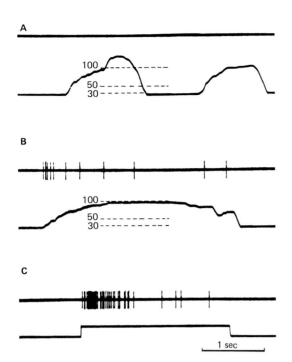

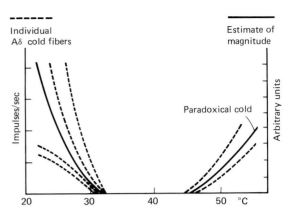

23–8 The rate of discharge of individual monkey Aδ cold fibers (**broken lines**) parallels human verbal estimations of the magnitude (**solid lines**) of cold stimuli of comparable intensities and durations (**left**). A heat stimulus applied to a cold receptor also elicits a response, but the human subject reports the sensation as cold (**right**).

23–7 The selective sensitivity of a mechanical nociceptor with a myelinated afferent fiber is revealed by the response of the receptor (**upper trace** in each part) to different types of stimuli (**lower trace** in each part). A blunt tip of 2 mm (**A**) elicited no response from this nociceptor, but the tip of a needle (**B**) produced a modest response. (In **A** and **B**, the lower trace shows the output of the calibrated probe in grams.) In contrast, a pinch with a serrated forceps (**C**) produced a brisk response. (Adapted from Perl, 1968.)

sickening burning sensation, which follows fast pain. Both types of pain can be felt in succession when, for example, the web between the fingers is pinched hard and quickly by the fingernails.

Thermal Sensation Is Mediated by Cold and Warm Receptors

Temperature sensitivity is punctate: separate hot and cold spots on the skin (each approximately 1 mm in diameter) correspond to discrete zones of innervation where thermal stimulation elicits the sensation of either warmth or cold. The threshold for eliciting a thermal sensation at these spots is considerably lower than at surrounding regions.

Cold receptors are connected to fibers that belong to the same bands of the fiber spectrum as the pain fibers, the Aδ and C fibers. The cold fibers discharge intensely when a cold stimulus is delivered, and the frequency of firing is proportional to the rate and extent of temperature lowering, as are the psychophysical responses (Figure 23–8).

A curious sensory illusion called *paradoxical cold* can be demonstrated by applying a heat stimulus of 45°C to

a cold spot on the skin (Figure 23–8). This stimulus is ordinarily painful when applied to diffusely innervated areas of skin, but when applied to a single cold spot it is experienced by the subject not as hot, but as cold. Normally, the cold receptors are excited by decreasing the temperature, and the range of their optimal activation is between 30° and 10°C. In this range they respond best to small decreases in temperature. However, beyond this range these receptors respond even to a heat stimulus. Thus, a stimulus of 45°C applied to a cold spot excites the cold receptors and causes them to fire more rapidly. This is another example of a labeled line code. Regardless of the mode of activation, activity in the cold fiber population elicits the sensation of cold.

There is also an interesting relation between the psychophysics of warmth and heat pain (Figure 23–9). Warmth is mediated by unmyelinated C warm fibers,

23–9 The rate of discharge of individual monkey C warm fibers (**broken lines**) and the human estimation of the magnitude (**solid line**) of heat stimuli differ when the temperature exceeds 45° and activates heat nociceptors instead.

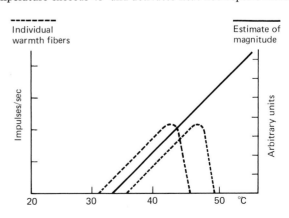

whereas the initial pain associated with intense heat is mediated by heat nociceptors (Aδ). Therefore, for warm stimuli (less than 45°C), there is a strong correlation between the discharge properties of warm fibers and estimations of warmth (Figure 23–9), but the correlation is only weak for hot stimuli (greater than 45°C). In contrast, the discharge of heat nociceptors (not shown) correlates well with perceived heat pain, but not with perceived warmth. Thermal receptors, like nociceptors, are free nerve endings.

Tactile Sensations Are Mediated by Slowly and Rapidly Adapting Mechanoreceptors

Tactile sensation, like the other somatic sensory modalities, is mediated by a single class of receptor, the mechanoreceptor. The axons of mechanoreceptors conduct action potentials in the Aβ range. These receptors can be divided into two major groups: the slowly adapting mechanoreceptors, which respond continuously to an enduring stimulus, and the rapidly adapting mechanoreceptors, which respond only at the onset (and perhaps also the termination) of a long-lasting stimulus.

Glabrous skin (such as that on the finger tips) contains two kinds of rapidly adapting mechanoreceptors, each of which has a special morphology. These mechanoreceptors are called the *Meissner* and the *Pacinian corpuscles*. The Meissner corpuscle is located in the dermal papillae, and the Pacinian corpuscle is located in the subcutaneous tissue (Figure 23–10). As we saw earlier, the properties of the accessory structure of the Pacinian corpuscle account for the rapid adaptation of its receptor potential.

Glabrous skin also contains two morphologically distinct kinds of slowly adapting mechanoreceptors, called the Merkel receptor and the Ruffini corpuscle. The Merkel receptor is located in the superficial portion of the dermis. It is an unusual skin receptor: ultrastructural studies suggest that a synapse is interposed between the transducing membrane and the primary afferent fibers. We do not know, however, whether this structure functions as a synapse physiologically.

The receptive field dimensions of different types of mechanoreceptors vary. Merkel receptors have receptive fields that are smaller than those of Ruffini corpuscles. Similarly, among the rapidly adapting receptors, the dimensions of the receptive fields of the Pacinian corpuscle are larger than those of the Meissner corpuscle (Figure 23–11). Mechanoreceptors with small receptive fields are more suitable for fine spatial discrimination than mechanoreceptors with large receptive fields.

Hairy skin, which covers most of the body, also contains Pacinian corpuscles, Ruffini corpuscles, and Merkel receptors (which have a somewhat different organization in hairy skin). The Meissner corpuscle is located in glabrous skin only. In its stead is the hair receptor, which has similar physiological properties.

What mechanical stimuli best activate the different types of mechanoreceptors? What sensations do these stimuli evoke? A simple way to activate both rapidly and slowly adapting mechanoreceptors is to present a long-lasting stimulus such as a steady skin indentation (Figure 23–12A). This stimulus first evokes the sensation of contact or tap, which may be mediated by both rapidly and slowly adapting receptors. After a few hundred millisec-

23–10 Glabrous skin contains four morphologically distinct types of mechanoreceptors. Two are rapidly adapting **(RA)** receptors: the Meissner corpuscles, which are located in dermal papillae; and the Pacinian corpuscles, which are located beneath glabrous skin (as well as hairy skin). The two slowly adapting **(SA)** mechanoreceptors are the Merkel receptor (also called **type I**) and the Ruffini corpuscle (also called **type II**).

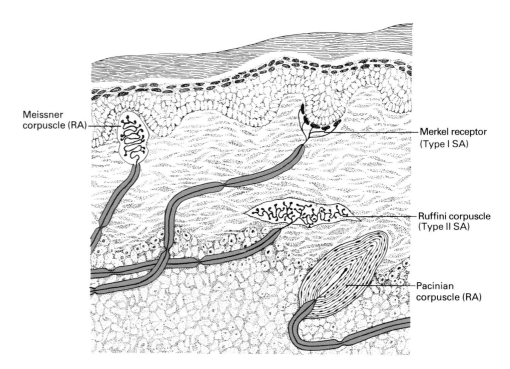

Meissner corpuscle (RA)

Merkel receptor (Type I SA)

Ruffini corpuscle (Type II SA)

Pacinian corpuscle (RA)

A Rapidly adapting
mechanoreceptors

B Slowly adapting
mechanoreceptors

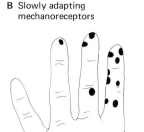

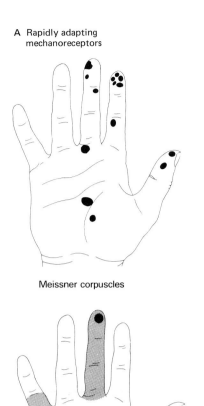

Meissner corpuscles

Merkel receptors

Pacinian corpuscles

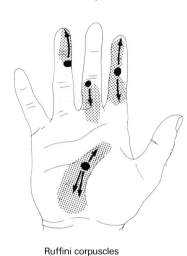

Ruffini corpuscles

23–11 The locations and shapes of some of the receptive fields in the glabrous skin area.
A. Rapidly adapting receptors. The receptive fields of Meissner corpuscles are smaller than those of Pacinian corpuscles. The receptive fields of Pacinian corpuscles have a zone of maximal sensitivity that is shown as a small dot within the **shaded** area.
B. Slowly adapting receptors. The receptive fields of Merkel receptors are smaller than those of Ruffini corpuscles. The directions of skin stretch that caused an increase in discharge of the Ruffini corpuscles are indicated by an **arrow** drawn over receptive field **(stippled area)**. (Adapted from Johansson and Vallbo, 1983).

onds, however, only slowly adapting receptors are active and now only a steady skin indentation is sensed.

Sinusoidal mechanical stimuli are particularly effective in distinguishing the sensitivities of different rapidly adapting mechanoreceptors (Figure 23–12B). This differential sensitivity of the rapidly adapting mechanoreceptors is best illustrated by plotting receptor threshold against stimulus frequency. Such studies have shown that the Meissner corpuscle is most sensitive to low-frequency sinusoidal mechanical stimuli, whereas the Pacinian corpuscle is most sensitive to high-frequency stimuli (Figure 23–13). The low-frequency stimuli to which the Meissner corpuscle is responsive are felt as gentle fluttering, which is well localized to the skin surface. In contrast, high-frequency sinusoidal mechanical stimulation, which excites the Pacinian corpuscle, evokes a diffuse, humming feeling localized to deeper tissues. This is the familiar sense of vibration.

Confirming the law of specific energies first formulated by Müller, we now know that different mechanoreceptors mediate different sensations. However, these sensory experiences are quite different from the tactile sensations evoked by complex natural stimuli characteristic of our daily experiences. Natural stimuli rarely activate a single type of receptor; rather, they activate different combinations of mechanoreceptor classes.

Proprioception Is Mediated by Muscle Afferent Fibers

Proprioception is the sense of balance, of position, and of movement of the limbs. Balance is largely mediated by the specialized receptors of the vestibular apparatus (discussed in Chapter 44). Here we shall consider (1) the sense of stationary position of the limbs *(limb position sense)* and (2) the sense of limb movement *(kinesthesia)*.

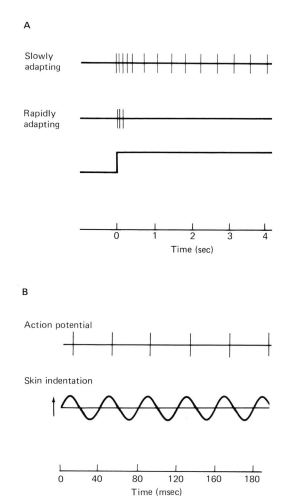

A

Slowly
adapting

Rapidly
adapting

B

Action potential

Skin indentation

23–12 Slowly adapting mechanoreceptors continue
responding to a continuous stimulus, whereas rapidly
adapting mechanoreceptors respond only at the beginning of
the stimulus. **A.** Responses of slowly and rapidly adapting
mechanoreceptors to a step indentation of the skin.
B. Response of a rapidly adapting mechanoreceptor to
sinusoidal mechanical stimuli. Note that the afferent fiber
response is a single action potential for each phase of the
stimulus.

Under most circumstances, proprioceptive sensations
of the limbs occur as a consequence of voluntary (or reflexive) movement. For this reason, proprioception of the
limb was long thought to depend on signals from brain
regions controlling limb movement, and therefore to differ from the other modalities of somatic sensation, which
are each mediated by peripheral receptors. This view derives from Hermann Helmholtz (see Boring, 1942, and
Sherrington, 1900), who over a century ago first called
attention to the importance of motor centers in evoking
sensation. According to this view, commands for movement that are issued by a motor center are also conveyed
to other parts of the brain so as to inform them about the
details of the commands that have just been issued. This
"sense of innervation" or "corollary discharge," as Helmholtz described it, would follow directly from the actions
of neurons in the central nervous system, not peripheral
receptors.

One way to test the role of corollary discharges in proprioception is to produce a disparity between what the
brain commands the muscles to do and what actually
happens. This can be done by altering the effectiveness
of the neural signals responsible for muscle contraction
by occluding circulation of the responding limb with a
blood pressure cuff inflated above systolic pressure. This
procedure gradually prevents action potential conduction
in the portion of afferent and efferent nerves distal to the
cuff. Guy Goodwin, David McClosky, and P. B. C. Matthews at Oxford University showed that as the nerve becomes anoxic, the ability to move the limb and to perceive its movement are differentially affected. The
perception of voluntary movement diminishes before the
movement itself, suggesting that conduction of action
potentials in afferent nerves is blocked before conduction
in efferent nerves innervating skeletal muscles. These
findings indicate that the senses of limb position and
movement are mediated by peripheral receptors, not by
central commands controlling the movement.

Another way of assessing whether proprioceptive sensations are mediated by receptors or by corollary discharges is to compare sensations evoked by passively im-

23–13 Idealized tuning curves show that Meissner
corpuscles are more sensitive to low-frequency
sinusoidal mechanical stimuli, whereas Pacinian corpuscles are
more sensitive to high-frequency stimuli. The **abscissa** shows
frequency of sinusoidal mechanical stimulus and the **ordinate**
indicates the magnitude of the threshold stimulus. In this case
the threshold corresponds to the lowest stimulus intensity that
evokes one action potential per cycle of the sinusoidal
stimulus.

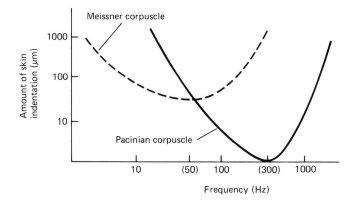

posed changes in limb position with those evoked by actively generated changes. Studies using this method have shown that limb position sense and kinesthesia are well developed in the absence of voluntary muscle contraction. For example, at rest, the angle of the knee joint can be evaluated to within 0.5°.

Three main types of peripheral receptors may signal the stationary position of the limb and the speed and direction of limb movement: (1) mechanoreceptors located in joint capsules, (2) cutaneous mechanoreceptors, and (3) mechanoreceptors in muscle that are specialized to transduce stretch of the muscle. During the past few years, P. R. Burgess and his colleagues at the University of Utah have carried out systematic psychophysical studies of limb position sense in humans, while examining the physiological properties of joint afferent fibers innervating the knee in separate experiments in cats. They found that knee joint afferents are not sensitive to joint angle over the midrange (when bent half-way to full flexion)—where static position sense is well developed—but rather are sensitive at extremes of joint angles. Moreover, individuals with artificial joints can have good static limb position sense. This evidence suggests that the joint afferents may not play a dominant role in sensing position of the limb at rest.

What role, if any, joint receptors have in the sense of limb movement is unclear. Patients who have undergone total hip replacement and who therefore have no innervation of their joints are nonetheless still able to detect the direction of passive limb movement; however, the threshold for movement detection is elevated compared with the threshold before surgery. As with joint receptors, cutaneous receptors are not necessary for accurate assessments of limb position or movement; for example, anesthetizing the skin around the knee joint has no effect on estimates of knee joint angle.

Matthews, Burgess, and their colleagues found that *we estimate joint angle from information about muscle length provided by muscle spindle receptors*. Matthews produced illusions of limb position and movement by vibrating the muscles of the limb. Strong vibration, in addition to activating Pacinian corpuscles, causes the length of the muscle to vary by a small amount; these vibrations powerfully excite specialized receptors in muscle called *muscle spindles*. Matthews found a considerable disparity between the actual limb position and the perceived position that a subject reported when the limb was vibrated (Figure 23–14). These illusions were always in the direction expected if muscle spindles mediate the illusion. Thus, vibration of the biceps increases muscle spindle activity within the biceps and the illusion is that the arm is in a more extended position.

As we shall see in Chapter 34, muscle spindle receptors have complex properties that are also controlled by efferent neurons from the central nervous system. The major function of the joint afferents seems to be to signal the extremes of limb position and to respond to pressure changes within the joint capsule. Other information

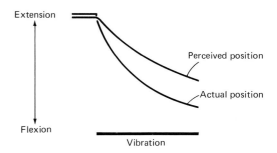

23–14 Upon vibration of the biceps tendon, the subject perceives his forearm to be somewhat more extended than the actual position. Since the muscle spindles contain stretch receptors that excite the motor neurons innervating the muscle, vibrating a muscle is similar to tapping on the tendon of a muscle: the stimulus causes the muscle to contract and the limb to move. Note that the illusion of the limb movement is in the direction of limb extension.

about muscle length is signaled by the receptors in the muscle spindle.

An Overall View

Our knowledge about many peripheral receptors is rather complete. Discriminative mechanoreception and proprioception depend upon encapsulated receptors, axons with fast conduction velocities, and receptor specificity. In contrast, the sensations of pain and temperature utilize free nerve endings and axons with slower conduction velocity (Table 23–2).

Each type of sensory receptor is tuned to different characteristics of the stimulus, ranging from steady indentation to high-frequency vibration for mechanosensation, and from cold to warm for thermal sensation. Natural stimuli are complex and generate neural activity that is fractionated into separate sensory channels by the filtering properties of the various receptors. At its point of entry into the nervous system, a sensory message already is transformed, and this transformation is only the

Table 23–2. Receptor Types Active in Various Sensations

Receptor type	Fiber group	Modality
Hair follicle	Aβ	Tactile
Meissner corpuscle	Aβ	Tactile
Ruffini corpuscle	Aβ	Tactile
Merkel receptor	Aβ	Tactile
Pacinian corpuscle	Aβ	Tactile
Free nerve ending	Aδ, C	Pain and temperature sense
Muscle spindle	Aα, Aβ	Proprioception
Joint receptors	Aβ	Extremes of joint angle; joint capsule pressure

beginning of the greater degree of abstraction that occurs later at higher levels within the central nervous system.

Selected Readings

Boivie, J. J. G., and Perl, E. R. 1975. Neural substrates of somatic sensation. In C. C. Hunt (ed.), MTP International Review of Science. Physiology, Series 1: Neurophysiology, Vol. 3. Baltimore: University Park Press, pp. 303–411.

Burgess, P. R., and Perl, E. R. 1973. Cutaneous mechanoreceptors and nociceptors. In A. Iggo (ed.), Handbook of Sensory Physiology, Vol 2: Somatosensory System. New York: Springer, pp. 29–78.

Burgess, P. R., Wei, J. Y., Clark, F. J., Simon, J. 1982. Signaling of kinesthetic information by peripheral sensory receptors. Annu. Rev. Neurosci. 5:171–187.

Goodwin, G. M., McCloskey, D. I., and Matthews, P. B. C. 1972. The contribution of muscle afferents to kinaesthesia shown by vibration induced illusions of movement and by the effects of paralysing joint afferents. Brain 95:705–748.

Iggo, A., and Andres, K. H. 1982. Morphology of cutaneous receptors. Annu. Rev. Neurosci. 5:1–31.

McCloskey, D. I. 1978. Kinesthetic sensibility. Physiol. Rev. 58:763–820.

Mountcastle, V. B. 1975. The view from within: Pathways to the study of perception. Johns Hopkins Med. J. 136:109–131.

Mountcastle, V. B. 1980. Sensory receptors and neural encoding: Introduction to sensory processes. In V. B. Mountcastle (ed.), Medical Physiology, 14th ed., Vol. 1. St. Louis: Mosby, pp. 327–347.

Stevens, S. S. 1961. The psychophysics of sensory function. In W. A. Rosenblith (ed.), Sensory Communication. Cambridge, Mass.: MIT Press, pp. 1–33.

Stevens, S. S. 1975. Psychophysics: Introduction to Its Perceptual, Neural, and Social Prospects. New York: Wiley.

Vallbo, Å. B., Hagbarth, K.-E., Torebjörk, H. E., and Wallin, B. G. 1979. Somatosensory, proprioceptive, and sympathetic activity in human peripheral nerves. Physiol. Rev. 59:919–957.

Willis, W. D., and Coggeshall, R. E. 1978. Sensory Mechanisms of the Spinal Cord. New York: Plenum Press.

References

Adrian, E. D., and Zotterman, Y. 1926. The impulses produced by sensory nerve-endings. Part 2. The response of a single end-organ. J. Physiol. (Lond.) 61:151–171.

Boring, E. G. 1942. Sensation and Perception in the History of Experimental Psychology. New York: Appleton-Century.

Boyd, I. A., and Davey, M. R. 1968. Composition of Peripheral Nerves. Edinburgh: E. and S. Livingstone Ltd.

Coggeshall, R. E., Applebaum, M. L., Fazen, M., Stubbs, T. B., III, and Sykes, M. T. 1975. Unmyelinated axons in human ventral roots, a possible explanation for the failure of dorsal rhizotomy to relieve pain. Brain 98:157–166.

Fechner, G. 1860. H. E. Adler (trans.). In D. H. Howes and E. G. Boring (eds.), Elements of Psychophysics, Vol. 1. New York: Holt, Rinehart and Winston, 1966.

Johansson, R. S., and Vallbo, A. B. 1983. Tactile sensory coding in the glabrous skin of the human hand. Trends Neurosci. 6(1):27–32.

Knibestöl, M., and Vallbo, Å. B. 1976. Stimulus-response functions of primary afferents and psychophysical intensity estimation on mechanical skin stimulation in the human hand. In Y. Zotterman (ed.), Sensory Functions of the Skin in Primates with Special Reference to Man. Oxford: Pergamon Press, pp. 201–213.

Loewenstein, W. R., and Mendelson, M. 1965. Components of receptor adaptation in a Pacinian corpuscle. J. Physiol. (Lond.) 177:377–397.

Perl, E. R. 1968. Myelinated afferent fibres innervating the primate skin and their response to noxious stimuli. J. Physiol. (Lond.) 197:593–615.

Sherrington, C. S. 1900. The muscular sense. In E. A. Schäfer (ed.), Text-book of Physiology, Vol. 2. Edinburgh: Pentland, pp. 1002–1025.

Stevens, S. S. 1953. On the brightness of lights and the loudness of sounds. Science 118:576.

Tanner, W. P., Jr., and Swets, J. A. 1954. A decision-making theory of visual detection. Psychol. Rev. 61:401–409.

Weber, E. H. 1846. Der Tastsinn und das Gemeingefühl. In R. Wagner (ed.), Handwörterbuch der Physiologie, Vol. III, Abt. 2. Braunschweig: Vieweg, pp. 481–588.

John H. Martin

Anatomical Substrates for Somatic Sensation

24

In the last chapter we saw that different somatic sensory receptors are sensitive to different stimulus qualities. This specificity is shared by the chain of central neurons that carries sensory information along the ascending somatic sensory pathways to the cerebral cortex. The afferent fibers from the various submodality-specific receptors connect to discrete regions in the spinal cord and in the brain stem. There, second-order neurons transmit sensory information to the thalamus; this information is then conveyed by the third-order cells of the thalamus to the cerebral cortex.

In this chapter we shall examine the structural organization of the peripheral and central neuronal pathways for somatic sensation. We shall consider only the projections from the arms, legs, and trunk that are conveyed through the spinal cord. The projection from the face, mediated by the trigeminal nerve, is discussed in Chapter 42.

The Area of Skin Innervated by a Single Dorsal Root Is Called a Dermatome

Information from the periphery is brought into the central nervous system by afferent nerve fibers that run together with efferent fibers in *peripheral nerves.* As the peripheral nerves approach the spinal cord they join together into *spinal nerves.* The afferent fibers in the spinal nerves separate from the efferent fibers and enter the spinal cord as the dorsal roots. Each dorsal root innervates a restricted peripheral region called a *dermatome* (Figure 24–1). At various points, called *plexuses,* located between the spinal cord and the periphery, the afferent fibers are regrouped so that each spinal nerve receives afferents from several peripheral

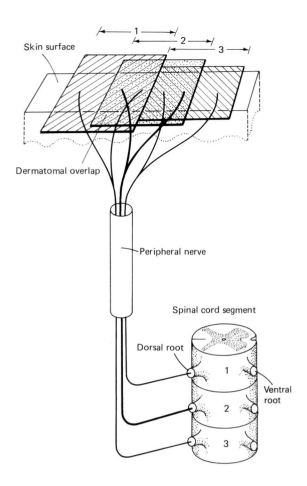

24–1 Each dorsal root innervates a particular area of skin called a dermatome. However, dermatomal boundaries are not clear-cut because fibers from several dorsal roots mix to some extent in the peripheral nerves and because more than one peripheral nerve sends afferents into each dorsal root (not shown). Thus, there is considerable overlap in the peripheral innervation of adjacent spinal cord segments.

nerves. As a result of this mixing of fibers, the area innervated by an individual dorsal root is less well defined than the area innervated by a single peripheral nerve. In fact, the areas innervated by adjacent dorsal roots overlap a good deal. Therefore, sectioning of the distal portion of a peripheral cutaneous nerve results in a circumscribed area of sensory loss in the skin. In contrast, damage to a spinal nerve or a dorsal root often results only in a modest sensory deficit.

Dermatomes are arranged in a highly ordered way on the body surface. It has been possible to map the distribution along the body surface of the dermatomes for all of the spinal segments by studying the sensibility and responsiveness that remain after injury to dorsal roots (Figure 24–2). Since the fibers within a dorsal root mediate several modalities of somatic sensation (tactile, limb proprioceptive, pain, and temperature sense), the boundaries of the dermatomes can be probed by using different stimuli. Tests used to locate the border between the area served by intact and injured dorsal roots reveal different dermatomal territories depending on the modality of the test stimulus. For example, dermatomes mapped with a pinprick (pain dermatomes) are smaller than those

mapped with light mechanical stimuli (tactile dermatomes). The areas are not congruent because the peripheral area served by large-diameter mechanoreceptive afferents of one dorsal root overlap extensively with similar afferents in adjacent dorsal roots. In contrast, the peripheral areas served by nociceptive afferents in adjacent dorsal roots overlap much less. Because of the differences in the size of the dermatomes for different modalities, injury to a single dorsal root is more likely to be noticed by examining sensibility for pain rather than sensibility for touch.

In addition to mapping with natural stimuli, a common method for identifying the peripheral distribution of dorsal root fibers is to examine the spatial distribution of the skin lesions in shingles (herpes zoster), a painful inflammation of dorsal root ganglia produced by a viral infection. Dermatomal maps vary when tested with different methods, as well as from individual to individual even when the same mapping technique is used. Despite this variability, dermatomal maps provide an important diagnostic tool for localizing levels of injury to the spinal cord and dorsal roots. For example, on the basis of the dermatomal map for the human forearm (Figure 24–3),

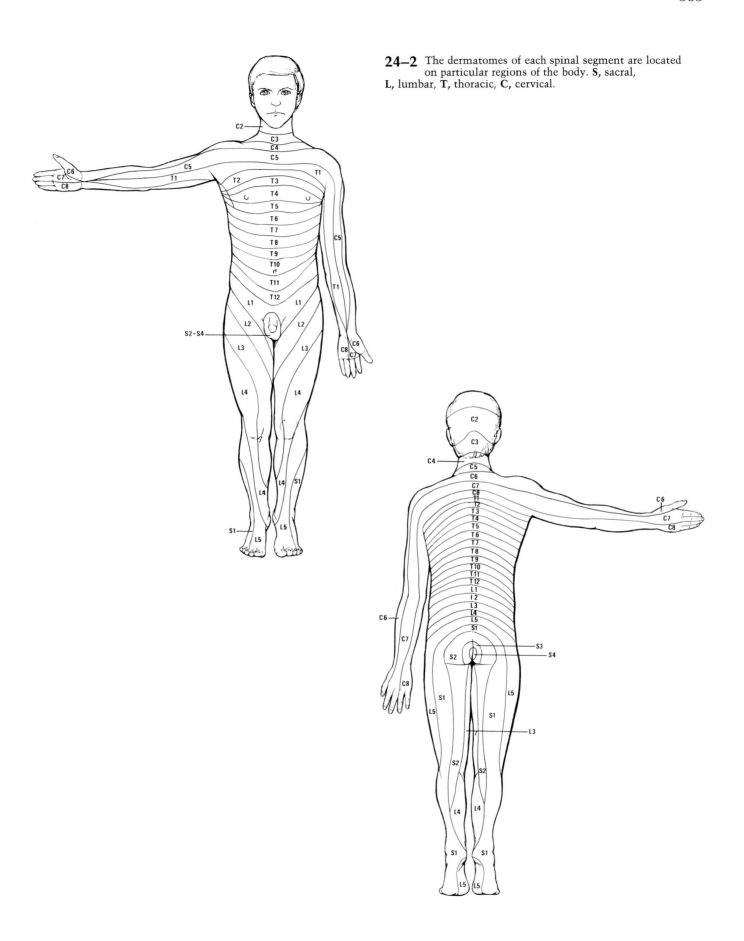

24–2 The dermatomes of each spinal segment are located on particular regions of the body. **S**, sacral, **L**, lumbar, **T**, thoracic, **C**, cervical.

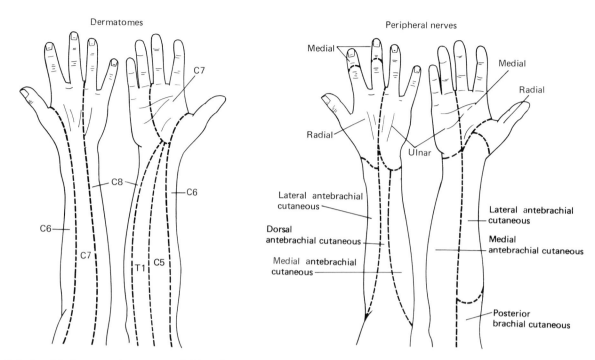

24–3 Relationship between dermatomes (left) and areas innervated by peripheral nerves (right) in the human forearm.

we know that sensory changes limited to the distal forearm and the fourth and fifth fingers may result from injury to the spinal cord at levels C8 and T1.

The segmental organization of the dorsal roots is preserved in the various ascending systems, considered in detail in Chapter 25. This is an example of one of the key principles of sensory organization: *there is an orderly topographic arrangement between adjacent regions of the receptive sheet and all of the sites in the nervous system that receive sensory projections.* This ordered mapping of the body surface onto central neural structures is called *somatotopy.* There are analogous organizational schemes for the visual system *(retinotopy)* and for the auditory system *(tonotopy).*

The Spinal Cord Is Organized into Gray and White Matter

To convey sensory information to the brain for perception, the somatic sensory pathways must first traverse the spinal cord. The spinal cord has three readily identifiable functions:

1. It is a relay for sensory information.
2. It carries both ascending afferent pathways and descending motor tracts that serve the trunk and limbs.
3. It contains the interneurons and motor neurons that control the movements of the trunk and the limbs.

In this chapter we shall focus on the sensory functions of the spinal cord.

As we saw in Chapter 20, a transverse section of the spinal cord shows that it is organized into a butterfly-shaped central gray area, where the cell bodies of spinal neurons are located, and a surrounding region of white matter that contains afferent and efferent axons, most of which are myelinated (Figure 24–4A).

Spinal Gray Matter Contains Nerve Cell Bodies

The butterfly-shaped gray matter is divided into a dorsal horn, an intermediate zone, and a ventral horn (Figure 24–4B). Each of these zones can be subdivided into nuclei. Six nuclei are particularly important (Figure 24–5A):

1. The *marginal zone*, which is located in the outermost region of the dorsal horn and serves as an important relay for pain and temperature sense.
2. The *substantia gelatinosa* of the dorsal horn, which integrates afferent information from unmyelinated afferent fibers.
3. The *nucleus proprius*, which is located in the base of the dorsal horn and integrates sensory information with information that descends from the brain.
4. *Clarke's nucleus*, or *cell column*, which lies in the intermediate zone and relays information about limb position and movement to the cerebellum.
5. The *intermediolateral nucleus*, or *cell column*, which is located in the intermediate zone and contains autonomic preganglionic neurons.
6. The *motor nuclei* of the ventral horn, which contain motor neurons that innervate the skeletal muscles.

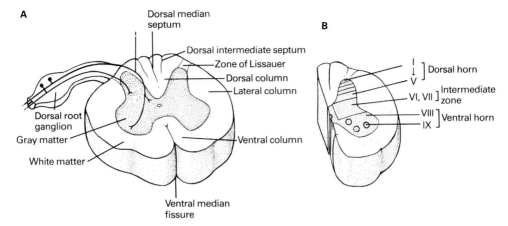

24–4 The white matter of the spinal cord is divided into columns, and the gray matter is divided into horns. **A.** General organization of a spinal segment. **B.** Schematic view of the spinal gray matter showing its three major divisions and the laminae of Rexed associated with each.

24–5 Nuclei and laminae of the spinal gray matter. In each part, the left-hand section is a low lumbar segment and the right-hand section is a thoracic segment. **A.** The important nuclei. **B.** Rexed's laminae. The lumbar (and sacral) segments innervate the lower limb and, as a consequence, have a larger area of gray matter than thoracic segments. Note also that lamina VI is not ordinarily present in thoracic segments.

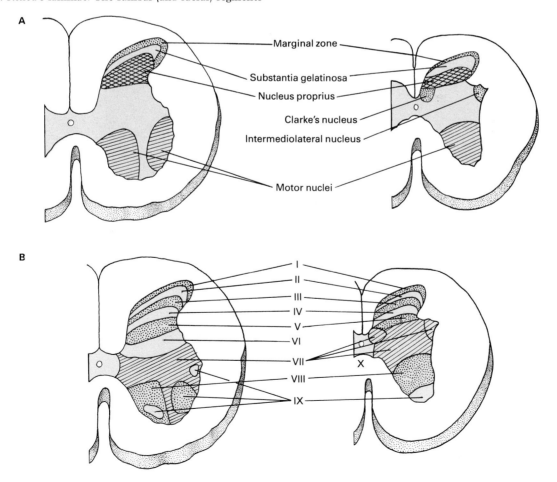

Table 24–1. Major Spinal Cord Nuclei and Corresponding Laminae and Regions

Nuclei	Laminae	Regions
Marginal zone	I	Dorsal horn
Substantia gelatinosa	II	Dorsal horn
Nucleus proprius	III, IV	Dorsal horn
Clarke's nucleus (T1-L2)	VII	Intermediate zone
Intermediolateral nucleus	VII	Intermediate zone
Motor nuclei	IX	Ventral horn

In 1952, Bror Rexed proposed a classification for understanding the organization of the gray matter of the spinal cord based on 10 layers or laminae. This classification proved useful because neurons in different layers were subsequently found to subserve different functions (Figures 24–4B and 24–5B). Laminae I–V are roughly equivalent to the dorsal horn, laminae VI and VII are roughly equivalent to the intermediate zone, and laminae VIII and IX are equivalent to the ventral horn. Lamina X consists of the gray matter surrounding the central canal. The major spinal cord nuclei and the laminae in which they are found are presented in Table 24–1.

Spinal White Matter Contains Myelinated Axons

The white matter is divided into three bilaterally paired columns, or funiculi (Figure 24–4A):

1. The *dorsal columns*, which lie medial to the dorsal horns, contain axons that relay somatic sensory information to the medulla.
2. The *lateral columns*, which lie lateral to the spinal gray matter, contain axons descending from the brain that control sensory, motor and autonomic functions as well as somatic sensory pathways ascending to the brain.
3. The *ventral columns*, which lie medial to the ventral horns, contain axons of the motor neurons that control the axial muscles of the body.

In addition to the major ascending (sensory) and descending (motor) tracts that make up these columns, the spinal cord contains pathways for the axons of propriospinal neurons that connect different regions of the spinal cord. (These interconnecting tracts are collectively called the *fasciculus proprius*.)

Dorsal Root Fibers Run in the White Matter and Arborize in the Gray Matter

Dorsal root fibers, whose cell bodies are in the dorsal root ganglia, enter the spinal cord at its dorsolateral margin. The largest cells have large myelinated axons that are up to 20 μm in diameter, and these fibers enter the spinal cord medially. The smallest cells have small unmyelinated axons less than 1 μm in diameter, which enter the spinal cord more laterally (Figure 24–4A).

After entering the spinal cord, the dorsal root fibers branch to ascend and descend in the white matter and arborize in the gray matter. Some ascending branches project to the medulla. The axons from large and small cells, carrying information from different somatic modalities, have different distributions. Collaterals of small-diameter fibers, which mediate pain and temperature sense, do not enter the gray matter immediately but pass into the *zone of Lissauer* (located dorsal and lateral to lamina I of the dorsal horn; Figure 24–4A). There the fibers bifurcate into branches that ascend and descend one to two segments and terminate in the superficial portion of the dorsal horn (Rexed's laminae I, II, and III). Collaterals of large-diameter fibers, which mediate tactile sense and limb proprioception, do not pass into the zone of Lissauer but enter the lateral aspect of the dorsal columns and enter the dorsal horn from its medial aspect (Figure 24–4A). Recently, A. R. Light and E. R. Perl, at the University of North Carolina, traced the pattern of termination of afferent fibers by following the anterograde transport of intra-axonally injected horseradish peroxidase (see Chapter 4). They found that small-diameter myelinated (Aδ) fibers terminate in layer I and the nucleus proprius, and large-diameter myelinated fibers terminate only in the nucleus proprius. Because axons of different diameters serve different somatic modalities, the neurons in the central nervous system that mediate pain and temperature senses are located in a different region of the dorsal horn from neurons that mediate tactile sense and limb proprioception.

The identity of some of the chemical transmitters that mediate the transfer of sensory information at primary afferent synapses in the spinal cord has recently been established. The majority of primary sensory neurons appear to release glutamate as a rapidly acting excitatory transmitter, independent of the sensory modality conveyed by the afferent fiber. In addition to releasing glutamate, many small-diameter sensory neurons also release peptide transmitters, notably substance P, somatostatin, and vasoactive intestinal polypeptide, which are thought to mediate slow synaptic potentials at synapses made in the dorsal horn. Unlike glutamate, which is released by afferent fibers that innervate diverse peripheral structures, peptides appear to be associated with distinct classes of sensory neurons. However, the precise relationship between sensory modality and the expression of particular peptide transmitters awaits demonstration. The physiological role of peptides at afferent synapses may be to alter the response of dorsal horn neurons to other synaptic inputs.

In addition to their role in perception, afferent fibers also mediate reflexes. Some large-diameter fibers terminate in motor nuclei (lamina IX) and mediate *stretch reflexes*, such as the knee-jerk reflex described in Chapters 2, 3, and 35. The knee-jerk reflex is an example of an *intrasegmental reflex*; it is generated by collaterals of afferent fibers that enter the spinal cord (through a dorsal root) and terminate in the gray matter of the same segment. In contrast, the scratch reflex, seen in cats and dogs after a flea bite, and postural reflexes following a perturbation in body position are examples of *interseg-mental reflexes*. These reflexes are mediated by collaterals associated with the ascending and descending branches of the afferent fibers.

Two Major Ascending Systems Convey Somatic Sensory Information to the Cerebral Cortex

There are two major ascending systems for somatic sensation: (1) the dorsal column–medial lemniscal system and (2) the anterolateral system. These systems relay afferent information to the brain for three purposes: perception, arousal, and motor control.

The *dorsal columns* relay information about somatic stimuli to the medulla. This tract runs ipsilaterally in the spinal cord. It originates both from the ascending axons of large-diameter primary afferent fibers and from the axons of neurons in the dorsal horn. The axons of the dorsal columns ascend to the caudal medulla where they synapse on the cells of the dorsal column nuclei. From there, by means of the medial lemniscus, a brain stem pathway, information is relayed first to the contralateral thalamus and then to the anterior parietal lobe. The dorsal column–medial lemniscal system mediates tactile sensation, including vibration sense, and proprioception from the contralateral side of the body. Proprioceptive information from the contralateral arm ascends in the dorsal column, whereas information from the contralateral leg ascends in the dorsal part of the lateral column, a region termed the dorsolateral funiculus.

The *anterolateral system* carries information chiefly about pain and temperature. It originates from cells in the dorsal horn. These cells send their axons to the contralateral side of the spinal cord and ascend in the anterolateral portion of the lateral column. In addition to pain and temperature, this ascending system also relays some tactile information. Because of this functional overlap with the dorsal columns, patients with a lesion involving the dorsal columns retain some residual crude tactile sensibility. As we saw in Chapter 23, the dorsal column–medial lemniscal system and the anterolateral system are examples of parallel ascending systems. Even though each subserves somewhat different functions, there is a degree of redundancy. Parallel pathways are advantageous for two reasons: they add subtlety and richness to a perceptual experience by allowing the same information to be handled in different ways, and they offer a measure of insurance. If one pathway is damaged, the others can provide residual perceptual capability.

The proprioceptive information from the limbs is used in two ways. First, it mediates reflex responses through a local circuit in the spinal cord. Some of this information is relayed through the spinocerebellar pathways to the cerebellum, which modulates the actions of reflexes and voluntary movement. (Because the cerebellum does not participate in perception, the spinocerebellar pathways will be considered with the motor system in Chapter 39.)

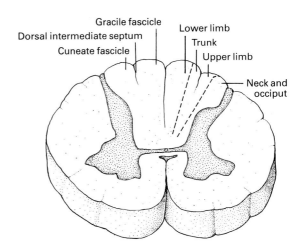

24–6 The somatotopic organization of the dorsal column is illustrated in this cross section through a high cervical spinal section.

Second, proprioceptive information projects to the cerebral cortex where it is used for the perception of limb position. The distinction between the information carried by the spinocerebellar tracts and that carried by the dorsal columns and the anterolateral system is important because it illustrates that not *all afferent or ascending information gives rise to sensation*. It is therefore useful to distinguish *afferent pathways*, which carry information into the nervous system that does not enter consciousness but contributes to movement, from *sensory pathways*, which carry information that contributes to conscious perception.

The Dorsal Column–Medial Lemniscal System Mediates Tactile Sense and Limb Proprioception

The dorsal columns are primarily composed of the central branches of dorsal root ganglion cells (primary afferent fibers), which ascend to the caudal medulla without synapsing. It has recently been shown, however, that about 15% of the fibers in the dorsal columns actually are ascending axons of dorsal horn neurons, and therefore are second-order cells. At upper spinal levels, the dorsal columns can be divided into two fascicles, the *gracile fascicle* and the *cuneate fascicle* (Figure 24–6). Input from the ipsilateral sacral, lumbar, and lower thoracic segments ascends medially in the gracile fascicle. This fascicle terminates at the level of the lower medulla, in the *gracile nucleus* (Figure 24–7; see also Figure 20–7). Input from the upper thoracic and cervical segments ascends laterally in the dorsal columns in the cuneate fascicle (Figure 24–6), which terminates in the *cuneate nucleus* of the lower medulla (Figures 24–7 and 20–7). The cuneate and gracile nuclei are located at about the same level in the caudal medulla and are referred to collectively as the *dorsal column nuclei*.

The fibers that leave the dorsal column nuclei arch

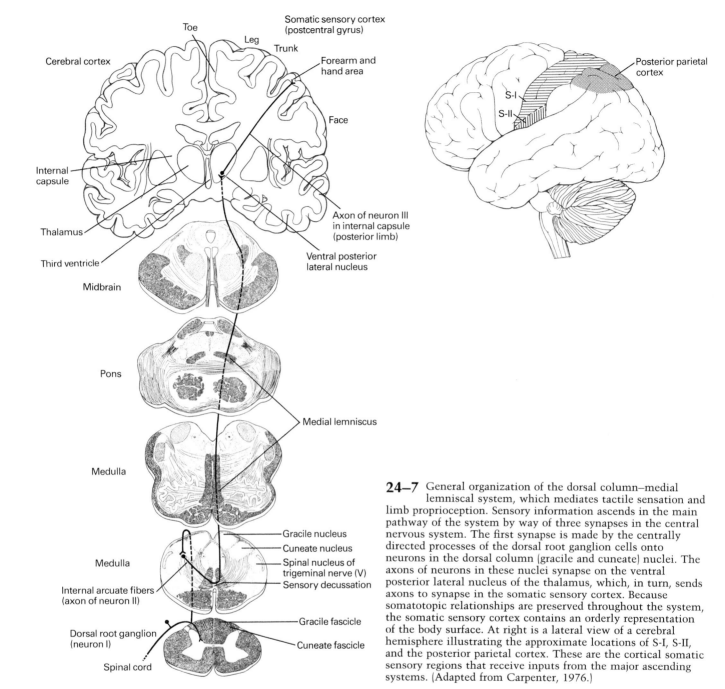

24–7 General organization of the dorsal column–medial lemniscal system, which mediates tactile sensation and limb proprioception. Sensory information ascends in the main pathway of the system by way of three synapses in the central nervous system. The first synapse is made by the centrally directed processes of the dorsal root ganglion cells onto neurons in the dorsal column (gracile and cuneate) nuclei. The axons of neurons in these nuclei synapse on the ventral posterior lateral nucleus of the thalamus, which, in turn, sends axons to synapse in the somatic sensory cortex. Because somatotopic relationships are preserved throughout the system, the somatic sensory cortex contains an orderly representation of the body surface. At right is a lateral view of a cerebral hemisphere illustrating the approximate locations of S-I, S-II, and the posterior parietal cortex. These are the cortical somatic sensory regions that receive inputs from the major ascending systems. (Adapted from Carpenter, 1976.)

across the midline and, for this reason, are called the *internal arcuate fibers.* As these fibers cross the midline, they collect into a discrete bundle, the *medial lemniscus,* and ascend to the thalamus (Figures 24–7, 24–8, and 20–8).

Whereas tactile information from the arms and legs is relayed by subdivisions of the dorsal columns—the gracile and cuneate fascicles, respectively—proprioceptive information from the arms and legs follows different paths to the medulla. The pathway for proprioceptive information from the arm is similar to that for tactile information (axons in the cuneate fascicle synapse on neurons in the cuneate nucleus, which project in the contralateral medial lemniscus). Proprioceptive information from the leg is relayed in the lateral column by the axons of neurons in Clarke's nucleus. These axons synapse on neurons in the caudal medulla that join the contralateral medial lemniscus. Sensory information from the face, which is innervated by the *trigeminal nerve,* also joins the medial lemniscus. The organization of the ascending trigeminal pathways will be discussed in Chapter 42.

In the medulla, the medial lemniscus lies above the medullary pyramids, at the approximate center of the re-

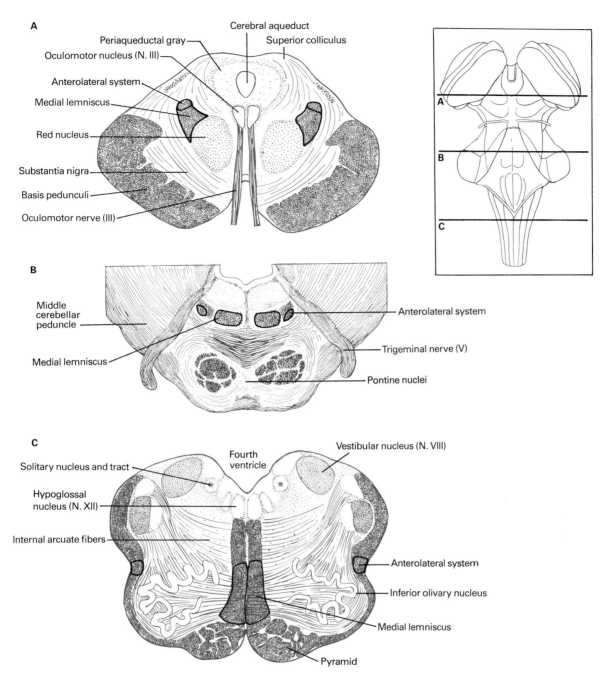

A
- Periaqueductal gray
- Cerebral aqueduct
- Superior colliculus
- Oculomotor nucleus (N. III)
- Anterolateral system
- Medial lemniscus
- Red nucleus
- Substantia nigra
- Basis pedunculi
- Oculomotor nerve (III)

B
- Middle cerebellar peduncle
- Medial lemniscus
- Anterolateral system
- Trigeminal nerve (V)
- Pontine nuclei

C
- Solitary nucleus and tract
- Fourth ventricle
- Vestibular nucleus (N. VIII)
- Hypoglossal nucleus (N. XII)
- Internal arcuate fibers
- Anterolateral system
- Inferior olivary nucleus
- Medial lemniscus
- Pyramid

24–8 The approximate locations of the medial lemniscus and anterolateral system in the brain stem. Inset shows dorsal view of the brain stem indicating the planes of section shown in parts A, B, and C: transverse sections through the midbrain, the pons, and the medulla. In the medulla and pons the medial lemniscus and anterolateral pathways are separate. In the midbrain they join together although their respective fibers remain segregated. The anterolateral system in the midbrain is predominantly composed of spinothalamic tract fibers. Most spinoreticular and spinotectal tract fibers have terminated at lower levels. From top to bottom: midbrain at the level of the superior colliculus, pons at the level of the genu of the facial nerve, and the rostral medulla.

ticular formation (Figure 24–8C). A characteristic feature of the reticular formation is that many of its neurons receive information from several sensory modalities and collectively project to many regions in the nervous system. This organization makes the reticular formation well suited to regulate arousal and the level of consciousness.

Like the dorsal columns, the medial lemniscus is somatotopically organized. However, the relationship of its somatotopic organization to the midline and the brain stem axes changes at different rostrocaudal levels. In the medulla, sensory information from the leg is located in the most ventral portion, and information from the face and arm, in the dorsal portion.

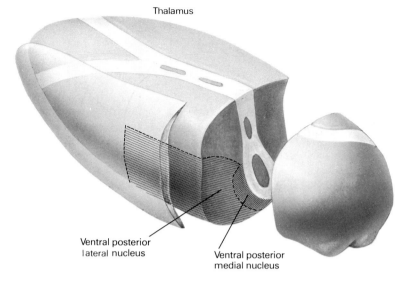

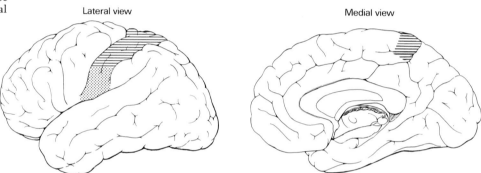

24–9 Location of somatic sensory thalamic nuclei and their projections to the primary somatic sensory cortex **(below).** The ventral posterior nucleus contains two major divisions: the lateral division, which relays somatic sensory information from the arms, trunk, and legs to the medial and superior portions of the postcentral gyrus **(hatching),** and the medial division, which relays information from the face to the lateral portion of the postcentral gyrus **(stippled).**

At the level of the pons (Figure 24–8B), the medial lemniscus has moved to a more lateral position within the reticular formation. Because the ventral portion of the medial lemniscus has moved farther laterally than the dorsal portion, sensory information from the face and arm is now medial to that from the leg. Farther rostrally in the midbrain (Figure 24–8A), the medial lemniscus is lateral to the red nucleus and dorsal to the substantia nigra, both of which serve motor functions. In the thalamus the fibers of the medial lemniscus synapse on neurons in the ventral posterior nucleus.

The thalamus plays a key role in transforming information that reaches the cerebral cortex. With rare exception, all afferent pathways projecting to the cerebral cortex do so through a relay nucleus in the thalamus. As we saw in Chapter 20, the lateral thalamus contains the nuclei that mediate specific sensory and motor functions.

The *ventral posterior nucleus* (Figure 24–9) mediates somatic sensation. The somatic sensory inputs from the trunk and limbs terminate on cells in the *lateral division* of the ventral posterior nucleus (*ventral posterior lateral nucleus*). Somatic sensory input from the face projects to the *medial division* of the ventral posterior nucleus (Figure 24–9). This thalamic region, which is called the *ventral posterior medial nucleus,* will be discussed in Chapter 42 together with the ascending trigeminal pathways.

Axons of the medial lemniscus that subserve a particular modality from a restricted body part form a bundle as they enter the thalamus and synapse on a row of cells in the ventral posterior lateral nucleus. These cells form a cylinder with its long axis oriented in the anterior–posterior direction. These thalamic neurons, which serve the same body part and modality as the bundle of medial lemniscal axons, project to a discrete sector of the cerebral cortex through the *posterior limb* of the *internal capsule.* The cortical region that receives this somatic sensory projection from the ventral posterior nucleus is located in the postcentral gyrus and is called the *primary somatic sensory cortex.* The projections from the medial and lateral divisions of the ventral posterior nucleus are directed to different parts of the postcentral gyrus (Figure 24–9), a reflection of the somatotopic organization of this portion of the cerebral cortex. This organizational feature of the primary somatic sensory cortex is considered in detail in Chapter 25. In the primary somatic sensory cortex, the axons from the thalamus terminate on pyramidal cells and excite them powerfully. In addition, these axons terminate on interneurons whose axons are oriented perpendicular to the surface and parallel to the apical dendrites of pyramidal cells. Thalamic axons conveying information about a particular body part or modality terminate on cortical neurons with axons or dendrites

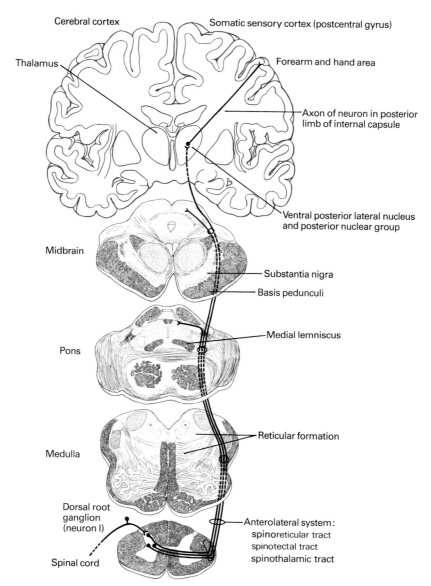

Cerebral cortex

Somatic sensory cortex (postcentral gyrus)

Thalamus

Forearm and hand area

Axon of neuron in posterior
limb of internal capsule

Ventral posterior lateral nucleus
and posterior nuclear group

Midbrain

Substantia nigra

Basis pedunculi

Pons

Medial lemniscus

Reticular formation

Medulla

Dorsal root
ganglion
(neuron I)

Anterolateral system:
spinoreticular tract
spinotectal tract
spinothalamic tract

Spinal cord

24–10 General organization of the anterolateral system. The three divisions of the anterolateral system—the spinothalamic tract, the spinoreticular tract, and the spinotectal tract—course rostrally in the anterolateral portions of the spinal cord white matter. There is a rough somatotopic organization to the anterolateral system. Sensory information from progressively more rostral spinal cord segments assumes a more ventral and medial position. (Adapted from Carpenter, 1976.)

oriented in narrow, vertically aligned columns. This feature represents an important principle of cortical organization, which will be discussed in the next chapter.

The Anterolateral System Mediates Pain and Temperature Sense

The anterolateral system (Figure 24–10) is the second major ascending system that mediates somatic sensation. It is actually composed of separate ascending pathways that, together, play a dominant role in pain and temperature sense and only a minor role in tactile sense and limb proprioception. This system differs from the dorsal column–medial lemniscal system in four respects: (1) The anterolateral system has a large contingent of uncrossed ascending fibers, whereas the dorsal column–medial lemniscal system does not. (2) Crossing in the anterolateral system occurs in the spinal cord, whereas the dorsal column–medial lemniscal system crosses in the medulla. (3) The cells of origin of the anterolateral system are located in the dorsal horn and therefore they are neurons that are postsynaptic to the primary afferent fibers; on the other hand, most axons in the dorsal columns are collaterals of primary afferent fibers. (4) Most axons in the medial lemniscus terminate in the thalamus, but anterolateral fibers terminate throughout the brain stem as well as the thalamus.

The anterolateral system contains three major pathways distinguished by their sites of termination: the spinothalamic (or neospinothalamic) tract, the spinoreticular (or paleospinothalamic) tract, and the spinotectal tract. The *spinothalamic* (or *neospinothalamic*) *tract* originates principally from cells in lamina I. Neurons that project from the spinal cord to the brain are called *projection* (or *relay*) *neurons* and differ from interneurons, whose axons ramify locally. The spinothalamic tract mediates fast pain, relayed from the periphery to the spinal cord by Aδ fibers. In contrast, the *spinoreticular* (or *paleospinothalamic*) *tract* is important in slow pain, which is mediated by C fibers. Axons of spinoreticular tract cells end on neurons in the reticular formation of the brain stem, which then relay information rostrally to the thalamus and other structures in the diencephalon. The spinoreticular tract also relays information to the *mesencephalic periaqueductal gray*, the region surrounding the cerebral aqueduct. This area is part of a descending pathway that regulates pain transmission (Chapter 26). The *spinotectal tract* terminates in the tectum of the midbrain (in the superior and inferior colliculi).

As fibers of the anterolateral system ascend through the brain stem, they are at first located on the lateral margin of the medulla and are therefore clearly separated from the medial lemniscus, which is located on the midline (Figures 24–8 and 24–10). They assume a position closer to the midline in the pons but are still separated from the medial lemniscus. In the midbrain, the fibers of the anterolateral septum join the medial lemniscus but they remain segregated laterally. At the level of the midbrain the anterolateral system contains mostly spinothalamic fibers because the spinoreticular and spinotectal fibers terminate at this or lower levels.

Whereas the medial lemniscus terminates chiefly in the ventral posterior nucleus, fibers of the anterolateral system synapse on neurons in three thalamic regions (Figure 24–9): the posterior nuclei, the intralaminar nuclei, and the ventral posterior lateral nucleus. The ventral posterior lateral nucleus in turn projects only to the somatic sensory cortical areas. In contrast, the intralaminar nuclei project more widely to areas of the brain stem and cortex. The posterior nuclei project to regions of the parietal lobe outside the somatic sensory areas.

The functional organization of the anterolateral system will be discussed in Chapter 26, but we can already see that the anterolateral and dorsal column–medial lemniscal systems are organized differently. This is demonstrated most dramatically by considering what occurs when the spinal cord is hemisected, as might happen after a serious automobile accident. In the arm, for example, tactile sense and proprioception, which are relayed by the dorsal columns, are lost on the ipsilateral side, whereas pain and temperature sense, which are relayed by the anterolateral system, are lost on the contralateral side of the body. This loss of pain and temperature sense begins a few segments below the level of the lesion because decussation occurs through a few segments.

The Primary Somatic Sensory Cortex Is Divided into Four Parts

Several cytoarchitectonically distinct regions in the anterior part of the parietal cortex receive somatic inputs. The information relayed to these cortical areas is important primarily in tactile sense and limb proprioception.

24–11 Two views show the location of the somatic sensory cortices and the posterior parietal association cortex. **A.** Lateral view of cerebral hemisphere illustrating somatic sensory receiving areas. **B.** Schematic section taken at level B of part **A**, perpendicular to the cortical surface. Brodmann's areas are shown for S-I (Brodmann's areas **3a, 3b, 1, 2**), part of the motor cortex (area **4**), and the posterior parietal cortex (areas **5** and **7**; only **5** is illustrated).

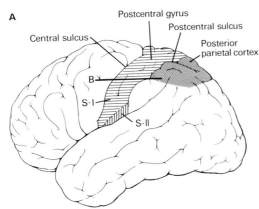

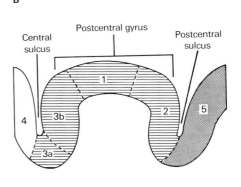

The role of the cerebral cortex in pain and temperature sense will be considered in Chapter 26.

The *primary somatic sensory cortex* (S-I) is located in the postcentral gyrus and in the depths of the central sulcus (Figure 24–11). It consists of four cytoarchitectonic areas: Brodmann's areas 1, 2, 3a, and 3b. Each of these cytoarchitectonic areas is important in somewhat different aspects of somatic sensation. Lateral and somewhat posterior to the primary somatic cortex is the *secondary somatic sensory cortex* (S-II), lying in the upper bank of the Sylvian fissure. S-II corresponds to the preinsular portion of Brodmann's area 2. Both S-I and S-II are somatotopically organized. The afferent inputs to S-I derive entirely from the contralateral body, whereas the inputs to S-II are bilateral. Direct thalamic projections to S-I and S-II arise chiefly from the ventral posterior nucleus. Also located deep within the Sylvian fissure, in the insular region, are sites that receive somatic sensory information. In addition to the postcentral gyrus and the cortex in the Sylvian fissure, a third cortical region that receives somatic inputs is located in the posterior parietal lobe (including Brodmann's area 5 and portions of area 7). This region is a higher order sensory cortex similar in function to association cortex; it relates sensory and motor processing and is concerned with integrating the different somatic sensory modalities necessary for perception (Figure 24–11).

Pyramidal Cells Are the Output Cells of the Cerebral Cortex

The neurons in the somatic sensory cortex that receive the thalamic input make four types of connections: intracortical, association, callosal, and subcortical.

Intracortical connections are made to neurons within the local cortical region. *Stellate cells*, one of two major cortical cell types, subserve this function. The other three types of connections are made by the second cell type, the *pyramidal cells*, which have axons that project out of the local cortical region.

Association connections communicate between different cortical regions *on the same side*. There are association connections among the four cytoarchitectonic regions of S-I (Brodmann's areas 1, 2, 3a, and 3b), and there is an association projection from S-I to the association area in the posterior parietal lobe (Brodmann's areas 5 and 7). Reciprocal association connections also exist between S-I and S-II and between these two somatic cortices and the motor cortex (which is located in the precentral gyrus and corresponds to Brodmann's area 4).

Callosal connections tie together symmetrical areas of the two hemispheres. In general, cortical areas (including the somatic sensory cortices) of each cerebral hemisphere are connected to the corresponding area in the other hemisphere via the commissural fiber tract, the *corpus callosum*. (Exceptions exist, however. For example, the cortical regions in each hemisphere that receive inputs

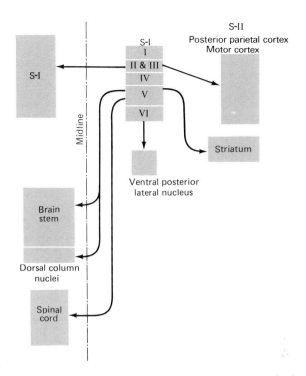

24–12 Projections from the different layers of the cerebral cortex of S-I have different destinations. Pyramidal cells in layers II and III project to other areas of cortex, whereas those in layers V and VI project to subcortical structures. Layer I contains few neurons; it consists mostly of dendrites from cortical neurons whose somata are located in deeper layers and axons of neurons from other parts of cortex and the brain stem. Layer IV contains interneurons that connect with other cortical layers.

from the distal limbs are not connected through the corpus callosum.)

Projection connections originate from cortical neurons and project to subcortical structures. Four major descending projections of the primary somatic sensory cortex are to the basal ganglia (striatum), the ventral posterior nucleus of the thalamus, the dorsal column nuclei, and the dorsal horn of the spinal cord. The projections to the thalamus and the spinal cord permit the cortical control of sensory inflow, an important principle of sensory organization.

Association, callosal, and projection fibers distribute information to other regions of the cortex and subcortical structures. Edward Jones and colleagues working at Washington University in St. Louis have shown that the cells of different layers of the cerebral cortex give rise to axons that terminate in different regions (Figure 24–12). For example, pyramidal cells located in layers II and III establish connections in S-II, in the posterior parietal association cortex, and in the motor cortex. Neurons in these layers also give rise to the callosal fibers destined for the contralateral cortex. The axons of the cells in layers V and VI are the projection fibers to subcortical struc-

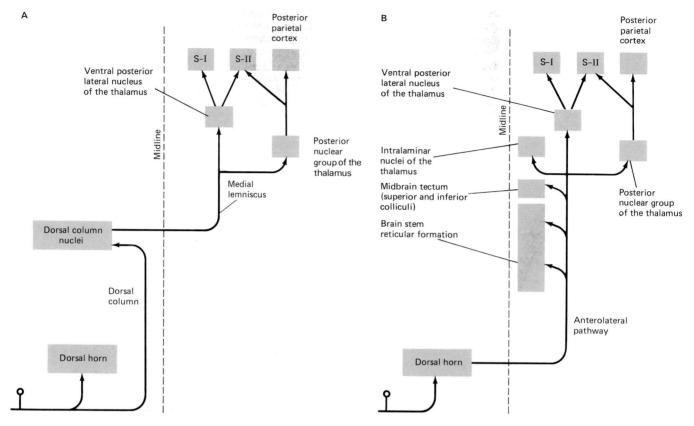

24–13 Summary diagram of the major ascending somatic sensory systems. **A.** Dorsal column–medial lemniscal system. **B.** Anterolateral system. A general understanding of the organization of these two ascending systems reveals key principles underlying the organization of sensory systems of the brain and provides a basis for localizing sites of injury following trauma. Both the dorsal column and anterolateral systems relay sensory information to the contralateral brain; however, decussation occurs at different levels. In the dorsal column–medial lemniscal system, second-order neurons have an axon that crosses the midline in the medulla. In contrast, the anterolateral system decussates in the spinal cord. These pathways also exhibit both a serial and parallel organization. The organization within each pathway is serial (i.e., an afferent fiber synapses on a neuron in the dorsal column nucleus, which synapses on a thalamic neuron). A parallel organization collectively describes the operation of the two systems. Sensory information distributes to both systems, each with somewhat different but overlapping functions. The dorsal column–medial lemniscal system mediates tactile sense and proprioception, whereas the anterolateral system mediates pain and temperature sense, and to a much lesser extent, tactile sensation.

Table 24–2. Major Ascending Somatic Sensory Systems

	Anterolateral	Dorsal column–medial lemniscus
Modalities	Pain Thermal Crude touch	Tactile Proprioception (of arm only)
Location in spinal cord	Anterolateral column	Dorsal column
Level of decussation	Spinal cord	Medulla
Brain stem terminations	Brain stem reticular formation Midbrain tectal region Ventral posterior lateral nucleus, posterior nuclear group of thalamus, intralaminar nuclei	Ventral posterior lateral nucleus and posterior nuclear group of thalamus
Cortical terminations	Primary and secondary somatic sensory cortices and posterior parietal cortex	Primary and secondary somatic sensory cortices and posterior parietal cortex

tures. Whereas neurons in layer V project to the brain stem, spinal cord, and striatum, layer VI pyramidal cells send out fibers that project only to the ventral posterior nucleus.

An Overall View

Afferent information from the body is relayed to the brain by two major ascending systems: the dorsal column–medial lemniscal system and the anterolateral pathways (Figure 24–13). These systems, which serve different functions, converge in the thalamus (Table 24–2). There, the ventral posterior lateral nucleus and the posterior nuclear group mediate the projection to the somatic sensory cortices, which include S-I, S-II, and the posterior parietal cortex. In these areas of cortex, afferent information is further processed for somatic perception.

Selected Readings

Brodal, A. 1981. Neurological Anatomy in Relation to Clinical Medicine. 3rd ed. New York: Oxford University Press.

Jahr, C. E., and Jessell, T. M. 1985. Synaptic transmission between dorsal root ganglion and dorsal horn neurons in culture: antagonism of monosynaptic EPSPs and glutamate excitation by kynurenate. J. Neurosci. (In Press).

Jones, E. G., Friedman, D. P., and Hendry, S. H. C. 1982. Thalamic basis of place- and modality-specific columns in monkey somatosensory cortex: A correlative anatomical and physiological study. J. Neurophysiol. 48:545–568.

Jones, E. G., and Powell, T. P. S. 1973. Anatomical organization of the somatosensory cortex. In A. Iggo (ed.), Handbook of Sensory Physiology, Vol. 2: Somatosensory System. New York: Springer, pp. 579–620.

Kuypers, H. G. J. M. 1973. The anatomical organization of the descending pathways and their contributions to motor control especially in primates. In J. E. Desmedt (ed.), New Developments in Electromyography and Clinical Neurophysiology, Vol. 3. Basel: Karger, pp. 38–68.

References

Brodmann, K. 1909. Vergleichende Lokalisationslehre der Grosshirnrinde in ihren Prinzipien dargestellt auf Grund des Zellenbaues. Leipzig: Barth.

Carpenter, M. B. 1976. Human Neuroanatomy, 7th ed. Baltimore: Williams & Wilkins.

Jones, E. G., and Wise, S. P. 1977. Size, laminar and columnar distribution of efferent cells in the sensory-motor cortex of monkeys. J. Comp. Neurol. 175:391–437.

Light, A. R., and Perl, E. R. 1979. Reexamination of the dorsal root projection to the spinal dorsal horn including observations on the differential termination of coarse and fine fibers. J. Comp. Neurol. 196:117–131.

Rexed, B. 1952. The cytoarchitectonic organization of the spinal cord in the cat. J. Comp. Neurol. 96:415–495.

Eric R. Kandel

Central Representation of Touch

25

The somatic sensory system allows us to perceive and recognize objects through touch, to read braille, and to experience pain or a change in temperature. This system is distinctive for two reasons. First, the receptors for somatic sensibility are not restricted to a small, well-delineated organ, like the eye for vision or the cochlea for hearing, but are distributed throughout the body. For this reason the somatic sensibilities are called the *skin* or the *body senses*. Second, the sensations mediated by the somatic sensory system are remarkably diverse; they include not only the four relatively elementary modalities—touch, proprioception, pain, and temperature sense—but also various submodalities. For example, we can distinguish subforms of tactile sensation such as superficial and deep touch (pressure), or static proprioception (position sense) and dynamic proprioception (kinesthesia). In addition, there are compound sensations, such as wetness, that are achieved by combining elementary modalities and submodalities in different ways.

How does neuronal activity within the somatic sensory system give rise to perception? In this chapter we shall consider this question by focusing on the mechanisms underlying tactile sensation. We shall first explore how we make tactile discriminations and why we do so better with our finger tips than with our toes or with the skin of our back. We shall next examine the degree to which the various modalities of somatic sensibility are segregated. Because this is the first system whose central projections we shall consider, this discussion will also provide an opportunity to see how the brain, and particularly the cerebral cortex, is organized to handle information coming from the outside world.

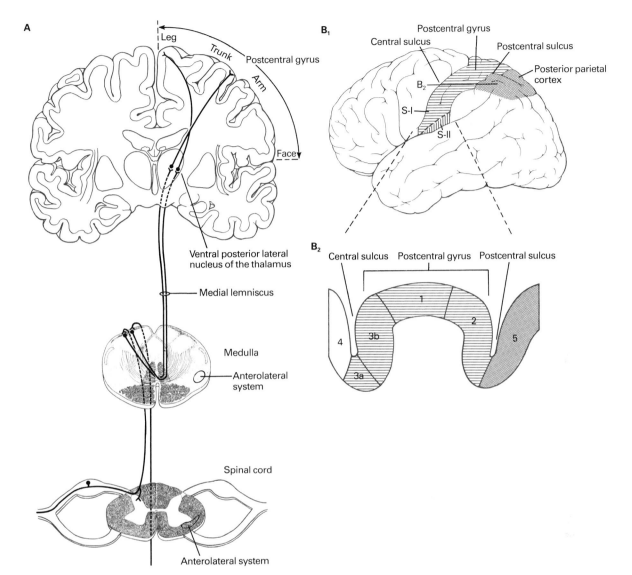

25–1 The dorsal column–medial lemniscal system connects the neurons of the dorsal root ganglia to those of the somatic sensory cortex by means of synapses in the medulla and thalamus. **A.** Information about somatic sensation is carried up through the spinal cord by the long axons of the dorsal root ganglion cells (or, in the case of facial sensation, by fibers in the trigeminal nerve). These axons terminate in the dorsal column nuclei of the medulla, the first relay of the somatic afferent pathway. In the medulla, a major crossing occurs as the axons of the cells in the dorsal column nuclei cross to the other side and ascend in the contralateral medulla to end in the ventral posterior lateral nucleus of the thalamus. This nucleus, in turn, sends out an extensive projection (radiation) to the primary somatic sensory cortex. The location of the spinothalamic tract of the anterolateral system is also indicated in the spinal cord and medulla. (Adapted from Brodal, 1981.) **B.** The somatic sensory cortex, located in the parietal lobe, has three major divisions: S-I, S-II and the posterior parietal cortex. **1:** The relationship of S-I to S-II, and to the higher order posterior parietal cortex (Brodmann's areas 5 and 7), is best seen from a lateral perspective of the surface of the cerebral cortex. **2:** The primary somatic cortex (S-I) is in turn subdivided into four distinct cytoarchitectonic regions. This sagittal section shows these four regions (Brodmann's areas 3a, 3b, 1, and 2) and illustrates their spatial relationship to area 4 of the motor cortex and area 5 of the posterior parietal cortex (area 7, the other subdivision of the posterior parietal cortex, is not shown).

Sensory Systems Transform Information at Specific Relay Points

Normal human somatic sensibility is usually subdivided into four major types: (1) *discriminative touch* (used to recognize size, shape, texture, and movement across the skin), (2) *proprioception* (the sense of static and dynamic position of limbs and body), (3) *pain* (slow and fast), and (4) *temperature sense* (warm and cold). Lesions of systems concerned with discriminative tactile sensibility often reveal a fifth modality: crude touch. This form of touch is thought to be dependent on central neural mechanisms that detect position but not movement of the eliciting stimulus. In contrast, discriminative touch is thought to

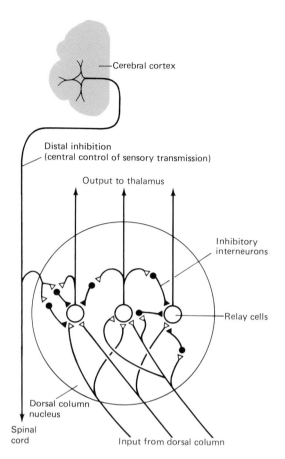

25–2 This cross-sectional view of a few cells in a dorsal column nucleus shows the types of neural activity that take place in this sensory relay. The projection (or relay) cells of this nucleus run to the thalamus. These cells receive convergent and divergent excitatory input from axons traveling in the dorsal columns. The projection cells also receive pre- and postsynaptic inhibitory input from interneurons activated by recurrent collateral axons as well as from neurons in the cerebral cortex. In this, as in subsequent figures, excitatory synapses are indicated by **open triangles,** inhibitory synapses by **filled triangles.**

be dependent on mechanisms that can also detect movement.

Most aspects of tactile and proprioceptive sensibility (except for crude touch and proprioception in the lower extremities) are carried by the dorsal column–medial lemniscal system and are therefore also called dorsal column–medial lemniscal modalities. Information about pain, warmth, cold, and crude tactile sensibility is carried primarily by the anterolateral system. Here we shall focus on the dorsal column–medial lemniscal sensibilities—in particular, touch. In the next chapter we shall consider the anterolateral system and the perception of pain.

The anatomical plan of tactile sensation is simple and can be briefly recapitulated. There are specific receptors for each submodality. For example, Meissner corpuscles respond to tactile stimuli applied to the skin, and the Pacinian corpuscles respond to vibration. Large myelinated

afferent fibers from these receptors in skin, subcutaneous tissues, and deep tissue enter the spinal cord via the dorsal roots. There, each axon sends a long ascending branch into the dorsal columns to synapse in the medulla with cells in the dorsal column nuclei (the gracile and cuneate nuclei). Somatic sensory information from the face and the rostral part of the head is carried by the trigeminal nerve. Axons of second-order sensory cells in the dorsal column nuclei cross the midline in the medulla. These axons then ascend through the brain stem on the opposite side as the medial lemniscus and form synapses with cells in the ventral posterior lateral nucleus of the thalamus (Figure 25–1A).

The third-order neurons in the thalamus send axons to the cerebral cortex (which run together with those from certain other thalamic nuclei) in the extensive *thalamocortical projection* or radiation. These fibers run through the internal capsule and terminate in the primary somatic sensory cortex (S-I), located in the postcentral gyrus of the parietal lobe. This area is subdivided into four distinct cytoarchitectonic regions, Brodmann's areas 1, 2, 3a, and 3b (Figure 25–1B). Most of the thalamic fibers terminate in areas 3a and 3b, which then project to areas 1 and 2. Third-order neurons from the thalamus also project to the adjacent cortex, called the secondary somatic sensory cortex (S-II). Unlike S-I, which receives input only from the contralateral part of the body, S-II receives input from both parts of the body. Here we shall be concerned primarily with S-I.

S-I projects to the posterior parietal cortex, Brodmann's areas 5 and 7. The posterior parietal cortex is a higher order sensory area that also receives an independent input from the thalamus.

As the anatomical plan of the somatic sensory system illustrates, all sensory systems consist of a series of relay or transfer nuclei within the brain. To understand what function these relays serve, it is necessary to combine the longitudinal analysis illustrated in Figure 25–1 with a segmental or cross-sectional analysis (Figure 25–2) that shows what happens to the flow of neural activity within each relay nucleus.

At each relay nucleus the *projection*, or relay, cells—the cells that project out of the nucleus to the next relay point—receive synaptic input from many incoming (afferent) axons; each afferent axon ends on many relay cells. Occasionally, as in some cells of the dorsal column nuclei, the synapses of some incoming fibers are so effective that one action potential in a single afferent fiber can discharge a relay cell. Such limited convergence allows information to be transmitted with high fidelity and with a high degree of spatial and temporal resolution. More commonly, however, there is extensive convergence and divergence of sensory input on relay cells. In addition to relay cells, the afferent fibers activate both excitatory and inhibitory interneurons. These interneurons allow sensory information to be processed as it passes from the projection neurons of one nucleus to those of the next. In some nuclei the afferent message ascends to the next level without change; in others, the information may be transformed into a new, more abstract pattern of activity.

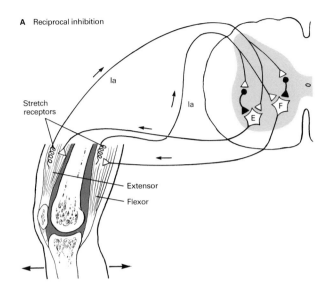

A Reciprocal inhibition

Stretch receptors

Ia

Ia

Extensor

Flexor

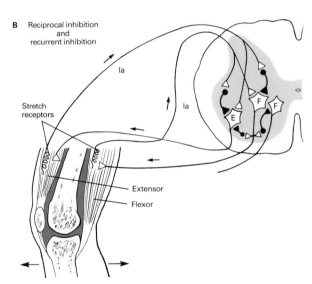

B Reciprocal inhibition and recurrent inhibition

Stretch receptors

Ia

Ia

Extensor

Flexor

25–3 This cross-sectional analysis of a motor nucleus in the spinal cord involved in the stretch reflex illustrates excitatory and inhibitory interactions similar to those that occur in sensory relay nuclei. **A.** Reciprocal inhibition produced by afferent neurons innervating agonist muscles serves to inhibit the antagonist motor neurons during excitation of agonist motor neurons. In this example, the Ia afferent fiber from an extensor excites the extensor (**E**) motor neurons while also exciting an inhibitory interneuron that acts on the flexor (**F**) motor neuron; the Ia afferent fiber that activates the flexor motor neuron does the converse.
B. Recurrent inhibition restricts excitation and prevents it from spreading to interconnected cells whose activity is either unnecessary or counterproductive. In this example, in addition to reciprocal inhibition, a series of inhibitory interneurons act on the various motor cells, so that when one set is excited, the others are inhibited. As a result, the contrast in activity between active and inactive cells is enhanced.

The processing of neural information at a sensory relay nucleus does not differ in principle from that which we encountered earlier in considering the motor relay nuclei in simple stretch reflexes (Chapter 2). In fact, we can gain additional insight into what happens at a sen-sory relay nucleus by examining once again a cross section of a motor nucleus in the spinal cord. There we encounter, in addition to the convergence and divergence of the excitatory synaptic input, two types of inhibitory pathways mediating (1) reciprocal, or feed-forward, inhibition and (2) recurrent, or feedback, inhibition (Figure 25–3).

Reciprocal inhibition in a motor system ensures that excitation of a synergist group of neurons (such as flexor motor neurons in a motor nucleus) leads to inhibition of the antagonist neurons (such as extensor motor neurons). Reciprocal inhibition is functionally economical and permits what Sherrington called a "singleness of action," ensuring that only one of two or more competing responses is expressed. By this means a strong tactile stimulus can override and block out other somatic sensibilities, including pain (see Chapter 26). Whereas reciprocal inhibition occurs only between antagonist groups of neurons, *recurrent*, or *feedback*, *inhibition* limits the spread of excitation among adjacent units, thereby functionally isolating cells that are anatomically near each other. The interesting feature of both types of inhibition is that both create contrast; there is a central excitatory zone of active neurons surrounded by an inhibitory annulus of less active neurons. As a result, the two types of inhibitory actions are often collectively called *lateral inhibition*.

These lateral inhibitory interactions—first noted in the analysis of motor nuclei in the spinal cord—turn out to be quite general: we shall encounter them repeatedly in our analysis of relay sensory nuclei in the sensory systems. Consider, for example, the dorsal column nuclei, the first relay in the somatic sensory system. There is no synaptic inhibition at the level of the peripheral receptor in the somatic sensory system. In contrast, in the dorsal column nuclei there are at least two types of feedback inhibition: (1) *local feedback inhibition* (of both the postsynaptic and presynaptic variety), which results from activity in relay cells within the dorsal column nuclei and leads, by means of collaterals from these cells, to inhibition of the surrounding relay cells; and (2) *distal feedback inhibition* (mostly presynaptic), which is exerted from remote sites onto the input coming into the relay cells. This inhibition is produced by the axons of neurons in the motor and somatic sensory cortices as well as those in the brain stem. Distal feedback illustrates still another principle in the organization of the sensory system: *central control of sensory transmission*. Higher areas of the brain are able to control the sensory inflow from the peripheral receptors into relay nuclei.

The Body Surface Is Mapped onto the Brain

Functional Analyses Localized Somatic Sensations to Specific Regions of Cortex

The earliest information about the function of the somatic sensory system came from the analysis of traumatic injuries of the spinal cord and disease states. Until penicillin became available during the 1940s, syphilis was a common chronic disease. One of the late consequences of syphilitic infection in the nervous system is a syndrome called *tabes dorsalis*, which affects the large-diameter fibers in the dorsal roots, the dorsal root ganglia, and the dorsal columns. Patients with tabes have severe deficits in tactile sensibility and in position sense but little deficit in temperature or pain perception.

Additional information about the somatic afferent systems comes from transection of the dorsal columns in experimental animals or following trauma in humans. This type of injury results in a chronic deficit in certain tactile discriminations such as detecting the direction of movement across the skin, the relative position of two cutaneous stimuli, and *two-point discrimination* (the minimum stimulus separation necessary for a subject to perceive two stimuli). The deficit is ipsilateral to the lesion (and, of course, occurs at levels below the lesion).

Transection of the dorsal columns does not change the threshold for painful stimuli, but transection of the anterolateral system results in prolonged (although not necessarily permanent) loss of pain sensation contralateral to the side of the lesion.

Experimental studies of the various somatic areas of the cortex have also provided valuable information about the functioning of the somatic sensory system. Total removal of S-I produces deficits in position sense and in the ability to discriminate size, roughness, and shape. Thermal and pain sensibilities are not abolished, but perception is altered even for these submodalities. In addition, Josephine Semmes and her colleagues at the NIH have used monkeys to study the functions of the different Brodmann areas concerned with somatic sensibility. By making small lesions in the hand region of each area, she found that lesions in area 3b produce deficits in the discrimination of texture as well as size and shape. In contrast, lesions in area 1 produce a selective defect in the ability to assess the texture of objects, whereas lesions in area 2 alter only the ability to differentiate the size and shape of objects. This is consistent with the idea that area 3b, which (together with 3a) is the initial and principal target for the afferent projections from the ventral posterior lateral nucleus of the thalamus, receives information about texture as well as about size and shape. Area 3b then projects to both areas 1 and 2. The projection to area 1 is concerned primarily with texture and that to area 2 is concerned with size and shape.

Removing S-II in monkeys prevents them from learning new tactile discriminations on the basis of shape. Damage to the posterior parietal cortex produces complex abnormalities in spatial orientation for the contralateral half of the body.

Modern Electrophysiological Studies Correlated Body Areas and Cortical Areas

Modern interest in the somatic sensory system started in 1920 with the work of E. D. Adrian and Yngve Zotterman on cutaneous and muscle receptors. This interest extended to the central nervous system in the late 1930s with the work of Wade Marshall, Clinton Woolsey, and

Philip Bard at the Johns Hopkins School of Medicine. Their important series of experiments began with a chance observation made in the course of studying the electrical activity of the cerebral cortex in the cat and monkey. Using large surface electrodes that record the activity of thousands of cells in an area of cortex several millimeters in extent, Marshall found that when a part of the animal's body surface was touched, a deflection could be recorded from the postcentral gyrus of the contralateral cerebral cortex, indicating that neurons in that part of the cortex were activated (Figure 25–4). These evoked potentials represent the electrical activity of populations of neurons activated by stimulating a point on the skin.

Later, Marshall joined Woolsey and Bard to map systematically the representation of the body surface on the postcentral gyrus. By connecting the points of maximal activity (that is, by relating a position on the body surface to a position of maximal electrical activity in the cortex), they could produce a coherent map of the body surface (Figures 25–5 and 25–6). Representations of the body surface and deep tissue exist not only in the cortex but also in the thalamus and the dorsal column nuclei.

Similar representations were found in the human cortex by the neurosurgeon Wilder Penfield during operations for epilepsy and other brain lesions. Working with locally anesthetized patients, Penfield stimulated the surface of the postcentral gyrus at various points in the area of S-I and asked the patients what they felt. This protocol was necessary to ascertain the focus of the epi-

25–4 With this experimental arrangement, a map of evoked potentials can be obtained in a monkey from the surface of the left postcentral gyrus of the cerebral cortex by applying stimuli to the body surface on the opposite side.

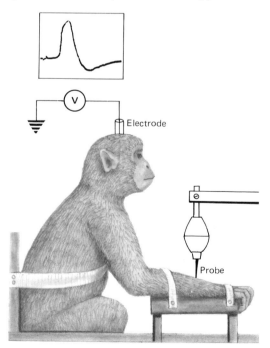

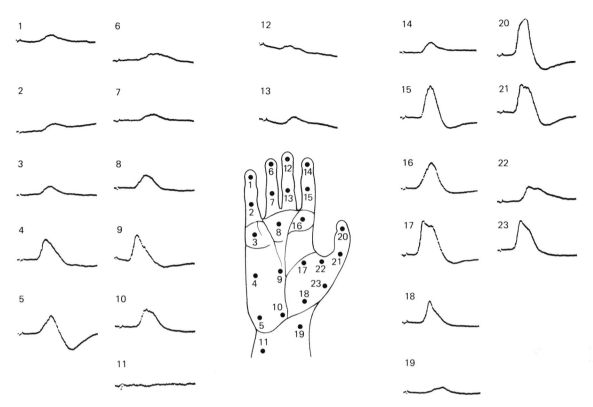

25-5 It is possible to determine which areas of the somatic sensory cortex respond maximally to tactile stimulation of different areas of the body surface by recording evoked potentials from a single spot in the cortex while varying the sites of stimulation on the body surface. In this experiment, a spot in the hand area of the left postcentral gyrus of a monkey responded very differently to a light tactile stimulus applied to various points on the right palm. (Adapted from Marshall, Woolsey, and Bard, 1941; Bard, 1938.)

lepsy and therefore to avoid unnecessary damage during surgery. Penfield found that stimulation produced tactile sensations—paresthesias (numbness, tingling) and pressure—in the corresponding part of the opposite side of the body. A transverse section through the somatic sensory cortex of the human brain based on these studies is shown in Figure 25–7; it illustrates the representation of the body in one hemisphere. The leg is represented most medially, followed by the trunk, arms, face, and finally, most laterally, the teeth, tongue, and esophagus.

Penfield's observations were important. First, they provided independent confirmation in humans of Marshall, Woolsey, and Bard's experimental mapping technique based on evoked potentials in animals. Second, Penfield's findings explained how a disturbance within the somatic sensory system can be readily localized clinically. They illustrated why neurology has been a precise diagnostic discipline, even though for many decades its practice relied on only the simplest tools—a wad of cotton, a safety pin, a tuning fork, and a hammer: the reason is that the brain is precisely organized in space and many regions of that space correspond to a particular function. By carefully diagnosing the disturbance of function, one can accurately infer the location of the lesion within the neural space of the patient.

To take a particularly dramatic example, before Penfield's contributions, the great British neurologist Hughlings Jackson had described a characteristic sensory epileptic attack that now bears his name. The Jacksonian seizure has as its early and sometimes only feature a sensory progression of numbness and paresthesia that begins at one locus and spreads throughout the body. The numbness might begin on the right side at the tip of the finger, spread to the hand, up the arm, down across the shoulder, into the back, and down the ipsilateral leg. The topography of this kind of sensory seizure can now be explained by the projection of the sensory information in the brain. The irritative focus of the seizure is in the opposite hemisphere, in this case the left, and specifically in the postcentral gyrus. In this gyrus the seizure is initiated laterally in the hand area and propagates medially in an orderly fashion.

Potentials from the somatic sensory cortex can now be recorded from the surface of the scalp in humans in a completely noninvasive manner by using computers to obtain an average of many evoked signals so that the evoked response can be resolved from background electrical activity. These evoked potentials provide information not only about the somatic sensory cortex but also about the ascending pathways in the spinal cord, brain stem, and thalamus. For example, in demyelinating disease, the evoked potentials in the cortex can reveal a delay due to slowing of conduction in the spinal cord and brain stem. (As we saw in Chapter 18, demyelination also

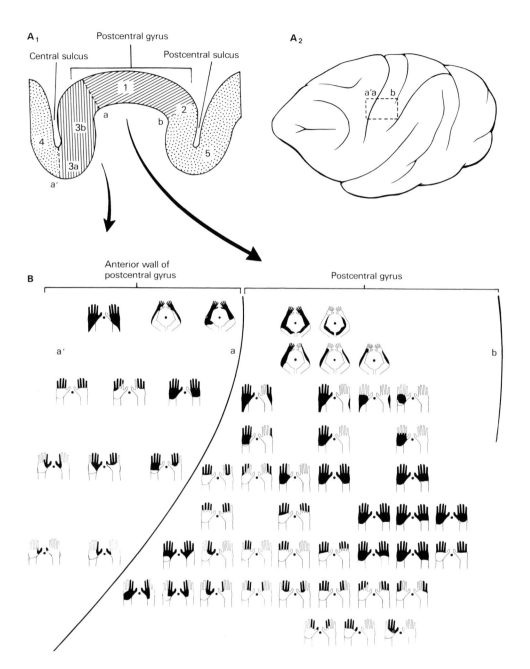

25–6 Marshall, Woolsey, and Bard mapped the projection of the monkey's right hand onto the postcentral gyrus of the left parietal lobe—the area we now call S-I—by examining the cortical responses to tactile stimulation of both the palmar and dorsal surface of the right hand. **A₁** illustrates a sagittal view of S-I showing the Brodmann subdivisions. **A₂** illustrates the location of the recording site in a lateral view of the brain. **B.** Maps based on recordings from what we now know to be Brodmann's areas 3b and 1. These maps reflect the responses evoked in different parts of these two areas by stimulation of the palmar and dorsal surfaces of the right hand (the two surfaces of the right hand are joined by **dots** in the figure). The hands illustrated on the left side of the figure (between lines a' and a) are from the representation of the hand region in the anterior wall of the postcentral gyrus (vertically hatched areas in part **A₁**, lying between lines a' and a). These areas correspond roughly to 3b and 3a in S-I. The hands on the right side of the figure (between a and b) are from the representation on the dorsal surface of the postcentral gyrus (diagonally hatched area in part **A₁**, lying between lines a and b). This area corresponds roughly to Brodmann's area 1 in S-I. (Adapted from Marshall, Woolsey, and Bard, 1941).

causes slowing of conduction in peripheral nerves by interfering with the saltatory propagation of action potentials.) A common cause for demyelination in the central nervous system is multiple sclerosis. Conduction can be slowed at an early stage of the disease when sensation is still normal. Thus, evoked responses can provide *clinical* information about sensory deficits that may not be detectable in a routine neurological examination.

Why Is the Map So Distorted?

The representation of the body surface in the cortex as revealed by evoked responses illustrates another important principle. The map in Figure 25–7 is drawn to scale; in it different parts of the body are represented in brain areas of different sizes. The face is large compared with the back of the head; the index finger is gigantic compared with the big toe.

As the homunculus in the human brain is a distorted picture of man, so is the body image of other species. Comparative studies by Woolsey and his colleagues show that the distortions parallel the importance of a particular part of the body surface for tactile sensibility (Figure 25–8). In humans, in whom the handling of tools and of language is so well developed, the hand and the tongue predominate, and both representations are large. However, in both humans and lower animals a coherent map of the body surface emerges only if one connects the points of maximal response. Each area in neural space is involved in both convergent and divergent relationships.

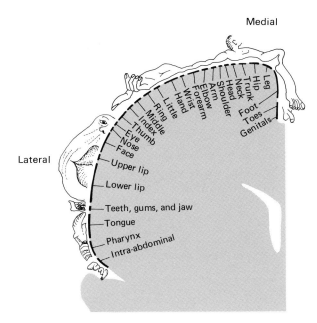

Medial

Lateral

25–7 The projection of the body surface onto a sagittal section of the postcentral gyrus of the parietal cortex of the human brain illustrates the orderly medial-to-lateral progression of the representation of the body surface. (Adapted from Penfield and Rasmussen, 1950.)

The distortions of the sensory maps obtained by studying evoked potentials also presented several puzzles. The contours of the map of each region of the body in Figure 25–6 are ill-defined. In addition, there is much overlap in the representation of various parts of the body. Given these two facts, how do we achieve the extraordinarily precise tactile sensibility of which we are capable? In the early maps for somatic sensibility, the various submodalities (deep pressure versus superficial touch, for example) were superimposable. Thus, all the receptors from each part of the body seemed to project to roughly the same area of cortex. Since we know that superficial sensations can be discriminated from deep ones, and touch can be perceived as being distinct from position sense, this also was puzzling.

Each Central Neuron Has a Specific Receptive Field

To try to resolve these problems, Vernon Mountcastle, Jerzy Rose, and their colleagues began to examine the somatic sensory system at the cellular level using extracellular microelectrodes (which became available in the late 1940s) to record the electrical responses of individual neurons. More recently, this work has been extended by Michael Merzenich, Jon Kaas, and their colleagues.

It is difficult to record intracellularly in the brain, where neurons are small and often inaccessible. Fortunately, it is possible to record from cells extracellularly for several hours without damage. Extracellular recordings reveal only the action potentials of the cell; they do not show synaptic activity except under rare circumstances. Nevertheless, a great deal has been learned by studying how sensory stimuli modulate the firing patterns of single cells.

Mountcastle and his colleagues found that neurons in the somatic sensory system are not silent but spontaneously active. Sensory stimuli therefore act to modulate ongoing neuronal activity in central nuclei and in the cerebral cortex. Moreover, the activity of a given cell cannot be modulated by stimuli applied to just any point on the body surface; rather, each cell responds only to stimulation of a specific area of the skin. Mountcastle called that area the *receptive field* of the cell, following the tradition established in the study of peripheral receptor cells. The receptive field of a cell is *that area on any receptive sheet where stimulation will either excite or inhibit the firing of that cell.* In anatomical terms, this refers to the area on the receptive sheet (in the somatic sensory system, the skin; in the visual system, the retina) that projects directly or indirectly onto the particular cell. In physiological terms, it refers to the area over which stimulation will either increase or decrease the firing rate of the cell. The receptive field is probably the most important concept of sensory physiology.

The restriction of a neuron's receptive field to a particular area has an important functional consequence. If we apply a probe to a point on the skin, the excited neurons are those connected to the afferent fibers that innervate

25–8 These highly schematic drawings of the body representation for somatic sensibility were obtained from studies of evoked potentials in the thalamus and cortex.

They reflect the relative importance of various body regions in the somatic sensibilities of the rabbit, cat, monkey, and humans.

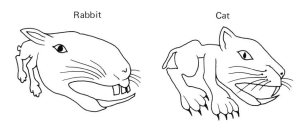

Rabbit   Cat

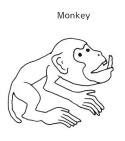

Monkey

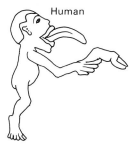

Human

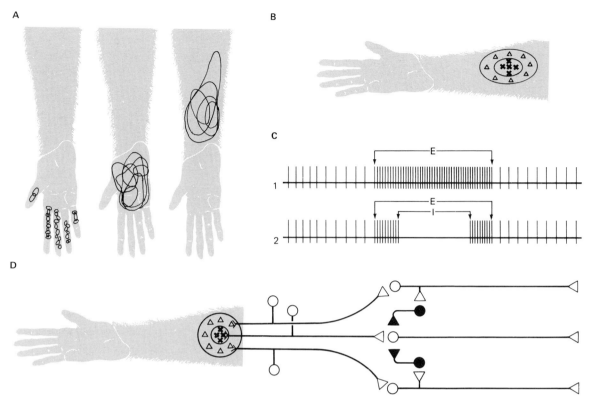

25–9 The sizes of the inhibitory and excitatory regions of the tactile receptive fields of cells in the thalamus and cortex that respond to tactile stimulation of the monkey.
A. Variations in receptive field size along the arm. The fields are small in the distal finger tips; they become larger in the hand and even larger proximally along the forearm.
B. Topographical relationship of the excitatory (**X**) and inhibitory (**Δ**) zones of the receptive fields for a neuron in the postcentral gyrus. Often the excitatory and inhibitory zones are coextensive, so that there is no inhibitory surround of the sort illustrated. **C.** Extracellular recordings from a single cell in the cortex illustrating the interaction of excitatory (**E**) and inhibitory (**I**) portions of the receptive field. In **trace 1** only the excitatory part of the receptive field is stimulated. In **trace 2**

the excitatory part is again stimulated; but now, with the stimulus still on the excitatory portion of the field, the inhibitory region on the skin is stimulated and the excitation is inhibited. When the stimulus is removed from the inhibitory region the excitatory stimulus reasserts its effectiveness.
D. Schema for an excitatory zone and inhibitory surround in a dorsal column nucleus. A stimulus applied to the skin activates a group of receptors that excite a group of cells in the nucleus. This central area of skin is part of the excitatory portion (**X**) of the receptive field of these cells. Stimulation of surrounding skin activates other cells that end on inhibitory interneurons and suppress the firing of the cells activated by the excitatory portion of the receptive field.

the point being stimulated. If we now move the probe to a new point, another population of neurons is activated. Thus, we consciously perceive that one point rather than another is being stimulated on the skin because one rather than the other population of neurons in the brain is active.

Mountcastle next described two other interesting features of receptive fields: their size distribution on the body surface and their fine structure.

Sizes of Receptive Fields Vary

The size of the receptive field on the body surface varies in precise correspondence with the distortion of the body surface in the map (Figure 25–9A). The areas of the skin that are most sensitive to touch and that therefore have the greatest cortical representation—the tips of the fingers and the tongue—have the smallest receptive fields

and the largest number of receptive fields per unit area of skin. Moving proximally along the arm, one finds a gradient of both receptive field sizes and density that parallels the gradient of innervation and is reflected in tactile sensibility. The distortions in the map of the body representation in the cerebral cortex (Figures 25–5, 25–6, and 25–7) are therefore due to innervation density: relatively more neural innervation and more cortical representation is given to areas of greater sensibility. As a result, the receptive fields are small in these areas of the body surface. The cortical magnification (the area of cortex devoted to a unit area of body surface) for the fingers as compared with the trunk is about 100:1, and the receptive fields of the trunk are about 100 times larger than those of the finger tips. Thus, cortical magnification and receptive field size are inversely related. It should now be understandable why finger tips can be used for reading braille, but elbows and shoulders cannot.

Receptive Fields Have a Fine Structure

Each receptive field has a fine-structural organization. First, there is a gradient within the excitatory portion of the receptive field that is reflected in the brain as a gradient of activity at each relay point, including the cortex. The discharge of the cell is greatest when a stimulus is applied to the center of the excitatory part of the receptive field; the discharge is weakest at the periphery. Superimposed upon this excitatory gradient is a gradient of inhibition, which is largely masked by the more powerful excitation. The inhibitory gradient is also greatest at the center and decreases toward the edge of the excitatory zone of the receptive field. Inhibition sometimes extends beyond the excitatory receptive field, giving rise to an *inhibitory surround* (Figure 25–9B through D). Under these circumstances, stimulation of the area surrounding the excitatory portion of the receptive field inhibits the cell. Thus, a stimulus in the excitatory portion of the receptive field sets up a gradient of activity in the brain and activates a population of cells—some greatly, some moderately, and some slightly. This active population is surrounded by a population of less active cells that serves to sharpen the peak of activity within the brain.

Lateral Inhibition Can Aid in Two-Point Discrimination

Fine tactile discrimination, such as reading braille, involves discriminating shape and contour. We can understand how this is accomplished by considering the simplest example of spatial discrimination: the ability to distinguish two closely placed point stimuli as two rather than as one. Clinically, this test is called two-point discrimination.

Mountcastle proposed a model for two-point discrimination based on the reconstruction of the neural events in the postcentral gyrus of the cortex produced by a light tactile stimulus delivered to the skin. According to this model, two stimuli applied to separate positions on the skin set up two excitatory gradients of activity at every

relay point in the somatic sensory system. The activity in each population of cells has a discrete peak. The inhibitory surround sharpens each peak and further enhances the distinction between the two peaks.

Consider a single-point stimulus. This stimulus activates several touch receptors that provide short trains of impulses in each of the first-order afferent fibers activated. These afferent fibers provoke a discharge in a group of cells in a dorsal column nucleus, and those cells activate another group of cells in the ventral posterior lateral nucleus of the thalamus, which in turn discharges a group of cells in the cortex. At each level of the central nervous system the population of cells that discharges impulses is confined to a restricted zone by two factors: (1) the specific anatomical connections that are excited by the particular receptors stimulated and (2) lateral inhibition. This inhibition is *not present at the level of the receptor but comes in at the dorsal column nuclei and is found at each subsequent relay step, so that in the brain the population excited by the stimulus is also surrounded by a ring of inhibition.* As a result of these two factors, the activated cells at each level may be regarded as forming an anatomical zone of excitatory discharge.

The *location* of the stimulus on the body surface is thus signaled in the nervous system by the firing of specific populations of neurons activated by the stimulus. Those populations are located at specific points in each relay nucleus as well as in the cerebral cortex. The *inten-*

25–10 Schematic diagram proposed by Mountcastle to illustrate how lateral inhibition enables two-point discrimination. **A.** Distribution of activity in a population of cells as illustrated in the three-dimensional neural space of the brain. The population is activated by stimulation of a *single* point of the skin. **B.** Distribution of cells activated by stimulation of *two* adjacent points. The activity of each point is indicated by the **dotted line.** The **solid line** indicates the sum of the activities at both points. **Curve 1** indicates the sum of activity in the presence of lateral inhibition; **curve 2** indicates the sum of activity without lateral inhibition. (Adapted from Mountcastle and Darian-Smith, 1968.)

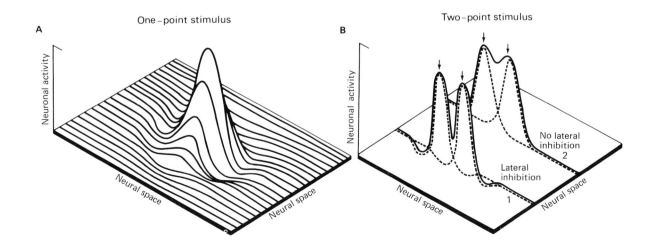

One-point stimulus

A

Neuronal activity

Neural space

Neural space

Two-point stimulus

B

Neuronal activity

No lateral inhibition 2

Lateral inhibition

Neural space

Neural space

1

sity of the stimulus is signaled by the frequency of firing of the specific populations and by the size of the active populations because a strong stimulus to the skin causes a higher frequency of firing and a wider excitation profile in these populations than a weak stimulus. Not all cells in this population respond in an identical manner. Cells at the center, which have the most powerful connections with the area being stimulated, discharge most effectively and with the shortest latency. Cells just off the center have a lower probability of firing and discharge fewer impulses with longer latency.

Because each point on the skin sets up a gradient of activity at each level in the nervous system, we can begin to see how the evolution of the receptive field along the ascending system can give rise to two-point discrimination. Each stimulus excites a set of cells that has a receptive field with a central excitatory zone surrounded by a weaker excitatory zone (Figure 25–10A). The weaker excitatory zone is further depressed by the inhibitory surround. When two stimuli are brought close together there is a summation of the surround inhibition of each field that affects the neurons activated in the area of the skin between the two stimuli. This summation of inhibition retards fusion of the excitatory zones set up by the two stimuli, thus preserving peaks of activity at the cortical level and enhancing the contrast between the two points (Figure 25–10B, 1). Lateral inhibition occurs in all sensory and motor systems. In each system and at each level, it functions to enhance contrast. It is easy to see how a neural organization such as this might lead to the ability to recognize pattern and contour.

Modality-Specific Labeled Communication Lines Are Organized into Columns

In addition to inhibition, another feature of cortical organization was revealed with microelectrodes that could not have been found with evoked responses. This feature explained the puzzling observation that the gross maps of the various submodalities for touch–pressure and position sense are topographically often the same. Cellular techniques have made it possible to investigate whether there is segregation on the cellular level; that is, are single cells sensitive to one or to several submodalities? Work has now been carried out on single neurons in the dorsal column nuclei, in the thalamus, and in the cortex. In each region, single nerve cells respond to only one submodality: cells respond specifically either to superficial touch stimuli or to deep pressure stimuli. There is even segregation between the superficial modalities, such as movement of hairs and steady indentation of skin. Moreover, cells responding to one submodality are located together and are segregated from cells responding to other submodalities. The most remarkable example of this grouping is evident in the cerebral cortex.

In a series of pioneering studies, Mountcastle explored the somatic sensory cortex for the distribution of the various submodalities. Because the cortex consists of six major cellular layers (see Chapter 20), he first looked for

a correlation between cell layer and submodality but found none. He then examined the submodalities with respect to vertical position in the cortex and found, to his surprise, that the cortex is organized into vertical columns or slabs running from the cortical surface to the white matter. Each neuron in such a vertical column is activated by the same submodality: some columns are activated by position of the joints, some by touch, and some by movement of hairs. In addition, the locations of the receptive fields of the neurons in a column are almost identical. Neurons lying within a vertical column therefore make up the elementary topographical and modality-specific unit of function. We shall soon see that columnar organization is quite general and reflects a basic organizational principle of the cerebral cortex.

Modality-Specific Columns Are Grouped into Domains

Kaas, Merzenich, and their colleagues, using microelectrodes that allow particularly fine resolution, have found that there are actually four independent and fairly complete maps in S-I, one for each of the Brodmann areas: 3a, 3b, 1, and 2 (Figure 25–11). The four representations are adjoining; they are parallel and correspond to each other in their medial-to-lateral representation. This explains why the earlier studies of Marshall, Woolsey, and Bard, and of Penfield (who used gross recording electrodes that sampled more than 1 mm of cortex) led to the inference that the somatic sensory map consists of only a *single* large representation, as in Figure 25–7. Each of these four architectonic areas has its own pattern of extrinsic connections and most areas are reciprocally interconnected. Still another map of the body surface is present in the secondary somatic cortex (S-II).

In any one area of the cortex, input from one or another submodality tends to dominate, but other submodalities are also present. For example, the cells in Brodmann's area 3a respond primarily to deep input, input from muscle stretch; cells in Brodmann's area 3b respond primarily to the activation of rapidly or slowly adapting cutaneous receptors; cells in Brodmann's area 2 respond primarily to deep pressure; and those in area 1 respond to the activation of rapidly adapting cutaneous receptors (Figure 25–12A). But additional submodalities exist within each region. Thus, for each digit in Brodmann's area 3b there are separate strips of unequal width for rapidly adapting and slowly adapting submodalities (800 μm for fast and 200 μm for slow). The inputs from these two receptors—the slowly and rapidly adapting skin receptors—are segregated into columns rather than being distributed as a mosaic (Figure 25–12B). Thus, within any one of the four architectonic areas of S-I there are, on the microscopic level, several interrelated maps of the body surface (Figure 25–12B).

In view of the importance of columnar organization of the cortex, what is the function of the six histological cell layers that are so prominent in the cross section of the cortex? Anatomical studies with various anatomical tracers have shown that different layers project to differ-

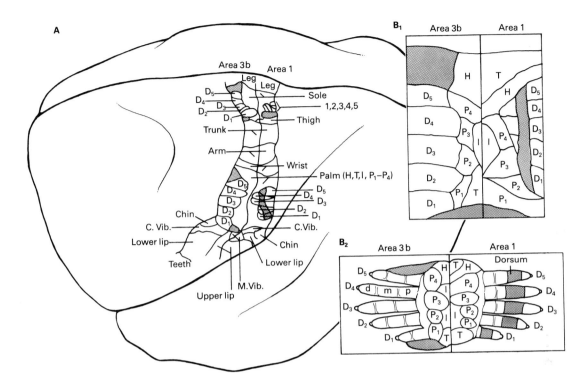

25–11 The mapping experiments of Kaas, Merzenich, and their colleagues indicate that each of the four subregions of S-I (areas 3a, 3b, 1 and 2) has its own representation. **A.** Dorsolateral view of the brain of an owl monkey shows that area 3b and area 1 each has its own cutaneous representation. The two representations, however, have many corresponding features. The representation of the hairy surfaces of the foot and hand are **shaded.** The digits of the hand and foot are **numbered. B.** Enlarged drawings of the representation of the glabrous pads of the palm in areas 3b and 1. **B₁** is an expanded and more detailed map of the hand areas of the particular monkey cortex illustrated in part **A. B₂** is an idealized map generated from similar studies on a large number of monkeys. The distortions in the palm reflect the relative representations of each area in the cortex. In both maps, the representation in area 1 is roughly a mirror image of the representation in area 3b. The palmar pads (**P**) are numbered in order (P_4 to P_1); there are two insular pads (**I**), one hypothenar pad (**H**), and two thenar pads (**T**). The five digital pads (**D**) also are numbered; distal, **d**, middle, **m**, proximal, **p**. (From Kaas et al., 1983.)

ent parts of the brain: layer VI projects back to the thalamus, layer V to subcortical structures, layer IV *receives* input from the thalamus, and layers II and III project to other somatic cortices. Thus, as we shall see again in the visual system, the cortical columns are computational modules that transform information coming from a particular point on the skin and distribute that transformed information to various regions of the brain.

Dynamic Properties of Receptors Are Matched to Those of Central Neurons

The finding that neurons of a given modality are grouped together suggests that there are specific and spatially segregated communication lines, or sensory channels, for various submodalities. Submodality-specific receptors and the axons of primary sensory neurons are connected to clusters of submodality-specific cells in the dorsal column nuclei and in the thalamus, and these then project to a submodality-specific column in the cortex.

We saw in Chapters 23 and 24 that the various mechanoreceptor cells differ in their dynamic response properties: some receptor cells adapt rapidly, others adapt

slowly. Given submodality-specific communication lines, how do the properties of the receptor at the beginning of the sensory line relate to the properties of the subsequent neurons in the brain with which the receptors communicate? Mountcastle and his colleagues examined this question and found that the various receptors are well matched to their central neurons. Rapidly adapting hair receptors connect to rapidly adapting neurons in the thalamus and the cortex. Slowly adapting joint receptors connect to neurons in the brain that adapt slowly. As a result, the dynamic response of a central neuron corresponds to that of the receptors to which it is connected, ensuring that the response of the receptor is faithfully transmitted to the cortex.

Thus, for sensory channels concerned with tactile sensibility, the sensitivity of the receptor sets the sensitivity for the whole communication line. In these channels, a major transformation of the stimulus is determined by the peripheral receptor. Indeed, psychophysical studies show that several elementary aspects of tactile perceptions in humans are determined by the response properties of the receptors. The subsequent relays in the sensory pathways are matched appropriately to the receptor and serve to preserve this initial abstraction.

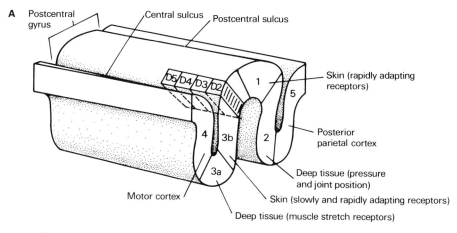

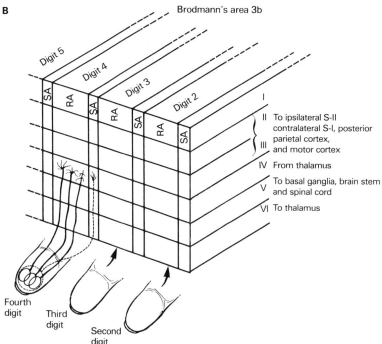

25–12 The somatic sensory cortex has a highly specific columnar organization. **A.** The various regions of the somatic sensory cortex—Brodmann's areas 3a, 3b, 1, and 2—receive their predominant projections from different receptors in the skin. Thus, area 3a receives predominant input from deep tissue from the stretch receptors of muscles, whereas area 3b receives input from the superficial skin, from both slowly and rapidly adapting receptors; area 1 receives superficial input primarily from rapidly adapting skin receptors, and area 2 from receptors in deep tissue that signal joint position and deep pressure. **B.** In addition to having a predominant projection from one receptor type, each of the Brodmann areas of the somatic sensory cortex is also organized vertically and horizontally. *Vertically*, the cortex is organized into columns that run from surface to white matter. Each column is specific for a submodality. The examples shown here are from Brodmann's area 3b and mediate rapidly adapting (**RA**) and slowly adapting (**SA**) tactile sensation. The columns for each part of the body (such as a given digit) are grouped together. *Horizontally*, the cortex is organized into layers that receive inputs from certain regions of the brain and project to other regions. (Adapted from Kaas et al., 1979.)

Considering the specificity that is characteristic of submodality channels, we might predict that eliciting a *single* action potential in a *single* receptor neuron would give rise to a quantum—an elementary unit—of tactile perception. Indeed, as we saw in Chapter 23, Å. B. Vallbo and his colleagues in Sweden have recently demonstrated that humans can perceive the activation of a single tactile receptor in the hand.

Feature Detection: Some Central Nerve Cells Have Complex Properties

In the hand area of the somatic sensory cortex of the monkey a few cells (about 6%) have properties that are more complex than those we have so far considered. These cells do not respond well to punctate stimuli on the receptive field, but respond briskly to movement of a

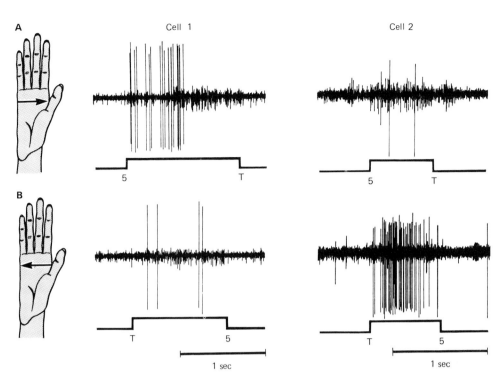

25–13 Some neurons in the somatic sensory cortex are directionally sensitive. These recordings are from two neurons in the hand area of the monkey cortex that have the same receptive field but opposite direction preferences. (Recordings came from the same electrode penetration.) **A.** Responses to movement of a sable hair brush from fifth digit (**5**) to thumb (**T**) across the interdigital pads of the palm. **B.** Responses to the same stimulus moving across the pads from T to 5. For cell **1,** movement from 5 to T evoked a strong response (Part **A**), while movement from T to 5 evoked a very weak response (Part **B**). The converse was true for cell **2.** (Adapted from Costanzo and Gardner, 1980.)

mechanical stimulus within the receptive field. Many of these cells are *directionally sensitive* and respond better to movement along the skin in one direction than in the reverse direction (Figure 25–13). Some neurons respond well to an edge placed on the skin in a certain (optimal) direction. These complex cells are not found in Brodmann's areas 3a and 3b, the primary target for the axons that project from the ventral posterior lateral nucleus of thalamus. They are found instead in the two posterior cortical regions: in area 1 and, particularly, in area 2. This suggests that these complex properties arise not from the receptor but from cortical processing of the incoming sensory information. (We shall encounter this idea again in considering the visual system.)

What is the function of cortical neurons with complex receptive field properties? Juhani Hyvärinen and Antti Poranen suggest that these cells become active during movements of the hand designed to explore the shape of an object and that they have a role in *stereognosis*—the capacity to appreciate three-dimensional structure.

The somatic sensory areas of the cortex project to the posterior parietal cortex (Brodmann's areas 5 and 7) (Figure 25–1B). In the posterior parietal cortex, cells have very complex properties, receive convergence from several separate modalities, and are often related to movement. There the mechanisms for tactile discrimination and position sense are integrated with visual information and used to probe *extrapersonal space,* the environment immediately surrounding the subject. It is in the posterior parietal cortex that the picture we have of our body is thought to arise.

An Overall View

What are the advantages of somatotopy? What are the benefits of having the sensory sheet represented in an orderly map in the brain? Topographical organization facilitates the orderly specification of intracortical connections and allows these connections to be short. Contrast enhancement of adjacent regions, which results from lateral inhibition and is important for two-point discrimination, is also achieved most economically by having a topographical representation. Such an arrangement permits the interneurons necessary for tuning receptive fields and for sharpening their contrast to be close together.

For touch, as for other sensory and motor modalities, signals from the periphery reach the cortex by several parallel pathways, each carrying information, some of which is redundant and some unique to its pathway. As a result, lesions of the medial lemniscus do not abolish tactile perception completely. Patients with these lesions still retain the capability for crude tactile discrimination, through pathways that ascend in the anterolateral column, although aspects of discriminative touch are lost or seriously impaired.

In addition to parallel ascending pathways, any given pathway often projects to more than one cortical area. Thus, there are five representations of the body surface in the posterior parietal cortex, one in S-II, and four in S-I. Why are there so many representations of the body surface? Somatic sensation involves the isolation and parallel analysis of different stimulus attributes in different cortical areas. Parallel processing in the brain is a form of processing that we shall encounter again. It should not be confused with redundancy, which it resembles. Redundancy is a cybernetic term that is used to denote duplication of components—such as multiple lighting, tracking, or ignition systems. The purpose of redundancy is to provide security—to ensure that one system will operate when the others break down. Although parallel processing also achieves a measure of security in the case of disease, this is not its primary purpose. Parallel processing is designed not to achieve multiplication of identical circuitry but to allow different neuronal pathways and brain relays to deal with the same sensory information in slightly different ways. Because of parallel processing, simple neuronal transformations, using signals based on synaptic excitation, synaptic inhibition, and action potentials, are able to endow our perceptions with richness.

Selected Readings

Brodal, A. 1981. Neurological Anatomy in Relation to Clinical Medicine, 3rd ed. New York: Oxford University Press, pp. 46–147.

Darian-Smith, I. 1982. Touch in primates. Annu. Rev. Psychol. 33:155–194.

Hyvärinen, J., and Poranen, A. 1978. Movement-sensitive and direction and orientation-selective cutaneous receptive fields in the hand area of the post-central gyrus in monkeys. J. Physiol. (Lond.) 283:523–537.

Kaas, J. H., Nelson, R. J., Sur, M., Lin, C.-S., and Merzenich, M. M. 1979. Multiple representations of the body within the primary somatosensory cortex of primates. Science 204:521–523.

Kaas, J. H., Nelson, R. J., Sur, M., and Merzenich, M. M. 1981. Organization of somatosensory cortex in primates. In F. O. Schmitt, F. G. Worden, G. Adelman, and S. G. Dennis (eds.), The Organization of the Cerebral Cortex. Cambridge, Mass.: MIT Press, pp. 237–261.

Mountcastle, V. B. 1975. The view from within: Pathways to the study of perception. Johns Hopkins Med. J. 136:109–131.

Mountcastle, V. B. 1976. The world around us: Neural command functions for selective attention. Neurosci. Res. Program Bull. [Suppl.] 14.

Mountcastle, V. B. 1984. Central nervous mechanisms in mechanoreceptive sensibility. In I. Darian-Smith (ed.), Handbook of Physiology, Section 1: The Nervous System, Vol. III, Sensory Processes. Bethesda, Md.: American Physiological Society, pp. 789–878.

Starr, A. 1978. Sensory evoked potentials in clinical disorders of the nervous system. Annu. Rev. Neurosci. 1:103–127.

Vallbo, Å. B., Olson, K. Å., Westberg, K.-G., and Clark, F. J. 1984. Microstimulation of single tactile afferents from the human hand: Sensory attributes related to unit type and properties of receptive field. Brain 107:727–749.

Werner, G., and Whitsel, B. L. 1973. Functional organization of the somatosensory cortex. In A. Iggo (ed.), Handbook of Sensory Physiology, Vol. 2: Somatosensory System. New York: Springer, pp. 621–700.

References

Adrian, E. D., and Zotterman, Y. 1926. The impulses produced by sensory nerve-endings. Part 2: The response of a single end-organ. J. Physiol. (Lond.) 61:151–171.

Bard, P. 1938. Studies on the cortical representation of somatic sensibility. Harvey Lect. 33:143–169.

Costanzo, R. M., and Gardner, E. P. 1980. A quantitative analysis of responses of direction-sensitive neurons in somatosensory cortex of awake monkeys. J. Neurophysiol. 43:1319–1341.

Hikosaka, O., Tanka, M., Sakamoto, M., and Iwamura, Y. 1985. Deficits in manipulative behavior induced by local injections of muscimol in the first somatosensory cortex of the conscious monkey. Brain Res. 325:375–380.

Jackson, J. H. 1931–1932. Selected Writings of John Hughlings Jackson. J. Taylor (ed.). London: Hodder and Stoughton.

Kaas, J. H., Merzenich, M. M., and Killackey, H. P. 1983. The reorganization of somatosensory cortex following peripheral nerve damage in adult and developing mammals. Annu. Rev. Neurosci. 6:325–356.

Marshall, W. H., Woolsey, C. N., and Bard, P. 1941. Observations on cortical somatic sensory mechanisms of cat and monkey. J. Neurophysiol. 4:1–24.

Mountcastle, V. B. 1957. Modality and topographic properties of single neurons of cat's somatic sensory cortex. J. Neurophysiol. 20:408–434.

Mountcastle, V. B., and Darian-Smith, I. 1968. Neural mechanisms in somesthesia. In V. B. Mountcastle (ed.), Medical Physiology, 12th ed., Vol. II. St. Louis: Mosby, pp. 1372–1423.

Norrsell, U. 1980. Behavioral studies of the somatosensory system. Physiol. Rev. 60:327–354.

Penfield, W., and Rasmussen, T. 1950. The Cerebral Cortex of Man. A Clinical Study of Localization of Function. New York: Macmillan.

Randolph, M., and Semmes, J. 1974. Behavioral consequences of selective subtotal ablations in the postcentral gyrus of Macaca mulatta. Brain Res. 70:55–70.

Sherrington, C. S. 1947. The Integrative Action of the Nervous System, 2nd ed. New Haven: Yale University Press.

Woolsey, C. N. 1958. Organization of somatic sensory and motor areas of the cerebral cortex. In H. F. Harlow and C. N. Woolsey (eds.), Biological and Biochemical Bases of Behavior. Madison: University of Wisconsin Press, pp. 63–81.

Dennis D. Kelly

Central Representations of Pain and Analgesia

26

Pain is a protective experience that we share with almost all animals. Because there is such an urgent and primitive quality about the array of sensations that we call painful (for example, pricking, burning, aching, stinging, and soreness), it is difficult to appreciate that the neural activity associated with pain, like that of other sensory systems, can be modulated by a wide range of behavioral experiences. Pain can be altered by drugs, acupuncture, and surgery, but it can also be altered by the joy of childbirth, the fear of a dentist, by stress, hypnosis, and many other forms of stimulation and ritual. The extraordinary plasticity of human pain suggests that neural mechanisms must exist that either modulate transmission in primary pain pathways or modify the organism's emotional reaction to pain. As we shall see, both types of modulatory activity occur in the nervous system.

Pain is more than a conspicuous sensory experience that warns of danger. Chronic pain represents a massive social problem and sustains a major industry. In the United States more than 2 million workers are incapacitated by pain at any given time, and compensation payments for pain exceed 2.5 billion dollars each year. Despite these social dimensions, until recently there has been little systematic animal experimentation dealing with pain and its relief. This may be partly due to a lag in the development of accurate psychophysical methods for assessing pain in animals. Clinical researchers were also uncertain about the fundamental relevance of animal research to human pain. Given the extraordinary psychological malleability of the human response to pain, there has been a reluctance to acknowledge that similar nonsensory factors might operate in the pain experience of animals. However, many of the neurons capable of influencing neural information associated with pain are found in phylogenetically conserved areas of the brain that line the walls of the medial and caudal portions of the ventricles: the limbic system, the thalamus, the hypothalamus, and the reticular core of the brain stem. This localization to phylogenetically conserved areas suggests that we share the capability for pain inhibition with many living species and that, therefore, the physiological properties of the system can be studied experimentally in animals. It also suggests that the pain inhibitory system evolved before the earliest hominids, and we may assume that it survived in the human brain because it offered a significant selective advantage. In this chapter, we shall first consider the mechanisms involved in the perception of pain and then examine those involved in suppressing it.

Pain Is Transmitted by Specific Neural Pathways

Receptors for Pain May Be Activated by Mechanical, Thermal, or Chemical Stimuli

Information related to pain is transduced by the morphologically least differentiated receptors in the skin: the free nerve endings. As with all neurons involved in somatic sensation, the cell bodies of the primary afferent pain neurons are located in the dorsal root ganglia. Some of these cell bodies give rise to myelinated axons, others to unmyelinated axons. Many of the nerve endings can be activated most efficiently by strong mechanical pressure and by extreme heat. This is particularly true for the Aδ fibers, nociceptive neurons with myelinated axons. The terminal regions of C fibers, whose axons are unmyelinated, are believed to be activated by a chemical released into the extracellular fluid as a result of tissue damage. The local release of a chemical intermediary might explain the burning pain that persists after a mechanical or thermal stimulus is removed.

Thus, pain is, in part, caused by chemoreceptors. Extracts from damaged tissue produce intense pain when injected into normal skin. Various substances cause pain when injected into skin, and each has been proposed as the chemical mediator of pain. Pain can be induced by acidic solutions as well as by histamine, the peptide bradykinin, serotonin, acetylcholine, and K^+. The response to K^+ is particularly interesting because most tissue damage results in an increase in extracellular K^+ concentration and there is a good correlation between pain intensity and local K^+ concentration. The neuronal response to chemical, mechanical, and thermal stimuli on nociceptive terminals is greatly enhanced by the local presence of prostaglandins, which appear to sensitize all classes of nociceptive receptors. Consequently, aspirin-like drugs that inhibit the synthesis of prostaglandins often reduce inflammatory pain at the site of its origin.

Primary Pain Afferents Terminate in the Dorsal Horn of the Spinal Cord

As we saw in Chapter 23, pain in humans is subserved by two distinct populations of peripheral afferent fibers.

One set consists of a portion of the small, thinly myelinated Aδ fibers that conduct at about 5–30 m/sec. Activation of these nociceptors is associated with sensations of sharp, pricking pain. These Aδ fibers are aroused primarily by noxious heat and mechanical stimuli. The other set of nociceptive fibers consists of small unmyelinated C fibers that conduct at 0.5–2 m/sec. Their free nerve endings are activated by a variety of high-intensity mechanical, chemical, and thermal (greater than 45°C) stimulation; they are therefore called *polymodal nociceptors*. These unmyelinated C fibers are widely distributed in deep tissues as well as skin (in the skin they are much more dense than Aδ fibers), and mediate long-lasting burning pain. A similar duality exists in peripheral populations of trigeminal neurons.

Upon entering the spinal cord in the lateral division of the dorsal root, the Aδ and C fibers bifurcate and ascend and descend for one to three segments, forming part of the tract of Lissauer, before synapsing on neurons in the dorsal horn. The two types of fibers terminate primarily in the outermost laminae of the dorsal horn, in the marginal zone, which corresponds to Rexed's lamina I, and in the substantia gelatinosa (lamina II). Some Aδ fibers project more deeply to terminate on lamina V cells as well. The laminar pattern of termination of Aδ and C primary afferents does not limit their direct influence to cells in those zones. Some neurons in lamina V have dendrites that extend to the outermost layers of the dorsal horn, and thus they could be excited directly there by primary afferent nociceptors that do not penetrate beyond the superficial layers.

Among the several potential neurotransmitters that have been identified within primary nociceptive afferent neurons, most attention has been focused on the 11-amino-acid peptide substance P (Arg-Pro-Lys-Pro-Gln-Gln-Phe-Phe-Gly-Leu-Met). This substance is released at the central synapses of some primary afferent neurons following electrical stimulation of their high-threshold (C-fiber) axon. The release is blocked when morphine is applied in concentrations known to elicit analgesia. Using immunohistochemical techniques, Tomas Hökfelt has localized this peptide to small unmyelinated primary pain afferents in the skin, in the smallest cells of the dorsal root ganglion, in the tract of Lissauer, and in laminae I, II, and III of the dorsal horn.

Like the large primary sensory neurons described in Chapter 3, the cells whose activity is related to pain have one axon that terminates in the spinal cord and another that terminates in the periphery. Recently, substance P, somatostatin, and other neuropeptides that have been localized in the C fibers have been found to be transported along both the central and the peripheral axons. They are also released from *both* central and peripheral terminals. By releasing substances into the skin, the small-diameter nociceptors may participate in local inflammatory and irritative reactions. It is conceivable that the sensory information received centrally via unmyelinated C fibers may be modulated in part by interactions between substances released at the peripheral terminals of nociceptive afferents and other chemical mediators in the skin.

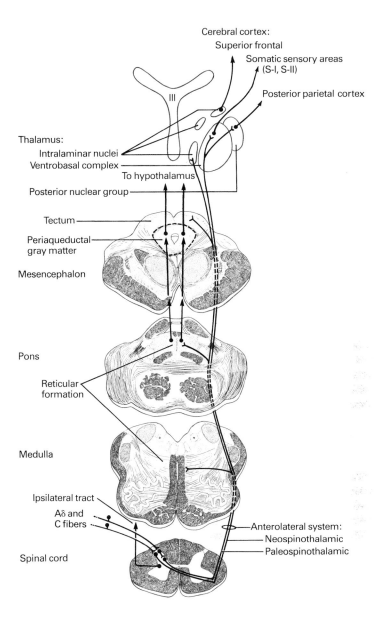

26–1 The anterolateral system of spinothalamic, spinoreticular, and spinotectal fibers conveys information about pain to several regions of the brain stem and diencephalon.

At Least Two Populations of Neurons in the Spinal Cord Transmit Information about Pain

Second-order neurons are either relay cells, whose axons project to the brain stem or thalamus, or interneurons that transfer information about pain to other interneurons or to relay cells (Figure 26–1). These second-order neurons receive Aδ and C fiber input from interneurons in the substantia gelatinosa.

Relay cells for pain are located in two regions of the dorsal horn, and their axons *ascend in the anterolateral quadrant* of the white matter. The axons of relay cells in Rexed's lamina I project directly to the thalamus. Because this part of the ascending pain projection is a recent phylogenetic development, it is often called the *neospinothalamic tract* (or the lateral spinothalamic tract because its axons are thought to be segregated laterally in the anterolateral quadrant). In contrast to the

neospinothalamic tract, relay cells located in deeper layers of the dorsal horn (especially layer V) make up the phylogenetically older *paleospinothalamic tract*. (Actually, few cells in the paleospinothalamic tract project directly to the thalamus. Most terminate in the reticular formation and are more appropriately considered as a spinoreticular tract.)

The pain projection pathways are collectively called the *anterolateral system* because they all ascend in the anterolateral portion of the lateral column. The anterolateral system, especially the neospinothalamic component, is primarily crossed in humans; however, a small but significant ipsilateral component also exists. These uncrossed fibers may be the reason pain returns in some patients despite an initially successful surgical section of anterolateral fibers.

Electrophysiological analysis of dorsal horn cells that receive nociceptive input and whose axons ascend in the anterolateral columns suggests that there are two general populations of spinal cord nociceptive neurons (Figure 26–2): (1) neurons in lamina I that are selectively activated by pain afferents, and (2) neurons in lamina V that receive input from mechanoreceptors and thermoreceptors as well as pain receptors. We shall consider these populations in turn.

The first group of ascending dorsal horn nociceptive neurons is located in lamina I. Edward Perl at the University of North Carolina has found that these neurons are vigorously excited by both noxious thermal and mechanical stimuli and are unaffected by touch or movement of hairs. These neurons send their axons to the anterolateral portion of the contralateral cervical cord and from there to the thalamus. As indicated in Figure 26–2, their axons form the *neospinothalamic* component of the anterolateral system and, as we shall see later, may be responsible for the fine localization of sharp or acute pain on the body surface. Although this is the type of pain most often studied in the laboratory, it is not the type that normally prompts patients to seek medical attention.

The second group of ascending dorsal horn nociceptive neurons in Figure 26–2 is located primarily in lamina V. These large cells respond to activity of all three of the main fiber components of the cutaneous nerves: Aβ, Aδ, and C fibers. As might be expected, they respond to both nonnoxious and noxious stimuli, and hence are called *multireceptive* or *wide dynamic range nociceptors*. The type of response to each of these fiber groups differs. Threshold touch stimuli produce a brief burst of firing in lamina V cells followed by brief inhibition. However, when large-fiber touch input is suppressed, there is a remarkable build-up in the activity of the same cell following C fiber stimulation, leading to prolonged afterdischarges and facilitation. The axons of these cells contribute to the paleospinothalamic and spinoreticular components of the anterolateral system, which seem to subserve the more diffuse, chronic types of pain that are of most importance to the practice of medicine.

Spinal Pain Projections to the Brain Stem Are Widespread

Only a small proportion of the fibers of the anterolateral system go to the thalamus. Most of the fibers synapse at brain stem levels below the thalamus, largely in the reticular formation of the brain stem tegmentum. In the brain stem, the anterolateral system of the spinal cord shows great divergence of terminations, which presumably underlies the capability of noxious stimuli to produce behavioral activation and alertness.

In addition to the direct spinothalamic and spinoreticular projections, there is a third projection, the *spinotectal tract*. Many anterolateral, pain-activated fibers from the spinal cord end at the level of the midbrain in the lower layers of the superior and inferior colliculi. Noxious stimuli give rise to evoked potentials in the tectum, and electrical stimulation of this area is particularly painful. Moreover,

from a phylogenetic standpoint, the midbrain tectum of reptiles is a well-developed somatic sensory relay nucleus, not unlike the thalamus of mammals.

An even larger number of anterolateral fibers enters the gray matter of the midbrain that surrounds the cerebral aqueduct, called the midbrain *periaqueductal gray matter* (medial projection in Figure 26–1). The periaqueductal gray region has strong reciprocal connections with the periventricular region of the diencephalon (through the dorsal longitudinal fasciculus) and, via the hypothalamus, with the limbic system. As we shall see later, current theories of pain consider the mesencephalic central gray as a probable convergent area of limbic forebrain and sensory information. This area may therefore be important in modulating pain input on the basis of emotional state.

Thalamic Relays Preserve the Duality of Ascending Pain Projections

The few truly spinothalamic fibers in the anterolateral system terminate in thalamic areas that generally reflect the separate projections of the neospinothalamic and paleospinothalamic neurons. The neospinothalamic neurons terminate in three nuclei of the posterior thalamus: the ventrobasal complex, the ventrocaudal parvocellular nucleus, and the posterior nuclear group.

The most somatotopically arrayed terminations from pathways innervating the trunk and extremities are in the *lateral part of the ventral posterior nucleus*. Fibers from the trigeminal nucleus, relaying somatic information from the face, terminate in the *medial part of the ventral posterior nucleus*. Together the lateral and ventral parts are referred to as the *ventrobasal complex*. Neurons of this portion of the thalamus project in a somatotopic manner to areas S-I and S-II of the somatic sensory cortex. However, less than 10% of neurons in the ventrobasal complex respond to noxious stimuli. As we have seen in Chapters 24 and 25, a numerically much larger input to the ventrobasal complex is the medial lemniscus, conveying information concerning touch and proprioception. As a result, this part of the thalamus is both a gateway to the somatic sensory cortical areas and the site where lemniscal fibers converge with a small but important part of the anterolateral system. This overlap is particularly marked in the ventral posterior lateral nucleus, where many spinothalamic fibers appear to be arranged like an archipelago in discrete clusters of terminals interspersed among the more regularly spaced somatotopic terminations of lemniscal axons from dorsal column nuclei.

In humans, the most important spinothalamic termination related to pain is a region immediately ventral to the tactile portion of the ventrobasal complex, called the *ventrocaudal parvocellular nucleus* because of the small size of these thalamic cells. Rolf Hassler in Germany has shown that stimulation of this small region in humans results in specific, localized pain referred to the contralateral side of the body. This pain resembles that elicited by stimulating the spinothalamic system at more caudal levels, suggesting that neurons in this part of the ventrobasal complex are especially important for localized pain.

A third area of neospinothalamic termination is the posterior nuclear group described physiologically by Gian F. Poggio and Vernon Mountcastle. This group lies in a zone between the mesencephalon and thalamus, caudal to the ventral posterior nucleus. Again, only some cells in this transitional region respond to noxious stimuli, but the neurons that do respond show exceptionally large receptive fields. Because such cells are not likely to provide information precise enough to localize the painful stimulus, Poggio and Mountcastle suggested that the simultaneous stimulation of mechanoreceptors that accompanies a painful stimulus may provide an alternative mechanism for localizing pain. The assumption that this group of nociceptive neurons is not well equipped to localize pain is supported by clinical observation of patients with lesions that interrupt the lemniscal system. These patients cannot localize painful stimuli well.

Paleospinothalamic fibers terminate in the nonspecific intralaminar nuclei, particularly the paracentral and central lateral nuclei. Mountcastle proposed that these projections on the intralaminar nuclei are responsible for slow, burning pain. In addition to spinothalamic fibers, the intralaminar nuclei also receive projections from the cerebellum, basal ganglia, and brain stem reticular tegmentum, and they project diffusely to the cortex.

Stereotaxically placed surgical lesions in the thalamus have been attempted often during the past 20 years to relieve the pain of patients suffering from advanced cancer. In one particularly informative study by Vernon Mark, Frank Ervin, and Paul Yakovlev, damage to the sensory relay nuclei (the ventrobasal complex) produced a loss of cutaneous touch and sharp pain (pinprick), but left deep chronic pain unaffected. Lesions of the intralaminar nuclei successfully relieved chronic deep pain but not cutaneous pain. These observations support the idea that the duality of pain initially noted in distinct populations of peripheral afferents is preserved even at the thalamic level.

Central Pain Syndrome: Surgery Intended to Relieve Existing Pain May Produce New Pain

In 1920 the British neurologist Henry Head studied 24 patients who had developed lesions in the lateral thalamus after a stroke. These patients showed an interesting combination of initial postural and motor deficits followed by exaggerated affective responses to somatic sensory stimuli. He called this sequence the *thalamic syndrome*, and later investigators have described the unusual and unpleasant sensory phenomena as *central pain*. In Head's patients, touch, cold, heat, and painful stimuli were felt as much more unpleasant on the side *opposite* the lesion than on the affected side. This is because the ascending somatic sensory pathways cross the midline in the spinal cord and brain stem. The two major

symptoms—motor deficits and exaggerated affective responses to somatic sensory stimuli—showed a similar somatotopic distribution but different time courses. The motor deficits were maximal at the time of vascular accident and diminished gradually, whereas the spontaneous pain and unpleasant sensory effect developed months later, while the patient was recovering from the earlier deficits. The central pain then persisted unaltered for years.

We now know that central pain can arise not only from pathological lesions in the thalamus but also from neurosurgical lesions placed anywhere along the nociceptive pathway, from spinal cord and brain stem to thalamus and cortex. Even when surgery is initially successful in alleviating the original pain, central pain can develop later in some patients. The new sensations are unpleasant and abnormal, often unlike anything the patients had ever felt before: spontaneous aching and shooting pain, numbness, cold, heaviness, burning, and other unsettling sensations that even the most articulate patients find difficult to describe. Central pain is particularly distressing emotionally, often more so than the pain the operation was intended to relieve.

Fortunately, pain following lesions along the nociceptive pathway develops in only a few patients. In the unpredictable instances in which central pain does develop, the symptoms are similar to those originally described by Head for the thalamic syndrome, irrespective of the level in the central nervous system of the triggering lesion.

The Gate Control Theory Emphasized the Modulation of Pain by Sensory and Emotional Stimuli

The gate control theory of pain was developed in the early 1960s by Ronald Melzack and Patrick Wall to account for some of the ways in which pain differs from other sensations. In particular, they were interested in the mechanisms by which other cutaneous stimuli and emotional states alter the level of pain felt. One site of interaction suggested by the theory is among the interneurons of the substantia gelatinosa in the spinal cord (laminae II and III; Figure 26–2). Melzack and Wall suggested that collateral input from the large myelinated Aβ touch fibers and collateral input from the smaller Aδ and C fibers have antagonistic effects on cells in the substantia gelatinosa. These gate cells, in turn, are presumed to regulate the firing of cells deeper in the dorsal horn, presumably in lamina V, that give rise to the paleospinothalamic tract. These investigators proposed that a higher central decoding mechanism monitors spinothalamic activity for a critical level at which, and above which, pain is felt. The brain is also assumed to exert descending control on this system, since cognitive factors are known to influence even spinal withdrawal reflexes. For example, a hot cup of tea is likely to be dropped; but if the cup is made of fine Wedgewood china, one is less apt to drop it, and may even manage jerkily to put it back on the table *before* shaking the hand.

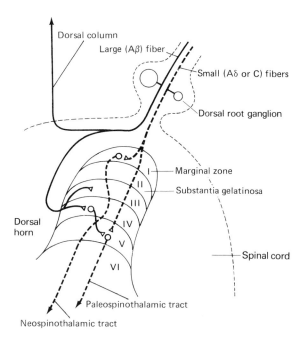

26–2 Schematic drawing of the dorsal horn of the spinal cord illustrating that the nociceptive neurons, whose axons form the ascending anterolateral system, are found in lamina I and lamina V of the dorsal horn. While neurons in the marginal layer (lamina I) receive input primarily from small Aδ and C fibers, there is greater convergence of large- and small-fiber input upon nociceptive neurons in lamina V. This difference is reflected in the electrophysiology of these cells. Many nociceptive neurons in the marginal layer do not respond to nonpainful touch stimuli, while those in the deeper layers display a wider dynamic range.

Although the anatomical possibility exists for large- and small-fiber interactions in the dorsal horn (Figure 26–2), there is relatively little physiological evidence for the gate control theory. At a spinal level, the gate control theory predicts that somatic stimulation will produce presynaptic inhibition on both the small- and large-diameter dorsal root fibers that synapse on spinothalamic neurons. To test this, David Whitehorn and Paul Burgess stimulated mechanoreceptive fibers and looked for evidence of presynaptic inhibition on nociceptive Aδ fibers. They found none. Only when nociceptors themselves were activated by noxious stimuli was any presynaptic inhibition seen on central nociceptive fibers. Similarly, presynaptic inhibition of large-diameter fibers was found only with gentle mechanical stimulation, the quality mediated by these fibers. Although disappointing for the gate control hypothesis, these negative results involving Aδ fibers are probably not definitive.

As several studies have failed to provide support for the gate control theory, it is appropriate to ask why the theory should be mentioned. There are two reasons. First, even if the theory is incorrect in detail, some of its clinical predictions are useful—for example, the suggestion that stimulation of the large-diameter dorsal column fibers should close the gate and thus diminish pain. Direct

or even transcutaneous electrical stimulation of sensory nerves, particularly the dorsal column—which by itself is felt as tingling—does provide pain relief for long periods. The second reason is that the gate control theory reversed the historical research emphasis on pain as solely an afferent sensory experience. Pain also disrupts ongoing behavior, demands immediate attention, and serves as a primary negative reinforcer in a variety of situations. It suppresses behavior upon which it is contingent and supports a broad repertoire of avoidance and escape responses. To emphasize only the sensory features of pain in the study of its neural bases and to ignore its unique affective and motivational properties is to confront only part of the problem. Similarly, to treat pain simply by trying to cut down the sensory input by pharmacological or surgical blocks disregards several useful modalities of treatment and can only delay the understanding of how the brain itself is organized to inhibit the perception of pain.

Pain Is Also Inhibited by Select Neural Pathways: The Mechanisms of Analgesia

It was once believed that sensory systems are fully reliable in their afferent transmission of signals and that central ascending pathways convey to the cortex with minimal transformations whatever messages are generated by sensory end-organs. Only when sensory impulses reached the cortex were they believed to be accessible to perceptual processing and modification by psychological factors. However, we now know that pain, like all other sensory information, can be modulated from its very point of origin through successive synaptic junctions in its central pathway. In this section, we shall briefly consider four convergent lines of research on inhibition of pain: (1) analgesia produced by direct brain stimulation, (2) the mapping of morphine-sensitive sites in the brain, (3) the characterization of the opiate receptor, and (4) the discovery of endogenous opiates.

Direct Electrical Stimulation of the Brain Produces Analgesia

Although it has been known for at least 30 years that central stimulation can elicit pain, only recently has it been shown that stimulation of the gray matter that surrounds the third ventricle, cerebral aqueduct, and fourth ventricle results in profound analgesia that is sufficient for abdominal surgery to be performed without discomforting an unanesthetized rat. Stimulation-produced analgesia is a specific antinociceptive effect and not a generalized sensory, motivational, or motor deficit. It is particularly interesting that stimulation-produced analgesia often has a restricted peripheral field. Subjects respond normally to noxious stimuli in the unaffected body areas. Moreover, subjects still respond to nonpainful stimuli such as touch and temperature within the circumscribed area of analgesia.

Stimulation-produced analgesia also exhibits another, as yet unexplained, feature first noted by David Mayer and John Liebeskind: the analgesia may continue for many minutes or even hours after stimulation. Fortunately, analgesic relief of chronic pain in patients has (after an initial latent period of 10–15 min) been seen to outlast a period of periaqueductal gray stimulation by over 24 hr. Although nociceptive neural activity can be suppressed by stimulating a number of brain regions, some of the best examples of pure analgesia unaccompanied by other behavioral reactions have been obtained from electrodes placed in the midbrain periaqueductal gray (particularly in the region of the serotonin-rich dorsal raphe nucleus) and in the medullary nucleus raphe magnus of the medulla. Although the periaqueductal gray receives nociceptive input from the anterolateral system, destroying it or perfusing it with the local anesthetic procaine (novocaine) does not increase pain thresholds. Thus, the periaqueductal gray matter is not an obligatory pain relay and stimulation-produced analgesia does not result from a temporary disruption of afferent transmission of pain information; rather, the stimulation appears to exert its effects through active inhibition of afferent input in the dorsal horn of the spinal cord and the trigeminal nerve nucleus.

This inhibition is selective. For example, stimulation of the periaqueductal gray completely inhibits responses of lamina V-type cells of the dorsal horn of the cat to intensely noxious peripheral stimuli, while the discharge of lamina IV-type cells, which are unrelated to pain, is unaffected. Furthermore, lesions of the dorsolateral column in the spinal cord—which interrupt serotonin-containing axons descending from cells in the medullary nucleus raphe magnus and terminating in the dorsal horn—block analgesia elicited from the periaqueductal gray matter.

Stimulation-Produced Analgesia Is Related to Opiate Analgesia

The sites and mechanisms of morphine's analgesic action seem to parallel the sites and mechanisms of stimulation-produced analgesia. Narcotic analgesic drugs exert a powerful, lamina-specific inhibition on spinal cord sensory interneurons remarkably similar to that just described for periaqueductal stimulation. Furthermore, recent work on opiate-sensitive receptor sites (outlined below) indicates that their distribution overlaps extensively with the areas whose stimulation results in analgesia. Microinjecting morphine directly into many of these sites, particularly the periaqueductal gray, results in profound analgesia.

Depletion of serotonin by prior administration of parachlorophenylalanine (which blocks the synthesis of serotonin) or by lesions of the raphe nuclei blocks the ability of both intracranial and systemic narcotics to diminish pain; stimulation-produced analgesia is similarly blocked by depletion of serotonin. Perhaps the most impressive

evidence linking stimulation-produced analgesia and opiate mechanisms has been developed by Huda Akil, David Mayer, and John Liebeskind. They found that naloxone, a specific narcotic antagonist, blocks not only morphine analgesia, but stimulation analgesia as well, although somewhat less reliably. Thus, a study of either one of these mechanisms may advance our understanding of the other.

Opiate Receptors Are Distributed Throughout the Nervous System

Morphine and related opiates exert their analgesic effects by interacting with specific postsynaptic receptors. Because the opiates demonstrate an extreme chemical specificity, the existence of specific opiate receptors had long been assumed by pharmacologists before these receptors were discovered almost simultaneously in the laboratories of Lars Terenius in Sweden, Solomon H. Snyder at Johns Hopkins, and Eric Simon at New York University. The procedures of these investigators were similar. Brain tissues were homogenized, and synaptosomes were extracted by means of differential centrifugation. The samples were then incubated in a solution of labeled opiates or antagonists with high specific activity and subsequently washed to remove loosely bound and unbound radioactivity. The binding that occurred, like the pharmacological activity of opiates, showed high stereospecificity. There was also a precise correlation between the pharmacological potency of various opiates in producing or antagonizing analgesia and their affinity for the binding sites. Potent opiates, such as morphine and levorphanol, demonstrated affinities in the nanomolar range, whereas weak opiates, such as meperidine, did not bind at these concentrations.

The in vitro identification of a cellular component with which opiates combine to produce their characteristic analgesic and euphoric effects raised the inevitable question of what normal physiological role these receptors play. It seemed unlikely that such highly specific receptors should have evolved in nature fortuitously only to interact with alkaloids from the opium poppy. On the contrary, as originally suggested by Paul Ehrlich, the more likely possibility is that many drug receptors are targets for endogenous ligands. Endogenously occurring morphinelike substances, which are members of the opioid peptide family (Chapter 13), are the ligands for these opiate receptors. The wide distribution of opiate receptors in the brain (Table 26–1) and their high density in regions not associated with analgesia suggest that the endogenous opioids operate in a variety of physiological roles in addition to pain modulation.

There Are Three Branches of Opioid Peptides

The first endogenous opiates to be characterized were the enkephalins, two small peptides isolated from pig brain in 1975 by John Hughes and Hans Kosterlitz in Scotland.

Table 26–1. Localization and Possible Functions of Opiate Receptors

Localization[a]	Functions influenced by opiates
Spinal cord	
Laminae I and II	Modulation of pain perception
Brain stem	
Substantia gelatinosa of spinal tract of caudal trigeminal nuclei	Modulation of pain perception
Nucleus of solitary tract, nucleus commissuralis, nucleus ambiguus	Taste, vagal reflexes, cough suppression, respiration, orthostatic hypotension, inhibition of gastric secretion, EEG synchronization and sleep induction
Area postrema	Nausea and vomiting, as in motion sickness
Locus ceruleus	Arousal, attentiveness, muscular inhibition during REM sleep
Habenula-interpeduncular nucleus-fasciculus retroflexus	Emotional behavior, site of interaction between limbic areas and basal ganglia
Pretectal area (medial and lateral optic nuclei)	Upward eye movements and pupillary reflexes
Superior colliculus	Orienting movements of head and eyes to sensory targets (visual, auditory and somatosensory)
Ventral nucleus of lateral geniculate	Central modulation of visual input
Dorsal, lateral, medial terminal nuclei of accessory optic pathway	Entrainment of endocrine rhythms by light, fine adjustment of head-eye coordination
Dorsal cochlear nucleus	Modulation of auditory input
Parabrachial nucleus	Respiration, coordination of breathing patterns with behavioral states, modulation of taste and pain perception
Diencephalon	
Infundibulum	Oxytocin and vasopressin secretion
Thalamus	
Medial lateral nucleus, internal and external laminae, intralaminar (centromedian) nuclei, periventricular nucleus	Modulation of pain and other somatic sensory perceptions, arousal, selective attention
Telencephalon	
Amygdala	Emotional behavior, autonomic expression of fear and other aversively motivated behaviors
Caudate, putamen, globus pallidus	Motor coordination, spatial-motor orientation
Nucleus accumbens	Locomotion, mediation of stimulant and opiate drug reinforcing properties
Subfornical organ	Water balance
Bed (interstitial) nucleus of stria terminalis	Olfactory control of male sexual behavior, emotional behavior

[a]Anatomical localization from Miller, R. J. and Pickel, V. M. 1980. The distribution and functions of the enkephalins. J. Histochem. Cytochem. 28:903–917.

These two opioid pentapeptides, *Met-enkephalin* (Tyr-Gly-Gly-Phe-Met-NH$_2$) and *Leu-enkephalin* (Tyr-Gly-Gly-Phe-Leu), are only mildly analgesic. When injected directly into the cerebral ventricles, they produce a brief analgesia of approximately 10 min in rats.

Since the original observations of Hughes and Kosterlitz, 18 distinct peptides with opioid activity have been discovered, all of which contain the sequence Tyr-Gly-Gly-Phe. With recombinant DNA techniques, it has been shown that each of these opioid peptides arises from one of three different polyprotein precursors. Each precursor has a molecular weight of about 28,000 and is the product of one of three distinct genes. The occurrence of a particular coding sequence in genomic DNA can be detected by probing a genomic library (a set of cloned DNA fragments representing the entire genome) with a radioactively labeled polynucleotide polymer containing the appropriate base sequence.

Sequences coding for opioid peptides in the genome were first discovered by using cDNA copied from mRNA isolated from tissues prolific in producing the peptides (for example, from the pituitary and the adrenal medulla). Later, polynucleotides were synthesized chemically that corresponded in base sequence to all possible genomic coding sequences for particular peptides, and these were used as hybridizing probes. By 1983, the three opioid polyprotein precursors and their mRNAs in the form of cDNA had been completely sequenced. In addition, the structure of much of the genomic DNA encoding the three messengers was understood.

Elucidation of the *proopiomelanocortin* branch of the opioid family tree resulted from the protein chemical studies of Edward Herbert at the University of Oregon and Choh Hao Li at the University of California at San Francisco and their co-workers. The proopiomelanocortin gene is expressed in the pituitary, and its peptide products are released into the blood stream in response to stress. The polyprotein is processed differently in different cells, however. Differences in processing have been studied most thoroughly in the rodent central nervous system. In the anterior pituitary, the predominant peptides produced from proopiomelanocortin are adrenocorticotropin (ACTH) and β-lipotropin (β-LPH) (Figure 26–3). In the intermediate lobe of the pituitary, adrenocorticotropin is converted to α-melanocyte-stimulating hormone (α-MSH) and corticotropinlike intermediate lobe peptide (CLIP); β-lipotropin is processed to γ-lipotropin and β-endorphin (β-END). Although humans do not have an intermediate lobe and do not produce CLIP and α-MSH, differential processing of peptide messengers undoubtedly is universal. The processing in neurons in the arcuate nucleus of the brain resembles that of the intermediate lobe.

Proenkephalin was the second branch of the opioid family to be analyzed, largely through the work of Sidney Udenfriend and his collaborators at the Roche Institute in New Jersey. In the early stages of studying this group of peptides, investigators were confused because it was believed that the products of the third branch, *prodynorphin*, were also derived from proenkephalin. The genes for both branches are expressed in a much wider distribution of tissues than is the proopiomelanocortin gene. In addition to the pituitary, enkephalins and dynorphins occur in many parts of the brain and spinal cord, and in the adrenal medulla. When the products of the genes encoding proenkephalin and prodynorphin were finally resolved, it was found that proenkephalin yields four copies of Met-enkephalin (Met-ENK), one copy of Leu-enkephalin (Leu-ENK), and several other opioid peptides, and that prodynorphin contains three copies of Leu-enkephalin and a series of peptides called dynorphins that are not found in the two other opioid precursors.

Prodynorphin was distinguished from proenkephalin by Shosaku Numa and his co-workers in Kyoto, who, since 1978, have carried out brilliant analyses of all three opioid genes. To distinguish these two branches, Numa synthesized the oligodeoxyribonucleotides corresponding to unique amino acid sequences in a dynorphin peptide as a probe for identifying and isolating the coding se-

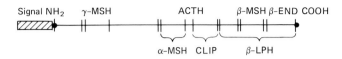

A Pro-OPIOMELANOCORTIN (POMC)

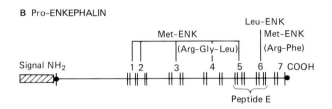

B Pro-ENKEPHALIN

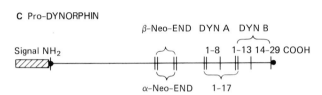

C Pro-DYNORPHIN

26–3 Schematic representation of the protein precursor structures of the three opioid peptide families.
A. Proopiomelanocortin branch (or POMC) was derived primarily from protein biochemical studies and later confirmed by DNA cloning methods. **B.** The Pro-enkephalin precursor structure (also known as Pro-enkephalin A) was determined by DNA cloning methods. **C.** The Pro-dynorphin precursor (also known as Pro-enkephalin B) was distinguished from the Pro-enkephalin branch through the work of Numa in Kyoto, Japan. The double vertical lines represent di-basic amino acid cleavage sites. (From Akil et al., 1984.)

quences of the third branch of the opioid family tree. Dynorphin is 200 times more potent than morphine. Avram Goldstein of Stanford University and colleagues gave this peptide its name from *dynamis* (Greek for power) and endorphin. Dynorphin is 13 amino acids long with the structure

Tyr-Gly-Gly-Phe-Leu-Arg-Arg-Ile-Arg-Pro-Lys-Leu-Lys.

Which of the other peptides function as endogenous analgesics? Several are extremely active: from the proopiomelanocortin branch, α-endorphin (amino acids 61–76), β-endorphin (61–91), and γ-endorphin (61–77) are active. The most potent is β-endorphin, which shows an even greater affinity for the opiate receptor than does morphine; it is 48 times more potent than morphine when injected intraventricularly and 3 times more potent when given intravenously. Unfortunately, chronic administration of β-endorphin produces progressively weaker analgesic effects (tolerance) and also results in withdrawal signs comparable to those of morphine (dependence). Nevertheless, the potential role of the enkephalins and endorphins in the therapeutic control of pain is of great interest to researchers.

In addition to their addictive properties, the relatively brief duration of the analgesia induced by these naturally occurring opiates is a major obstacle to their clinical use. The enkephalins also appear to have epileptogenic effects (which are naloxone reversible) on the rat's cerebral cortex, and intracerebral injections of β-endorphin lead to a pronounced catatonic posturing.

Different Classes of Opiate Receptors Mediate Different Actions

Many opiate actions, including analgesia, appear to be mediated on a cellular level by different classes of opiate receptors. The concept of receptor subtypes is not unique to the opioids, as illustrated by the α and β receptors of norepinephrine and the nicotinic and muscarinic receptors of acetylcholine.

Initially W. R. Martin and co-workers proposed three classes of opiate receptors named after the drugs whose different actions and affinities prompted the subclass hypothesis: μ (morphine), κ (ketocyclazocine), and σ (SKF 10, 047, then an experimental compound). When the enkephalins were subsequently described, a δ receptor was proposed to account for their selective actions, and, for similar reasons, an ε receptor was proposed for β-endorphin.

What is the relationship of receptor type to physiological response? Analyses of opiate receptor subtypes suggest that the receptors responsible for producing respiratory depression after opiate administration are different from those responsible for analgesia. From the distribution of receptor types within the central nervous system, and the structure–activity relationships of opioids, it appears that the μ receptors are involved in pain inhibition. If so, this is particularly important for interpreting studies (such as those reviewed above on stimulation-produced analgesia) in which naloxone has been used as a probe to assess opioid involvement, because naloxone is not an equally effective antagonist of all opiate receptor subtypes. In fact, at the δ receptor preferred by enkephalins, the affinity of naloxone is 10 times lower than at the μ receptor, which is preferred by morphine. The affinity of naloxone is even lower at the κ receptor.

Spinal Pain Transmission Neurons Are Subject to Descending Control

The evidence summarized in the preceding sections suggests that opiate, stimulation-produced, and endorphin analgesias may share a common physiological substrate. As noted above, an optimal site for eliciting stimulation-produced analgesia appears to be the midbrain periaqueductal gray matter in or near the serotonergic dorsal raphe nucleus, as well as in the gray matter that extends rostrally into the diencephalic periventricular area. These observations may be relevant clinically since visceral as well as somatic pain can be inhibited by stimulating this region. Moreover, anatomical tracer studies have demonstrated widespread projections from this periventricular–periaqueductal area, of which the following are of

particular interest: (1) descending connections to the medullary reticular nuclei as well as to the nucleus raphe magnus and the adjacent nucleus reticularis paragigantocellularis (both important sites for stimulation-produced analgesia), all of which project to the spinal cord; and (2) ascending projections to the intralaminar nuclei of the thalamus in a pattern similar to that known for the spinothalamic tract. The descending fibers probably form part of a control system that modulates pain transmission in the dorsal horn of the spinal cord via the raphe nuclei in the midline of the medullary reticular formation (Figure 26–4A). From the nucleus raphe magnus, serotonergic or monoaminergic fibers descend through the dorsolateral funiculus of the spinal cord to end in the substantia gelatinosa. There the raphe spinal neurons may synapse with enkephalinergic interneurons that inhibit neurons normally responsible for the onward transmission of noxious information (Figure 26–4B). This model would explain why stimulation of the periaqueductal gray area can block the upward transmission of pain and why transection of the dorsolateral funiculus can block stimulation-produced analgesia as well as attenuate analgesia induced by systemic morphine injections.

Leslie Iversen and Thomas Jessell have suggested that enkephalinergic neurons in the substantia gelatinosa may modulate pain transmission by inhibiting primary afferent Aδ and C fibers presynaptically at their first central synapse. The evidence for this hypothesis, illustrated in Figure 26–4B, is that when the dorsal root is sectioned (at the broken line) the opiate receptors previously present in the dorsal horn of the cord disappear, while there is a slight build-up in enkephalin concentrations. This finding suggests that the opiate receptors are located on the primary afferent cells themselves and that enkephalin-containing neurons, intrinsic to the dorsal horn and thus spared by dorsal root section, may make presynaptic contact on them.

The work of Ann Mudge, Susan Leeman, and Gerald Fischbach at Harvard University has supported the idea that the mechanisms of analgesia may involve presynaptic inhibition of the sensory nociceptive neurons. Specifically, enkephalin inhibits calcium influx into cultured sensory neurons by modulating voltage-sensitive channels. Blockage of Ca^{++} influx into sensory cell terminals could block the release of substance P or other transmitter substances used by nociceptive neurons.

Behavioral Stress Can Induce Analgesia via Both Opioid and Non-Opioid Mechanisms

An important part of an organism's response to emergency situations is a reduction in sensitivity to pain. In meeting the behavioral demands prompted by exposure to stressful situations, such as those involving predation, defense, dominance, or adaptation to an extreme environmental demand, an organism's normal reactions to pain could prove disadvantageous. Pain normally promotes a set of reflex withdrawals, escape, rest, and other recuper-

A

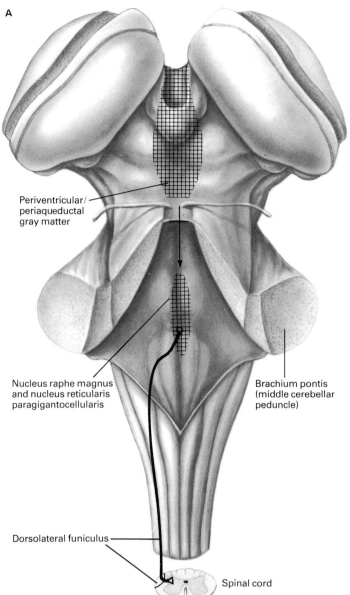

Periventricular/periaqueductal gray matter

Nucleus raphe magnus and nucleus reticularis paragigantocellularis

Brachium pontis (middle cerebellar peduncle)

Dorsolateral funiculus

Spinal cord

B

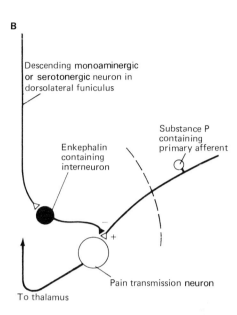

Descending monoaminergic or serotonergic neuron in dorsolateral funiculus

Enkephalin containing interneuron

Substance P containing primary afferent

Pain transmission neuron

To thalamus

26–4 Models have been proposed for the descending control of pain transmission neurons. **A.** Descending pain modulatory system described by Fields and Basbaum. Neurons in the periventricular and periaqueductal gray matter excite those in the nucleus raphe magnus in the medullary reticular formation. From here, serotonergic fibers descend in the dorsolateral funiculus of the spinal cord to terminate in the substantia gelatinosa, where they are believed to activate (or disinhibit) enkephalinergic inhibitory interneurons. **B.** Cellular model proposed by Jessell and Iversen to account for modulation of pain transmission neurons in the dorsal horn of the spinal cord by descending monoaminergic and/or serotonergic neurons of the brain stem. Enkephalinergic interneurons may exert presynaptic inhibitory control over incoming substance P-containing primary afferent fibers concerned with pain.

ative behaviors. During the stressful encounter these reactions to pain might be suppressed automatically in favor of more adaptive behavior. For example, when a laboratory animal is exposed to a novel and severe stress agent, such as an inescapable electric shock to the foot or a brief, forced swim in cold water, its sensitivity to other painful stimuli is reduced. The time course of stress-induced analgesia may range from minutes to hours, depending on the type of stress agent employed, its severity, and the method selected to measure pain thresholds. Repeated exposures to the same stress agent lead to a progressive decline in the analgesic response, in much the same manner that the pituitary–adrenal responses to stress show adaptation.

If an organism's natural response to emergency situations includes a diminished sensitivity to pain, then it seems reasonable that the pain inhibitory system we have considered above, which utilizes opioid peptides, might be involved. However, there is evidence that stress can induce both opioid and non-opioid forms of analgesia.

Studies of the neural and hormonal mechanisms that might account for how stress induces analgesia have shown that virtually every physical stress agent increases plasma levels of β-endorphin as well as adrenocorticotropin and corticosterone; but not all stress agents produce analgesia. Although analgesic stress agents produce profound hormonal responses and a wide range of behavioral deficits, many other stress agents prompt similar plasma elevations in stress hormones without inducing either analgesia or behavioral deficits. Some laboratory examples of stress-induced analgesia are sensitive to opiate receptor blockade by naloxone, but others are not. Some forms of stress-induced analgesia are attenuated by removal of the pituitary, others are enhanced, and many are simply unaffected by the operation.

Nevertheless, there is strong intuitive support for the existence of stress-induced analgesia in humans. Soldiers wounded in battle and athletes injured in sports sometimes report that they do not feel pain. Perhaps, as in the laboratory, stress induces analgesia only in the most extreme or life-threatening situations. We can find extraordinary and century-old expression of this idea in the writings of David Livingstone, the Scottish missionary and explorer of Africa. On an early journey to find the source of the Nile, Livingstone was attacked by a lion that crushed his shoulder:

. . . I heard a shout. Starting, and looking half round, I saw the lion just in the act of springing upon me. I was upon a little height; he caught my shoulder as he sprang, and we both came to the ground below together. Growling horribly close to my ear, he shook me as a terrier does a rat. The shock produced a stupor similar to that which seems to be felt by a mouse after the first shake of the cat. It caused a sort of dreaminess in which there was no sense of pain nor feeling of terror, though quite conscious of all that was happening. It was like what patients partially under the influence of chloroform describe, who see all the operation, but feel not the knife. This singular condition was not the result of any mental process. The shake annihilated fear, and allowed no sense of horror in looking round at the beast. This peculiar state is probably produced in all animals killed by the carnivora; and if so, is a merciful provision by our benevolent creator for lessening the pain of death.

(David Livingstone, *Missionary Travels*, 1857)

An Overall View

Matching the complex experience of pain is the complexity of its several submodalities. Nevertheless, like other sensory modalities, the pain system is based on the orderly neuroanatomical arrangement of fibers connecting the periphery with higher central nervous system structures. In addition, clinical observations, pharmacological study of narcotics, and the discovery of the opioid family of peptides all converge to suggest that the brain also contains a neuronal system, which includes the periaqueductal gray region, that serves to suppress pain.

Opioid peptides are the best candidates for chemical messengers in this modulatory system. Like other chemical messengers, the opioid peptides participate in additional physiological processes. Perhaps other sensory systems, as well, are regulated by similar modulatory systems with characteristic transmitter biochemistry.

Selected Readings

Akil, H., Watson, S. J., Young, E., Lewis, M. E., Khachaturian, H., and Walker, J. M. 1984. Endogenous opioids: Biology and function. Annu. Rev. Neurosci. 7:223–255.

Basbaum, A. I., and Fields, H. L. 1984. Endogenous pain control systems: Brainstem spinal pathways and endorphin circuitry. Annu. Rev. Neurosci. 7:309–338.

Bowsher, D. 1976. Role of the reticular formation in responses to noxious stimulation. Pain 2:361–378.

Cassinari, V., and Pagni, C. A. 1969. Central Pain, A Neurosurgical Survey. Cambridge, Mass.: Harvard University Press.

Dubner, R., and Bennett, G. J. 1983. Spinal and trigeminal mechanisms of nociception. Annu. Rev. Neurosci. 6:381–418.

Herbert E., Oates, E., Martens, G., Comb, M., Rosen, H., and Uhler, M. 1983. Generation of diversity and evolution of opioid peptides. Cold Spring Harbor Symp. Quant. Biol. 48:375–384.

Kakidani, H., Furutani, Y., Takahashi, H., Noda, M., Morimoto, Y., Hirose, T., Asai, M., Inayama, S., Nakanishi, S., and Numa, S. 1982. Cloning and sequence analysis of cDNA for porcine β-neo-endorphin/dynorphin precursor. Nature 298:245–249.

Kilpatrick, D. L., Jones, B. N., Lewis, R. V., Stern, A. S., Kojima, K., Shively, J. E., and Udenfriend, S. 1982. An 18,200-dalton adrenal protein that contains four [Met]enkephalin sequences. Proc. Natl. Acad. Sci. U.S.A. 79:3057–3061.

Noda, M., Teranishi, Y., Takahashi, H., Toyosato, M., Notake, M., Nakanishi, S., and Numa, S. 1982. Isolation and structural organization of the human preproenkephalin gene. Nature 297:431–434.

Pasternak, G. W. 1981. Opiate, enkephalin, and endorphin analgesia: Relations to a single subpopulation of opiate receptors. Neurology 31:1311–1315.

Terman, G. W., Shavit, Y., Lewis, J. W., Cannon, J. T., and Liebeskind, J. C. 1984. Intrinsic mechanisms of pain inhibition: Activation by stress. Science 226:1270–1277.

Watkins, L. R., and Mayer, D. J. 1982. Organization of endogenous opiate and nonopiate pain control systems. Science 216:1185–1192.

Yaksh, T. L., and Hammond, D. L. 1982. Peripheral and central substrates involved in the rostrad transmission of nociceptive information. Pain 13:1–85.

References

Akil, H., Mayer, D. J., and Liebeskind, J. C. 1976. Antagonism of stimulation-produced analgesia by naloxone, a narcotic antagonist. Science 191:961–962.

Christensen, B. N., and Perl, E. R. 1970. Spinal neurons specifically excited by noxious or thermal stimuli: Marginal zone of the dorsal horn. J. Neurophysiol. 33:293–307.

Ehrlich, P. 1909. On Partial Functions of the Cell. Nobel Lecture. Les Prix Nobelen 1908. Stockholm.

Fields, H. L., and Basbaum, A. I. 1978. Brainstem control of spinal pain-transmission neurons. Annu. Rev. Physiol. 40:217–248.

Goldstein, A., Tachibana, S., Lowney, L. I., Hunkapiller, M., and Hood, L. 1979. Dynorphin-(1–13), an extraordinarily potent opioid peptide. Proc. Natl. Acad. Sci. U.S.A. 76:6666–6670.

Hassler, R. 1970. Dichotomy of facial pain conduction in the diencephalon. In R. Hassler and A. E. Walker (eds.), Trigeminal Neuralgia. Pathogenesis and Pathophysiology. Philadelphia: Saunders, pp. 123–138.

Head, H. 1920. Studies in Neurology, Vol. 2, Part IV, The Brain. London: Oxford University Press, pp. 533–800.

Hökfelt, T., Kellerth, J. O., Nilsson, G., and Pernow, B. 1975. Substance P: Localization in the central nervous system and in some primary sensory neurons. Science 190:889–890.

Hughes, J., Smith, T. W., Kosterlitz, H. W., Fothergill, L. A., Morgan, B. A., and Morris, H. R. 1975. Identification of two related pentapeptides from the brain with potent opiate agonist activity. Nature 258:577–579.

Jessell, T. M., and Iversen, L. L. 1977. Opiate analgesics inhibit substance P release from rat trigeminal nucleus. Nature 268:549–551.

Mark, V. H., Ervin, F. R., and Yakovlev, P. I. 1963. Stereotactic thalamotomy. III. The verification of anatomical lesion sites in the human thalamus. Arch. Neurol. 8:528–538.

Martin, W. R., Eades, C. G., Thompson, J. A., Huppler, R. E., and Gilbert, P. E. 1976. The effects of morphine- and nalorphine-like drugs in the nondependent and morphine-dependent chronic spinal dog. J. Pharmacol. Exp. Ther. 197:517–532.

Mayer, D. J., and Liebeskind, J. C. 1974. Pain reduction by focal electrical stimulation of the brain: An anatomical and behavioral analysis. Brain Res. 68:73–93.

Melzack, R., and Wall, P. D. 1965. Pain mechanisms: A new theory. Science 150:971–979.

Mudge, A. W., Leeman, S. E., and Fischbach, G. D. 1979. Enkephalin inhibits release of substance P from sensory neurons in culture and decreases action potential duration. Proc. Natl. Acad. Sci. U.S.A. 76:526–530.

Nakanishi, S., Teranishi, Y., Watanabe, Y., Notake, M., Noda, M., Kakidani, H., Jingami, H., and Numa, S. 1981. Isolation and characterization of the bovine corticotropin/β-lipotropin precursor gene. Eur. J. Biochem. 115:429–438.

Poggio, G. F., and Mountcastle, V. B. 1960. A study of the functional contributions of the lemniscal and spinothalamic systems to somatic sensibility. Central nervous mechanisms in pain. Bull. Johns Hopkins Hosp. 106:266–316.

Poggio, G. F., and Mountcastle, V. B. 1963. The functional properties of ventrobasal thalamic neurons studied in unanesthetized monkeys. J. Neurophysiol. 26:775–806.

Simon, E. J., Hiller, J. M., and Edelman, I. 1973. Stereospecific binding of the potent narcotic analgesia [^{3}H]etorphine to rat-brain homogenate. Proc. Natl. Acad. Sci. U.S.A. 70:1947–1949.

Snyder, S. H. 1980. Brain peptides as neurotransmitters. Science 209:976–983.

Terenius, L. 1973. Characteristics of the "receptor" for narcotic analgesics in synaptic plasma membrane fraction from rat brain. Acta Pharmacol. Toxicol. 33:377–384.

Whitehorn, D., and Burgess, P. R. 1973. Changes in polarization of central branches of myelinated mechanoreceptor and nociceptor fibers during noxious and innocuous stimulation of the skin. J. Neurophysiol. 36:226–237.

Craig H. Bailey and Peter Gouras

The Retina and Phototransduction

27

In this chapter, the first of four devoted to the visual system, we shall examine the retina—a remarkable sensory structure. We shall concentrate on two aspects of retinal function: the biochemical processes involved in photoreception; and the physiological events and structures involved in the processing of visual information.

Unlike somatic receptors of the skin, such as the touch corpuscles, or even the cochlea in the ear, the retina is not a peripheral organ, but a part of the central nervous system. Skin receptors and the cochlea derive embryologically from conventional ectoderm. In contrast, the retina is derived from neuroectoderm, the specialized part of the ectoderm that gives rise to the brain. Indeed, the structural organization and physiological diversity of the cellular components of the retina are sufficiently complex to warrant our considering the retina as a small brain.

There Are Two Types of Photoreceptors: Rods and Cones

Figure 27–1 is a highly schematic illustration of the eye and retina. A surprising feature of the retina is that light must travel through the most proximal layers before it strikes the photoreceptors, the first neural element in the visual pathway. The proximal neural layers, however, are relatively transparent, allowing most light to enter the photoreceptors unabsorbed and undistorted. (The terms *proximal*, or *inner*, and *distal*, or *outer*, are used in relation to the three-dimensional center of the eye.)

In the *fovea*, the area of the retina that has the greatest spatial resolution, the intervening neural layers have been shifted to the side, enabling the photoreceptors, mostly cones, to receive the optical

27–1 In most of the retina, light must first pass through overlying layers of nerve cells and their processes before it reaches the photoreceptors. However, in the center of the fovea, the foveola, these proximal neural elements are shifted to the side; light therefore has a direct pathway to the photoreceptors in this region. An enlarged drawing of the back of the retina is shown on the right.

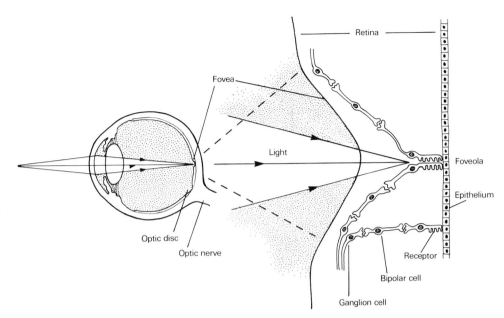

image in its clearest form. This is most pronounced in the center of the fovea, the *foveola*, where only photoreceptors are present. Nasal to the fovea is the *blind spot*, where the optic nerve fibers leave the retina. This region, where the optic nerve fibers come together, is also called the optic disc. The blind spot has no photoreceptors and consequently no vision. (See Figure 28–5.)

The human retina contains two types of photoreceptors, rods and cones. *Cones* detect form and color, and are responsible for day vision. *Rods* mediate night vision; they function in the dim light that is present at dusk or in the dark. Under these conditions most stimuli are too weak to excite the cone system.

In 1866, the German histologist Max Schultze first proposed the duplicity theory, according to which the two functionally distinct photoreceptor systems process visual information at different levels of ambient illumination. The distinctive characteristics of the two systems are due partly to the properties of the receptors (the rods and cones) and partly to the pattern of connections that rods and cones make with other neural elements in the retina (Table 27–1). Except in the fovea, there are 10 times more rods (10^8) than cones in the retina. Nevertheless, cones are much more important to vision because their loss produces legal blindness, whereas total loss of rods produces only night blindness. (Night vision is virtually unnecessary in modern society.) Rods differ from cones structurally in having longer photoreceptor (outer) segments that allow them to capture more light. Rods are also sensitive to light rays approaching their long axis at a wide angle, whereas cones are directionally selective and are more sensitive to direct axial rays. Because the outer segments of rod cells are longer than those of cones, rod cells are affected more by scattered light, leading to greater sensitivity but poorer spatial resolution. Rods have a slower response time than cones, which also facilitates their ability to detect small amounts of light. In addition, the rod system is convergent; many rods synapse on the same interneuron—the bipolar cell. This arrangement increases the ability of the rod system to detect light, but again at the expense of image quality. On the other hand, because cones are less sensitive, have

Table 27–1. Properties of Rod and Cone Systems

Rods	Cones
More photopigment	Less photopigment
Slow response: long integration time	Fast response: short integration time
High amplification, single quantum detection	Probably less amplification
Saturating response	Nonsaturating response
Not directionally selective	Directionally selective
Highly convergent retinal pathways	Less convergent retinal pathways
High sensitivity	Low sensitivity
Low acuity	High acuity
Achromatic: one type of pigment	Chromatic: three types of pigment

a faster response time, and are connected to more individualized neural channels, the cone system provides greater spatial and temporal resolution. As we shall see in Chapter 30, three distinct types of cones, each sensitive to a different range of wavelengths, mediate color vision.

Rods and Cones Differ in Structure and Function

What are the structural differences between the rods and cones? Both types of photoreceptors are differentiated into three major parts: an *outer segment*, an *inner segment*, and a *synaptic terminal* (Figure 27–2). The outer segments are specialized for photoreception. In both rods and cones the outer segments connect to the inner segments through a thin cytoplasmic bridge. This bridge contains a modified cilium with nine pairs of microtubules but lacks the central two pairs characteristic of other cilia. The inner segment is continuous with the terminal portion of the receptor cell that forms synaptic contacts with the next neural elements in the retinal pathway. The inner segment contains the nucleus and numerous mitochondria and ribosomes as well as a normal complement of other cytoplasmic inclusions.

The outer segments of rods and cones contain an elaborate system of stacked membranous discs, which develop as a series of invaginations of the cell's outer membrane. In rods, most of these discs eventually pinch off and become separated from the outer membrane, whereas in cones, the discs remain connected with the surface membrane.

What is the function of these elaborate morphological specializations? The membranes of the discs of the outer segment contain the *visual photopigments*. Each pigment molecule is oriented within the disc membrane to maximize the absorption of a photon from a stream of light traversing the outer segment axially. The light-catching potential of rods and cones is further enhanced because the pigment-bearing discs are stacked vertically, allowing light that escapes one disc to be caught by the pigment in another.

In 1963, Bernard Droz, now working in Saclay, France, observed from autoradiographic studies that the outer segments of rod cells undergo constant renewal as the discs migrate outward from the base to the tips of the outer segments. Also using autoradiography with radio-labeled amino acids, Richard Young at the University of California at Los Angeles found that during 1 hr as many as three or four discs are synthesized! The discarded tips of the outer segments of the rods are removed by the phagocytotic activity of the contiguous (retinal) pigment epithelial cells. Although renewal and phagocytosis of the outer segment membranes of the cones also occurs, the migration of membranous material has not yet been detected by autoradiography.

Phagocytotic removal of the growing outer segments occurs with a circadian (approximately 24 hr) rhythm. Rod tips are phagocytized in the morning by a mechanism triggered by light; cone phagocytosis occurs in the

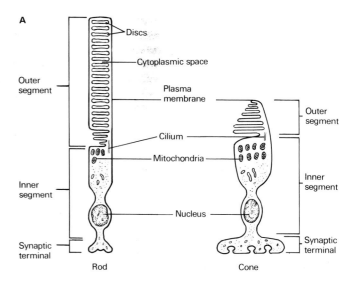

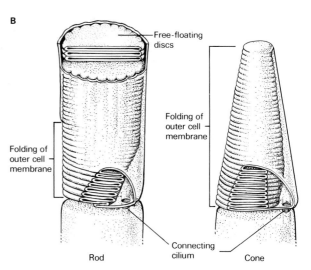

27–2 The two types of photoreceptors, rods and cones, have characteristic structures. **A.** Both rod and cone cells are differentiated into inner and outer segments connected by a cilium. The inner segments of both cell types contain the nucleus and most of the cell's biosynthetic machinery and are continuous with the synaptic terminals. The outer segments of the membranous discs contain the light transducing apparatus. The membranous discs in the outer segments of rod cells are separated from the plasma membrane, whereas the discs of cone cells are not. (Adapted from O'Brien, 1982.) **B.** The outer segments of rod and cone cells are concerned with visual transduction. In both receptors, discs are formed by infolding of plasma membrane. In rods the folds pinch off so that discs become free floating within the outer segment. Cone discs persist as folds and are in contact with the extracellular space. (From Young, 1970.)

evening and is triggered by darkness. As we shall see in Chapter 32, turnover of sensory receptor cells also occurs in the taste and smell systems. Normal turnover of rod and cone outer segments may be impaired in certain retinal diseases such as *retinitis pigmentosa*. In a rat with this disease, cellular debris accumulates between the distal tip of the receptors and the pigment epithelium, suggesting that normal phagocytotic activity of the epithelial cells is disturbed.

Excitation of Rod Cells Involves the Breakdown of Rhodopsin

How is light absorbed and subsequently transduced into electrical signals? We shall first consider the excitation of rod cells. The rod cells are sensitive to light because they contain a visual pigment, *rhodopsin*, which is capable of absorbing photons. There are about 10^9 rhodopsin molecules in the outer segment of each rod photoreceptor cell, and these molecules are arranged as monomolecular layers in the discs of the outer segment. Each rhodopsin molecule has two essential components: retinal and opsin. *Retinal*, the aldehyde form of vitamin A, is a chromophore, a light-absorbing molecule. It is attached to *opsin*, a protein found in different chemical forms.

Retinal can assume two different three-dimensional (isomeric) conformations, and each form is significant for a different phase of the visual cycle: (1) The bent 11-*cis* isomer is the form of retinal that binds to opsin. Retinal retains the 11-*cis* configuration provided it remains in the dark (Figure 27–3). (2) The all-*trans* form has a straight carbon–carbon backbone and does not bind opsin.

The sequence of reactions that underlie the visual cycle was worked out by George Wald at Harvard University. In the first step, the absorption of light by rhodopsin causes retinal to change from the 11-*cis* to the all-*trans* form. *This reaction is the only light-dependent stage in visual excitation.*

Once all-*trans*-retinal is formed, opsin proceeds through a series of unstable intermediates, which can no longer bind retinal. As a result, all-*trans*-retinal separates from opsin. In order to be reused for the synthesis of rhodopsin, the *trans*-retinal must be re-isomerized to the *cis*-form, a reaction thought to take place in the neighboring retinal (pigment) epithelium. Since retinal is not very soluble in water, and in addition is toxic to cell membranes, its movement from the outer segment of the rods to the retinal epithelium is mediated by a special transport protein. All-*trans*-retinal is reduced to all-*trans*-retinol (vitamin A), re-isomerized, and esterified in the retinal epithelium. The esters serve as precursors for 11-*cis*-retinal.

After exposure to a continuous bright light, such as that found at the beach on a summer day, most of the rhodopsin in the rods is broken down, driving much of the *trans*-retinal into the retinal epithelium and making the rods much less sensitive to light. If the rods are then exposed to darkness, retinal returns to the outer segment in the form of the *cis*-isomer to be used in the resynthesis of new rhodopsin. After exposure to a very bright light, when most of the rhodopsin in the rods has been broken down, it takes almost 1 hr for the total resynthesis of rhodopsin. This rise and fall of rhodopsin concentration in rod outer segments is called *photochemical adaptation*. The electrical response of the rods is also reduced after exposure to bright light, a phenomenon called *neural adaptation*. In general, neural adaptation is much quicker than photochemical adaptation. Together these two processes tend to regulate the sensitivity of the rods to the ambient level of illumination. A nutritional deficiency in vitamin A at first reduces vision by causing night blindness. If prolonged, the absence of vitamin A can lead to deterioration of receptor outer segments and cause total blindness.

Excitation of Cone Cells Involves the Breakdown of Cone Opsin

Like rhodopsin, the visual pigments found in cone cells are composed of two parts, a protein called *cone opsin* and a light-absorbing molecule that, as in rods, appears to be 11-*cis*-retinal. Unlike rod cells, however, there are three types of cone cells in the retina of primates, each of which contains a different cone opsin and therefore absorbs light best in a different part of the visible spectrum. In each cone cell the sensitivity of the retinal molecule to a particular wavelength of light is determined by the type of opsin to which the retinal is bound. Each of the three opsins interacts with retinal in a different way, probably because of differences in the number and distribution of electrical charges on the protein. This makes each of the three classes of cone photoreceptors more sensitive to a particular part of the visible spectrum and establishes normal human trivariant color vision (see Chapter 30). The decomposition and regeneration of the cone visual pigments are believed to occur by a mechanism like that of rhodopsin, but much more rapidly.

Light Is Transduced into Electrical Signals by A Second-Messenger System

The conformational changes resulting from the breakdown of rhodopsin in rods and of cone opsins in cones produce a change in the permeability of the external membrane of the outer segment, causing the closure of Na^+ channels that are open in the dark. The closure of the Na^+ channels leads to a hyperpolarization of the photoreceptor from -30 to -70 mV, leading to a decrease in the amount of transmitter released at its synaptic terminal. The surprising discovery that light inhibits (hyperpolarizes) and darkness excites (depolarizes) photo-receptor cells was made by Tsuneo Tomita in Japan.

As we have seen, in rod cells most of the rhodopsin is not located in the external (plasma) membrane but rather in the membrane of the disc within the cell. Nonetheless, photoisomerization of the 11-*cis*-retinal chromophore of rhodopsin to the all-*trans* form leads to the hyperpolarization of the external membrane of the photoreceptor neuron, which is essential for signaling. Indeed, this process is characterized by remarkable amplification. Absorption of a single photon by a single molecule of rhodopsin leads to the closure of several hundred Na^+ channels! How is this accomplished? Presumably, a chemical messenger—a transmitter or an

348

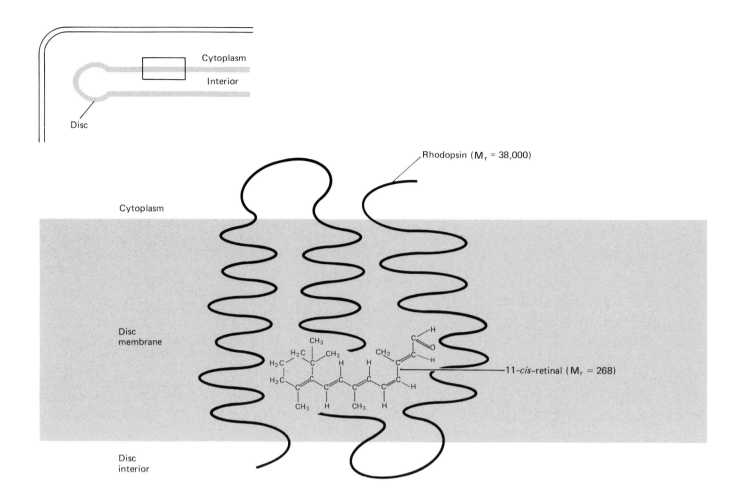

11-*cis*-retinal

All-*trans*-retinal

27–3 The absorption of light by rod cells results in a three-dimensional change in the structure of the retinal chromophore of rhodopsin. The protein portion of rhodopsin has recently been cloned by Jeremy Nathans and David Hogness of Stanford. It has 348 amino acids and a molecular weight of about 38,000. It is thought to loop back and forth seven times across the lipid bilayer of the rod disc plasma membrane, with the N terminus lying on the external face of the membrane and the C terminus on the cytoplasmic face (only three such loops are indicated schematically on this drawing). Rhodopsin contains 11-*cis*-retinal, the site where light acts on the visual pigment. The absorption of a photon of light by the chromophore is translated into atomic motion. Specifically, a rotation occurs around the 11-*cis* double bond, allowing retinal to return to its more stable all-*trans* configuration. This reaction is the molecular mechanism underlying vision.

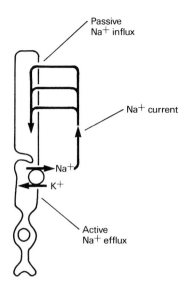

27–4 The dark current flows longitudinally through rods and cones in the dark because of the continuous passive leakage of Na$^+$ into the cell through the high conductance pathway for Na$^+$ in the outer segment. Ion pumps in the inner segment utilize metabolic energy to extrude Na$^+$ and consequently drive the dark current. Light blocks the Na$^+$ conductance channels in the outer segment and reduces or stops this dark current. (Adapted from O'Brien, 1982.)

ion—carries information from the disc membrane to the external membrane. Evidence points strongly to the participation of the second messenger, cyclic GMP. Cyclic GMP is thought to keep Na$^+$ channels open in the dark, thereby depolarizing the membrane. Light activates a *phosphodiesterase*, an enzyme that hydrolyzes cyclic GMP, closes the Na$^+$ channels, and hyperpolarizes the cell. This model has now been tested directly. Evgeniy Fesenko and his colleagues in the Soviet Union have used patch clamp techniques to expose the inside surface of a cell-free patch of rod membrane to a solution containing cyclic GMP and found that it rapidly opens Na$^+$ channels. Conversely, removal of cyclic GMP, as occurs with rapid hydrolysis of cyclic GMP produced by light, closes the Na$^+$ channels.

This process has the required amplification. A single photoexcited rhodopsin molecule activates several hundred molecules of phosphodiesterase, which acts like the catalytic subunit of adenylate cyclase described in Chapter 14. The photoactivation of the phosphodiesterase (an intrinsic membrane protein) is mediated by *transducin*, a peripheral membrane protein whose activation requires the exchange of GTP for GDP. The phosphodiesterase and the guanine nucleotide binding protein make up a large proportion of the protein in the retina other than rhodopsin. In its dependence on GTP and its sensitivity to cholera toxin, transducin is analogous to the G-proteins, the coupling factors that regulate the cyclase. More direct evidence that transducin and the G-proteins belong to the same family of transmembrane signal-coupling protein is, first, that monoclonal antibod-

ies raised against transducin bind the G-proteins and, second, that studies with recombinant DNA reveal extensive homology in the amino acid sequences of transducin and the G-proteins. All of these similarities suggest that the two proteins belong to the same family of transmembrane signal-coupling proteins and that the activation of cyclic guanosine monophosphate phosphodiesterase by light resembles the activation of adenylate cyclase by hormones or transmitters.

How does closure of Na$^+$ channels hyperpolarize the photoreceptor cell? In the dark state, an inward leakage of Na$^+$ through open channels in the outer segment keeps the resting membrane potential of the photoreceptor cells at a relatively low value (−30 mV); thus, there is a continuous passive flow of Na$^+$ current into the outer segment. The Na$^+$ is actively extruded from the inner segment. This produces a continuous flow of Na$^+$ current into and out of the photoreceptor (called the *dark current*). Light closes Na$^+$ channels, removes the depolarizing influence of inwardly flowing Na$^+$ ions, and allows the membrane to move toward the equilibrium potential of other ions (primarily K$^+$), thereby slowing or stopping the dark current (Figure 27–4). The net result is a hyperpolarizing response in the photoreceptor.

We shall next consider how the retina signals excitation through predominantly hyperpolarizing or inhibitory responses.

Visual Information Is Processed by Five Major Classes of Neurons in the Retina

The synaptic events subsequently involved in the transfer of information from the receptor cells to other neurons in the retina have been well documented.

Although there are many subclasses of neurons, the vertebrate retina consists of only five major classes: receptor cells, bipolar cells, horizontal cells, amacrine cells, and ganglion cells.

Both types of *receptor cells*, rods and cones, make direct synaptic contact with a class of interneurons called the *bipolar cells*, which connect the receptor cells with the *ganglion cells*. The ganglion cells are the projection neurons of the retina; they relay visual information to the central nervous system by projecting to the lateral geniculate nucleus and the superior colliculus as well as to brain stem nuclei. Modulating the flow of information from receptor to bipolar to ganglion cells are two classes of interneurons: the *horizontal cells* and the *amacrine cells*. The horizontal cells mediate lateral interactions between receptor and bipolar cells. The *amacrine cells* mediate lateral interactions between bipolar cells and ganglion cells.

The cell bodies of these five classes of neurons are found in three layers: (1) the *outer nuclear layer* (receptors), (2) the *inner nuclear layer* (bipolar, horizontal, and amacrine), and (3) the *ganglion cell layer* (ganglion). The processes of these five major cell classes interact in two distinct synaptic layers: the *outer plexiform layer* con-

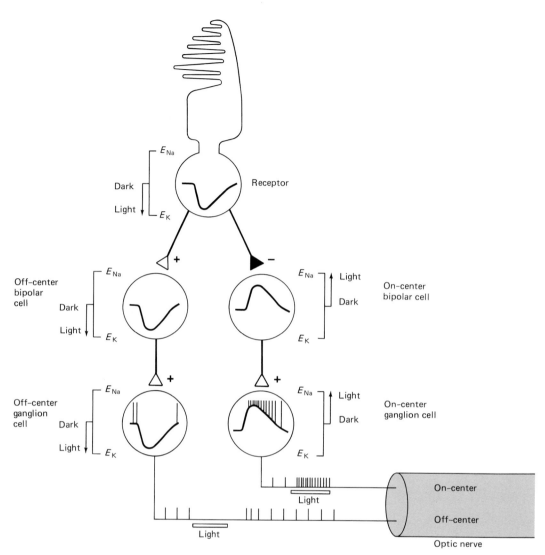

27–5 A single cone photoreceptor synapses on two separate bipolar cell channels: one is excited by light activation of this cone (on-center, or depolarizing bipolar cell), and the other is inhibited by light activation of this cone (off-center, or hyperpolarizing bipolar cell). The critical factor in this circuit is a transmitter substance that has opposite effects on the membrane voltage of these two bipolar cells. The cone forms an excitatory or "sign-preserving" synapse on the off-center bipolar cell and an inhibitory or "sign-reversing" synapse on the on-center bipolar cell. Note that this "excitatory" or "inhibitory" effect is the result of transmitter release, which takes place in the dark; when the receptive field of the cone is illuminated, the *decrease* in transmitter results in excitation (or disinhibition) of the on-center cell and inhibition (or disfacilitation) of the off-center cell.

tains the processes of receptor, bipolar, and horizontal cells; the *inner plexiform layer* contains the processes of bipolar, amacrine, and ganglion cells.

The flow of information from receptor to ganglion cells can best be followed by considering two major pathways available in the retina. The first is the simplest and is a direct route from receptor to bipolar to ganglion cell. This pathway carries information from nearby receptors to ganglion cells. In the second pathway, the surrounding horizontal cells integrate and transfer information from distant receptor cells to the bipolar–ganglion cell pathway.

There Are Distinct On-Center and Off-Center Pathways

We have considered above how light produces a decreased Na^+ conductance in photoreceptors and how this permeability change results in the production of graded, hyperpolarizing responses. We shall now consider how these hyperpolarizing receptor potentials are transmitted synaptically to the next elements in the visual pathway and how excitation is generated in the ganglion cells (the neurons ultimately responsible for transmitting information to the brain). Some of the essential features of retinal function can be best illustrated by examining the events that occur in the direct receptor–bipolar–ganglion pathway.

Rods and cones do not normally generate action potentials and are exceptions to the general model of the neuron we considered in Chapter 2. Their synaptic terminals (the output component where transmitter is released) are close to the input component, so that slight changes in membrane potential affect transmitter release.

In the dark the photoreceptor is depolarized and the terminals continually release a chemical transmitter that affects the bipolar cells. The cones synapse with two types of bipolar cells, *on-center* and *off-center*, each of which responds differently to the same transmitter released by a single cone. The on-center cell is inhibited by the transmitter, so that a decrease in the amount of transmitter released disinhibits, or excites, the cell. *Disinhibition*, or the removal of the constraints on excitation, is a fundamental mechanism in the nervous system. The off-center cell is excited by the transmitter, and a decrease in transmitter release disfacilitates or inhibits the cell. The two kinds of responses occur because the transmitter released by cones (thought to be glutamate) produces opposite results in the two types of bipolar cells. The cone transmitter hyperpolarizes and inhibits the on-center type by what is thought to be a closure of Na^+ channels, and depolarizes and excites the off-center type by opening Na^+ channels. Each cone photoreceptor can synapse on both on-center and off-center bipolars (Figure 27–5). An *on-center* bipolar cell is depolarized (excited) by direct illumination of the cone. An *off-center* bipolar cell is hyperpolarized (inhibited) by direct illumination of the same cone (Figure 27–5). Each type of bipolar cell in turn connects with a parallel set of ganglion cells, called correspondingly on- and off-center ganglion cells, with corresponding response properties.

This survey of retinal function reveals four unusual features of neuronal organization:

1. The response of receptor cells to light is a hyperpolarization mediated by a closure of Na^+ channels that are open in the dark. Photoreceptors are normally excited (i.e., tonically depolarized) in the dark by the flow of Na^+ current (the dark current). Light modulates this dark current to produce a hyperpolarizing response.
2. Synapses made by photoreceptors onto bipolar cells *do not* have a clear threshold for transmitter release. The photoreceptor synapses constantly release transmitter, and slight changes in membrane potential modulate this spontaneous release. Thus, retinal synapses release transmitter spontaneously just as some nerve cells have spontaneous activity. This release establishes a background of activity that can be modulated by information from other cells. Because the receptor cells are tonically depolarized in the dark, they are exquisitely sensitive. Very small voltage changes at the photoreceptor terminals can affect transmitter release.

3. A single species of transmitter released by the photoreceptors inhibits certain bipolar cells (on-center or depolarizing bipolar cells) and excites others (off-center or hyperpolarizing bipolar cells). Thus, the retina illustrates nicely a principle we encountered earlier (Chapter 14): the sign of transmitter action is determined not by the chemical nature of the transmitter but by the properties of the receptor in the postsynaptic membrane and the ion channels controlled by the receptor.
4. All of the distal cells in the visual pathway (i.e., receptor, bipolar, and, as we shall see below, horizontal cells) carry their information without the aid of action potentials. The primary function of action potentials is to carry information rapidly and reliably over long distances. Because the distances between the input and output components of the retinal cells are short, information can be transmitted passively along them.

The On-Center and Off-Center Pathways Use Both Electrical and Chemical Synapses

The retina contains electrical synapses (gap junctions) between both the terminals of receptor neurons and their inner segments. The horizontal cells also are extensively interconnected electrically. However, as in the rest of the brain, the predominant type of synapse in the retina is chemical. Particularly interesting is a variant called the *ribbon synapse*, found at the terminals of photoreceptors in the outer plexiform layer (Figure 27–6). Ribbon synapses differ in three ways from most other synapses considered so far. First, the presynaptic terminal contains an unusual modification of the active zone called the *presynaptic ribbon* (Figure 27–6B, arrows). This electron-dense ribbon lies perpendicular to the presynaptic membrane and is intimately associated with synaptic vesicles, probably serving to orient the vesicles toward the presynaptic membrane for exocytotic release. Second, a *single presynaptic terminal ends on three postsynaptic elements* (called a *triad*). Typically, two different postsynaptic neurons contribute to this arrangement: two horizontal cell processes occupy the two lateral positions and a single bipolar cell process occupies the central position. Finally, the three postsynaptic processes invaginate the presynaptic membrane. Ribbon synapses are occasionally found in the inner plexiform layer, where bipolar cells are the presynaptic neurons. These contacts typically have either a pair of amacrine cell processes or an amacrine process and a ganglion cell process as the postsynaptic elements.

The two classes of bipolar cells—depolarizing or on-center and hyperpolarizing or off-center—are morphologically distinct. The on-center bipolar cell is activated at the photoreceptor ribbon synapse and therefore is also called an *invaginating bipolar cell*. The off-center bipolar cells are activated at *flat contacts*. Unlike the receptor ribbon synapse, they have no presynaptic ribbon and only a single (noninvaginating) postsynaptic element (Figure 27–6A).

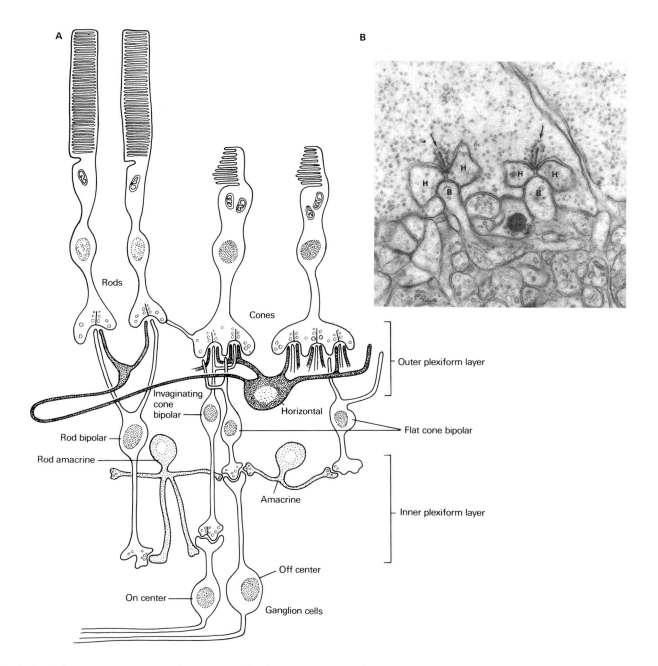

A

Rods

Cones

Outer plexiform layer

Invaginating
cone
bipolar

Horizontal

Flat cone bipolar

Rod bipolar

Rod amacrine

Amacrine

Inner plexiform layer

Off center

On center

Ganglion cells

B

27–6 Retinal synapses are organized in an outer plexiform layer and an inner plexiform layer. **A.** In the outer plexiform layer, synaptic terminals of rods (called *spherules*) and cones (called *pedicles*) are presynaptic to bipolar and horizontal cells. The retinal pathways for rod and cone signals are relatively independent until the ganglion cell layer, where both systems share the same output neurons. These signals are not completely independent because electrical synapses occur between processes that extend from cone pedicles to rods. There is only one type of rod bipolar cell, but there are at least two different classes of cone bipolar cells: *invaginating* and *flat*. The invaginating cone bipolar cells send their dendrites into invaginations in the cone pedicle, where they form the central element of three processes in each invagination centered on a *synaptic ribbon*. The two lateral elements in this "triad" relationship are dendrites of horizontal cells. Horizontal cell dendrites are both post- and presynaptic to cone pedicles; an axon terminal arborization of some of these horizontal cells forms a similar dendritic arrangement in rod spherules. The flat cone bipolar cells contact the base of the pedicle. Flat cone bipolar cells are considered to be off-center cells that synapse with off-center ganglion cells in the outer part of the inner plexiform layer. Invaginating cone bipolar cells are considered to be on-center cells that synapse with on-center ganglion cells in the inner part of the inner plexiform layer. Rod bipolar cells synapse in the innermost part of the inner plexiform layer with a specific amacrine cell interneuron; they do not appear to synapse directly on ganglion cells. **B.** Ribbon synapses at the photoreceptor terminal are characterized by an electron-dense ribbon (**arrows**) around which vesicles are clustered. One bipolar cell (**B**) and two horizontal cell (**H**) processes invaginate the presynaptic membrane. (Part **B** from Dowling, 1979.)

Helga Kolb and her colleagues have been able to distinguish between on-center and off-center ganglion cells through the intracellular injection of fluorescent dyes into ganglion cells in the cat. The dendritic processes of off-center ganglion cells are confined to the distal regions of the inner plexiform layer, whereas the dendritic processes of on-center ganglion cells branch primarily within the proximal levels of the inner plexiform layer. This layering of on- and off-center ganglion cell processes parallels the differential distribution of the terminals of depolarizing and hyperpolarizing bipolar cells.

There Are Three Parallel Systems of Ganglion Cells

In addition to differences in the location of the dendritic processes of on- and off-center ganglion cells, each retinal region has several morphologically and functionally distinct subsets of ganglion cells that subserve the same photoreceptors in parallel. The cat retina has been particularly well studied and has been found to contain three subsets of ganglion cells—the X, Y, and W cells. The X cells have medium-sized cell bodies and small dendritic fields, and participate in high-acuity vision. The Y cells have the largest cell bodies, a large dendritic arborization, and rapidly conducting axons. The Y cells respond only to large targets and are important in the initial analysis of crude form. The W cells have small cell bodies and large dendritic arborizations; these cells project to the superior colliculus and are involved in head and eye movement. Similar categories of ganglion cells exist in the primate retina. We shall return to a more detailed consideration of these cell types in Chapters 28 and 29.

Horizontal Cells Are Local Interneurons in the Outer Plexiform Layer That Contribute to Center–Surround Antagonism

The activation of bipolar cells at photoreceptor terminals (through either ribbon synapses or flat contacts) leads to the excitation of some ganglion cells in the inner plexiform layer and the inhibition of other ganglion cells. Bipolar cells are activated by *nearby* receptors but may also be affected by more distant receptors through interconnections with horizontal cells. Since horizontal cells are in turn electrically interconnected, their lateral extent is greatly increased and their effective range of influence thereby enlarged. (The considerable lateral projections of a single horizontal cell are shown in Figure 27–6A.)

What functions do the horizontal cells have in determining the receptive field properties of the retinal ganglion cells? The receptive field of any visual cell is that area of the retina which when stimulated can influence the cell's response. We have already considered the responses of retinal ganglion cells to direct illumination that derive from the direct receptor–bipolar–ganglion cell connections. As a result of horizontal cell modulation, a ganglion cell can acquire additional, more complex re-

sponse properties. For example, the response to direct light on the center of its receptive field is antagonized by direct light on the surround of its receptive field. This phenomenon, called *center–surround antagonism*, is important for detecting borders independent of the level of illumination. The existence of an antagonistic enhancement mechanism for sharpening contrast was first suggested by the physicist Ernst Mach in the nineteenth century. Center–surround antagonism was first demonstrated in 1949 in the eye of the horseshoe crab, *Limulus*, by H. Keffer Hartline, then at Johns Hopkins University (for which he was awarded the Nobel Prize in Physiology and Medicine). In 1953, Stephen Kuffler discovered that in the vertebrate retina there are two parallel ganglion cell systems with center–surround antagonism: an on-center system and an off-center system.

Antagonistic interactions between neighboring retinal areas are thought to be mediated by horizontal cells. How this might work was first indicated by Dennis Baylor, Michael Fuortes, and P. M. O'Bryan at the National Institutes of Health; they found that horizontal cells mediate antagonistic interactions between neighboring cones (Figure 27–7). The cones release a transmitter that depolarizes horizontal cells, which, in turn, release a transmitter that hyperpolarizes neighboring cones. Therefore, the hyperpolarization of some cones by light leads to the depolarization of neighboring cones by means of horizontal interneurons. Thus, horizontal cells make the darkness *darker* in the neighboring cones that are illuminated only weakly or not at all. Recent evidence suggests that dopamine in the fish retina and γ-aminobutyric acid (GABA) in the turtle retina can uncouple the gap junctions between horizontal cells and thereby modulate the distance across the retina over which horizontal cells can exert their antagonistic interactions among photoreceptors.

Here we can begin to see how an interneuron such as the horizontal cell uses inhibition to form and modify the neural representation of the external world on the retina. The action of horizontal cells in the retina is the first step in a chain of events that is repeated successively at higher levels of the visual system to increase contrast between brightness and darkness and to make it easier for us to distinguish contours.

Amacrine Cells Are Local Interneurons in the Inner Plexiform Layer That Mediate Antagonistic Interactions

In the outer nuclear layer there is only one cell, a photoreceptor subserving a particular area of visual space. In contrast, in the inner nuclear layer there are at least two bipolar cells subserving the *same* area of visual space for the cone system alone. One bipolar cell is an on-center cell; it carries information from the cone system to the inner part of the inner plexiform layer and synapses with on-center ganglion cells. The other bipolar cell is an off-center cell; it carries information from the cone system to off-center ganglion cells within the outer part of the

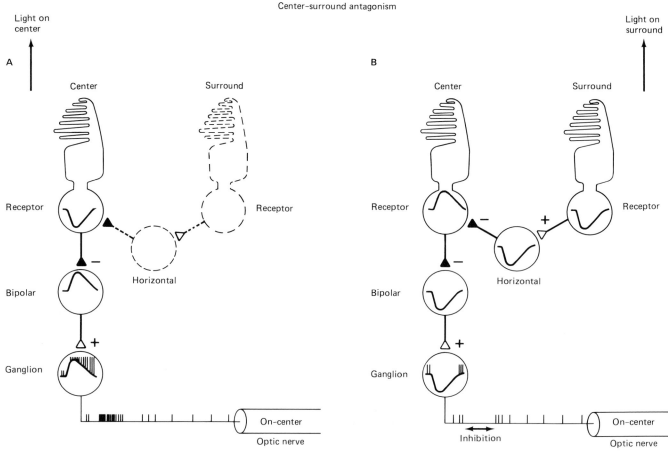

27–7 In center–surround antagonism, the response of a ganglion cell to direct light on the center of its receptive field (**A**) is antagonized by direct light on the surround of its receptor field (**B**). This antagonistic interaction between neighboring retinal areas is mediated by the inhibitory action of a horizontal cell. **A.** Direct illumination produces a hyperpolarization in the photoreceptor leading to a depolarization at the bipolar cell and excitation of the on-center ganglion cell. **B.** Direct light applied to a distant receptor affects this on-center pathway in an opposing fashion. Illumination of one distant receptor results in the hyperpolarization of a horizontal cell, which now produces a depolarization of the nearby receptor and subsequent hyperpolarization of the same ganglion cell.

inner plexiform layer. The processes of amacrine cells, found only in the inner plexiform layer, mediate antagonistic interactions between on-center and off-center channels. Some amacrine cells have small dendritic fields and mediate interactions between X-type ganglion cells, which have a relatively restricted dendritic spread. Other amacrine cells that have a more extensive dendritic network probably mediate the antagonistic interactions, transient responsiveness, and nonlinear behavior of the large, or Y-type, ganglion cells. Other amacrine cells are used to confer directional selectivity on another subset of ganglion cells. The rod system uses a unique amacrine cell interneuron to transmit its information to ganglion cells.

The great multiplicity of neural channels subserving the same area of visual space in the inner plexiform layer leads to a richer constellation of amacrine interneurons in this layer than horizontal cells in the outer plexiform layer; thus, the inner plexiform layer is larger than the outer plexiform layer.

As we shall see in later chapters, antagonistic interactions mediated by interneurons are used at all levels of the visual pathway to build up a large variety of responses needed to detect color and form in the external world and to construct its representation in the brain.

An Overall View

The absorption of light and its subsequent transduction into electrical signals is carried out by the photoreceptors. Visual information is then transferred from the receptors to the ganglion cells via the bipolar cells. The ganglion cells in turn project to the brain. Two types of interneurons (horizontal cells and amacrine cells) integrate and modulate the activity of both the bipolar neurons and the ganglion cells. Thus, the retina functions as a small brain. The retina is simpler than the brain because it uses only five basic neuronal types. Nonetheless, it can generate complicated receptive field properties that reflect considerable transformation of visual information.

Selected Readings

Barlow, H. B., Hill, R. M., and Levick, W. R. 1964. Retinal ganglion cells responding selectively to direction and speed of image motion. J. Physiol. (Lond.) 173:377–407.

Biernbaum, M. S., and Bowndes, M. D. 1985. Light-induced changes in GTP and ATP in frog rod photoreceptors. Comparison with recovery of dark current and light sensitivity during dark adaptation. J. Gen. Physiol. 85:107–121.

Daw, N. W., Ariel, M., and Caldwell, J. H. 1982. Function of neurotransmitters in the retina. Retina 2:322–331.

Dowling, J. E. 1979. Information processing by local circuits: The vertebrate retina as a model system. In F. O. Schmitt and F. G. Worden (eds.), The Neurosciences; Fourth Study Program. Cambridge, Mass.: MIT Press, pp. 163–181.

Enroth-Cugell, C., and Robson, J. G. 1966. The contrast sensitivity of retinal ganglion cells of the cat. J. Physiol. (Lond.) 187:517–552.

Fesenko, E., Kolesnikov, S. S., and Lyubarsky, A. L. 1985. Induction by cyclic GMP of cationic conductance in plasma membrane of retinal rod outer segment. Nature 313:310–313.

Gouras, P. 1969. Antidromic responses of orthodromically identified ganglion cells in monkey retina. J. Physiol. (Lond.) 204:407–419.

Hecht, S. 1937. Rods, cones, and the chemical basis of vision. Physiol. Rev. 17:239–290.

Holtzman, E., and Mercurio, A. M. 1980. Membrane circulation in neurons and photoreceptors: Some unresolved issues. Int. Rev. Cytol. 67:1–67.

Hurley, J. B., Simon, M. I., Teplow, D. B., Robishaw, J. D., and Gilman, A. G. 1984. Homologies between signal transducing G proteins and ras gene products. Science 226:860–862.

Kaneko, A. 1970. Physiological and morphological identification of horizontal, bipolar and amacrine cells in goldfish retina. J. Physiol. (Lond.) 207:623–633.

Kolb, H., Mariani, A., and Gallego, A. 1980. A second type of horizontal cell in the monkey retina. J. Comp. Neurol. 189:31–44.

Levick, W. R., and Thibos, L. N. 1981. Receptive fields of cat ganglion cells: Classification and construction. In N. Osborne and G. Chader (eds.), Progress in Retinal Research. Oxford: Pergamon Press, pp. 267–319.

Lewin, R. 1985. Unexpected progress in photoreception. Science 227:500–503.

Mariani, A. P. 1984. Bipolar cells in monkey retina selective for the cones likely to be blue-sensitive. Nature 308:184–186.

O'Brien, D. F. 1982. The chemistry of vision. Science 218:961–966.

Piccolino, M., Neyton, J., Witkovsky, P., and Gerschenfeld, H. M. 1982. γ-Aminobutyric and antagonists decrease junctional communication between L-horizontal cells of the retina. Proc. Natl. Acad. Sci. U.S.A. 79:3671–3675.

Rodieck, R. W. 1973. The Vertebrate Retina—Principles of Structure and Function. San Francisco: Freeman.

Stryer, L. 1983. Transducin and the cyclic GMP phosphodiesterase—Amplifier protein in vision. Cold Spring Harbor Symp. Quant. Biol. 48:841–852.

Teranishi, T., Negishi, K., and Kato, S. 1983. Dopamine modulates S potential amplitude and dye-coupling between external horizontal cells in carp retina. Nature 301:243–246.

Wassle, H., Reichl, L., and Boycott, B. B. 1981. Dendritic territories of cat retinal ganglion cells. Nature 292:344–345.

Werblin, F., and Dowling, J. E. 1969. Organization of the retina of the mud puppy, Necturas maculosus. II. Intracellular recording. J. Neurophysiol. 32:339–355.

Witt, P. L., Hamm, H. E., and Bownds, M. D. 1984. Preparation and characterization of monoclonal antibodies to several frog outer segment proteins. J. Gen. Physiol. 84:251–263.

Yau, K. W., and Nakatani, K. 1985. Light-induced reduction of cytoplasmic free Ca^{++} in retinal rod outer segment. Nature 313:579–582.

References

Baylor, D. A., Fuortes, M. G. F., and O'Bryan, P. M. 1971. Receptive fields of cones in the retina of the turtle. J. Physiol. (Lond.) 214:265–294.

Droz, B. 1963. Dynamic condition of proteins in the visual cells of rats and mice as shown by radioautography with labeled amino acids. Anat. Rec. 145:157–166.

George, J. S., and Hagins, W. A. 1983. Control of Ca^{++} on rod outer segment disks by light and cyclic GMP. Nature 303:344–348.

Hartline, H. K. 1949. Inhibition of activity of visual receptors by illuminating nearby retinal elements in the Limulus eye. Fed. Proc. 8:69.

Kuffler, S. W. 1953. Discharge patterns and functional organization of mammalian retina. J. Neurophysiol. 16:37–68.

Mach, E. 1866. Ueber den physiologischen Effect räumlich vertheilter Lichtreize, II. Sitzber. Akad. Wiss. Wien (Mathnat. Kl.), Abt. 2, 54:131–144.

Nathans, J., and Hogness, D. S. 1984. Isolation and nucleotide sequence of the gene encoding human rhodopsin. Proc. Natl. Acad. Sci. U.S.A. 81:4851–4855.

Nelson, R., Famiglietti, E. V., Jr., and Kolb, H. 1978. Intracellular staining reveals different levels of stratification for on- and off-center ganglion cells in cat retina. J. Neurophysiol. 41:472–483.

Schultze, M. 1866. Zur Anatomie und Physiologie der Retina. Arch. Mikrouk. Anta. 2:175–286.

Tomita, T. 1976. Electrophysiological studies of retinal cell function. Invest. Ophthalmol. 15:171–187.

Wald, G. 1968. Molecular basis of visual excitation. Science 162:230–239.

Young, R. W. 1970. Visual cells. Sci. Am. 223(4):80–91.

James P. Kelly

Anatomy of the Central Visual Pathways

28

In this chapter we shall examine the structure of the visual pathway from the retina to the thalamus and then to the visual cortex. We shall begin by considering the different types of retinal ganglion cells, and how the visual field is projected upon the retina. We shall next consider how the retinal ganglion cell axons are arranged in the optic nerve and in the optic tract, and the topographic manner in which these axons terminate in the lateral geniculate nucleus of the thalamus. This topography is extremely important because lesions in different parts of the visual pathway produce characteristic deficits of sight in the visual field. Once the topography of the visual pathway is known, it is possible to deduce the location of a lesion in the central nervous system that could produce particular types of visual field aberrations. Finally, we shall discuss the structure of the primary visual cortex, where the axons from the lateral geniculate nucleus terminate. To appreciate the role of the visual cortex in visual perception it is necessary to understand its three-dimensional structure. Studies of the visual cortex have provided important hints about the mechanisms used by the cerebral cortex in processing sensory input of all kinds to generate a perception of the world around us.

The Visual Field Is the Projection of the Visual World on the Retina

The axons of all three types of ganglion cells—Y, X, and W cells—exit from the retina by streaming toward the *optic disc,* the region where they become myelinated and join other axons to form the *optic nerve.* The optic nerves from each eye join at the *optic chiasm.* There, fibers destined for particular regions in the brain stem are sorted out. This sort-

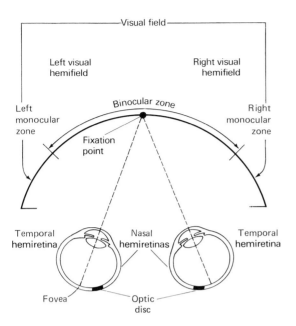

28-1 The left visual field and the right visual field overlap in the binocular zone; light from the binocular zone strikes both eyes, whereas light from the monocular zone strikes only the eye on the same side. The optic disc, which is free of photoreceptors, is the region where the ganglion cell axons leave the retina.

28-2 The lens of the eye projects an inverted image on the retina. **A.** The formation of an inverted image by a camera lens. **B.** The major structural features of the eye and its formation of an inverted image. (Adapted from Wald, in Groves and Schlesinger, 1979.)

ing process can best be understood in terms of the *visual fields,* or the way in which the visual world is projected onto the retina (Figure 28–1). The concept of a visual field is important in clinical medicine because lesions of the visual system produce characteristic defects in vision that are best described in terms of the gaps they produce in the visual field.

The regions of the retina are named with reference to the midline: the *nasal hemiretina* lies medial to the fovea, whereas the *temporal hemiretina* lies lateral to the fovea. Each half of the retina can also be divided into a *dorsal* and a *ventral* quadrant. The reason that we have two frontally placed eyes is to promote depth perception, a subject that is discussed in Appendix II.

The visual field is the field of view of the external world seen by the two eyes without movement of the head. To understand the visual field in optical terms, imagine that the foveas of both eyes are fixed on a single point in space. It is then possible to define a *left* and a *right* half of the visual field. The left half of the visual field projects on the nasal hemiretina of the left eye and on the temporal hemiretina of the right eye. Light originating in the central region of the visual field will strike *both* eyes; this area is called the *binocular zone* of the visual field. In either half of the visual field there is also a *monocular zone*, where light strikes only the eye on the same side.

Two important sets of terminology for the visual system should be clarified at the outset. Confusion might occur because the lens of the eye inverts the visual world upon the retina. This is illustrated in Figure 28–2, a schematic view of the eye from a lateral perspective. Notice that the superior half of the visual field is projected onto the inferior (or ventral) half of the retina, whereas the

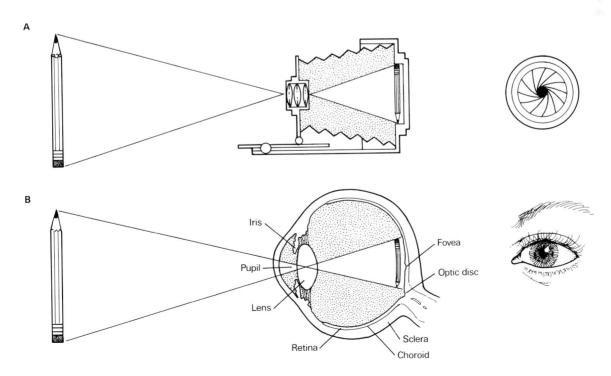

inferior half of the visual field is projected onto the superior (or dorsal) half of the retina. Similarly, the nasal portion of the visual field projects on the temporal retina. We see the world in its correct orientation because higher levels of the brain take this inversion into account and compensate for it. When speaking about the visual system, it is important, therefore, to distinguish between the visual field—which is in the external world—and a region of the *retina*. For example, suppose an individual sustained damage to the *inferior half of the retina* of one eye. This would cause a monocular deficit in the *superior half of the visual field.*

It is also important to distinguish the nasal and temporal halves of the *retina* from the nasal and temporal halves of the *visual field.* Consider the projection of a point in the binocular zone of the right visual hemifield upon the two retinas (Figure 28–3). Light originating from this point falls upon the temporal hemiretina of the left eye and the nasal hemiretina of the right eye. The optic nerves from each side join at the *optic chiasm*, where the fibers from the nasal half of each retina cross to the opposite side. The axons arising from ganglion cells in the temporal hemiretina do not cross. The left optic tract, therefore, is composed of axons from the left

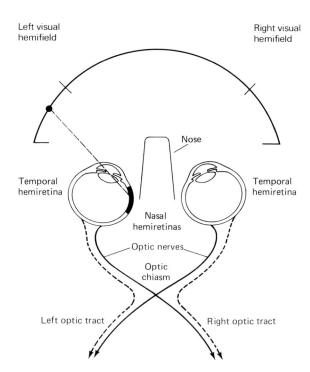

28–4 Light coming from the left monocular zone does not project upon the contralateral retina because it is blocked by the nose. Thus, the temporal portion of each visual hemifield projects only upon the nasal hemiretina of the eye on the same side.

28–3 Light from the right binocular zone falls on the left temporal hemiretina and the right nasal hemiretina. Because fibers from the nasal hemiretina of each eye cross to the opposite side at the optic chiasm, the left optic tract carries axons from the left temporal hemiretina and the right nasal hemiretina, and therefore contains a complete representation of the right hemifield of vision.

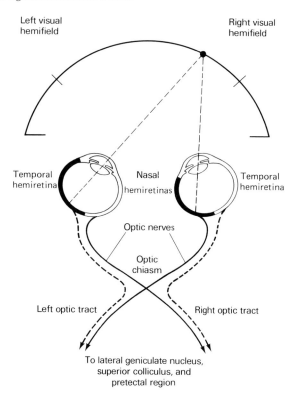

temporal hemiretina and the right nasal hemiretina. In other words, the *left optic tract* contains a complete representation of the *right hemifield* of vision. The axons in the optic tract synapse in the lateral geniculate nucleus of the thalamus, a structure that will be considered in some detail below. Cells in the lateral geniculate nucleus, in turn, send their axons to the visual cortex. This arrangement illustrates a key principle: *At the initial stages of visual processing each half of the brain is concerned with the contralateral hemifield of vision.* This pattern of organization begins with the segregation of axons in the optic chiasm, where fibers from the two eyes dealing with identical parts of the visual field are brought together (Figure 28–3). In essence, this is similar to the somatic sensory system, in which each hemisphere mediates sensation on the contralateral side of the body.

Let us now examine the projections in the brain of the monocular portion of each hemifield (Figure 28–4). The temporal portion of each hemifield projects only onto the nasal hemiretina of the eye on the same side because the nose blocks light coming from this region from reaching the eye on the opposite side. The monocular portion of the visual field is called the *temporal crescent* because it constitutes the crescent-shaped temporal extreme of each visual field. Since there is no binocular overlap in this region, vision is lost in the entire temporal crescent if the eye is severely damaged.

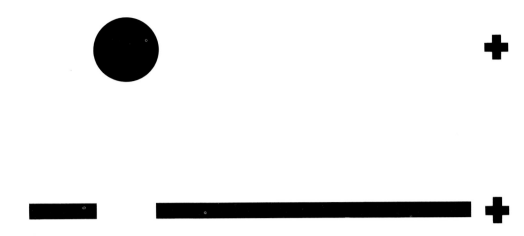

28–5 The blind spot in the left eye is located by shutting the right eye and fixating the **upper cross** with the left eye. If the book is held about 1.5 ft from the eye and its distance moved back and forth slightly, the **circle** on the left disappears since it is imaged on the blind spot. If the left eye fixates on the **lower cross,** the **gap in the black line** falls on the blind spot and the **black line** is seen as continuous because the gap is imaged on the blind spot. (Adapted from Hurvich, 1981.)

The optic disc, the region of the retina where the ganglion cell axons exit, contains no photoreceptors and therefore is insensitive to light. The optic disc lies medial to the fovea in both eyes (Figure 28–1). Consequently, light coming from a single point in the binocular zone never strikes both optic discs, so that we are normally unaware of this blind spot. The blind spot of the left eye can be demonstrated by closing the right eye and looking at the figure with the left eye (Figure 28–5). When the upper cross on the right of Figure 28–5 is viewed only with the fovea of the left eye at the appropriate distance (directly in front at about one and a half feet), the spot on the left disappears because it is projected medially from the left visual hemifield onto the optic disc of the left eye. This exercise demonstrates what blind people experience—not blackness, but simply nothing. It also reveals why large regions of the peripheral retina can be deprived of vision and go unnoticed. In these instances, no large dark zone appears in the periphery, and it is usually by accidents such as bumping into an unnoticed object, or by clinical testing of the visual fields, that the absence of sight is noticed.

The Lateral Geniculate Nucleus Is Composed of Six Cellular Layers

A substantial number of the fibers in the optic tract terminate in the *lateral geniculate nucleus*, a knee-shaped structure in the posterior aspect of the thalamus. In this nucleus there is an orderly representation of the contralateral visual hemifield. Ganglion cells at different loci in the retina project upon distinct visuotopic points in the lateral geniculate nucleus. However, all parts of the retina are not represented equally; proportionally much more of the nucleus is devoted to the representation of

the central area than to the periphery of the retina. Regions with increased ganglion cell density send more axons to the brain and consequently dominate a greater portion of the central representation of the retina.

In primates, the lateral geniculate nucleus consists of six layers of neurons separated by intervening layers of axons and dendrites. The layers are numbered from 6 most dorsally to 1 most ventrally (Figure 28–6). An individual layer in the nucleus receives input from one eye only: fibers from the contralateral nasal retina contact layers 6, 4, and 1; fibers from the ipsilateral temporal retina contact layers 5, 3, and 2. Thus, the complementary halves of the retina in both eyes each contact individual layers in a topographically ordered way, so that each layer contains a representation of the contralateral visual hemifield. These representations are stacked on top of one another in the layers of the nucleus. As a result, there are six maps of the contralateral hemifield in vertical register. The layers of the lateral geniculate nucleus that receive input from the contralateral eye contain a complete representation of the contralateral visual hemifield. The layers that receive input from the ipsilateral eye contain a representation of only a portion of the contralateral hemifield because they receive no input from the temporal crescent of the visual field. The two most ventral layers (1 and 2) of the lateral geniculate nucleus contain relatively large cells and are termed the *magnocellular* layers, in contrast to the four dorsal, or *parvocellular*, layers.

The *projection cells* of the layer send their axons on to the visual cortex. Using the electron microscope it is possible to determine the types of synapses formed by retinal ganglion cell axons on these cells in the lateral geniculate nucleus. This has been carried out in the cat by placing a lesion in the appropriate part of the retina and then searching for the types of synapses that degen-

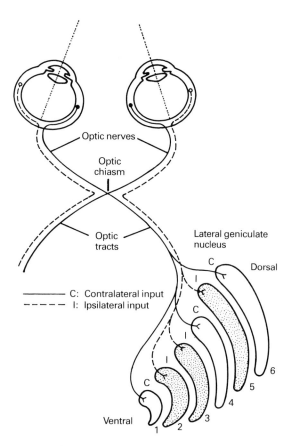

28–6 Contralateral input (**C**) and ipsilateral input (**I**) project to different layers of the lateral geniculate nucleus to create a representation of the contralateral visual hemifield.

erate in the lateral geniculate nucleus. By this means, a large, pale terminal containing round synaptic vesicles has been found to contact the dendrites of a small number of projection cells. Murray Sherman and his colleagues at the State University of New York at Stony Brook have found that the axons of Y ganglion cells of a particular region of retina project to a specific portion of the cat's lateral geniculate nucleus that deals with input from that region of retina. There the Y ganglion cells terminate in more than one layer of the lateral geniculate nucleus. In so doing, the axons pass through intervening layers without branching extensively, but in the target layers the axons branch widely (Figure 28–7).

In contrast, the X ganglion cells have thinner axons than the Y cells, but the most characteristic difference between the two is that X cells have a small, vertically oriented terminal zone that is only one-third the width of the Y terminal zone (Figure 28–7). Therefore, the structural differences observed between these two cell types in the retina are preserved in the lateral geniculate nucleus: Y ganglion cells have widely spread dendritic trees in the retina that give them large receptive fields and a relatively large terminal zone in the lateral geniculate nucleus, whereas X ganglion cells have narrow dendritic trees in the retina, smaller receptive fields, and narrow terminal zones in the lateral geniculate nucleus. The physiological properties of the different types of ganglion cells will be discussed in detail in Chapter 29, but it might already be intuitively evident that the narrow dendritic fields of the X cells would best subserve the resolution of the fine detail of form while Y cells would be better detectors of large objects and for movement.

28–7 The terminal zones of ganglion cell axons in the dorsal layers of the lateral geniculate nucleus are demonstrated by the intracellular injection of horseradish peroxidase. **A.** Axons of Y cells have large, wide terminal zones in the target layers. **B.** Axons of X cells have smaller, vertically oriented terminal zones. (Adapted from Sur and Sherman, 1982.)

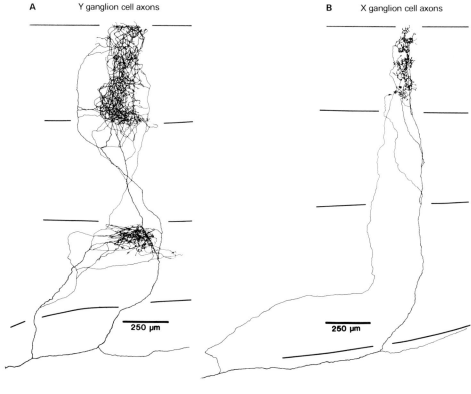

A   Y ganglion cell axons

B   X ganglion cell axons

250 μm

250 μm

The retina also projects to sites other than the lateral geniculate nucleus, notably the superior colliculus of the midbrain—a structure important for the control of eye movement. The Y cells have branching axons that project to both the superior colliculus and the lateral geniculate nucleus. Most W cells project to the superior colliculus.

The Superior Colliculus and Pretectum Are Visual Reflex Centers

Superior Colliculus

The superior colliculus has two distinct sources of visual input: direct input from the retina, and indirect input from the visual cortex. The location of the superior colliculus is shown in Figure 28–8. It is composed of several layers of cells. The superficial layers are dominated by visual inputs; the deepest layers receive inputs primarily from the somatic sensory and auditory systems.

Axons from cells in the superior colliculus are distributed to several areas. Some of these axons cross the midline and descend in the brain stem adjacent to the ventricle as the *tectospinal tract*. This tract is probably important for the reflex control of head and neck movements. Although there are few direct connections between neurons in the superior colliculus and the motor nuclei innervating the extraocular muscles, the superior colliculus has an important influence on the activity of these motor nuclei. For example, the superior colliculus is used to orient the head and eyes toward the source of a visual stimulus. As we shall see in Chapter 43, the superior colliculus is crucial for the performance of rapid eye movements.

Tectopontine axons also arise from the superior colliculus and synapse upon cells in the pontine nuclei. This pathway is an important part of the mechanism for relaying visual input to the cerebellum.

Pretectal Region

Another important visual reflex center, the *pretectal area*, lies just rostral to the superior colliculus, where the midbrain fuses with the thalamus (Figure 28–9). This

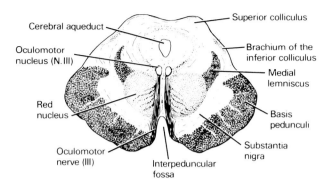

28–8 This myelin-stained section through the superior colliculus shows its location in relation to other brain structures.

region mediates pupillary light reflexes. Pupillary reflexes are significant clinically, so it is necessary to understand the pathways that underlie them. Light shone upon one eye causes a constriction of the pupil in that eye (the *direct response*) as well as a constriction of the pupil in the other eye (the *consensual response*). Certain retinal ganglion cells respond to the change in overall luminance of the visual field. These cells send their axons through the optic nerve and tract to synapse in the pretectal region. Axons from the pretectal area then project bilaterally to preganglionic parasympathetic neurons in the region immediately adjacent to the somatic motor neurons of the third nerve nucleus. Preganglionic neurons in this region send axons out of the brain with the third nerve to innervate the *ciliary ganglion*, where the postganglionic neurons innervating the smooth muscle of the pupillary sphincter are found.

Testing of pupillary reflexes provides important information about the functional state of the afferent and efferent pathways mediating them. As an example, imagine that light shone in the left eye of a patient elicits a consensual response, but not a direct one. This would mean that the afferent limb of the reflex is intact, but the efferent limb to the left eye is damaged, possibly by a lesion of the third nerve. If the optic nerve is lesioned unilater-

28–9 This myelin-stained section through the junction of the midbrain and thalamus shows the location of the pretectal region. (Adapted from Carpenter, 1976.)

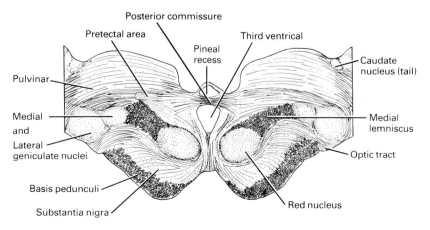

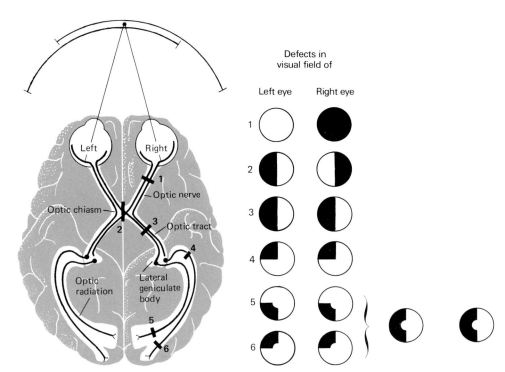

28–10 The level of a lesion in the visual pathway is indicated by the specific visual field deficits it causes. The **numbered bars** along the visual pathway indicate the sites of lesions. The visual field defects (**blackened areas**) that result from each lesioned site are shown in the accompanying visual field maps. **1:** A lesion of the right optic nerve causes a total loss of vision in the right eye. **2:** A lesion of the optic chiasm causes a bitemporal hemianopsia, a loss of vision in the temporal halves of both visual fields. Because the chiasm carries crossing fibers from both eyes, this is the only lesion in the visual system that causes a nonhomonymous deficit in vision, a deficit in two *different* parts of the visual field as a consequence of a single lesion. **3:** A lesion of the optic tract causes a complete homonymous contralateral hemianopsia, a complete loss of vision in the opposite half of the visual field. **4:** After leaving the lateral geniculate nucleus, the fibers representing both retinas mix in the optic radiation, although this is not indicated in the figure. A lesion of the optic

radiation fibers that curve into the temporal lobe (Meyer's loop) causes an upper contralateral quadrantic anopsia, a loss of vision in the upper quadrant of the visual field of both eyes on the opposite side. **5 and 6:** Partial lesions of the visual cortex lead to partial field deficits on the opposite side. A lesion in the upper bank of the calcarine cortex (**5**) causes a partial deficit in the inferior quadrant of the visual field on the opposite side. A lesion in the lower bank of the calcarine cortex (**6**) causes a partial deficit in the superior quadrant of the visual field of both eyes on the opposite side. A more extensive lesion of the visual cortex, including parts of both banks of the calcarine cortex, would cause a more extensive loss of vision in the contralateral hemifield. After cortical lesions, the central area of vision, or the macular area, is spared (**5 and 6**), probably because the representation of the macula is so extensive that a single lesion is unlikely to destroy the entire representation; the representation of the periphery of the visual field is smaller, and hence more easily destroyed by a single lesion.

ally, light shone in the affected eye causes no change in either pupil, whereas light shone in the intact eye elicits both a direct and a consensual response. In an unconscious patient, the absence of pupillary light reflexes indicates that massive damage to the midbrain has occurred.

Lesions in the Visual Pathway Cause Predictable Changes in Sight

Before examining the structure of the visual cortex in detail, let us consider the deficits produced by lesions at various levels along the visual pathway leading up to the visual cortex. After section of the optic nerve, the visual field is seen monocularly by the eye on the intact side.

The temporal crescent is normally seen only by the nasal hemiretina on the same side (Figure 28–4). An individual with optic nerve section would therefore be blind in the temporal crescent on the lesioned side. Removal of binocular input in this way would also affect *stereopsis,* which allows us to perceive spatial depth and is based upon binocular interactions.

Destruction of the fibers crossing in the optic chiasm would remove input from the temporal portions of both halves of the visual field. The deficit produced by this lesion is called *bitemporal hemianopsia* and occurs because fibers arising from the nasal half of each retina have been destroyed. This kind of damage is most commonly caused by an expanding tumor of the pituitary gland that compresses the chiasm.

Destruction of one optic tract produces a *complete homonymous hemianopsia*, that is, a loss of vision in the entire contralateral visual hemifield. Thus, destruction of the right tract causes a *left homonymous hemianopsia:* loss of vision mediated by the left nasal and right temporal hemiretinas. Finally, a lesion of the optic radiation or the visual cortex, where the fibers are more spread out, produces an *incomplete* or *quadrantic field defect* in the related part of the contralateral half of the visual field. The visual field deficits caused by lesions at various levels of the visual pathway are summarized in Figure 28–10.

The Primary Visual Cortex Has a Characteristic Cellular Architecture

The *primary visual cortex*, also called the *striate cortex* (Brodmann's area 17), is located in the occipital lobe. It receives the axons from the projection cells of the lateral geniculate nucleus. These axons are collectively termed the *optic radiation*. After sweeping around the lateral ventricle, the fibers of the optic radiation are found on the lateral surface of both the temporal and occipital horns of the lateral ventricle (Figure 28–11). Fibers representing the inferior parts of the retina swing in a broad arc over the temporal horn of the ventricle and loop into the temporal lobe before turning caudally to reach the occipital pole. This group of fibers, called *Meyer's loop*, accounts for the fact that unilateral lesions in the temporal lobe affect vision in the *superior* quadrant of the contralateral visual hemifield. The geniculocortical fibers relaying input from the inferior half of the retina terminate in the inferior bank of the cortex lining the calcarine fissure, whereas the fibers relaying input from the superior half of the retina terminate in the superior bank (Figure 28–12). Consequently, a lesion in the *inferior* bank of the calcarine cortex causes a defect in the *superior* half of the contralateral visual field.

The visual cortex is about 3 mm thick and consists of several alternating layers of fibers and cells stretching from the pial surface to the underlying white matter. The separate layers of the visual cortex perform different tasks. In the primate visual cortex, axons from the lateral geniculate nucleus terminate mostly in layer IV. We can study the pattern of termination of these axons by making use of *transneuronal transport* of radioactively labeled proteins, a process described for cells in the visual pathway by Bernice Grafstein at Cornell University Medical School. She found that if a tritiated precursor is injected into the eye, it is incorporated into proteins by the retinal ganglion cells, and some of these proteins are transported along ganglion cell axons to synaptic terminals in the lateral geniculate nucleus. A small fraction of the labeled material in the retinal terminals reaches the postsynaptic neurons of the lateral geniculate nucleus and is then transported to the terminals of the projection cells in the visual cortex. It is not yet known whether intact proteins are released from one cell and taken up

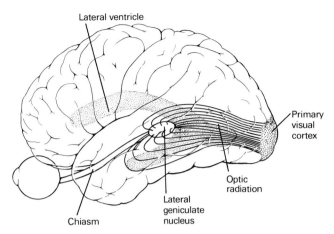

28–11 Course of the fibers of the optic radiation as they sweep around the lateral ventricle to reach the primary visual cortex. (Adapted from Brodal, 1981.)

by the next, or whether breakdown products are transferred at the synapses. The end result, however, is that regions of the cortex receiving input from the injected eye are selectively labeled.

Torsten Wiesel and David Hubel, whose physiological studies of the visual cortex will be discussed in Chapter 29, used transsynaptic transport, in collaboration with Dominic Lam, to study the architecture of the inputs from the lateral geniculate nucleus to the primary visual cortex. They injected one eye in a series of monkeys with a radioactive amino acid and, using autoradiography, found that only those layers of the lateral geniculate nucleus that receive input from the injected eye are labeled. In autoradiographs of the visual cortex from the same animals, they found that the pattern of thalamic input to the cortex has a strikingly regular array (Figure 28–13).

28–12 Fibers that relay input from the inferior half of the retina terminate in the inferior bank of the calcarine cortex; those that relay input from the superior half of the retina terminate in the superior bank.

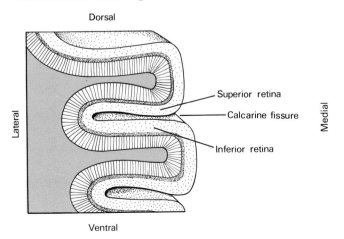

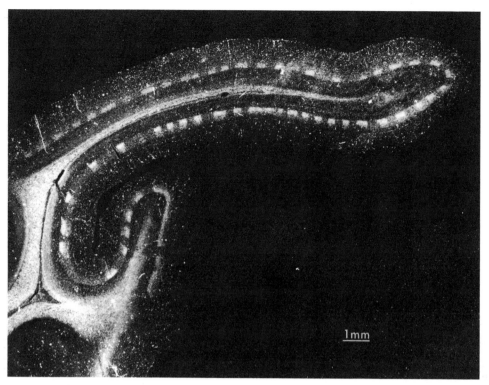

28–13 This dark-field autoradiograph of the primary visual cortex in an adult monkey demonstrates the thalamic input to the cortex (labeled by injection of tritiated proline and fucose in the ipsilateral eye 2 weeks before). Labeled areas show as **white**. The section passes for the most part in a plane perpendicular to the surface; part of the exposed surface of the primary visual cortex and the buried part immediately beneath are shown; some of the buried part had fallen away during sectioning. In all, some 56 columns can be counted in layer IVc. This section cuts through the gray matter of the cortex twice. Beginning at the pial surface (top of the figure) the section then goes through the gray matter and reaches layer IV, where the patches of label appear as bright bands. The section goes deeper through the gray matter to the underlying white matter, where labeled axons are evident. The section continues through the gray matter on the opposite side of the gyrus, through another band of columns in layer IV, and then reaches the pial surface. (From Hubel and Wiesel, 1977.)

Layer IV of the visual cortex is divided into three major sublayers: IVa, IVb, and IVc. In layer IVc, patches of cortex that mediate input from the injected eye are heavily labeled, and they alternate with adjacent unlabeled patches that mediate input from the uninjected eye. Therefore, cells in layer IVc receive input from either one eye or the other via the separate layers of the lateral geniculate nucleus; the output from layer IVc goes to the layers above and below it, where signals from both eyes converge upon individual cells. These clusters of terminals relaying input from each eye to separate zones within layer IV are the anatomical basis for the ocular dominance columns that will be described in Chapters 29 and 57.

The wiring pattern of the cells in each of the cortical layers is complex, but it is possible to recognize certain consistent patterns, especially when individual neurons are labeled intracellularly with horseradish peroxidase injected through a recording micropipette. Using this label, Charles Gilbert and Torsten Wiesel, now at Rockefeller University were able to correlate the morphology, physiology, and local axonal connections of individual cortical neurons.

Neurons in layer IVc that receive input from the lateral geniculate nucleus send their axons superficially to layers II and III. These layers, in turn, have local connections with the underlying layer V. Layer V cells connect with layer VI, which completes the local circuit with connections to layer IV. Each of these layers, however, also makes strong connections with other regions of the brain, so that information can leave this loop from any layer. Stellate cells appear to be concerned almost exclusively with the local integration of cortical activity, whereas pyramidal cells give rise to axons that leave Brodmann's area 17 and project to adjacent portions of the cortex or the brain stem.

The connections established by pyramidal cells with regions outside area 17 have been studied by retrograde tracing with peroxidase. The results of the studies can be summarized as follows: Cells in layers II and III project to higher visual areas, such as Brodmann's areas 18 and the medial temporal lobe. In primates, these areas do not receive strong direct connections from the lateral geniculate nucleus but, rather, receive the output of area 17. Cells in layer V project to the superior colliculus. The superior colliculus, therefore, integrates visual input re-

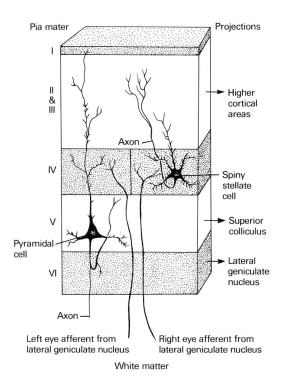

28–14 The afferent and efferent connections of the primary visual cortex are made in specific layers of cortex.

ceived directly from the retina with input derived from the visual cortex. Cells in layer VI project back to the lateral geniculate nucleus. Thus, this layer exerts a feedback control over visual input reaching the cortex from the thalamus.

The connections of the cortical layers in the primary visual area are illustrated in Figure 28–14. Visual input arrives in layer IV, and, after intracortical processing (through local cortical loops), is forwarded to higher cortical areas via layers II and III, to the superior colliculus via layer V, and back to the lateral geniculate nucleus via layer VI. Layer I contains mostly axons running parallel to the surface of the cortex. Its function may be to relate separate parts of area 17.

An Overall View

The degree of specificity in the central connections of the visual system is remarkable. Separate regions in the retina project upon the lateral geniculate nucleus in such a way that a complete representation of the contralateral visual hemifield is established in the thalamus. Furthermore, distinct cell types occupying the same retinal locus project their axons to different targets in the brain stem; some cells project to the thalamus, some to the midbrain, others to both. The lateral geniculate nucleus is mapped onto the primary visual cortex (Brodmann's area 17) in a point-to-point manner, since each geniculate axon terminates in and contacts only a small part of layer IV.

Cells in layer IV and in the other layers of area 17 have their own highly stereotyped patterns of connections.

One of the central problems in neurobiology is to understand how these intricate networks of synaptic connections arise during development. To appreciate the magnitude of the problem, remember that there are more than a million fibers in each optic nerve. An individual fiber must find its small target in the midst of the several million cells in the lateral geniculate nucleus; the geniculate neurons must then find their targets among the billions of cortical cells. The processes governing the formation of these specific connections are an intriguing subject that will be considered later in Chapter 57 in relation to the visual system and other systems of the brain.

Selected Readings

Brodal, A. 1981. Neurological Anatomy in Relation to Clinical Medicine, 3rd ed. New York: Oxford University Press, chap. 8.

Gilbert, C. D., and Wiesel, T. N. 1979. Morphology and intracortical projections of functionally characterised neurones in the cat visual cortex. Nature 280:120–125.

Grafstein, B., and Laureno, R. 1973. Transport of radioactivity from eye to visual cortex in the mouse. Exp. Neurol. 39:44–57.

Hubel, D. H., and Wiesel, T. N. 1972. Laminar and columnar distribution of geniculo-cortical fibers in the macaque monkey. J. Comp. Neurol. 146:421–450.

Hubel, D. H., and Wiesel, T. N. 1977. Ferrier Lecture: Functional architecture of macaque monkey visual cortex. Proc. R. Soc. Lond. [Biol.] 198:1–59.

Wiesel, T. N., Hubel, D. H., and Lam, D. M. K. 1974. Autoradiographic demonstration of ocular-dominance columns in the monkey striate cortex by means of transneuronal transport. Brain Res. 79:273–279.

References

Boycott, B. B., and Wässle, H. 1974. The morphological types of ganglion cells of the domestic cat's retina. J. Physiol. (Lond.) 240:397–419.

Carpenter, M. B. 1976. Human Neuroanatomy, 7th ed. Baltimore: Williams & Wilkins.

Groves, P., and Schlesinger, K. 1979. An Introduction to Biological Psychology. Dubuque, Iowa: W. C. Brown.

Hurvich, L. M. 1981. Color Vision. Sunderland, Mass.: Sinauer.

Sur, M., and Sherman, S. M. 1982. Retinogeniculate terminations in cats: Morphological differences between X and Y cell axons. Science 218:389–391.

Eric R. Kandel

Processing of Form and Movement in the Visual System

29

What does it mean, to see? The plain man's answer (and Aristotle's, too) would be, to know what is where by looking. In other words, vision is the process of discovering from images what is present in the world, and where it is. Vision is therefore, first and foremost, an information processing task, but we cannot think of it just as a process. For if we are capable of knowing what is where in the world, our brains must somehow be capable of *representing* this information—in all its profusion of color and form, beauty, motion, and detail. The study of vision must therefore include not only the study of how to extract from images the various aspects of the world that are useful to us, but also an inquiry into the nature of the internal representations by which we capture this information and thus make it available as a basis for decisions about our thoughts and actions.

(David Marr, *Vision*, 1982)

We are remarkably visual animals. Much of our conception of the world and our memory of it is based on sight. How do we perceive visual images? And, how do we perceive the movement of these visual images in space? How do we distinguish color? In this chapter and the next we shall examine research that is addressed to these questions.

Most of what we know about the functional organization of the visual system derives from experiments first with evoked responses and later with single-cell recordings. Because these methods are similar to those used by Marshall, Woolsey, and Bard and by Mountcastle in investigating the somatic sensory system, we are in a good position to compare these two sensory systems. The similarities may in turn lead us to some general principles governing the transformation of sensory information in the brain and the organization and functioning of the cerebral cortex. We should also look for differences between the two systems. For example, the visual system is numerically the most complex of all sensory systems. Whereas the auditory nerve contains about 30,000 fibers, the optic nerve contains 1 million. There are more optic nerve fibers than there are dorsal root ganglion cells in all the segments of the spinal cord!

The Superior Colliculus Participates in Visually Guided Saccadic Eye Movements

In Chapter 27 we saw that the retina has three classes of output neurons: cells with small cell bodies (W), medium-size cells (X), and large cells (Y). These three classes of ganglion cells have distinctive projections. The X cells project only to the lateral geniculate nucleus. The Y cells project both to the lateral geniculate nucleus (but to layers that do not receive input from X cells), and, to a lesser degree, to the superior colliculus. The W cells project almost exclusively to the superior colliculus. Let us first consider the projection of the Y and W cells to the superior colliculus.

In addition to receiving input from almost all of the W and many Y ganglion cells from the contralateral retina, the colliculus also receives visual input indirectly, from the visual cortex. This information is brought together in the colliculus with somatic and auditory information so that sensory responses can be coordinated with the movements of the head and eyes toward a stimulus in the environment. Thus, in addition to the visual representation, the superior colliculus also contains maps of the body surface and of the localization of sound in space. However, the map for somatic sensation in the colliculus is quite different from that in the somatic sensory cortex. In the colliculus the size of the central somatic representation is not determined by tactile importance, as reflected in peripheral innervation density, but rather by the visual map. Structures close to the eye such as the nose and face receive greater representation than do distal structures (such as the finger tips) concerned with fine tactile discrimination. A given location in the colliculus is thought to represent a given point in visual space around the animal. Several modalities can activate that location in the colliculus and result in movement oriented toward the stimulus.

The superior colliculus uses this sensory information to control visually guided saccadic eye movements, a function it carries out in conjunction with a region of the frontal cortex called the *frontal eye fields* (which we shall consider in Chapter 43). Peter Schiller and his colleagues at the Massachusetts Institute of Technology found that the superior colliculus is responsible for rapid, reflexlike saccadic eye movements that are elicited by easily discernible visual stimuli. The colliculus receives information about these stimuli from the Y cells, which are thought to be concerned with movement, with visual attention, and with identifying the broad visual outlines of objects. In contrast, the frontal eye fields are concerned with generating saccadic eye movements to complex vi-

sual stimuli and receive input from the primary visual cortex by means of the pathway of X cells, a pathway that is important for fine visual discrimination.

The Retina Is Mapped in the Lateral Geniculate Nucleus and Visual Cortex

As we saw in Chapter 28, fibers from the *right half of the retina of each eye* (the nasal hemiretina of the left eye and the temporal hemiretina of the right eye) project information about the left visual hemifield to the *right lateral geniculate nucleus* via both the optic nerve and the right optic tract. Similarly, the left hemiretina projects information about the right visual field to the left lateral geniculate nucleus (Figure 29–1). From the lateral geniculate nucleus, neurons project via the *optic radiation* to the *primary visual cortex* (Brodmann's area 17, or visual area I). This area is also called the *striate cortex* because it contains a prominent stripe of white matter, the *stria of Gennari*, which is produced by the massive termination in layer IV of the myelinated afferent fibers from the lateral geniculate nucleus. The primary visual cortex on each side receives information only from the opposite visual hemifield. From the primary visual cortex, neurons project to the higher order, *extrastriate* cortex (Brodmann's area 18). Neurons from area 17 also project to the superior colliculus and back to the lateral geniculate nucleus (another example of central control of sensory input). From area 18, neurons project to the *medial temporal cortex* (area 19), to the *inferotemporal cortex* (areas 20 and 21), and to the *posterior parietal cortex* (area 7). The inferotemporal cortex and area 18 also receive input from the *pulvinar* of the thalamus.

Modern physiological studies of the visual system began in 1941 with the experiments of Wade Marshall and Samuel Talbot. They used small spots of light projected through an operating ophthalmoscope to stimulate various parts of the retina. (With current methods, which are technically much simpler than an operating ophthalmoscope and give excellent spatial resolution, light patterns are indirectly projected onto the retina by directing a light source at an angle to a screen in front of the subject, as illustrated in Figure 29–2). Marshall and Talbot found that the primary visual cortex contains a map of the retina in which neighborhood relations are preserved. Continuous areas of the retina are represented as continuous areas of cortex. Subsequent work has shown that there are additional representations of the retina beyond the striate cortex! Some of these are complete representations but others are only partial. For example, there are six representations in the occipital lobe alone: one in the primary visual cortex, area 17 (V1), four in area 18 (V2, V3, V3a, V4), and one in the middle temporal area (MT), at the border between the temporal and occipital lobes (V5). There is also a representation in the adjacent inferotemporal cortex (areas 20 and 21), and one in the posterior parietal cortex (area 7a), an area of cortex concerned with integrating somatic and visual sensations.

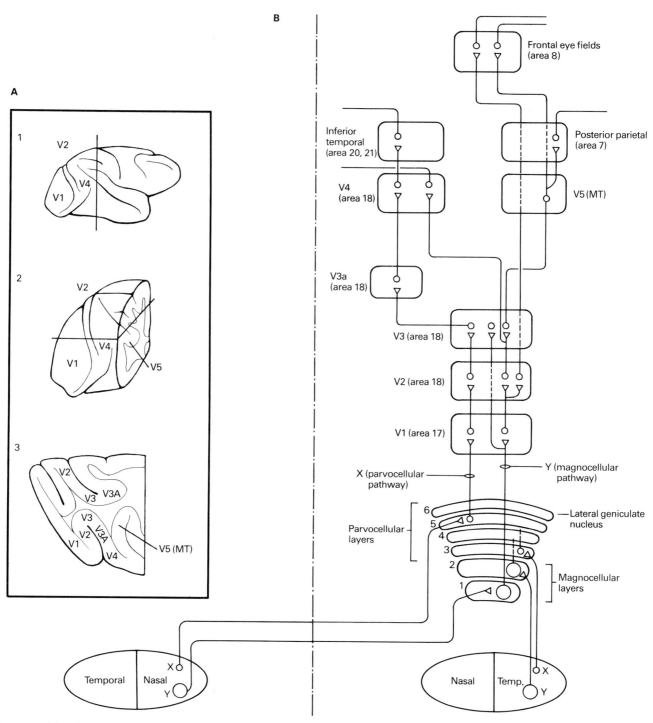

29–1 Highly schematic diagrams of the visual projections from the retina to the various visual areas of the cerebral cortex.

A. Visual cortical areas in the macaque monkey, as seen in the intact hemisphere (**A₁, A₂**), and in histological sections (**A₃**).

A₁. A lateral view of the right hemisphere, showing the exposed portions of visual areas V1, V2, and V4. Vertical line indicates the location of a cut in the coronal plane made to provide the view in **A₂**.

A₂. An expanded view, from an anterolateral angle, of the occipital lobe, showing areas V1, V2, V4, and V5, which lies in the buried middle temporal area, **MT**, in the superior temporal sulcus at the rostral border of the occipital lobe.

A₃. A horizontal section through the occipital lobe, showing the approximate locations of known visual areas at this level.

B. Diagram of the visual pathways emphasizing two key factors in their organization. First, there are discrete levels, suggesting a hierarchy of processing. Second, there are major pathways by which aspects of visual information can be processed in parallel. At least two major parallel pathways have been identified: the X (parvocellular) pathway and the Y (magnocellular) pathway. As we shall see later, the first is concerned primarily with detail, form, and color, and the second, primarily with movement, with visual attention, and with the gross features of the stimulus. (Adapted from Van Essen, 1979.)

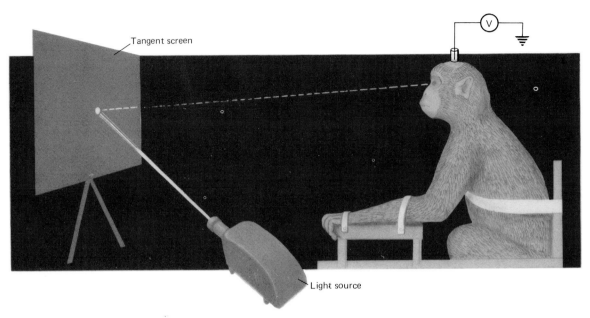

Tangent screen

Light source

29–2 Patterns of light are used to stimulate a particular small region of the retina in order to trace its projection to the visual cortex. The eyes of an anesthetized, light-adapted monkey focus on a screen onto which various patterns of light are projected, while an electrode records the responses from a single cell in the visual pathway.

These representations differ with respect both to the precision of the retinotopic map and to the stimulus attributes with which the cells seem to be concerned. In addition, maps of the retina are found within each layer of the lateral geniculate nucleus (as we saw in Chapter 28, the map in each of these layers is in register with the maps in the layers above and below it). Thus, in the visual system, we encounter again an organizational feature that we first noted in the somatic sensory system: through the recreation of various representations of its receptive sheet, the visual system allows us to perceive features of the external world.

As in the somatic sensory system, there are distortions in the retinal projection. For example, the area of the retina capable of the greatest acuity, the *fovea* (Figure 29–3), also has the greatest density of nerve cells and is

29–3 Visual acuity is greatest in the region of the fovea. This graph of visual acuity as a function of position in the visual field illustrates that acuity drops off sharply on both the temporal and nasal sides of the fovea. The blind spot, created by the origin (head) of the optic nerve as it leaves the retina, has no photoreceptors. (From Schmidt and Thews, 1983.)

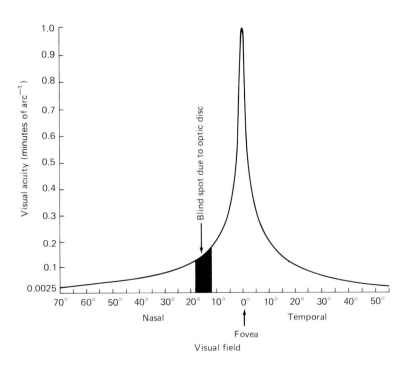

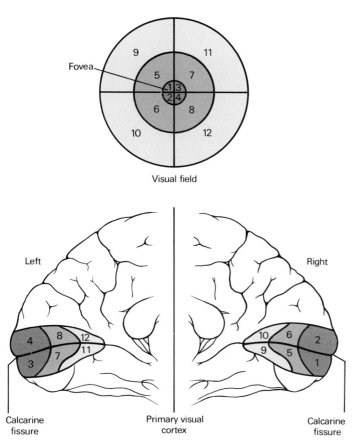

29–4 Brodmann's area 17, the primary visual cortex (or V1), contains an orderly map of the visual field. In humans, this cortex is located at the posterior pole of the cerebral hemisphere and lies almost exclusively on the medial surface. (In some people, its position is shifted so that part of it extends onto the lateral surface.) The various parts of the visual field **(top)** are numbered to match the corresponding areas in the primary visual cortex **(bottom)** devoted to their representation. Each half of the visual field is mapped to the contralateral hemisphere. The upper fields are mapped below the fundus of the calcarine fissure, and the lower fields above it. The striking aspect of this map is that representation of the fovea and the central region of the visual field is greatly magnified as compared with the representations of the more peripheral regions. (From Berne and Levy, 1983.)

represented in enormous detail in many of these maps: about half of the neural mass in the lateral geniculate nucleus and in the primary visual cortex (area 17) represents the fovea and the parafoveal region (Figure 29–4). The much larger peripheral portions of the retina are less well represented. Visual acuity requires detailed analysis and, therefore, many neurons. Because the eye is a globe that must rotate in its socket, the retina cannot have more area devoted to the center than to the periphery. To compensate for this restriction, the retinal ganglion cells in and near the fovea are densely packed. These optical considerations do not apply beyond the retina. Therefore, the lateral geniculate nucleus and the primary visual cortex can maintain a fairly homogeneous density of neurons by committing a larger area to the fovea than to the peripheral parts of the retina. The ratio of the area in the primary visual cortex (or in the lateral geniculate nucleus) to the area in the retina representing one degree of the visual field is called the *magnification factor.*

Receptive Fields of Neurons in Various Parts of the Visual System Have Different Properties

The next stage in the study of the mammalian visual system, after the work of Marshall and Talbot, came in 1952 when Stephen Kuffler, then at Johns Hopkins University, recorded the activity of single retinal ganglion

cells. He found that these cells are never silent, even in the dark, but that light modulates their spontaneous activity. Each cell responded to light, and the most effective stimulus for each cell was a spot of light directed to a specific area of the retina. Kuffler called this area the *receptive field* of the cell. The receptive field of a single cell in any part of the visual system is *that area in the retina where stimulation with light causes either excitation or inhibition of the cell's firing pattern.*

Using small spots of light to probe the properties of these receptive fields, Kuffler found that the receptive fields of the retinal ganglion cells are roughly circular, and that they vary in size across the retina. In the foveal region of the retina, where visual acuity is greatest (Figure 29–3), the receptive fields are very small, with centers that are only a few minutes of arc; at the periphery of the retina, where the acuity is low, the fields are larger, with centers of 3° to 5° (1° on the retina is equal to about 0.25 mm). Moreover, each field is not homogeneous throughout but has a fine structure. On the basis of this fine structure, Kuffler classified the cells into two large groups: on-center and off-center ganglion cells (Figure 29–5). The two types of cells are present in approximately equal numbers. On-center cells have receptive fields with a central excitatory zone and an inhibitory surround. Shining a spot of light on the center of the field causes an increase in the spontaneous firing of an on-center cell. In contrast, a light stimulus that encircles

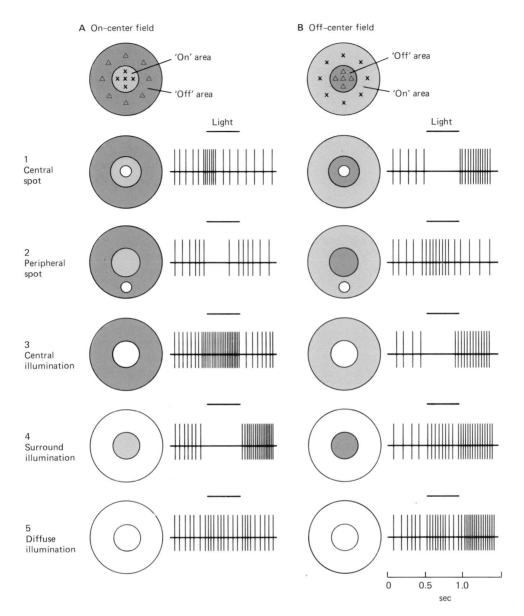

29–5 Neurons in the retina have two major classes of receptive fields: on-center and off-center. Electrical recordings of the activity of on-center and off-center retinal ganglion cells illustrate that both types of neurons respond optimally to *light contrast.* This is revealed by the difference in their responses to various types of illumination. **X,** excitatory zone; △, inhibitory zone. Duration of illumination is indicated by **bar** above each extracellular record. **A.** An *on-center* cell responds best when the entire central part of its receptive field is illuminated but the illumination does not extend beyond this central region (**3**). Such a cell also responds, but less vigorously, when only a portion of its central field is illuminated by a spot of light (**1**). Illumination of the surrounding area with a spot of light (**2**) or an annulus (**4**) reduces or suppresses the discharges and causes a response when the light is turned off. Diffuse illumination of the entire receptive field (**5**) elicits a relatively weak discharge because center and surround oppose each other's effects. **B.** The spontaneous firing of a cell with an *off-center* receptive field is suppressed when the central area of its field is illuminated (**1, 3**) and accelerated when the stimulus is turned off. Light shone onto the surround of an off-center receptive field excites the cell (**2, 4**). In this and subsequent figures the light stimulus is indicated as the white portion of the receptive field. (Adapted from Kuffler, 1952.)

this central zone inhibits the cell's firing. Thus, the most effective excitatory stimulus for this cell is a spot of light on the center of its receptive field, and the most effective inhibitory stimulus is a ring of light on the surround of the receptive field. The opposite is true for cells with off-center fields, which consist of an excitatory surround and an inhibitory center. Diffuse light over the whole of either type of receptive field (center plus surround) is much less effective in activating the cell. Here, on the level of the retinal ganglion cells, we find a key principle in the organization of the visual system: *the cells in the visual system read contrasts.*

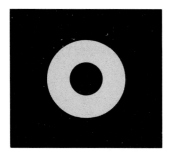 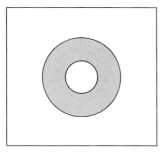

29–6 This visual illusion illustrates that the appearance of an object depends not on the intensity of the light source but on the contrast between the object and its surround. The gray rings in the two parts of the figure are identical in hue, but their brightness appears to vary with the contrast provided by their background. (From Brown and Herrnstein, 1975.)

The center–surround structure of the receptive field is an example of an antagonistic, or opponent, organization like that used by the somatic sensory system for two-point discrimination. We shall encounter this organization again in considering color vision in Chapter 30. For both black and white objects, the opponent organization of the receptive field is important in understanding why the appearance of an object does not depend significantly on the intensity of the light source that illuminates it, but on *spatial contrast*, the contrast between the object and its surroundings. For example, a gray ring looks much lighter against a black background than against a white background (Figure 29–6). A similar principle holds for color.

The Ganglion Cells of the Retina Project Information to the Lateral Geniculate Nucleus by Means of Several Independent Channels

Following up on Kuffler's work, Malcolm Slaughter and Robert Miller found that the on-center ganglion cells in the retina can be selectively and reversibly blocked by DL-2-amino-4-phosphonobutyric acid. This drug blocks a class of receptors for glutamic acid, which is thought to be the chemical transmitter of the photoreceptors. It acts by blocking the on-center bipolar cells and the on-center amacrine cells without interfering in any way with the center–surround organization of the off-center cells. Thus, the on- and off-center ganglion cells represent independent, parallel retinal *channels* that project separately to the lateral geniculate nucleus.

Moreover, as work by Christina Enroth-Cugell and John Robson of Northwestern University, and subsequently that of others, has shown, each of these two channels has subcomponents consistent with the three morphological classes of retinal ganglion cells—X, Y, and W. The W cells constitute 10% of the total ganglion cells in the retina. As we have seen, most of them project to the superior colliculus, and we shall not consider them further because they are concerned with head and eye

movement. Here we shall focus on the X and Y systems because they are concerned with the detection of form and movement.

Y cells (10% of the total) have large cell bodies, extensive dendritic trees, and thick, rapidly conducting axons that project primarily to the lateral geniculate nucleus but also to the superior colliculus. The Y cells respond *transiently* and only to large targets, particularly moving ones. These cells are thought to accomplish the initial analysis of crude form and to direct one's eyes and one's attention to objects moving in the visual field. In contrast, X cells (80% of the total) have medium-size cell bodies and small dendritic arbors, and are concentrated in the foveal region of the retina. The axons of the X cells conduct more slowly and project only to the lateral geniculate nucleus. X cells have smaller receptive fields than Y cells, respond better to small than to large targets, and do so in a *sustained* way. The X cells are thought to be involved in the detailed high-resolution analysis of the visual image. They are also involved in the analysis of color (Chapter 30).

Thus, the pathway from the retina to the lateral geniculate nucleus contains independent, opponent organized channels: one on-center and the other off-center. Each of these in turn is subdivided into X and Y channels: one pathway for the initial analysis of movement and the gross structure of the visual image (Y), the other for the analysis of its fine structure (X). The existence of these four channels is another example of the principle that we encountered earlier: *parallel processing*. A single locus in the retina abstracts several types of information from the visual world, and the information from this locus is projected to different cells and sometimes even to different regions in the central nervous system.

Because seven to eight relay points have been analyzed in the visual system, a more detailed longitudinal analysis can be carried out here than in the somatic sensory system. By knowing the organization of the receptive fields in the retina, we can now determine how the receptive fields are transformed at each sequential relay point in the higher reaches of the visual system. This is the task that David Hubel and Torsten Wiesel at Harvard Medical School set for themselves.

The Lateral Geniculate Nucleus Enhances the Antagonisms between the Center and the Surround

Hubel and Wiesel first examined the lateral geniculate nucleus. As you will recall from Chapter 28, each layer of the lateral geniculate nucleus is organized simply and receives input from only one eye: layers 2, 3, and 5 from the ipsilateral eye; and layers 1, 4, and 6 from the contralateral eye. Layers 1 and 2 have large cells and are therefore called the *magnocellular* layers, whereas layers 3, 4, 5, and 6 have small cells and are called the *parvocellular* layers.

The cells in the lateral geniculate nucleus have two interesting properties. First, relatively few of them are local inhibitory interneurons with short axons. Most neurons in the lateral geniculate nucleus are relay cells that project to the cerebral cortex. In the lateral geniculate nucleus, the principal cells interact extensively with one another by means of dendrodendritic contacts, thus reducing the need for interneurons. Second, each neuron in the lateral geniculate nucleus receives input from only a few retinal ganglion cells. Consistent with this simple anatomical arrangement, the receptive fields in the lateral geniculate nucleus are straightforward and resemble those found in the retina (Figure 29–7A). Cells have concentric receptive fields that are several degrees in diameter. The cells are on-center and off-center, and the most effective stimuli are small spots of light; the effect of diffuse light is much weaker.

Not surprisingly, the on- and off-center systems in the lateral geniculate nucleus receive their input from the on- and off-center systems in the retina and, again, the two systems in the lateral geniculate nucleus are as independent as those in the retina. Similarly, each on- and off-center channel has X and Y pathways, but evidence suggests that in the lateral geniculate these pathways *become segregated anatomically*. The Y cells, concerned with gross features of the stimulus and with its movement, project exclusively to the large-cell (magnocellular) layers of the lateral geniculate nucleus (layers 1 and 2), whereas the X cells, concerned with detail, project to both the small-cell (parvocellular) and the large-cell layers. As a result, these two parallel information-processing pathways are often referred to as the X-parvocellular pathway and the Y-magnocellular pathway.

The only major difference between cells in the lateral geniculate nucleus and those in the retina is that the antagonisms between the surround and the center are slightly enhanced in the geniculate cells. Although there seems to be no significant transformation of the receptive field properties, it is quite likely that the lateral geniculate nucleus serves at least two other functions. The basis for both of these functions is that in this nucleus the input from the two eyes is distributed in discrete layers. First, the anatomical segregation of the X and Y pathways to different layers of the lateral geniculate nucleus presumably facilitates the projection of these pathways to different layers in area 17. Second, there is also important input into the lateral geniculate nucleus from the visual cortex. Indeed, more fibers actually project to the lateral geniculate nucleus from layer VI of the primary visual cortex than from the retina! The separation of the retinal input into layers may allow these higher regions of the brain to modulate selectively the synaptic transmission of specific populations of nerve cells in the nucleus. For example, the optic tract axons ending on the projection neurons of the lateral geniculate nucleus can be powerfully modulated by presynaptic inhibition. This modulation is thought to be important for controlling the flow of visual information during behavioral arousal and during the transition from sleep to wakefulness. It could be exerted on the cells of some layers and not on others, thereby achieving a selectivity of action.

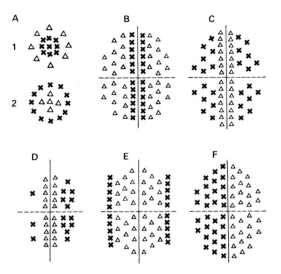

29–7 Comparison of the receptive fields of neurons in the retina and in the lateral geniculate nucleus with those of simple cortical cells in area 17. **A.** Cells of the retina and lateral geniculate fall into two classes: on-center (**1**) and off-center (**2**). **B–F.** Neurons of the primary visual cortex also fall into two major classes: simple and complex. Each of these classes, moreover, has several subclasses. This is illustrated here for simple cells. Despite this variety, however, all simple cells are characterized by three features: (1) specific retinal position, (2) their discrete excitatory (**x**) and inhibitory (Δ) zones, and (3) specific axis of orientation. For simplicity, only receptive fields with a vertical axis of orientation from 12 to 6 o'clock are shown in this figure; each has a rectilinear configuration. In fact, each region of the retina is represented in area 17, not only for this but for all axes of orientation—vertical, horizontal, and various obliques. (Adapted from Hubel and Wiesel, 1962.)

The Primary Visual Cortex Transforms the Visual Message in Various Ways

The primary visual cortex (Brodmann's area 17) contains a complete representation of the contralateral visual hemifield (Figure 29–4), much as does the lateral geniculate nucleus. However, the structure of the primary visual cortex is much more complex than that of the lateral geniculate nucleus. Most of the input from the lateral geniculate nucleus comes into layer IV of the cortex, where it ends on small stellate cells that convey it to the cortical layers above and below. Layer IV is divided into three subregions (a, b, c). Most of the input comes into IVc. The spatial segregation of the X and Y channels that we first encountered in the lateral geniculate nucleus is carried through into the primary visual cortex. The X cells (from the parvocellular layers of the lateral geniculate nucleus) terminate primarily in a strip of layer IVc called IVc-β (although some branches also terminate in layers IVa and VI); the Y cells terminate above this zone in a strip called IVc-α (see Figure 29–11).

In layer IVc, most of the stellate cells have concentric receptive fields of the on-center and off-center variety that we encountered in the lateral geniculate nucleus.

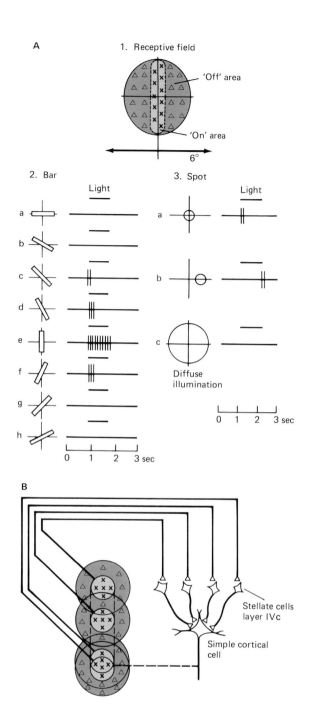

29-8 The receptive field of a simple cell in the primary visual cortex has clearly delineated excitatory (**X**) and inhibitory (△) zones with a specific axis of orientation. **A.** Properties of the receptive field. **1.** The receptive field has a narrow central excitatory area flanked by symmetrical inhibitory areas. **2.** The best stimulus for this cell is a vertically oriented light bar (1° × 8°) in the center of its receptive field (**record e**). Other orientations (rotated clockwise) are less effective or ineffective. **3.** In contrast to a vertical bar, a small spot of light in the excitatory center of the field (**record a**) gives only a weak excitatory response. A small spot in the inhibitory area (**record b**) gives a weak inhibitory response. Diffuse light (**record c**) is ineffective. (Period of illumination is marked by a **bar** above each extracellular record.) (Adapted from Hubel and Wiesel, 1959.) **B.** Hubel and Wiesel's scheme for explaining simple receptive fields. According to this scheme, a simple cortical neuron, such as that illustrated here, receives convergent excitatory connections from four or more cells in layer IV of the primary visual cortex that have similar center–surround organization and similar retinal positions but that are slightly displaced along a vertical line in the retina. The receptive field of the cortical cell, then, has an elongated excitatory region, indicated by the **broken rectangular outline** in the receptive field diagram. A bar of light that falls on this elongated excitatory region of the simple cortical cell activates several stellate cells in layer IV, and this excites the simple cortical neuron. (Adapted from Hubel and Wiesel, 1962.)

However, paralleling the increase in anatomical complexity, Hubel and Wiesel found that above and below layer IVc there is an increase in complexity of the stimulus requirements needed for cells to respond. Their most astonishing finding was that small spots of light, which are so effective in the retina, the lateral geniculate nucleus, and layer IVc, often are not effective stimuli for exciting cells in other areas of the primary visual cortex, with the exception of certain peg-like cell clusters, which we shall consider below. Most of the cells in layers above and below layer IVc do not have circular receptive fields. An effective stimulus for these cells must have linear properties (Figures 29–7, B–F, 29–8, and 29–

9): it must be a line, a bar, or something else with an edge. Hubel and Wiesel categorized the cortical cells in area 17 that lie above or below layer IVc into two major groups: simple and complex.

Simple cells resemble cells of the lateral geniculate nucleus and have discrete antagonist excitatory and inhibitory zones, but these zones are larger than those of retinal ganglion cells or geniculate cells (Figure 29–7, B–F). However, instead of circular excitatory and inhibitory zones, their subdivisions consist of parallel straight lines with a specific axis of orientation. For example, a cell may have a rectangular excitatory zone (with its long axis running from 12 to 6 o'clock) flanked on each side by

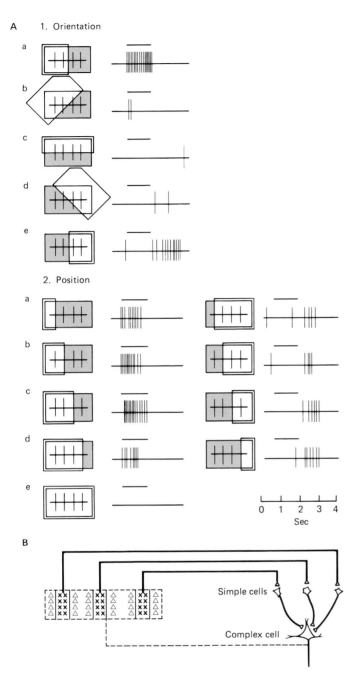

29–9 The receptive field of a complex cell in the primary visual cortex has no clearly defined excitatory or inhibitory zones. **A.** The cell responds best to a vertical edge; orientation is important but position within the field is not critical. **1:** Orientation. With light on the left and dark on the right (**record a**), there is an excitatory response. With light on the right (**record e**), there is an inhibitory response. Orientation other than vertical is less effective. **2:** Position of border within field. A vertical edge of light placed at any point within the field from the right produces an excitatory response. Coming from the left it produces an inhibitory response (**records a** to **d**). Illumination of the entire receptive field (**record e**) gives no response. (Illumination is indicated in each case by the **bar** above records). **B.** According to Hubel and Wiesel's hierarchical scheme for explaining the properties of complex receptive fields, a complex cortical neuron, such as the one illustrated here, receives convergent excitatory connections from several simple cortical cells that have a vertical axis of orientation, a central excitatory zone (**x**) with two flanking inhibitory regions (Δ), and retinal positions that are slightly displaced along a horizontal line in the retina. (Adapted from Hubel and Wiesel, 1962.)

rectangular inhibitory zones (Figure 29–8A). The effective stimulus for this field must have the correct position on the retina, the correct linear properties (in this case a bar), and a specific axis of orientation (in this case vertical, running from 12 to 6 o'clock). The best stimulus is one that coincides with the boundaries of the subdivisions of the particular receptive field. For the cell described above, a horizontally or even an obliquely placed stimulus is ineffective. Other cells in the cortex have similar retinal positions and receptive field shapes, but their axes of orientation are horizontal or oblique. *By this means, every retinal position is represented for every axis of orientation.* As a first approximation, Hubel and

Wiesel suggested that the properties of a simple cortical receptive field could be generated by appropriate connections from the stellate cells in layer IVc in the primary visual cortex—the cells that receive direct input from the lateral geniculate nucleus (Figure 29–8B).

The receptive fields of *complex cells* are usually larger than those of simple cells but also have a critical axis of orientation (Figure 29–9A). The position of the stimulus within the receptive field is not crucial, however, because there are no clearly defined excitatory or inhibitory zones. For certain cells, movement across the receptive field is a particularly good stimulus. Although some complex cells receive their connections directly from

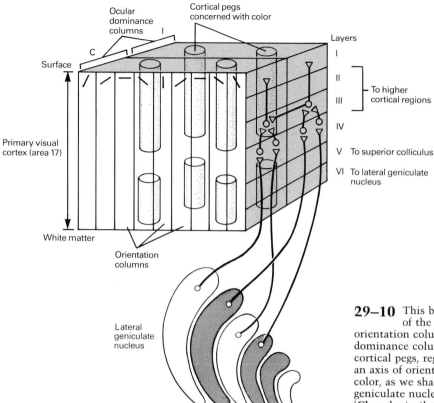

29-10 This basic cortical module (hypercolumn) in area 17 of the visual cortex contains a complete set of orientation columns representing 360° and a set of ocular dominance columns. Each hypercolumn also contains several cortical pegs, regions of cortex in which the cells do not have an axis of orientation. The cells in the pegs are concerned with color, as we shall see in Chapter 30. Each layer of the lateral geniculate nucleus receives input from either the contralateral (**C**) or the ipsilateral (**I**) eye and projects in turn to the ipsilateral or the contralateral ocular dominance columns.

cells of layer IVc, Hubel and Wiesel have proposed that a significant input to the complex cells comes from a family of simple cortical cells that have the same axis of orientation but slightly different positions (Figure 29–9B).

The Primary Visual Cortex Is Organized into Columns

Like the somatic sensory cortex, the primary visual (or striate) cortex is organized into narrow columns, running from the pial surface to the white matter. Each column is about 30–100 μm wide and 2 mm deep, and each column contains cells in layer IVc with concentric receptive fields. Above and below there are many simple cells with almost identical retinal positions and identical axes of orientation. Each column contains complex cells. The properties of these complex cells in a column could most easily be explained by postulating that each complex cell receives direct connections from the simple cells in the column.

In the visual system, columns seem to serve as anatomical devices for bringing cells together to generate, by means of their interconnections, a new level of abstraction of visual information. For instance, the columns allow cortical cells to generate *linear* (geometric) receptive field properties from a geniculate input that responds best to small spots of light.

The discovery of columns in the various sensory systems is perhaps the most important single advance in cortical physiology in the past several decades and has raised new questions that have led to a family of new discoveries. For example, given that cells with the same axis of orientation tend to be grouped into columns, how are columns of cells with *different* axes of orientation organized in relation to one another? Are they randomly organized or is there some order to their organization? Detailed mapping of sets of adjacent columns by Hubel and Wiesel, using tangential penetrations with microelectrodes, has revealed a very precise organization with an orderly shift in axis of orientation from one column to the next. Every 30–100 μm, the electrode encounters a new column and a shift in axis of orientation of about 10° (Figure 29–10). These systematic shifts are occasionally interrupted by peg-shaped regions of cortex that have been described by Margaret Livingstone and Hubel. These regions receive direct connections from the lateral geniculate nucleus. The cells in the cortical pegs, as we shall see later, are concerned not with orientation but with color.

In addition to columns devoted to axis of orientation and pegs related to color, there are also independent alternating columns devoted to the left or the right eye, as we saw in Chapter 28. These columns are concerned with ocular dominance properties that are important for

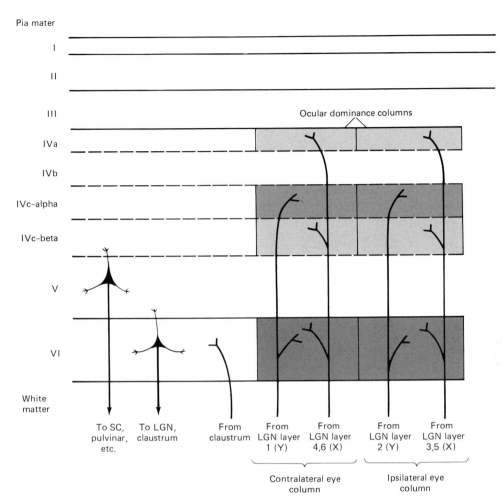

Pia mater

I

II

III

IVa

IVb

IVc-alpha

IVc-beta

V

VI

White matter

Ocular dominance columns

To SC, pulvinar, etc.

To LGN, claustrum

From claustrum

From LGN layer 1 (Y)

From LGN layer 4,6 (X)

From LGN layer 2 (Y)

From LGN layer 3,5 (X)

Contralateral eye column

Ipsilateral eye column

29–11 The primary visual cortex receives connections from the various layers of the lateral geniculate nucleus and from the claustrum (a thin nucleus that lies just below the insular cortex). Projections from the magnocellular layers of the lateral geniculate nucleus terminate in layer IVc-α (and to a lesser degree in VI), whereas those from the parvocellular layers terminate in layer IVc-β (and to a lesser degree in IVa and VI). Input representing one or the other eye is segregated into separate ocular dominance columns. Contralateral and ipsilateral eye columns (vertically oriented columns 500 μm wide and several millimeters long) lie next to one another in a regular array. The cortex, in turn, sends an important projection back to the lateral geniculate nucleus (**LGN**), as well as to the claustrum, superior colliculus (**SC**), pulvinar, and other structures. Projections to the superior colliculus and pulvinar derive from the pyramidal cells of layer V. Those to the lateral geniculate nucleus and claustrum derive from the pyramidal cells of layer VI. (From Berne and Levy, 1983.)

binocular interaction and depth perception. This set of columns again is formed in a very orderly manner in the primary visual cortex. The axons of the cells from the lateral geniculate nucleus terminate on small stellate cells in layer IVc of the primary visual cortex in a systematic way: fibers from layers 1, 4, 6 of the lateral geniculate nucleus alternate with fibers from layers 2, 3, 5 to terminate on adjacent patches of stellate cells (see Chapter 28). These alternate patches represent the contralateral eye (1, 4, 6) and the ipsilateral eye (2, 3, 5). The relationship between the orientation columns, the independent ocular dominance columns, and the cortical pegs is illustrated in Figure 29–10. (There are probably also columns for other aspects of vision.)

Hubel and Wiesel have used the term *hypercolumn* to refer to the whole set of columns for analyzing lines of all orientations from a particular region in space via *both* eyes. Each small region of the primary visual cortex, about 1 mm² at the surface, contains a complete sequence of ocular dominance columns and orientation columns, suggesting that the cortex has the repetitive structure of a crystal. All the neural action necessary for analyzing each small region of the visual field is repeated regularly and precisely over the surface of the primary visual cortex. Each hypercolumn is an elementary computational unit that represents the machinery necessary for analyzing a given area of the visual field. This regularity illustrates nicely the *modular organization characteristic of the cerebral cortex*. Its repeating organization ensures that all orientations (and other visual operations) occur at least once for each module and, therefore, once for each area of the visual field.

Besides being divided into columns, the cortex is also divided into six layers (Figures 29–10 and 29–11). Therefore, the cells of each layer in a column have slightly different inputs and slightly different outputs. The organization of the output connections from the primary visual cortex is similar to that of the somatic sensory cortex. The cells in layers II and III make association connections and project to higher visual cortical regions. Neurons in layers II and III also make callosal connections, but only from regions of the primary visual cortex that subserve vision along the midline of the visual field. Therefore, hypercolumns are arranged with input and output connections appropriate for their function as elementary computational devices. They receive a varied input, transform it, and project it to a number of different regions of the brain. Modular organization is present in all sensory cortices and may represent a simple method for developmental processes to construct a sensory representation.

It is apparent from these studies that the primary visual cortex has two major functions: (1) It decomposes the visual world (for each part of the visual field) into short line segments of various orientations, an early step in the process thought to be necessary for discrimination of form and movement. (2) It combines the input from the two eyes, a step in a sequence of transformations necessary for depth perception.

Simple and Complex Cells May Contribute to Positional Invariance in Perception

The elementary modules of the primary visual cortex have both simple and complex cells. What is their function? Hubel and Wiesel suggest that the interaction between simple and complex cells may be important for the perception of form no matter where the form falls on the retina. Consider an object with vertical edges that is located in front of you. The vertical edge (or the line) will excite a population of simple cells and a population of complex ones, each with a vertical axis of orientation. A slight saccadic movement of your eye or a movement of the object will call into play a new population of simple cells because these cells are very sensitive to the exact position of the line in the receptive field. However, for a small movement, the stimulus will still excite the original population of complex cells because these cells have larger receptive fields without clearly delineated regions and are responsive to movement within the receptive field. By generalizing orientation over a range of positions, the complex cells provide an elementary example of a psychophysical mechanism for *positional invariance*, the ability to recognize the same feature anywhere in the visual field. Moreover, as a population, both simple and complex cells in area 17 receive contributions from the X and Y pathways. Cells receiving input from the Y pathway seem to be concerned with the gross outlines and attentional aspects of the stimulus. These cells could contribute to the initial stages of what the theoretical biologist David Marr called the *primal sketch*, the initial visual approximation of gross stimulus shape and contour. In contrast, the subcategory of simple and com-

plex cells that receives input primarily from the X pathway might be concerned with the initial fine-grain analysis of detail and pattern.

Cells in the Higher Order Visual Cortices Elaborate the Visual Message Further

A great deal is known about the response properties of cells in area 17, but much less is known about the higher order visual cortices, the six visual representations that are present in area 18 and beyond. These areas receive input from area 17 and process the information further. The stimulus requirements for exciting cells in area 18 are much more complex than those for exciting cells in area 17. In the simplest cases, cells have properties that are classified as *hypercomplex* (Figure 29–12). (These properties are seen in simple and complex cells in area 17, but they seem to be more prevalent in cells of area 18.) Among cells with hypercomplex properties, a hierarchy can be discerned, with lower order and higher order cells. Some cells with hypercomplex properties respond well to a bar of light in the excitatory part of the receptive field as long as it is *stopped;* that is, it does not extend beyond the excitatory receptive field in *one specific* direction (Figure 29–12A). Hubel and Wiesel have suggested that these hypercomplex cells receive the convergent input from two complex cells with similar properties, one being excitatory, the other inhibitory (Figure 29–12A, 2). Together, they would create a receptive field consisting of adjacent excitatory and inhibitory halves.

Other cells with hypercomplex properties respond best to a bar of light that passes over the middle of the receptive field but does not extend to *either* of the two lateral inhibitory areas (Figure 29–12B). A narrow bar of light causes the higher order hypercomplex cell to discharge, but the cell decreases its firing in response to a bar of light that is wider than the receptive field because the bar encroaches on the inhibitory areas. Thus, whereas some hypercomplex cells deal with edges that stop in one direction (they can, for example, signal a corner moving in one direction over part of the retina), other hypercomplex cells are even more specific. They signal that there is a small bar moving over a part of the retina that is not wider than an amount specified by the inhibitory component of the receptive fields. Hubel and Wiesel have suggested that these cells with hypercomplex properties might receive convergence from three cells with a complex receptive field having the same axis of orientation (a central excitatory one and two lateral inhibitory ones), and whose fields are lined up one below the other (Figure 29–12B, 2). Helen Sherk and Simon Levay have now shown that some of the inhibitory connections necessary for end-stopping come not from complex cortical cells but from cells in the *claustrum*.

Thus, although this hierarchical arrangement is thought to be correct in principle, it is almost certainly not correct in its detail. For example, even some simple cells have receptive fields with hypercomplex properties, and their excitation is restricted (stopped) either unilat-

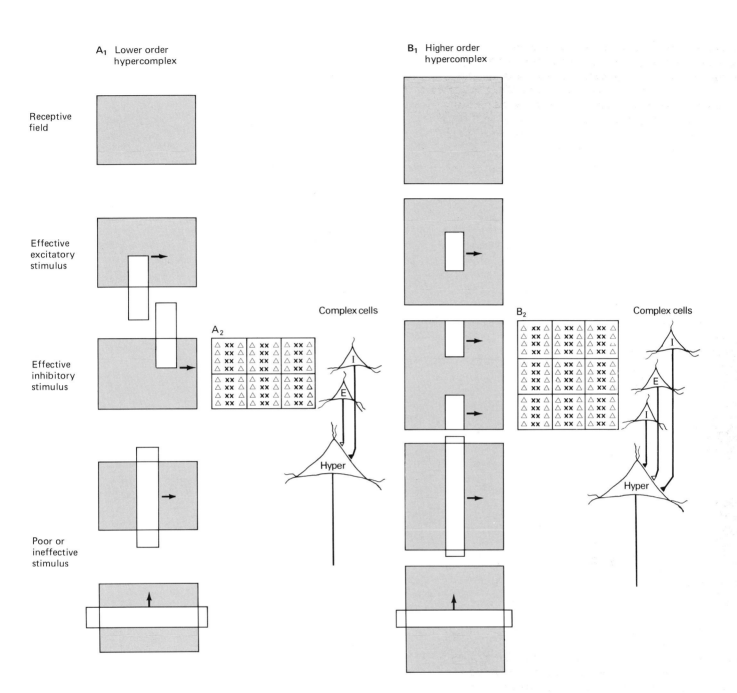

A₁ Lower order hypercomplex

B₁ Higher order hypercomplex

Receptive field

Effective excitatory stimulus

Effective inhibitory stimulus

Poor or ineffective stimulus

Complex cells

A₂

B₂

Complex cells

29–12 The receptive fields of cells in Brodmann's area 18 of the higher order visual cortex often have hypercomplex properties. **A.** A single end-stopped (lower order) cell. **1:** The stimulus excites only if it remains restricted to the lower half of the receptive field. If the stimulus extends into the upper half of the receptive field, it can become inhibitory. In contrast, the stimulus can extend below the lower half without altering the cell's response properties. **2:** Hubel and Wiesel's suggestion of one way for generating such a cell with hypercomplex properties. According to this scheme, two complex cells that have similar receptive field properties (**x,** excitatory; Δ, inhibitory) and axes of orientation, but with their fields lined up one below the other, converge on a common lower order hypercomplex cell. One complex cell excites (**E**) the hypercomplex cell; the other complex cell inhibits (**I**) it. **(B).** Double-stopped (higher order) hypercomplex cell. **1:** In this cell, the stimulus is effective in exciting the cell only if it is restricted to the middle region of the receptive field. If the stimulus extends either into the upper or lower regions of the field it becomes inhibitory. **2:** Hubel and Wiesel's scheme for generating the receptive field of the cell. Three complex cells with similar receptive field properties, and with their fields lined up one below the other, converge on a common higher order complex cell. Two of the complex cells are inhibitory; the central one is excitatory. Some of the inhibitory connections responsible for end-stopping come from neurons located in the claustrum. The **white area** is the light stimulus. The **arrow** indicates direction of movement. The various schemes outlined here and in Figures 29–8 and 29–9 are by no means unique to the processing of form and movement in the visual system. They represent the simplest way by which direct interconnections between cells could generate higher order properties. (Adapted from Hubel and Wiesel, 1965.)

380

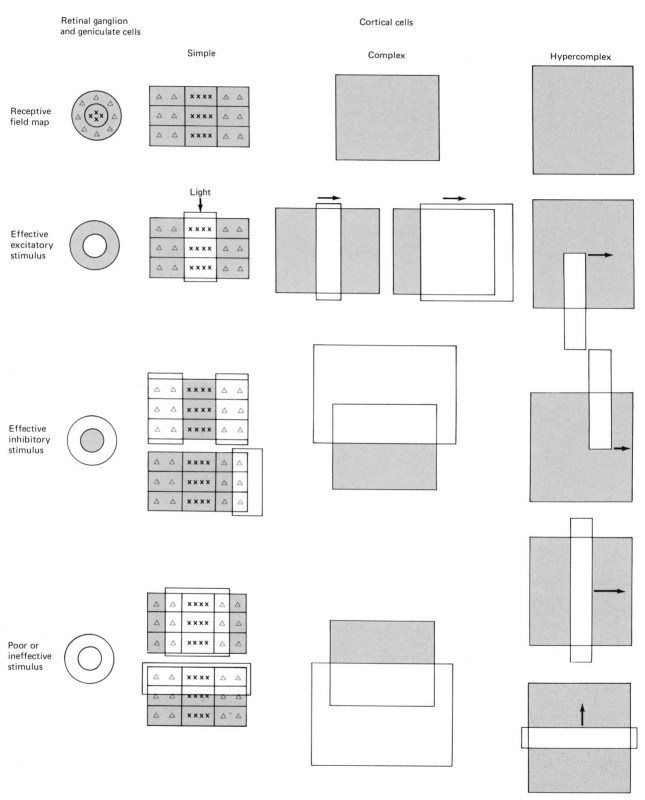

29–13 The receptive field properties of neurons in the retina and lateral geniculate nucleus and those in the primary visual cortex contribute to a hierarchy of visual abstraction. Retinal ganglion and lateral geniculate cells respond mainly to brightness contrast; simple and complex cortical cells respond to shapes, lines, edges, and boundaries. **X,** excitatory zone; △, inhibitory zone; **white area,** light stimulus. **Arrows** indicate direction of movement. (Adapted from Hubel and Wiesel, 1962; Kuffler, Nicholls, and Martin, 1984.)

erally or bilaterally. In addition, not all cells with complex receptive fields receive their input from simple cortical cells; some complex cells can receive their input directly from the concentric receptive field cells in layer IVc. Finally, we have considered only two representative examples here. Within each category of cells (particularly among the hypercomplex cells), there is a large variety of subtypes.

Some Feature Abstraction Could Be Accomplished by Progressive Convergence

On the basis of these data, Hubel and Wiesel have proposed that the cells in areas 17 and 18 are the early building blocks of perception and that they operate by a principle of increasing convergence. In its simplest form, this scheme suggests that each hypercomplex cell surveys the activity of a group of complex cells, which in turn surveys the activity of a group of simple cells. The simple cells survey the activity of a group of geniculate cells, which themselves survey the activity of a group of ganglion cells. The ganglion cells survey the activity of bipolar cells that survey a group of receptors. *At each level, each cell sees more than do the cells at the lower levels, and higher cells have a greater capacity for abstraction.*

Hubel and Wiesel postulated that, as a first approach, one can view the part of the visual system that they have analyzed as a hierarchy of relay points, each of which is involved in increasing visual abstraction (Figure 29–13). At the lowest level of the system, the level of the retinal ganglion and the geniculate cells, neurons respond primarily to brightness contrast. As we move up the hierarchy to the simple and complex cells of the cortex, cells begin to respond to line segments and boundaries. The hypercomplex cells respond to changes in boundaries. Thus, as we progress up the system, the stimulus requirements necessary to activate a cell become more precise. In the retina and the lateral geniculate nucleus, position is important. In simple cells, in addition to position, the axis of orientation is important. In complex cells, whose receptive fields are larger, the axis of orientation is still important, but these cells have a more generalized ability to detect orientation over a range of positions. In hypercomplex cells, edges and corners become important.

Visual Perception Also Involves Parallel Processing

There is an unresolved question that is now receiving increasing attention: How far can this hierarchy go? Is there a special supercomplex cell or cell group on top of the hierarchical processing for each familiar face? (Is there a grandmother cell?) Is there a group of cells that observe the hyper-hypercomplex cells and make us aware of the total pattern? If so, is there a still higher group in the hierarchy that looks at combinations of complex patterns as they enter our awareness?

There may indeed be other higher order cells combining the computational results of the inferotemporal, extrastriate, and striate cortices to produce even more elaborate abstractions. However, to discern the relatively simple features we have thus far considered has already required an enormous proportion of visual brain. It would appear curious to attribute progressively more important processing to a relatively small group of cells and expect of them this tremendously complex abstraction. An alternative to this supposition is that in addition to a hierarchical organization there is, from the very earliest stages in the retina onward, extensive parallel processing so that single cells do not by themselves serve to represent complete perceptions but only selected aspects of the percept. To represent a familiar face or a landscape may therefore require parallel as well as hierarchical processing, that is, activity in cells in different areas in the inferotemporal, posterior parietal, peristriate, and striate cortices, with the cells in each area coding for a particular aspect of the stimulus: shape, depth, movement, and color. At this level of visual recognition, cells in many parallel visual areas are likely to be involved, and their simultaneous activity may serve as the feature detector. The states of the parts taken separately may not represent the whole; rather, the relationship among them may be the important factor. An analogy can be found in the individual silver halide grains of a photograph: the grains themselves do not represent the photograph of a face, but the ensemble of grains does.

Although our understanding of how the visual system generates perception of form and movement is still very rudimentary, there is in fact considerable support for the idea that visual perception depends on a combination of hierarchical and parallel processing.

First, there is clinical evidence for parallel processing. There are patients, for example, who have loss of color vision (achromatopsia) or loss of vision for motion because of localized damage to the cerebral cortex, but who nonetheless have reasonably good vision for form and pattern. The realization that different aspects of visual perception may be separately localized dates to the turn of the century, when Sigmund Freud first introduced the term *agnosia* to describe the inability of certain patients to recognize visual objects not because of a sensory deficit but because of the inability to combine components of visual impressions into a complete pattern. The agnosias are thought to represent defects in higher visual function and can be remarkably specific (Table 29–1). For example, in one form of agnosia, the patient is unable to scan an image appropriately, but instead concentrates eye movement on distinctive features of the image such as the nose and mouth of a face. In addition to agnosia for color or visual motion, patients can have agnosia even for familiar inanimate objects. Most patients with agnosia for faces (*prosopagnosia*) cannot recognize people whom they know well. In a famous case recently described by Oliver Sacks at the Albert Einstein College of Medicine, a man mistook his wife for a hat! Patients with prosopagnosia may not even recognize their own

Table 29–1. The Visual Agnosias

Type	Deficit	Most probable lesion site
Agnosia for form and pattern		
Object agnosia	Naming, using, or recognizing real objects	Areas 18, 20, 21 on left and corpus callosum
Agnosia for drawings	Recognition of drawn objects	Areas 18, 20, 21 on right
Prosopagnosia	Recognition of faces	Areas 20, 21 on right
Agnosia for color		
Color agnosia	Association of colors with objects	Area 18 on right
Color anomia	Naming colors	Speech zones or connections from areas 18, 37
Achromatopsia	Distinguishing hues	Areas 18, 37
Agnosia for depth and movement		
Visual spatial agnosia	Stereoscopic vision, topographical concepts	Areas 18, 37 on right
Movement agnosia	Discerning movement of object	Bilateral medial-temporal area (junction of occipital and temporal cortex)

Source: Modified from Kolb and Whishaw, 1980.

faces in the mirror. This clinical evidence supports a parallel processing scheme.

Second, as we have seen, starting with the retina, visual information is carried to the lateral geniculate nucleus and then to area 17 of the cortex by two parallel systems, the X and Y pathways (and probably by others). Beyond area 17 both the X and the Y systems also project to higher visual regions. Semir Zeki at University College London has found that area 17 sends at least four separate projections to area 18 and one to the nearby medial temporal area (a portion of area 19). Each of these projections contains a topographically ordered map of the retina. The cells in each of the five regions have different functional properties—a finding that supports the idea that each region handles a different aspect of visual information. For example, region V4 in area 18 contains cells that are particularly concerned with color, and region V5 in the medial temporal area contains cells that code for the three-dimensional movement of an object, but not for the object's color or form; still other areas code for the binocular disparity necessary for depth perception.

On the basis of these findings, David Van Essen and John Maunsell at the California Institute of Technology and Mortimer Mischkin and Leslie Ungerleider at the National Institutes of Health have proposed that area 17 gives rise to at least two major pathways that project to different extrastriate areas and that process functionally distinct aspects of the visual stimulus (Figure 29–1). One pathway, thought to be the continuation of the X pathway, projects from area 17 to V2, then to V3, V3A, V4, and to the inferotemporal cortex. This pathway is primarily concerned with the perception of form and color (each of which is thought to be handled by a specific cortical subsystem). The other, thought to be the continuation of the Y pathway, projects from area 17 to V2 and to V3, then to V5, and to the posterior parietal cortex. This pathway is concerned with the perception of

movement and with the attentional aspects of the stimulus. These two pathways are interconnected at various levels, and the interconnections among them and other parallel pathways are thought to be capable of generating a large variety of response types suitable for analyzing in almost endless detail the intricacies of the visual world.

An Overall View

There are similarities and differences between the somatic sensory and visual systems. Both are modality specific, topographically organized, and have a modular organization consisting of columns. However, in the somatic sensory system the receptor at the periphery sets the sensitivity for the system—at least for certain dimensions of the stimulus. There is relatively little change in the receptive field until we go beyond the primary somatic sensory cortex. In contrast, in the visual system complex transformation of neural information occurs at all levels in the system, and progressively greater abstraction occurs as information ascends into the higher centers. Thus, whereas aspects of tactile perception literally reside in the hand of the perceiver, visual perception resides largely in the abstracting capabilities of the neurons of the brain.

Selected Readings

Freud, S. 1891. Zur Auffassung der Aphasien: Eine kritische Studie. E. Stengel (trans.), On Aphasia. A Critical Study. London: Imago, 1953.

Hubel, D. H., and Wiesel, T. N. 1977. Ferrier Lecture: Functional architecture of macaque monkey visual cortex. Proc. R. Soc. Lond. [Biol.] 198:1–59.

Hubel, D. H., and Wiesel, T. N. 1979. Brain mechanisms of vision. Sci. Am. 241(3):150–162.

Kuffler, S. W. 1952. Neurons in the retina: Organization, inhibition and excitation problems. Cold Spring Harbor Symp. Quant. Biol. 17:281–292.

Marr, D. 1982. Vision. San Francisco: Freeman.

Sacks, O. 1983. The man who mistook his wife for a hat. London Review of Books, May 19, pp. 3–5.

Schiller, P. H. 1982. Central connections of the retinal ON and OFF pathways. Nature 297:580–583.

Stone, J., Dreher, B., and Leventhal, A. 1979. Hierarchical and parallel mechanisms in the organization of visual cortex. Brain Res. Rev. 1:345–394.

Van Essen, D. C., and Maunsell, J. H. R. 1983. Hierarchical organization and functional streams in the visual cortex. Trends Neurosci. 6:370–375.

Zeki, S. M. 1976. The functional organization of projections from striate to prestriate visual cortex in the rhesus monkey. Cold Spring Harbor Symp. Quant. Biol. 40:591–600.

References

Berne, R. M., and Levy, M. N. (eds.). 1983. Physiology. St. Louis: Mosby.

Brown, R., and Herrnstein, R. J. 1975. Psychology. Boston: Little, Brown.

Cleland, B. G., Dubin, M. W., and Levick, W. R. 1971. Sustained and transient neurones in the cat's retina and lateral geniculate nucleus. J. Physiol. (Lond.) 217:473–496.

Cowey, A. 1981. Why are there so many visual areas? In F. O. Schmitt, F. G. Worden, G. Adelman, and S. G. Dennis (eds.), The Organization of the Cerebral Cortex. Cambridge, Mass.: MIT Press, pp. 395–413.

Enroth-Cugell, C., and Robson, J. G. 1966. The contrast sensitivity of retinal ganglion cells of the cat. J. Physiol. (Lond.) 187:517–552.

Ferster, D., and Lindstrom, S. 1983. An intracellular analysis of geniculo-cortical connectivity in Area 17 of the cat. J. Physiol. (Lond.) 324:181–215.

Gross, C. G. 1973. Visual functions of inferotemporal cortex. In R. Jung (ed.), Handbook of Sensory Physiology, Vol. 7, Pt. 3B. Berlin: Springer, pp. 451–482.

Hecaen, H., and Albert, M. L. 1978. Human Neuropsychology. New York: Wiley.

Hubel, D. H., and Wiesel, T. N. 1959. Receptive fields of single neurones in the cat's striate cortex. J. Physiol. (Lond.) 148:574–591.

Hubel, D. H., and Wiesel, T. N. 1962. Receptive fields, binocular interaction and functional architecture in the cat's visual cortex. J. Physiol. (Lond.) 160:106–154.

Hubel, D. H., and Wiesel, T. N. 1965. Binocular interaction in striate cortex of kittens reared with artificial squint. J. Neurophysiol. 28:1041–1059.

Kolb, B., and Whishaw, I. Q. 1980. Fundamentals of Human Neuropsychology. San Francisco: Freeman.

Kuffler, S. W., Nicholls, J. G., and Martin, A. R. 1984. From Neuron to Brain: A Cellular Approach to the Function of the Nervous System, 2nd ed. Sunderland, Mass.: Sinauer.

Livingstone, M. S., and Hubel, D. H. 1984. Anatomy and physiology of a color system in the primate visual cortex. J. Neurosci. 4:309–356.

Marshall, W. H., and Talbot, S. A. 1942. Recent evidence for neural mechanisms in vision leading to a general theory of sensory acuity. In H. Klüver (ed.), Visual Mechanisms. Lancaster, Pa.: Cattell, pp. 117–164.

Marshall, W. H., Woolsey, C. N., and Bard, P. 1941. Observations on cortical somatic sensory mechanisms of cat and monkey. J. Neurophysiol. 4:1–24.

Mountcastle, V. B. 1975. The view from within: Pathways to the study of perception. Johns Hopkins Med. J. 136:109–131.

Mountcastle, V. B. 1976. The world around us: Neural command functions for selective attention. Neurosci. Res. Program Bull. [Suppl.] 14.

Moushon, J. A., Adelson, E. H., Gizzi, M. S., and Newsome, W. T. 1985. The analysis of moving visual patterns. In C. Chagas, R. Gattass, and C. Gross (eds.), Pattern Recognition Mechanisms. Rome: Vatican Press (in press).

Schiller, P. H. 1983. Parallel channels in vision and visually guided eye movements. Arvo Abstracts.

Schiller, P. H., True, S. D., and Conway, J. L. 1980. Deficits in eye movements following frontal eye-field and superior colliculus ablations. J. Neurophysiol. 44:1175–1189.

Schmidt, R. F., and Thews, G. (eds.). 1983. Human Physiology. M. A. Biederman-Thorson (trans.). Berlin: Springer.

Sherk, H., and Levay, S. 1983. Contribution of the corticoclaustral loop to the receptive field properties in area 17 of the cat. J. Neurosci. 11:2121–2127.

Slaughter, M. M., and Miller, R. F. 1981. 2-Amino-4-phosphonobutyric acid: A new pharmacological tool for retina research. Science 211:182–185.

Talbot, S. A., and Marshall, W. H. 1941. Physiological studies on neural mechanisms of visual localization and discrimination. Am. J. Ophthalmol. 24:1255–1264.

Ungerleider, L. G., and Mishkin, M. 1982. Two cortical visual systems. In D. J. Ingle, M. A. Goodale, and R. J. W. Mansfield (eds.), Analysis of Visual Behavior. Cambridge, Mass.: MIT Press, pp. 549–586.

Van Essen, D. C. 1979. Visual areas of the mammalian cerebral cortex. Annu. Rev. Neurosci. 2:227–263.

Peter Gouras

Color Vision

30

Perception of color greatly enriches visual experience. Beyond its esthetic value, color vision is of great practical value for detecting patterns and objects that would be elusive in a world devoid of color. Although color depends on the physical parameters of light, its perception, like the perception of pattern, is a sophisticated abstraction by neurons within the brain of the physical parameters of the light reflected by objects. It is this abstraction that creates the experience of color and attributes it to the objects we see. Color perception has evolved from simple brightness perception (which we considered in Chapter 29) and serves to enhance contrast. It does so by discriminating between differences in the wavelength of the light reflected from an object and that of the light reflected from its background in an environment where gradients of light energy are often small.

Color vision *does not* simply detect the wavelength composition of light reflected from an object's surface; rather, it analyzes an object in relation to its background. This is why color is not experienced when the eye is bathed in a uniform field of color devoid of any pattern. The best example of this is "graying out," a temporary but total absence of vision experienced by pilots in cockpits under a cloudless, blue sky. A more common and persuasive example of graying out is that a point source of white light—a source of light with a particular balance of all wavelengths—can appear almost any color. Furthermore, totally different wavelength combinations can produce identical colors (a mixture of red and green can match a spectrally different yellow), and different colors can sometimes be produced by identical combinations of wavelengths. Against the proper background, a white object can appear to be pink, pale green, or yet another color. The colors we see in objects are

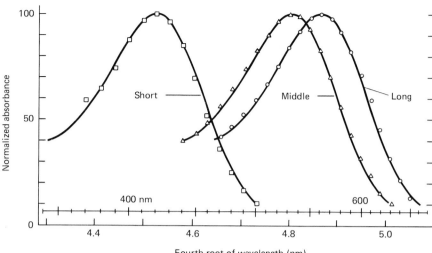

30–1 The mean absorbance spectra of the outer segments of the three human cone photoreceptor mechanisms, designated short-, middle-, and long-wavelength sensitive. The short wavelength mechanism contributes to the perception of blue, the middle to green, and the long to red. The abscissa is an empirically derived scale that makes the shapes but not the positions of the three absorbance spectra identical. (Adapted from Dartnall, Bowmaker, and Mollon, 1983.)

those that best set them off from their background under the existing lighting conditions.

In this chapter we shall first consider the photoreceptor systems required for color discrimination and then review the spectrophotometric and psychophysical data indicating that we use three different cone systems to see all colors. We shall then consider the physiological mechanisms involved in color vision and the diseases that produce color blindness.

Cones Have Three Different Pigments

The human eye is sensitive to wavelengths of light that range from 400 to 700 nm. Throughout this range, the colors change gradually from blue, through green, to red. At the beginning of the nineteenth century, Thomas Young, an English physician, proposed a three-variable, or *trichromatic theory of color vision* based upon the action of three different retinal receptors. He argued that there are three classes of light-absorbing responding elements with overlapping absorption spectra and that excitation of each of them is transmitted separately to the brain. In the brain they are combined to generate the variety of colors that we encounter in the world. Young's simple but sophisticated hypothesis received independent support 50 years later when James Clerk Maxwell, the British physicist (then in his twenties), and Hermann von Helmholtz, the German physiologist, independently demonstrated that all the colors we see can be completely matched by mixtures of three suitably chosen spectral lights. A wide assortment of three such lights can be used.

This hypothesis of color vision was confirmed in 1964 when Edward MacNichol and his colleagues at Johns Hopkins University and George Wald at Harvard University measured directly the absorption spectrum of visual pigments of single cones in humans, the first stage in color vision. They found that individual cones contain only one of three pigments: (1) a pigment primarily sensitive to short wavelengths (S) in the visible spectrum, which makes a strong contribution to the perception of

blue; (2) a pigment for middle wavelengths (M), which makes a strong contribution to the perception of green; or (3) a pigment for longer wavelengths (L), which makes a strong contribution to the perception of red. Recent measurements show that the peak absorbances of these pigments (in nm) are 420 for S, 531 for M, and 558 for L (Figure 30–1).

Similar results were obtained from psychophysical experiments that measured the spectral properties of these three mechanisms by using the subject's response to visual stimuli, the final stage of color vision (Figure 30–2).

30–2 The spectral sensitivity curves of the three human cone mechanisms obtained by isolating each separately in subjects who lack one or more of them in their retinas, i.e., so-called color-deficient individuals. The different vertical positions of the three curves reflect the overall impact of these photoreceptors on visual functions and to a great extent their relative numbers in the normal retina. The ordinate scale is logarithmic rather than linear because of the relatively great range of vision. (Adapted from Smith and Pokorny, 1975.)

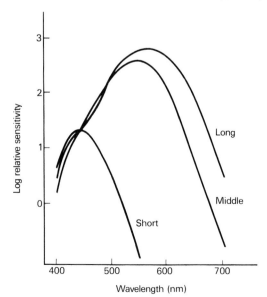

To obtain the best psychophysical data, subjects who had specific genetic defects in their photoreceptors were examined. As we shall see later, some people have only two cone pigments (dichromats), and others only one (monochromats). In patients with these genetic defects, the psychophysical measurement of the spectral sensitivities of the remaining mechanisms is greatly facilitated.

As Figures 30–1 and 30–2 illustrate, the short wavelength cone mechanism is located on the absorption spectrum at some distance from the other two mechanisms, which have their peak sensitivities near one another in the yellow region of the spectrum. This gives the short wavelength cones a greater latitude for spectral contrast. Chromatic aberration, however, blurs the optical image in this spectral region (see Appendix II). Consequently, the short-wavelength mechanism is not found in the central fovea, where resolution of fine detail is maximal (because of the fine receptive field sizes of the foveal cones). Thus, in the central fovea, color vision is *dichromatic*. Single photoreceptors are color blind. Color vision depends on the comparison of the outputs of different cones. As a result, color deteriorates when objects become so small as to stimulate only single cones. Color vision therefore is not designed to discriminate fine spatial detail but to detect relatively large objects against backgrounds that could make these objects invisible.

Good Color Discrimination Requires Three Photoreceptor Systems

Why do we need more than one cone pigment for color? With *one set of cones* we would detect objects only as more or less bright because we could detect an object only if it reflected more or less light energy than its background. A single set of cones could not distinguish between different wavelengths of light, even though it might be more sensitive to some wavelengths than to others. A system with only one set of cones is unable to distinguish changes in energy from changes in wavelength (Figure 30–3A). Objects are either more or less *bright*.

We can simulate a single-photoreceptor system by adapting to dim light and relying completely on rod vision, which is color blind. All the objects seen with rod vision have brightnesses different from their background but are achromatic (colorless) because we are using only a single set of photoreceptors. Many objects that reflect spectrally different wavelengths from their background but have identical brightnesses are invisible under these conditions. A full moon looks yellow only because its brightness is sufficient to excite cones.

Color vision requires two sets of photoreceptors. A stimulus that may be indistinguishable on the basis of energy for one set is usually distinguishable on the basis of energy for the other. A two-receptor system allows us to see *two* brightnesses for every object, corresponding to two distinct photopigment processes. The perception of color is achieved by comparing the two brightnesses. If the object reflects primarily light of a long wavelength, it favors a higher reading in the long-wavelength cone system, and the object appears yellow. If the object reflects primarily shorter wavelengths, it favors a higher reading in the short-wavelength system and is perceived as blue. If the object reflects long and short wavelengths equally, we perceive it as white if the level of excitation is strong, or black if the excitation is weak.

A two-receptor, or dichromatic, system may have been a first step in the evolution of color vision. Many spectral combinations between object and background can nevertheless be invisible to a dichromatic system. An object reflecting both ends of the spectrum in a midspectral background could be undetectable (Figure 30–3B). This object could produce the same output from both types of photoreceptors as does the background stimulus. It would therefore be invisible to both of these photoreceptors. Theoretically, there are infinite combinations of these possibilities. A three-receptor, or trichromatic system greatly reduces such ambiguities and creates new color sensations, such as red and green (Figure 30–3C). Although some birds may employ tetrachromacy, the evolutionary evidence suggests that any further augmentation of receptor systems yields diminishing returns.

Color Experience Is Composed of Impressions of Hue, Saturation, and Brightness

The use of three photoreceptors to detect objects is not equivalent to using them to see colors. The honeybee and other animals detect objects using three photoreceptor systems but may never see the colors of these objects if the input from these receptors is not mixed to allow for color contrast, the essential feature of color perception in higher animals. For example, a neuron designed to detect an object brighter (or darker) than the background could be excited by activity in any one of the three photoreceptor systems. Such a cell would be sensitive to the presence of an object in the external world and would share the benefits of a trichromatic detector system but might not contribute to color vision. A color detector must be able to distinguish how much each of the three cone mechanisms is activated by the object.

Added to its esthetic importance, color vision endows animals with great perceptual capabilities, and this presumably has great survival value. Think for a moment of a black and white version of a work by a colorist such as Turner, Monet, or Renoir; so many nuances of contrasting shapes are lost by an achromatic copy of the painting! This high degree of discrimination in color vision can actually be understood in quantitative terms. The subjective experience of color can be broken down into three semi-independent sensibilities: hue, saturation, and brightness. All color experience is composed of these three psychological impressions.

Hue has the strongest effect on color and is the major determinant of principal colors (red, yellow, green, and blue). Hue is what we ordinarily mean by color. This

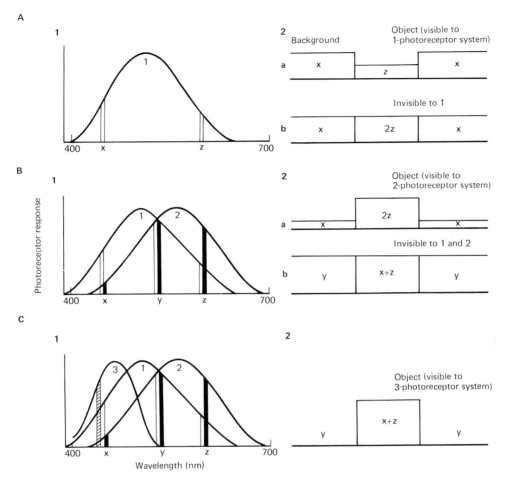

30–3 Discrimination of objects by a three-photoreceptor system is clearly superior to that by systems with only one or two photoreceptors. **1:** The spectral response function of each photoreceptor system, with wavelength on the **abscissa** (400 nm, violet, to 700 nm, deep red) and relative response on the **ordinate. 2:** Hypothetical spectral reflectances (color) of an object **(middle rectangle)** and the background **(flanking regions)** against which it can be seen (the color of the object is different from its background). In all cases the spectral characteristic of this reflected signal is shown by its position on the abscissa on the left.

A. Single-photoreceptor system. **1:** Object **z** affects photoreceptor 1 about one-half as much as the background **x. 2a:** Therefore, photoreceptor 1 will be stimulated about one-half as much by the object as by the background; consequently, object **z** will appear dark in a bright background. **2b:** If object **z** reflects sunlight about twice as much as the background, however, it will become totally invisible to photoreceptor 1 since the response will be about **z,** which is identical to the

response generated by background **x.** Even though this object **(2z)** is spectrally quite different from its background, it cannot be detected by a single-photoreceptor system under these particular conditions.

B. Two sets of photoreceptors, each with a different spectral response. **1:** Objects invisible to photoreceptor 1 are usually visible to photoreceptor 2. **2a:** An object **2z,** which is invisible to photoreceptor 1, is strongly visible to photoreceptor 2. **2b:** There is, however, a possibility that some unusual objects could be bispectrally reflectant, such as object **(x + z).** Such an object would stimulate both photoreceptors 1 and 2 exactly the same as background **y** and consequently be invisible to both photoreceptors. One can work this out by showing that **x + z = y** for both photoreceptors 1 and 2.

C. Trichromatic system. This system would be tougher to fool than the others, at least under natural light. Both **y** and **z** affect photoreceptors 1 and 2, but only **y** affects photoreceptor 3; therefore, object **(x + z)** will be a bright object in a dark background to photoreceptor 3.

impression is determined by the proportion in which the three cone mechanisms are activated by the object and its background. The brain must keep track of how much *each* of the three photoreceptor systems contributes to the detection of an object. Most of us have names for only a restricted number of hues, but actually about 200 varieties can be distinguished.

The second distinct quality of color is *saturation,* which reflects how much a hue has been diluted by grayness; this is determined by the degree to which all three cone mechanisms are stimulated in common by the object and by the background. At short and long wavelengths there are about 20 distinguishable steps of saturation for each hue. In the midspectral region (530–590 nm) there are only about 6 distinguishable steps of saturation.

The third quality of color, *brightness*, is a sensation shared with achromatic visual systems. It is due to the total effect on all three cone mechanisms of an object relative to its background. We shall see later that one of the three cone mechanisms (the so-called short-wavelength cone mechanism) makes little or no contribution to brightness. It is the brightness factor that turns orange into brown and gray into black or white. There are about 500 distinguishable steps of brightness for every hue and grade of saturation. In contrast to achromatic vision, with only 500 steps, color vision has more than 1 million gradations with which to detect the contours of shapes in the external world (500 for brightness × 200 for hue × 20 for saturation). It is no wonder that natural selection made use of color vision!

Color Vision Is Best Explained by Combining Trichromacy with Color Opponent Interactions

As we have seen, the trichromatic theory of color vision advanced by Young and Helmholtz attributes color perception to the activity of three primary cone mechanisms. According to this theory, the message generated in these cone mechanisms reaches the cortex in independent, parallel channels without significant convergence or mixing of common elements. At the cortex these three outputs are compared for color vision. This theory explains a large variety of data concerned with the mixing of colors. For example, the mixture of two (such as what we perceive as green and red) is seen as yellow and the

mixture of all three (what we perceive as blue, green, and red) is seen as white. The trichromacy theory has found striking support in the discovery of three cone pigments capable of responding best to those parts of the spectrum that contribute importantly to our perception of blue (S), green (M), and red (L).

However, trichromacy alone fails to explain a variety of color phenomena encountered in nature. In particular, it fails to explain why certain color combinations cancel one another, but others do not. For example, we can never perceive reddish green or bluish yellow colors even though we can readily perceive reddish blue (magenta), reddish yellow (orange), greenish yellow, or bluish green (cyan). Red and green lights can be mixed so that all traces of the original redness or greenness are lost and a pure yellow is seen; analogously, yellow and blue can be mixed to produce a pure white without any trace of the original blue or yellow. This perceptual cancellation of colors led the German physiologist Ewald Hering to propose the *opponent process theory*, whereby certain colors (opponent colors) are mutually inhibitory. According to this theory there are three primary color pairs, which are coupled in a mutually inhibitory opponent fashion: red–green, yellow–blue, and white–black. Hering postulated that these three color pairs are represented in the retina in three color opponent channels. One was thought to respond in one direction (excitation or inhibition) to red and in the opposite direction to green. When properly balanced with the precise mixture of red and green, this channel would produce no output. A second channel was thought to oppose the sensations of yellow and blue; a third to oppose white with black (Figure 30–4A).

30–4 Color opponency and color contrast are two unique forms of interactions between color sensations in human vision. **A.** The concept of color opponency is based on the Hering theory of color vision. Redness and greenness, yellowness and blueness, and whiteness and blackness antagonize each other in contributing to color *within* the confines of an object. The underlying physiological explanation is that L cones antagonize M cones and vice versa, and S cones antagonize M and L cones and vice versa within the receptive fields of neurons. Such opponent cone interactions are seen in single neurons in the retina and the lateral geniculate nucleus of primates. **B.** The concept of simultaneous color contrast led

to E. H. Land's retinex theory of color vision. Here redness and greenness act synergistically *across* the contours of an object within its background; similarly yellowness and blueness and whiteness and blackness enhance each other. The underlying physiological explanation comes from the existence of so-called double-opponent cells, in which L cones on one side of an edge of contrast enhance M cone activity on the other side of the edge; a similar phenomenon occurs for S versus L and M cone activity for yellow–blue contrasts. In contrast to single opponent cone interactions, double-opponent neurons have been found only in the visual cortex.

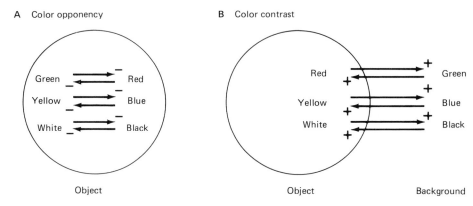

The extensive studies of Dorothea Jameson and Leo Hurvich at the University of Pennsylvania have supported the idea (first advanced in 1905 by the German physiologist Johannes von Kries, a student of Helmholtz) that the opponent process and the trichromatic theories need to be combined to explain fully the perception of color in everyday life (and that, in fact, there is no conflict between the theories!). Jameson and Hurvich therefore proposed that color vision must occur in stages. At the first stage, at the level of the cones, color vision is trichromatic (as indeed the findings of three spectrally different cones now show so clearly). At subsequent stages, the signals are transformed into opponent color form. This formulation predicts that the output of the long- and medium-wavelength cone systems should interact in the visual system to form a green–red opponent processing system, and the short- and long-wavelength cone systems should interact to form the blue–yellow opponent system.

Support for this theory was obtained when the Scandinavian physiologist Gunnar Svaetichin recorded from horizontal cells in the fish retina and found that they were hyperpolarized by one cone mechanism and depolarized by another cone mechanism. Svaetichin's discovery provided the first evidence that "opponent" interactions between cone mechanisms occur in the visual system. Subsequent studies have shown that cone opponent interactions are common in all animals with color vision. Later studies by Russell De Valois of the University of California at Berkeley and David Hubel and Torsten Wiesel of Harvard University demonstrated that similar cells could occur both in the retina and lateral geniculate nucleus of primates. Many cells in the primate retina and the lateral geniculate nucleus come in pairs: some show antagonism between the long-wavelength and middle-wavelength cone mechanisms, and others show antagonism between short-wavelength cones and the other two cone mechanisms. Thus cells in the first class are hyperpolarized (or depolarized) by long wavelengths (red light), depolarized (or hyperpolarized) by middle wavelengths (green light), and give no response to yellow (red plus green) light. The second class is hyperpolarized (or depolarized) by yellow light and depolarized (or hyperpolarized) by blue light. These neurons resemble Hering's red–green and yellow–blue color opponent channels. As we shall see below, however, the information that each retinal or lateral geniculate cell transmits about color is ambiguous (see Figure 30–5). Although the cells of the retina and lateral geniculate initiate the color coding process, cells specifically sensitive to color (hue) exist only in visual cortex where the information from several pairs of cone opponent geniculate cells are sampled simultaneously.

The color opponent theory explains why certain colors *within* the boundaries of a perceived object can cancel one another (Figure 30–4A). An additional factor must be incorporated into this model to explain simultaneous color contrast, a fact that Hering was aware of. In the phenomenon of simultaneous color contrast, what are opposing cone mechanisms within the boundaries of objects now become facilitatory to each other across boundaries of objects (Figure 30–4B). A gray object seen in a background of red has a green tinge; in a background of green, it has a red tinge.

Finally a theory of color needs to explain *color constancy*. A lemon, for example, remains yellow whether viewed in sunlight (which is whitish), or with the light from a tungsten filament bulb (which is reddish), or by fluorescent (bluish) light. Color constancy is not foolproof, however, as anyone can testify who has bought paint or a dress in artificial light and later is startled to see it in daylight as a different shade of color.

Edwin Land, the inventor of the Polaroid camera and the founder of the Polaroid Corporation, has developed a model that sees the same color in objects as we do despite enormous changes in the spectral composition of the light illuminating a scene. He has called this model the *retinex* (retina + cortex) model.

Land also demonstrated by ingenious psychophysical experiments how important an object's background can be in determining its color. He showed that objects reflecting an identical composition of wavelengths from their surfaces can have totally different colors if their backgrounds are different. Land's model predicts the colors of objects by comparing brightness contrasts across the contours of objects in a scene and does so independently for each of the three cone mechanisms. Each brightness value for a cone mechanism, for each contour, is normalized to the brightest object in the scene. By comparing these three brightness values of an object for each of the three cone mechanisms, the object's color can be accurately predicted. Thus, before obtaining the information necessary to determine the colors of objects in the scene, the retinex model requires that the visual system serially scan every contour in a visual scene separately for each cone mechanism.

The psychophysical experiments illustrating color contrast and color constancy provide an important conceptual framework for the analysis of the neural mechanisms of color vision. To be informative, analysis on the level of single nerve cells must address two of the central questions in the study of color vision: (1) Do the higher stages of the visual system encode color in an opponent process as predicted by modern psychophysical theories of vision? (2) How does the visual system account for color contrast and constancy?

Color Is Coded by Single-Opponent and Double-Opponent Cells

As we saw in Chapter 29, the cells in the retina, the lateral geniculate nucleus, and the visual cortex of primates that code for pattern use a spatially opponent mechanism that is sensitive to brightness contrast. Two sets of cones (or two sets of rods) are connected to a single cell in a spatially separate concentric center–surround fashion. One family of cones together subserves the center of the cell's receptive field and another set of cones subserves

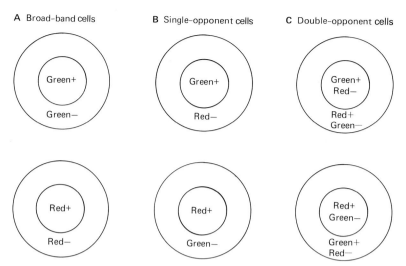

30–5 Two of the three cone mechanisms known to exist in the human retina can be combined to form different types of visual neurons. **A.** The broad-band system responds similarly to *all* parts of the visible spectrum although it is somewhat more sensitive to one part of the spectrum. These neurons are color blind and transmit information only about brightness contrast. The reason for this is that they have the same cone mechanism in the center and the surround of their receptive field. Such cells, integrating signals from only *one* cone mechanism, have never been found in the primate but are common in the cat visual system. **B.** The single-opponent neurons are common in the primate retina and lateral geniculate nucleus. These cells transmit information about *both* brightness and color (see Figure 30–6). **C.** The double-opponent neurons are sensitive only to color (hue) contrast. They are found in primate primary visual cortex and seem to be formed from single-opponent geniculate neurons (see Figure 30–7).

the surround (both sets of cones respond identically to all wavelengths). This system is designed to detect contrast between light and dark. A spot of light on the center excites the cell. Simultaneous stimulation of the center and surround leads to mutual antagonisms. Diffuse light is a poor stimulus (see Figure 29–5). This system, called a *broad-band system*, does not contribute to the perception of color.

Early studies of primates revealed that the responses of many cells to spectral lights and to white light differ, regardless of the effective energy of the stimulus. These cells show two sets of opponent mechanisms. In one class of cells a *single-opponent* receptive field mechanism is used to detect *brightness* differences across contours (Figure 30–3). In primates, the receptors converge on cells in the retina to give rise to single-opponent cells and all the subsequent color-sensitive cells in the retina and lateral geniculate nucleus are all of this variety. A second class of cells, found only in the cortex in primates, uses a *double-opponent* mechanism to abstract the basic sensations that we associate with color (hue) by comparing the activities of each of these receptor mechanisms across contours. The double-opponent cells are thought to be formed by the convergence of single-opponent color cells. We shall consider each of these in turn.

Single-opponent cells typically have a small receptive field center mediated by one cone mechanism and a larger, concentrically organized surround mediated by a different cone mechanism (Figure 30–5). These cells transmit information about *both* brightness and color.

The color signal is present only when the stimuli are large enough to stimulate *both* the center and surround of the cell's receptive field. When this occurs the cell no longer responds to the effective energy in the stimulus, but becomes spectrally selective, responding to the *difference* between the absorption spectrum of the center cone mechanism and the absorption spectrum of the surround cone mechanism. A long-wavelength cone on-center cell with a medium-wavelength cone surround is excited only by red and inhibited by green light; a medium-wavelength cone on-center cell with long-wavelength cone surround is excited by green and inhibited by red light (Figure 30–5). This resembles the red–green opponent channel of Hering. Other cells resemble the yellow–blue opponent channel of Hering. In the retina and the lateral geniculate nucleus, there are four types of red–green opponent cells: a red on-center cell with a green inhibitory surround; a green on-center cell with a red inhibitory surround; a red off-center cell with a green excitatory surround; and a green off-center cell with a red excitatory surround.

Single-opponent cells are ambiguous for color and brightness. It is impossible to know, for example, whether a strong excitatory response in a red on-center cell with a green inhibitory surround is due to a small bright spot or a large red spot (Figure 30–6). To distinguish this, the visual cortex probably decodes this message by tapping the parallel responses of other cells subserving the same areas of visual space. Double-opponent cells can do this, and they do so in a circuit that is highly selective for color contrast (Figure 30–6). One type of

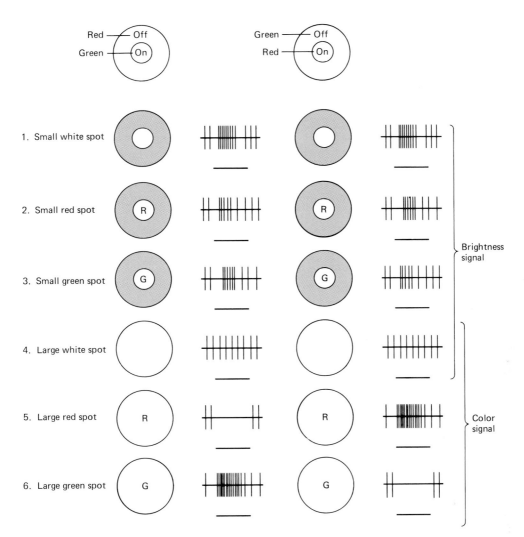

30–6 The receptive fields of single-opponent color- and brightness-sensitive cortical cells are concentrically organized with on-center and off-surround (see Figure 29–5). These two typical cells in primate (monkey) retina differ from broad band cells in having the center and surround responses mediated by *different* cone mechanisms. The cell on the left has the center mechanism mediated by the green-sensitive cones and the surround by the red-sensitive cones; the cell on the right shows the reverse arrangement: red center, green surround. The red and green sensitive cones respond to *all* spectral lights as well as to white light. The response of these cells to white light is similar to that of the retinal ganglion cells that we considered in Chapter 29. They are excited by small centered white spots and are unresponsive to large white spots. Small centered red or green spots act like weaker white spots. Larger colored spots show the color selectivity of these cells. A large red spot inhibits the cell on the left and excites the cell on the right; a large green spot does exactly the opposite. The light stimulus is indicated by the **bar** below each oscilloscope trace. **Outer circles** indicate receptive fields of the geniculate fibers. **Inner circles** distinguish center from surround in the concentric cell's field.

double-opponent cell is excited by the long-wavelength cone mechanism and inhibited by the medium-wavelength cone mechanism in its receptive field center, and excited by the medium-wavelength cone mechanism and inhibited by the long-wavelength cone mechanism in the surround. This receptive field combines color opponency in the center and color contrast in the surround. Such a cell responds best to a red spot on a green surround. Other cells respond best to a green spot in a red surround or a blue spot in a yellow surround.

The neural circuit that is used to generate double-opponent cortical cells from single-opponent lateral geniculate cells is not known, but a reasonable possibility is shown in Figure 30–7B. The uniqueness of this circuit is the arrangement of excitatory and inhibitory inputs onto the cortical cell from the appropriate lateral geniculate cells and the assumption that the center of cortical double-opponent cells equals the size of both the center and surround of single-opponent geniculate cells.

The existence of such double-opponent cells was first discovered by Nigel Daw in studies of the retinal ganglion cells in goldfish. These cells were then found in primates by Charles Michael at Yale University and by Peter Gouras and Jurgen Kruger at Columbia University.

Double-opponent cells provide an explanation for both simultaneous color contrast and color constancy. For ex-

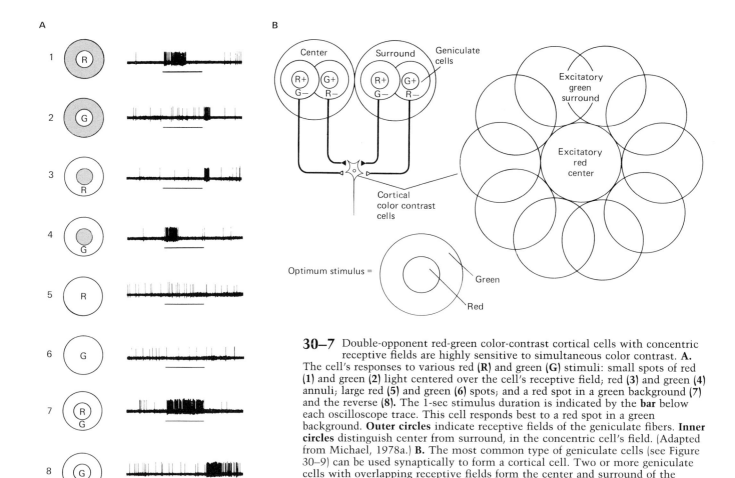

30–7 Double-opponent red-green color-contrast cortical cells with concentric receptive fields are highly sensitive to simultaneous color contrast. **A.** The cell's responses to various red (**R**) and green (**G**) stimuli: small spots of red (**1**) and green (**2**) light centered over the cell's receptive field; red (**3**) and green (**4**) annuli; large red (**5**) and green (**6**) spots; and a red spot in a green background (**7**) and the reverse (**8**). The 1-sec stimulus duration is indicated by the **bar** below each oscilloscope trace. This cell responds best to a red spot in a green background. **Outer circles** indicate receptive fields of the geniculate fibers. **Inner circles** distinguish center from surround, in the concentric cell's field. (Adapted from Michael, 1978a.) **B.** The most common type of geniculate cells (see Figure 30–9) can be used synaptically to form a cortical cell. Two or more geniculate cells with overlapping receptive fields form the center and surround of the concentrically organized color contrast cortical cell.

ample, putting a green light in the surround of a double-opponent cell with a red center and green surround induces a centerlike (redness) response. Increasing only the long-wavelength component in the ambient illumination of an entire visual scene, such as occurs during a shift from fluorescent to incandescent illumination, will have little effect on a double-opponent cell since the increased long-wavelength illumination of the center will be cancelled by the same increase in long wavelengths illuminating the surround.

Many Double-Opponent Cells Have Receptive Fields That Are Not Oriented

Recently, David Hubel and Margaret Livingstone have explored area 17 and have found that double-opponent cells are heavily concentrated in peglike structures (called *blobs*) that have a function similar to cortical columns. Cortical pegs consist of cells that have circular receptive fields with no specific axis of orientation. The pegs are interspersed between columns of well-tuned orientation-selective cells. The cortical pegs (Figure 30–8) extend through the upper layers (II and III) of area 17 as well as through the lower layers (IVb, V, and VI). The

pegs in the lower layers are in register with those of the upper layers; both are centered along ocular dominance columns to which their long axis is parallel. These peg regions receive a direct input from the lateral geniculate nucleus. Cells within these peg regions project directly out of area 17 to stripelike regions in area 18.

Livingstone and Hubel believe that the cells in the cortical pegs represent a separate system for color—a system that is independent of and parallel with the columnar system of orientation-sensitive cells that is concerned with contours, forms, and movements. In support of this idea, the cortical pegs in area 17 have been found to receive a separate input from the lateral geniculate nucleus and in turn to project to special regions in area 18 called V2, which in turn project to an area called V4, which Semir Zeki, at University College London, has shown is particularly concerned with color.

Double-opponent cells with orientation selectivity have also been found in striate and peristriate visual cortex where they contribute to cortical columns. These cells might be formed from double-opponent concentrically organized cells (Figure 30–9), just as concentrically organized brightness contrast cells can be used to form orientation-selective simple cells (Figure 29–9). Using

30–8 The modular organization of the primary visual cortex includes the cortical pegs (also called blobs) that contain concentrically organized double-opponent cells concerned with simultaneous color contrast. These pegs, located in the ipsilateral (**I**) or contralateral (**C**) ocular dominance columns, make up a system that is parallel to the vertical columns, whose cells are concerned with edges and contours. (Adapted from Livingstone and Hubel, 1984.)

30–9 Some simple cells in the primary visual cortex that have double-opponent red–green color contrast also exhibit orientation selectivity. **A.** The cell's responses to red (**R**) and green (**G**) bars with various orientations: red (**1**) or green (**2**) bars placed in the center of the cell's receptive field; red bars (**3**) or green bars (**4**) in the surround of the cell's receptive field; and a red central bar flanked by green surround bars (**5**) or the reverse (**6**). The 1-sec stimulus duration is indicated by the **bar** below each oscilloscope trace. This cell responds best to a red horizontal bar flanked by green bars. **B.** The cortical concentric color contrast cells (see Figure 30–5) can be used synaptically to form such a cortical cell. **Outer circles** indicate receptive fields of the geniculate fibers. **Inner circles** distinguish center from surround in the concentric cell's field. (Adapted from Michael, 1978b.)

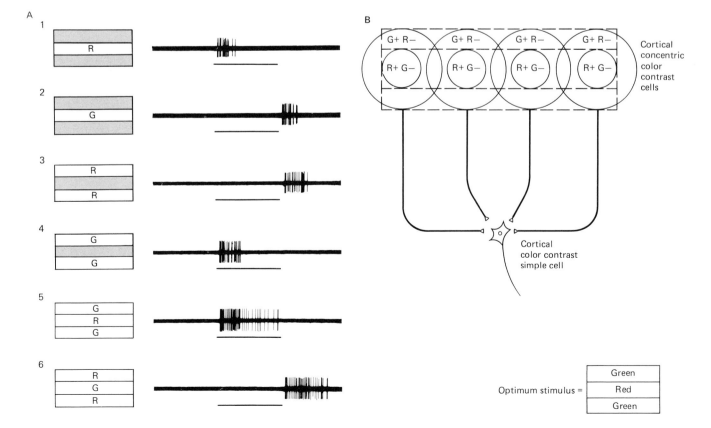

double-opponent simple cells, double-opponent complex and hypercomplex cells can be formed, allowing color (hue) contrast to have a similar repertoire of cortical neurons as that of brightness contrast.

Is Color Analyzed Independently of Form?

How are the three independent abstractions of color vision incorporated into a single image of an object that has a specific hue, saturation, and brightness? The answer to this question is not known, in part because it also requires prior understanding of how we perceive the shape of an object. One theory proposed by Zeki is that the color of an object is analyzed independently of form: the color of an object is analyzed in one set of areas in the brain, while its shape is analyzed in another. This bold idea receives support from three different sources. One is the finding that the entire visual field is mapped repeatedly in different areas of peristriate cortex. Furthermore, certain patients show a selective cortical defect for color vision but can still discern forms (presumably only by brightness contrast). Finally, the recent evidence of Livingstone and Hubel shows that some components of neural systems concerned with color are parallel to and independent from those concerned with form.

Others favor the view that form and color are abstracted in all subareas of the visual cortex. Understanding how color and form are processed will provide a much deeper insight into the operation of the cerebral cortex.

Color Blindness Can Be Caused by Genetic Defects in the Photoreceptor or by Retinal Disease

Although most of us agree on the colors we see because we are using similar neural circuits to see them, some people disagree and have been called color defective by the rest of us. This deficit can result from either inherited or acquired factors. Most forms of color blindness are listed in Table 30–1. In general, they involve either a loss of one or more of the three cone mechanisms or a change in the absorption spectrum of one or more of the photopigments within these cones. The adjectives *protan*, *deutan*, and *tritan* refer to the long-wavelength, medium-wavelength, and short-wavelength mechanisms, respectively. The suffixes *-opia* and *-omalous* refer, respectively, to a total loss or a moderate defect of each of these three mechanisms. Some people lose two (usually the L and M) or all three cone mechanisms and consequently have no color vision at all (achromats). It is noteworthy that the genes for the L and M cone mechanisms are on the X (sex-linked) chromosome, whereas that for the blue is autosomal. Jeremy Nathans and David Hogness of Stanford University have recently isolated each of these three genes, making it possible to obtain their nucleotide sequence and to derive the amino acid sequences of the protein of the three color pigments.

Acquired defects of color vision are more complex, but an old clinical rule, occasionally disobeyed, states that

Table 30–1. Classification and Incidence of Defects in Color Vision

Classification	Incidence (% males)
Congenital	
Trichromats (three cones present)	
Normal	91.2
Anomalous	
Protanomaly (L-cone pigment abnormal)	1.3
Deuteranomaly (M-cone pigment abnormal)	5.0
Tritanomaly (S-cone pigment abnormal)	0.001
Dichromats (two cones present)	
Protanopia (L-cone absent)	1.3
Deuteranopia (M-cone absent)	1.2
Tritanopia (S-cone absent)	0.001
Monochromats (achromats)	
Typical (all cones absent)	0.00001
Atypical (two cones absent)	0.000001
Acquired	
Tritanopia: outer retinal layer disease	
Protan-deutan defects: inner retinal layer disease	

diseases of the outer retinal layers tend to produce tritanopia, whereas diseases of the inner layers and optic nerve produce protan-deutan defects. The protan-deutan defects are presumably associated with disease of the inner layer because of the great number of axons that subserve the L and M cones, many of which are very fine and are likely to be affected by any disease state of the inner layer.

Although color vision involves larger numbers of extraretinal than retinal cells, most of the defects, especially the genetic ones, involve only photoreceptors. This is undoubtedly due to the fact that the genes that code for photoreceptors are more dedicated to color vision than are those that code for the neural circuitry that processes the information provided by these photoreceptors. The genes involved in this neural circuitry must code for mechanisms common to much of the brain, and consequently mutations in them have a greater chance of being lethal. Most of the genetic information that codes for color vision involves neural mechanisms common to all of the nervous system.

An Overall View

Our consideration of color vision shows how subsets of neural circuits can abstract different aspects of information from the spatiotemporal distribution of light energy in the external world. The only way in which we can see anything is by brightness contrast (effective light energy) and by spectral contrast (wavelength) formed by an object relative to its background. Brightness contrast is abstracted by one subset of neurons, spectral contrast by another subset. The commitment to one or the other form of contrast detection does not appear to occur until the visual cortex, at least in primates. At earlier levels the same subset of neurons transmits both forms of information. It is impossible to tell either the color or the brightness of an object within the receptive field of a retinal or geniculate neuron by detecting its discharges; the message is contained in the ensemble of neurons detecting that object. In the visual cortex the discharges of a single neuron indicate the color contrast (hue) of an object but not its brightness; another neuron abstracts its brightness. Again, the message for both brightness and color is contained in the ensemble of neurons, but now brightness and color can vary independently of each other. By having enormous numbers of neurons at its disposal, the cerebral cortex allows different aspects of the retinal image to be processed by independent subsets of neurons offering a greater range of visual impressions.

Selected Readings

Boynton, R. M. 1979. Human Color Vision. New York: Holt, Rinehart and Winston.

Daw, N. W. 1984. The psychology and physiology of colour vision. Trends Neurosci. 7(9):330–335.

Gouras, P. 1984. Color vision. In N. N. Osborne and G. J. Chader (eds.), Progress in Retinal Research, Vol. 3. Oxford: Pergamon Press, pp. 227–261.

Hurvich, L. M. 1972. Color vision deficiencies. In D. Jameson and L. M. Hurvich (eds.), Handbook of Sensory Physiology, Vol. 7, Part 4. Visual Psychophysics. Berlin: Springer, pp. 582–624.

Land, E. H. 1977. The retinex theory of color vision. Sci. Am. 237(6):108–128.

Stiles, W. S. 1978. Mechanisms of Colour Vision. New York: Academic Press.

Wald, G. 1964. The receptors of human color vision. Science 145:1007–1016.

References

Dartnall, H. J. A., Bowmaker, J. K., and Mollon, J. D. 1983. Microspectrophotometry of human photoreceptors. In J. D. Mollon and L. T. Sharpe (eds.), Colour Vision: Physiology and Psychophysics. New York: Academic Press, pp. 69–80.

Daw, N. W. 1968. Colour-coded ganglion cells in the goldfish retina: Extension of their receptive fields by means of new stimuli. J. Physiol. (Lond.) 197:567–592.

De Valois, R. L. 1960. Color vision mechanisms in the monkey. J. Gen. Physiol. [Suppl. 2] 43:115–128.

Gouras, P., and Krüger, J. 1979. Responses of cells in foveal visual cortex of the monkey to pure color contrast. J. Neurophysiol. 42:850–860.

Gouras, P., and Zrenner, E. 1981. Color vision: A review from a neurophysiological perspective. In D. Ottoson (ed.), Progress in Sensory Physiology 1. Berlin: Springer, pp. 139–179.

Helmholtz, H. von. 1911. The Sensations of Vision. In J. P. C. Southall (ed. and trans.), Helmholtz's Treatise on Physiological Optics, Vol. 2. Wash., D. C.: Optical Society of America, 1924. Translated from the 3rd German edition.

Hering, E. 1964. Outlines of a Theory of the Light Sense. L. M. Hurvich and D. Jameson (trans.). Cambridge, Mass.: Harvard University Press.

Hubel, D. H., and Livingstone, M. S. 1981. Regions of poor orientation tuning coincide with patches of cytochrome oxidase staining in monkey striate cortex. Soc. Neurosci. Abstr. 7:357.

Hubel, D. H., and Wiesel, T. N. 1972. Laminar and columnar distribution of geniculo-cortical fibers in the macaque monkey. J. Comp. Neurol. 146:421–450.

Hubel, D. H., and Wiesel, T. N. 1977. Ferrier Lecture: Functional architecture of macaque monkey visual cortex. Proc. R. Soc. Lond. [Biol.] 198:1–59.

Kries, J. von. 1911. Appendix I. Normal and anomalous colour systems. In J. P. C. Southall (ed. and trans.), Helmholtz's Treatise on Physiological Optics, Vol. 2, pp. 395–425. Wash., D. C.: Optical Society of America, 1924. Translated from the 3rd German edition.

Livingstone, M. S., and Hubel, D. H. 1984. Anatomy and physiology of a color system in the primate visual cortex. J. Neurosci. 4:309–356.

Marks, W. B., Dobelle, W. H., and MacNichol, E. F., Jr. 1964. Visual pigments of single primate cones. Science 143:1181–1183.

Michael, C. R. 1978a. Color vision mechanisms in monkey striate cortex: Dual-opponent cells with concentric receptive fields. J. Neurophysiol. 41:572–588.

Michael, C. R. 1978b. Color vision mechanisms in monkey striate cortex: Simple cells with dual opponent-color receptive fields. J. Neurophysiol. 41:1233–1249.

Nathans, J., and Hogness, D. S. 1984. Isolation and nucleotide sequence of the gene encoding human rhodopsin. Proc. Natl. Acad. Sci. U.S.A. 81:4851–4855.

Niven, W. D., ed. 1890. The Scientific Papers of James Clerk Maxwell. Cambridge: The University Press.

Pokorny, J., Smith, V. C., Verriest, and G., Pinckers, A. J. L. G. 1979. Congenital and Acquired Color Vision Defects. New York: Grune & Stratton.

Smith, V. C., and Pokorny, J. 1975. Spectral sensitivity of the foveal cone photopigments between 400 and 500 nm. Vision Res. 15:161–171.

Svaetichin, G., and MacNichol, E. F., Jr. 1958. Retinal mechanisms for chromatic and achromatic vision. Ann. N. Y. Acad. Sci. 74:385–404.

Young, T. 1802. The Bakerian Lecture. On the theory of light and colours. Phil. Trans. R. Soc. Lond., pp. 12–48.

Zeki, S. 1980. The representation of colours in the cerebral cortex. Nature 284:412–418.

James P. Kelly

Auditory System

31

The auditory system, the afferent limb of human communication, evolved to detect sounds that are of particular interest to us (such as those of human speech) and to detect these sounds even in an environment filled with distracting noises. A concert hall illustrates the auditory system's ability to analyze the environment. The sounds of musical instruments, the voices of the audience, and the rustle of clothing all intermingle. However, the auditory system enables us to distinguish the separate parts of this intricate mixture of sounds and to attend to those that are most significant. The frequency analysis performed by the auditory system enables animals in the wild to detect subtle signals important to both predators and prey; this frequency analysis is also ideal for the analysis of human sounds, such as speech.

Over 100 years ago, the physicist Georg Ohm, who gave his name to Ohm's law, recognized the basic principle governing the function of the ear. He proposed that complex sounds are broken down into simple and discrete vibrations for subsequent analysis by the brain. In effect, Ohm suggested that the ear performs a type of analysis described several years earlier by the French mathematician Jean Fourier. According to Fourier, even the most complex waveforms can be described by the sum of many simpler sine waves and cosine waves of appropriate phases and amplitudes. The results of modern research have confirmed Ohm's original idea that the auditory system performs a Fourier analysis of air-borne sounds by breaking them down into basic frequency components of different phases and amplitudes. This chapter is devoted to the mechanisms used by the ear to transform incoming sounds—the Fourier analysis—and the means by which sounds such as speech are received by the ear and interpreted by the brain.

We shall begin by considering the peripheral conductive apparatus, which consists of three parts: the outer ear, the middle ear, and the inner ear. We shall then focus on the *cochlea* (Latin, snail shell), a spiral bony canal that is filled with fluid and contains the sensory transduction apparatus: the *organ of Corti*. Finally, we shall examine the organization and function of pathways in the central nervous system associated with hearing. (Other aspects of the auditory system will be considered in Chapter 44 in the discussion of the vestibular system.)

The Conductive Apparatus Transforms Acoustic Waves into Mechanical Vibrations

To understand the physical nature of sound, consider a simple sinusoidal wave (Figure 31–1), which consists of regularly alternating condensations and rarefactions (increased and decreased pressure, respectively) of the air. The *frequency* of the wave, measured in cycles per second or hertz (Hz), determines its pitch. The human ear is sensitive to a wide range of sound frequencies, from about 20 to 15,000 Hz. For example, middle C on a piano keyboard has a fundamental frequency of 523 Hz.

The *amplitude* of the wave is correlated with its perceived loudness, and a special scale, the decibel scale, is used to measure the amplitude of pressure waves. The decibel (dB) is a logarithmic ratio defined as follows:

Sound Pressure Level (SPL) in decibels $= 20 \log_{10} P_t/P_r$

where P_t is the test pressure and P_r is the reference pressure (2×10^{-4} dynes/cm^2). This logarithmic scale was devised by Alexander Graham Bell, because he noted that the Weber-Fechner law (Chapter 23) applied to hearing. Equal increases in sound pressure level, measured in decibels, correspond to equal increases in subjective loudness regardless of the absolute value of the sound pressure level. The reference pressure (P_r) in the equation above is the sound pressure required to make a sound between 1000 and 3000 Hz just audible to average listeners (human hearing is most acute in this range). A test sound pressure (P_t) ten times more intense would have a sound pressure level of 20 dB ($P_t/P_r = 10$, therefore 20 $\log_{10} 10 = 20$). Similarly, a test sound 100 times P_r would correspond to a sound pressure level of 40 dB. For reference, conversational speech is about 65 dB in sound pressure level. The range of sound over which the ear responds is about 120 dB, so that the loudest sound that can be heard without physical discomfort is 1 million times louder than the faintest sound that the ear can detect. Sound pressure levels greater than 100 dB may damage the sensory apparatus of the cochlea. The extent of this damage is dependent on the intensity of the sounds, their frequency, and the duration of exposure.

Air-borne sounds travel through the external auditory meatus (Latin, opening), the external ear canal, to reach the *tympanic* (Latin, drum) *membrane*, causing it to vibrate. This vibration is conveyed to the middle ear where there are a series of small bones called *ossicles*, one of which, the *malleus* (Latin, hammer), is attached to the tympanic membrane. The vibration of the malleus is transmitted to an opening in the cochlea, called the *oval window*, by the remaining two ossicles, the *incus* (Latin, anvil) and the *stapes* (Latin, stirrup) (Figure 31–2). The major components of the middle ear, the tympanic membrane and the ossicles, function to make more efficient the transmission of sounds from air in the outer ear to the fluid-filled cochlea of the inner ear. If the middle ear were absent, sounds would reach the fluid at the oval window directly, and most of the sound energy would be reflected because fluid has a higher acoustic impedance than air. As a result, the sound pressure level required for hearing would be elevated. There is therefore a problem in impedance-matching between air-borne sounds and fluid motion within the cochlea. The tympanic membrane and the ossicles help to counteract this problem.

The area of the tympanic membrane is greater than the area of the oval window, and as a consequence the total pressure (force/unit area) acting on the smaller oval window is increased. At frequencies near 1 kHz (1 kHz = 1000 Hz), the ossicles also act as a lever system to increase the pressure on the round window, but this ef-

31–1 As a sinusoidal sound wave propagates through space, the ambient pressure in the air is measured with a microphone probe at a fixed point. The speed of sound is a constant in air (approximately 340 m/sec) and is related to both the wavelength (λ) and frequency (f) of the wave as shown in the equation in the figure. The tympanic membrane of the ear moves in response to the alternating condensations (peaks) and rarefactions (troughs) of the sound wave.

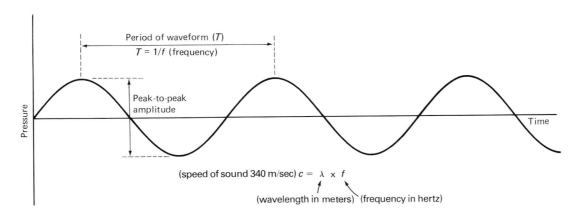

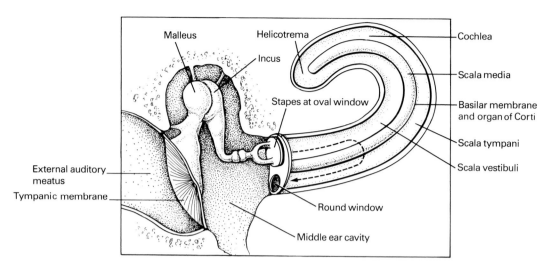

31–2 The auditory periphery consists of (1) the external ear (which includes the pinna, the external auditory meatus, and the tympanic membrane), (2) the middle ear (which contains the three ossicles: the malleus, the incus, and the stapes), and (3) the internal ear, which is composed of the cochlea and the vestibular apparatus (Chapter 44). The tympanic membrane is joined to a chain of ossicles. Motion of the tympanic membrane causes motion of the stapes, which in turn sets up a propagated wave in the fluid-filled cochlea. The cochlea, a spiral bony canal, contains three compartments: (1) the *scala tympani*, (2) the *scala vestibuli*, and (3) the *scala media*, or the cochlear duct that contains the basilar

membrane. Changes in fluid pressure in the cochlea are possible because both the oval window of the scala tympani, into which the stapes fits, and the round window of the scala vestibuli are flexible membranes. As a result, pushing the oval window inward causes the round window to bulge into the middle ear cavity. The compartment of the oval window (the scala tympani) and that of the round window (the scala vestibuli) communicate with each other at the helicotrema, so that the perilymph in the two compartments is continuous. The basilar membrane, which makes up the floor of the scala media, separates the two compartments over much of their length and is set in motion by the pressure waves.

fect is reduced at both higher and lower frequencies because the tympanic membrane does not vibrate as a uniform plate, and therefore the ossicles cannot be viewed as a simple lever system. They are probably also arranged to reduce inertial motion of the conductive apparatus that might occur as a result of head movements.

The cochlea spirals for two-and-a-half turns around a central pillar called the *modiolus* (Latin, pillar or hub). In Figure 31–2, the cochlea has been uncoiled for purposes of illustration. Here we can clearly see that the cochlea has three compartments or *scalae* (Latin, staircase). These are: (1) the *scala tympani*, which follows the outer contours of the spiral cochlea; (2) the *scala vestibuli*, which follows the inner contours and is continuous with the scala tympani at the *helicotrema* (Latin, spiral hole); and, lying between these two, (3) the *scala media* (or the cochlear duct), which extends like a gloved finger into the spiral channel and ends blindly near its apex.

Sound entering the ear causes the stapes to oscillate, and these oscillations transmit energy to each of the three compartments. The pressure transmission works as follows. When the stapes oscillates it pushes into and out of the cochlea and puts varying pressure on the fluid in the scala vestibuli. Because fluid is incompressible, the pressure wave causes an alternating outward and inward movement of the membrane of the round window of the scala tympani. Moreover, because the two compartments are almost entirely separated by the scala media, the pressure waves set up by the oscillating movement of the

stapes also cause oscillating movements of the scala media and of the basilar membrane (the floor of the scala media). Since the organ of Corti, the sensory transduction apparatus in the scala media, rests on the basilar membrane, it is also stimulated by this movement.

Thus, the cochlear compartments are arranged to convert the differential pressure between the scala vestibuli and scala tympani into oscillating movements of the basilar membrane that excite and inhibit the sensory transducing cells in the scala media.

Sounds can also bypass the middle ear and reach the cochlea directly by *bone conduction*, that is, by vibration of the entire temporal bone. This is an inefficient means of energy transfer, and becomes important only as a part of audiological diagnosis when the auditory system is malfunctioning. In *otosclerosis*, for example, the footplate of the stapes becomes locked in place due to the growth of the bone around the annular ligament which binds the stapes to the oval window. During the nineteenth century, Heinrich Rinne developed a test to reveal this and other types of hearing abnormalities.

Rinne's test compares a hearing-impaired patient's ability to detect air-conducted and bone-conducted sounds. A tuning fork is struck so as to vibrate and then is held near the patient's ear. When the patient can no longer hear the sound produced by the fork because the amplitude of its vibration has decreased, the stem of the fork is placed against the mastoid process of the temporal bone behind the ear. If the patient once again hears the vibration, this indicates that hearing by bone conduction is more sensitive than that by air conduction and implies some disruption of the conductive apparatus (for example, otosclerosis). Using Rinne's test, it is possible to distinguish two broad classes of deafness: (1) conductive deafness, caused by damage to the middle ear, and (2) sensorineural deafness, caused by damage to the cochlea, the eighth nerve, or the central auditory pathway. In conductive deafness, as we have seen, bone conduction is unimpaired. In sensorineural deafness, hearing by both bone and air conduction is impaired. The distinction is clinically important because modern surgical procedures can readily repair many conductive lesions.

The Cochlea Transduces Changes in Fluid Pressure into Neural Activity

The sensory receptor cells of the ear, the *hair cells,* are contained within the organ of Corti. When the oscillating motion of the stapes causes changes in fluid pressure within the cochlea, it initiates, in turn, motion of a particular portion of the basilar membrane and therefore of particular hair cells (Figure 31–2).

How do the vibrations produced by different sounds modulate the excitation of different hair cells at different points along the basilar membrane? A cross section of the cochlea shows the hair cells as they are located in the organ of the Corti (Figure 31–3). There are three rows of outer hair cells and one row of inner hair cells. The terms *inner* and *outer* refer to the relative proximity of the hair cells to the modiolus, the bony hub of the cochlea. On the apical surface of each hair cell is a bundle of "hairs" or *stereocilia* (Figure 31–4). These are filled with parallel arrays of cross-bridged actin filaments and consequently are stiff (the prefix *stereo* is Greek for solid). The stereocilia of most of the hair cells project into the overlying *tectorial membrane.* Because the tips of the stereocilia are embedded in the tectorial membrane, they are fixed and cannot move freely, as can the base of the hair cell, which rests on the basilar membrane. Therefore, when the basilar membrane moves, the resulting movement of the basal part of the hair cells is thought to cause the stereocilia to bend and undergo an angular displacement in relation to their fixed tips (Figure 31–5).

Thus, when a given sound produces an oscillatory movement of the basilar membrane, the back-and-forth angular displacement of the stereocilia alternately opens and closes *transduction channels* of the hair cell, resulting in sinusoidal (depolarizing–hyperpolarizing) potential changes in the hair cell that are the same frequency as those of the sound stimulus.

In addition to having an input component at its apical end (from which the stereocilia arise), the hair cell has specialized machinery for releasing chemical transmitter at its basal end. Here the cells are contacted by the peripheral axons of the bipolar neurons whose cell bodies lie in the spiral ganglion and whose central axons give rise to the auditory nerve.

Motion of the stereocilia in *one direction* produces an inward current, carried by cations, that depolarizes the hair cell and causes it to release chemical transmitter at its basal surface. The transmitter excites the afferent endings of neurons in the spiral ganglion and initiates action potentials in their central processes in the auditory nerve. Motion of the stereocilia in the *opposite* direction hyperpolarizes the hair cell, and shuts off transmitter release and the firing of the auditory nerve fiber. In this way, the oscillatory movement of the basilar

31–3 The cochlea contains the organ of Corti, which rests on the basilar membrane and contains hair cells that are surrounded by an elaborate network of supporting cells. There are two types of hair cells: inner hair cells and outer hair cells. The hair cells are innervated at their bases by afferent fibers. These nerve fibers have cell bodies in the spiral ganglion. Efferent fibers from the central nervous system synapse on afferent terminals beneath the inner hair cells and on the bases of the outer hair cells. The hair cells project their apical sterocilia toward the overlying tectorial membrane and make contact with it. (Adapted from Wersäll, Flock, and Lundquist, 1965.)

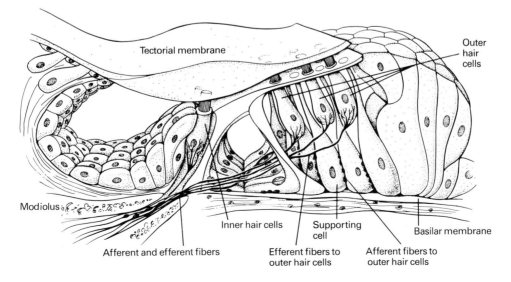

A Inner hair cells

B Outer hair cells

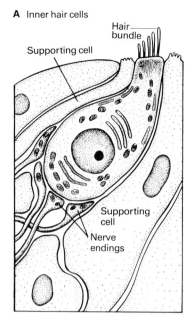
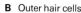
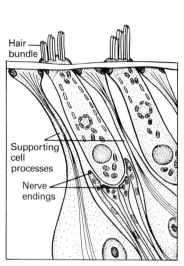

31–4 Although there are two different types of hair cells in the organ of Corti, physiological differences between them are not completely understood. **A.** Inner hair cells. **B.** Outer hair cells. The inner hair cells are innervated at their bases by about 10 afferent fibers, each of which innervates only 1 inner hair cell. The outer hair cells are innervated by several afferent fibers, each of which innervates many outer hair cells. The hair cells release transmitter at the basal end where they synapse upon and excite the axons of the spiral ganglion. Both types of hair cells are surrounded by supporting cells to which they are joined, at their apical surfaces, by tight junctions. The magnification in **B** is lower, so that the outer hair cells, which are actually larger than the inner hair cells, appear smaller. (Adapted from Miller and Towe, 1979.)

membrane produced by sound leads to oscillatory displacement of the stereocilia and sinusoidal changes in the membrane potential of the hair cells, which cause oscillatory release of transmitter by the hair cell and firing of axons in the auditory nerve.

Different Regions of the Cochlea Are Selectively Responsive to Different Frequencies of Sound

Given that hair cells respond to movement of their hair bundle, how does the vibration of the basilar membrane encode different frequencies of sound? This question was asked in the nineteenth century by Herman von Helmholtz, who discovered two interesting features of the basilar membrane. First, Helmholtz noted that the basilar membrane has cross striations much like the strings of a piano. Second, he noted that, again like a piano, the basilar membrane is not uniform but varies in width. It is narrow (100 μm) and stiff near the oval win-

dow, and wider (500 μm) and more flexible near the apex of the cochlea (Figure 31–6). With characteristic insight (he provided a mathematical formulation of the law of conservation of energy while he was a surgical resident in the army), Helmholtz proposed that the cross striations of different portions of the basilar membrane resonate with different frequencies of sound, much as piano strings of different length and stiffness resonate with different frequencies. The cross striations of the stiff part of the basilar membrane at the base near the oval window would, in this view, resonate with high frequencies (about 15,000 Hz), while the striations in the flexible part of the membrane near the apex would resonate with low frequencies (about 100 Hz). Between these extreme frequencies, there is a continuous spectrum of resonance, running from high at the base of the cochlea to low nearer the apex. According to this *resonance theory*, different frequencies of sound are encoded to different positions of the basilar membrane.

31–5 According to a common theory of cochlear function, deflection of the basilar membrane results in bending of hair cell stereocilia; this shearing force of the hair cells probably causes a conductance change at the apical surface of

the cell, a current flow, and resultant voltage change. **A.** Basilar membrane at rest. **B.** Basilar membrane deflection and angular displacement of stereocilia. (Adapted from Miller and Towe, 1979.)

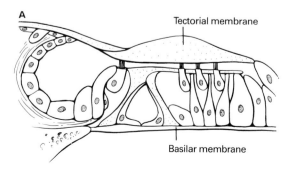
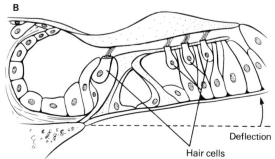

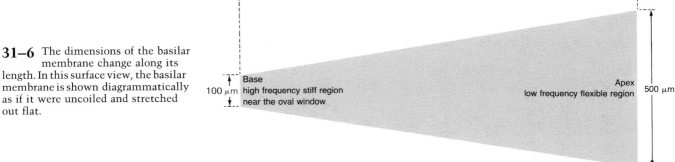

31–6 The dimensions of the basilar membrane change along its length. In this surface view, the basilar membrane is shown diagrammatically as if it were uncoiled and stretched out flat.

33 mm

100 μm   Base
high frequency stiff region
near the oval window

Apex
low frequency flexible region   500 μm

In the 1920s and 1930s, Georg von Békésy, who later won the Nobel Prize for this research, tested Helmholtz's idea directly by examining the pattern of mechanical vibrations in the cochlea. He sealed a microscope objective into a hole in the bony wall of the cochlea and measured the amplitude and phase of basilar membrane motion in response to sound. Von Békésy found—in contradiction to the resonance hypothesis—that each sound does not lead to the resonance of only one narrow segment of the basilar membrane but initiates a *traveling wave* along the length of the cochlea that starts at the oval window. The wave passes along the cochlea from the stapes to the helicotrema much like snapping a rope tied at one end to a post causes a wave to pass along it. The waves are called *traveling* because the stapes is in continuous oscillation during a sound, and as a result there is a continuous succession of waves along the basilar membrane (Figures 31–1 and 31–7). As Figure 31–7 illustrates, stimulation at a single frequency causes a very broad region of the basilar membrane to move. Different frequencies of sound produce different traveling waves and these, in turn, have *peak* amplitudes at different points along the basilar membrane. The variation in the mechanical properties of the basilar membrane along the length of the cochlea accounts for the fact that different regions of the basilar membrane vibrate maximally at different frequencies. At low frequencies, the peak amplitude of the motion is near the apex of the cochlea, in the region of the helicotrema. As the frequency of the stimulus increases, the peak amplitude of motion moves progressively toward the base of the cochlea. Each frequency, therefore, has its peak amplitude at a different position, and there is a logarithmic representation of frequencies along the basilar membrane. In fact, the peak motion of the basilar membrane in response to sounds of different frequencies occurs at exactly the points predicted by Helmholtz's resonance theory! Although the wave travels, the envelope produced by a given frequency is invariant in its position along the basilar membrane. The hair cells situated at the site where the oscillation is maximal are most excited, so that different frequencies excite different hair cells located at different positions along the basilar membrane. A sound composed of many frequencies will cause many different points along the basilar membrane to vibrate and will excite hair cells at all of these points. The central nervous system, therefore, re-

31–7 Plots of data from von Békésy's experiments on the mechanics of the basilar membrane show that the peak amplitude of the traveling wave occurs at different points for sounds of different frequencies. Modern measurements show that these curves reflect only the overall envelope of motion of a complex wave along the basilar membrane. The peak motion is sharp and restricted in distribution, although the exact waveform of the motion has not yet been established with certainty. (Adapted from von Békésy, 1960.)

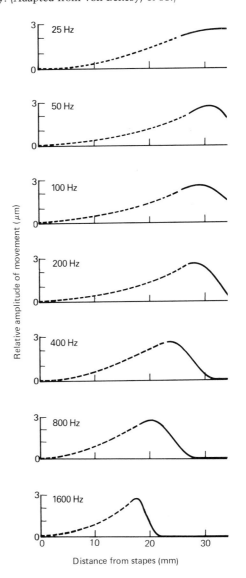

ceives information not about sound per se, but rather about the pattern of motion of the basilar membrane and associated structures in the organ of Corti.

Because von Békésy's measurements were made in cadavers, they proved, however, not to be a completely accurate reflection of the type of movement actually occurring in the living cochlea. Several subsequent investigators have examined the mechanical response of the basilar membrane with the Mossbauer technique and with laser interferometry, modern techniques that are capable of measuring the amplitude of basilar membrane motion with a resolution of about 10^{-9} cm. These studies indicate that the normal response is much more sharply tuned and larger in amplitude than the response von Békésy observed. The peak region of basilar membrane motion in response to a single frequency of sound probably extends only the width of a few hair cells.

Individual Hair Cells at Different Points along the Basilar Membrane Are Tuned Electrically as well as Mechanically

Until recently it was thought that frequency selectivity is determined only by variations in the mechanical properties of the basilar membrane itself and not by differences in the properties of the hair cells along the basilar membrane (Figure 31–7). According to this view, different hair cells respond not because they differ fundamentally from one another but only because they are located at different positions along the basilar membrane.

In fact, hair cells at different points along the basilar membrane are not identical but differ from one another in their electromechanical properties, and these variations probably play a further role in determining frequency selectivity. At the base of the cochlea, where the basilar membrane is narrow and stiff, the outer hair cells and their stereocilia are short and stiff. Where the basilar membrane is more flexible in the apex, the hair cells and their stereocilia are more than twice as long and more flexible than those in the base. Thus, part of the frequency selectivity of the cochlea may be due to the variation in the structure of the hair cells with the result that the hair cells are tuned mechanically; they have a *mechanical resonance*. Different sound waves activate different regions of the basilar membrane and activate different populations of mechanically tuned hair cells.

Recently, A.C. Crawford and R. Fettiplace in England and Richard Lewis and Albert Hudspeth of the University of California at San Francisco have discovered that the hair cells of certain lower vertebrates, in addition to being tuned mechanically, are tuned electrically *(electrical resonance)*. The hair cell membrane shows spontaneous oscillations in membrane potential. The frequencies of these oscillations differ in different hair cells according to their position along the basilar membrane. In each case the characteristic frequency of the spontaneous electrical oscillation matches the frequency at which the cell is most responsive to mechanical stimuli (its *mechanical resonance*). As the mechanical activation opens and closes the transduction channels, the potential

changes in the hair cells act to amplify the spontaneous voltage oscillations. This can be shown experimentally by artificially passing depolarizing or hyperpolarizing currents into the hair cell (Figure 31–8).

How is this electrical resonance achieved? Lewis and Hudspeth have found that three different currents interact to produce the electrical resonance: a Ca^{++} current, a Ca^{++}-activated K^+ current, and a delayed K^+ current. The depolarizing phase is due to a depolarizing influx of Ca^{++} that in turn activates, with a delay, the two hyperpolarizing K^+ currents. As the hyperpolarization wears off, the Ca^{++} current is again turned on, depolarizes the membrane again, and once more activates two hyperpolarizing currents. This interaction of inward and outward current produces spontaneous voltage fluctuations around the resting potential. As the mechanical stimulus depolarizes and hyperpolarizes the cell, it increases and decreases the spontaneous oscillation of the Ca^{++} and K^+ currents, which have different kinetics for different hair cells, and hence different frequencies of oscillation.

The mechanical resonance of the hair cell (determined by the physical properties of the hair cell and its stereocilia) is therefore coupled to its electrical resonance (determined by the electrical membrane characteristics of the cell). These resonances reinforce one another to establish the selective frequency tuning of the hair cell (Figure 31–8). Sound stimuli give rise to traveling waves that produce the mechanical resonance of the hair cell and excite it. This excitation in turn amplifies the electrical resonance because in each cell both the electrical and mechanical oscillations are tuned to a certain narrow range of frequencies, and only these frequencies elicit large oscillatory potential responses. The coupling of these resonance frequencies, therefore, causes the hair cell to behave as an amplifier, and optimizes the ability of the cell to transduce the mechanical stimuli of certain frequencies into electrical signals.

The Cochlea Is Innervated by Fibers of the Eighth Nerve

The hair cells release transmitter to activate the peripheral axons of the cells of the *spiral ganglion* that innervate them. The central processes of these cells make up the auditory nerve. This ganglion is composed of myelinated bipolar neurons lying in the modiolus of the cochlea. In the human cochlea, there are about 30,000 spiral ganglion cells. The peripheral processes of these cells run toward the organ of Corti. Ninety percent of the fibers innervate the inner hair cells; each inner hair cell (there are approximately 3000 in each cochlea) receives contacts from about 10 fibers and each fiber contacts only 1 inner hair cell. Each of the remaining 10% of the peripherally directed fibers diverges to innervate many outer hair cells. Efferent fibers coming from the central nervous system also synapse on outer hair cells and on the afferent axons innervating inner hair cells, but the function of the efferent fibers remains unknown.

In view of the fact that the majority of spiral ganglion cells innervate a restricted portion of the cochlea only a

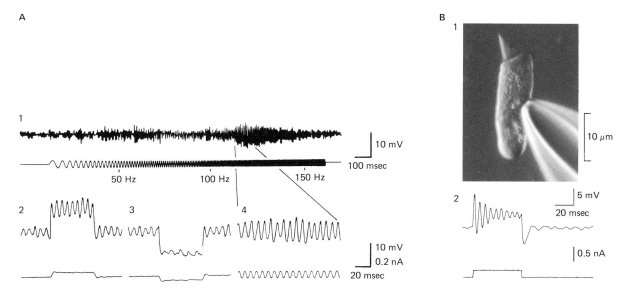

31–8 Recordings from single hair cells demonstrate the similarity between the mechanical and electrical resonances of the hair cells. **A.** Recordings from a hair cell in the excised saccular macula, made with a conventional intracellular microelectrode. **1:** A sound signal that varies in frequency from 0 to 170 Hz produces mechanical stimulation of the hair bundle with ± 0.03 μm deflections (**lower trace**) and evokes a maximal receptor potential (**upper trace**) at 120 Hz, with a secondary peak at about half that frequency (60 Hz). As this record shows, there are spontaneous oscillations before and after the frequency sweep. These spontaneous oscillations occur at about 125 Hz. **2:** Depolarization of the cell by injection of a constant-current pulse (**lower trace**) increased the frequency of these spontaneous voltage oscillations (**upper trace**) to 140 Hz from the spontaneous rate of 125 Hz at resting potential (– 66 mV). The spontaneous voltage oscillations that constitute the resting electrical resonance of the hair cell can

be seen in the **upper trace** before and after the current pulse. **3:** Hyperpolarizing current, conversely, lowered the frequency of membrane potential oscillation to 91 Hz. **4:** A segment of the cell's response to the frequency sweep near the characteristic frequency in **1** is displayed on a faster time scale. The characteristic frequency of the cell's response to mechanical stimulation is near the frequency of spontaneous oscillation in **2** and **3**. The **lower trace** in **4** is the frequency of the mechanical stimulus. **B.** Voltage oscillations in a solitary hair cell. **1:** Differential-interference contrast photomicrograph of a solitary hair cell from the bullfrog's sacculus, in contact with the tip of a recording pipette. **2:** Injection of a small depolarizing current (**lower trace**) evoked membrane potential oscillations in a solitary cell (**upper trace**). Depolarization increases the frequency from 137 Hz at the resting potential of – 62 mV to 195 Hz. (From Lewis and Hudspeth, 1983.)

single hair cell in extent, it is not surprising that auditory nerve fibers, the centrally directed branches of the ganglion cells, display a frequency-dependent response to sound. A *tuning curve* can be established by measuring the number of impulses produced by a single auditory nerve fiber in response to brief pulses of sound at various frequencies. Tuning curves are plots of the amplitude of sound required to produce a detectable response versus the frequency of the sound stimulus. An individual fiber responds to a range of frequencies since a substantial portion of the basilar membrane moves in response to a single frequency of sound even at moderate intensities (Figure 31–7). A single fiber, however, is most sensitive to a particular frequency, its *characteristic frequency*. This property is directly related to the location of the hair cell that the fiber innervates: fibers innervating hair cells near the oval window at the base of the cochlea have high characteristic frequencies, whereas those innervating hair cells near the apex of the cochlea have low characteristic frequencies. A sample tuning curve for an auditory nerve fiber with a 2-kHz characteristic frequency is shown in Figure 31–9.

The temporal pattern of the response to a brief tone burst at the characteristic frequency is similar from one au-

ditory nerve fiber to the next. There is an initial phasic increase in firing above the spontaneous level, followed by a maintained tonic discharge that persists for the duration of the tone. When the tone is turned off, there is a transient decrease in firing below the spontaneous level before the fiber returns to its resting state (Figure 31–10).

An interesting feature of the responses of individual auditory nerve fibers is that they are not consistent. A particular stimulus does not always elicit precisely the same response upon repeated presentation. A useful way to study these responses, therefore, is to indicate their average characteristics. This can be done by preparing a poststimulus time histogram of the averaged responses of a single auditory nerve fiber to many stimuli; this type of analysis was pioneered by Nelson Kiang at the Massachusetts Institute of Technology. A *poststimulus time histogram* is a plot of the number of spikes versus time, relative to the beginning of the stimulus. Each stimulus is repeated many times to obtain the average response (Figure 31–11). The stimulus was a 5000-Hz tone, 250 msec in duration, that was repeatedly presented twice every second for a 2-min period to produce each histogram. The amplitude of the stimulus was decreased in successive 10-dB steps from the lowest histogram to the

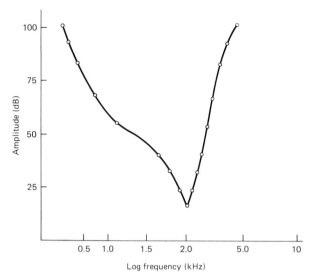

31–9 The tuning curve for an eighth-nerve fiber shows its sensitivity to a stimulus at its characteristic frequency of 2 kHz. The fiber gives a response that is just detectable when stimulated with a 2-kHz tone at about 15 dB. If the amplitude of the 2-kHz tone is increased then the fiber gives a more pronounced response. At another frequency, about 4 kHz, a much louder sound of nearly 80 dB is required to get a just detectable response.

uppermost. The envelope of the lowest histogram is similar to the model curve of Figure 31–10. There is an initial onset burst, followed by a constant level of firing, and finally a period of reduced activity after the tone is turned off. As the amplitude of the stimulus is decreased, the time structure and magnitude of the cell's response become progressively degraded.

Some fibers with low characteristic frequencies (less than 4000 Hz or so) can actually *phase lock* to a pure tone stimulus. These neurons tend to fire at a particular time during each cycle of the sinusoid. Consequently, such fibers can indicate the frequency of a stimulus on the basis of a *place principle*, because they innervate hair cells in a particular region of the cochlea, and also on the basis of a *volley principle*, since their discharges occur with a predictable relationship to the stimulating waveform.

31–10 An eighth-nerve fiber responds to a pure tone at its characteristic frequency for the duration of the tone burst; when the tone ceases there is a transient decrease to below the spontaneous firing level.

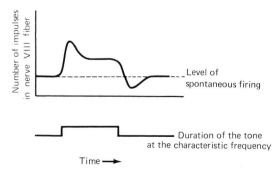

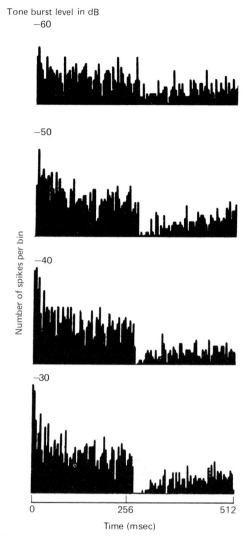

31–11 Poststimulus time histograms show the response patterns of an auditory nerve fiber to tone bursts as a function of stimulus level. Zero time of each histogram is 2.5 msec before the onset of the electrical input to the earphone. The stimuli were tone bursts at about 5000 Hz (the characteristic frequency of the unit), 250 msec duration, with a 2.5-msec rise–fall time. The stimulus was followed by a quiet period lasting 250 msec, then was repeated again, over a period of 2 min. The entire sample period is divided into a number of small time units, or bins, and the number of spikes occurring in each bin was measured. The important pattern to observe is the initial phasic increase in firing correlated with the onset of the stimulus, the maintained discharge during the course of the stimulus, and the decrease in activity following termination. There is a gradual return to baseline activity during the interstimulus interval. (Adapted from Kiang, 1965.)

The Central Auditory Pathways Are Organized Tonotopically

Auditory fibers in the eighth nerve terminate in the *cochlear nucleus*, lying on the external aspect of the restiform body (Figure 31–12). The organization of the co-

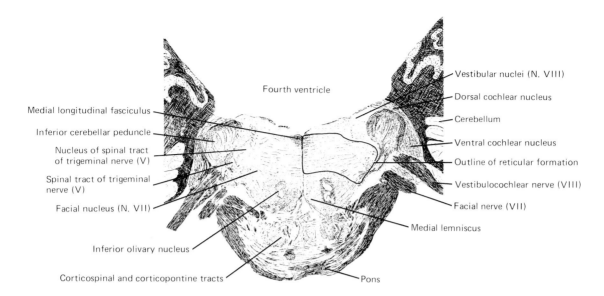

Fourth ventricle

Vestibular nuclei (N. VIII)

Dorsal cochlear nucleus

Medial longitudinal fasciculus

Cerebellum

Inferior cerebellar peduncle

Ventral cochlear nucleus

Nucleus of spinal tract of trigeminal nerve (V)

Outline of reticular formation

Spinal tract of trigeminal nerve (V)

Vestibulocochlear nerve (VIII)

Facial nucleus (N. VII)

Facial nerve (VII)

Medial lemniscus

Inferior olivary nucleus

Corticospinal and corticopontine tracts

Pons

chlear nucleus was analyzed very thoroughly in the 1930s by Rafael Lorente de Nó, a student of Santiago Ramón y Cajal, using the Golgi method. He found that the cochlear nucleus is divided into a *dorsal division* and a *ventral division.* The entering auditory nerve fibers pierce the ventral division of the cochlear nucleus at about the middle of its rostrocaudal extent, thereby separating the ventral division into an *anteroventral cochlear nucleus* and a *posteroventral cochlear nucleus.* Each auditory nerve fiber branches as it enters the cochlear nucleus. An *ascending branch* innervates the anteroventral nucleus, and a *descending branch* innervates the posteroventral cochlear nucleus along with the dorsal cochlear nucleus. The various subdivisions of the cochlear nucleus contain morphologically different cell types. It appears that each auditory nerve fiber makes a different type of synaptic contact with distinct cell classes in each division of the cochlear nucleus.

In view of the cellular diversity of the cochlear nucleus, it is reasonable to expect that a variety of physiological response types might be found within it. In addition to cells that respond to tone bursts in a manner very similar to the primary auditory nerve fibers, there are cells that respond only to the *onset* of the stimulus, cells whose rate of firing *builds up* slowly during the course of the stimulus, and others that *pause,* showing no response to the onset of the stimulus. These physiologically different cell types are located in different parts of the cochlear nucleus. Therefore, they probably correspond to particular morphological cell types, but proof of this correspondence is not yet complete.

The most important principle governing the topography of the cochlear nucleus is the *tonotopic organization* of its cells and axons (Figure 31–13). Primary auditory axons that innervate the base of the cochlea penetrate deeply into the nucleus before branching to terminate in its three principal divisions. Primary axons that innervate the apex of the cochlea branch at more superficial levels in the nucleus. Between these two extremes, fibers

31–12 This myelin-stained section through the lower pons shows the location of the cochlear nucleus. It lies on the external aspect of the restiform body. (Adapted from Ranson and Clark, 1953.)

that innervate the middle region of the cochlea terminate in an ordered array. Consequently, each part of the cochlear nucleus shows tonotopic order. This can be shown by making a long penetration with a microelectrode through the nucleus while recording the characteristic frequency of each cell encountered. If the path of the electrode is marked, then the location of each cell recorded from can be identified in the nucleus. Studies of this kind have demonstrated that all of the central auditory nuclei, including the auditory cortex, are organized on a tonotopic basis.

31–13 The three divisions of the cochlear nucleus receive input from the eighth nerve. The nerve fibers are arranged in an orderly sequence, so that a tonotopic map is established in the nucleus.

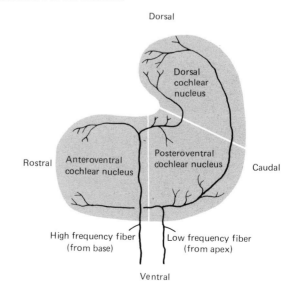

Dorsal

Dorsal cochlear nucleus

Rostral

Anteroventral cochlear nucleus

Posteroventral cochlear nucleus

Caudal

High frequency fiber (from base)

Low frequency fiber (from apex)

Ventral

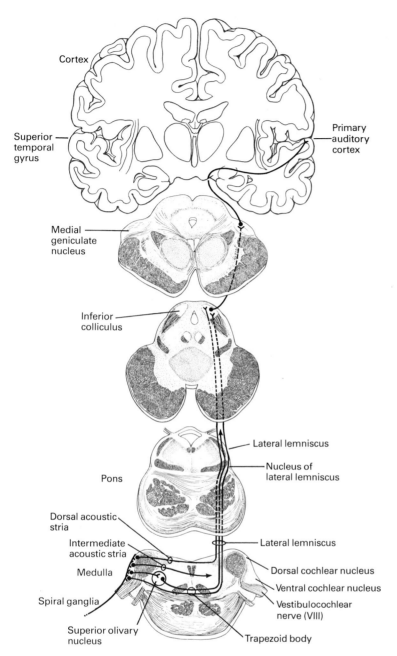

31–14 The central auditory pathways extend from the cochlear nucleus to the primary auditory cortex. Postsynaptic neurons in the cochlear nucleus send their axons to other centers in the brain via three main pathways: the dorsal acoustic stria, the intermediate acoustic stria, and the trapezoid body. The first binaural interactions occur in the superior olivary nucleus, which receives input via the trapezoid body. The medial and lateral divisions of the superior olivary complex are probably involved in the localization of sounds in space. Postsynaptic axons from the superior olive, along with axons from the cochlear nuclei, form the lateral lemniscus, which ascends to the midbrain. Axons relaying input from both ears are found in each lateral lemniscus. The axons synapse in the inferior colliculus, and postsynaptic cells in the colliculus send their axons to the medial geniculate nucleus of the thalamus. The geniculate axons terminate in the superior temporal gyrus (Brodmann's areas 41 and 42), also called the primary auditory cortex. (Adapted from Brodal, 1981.)

Each Cochlea Is Bilaterally Represented in the Brain

The ascending connections of the cochlear nuclei are complex because there are several brain stem auditory nuclei that receive input from the cochlear nuclei and myriad possibilities for interconnections among the relay nuclei. In the following account, the essential points will be stressed at the expense of detail.

The axons of cells in the cochlear nucleus stream out along three pathways: the *dorsal acoustic stria*, the *intermediate acoustic stria*, and the *trapezoid body* (Figure 31–14). By far the most important pathway is the trapezoid body. It contains fibers destined for the *superior olivary nucleus* on both sides of the brain stem.

The *medial superior olive* is an interesting structure. It is thought to be concerned with sound localization on the basis of time differences. William Stotler found that this nucleus is composed of spindle-shaped cells with one medial and one lateral dendrite, and that these dendrites receive input from the contralateral and ipsilateral cochlear nuclei, respectively. Subsequently, Jay Goldberg and his colleagues at the University of Chicago demonstrated that these *binaural cells* in the medial superior olive are very sensitive to differences in the time of arrival of auditory stimuli to the two ears. *Time difference* is one of the cues used to localize sounds in space, since a sound coming from one side reaches the ear on that side first and the ear on the other side a few tenths of a millisecond later.

The *lateral superior olive* is also concerned with localizing sounds in space, but by another mechanism. Cells in this nucleus detect interaural *differences in sound intensity.* When a high-frequency sound coming from one side reaches the ear, some of the sound energy is reflected by the head. As a result, the sound reaching the ear on the other side is a few decibels lower in amplitude. The binaural cells in the lateral superior olive are maximally stimulated by sounds of a particular frequency, but the sound amplitude presented to the two ears must be different. Nearly all the neurons in this nucleus are excited by inputs from the ipsilateral cochlear nucleus and inhibited, via an interneuron, by inputs from the contralateral cochlear nucleus. When this inhibition is reduced, by diminishing the input to the contralateral ear, the cells give a maximal response.

Axons arising from the superior olivary complex, along with crossed and uncrossed axons from the cochlear nucleus, run together to form the *lateral lemniscus.* Thus, from the outset there is extensive bilateral representation of each ear in the central nervous system. Consequently, *lesions of the central auditory pathway do not cause monaural disability.* The lateral lemniscus courses through the *nuclei of the lateral lemniscus,* where some fibers synapse. Here again there is extensive crossing between the two sides via *Probst's commissure.* All fibers in the lateral lemniscus eventually synapse in the *inferior colliculus.* The cells of the inferior colliculus receive binaural input, and are arranged in tonotopic order. The strategic difference between the inferior colliculus and the superior colliculus should be emphasized. The superior colliculus is a visual reflex center; it is not part of the perceptual pathway leading to the visual cortex. The inferior colliculus, on the other hand, is an integral part of the pathway leading to the auditory cortex. Most of the cells in the inferior colliculus send their axons to the *medial geniculate nucleus* of the thalamus on the same side of the brain, but a few project contralaterally. The cells in the medial geniculate nucleus send their axons to the homolateral *primary auditory cortex* located in the superior temporal gyrus (Brodmann's areas 41 and 42).

John Brugge and his colleagues at the University of Wisconsin have found that the primary auditory cortex contains several distinct tonotopic maps of the frequency spectrum. This is analogous to the multiple representations of the periphery seen in the somatic sensory cortex and the visual cortex. The different layers of the auditory cortex establish patterns of connections with other regions of the brain in a manner that is similar to other primary cortical areas. Layer VI, for example, projects back to the medial geniculate nucleus, and layer V projects to the inferior colliculus.

Three aspects of the organization of the auditory cortex deserve mention. First, the auditory cortex is organized on a columnar basis. In long tangential microelectrode penetrations through the cortex, binaural cells can be found clustered into two alternating columnar groups, *summation columns* and *suppression columns.* These columns run from the pial surface to the underlying white matter, and most cells within a column display

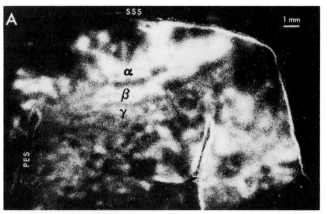

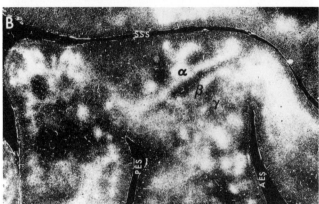

31–15 The topographic distribution of callosal axon terminals in the cat can be seen in tissue sections cut parallel to the cortical surface, which had been flattened by gently pressing it onto a glass plate. **A.** Autoradiograph of a tissue section in which callosal axon terminals were labeled with proline. One day before the animal was killed, ³H-proline was injected into each of 37 sites in the left hemisphere. **B.** Photomicrograph of degenerating callosal axon terminals. One week earlier, the corpus callosum was completely cut. α and β are the two major bands of callosal terminals. Note that these bands are irregular in outline and somewhat similar in appearance to the ocular dominance columns in the visual cortex (Chapter 29). Several prominent sulci in the cat's brain are also indicated: SSS, superior sylvian sulcus; PES, posterior ectosylvian sulcus; AES, anterior ectosylvian sulcus. (Photograph courtesy of Dr. J. Brugge.)

similar binaural interactions. In summation columns, the binaural response of the cells is greater than either monaural response. In suppression columns, one ear is dominant, and sound stimuli reaching this ear elicit a response that is greater than the binaural response. The physiological significance of these columns is not yet well understood.

The second significant point about the auditory cortex is its pattern of callosal connections. These connections can be studied by analyzing radioactive amino acid transport from one auditory cortex to its counterpart in the opposite hemisphere. Cortical bands that receive callosal connections are interspersed with zones that do not receive them (Figure 31–15). These bands branch and occasionally appear to join one another in a manner similar to the ocular dominance columns (see Chapter 29).

A third point of interest relates to lesions of the auditory cortex. Because there is extensive bilateral representation of each ear in both hemispheres, unilateral lesions of the auditory cortex do not disrupt the *perception of sound frequency* dramatically. But such lesions *do affect* the ability to *localize sounds in space*. An individual hemisphere is concerned principally with localizing sounds coming from the contralateral auditory hemifield; that is, the auditory cortex on the right side is important for localizing sounds arising from the left hemifield. To localize the position of a sound source, the auditory cortex utilizes the cues of interaural differences in sound intensity and interaural differences in the time of sound arrival only. Large lesions of the auditory cortex begin to affect sound-localizing ability to a significant extent. In this way, the auditory cortex differs from the primary visual cortex, where even small lesions produce noticeable deficits in the perception of the visual field.

The auditory system has an extensive set of *distal feedback connections*. Some cells in the auditory cortex send their axons back to the medial geniculate nucleus, and some back to the inferior colliculus. The inferior colliculus in turn sends recurrent fibers to the cochlear nucleus. A cluster of cells located near the superior olivary nucleus gives rise to the efferent *olivocochlear bundle*, which terminates either on the hair cells of the cochlea directly, or on the afferent fibers innervating them. Although the function of the recurrent connections is not fully understood, they are thought to be important for regulating selective attention to particular sounds.

An Overall View

The auditory system is equipped with a mechanical device, the cochlea, that performs a Fourier analysis on incoming sounds, breaking them down into simpler frequency components. The hair cells of the cochlea are tuned both mechanically and electrically, properties that enable them to transduce particular frequencies of sound into activity in auditory nerve fibers. The auditory pathways of the brain provide us with the ability to detect sounds of different pitch, loudness, and points of origin in space. We also have the ability to attend selectively to sounds of particular interest. Thus, the auditory system provides us with all the sensory capacities necessary to analyze complex sounds such as human speech.

Selected Readings

Brodal, A. 1981. Neurological Anatomy in Relation to Clinical Medicine, 3rd ed. New York: Oxford University Press, chap. 9.

See the following reviews in I. Darian-Smith (ed.), 1984, Handbook of Physiology; The Nervous System, Vol. III, Sensory Processes. Bethesda, Md.: American Physiological Society.

Aitkin, L. M., Irvine, D. R. F., and Webster, W. R. Central neural mechanisms of hearing, pp. 675–737.

Dallos, P. Peripheral mechanisms of hearing, pp. 595–637.

Green, D. M., and Wier, C. C. Auditory perception, pp. 557–594.

Kiang, N. Y. S. Peripheral neural processing of auditory information, pp. 639–674.

Goldstein, M. H., Jr. 1980. The auditory periphery. In V. B. Mountcastle (ed.), Medical Physiology, 14th ed. Vol. 1. St. Louis: Mosby, pp. 428–456.

Helmholtz, H. L. F. von. 1877. On the Sensations of Tone (2nd English ed.). New York: Dover, 1954.

Hudspeth, A. J. 1983. Transduction and tuning by vertebrate hair cells. Trends Neurosci. 6(9):366–369.

Imig, T. J., and Adrian, H. O. 1977. Binaural columns in the primary field (AI) of cat auditory cortex. Brain Res. 138:241–257.

Imig, T. J., and Brugge, J. F. 1978. Sources and terminations of callosal axons related to binaural and frequency maps in primary auditory cortex of the cat. J. Comp. Neurol. 182:637–660.

Khanna, S. M., and Leonard, D. G. B. 1982. Basilar membrane tuning in the cat cochlea. Science 215:305–306.

Kiang, N. Y.-S. 1965. Discharge Patterns of Single Fibers in the Cat's Auditory Nerve. Cambridge, Mass.: MIT Press.

Lorente de Nó, R. 1933. Anatomy of the eighth nerve. III. General plan of structure of the primary cochlear nuclei. Laryngoscope 43:327–350.

Merzenich, M. M., and Reid, M. D. 1974. Representation of the cochlea within the inferior colliculus of the cat. Brain Res. 77:397–415.

Morest, D. K. 1964. The laminar structure of the inferior colliculus of the cat. Anat. Rec. 148:314.

Rhode, W. S. 1971. Observations of the vibration of the basilar membrane in squirrel monkeys using the Mössbauer technique. J. Acoust. Soc. Am. 49:1218–1231.

References

Brugge, J. F., and Merzenich, M. M. 1973. Responses of neurons in the auditory cortex of the macaque monkey to monaural and binaural stimulation. J. Neurophysiol. 36:1138–1158.

Crawford, A. C., and Fettiplace, R. 1981. An electrical tuning mechanism in turtle cochlear hair cells. J. Physiol. (Lond.) 312:377–412.

Goldberg, J. M., and Brown, P. B. 1969. Response of binaural neurons of dog superior olivary complex to dichotic tonal stimuli: Some physiological mechanisms of sound localization. J. Neurophysiol. 32:613–636.

Lewis, R. S., and Hudspeth, A. J. 1983. Frequency tuning and ionic conductances in hair cells of the bullfrog's sacculus. In R. Klinke and R. Hartmann (eds.), Hearing—Physiological Bases and Psychophysics. Berlin: Springer, pp. 17–24.

Miller, J. M., and Towe, A. L. 1979. Audition: Structural and acoustical properties. In T. Ruch and H. D. Patton (eds.), Physiology and Biophysics, Vol. 1. The Brain and Neural Function, 20th ed. Philadelphia: Saunders, pp. 339–375.

Ranson, S. W., and Clark, S. L. 1953. The Anatomy of the Nervous System: Its Development and Function, 9th ed. Philadelphia: Saunders.

Stotler, W. A. 1953. An experimental study of the cells and connections of the superior olivary complex of the cat. J. Comp. Neurol. 98:401–431.

von Békésy, G. 1960. Experiments in Hearing. New York: McGraw-Hill.

Wersäll, J., Flock, Å., and Lundquist, P.-G. 1965. Structural basis for directional sensitivity in cochlear and vestibular sensory receptors. Cold Spring Harbor Symp. Quant. Biol. 30:115–132.

Vincent F. Castellucci

The Chemical Senses: Taste and Smell

32

And soon, mechanically, weary after a dull day with the prospect of a depressing morrow, I raised to my lips a spoonful of the tea in which I had soaked a morsel of the cake. No sooner had the warm liquid, and the crumbs with it, touched my palate than a shudder ran through my whole body, and I stopped, intent upon the extraordinary changes that were taking place. . . . I was conscious that it was connected with the taste of tea and cake, but that it infinitely transcended those savors, could not, indeed, be of the same nature of theirs.

. . .When from a long-distant past nothing subsists, after the people are dead, after the things are broken and scattered, still, alone, more fragile, but with more vitality, more unsubstantial, more persistent, more faithful, the smell and taste of things remain poised a long time, like souls, ready to remind us . . .

Proust, *Remembrance of Things Past*

We are continuously bombarded by molecules released into our environment. They signal pleasure or danger and inform us about food, drink, or the presence of something to seek or avoid. Unlike the senses we have so far considered (somatic sensitivity, vision, and hearing), which tell us about the external world, taste and smell have a special dual role. Taste and smell also inform us about the external world, but in addition they connect that perception with privileged information about our internal environment, its needs, and its satisfactions: hunger, thirst, sex, and satiety.

Taste and smell are phylogenetically primitive sensibilities. The sense of smell, for example, is unique among the sensory systems in that its central connections first project to phylogenetically older portions of the cerebral cortex before going to the thalamus and neocortex. Taste and smell also have access to neural circuitry that controls both feeling states of the body and certain memories. As illustrated by the passage from Proust quoted above, special memories spring to mind in response to a particular taste, a special aroma.

Even simple organisms have chemical senses and respond to chemical messages. For each animal, the task is fundamentally the same. A molecule or a mixture of molecules activates a specific receptor, and a message is generated and transmitted to subsequent groups of cells to be decoded and analyzed so that an appropriate response is emitted.

In this chapter we shall consider how chemical messages are received by the organs of taste and smell and how this information is conveyed to our consciousness; in so doing we shall examine the ways chemical messages are coded by the nervous system. We shall also look at aspects of the behavioral importance of the chemical senses.

Taste Receptors in the Tongue Are Specialized for Certain Taste Qualities

Four Basic Taste Qualities Can Be Delineated

Students of wine insist that they can distinguish more than 100 different components of taste in a wine. The sensation of wine or of food is based on the activation not only of taste receptors but also of olfactory receptors stimulated by the bouquet of the wine or the aroma of the food. Even when we restrict our perspective to taste

alone, food or drink is capable of activating many taste sensations. It was the German psychophysicist Hans Henning who first showed in 1927 that richness in tasting is achieved by a combinatorial mechanism. In controlled psychophysical experiments, he found that all tastes can be accounted for by combinations of four basic qualities: bitter, salty, sour, and sweet.

How are these basic qualities perceived? The oral cavity, especially the tongue, contains gustatory receptors that are preferentially sensitive to the chemical configuration of certain molecules present in the surrounding fluids. Not all of the four qualities can be perceived equally well by all parts of the oral cavity. For example, the ability to recognize each of the four qualities is differentially distributed on the tongue. Thus, although the tip is responsive to all four qualities, it is particularly sensitive to sweet and salty tastes. The lateral part of the tongue is responsive to sour tastes. The back of the tongue is responsive to bitter tastes. Actually, the bitter taste threshold is higher in the back than in the front, but receptors on the soft palate have the lowest threshold; this gives the illusion that the bitter threshold is lowest in the back of the mouth (Figure 32–1A).

Transduction Requires the Binding of Molecules to Specific Receptors on Taste Cells

A molecule that stimulates a particular taste sensation binds to the cell membrane of a receptor cell at specific recognition (receptor) sites (Figure 32–2). These sites rec-

32–1 Taste sensitivity, cranial nerve innervation, and papilla type differ in different regions of the human tongue. **A.** Lowest threshold regions for sweet, salty, sour, and bitter tastes in the human tongue. **B.** Innervation pattern of the tongue. The taste buds of the anterior two-thirds of the tongue are innervated by the afferent fibers that travel in a branch of the facial nerve (VII) called the chorda tympani. The taste buds

of the posterior third of the tongue are innervated by afferent fibers that travel in the lingual branch of the glossopharyngeal nerve (IX). **C.** Schematic cross sections of the main types of taste papillae. **Arrows** from part **B** indicate the areas on the tongue where each type predominates. (Adapted from Shepherd, 1983.)

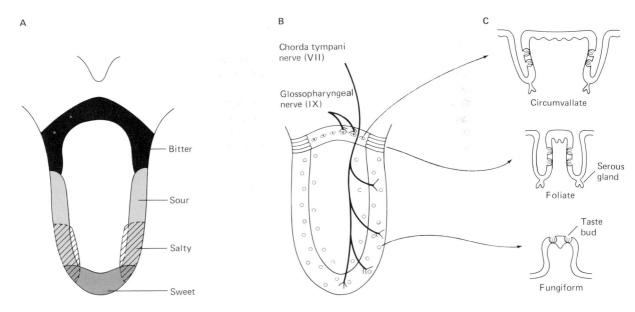

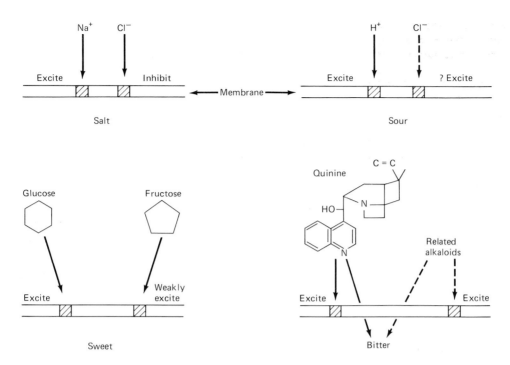

32–2 These simplified models illustrate hypothetical transducer mechanisms in the membranes of taste bud cells for reception of the four taste modalities. Salt perception is elicited by NaCl, which, according to this scheme, produces a biphasic response, with Na$^+$ exciting the receptor cell and Cl$^-$ inhibiting it. Acids stimulate the receptors that recognize sour sensation, with protons (H$^+$) and possibly also anions (Cl$^-$) exciting the receptors. Sugars excite the sweet receptors; quinine and related alkaloids (natural nitrogenous substances found in plants) excite the bitter receptors. In the case of bitter taste, the substance may not simply act on an external membrane receptor but may also be taken up into the cell to produce its effect. (Adapted from Murray, 1973.)

ognize the configuration of that molecule. Binding of the molecule to the recognition site produces a change in ion channels and a corresponding change in membrane potential. When a certain voltage threshold is reached, an action potential is triggered in the afferent fiber that synapses on the receptor cell. The *salt* taste is produced in its purest form by NaCl. *Sourness* is produced by acids. The active component for inorganic acids is the proton, but for organic acids sourness may also depend on the anion. *Sweetness* is believed to depend on the stereochemical configuration of glucose; the organic molecules with related conformations also can stimulate the specific membrane receptors for sweetness. Up to five different types of sweet receptors are currently recognized. The *bitter* taste is elicited by quinine or by toxic plants and other poisonous substances. It is not known what functional groups are responsible for the sensation of bitterness.

Taste Receptor Cells Contained in Papillae Are Embedded in Taste Buds

Gustatory receptor cells are not present in the tongue as isolated free nerve endings. Rather, these receptors are modified epithelial cells that are bundled into groups of about 50 and contained in a complex sensory organ called a *taste bud*. In turn, specialized structures called papillae contain clusters of taste buds. Each taste bud contains two other types of cells: *supporting cells* and *basal cells* (Figure 32–3). The taste receptor cells are constantly turning over at a rate of once every 10 days. To keep pace with the continual degeneration of the receptors, basal cells differentiate into supporting cells, which in turn continuously differentiate into receptor cells. The bud is embedded in the epithelium of the tongue and connected to the tongue's surface by a minute canal called a *taste pore*. Small processes *(microvilli)*, thought to be the sites of sensory transduction, extend from the apical surface of each taste receptor. The microvilli emerge through the taste pore to contact the saliva covering the tongue.

Each receptor cell is innervated at its base by an afferent nerve fiber. The contact between the receptor and the afferent nerve fiber has all the characteristics of a chemical synapse: vesicles cluster in the receptor cell, and the nerve terminal membranes straighten out where the terminal comes into apposition with the membrane of the receptor cell (Figure 32–3B). An afferent fiber branches many times before reaching the base of the taste bud, so that one fiber often innervates several taste buds and many receptor cells within each taste bud. Thus, the electrical activity recorded from a single afferent fiber represents the signals from many receptors.

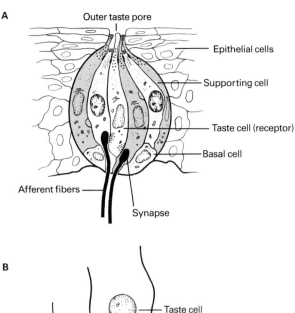

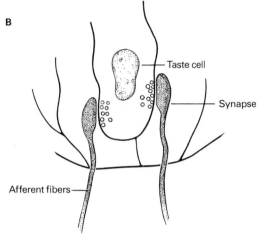

32–3 Taste receptor cells are contained in taste buds.
    A. The taste bud contains three types of cells: basal, supporting, and receptor cells. There is a continuous turnover of receptor cells to keep pace with their continual degeneration. Basal cells differentiate into supporting cells, which in turn give rise to new taste cells. Taste cells are innervated at their base. **B.** The contact between the receptor cell and the afferent nerve has the characteristics of a chemical synapse: clustering of vesicles and parallel membranes at the zone of apposition. (Adapted from Murray, 1973.)

The taste buds in the anterior two-thirds of the tongue (Figure 32–1B) are innervated by afferent fibers that travel in the chorda tympani, a branch of the facial nerve (cranial nerve VII). The cell bodies of these fibers lie in the geniculate ganglion. The taste buds of the posterior third of the tongue (Figure 32–1B) are innervated by afferent fibers that travel in the lingual branch of the glossopharyngeal nerve (cranial nerve IX) with cell bodies in the petrosal ganglion. Innervation of the taste bud is crucial for the maintenance of the receptor cells. If the chorda tympani nerve is severed, for example, all of the taste buds innervated by the nerve degenerate. Bruce Oakley and his colleagues at the University of Michigan have shown that, if normal axonal transport in the afferent nerve is blocked, taste buds start to degenerate.

Humans have three types of papillae: fungiform, foliate, and circumvallate (Figure 32–1C). *Fungiform papillae* look like small, blunt mushrooms. Several hundred of them are located on the anterior two thirds of the tongue. Each fungiform papilla contains one to five taste buds on its dorsal surface, and its receptors respond primarily to *sweet and salty*, but also to *sour stimuli*. The chorda tympani innervates the fungiform papillae. The *foliate papillae* form folds or leaves on the posterior edge of the tongue and respond best to *sour stimuli*. The *circumvallate papillae*, large round structures surrounded by a groove, are located in the posterior third of the tongue and respond primarily to *bitter stimuli*. Thousands of taste buds are located in the folds of foliate papillae or the grooves of the circumvallate papillae; they are innervated by the glossopharyngeal nerve.

In addition to the tongue, there are also taste buds in the epiglottis, in the upper third of the esophagus, and on the palate. The taste buds on the palate are innervated by the greater superficial petrosal branch of cranial nerve VII, and the buds on the epiglottis and esophagus by the superior laryngeal nerve—a branch of the vagus nerve (cranial nerve X). In young children, the mucosa of the cheeks contains some taste buds.

The Central Pathway of the Taste System Involves Distinct Representations in the Thalamus and Cortex

The flow of gustatory information can be traced from the taste buds of the oral cavity to the cerebral cortex. As with somatic, visual, and auditory information that enters conscious perception, information for taste reaches the cerebral cortex by first being relayed in the thalamus. Unlike the other sensory pathways, however, including the somatic sensory pathway from the tongue, the gustatory pathway is distinctive in that most of its fibers are uncrossed.

The first synapse of the taste system is, as we have seen, in the taste bud itself. Here, individual receptor cells synapse on the terminals of the taste afferents (Figure 32–4). The afferent fibers from the taste buds run in cranial nerves VII, IX, and X and enter the solitary tract of the medulla. All the afferent fibers then synapse on a thin column of cells in the rostral part of the *solitary nuclear complex* called the *gustatory nucleus*. The solitary nuclear complex is an important visceral relay nucleus because neurons in its caudal part relay afferent information from the gut, lungs, and cardiovascular system to more rostral brain stem nuclei.

The cells of the gustatory nucleus, in turn, project primarily ipsilaterally to the thalamus and end on the small-cell (parvocellular) part of the *ventral posterior medial nucleus*. There, the cells subserving taste are grouped separately from neurons related to other sensory modalities of the tongue. The neurons of this nucleus then project to the postcentral gyrus of the cerebral cortex. This cortical gustatory area lies ventral and rostral to the somesthetic representation of the tongue. Thus,

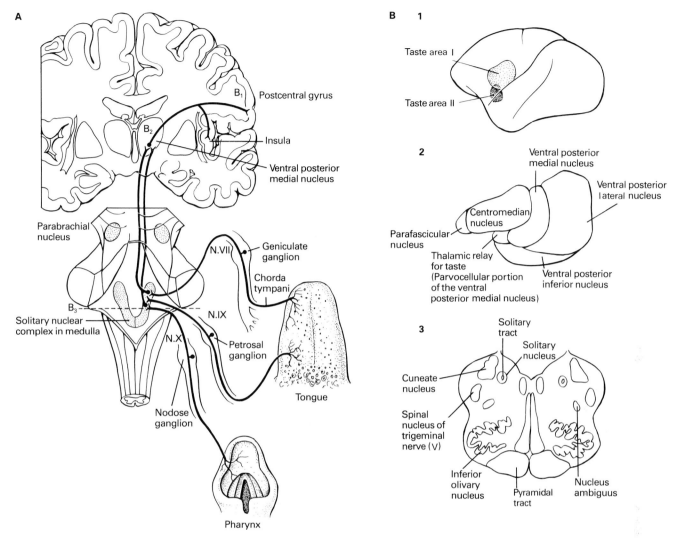

32-4 Taste information is transmitted from the taste buds in the tongue to the cerebral cortex via synapses in the brain stem and thalamus. **A.** Tongue innervation and central pathway of the taste system derived from studies in the monkey. **B.** Details of areas numbered in **A. 1.** Composite maps for projection areas for the chorda tympani and glossopharyngeal nerves. **Stippled region** delineates taste area I.

Solid area is in the insular projection area projected onto the lateral surface of the hemisphere. 2. Coronal section through the thalamus at the level of the gustatory thalamic relay, the parvocellular portion of the ventral posterior medial nucleus. 3. Cross section through the medulla showing the solitary tract and the location of the solitary nucleus. (Adapted from Burton and Benjamin, 1971.)

gustatory information, which is represented in a distinct area in the thalamus, also has a distinct representation in the cortex. Another cortical gustatory area is located in the insular cortex. Lesions of the cortical gustatory areas, the small-cell part of the ventral posterior medial nucleus, or the rostral part of the solitary nucleus impair taste sensibility.

From the medulla, the gustatory pathway also projects largely ipsilaterally to the pontine taste area (parabrachial nuclei), which in turn projects to the limbic system and the hypothalamus. This part of the gustatory pathway may be important for the affective qualities of taste perception.

Taste Sensation Is Coded by Labeled Lines and Patterns of Activity across Labeled Lines

How can we distinguish various types of gustatory stimuli? Does each primary quality (bitter, salty, sour, and sweet) have a "private line" that carries its specific message from the receptors in the taste buds to successive taste centers of the central nervous system? Does a single taste afferent specifically recognize a sugar molecule as being sweet rather than bitter? If so, is this specificity for the quality maintained through the medulla, the thalamus, and the cortex, as is the case for somatic information from the tongue such as touch?

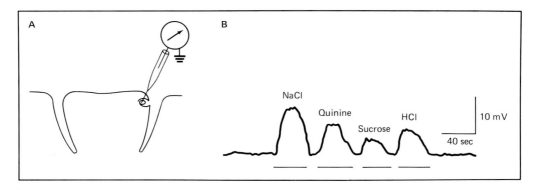

32–5 Receptor potentials recorded from a hamster taste receptor show that it responds to four types of stimuli applied to the tongue surface. **A.** Recording setup. **B.** Typical responses to each of the four basic taste sensations. (From Kimura and Beidler, 1961.)

These questions were first rigorously examined in 1941, when Carl Pfaffmann, then a doctoral student in Edgar Adrian's laboratory at Cambridge University, began a series of cellular studies on the taste system designed to explore the physiological basis of the four basic taste sensations. In a now classic experiment, Pfaffmann recorded from single fibers in the chorda tympani of the cat and found, surprisingly, that a single fiber responds not to one but to several different chemical stimuli. For example, fibers that respond to salt also respond to acid, and fibers that respond to acid also respond to bitterness. Each taste is not simply carried by a set of fibers that respond only to that *one* taste quality; rather, each taste seems to involve a comparison of the pattern of activation in all fibers of the population. Pfaffmann's experiments led to the formulation of the *across-fiber pattern coding theory* for taste perception. According to this theory a central comparator set of neurons receives input from a whole population of taste elements and reads out, or decodes, the pattern of activity generated within the population by each taste stimulus.

Since a given taste fiber receives synaptic signals within the taste bud from several receptor cells, Pfaffmann's discovery raised a further question: Is the response of the afferent fiber polysensory because it innervates several receptors, each of which responds exclusively to only one type of basic taste? Or can each receptor cell respond to more than one chemical stimulus? To answer this question, Katsumi Kimura and Lloyd Beidler at the University of Florida in Tallahassee obtained intracellular recordings from individual receptor cells in the 1960s. They found that even individual taste receptor cells respond not only to one but to two, three, or even all four taste qualities (Figure 32–5). The taste receptors respond to stimuli with graded receptor potentials much like those of the Pacinian corpuscle and other receptor cells. As the concentration of the taste molecule increases, the response becomes larger.

These results strengthened the idea that taste perception is encoded in the pattern generated by all the active fibers in the population. According to this scheme, specific receptor cells in taste buds and afferent fibers each have their preferred stimulus, but at each level there is significant responsiveness to other stimulus types.

Recent, more detailed experiments by Pfaffmann's students, Marion Frank, David Smith, and their colleagues, indicate that taste perception also has an important labeled line component. Even though no fiber ever shows an *absolute sensitivity* to one taste, almost all fibers show much greater sensitivity to one taste than to the others (Figure 32–6). More important, the most effective stimulus predicts the order of effectiveness of other stimuli. Thus, although the neurons in the taste system are broadly rather than finely discriminating, they clearly are able to discriminate. The fact that they are preferentially responsive to one of the four basic taste qualities indicates that particular tastes are carried along specific pathways akin to the labeled lines prominent in other sensory systems.

Because the discrimination is broad, however, ambiguities could arise in the thalamus and cortex if the cells in these regions were given only the information carried by each labeled line. For example, although one fiber is highly selective for sugar, another fiber not primarily responsive to sugar might also increase its rate of firing as the concentration of sugar is increased. As a result, if sufficiently different concentrations of test chemicals are present simultaneously on different areas of the tongue, both the sugar-sensitive neuron and the relatively sugar-insensitive neuron might respond at the same frequency. The sugar-sensitive neuron might double its firing frequency with an increase in sugar of just 10% above threshold. The sugar-insensitive cell might double its frequency with a 100% increase. The nervous system therefore could not infer an absolute concentration of sweetness by reading only fibers that double their rate of firing, because that same doubling can be achieved by nonsweet fibers in response to a high concentration of sugar. For unambiguous coding of sweetness, higher regions of the brain must read activity not only in the line labeled for sweet, but also in the line la-

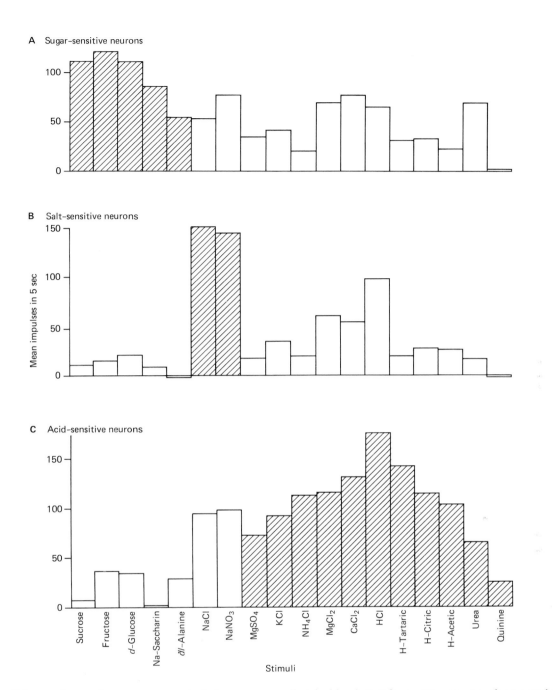

32–6 Three different classes of neurons are particularly sensitive to different types of stimuli. Mean response of each neuronal class is shown for each of 18 stimulus compounds. **A.** Sugar-sensitive neurons are predominantly sensitive to sucrose and other sweet-tasting compounds **(hatched bars). B.** Salt-sensitive neurons show a preference for sodium salts **(hatched bars). C.** Acid-sensitive neurons are most sensitive to nonsodium salts and acids **(hatched bars).** (From Smith et al., 1983.)

beled for the other qualities of taste. Thus, although taste is based on labeled lines, the broad potential for responsiveness of each channel requires that the information for a given taste be determined not only by the output of the line specific for that taste but also by comparison of the activity in that line with the activities in other lines (Figure 32–7).

Viewed from this perspective, the coding in taste resembles the coding in other sensory systems. In the auditory system afferent fibers and cortical cells have a preferred frequency but also respond to other frequencies. Late steps in the processing of audition must involve a comparison of the activity of different cells with different preferred frequencies. Similarly, the three different

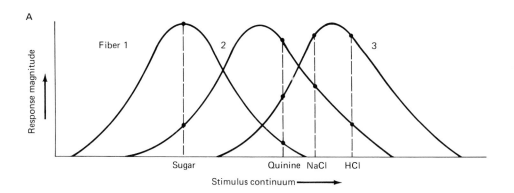

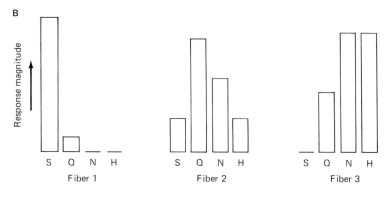

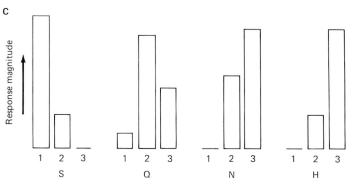

32–7 Because each channel in the taste system is broadly tuned, a given taste is not determined by the output of one labeled line but by a comparison of the activity in that line with the activities in other lines.

A. To illustrate this concept, let us consider idealized response curves of three hypothetical afferent fiber types (**1, 2, 3**) along a continuous stimulus dimension. We can select four stimuli along this stimulus dimension: sugar (**S**), quinine (**Q**), NaCl (**N**), and HCl (**H**). The responsiveness of a cell type to one of these stimuli is indicated by the intersection of the response curve (**solid line**) and the ordinate (**broken line**) erected at the chosen stimulus.

B. One neuron cannot adequately represent a stimulus because there is ambiguity at times. For example, fibers 1 and 3 cannot distinguish **N** from **H**. Fiber **2** cannot distinguish **S** from **H**.

C. Across-fiber patterns, however, are unique for each stimulus. (Adapted from Erickson, 1968.)

photopigments in the photoreceptors are broadly tuned across the visual spectrum. Although each photopigment has a peak at three specific points in the continuum of wavelengths, activity in any one receptor alone is inadequate to provide information about color discrimination. Thus, as we have seen, color information comes not from stimulation of an individual cone system but from the analysis of the outputs of all three cone systems. Indeed, even in the recognition of form in the absence of color, the visual system reads contrast. What appeared initially to be a mechanism of coding peculiar to taste—analysis across fibers—is now also seen as an analysis of contrast that is characteristic of other sensory systems. All sensory systems use a modified labeled line code for perception; all higher relays must compare the activities of different pathways.

Both Inborn and Learned Taste Preferences Are Important for Behavior

Taste and smell exercise profound control over food and water intake. An observation that first called attention to this aspect of taste perception was the discovery of *specific hunger* by Curt Richter in 1940. A psychologist at the Johns Hopkins Medical School, Richter reported that animals have an inborn ability to compensate for deficiencies in their diet by selecting foods that contain the missing nutrient. Most dramatic was the discovery of an *innate hunger for salt*. Richter encountered this hunger in a child whose adrenal cortex had been destroyed by a tumor. As a result, the child had lost the ability to secrete adrenal cortical hormones that maintain normal salt balance in the body, and thus was constantly deprived of salt. He lost much of his salt in urine and maintained little in the body. Richter found that, given unlimited access to food, this child compensated for his salt deficiency by an extraordinary craving for salt. Richter also found a similar craving in rats whose adrenal glands were surgically removed. Recently, Robert Contreras at Yale University found that removal of the adrenal gland makes the salt receptors in the tongue less sensitive to salt.

Certain Aspects of Taste Perception Are Genetically Determined

Some differences in the ability to taste are genetic. For example, the aromatic sulfur-containing compound phenylthiourea produces a bitter taste, which is due to the N—C≡S group. Sensitivity to this molecule is genetically determined. On the basis of their ability to sense phenylthiourea as bitter, people can be divided into either "tasters" or "nontasters." Nontasters can perceive sweet, sour, salty, and all bitter substances except those containing the N—C≡S group. The difference between nontasters and tasters is thought to result from the presence or absence of a particular receptor protein on the surface of the tongue. The ability to taste phenylthiourea is a dominant trait, which is either homozygous or heterozygous. Nontasters carry two recessive genes.

A more serious genetic disorder of taste is familial dysautonomia, a neurological disease characterized by a variety of autonomic disturbances. In this disease, most of the gustatory papillae and taste buds are absent.

Taste-Aversion Learning Is Demonstrated by the "Sauce Béarnaise" Phenomenon

Hunger for salt and for certain other foods is inborn, but we also learn to prefer some foods and to avoid others. A particularly powerful demonstration of this phenomenon has come from the work of John Garcia at the University of California at Los Angeles. In experiments we shall consider again later, Garcia exposed rats to two stimuli: a specific taste and an auditory stimulus, a tone. He paired the two stimuli with a mild poison that produced nausea. Even though the poison was paired with both the taste of the food and the tone, only the taste became aversive. From then on, the animal invariably avoided food with that particular taste. In a complementary experiment, Garcia gave rats the same two stimuli (taste of food and tone) but now paired them with a shock to the foot. Only the tone and not the taste became aversive.

This experiment illustrates that animals have evolved brain mechanisms that enable them to associate taste (and not other sensory modalities) with nausea and stomach illness. The evolutionary advantage that this specific learning ability would provide is obvious: animals that are poisoned by a distinctively flavored food and survive do well not to eat it again.

Food avoidance learning is not unique to lower animals but occurs commonly in our own everyday life, as the psychologist Martin Seligman has described so vividly:

Sauce Béarnaise is an egg-thickened, tarragon-flavored concoction, and it used to be my favorite sauce. It now tastes awful to me. This happened several years ago, when I felt the effects of the stomach flu about six hours after eating filet mignon with sauce Béarnaise. I became violently ill and spent most of the night vomiting. The next time I had sauce Béarnaise, I couldn't bear the taste of it. At the time, I had no ready way to account for the change, although it seemed to fit a classical conditioning paradigm: conditioned stimulus (sauce) paired with unconditioned stimulus (illness) and unconditioned response (vomiting) yields conditioned response (nauseating taste). But if this was classical conditioning, it violated at least two Pavlovian laws: The delay between tasting the sauce and vomiting was about 6 hours, and classical conditioning isn't supposed to bridge time gaps like that. In addition, neither the filet mignon, nor the white plate off which I ate the sauce, nor *Tristan und Isolde*, the opera that I listened to in the interpolated time, nor my wife, Kerry, became aversive. Only the sauce Béarnaise did. Moreover, unlike much of classical conditioning, it could not be seen as a "cognitive" phenomenon, involving expectations. For I soon found out that the sauce had not caused the vomiting and that a stomach flu had . . . . Yet in spite of this knowledge, I could not later inhibit my aversion.

(Martin Seligman, in *Biological Boundaries of Learning*)

Olfactory Receptors Have Receptor Sites Specialized for Certain Odors

There Are at Least Seven Primary Odors, Probably More

The discriminative capability of the olfactory system is remarkable: humans (by no means the most accomplished sensors among animals) can distinguish between thousands of odoriferous chemicals. Moreover, the olfactory system is extremely sensitive. We can detect the presence of as few as 10^8 molecules of an odorant in a room. Dogs, of course, are much more sensitive. A well-trained dog can be taught rapidly to recognize the distinctive odor of a single person. However, the threshold for detection of an odor is much lower than the threshold for specific recognition. At very low concentrations of an odor, the sensation is unspecific; only at higher concentrations can the odor be identified precisely.

One of the most serious problems in the study of olfaction has been to define the odorant molecules and to classify chemicals into a set of primary odors. One might intuitively think that all similar molecular structures are experienced as similar odors. On the basis of Henning's success with primary tastes, John Amoore and his colleagues examined over 600 odoriferous substances and proposed that there are at least 7 primary odors: camphoraceous, musk, floral, peppermint, ethereal, pungent, and putrid (Figure 32–8). All of the substances within a particular category have common molecular configurations. Although many odors fall within these seven categories, there are, nonetheless, many exceptions to Amoore's scheme: similar odors are not always produced by molecules with similar structures.

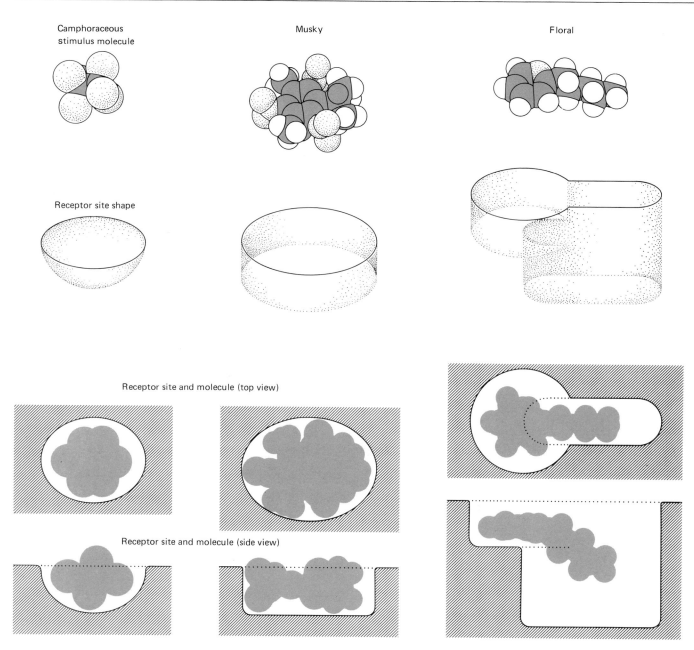

32–8 According to the stereochemical theory of odor, there are seven primary odors, and there are receptor sites of a distinct shape and size to match each of these odors; each site accepts only molecules of the appropriate configuration.

Molecules representative of each odor and their receptor sites are shown. Note that pungent and putrid molecules fit because of charge, not shape. (From Amoore, Johnston, and Rubin, 1964.)

Olfactory Receptors Lie within the Olfactory Epithelium

The sense of smell is carried by olfactory receptors that lie deep within the nasal cavity. In humans, the receptors are confined to a yellowish brown patch of specialized epithe-lium, the olfactory epithelium, covering roughly 5 cm² of the dorsal recess of the nasal cavity (Figure 32–9). This epi-thelium contains three types of cells: the *receptor*, the *supporting*, and the *basal* cells (Figure 32–10). The recep-tor cells are themselves bipolar neurons that have a short peripheral process and a long central process.

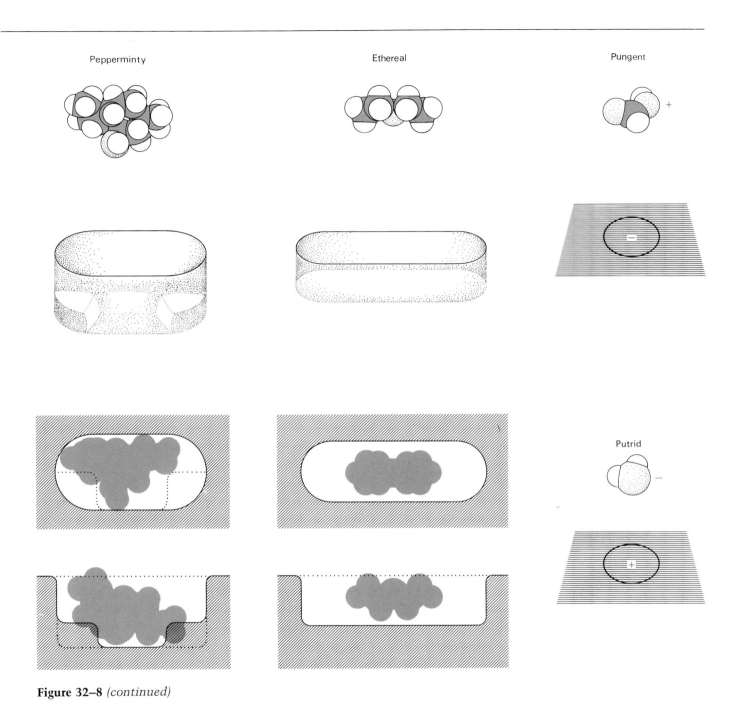

Figure 32–8 *(continued)*

The *short peripheral* process extends to the surface of the mucosa, where it expands into a small knob that gives rise to several cilia. These cilia form a dense mat at the mucosal surface and are thought to interact with odor-producing molecules. The *longer central* process, an unmyelinated axon, runs from the nasal cavity to the part of the brain called the *olfactory bulb*. Between 10 and 100 of these axons form a bundle that is surrounded by Schwann cell processes. Collectively, these bundles of axons are known as the *olfactory nerve*, the first cranial nerve. To reach the bulb the axon goes through the cribriform plate of the ethmoid bone. The olfactory bulb is a

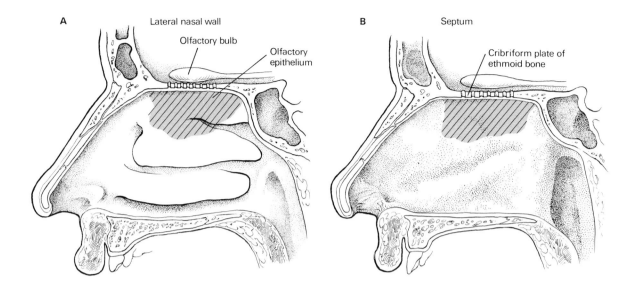

A   Lateral nasal wall

Olfactory bulb

Olfactory
epithelium

B   Septum

Cribriform plate of
ethmoid bone

32–9   The location of the olfactory epithelium in the nasal cavity is shown by the **striped** area. The olfactory bulb is a small, flattened ovoid body that rests on the cribriform plate of the ethmoid bone. **A.** Lateral nasal wall. **B.** Septum.

32–10   The vertebrate olfactory epithelium contains receptor, supporting, and basal cells. (From Andres, 1966.)

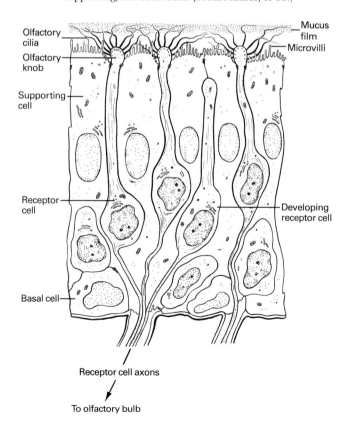

Olfactory cilia

Olfactory knob

Supporting cell

Receptor cell

Basal cell

Mucus film

Microvilli

Developing receptor cell

Receptor cell axons

To olfactory bulb

part of the central nervous system that develops from the telencephalon. There are two symmetrical olfactory bulbs serving the olfactory mucosa of the two nasal cavities. Thus, unlike the other sensory modalities, the olfactory pathway is distinguished by the fact that *the first synapse is in the telencephalon.*

There are more than 100 million olfactory receptor cells. Like taste receptors, the olfactory receptors turn over rapidly; they are generated anew every 60 days from precursor basal cells. The regeneration of the olfactory receptor is even more remarkable than that of the taste receptor because the olfactory receptor cells are neurons and have axons. Indeed, they are the only known neurons of the adult nervous system that are capable of mitotic division. The developing cell must send its newly formed dendrite toward the mucosal surface and its axon in the opposite direction to synapse appropriately in the olfactory bulb.

Neuronal Coding for Olfaction Involves a Novel Use of Neural Space

As in taste reception, odoriferous molecules stimulate olfactory cells by first being absorbed into the mucous layer. The molecules then diffuse to the cilia of the receptor neurons and bind to specific molecular recognition sites having a distinct shape and size. The binding of a specific odorant to a molecular recognition site on the receptor cell is thought to open ion channels specific to Na$^+$ and K$^+$ and thereby to generate a depolarizing receptor potential. The receptor cells are spontaneously active. The receptor potential produced by appropriate olfactory stimulation causes an increase in the rate of impulse firing, which is graded; strong olfactory stimulation increases the receptor potential and the frequency of firing (Figures 32–11 and 32–12). The epithelial supporting cells that surround the receptor also respond to odor stimulation with a small depolarization or hyperpolarization, but these cells do not generate action po-

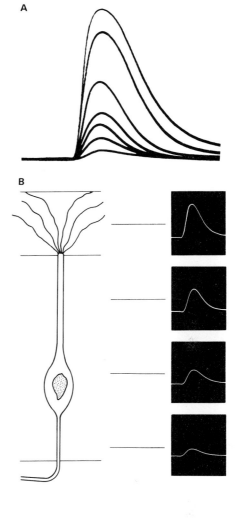

32–11 Electroolfactogram recordings represent the evoked activity of many receptor cells recorded extracellularly. **A.** The amplitude of the electroolfactogram increases with increasing intensities of odor stimulation. **B.** Recordings at different depths of the olfactory mucosa (Figure 32–10) show that the largest response is obtained in the outermost layer; this provides evidence that the activity being recorded is produced by the cilia. (Adapted from Ottoson, 1971.)

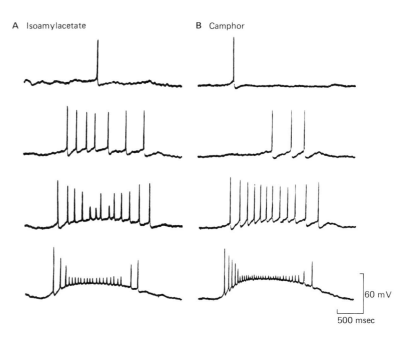

32–12 Intracellular recordings from an olfactory receptor. The rate of impulse firing of the receptor increases with increasing concentrations (**from top trace down**) of odorant molecules. **A.** Responses to increasing concentrations of isoamylacetate. **B.** Responses to increasing concentrations of camphor. (From Trotier and MacLeod, 1983.)

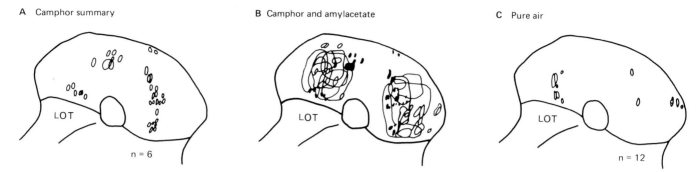

A Camphor summary

B Camphor and amylacetate

C Pure air

LOT

LOT

LOT

n = 6

n = 12

32–13 Different odors elicit different degrees of activity in different regions of the olfactory bulb. Density patterns of 2-deoxyglucose label produced in the glomerular layer of the olfactory bulb by stimulation with camphor odor are compared with those produced by amylacetate odor and

pure air. **A.** Summary map of 6 experiments using camphor. **B.** Comparison of summary maps of camphor (**dark areas**) and amylacetate. **C.** Summary map of 12 experiments using filtered air as a stimulus. LOT, lateral olfactory tract. (Adapted from Stewart, Kauer, and Shepherd, 1979.)

tentials. Their graded potentials may be related to the production of mucus.

How is a specific molecule recognized by the organism? Outside of the laboratory we almost always encounter not a single type but a complex mixture of many odorant molecules that potentiate or interfere with each other. How do we recognize one from another? Are there specific receptors for each of the seven or more primary odors? Recent electrophysiological studies by Gordon Shepherd and Thomas Getchell at Yale, using controlled step pulses of odor, indicate that single receptors are often rather well tuned to chemicals of one or even two

32–14 The olfactory bulbs are small, flattened ovoid bodies that rest on the cribriform plate of the ethmoid bone. They are connected to each other by the anterior commissure. (From Ottoson, 1983.)

categories. Using autoradiography with radiolabeled 2-deoxyglucose to map the metabolic activity of neurons, Shepherd and his colleagues William Stewart and John Kauer determined which cells in the olfactory bulb respond to specific odors and thereby provided evidence for a labeled line mechanism similar to that of the taste system. They found that different odors elicit different degrees of activity in different regions of the olfactory bulb. Thus, as in other sensory systems, coding must occur in modified labeled line pathways. In the case of the olfactory nerve, labeled pathways distribute activity to different areas of the olfactory bulb (Figure 32–13).

A corollary of this finding is that neural space is used for a somewhat different purpose in the olfactory system than in other sensory systems. In somatic sensation and vision, the central relays must represent the receptive sheet topographically: neighborhood relations must be preserved. However, the receptive sheet of olfaction has

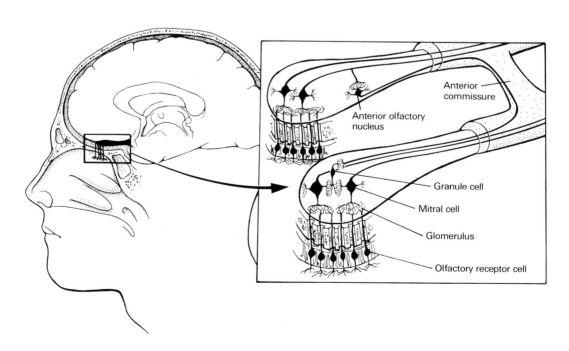

Anterior commissure

Anterior olfactory nucleus

Granule cell

Mitral cell

Glomerulus

Olfactory receptor cell

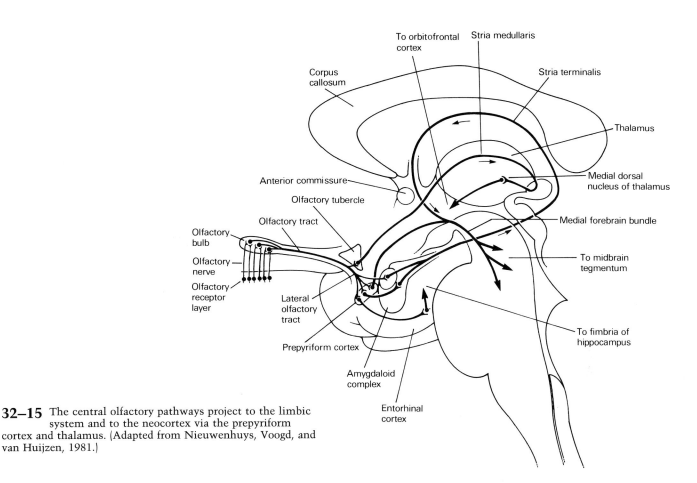

32–15 The central olfactory pathways project to the limbic system and to the neocortex via the prepyriform cortex and thalamus. (Adapted from Nieuwenhuys, Voogd, and van Huijzen, 1981.)

no intrinsic spatial map; rather, we localize olfactory stimuli in space by turning our head. The bulb and higher centers, therefore, use different spatial subregions to represent different odors. Unlike other sensory systems in which central localization is represented topographically as spatial coordinates to the physical world, the bulb and higher centers use their own neural space not to represent the physical space of the outside world, but to order the representation of different basic odors.

The Olfactory System Projects to the Paleocortex Before Relaying to the Neocortex via the Thalamus

What structures in the central nervous system receive information about smell? The small unmyelinated axons of the olfactory receptor neurons terminate in the olfactory bulb, the first relay in the olfactory system (Figures 32–14 and 32–15). Within the olfactory bulb the axons of the olfactory receptors synapse (in specialized spherical synaptic areas called *glomeruli*) with various types of cells, particularly the large mitral cells and the smaller tufted cells that are its main output cells (Figure 32–16). The axons of the mitral and the tufted cells pass in the olfactory tract and are distributed to the secondary olfactory areas called the *olfactory cortex*. This cortex is di-

vided into five parts: (1) the anterior olfactory nucleus (which connects the two olfactory bulbs through a portion of the anterior commissure; Figure 32–14), (2) the olfactory tubercle, (3) the prepyriform cortex (the main olfactory discrimination region), (4) the cortical nucleus of the amygdala, and (5) the entorhinal area, which in turn projects to the hippocampus (Figure 32–15). All of these cortical areas are part of the subdivision of the primitive allocortex called the paleocortex.

It is clear, however, that olfactory processing does not end with the paleocortex. As is the case with all sensory systems, olfactory information is ultimately relayed to the thalamus and the neocortex. The olfactory tubercle projects to the medial dorsal nucleus of the thalamus. This thalamic nucleus in turn projects to the orbitofrontal cortex, that part of the cortex thought to be involved in conscious perception of smell. As in the taste pathway, therefore, the olfactory system has two separate projections, one to the limbic system (the amygdala and hippocampus), the other to the thalamus and neocortex. The amygdala are also relay centers that connect the olfactory cortex to the hypothalamus and the tegmentum of the midbrain. This limbic pathway is thought to mediate the affective component of odoriferous stimuli. In contrast, the thalamus–neocortex projection is involved in the conscious perception of smell. People with lesions

A

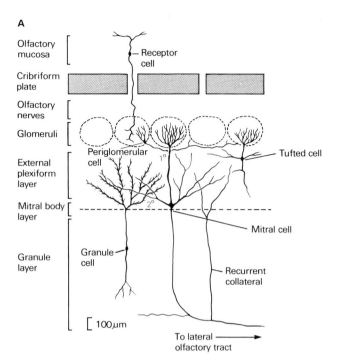

B

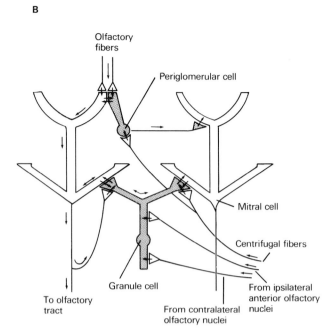

32–16 The mammalian olfactory bulb is organized in layers of cells. **A.** Neuronal elements. The mitral cell, which resembles a bishop's miter in outline, has primary (**1°**) and secondary (**2°**) dendrites and recurrent axon collaterals. There are also tufted cells, periglomerular cells, and granule cells. The bulb is divided into five layers according to the distribution of these elements. (Adapted from Cajal, 1909, and Shepherd, 1972.) **B.** Basic circuit diagram. The olfactory axons terminate in a layer of spherical structures of the neuropil called glomeruli, where they synapse with the mitral cells, the tufted cells, and small inhibitory interneurons called the periglomerular cells. The dendrites of mitral cells and periglomerular cells are synaptically connected. Periglomerular cells distribute their axons to neighboring glomeruli. Secondary dendrites of the mitral cells make and receive synaptic contacts with the dendrites of granule cells. The inhibitory interneurons (periglomerular and granule cells) provide a curtain of inhibition that must be penetrated by the peaks of excitation provided by odorant stimuli. The output of the bulb is carried by the axons of the mitral cells and the tufted cells. Various centrifugal fibers from the central nervous system act directly on the periglomerular and granule cells. (From Shepherd, 1972.)

of the orbitofrontal cortex cannot discriminate odors. Thus, we have in the olfactory system another example of parallel processing.

Abnormalities of Olfaction Vary Greatly in Degree of Sensory Loss

Olfactory acuity varies enormously from person to person. Sensitivity may vary as much as 1000-fold even among people with no obvious abnormality. In the medical literature the term *hyposmia* (diminished sense of smell) is favored for milder olfactory defects that are comparatively general in extent, such as occur during the common head cold. General hyposmia occurs in conjunction with cystic fibrosis of the pancreas and Parkinson's disease. Hyposmia is also found in patients with untreated adrenal insufficiency. *Specific anosmia,* a common olfactory abnormality, is a lowered sensitivity to a single odorant or a few related compounds while perception of most other odors remains normal.

Total loss or an absence of the sense of smell is known as *general anosmia* or simply *anosmia.* The olfactory nerve is utterly inoperative for one or another reason, such as mechanical blockage of the airway, infection, chemical interference with olfactory receptors, or tumor. Olfactory hallucinations, of repugnant smells (cacosmia) occur as part of so-called uncinate fits. This symptom generally indicates an epileptogenic focus in the anterior medial portion of the temporal lobe, where the prepyriform and entorhinal cortices are located. The sense of smell may also diminish during the later decades of life. For example, the threshold for detecting various odorants, including cherry, grape, and lemon, is considerably higher in older people.

An Overall View

Taste and smell are fascinating because they are so vivid emotionally and perceptually and so important nutritionally for the regulation of bodily function. For these reasons, taste and smell were for many years thought to be different from the other senses; however, modern studies have shown that this is not so. The same general rules for coding that we have encountered in the other senses—modified labeled lines, analysis of contrast, and parallel processing—also apply to taste and smell. Thus all sensory systems rely on the same basic principles of processing and organization, not only in humans, but throughout much of phylogeny. Even in the mechanisms of perception, evolution has been remarkably conservative.

Selected Readings

Beidler, L. M. (ed.) 1971. Handbook of Sensory Physiology, Vol. IV: Chemical Senses. Berlin: Springer.

Beidler, L. M. 1980. The chemical senses: Gustation and olfaction. In V. B. Mountcastle (ed.), Medical Physiology, 14th ed., Vol. 1. St. Louis: Mosby, pp. 586–602.

Cajal, S. R. 1909. Histologie du Système Nerveux de l'Homme & des Vertébrés, Vol. 1. L. Azoulay (trans.). Madrid: Instituto Ramón y Cajal, 1952.

Carpenter, M. B., and Sutin, J. 1983. Human Neuroanatomy, 8th ed. Baltimore: Williams & Wilkins.

Engen, T. 1982. The Perception of Odors. New York: Academic Press.

McBurney, D. H. 1984. Taste and olfaction: Sensory discrimination. In I. Darian-Smith (ed.), Handbook of Physiology, Section 1: The Nervous System, Vol. III, Sensory Processes. Bethesda, Md.: American Physiological Society, pp. 1067–1086.

Netter, F. H. 1983. The CIBA Collection of Medical Illustrations. Vol. 1, Nervous System, Part I, Anatomy and Physiology. West Caldwell, N.J.: CIBA.

Nieuwenhuys, R., Voogd, J., and van Huijzen, Chr. 1981. The Human Central Nervous System: A Synopsis and Atlas. Berlin: Springer, pp. 1–253.

Norgren, R. 1984. Central neural mechanisms of taste. In I. Darian-Smith (ed.), Handbook of Physiology, Section 1: The Nervous System, Vol. III, Sensory Processes. Bethesda, Md.: American Physiological Society, pp. 1087–1128.

Ottoson, D. 1983. Physiology of the Nervous System. New York: Oxford University Press.

Pfaff, D. W. (ed.) Taste, Olfaction, and the Central Nervous System. New York: Rockefeller University Press, 1985.

Shepherd, G. M. 1983. Neurobiology. New York: Oxford University Press, chap. 12.

References

Amoore, J. E., Johnston, J. W., Jr., and Rubin, M. 1964. The stereochemical theory of odor. Sci. Am. 210(2):42–49.

Andres, K. H. 1966. Der Feinbau der Regio olfactoria von Makrosmatikern. Z. Zellforsch. 69:140–154.

Burton, H., and Benjamin, R. M. 1971. Central projections of the gustatory system. In L. M. Beidler (ed.), Handbook of Sensory Physiology, Vol. IV: Chemical Senses, Part 2, Taste. Berlin: Springer, pp. 148–164.

Contreras, R. J., 1977. Changes in gustatory nerve discharges with sodium deficiency: A single unit analysis. Brain Res. 121:373–378.

Erickson, R. P. 1968. Stimulus coding in topographic and nontopographic afferent modalities: On the significance of the activity of individual sensory neurons. Psychol. Rev. 75:447–465.

Frank, M. 1973. An analysis of hamster afferent taste nerve response functions. J. Gen. Physiol. 61:588–618.

Frisch, D. 1967. Ultrastructure of mouse olfactory mucosa. Am. J. Anat. 121:87–119.

Garcia, J., Hankins, W. G., and Rusiniak, K. W. 1974. Behavioral regulation of the milieu interne in man and rat. Science 185:824–831.

Getchell, T. V. 1977. Analysis of intracellular recordings from salamander olfactory epithelium. Brain Res. 123:275–286.

Getchell, T. V., and Shepherd, G. M. 1978. Responses of olfactory receptor cells to step pulses of odour at different concentrations in the salamander. J. Physiol. (Lond.) 282:521–540.

Henning, H. 1922. Psychologische Studien au Geschmackssinn. Handbh. Biol. Arbeitsmeth. 6A:627–740.

Kimura, K., and Beidler, L. M. 1961. Microelectrode study of taste receptors of rat and hamster. J. Cell. Comp. Physiol. 58:131–139.

Mathews, D. F. 1972. Response patterns of single neurons in the tortoise olfactory epithelium and olfactory bulb. J. Gen. Physiol. 60:166–180.

Moulton, D. G. 1976. Spatial patterning of response to odors in the peripheral olfactory system. Physiol. Rev. 56:578–593.

Murray, R. G. 1973. The ultrastructure of taste buds. In I. Friedmann (ed.), The Ultrastructure of Sensory Organs. New York: American Elsevier, pp. 1–81.

Ottoson, D. 1971. The electro-olfactogram. In L. M. Beidler (ed.), Handbook of Sensory Physiology, Vol. IV. Chemical Senses, Part 1, Olfaction. Berlin: Springer, pp. 95–131.

Ozeki, M., and Sato, M. 1972. Responses of gustatory cells in the tongue of rat to stimuli representing four taste qualities. Comp. Biochem. Physiol. 41A:391–407.

Pfaffmann, C. 1941. Gustatory afferent impulses. J. Cell. Comp. Physiol. 17:243–258.

Pfaffmann, C. 1955. Gustatory nerve impulses in rat, cat and rabbit. J. Neurophysiol. 18:429–440.

Richter, C. P. 1942. Total self regulatory functions in animals and human beings. Harvey Lect. 38:63–103.

Roper, S. 1983. Regenerative impulses in taste cells. Science 220:1311–1312.

Schiffman, S. S. 1983. Taste and smell in disease. N. Engl. J. Med. 308:1337–1343.

Scott, T. R., Jr., and Erickson, R. P. 1971. Synaptic processing of taste-quality information in thalamus of the rat. J. Neurophysiol. 34:868–884.

Seligman, M. E. P., and Hager, J. L. 1972. Biological Boundaries of Learning. Englewood Cliffs, N.J.: Prentice-Hall.

Shepherd, G. M. 1972. Synaptic organization of the mammalian olfactory bulb. Physiol. Rev. 52:864–917.

Sloan, H. E., Hughes, S. E., and Oakley, B. 1983. Chronic impairment of axonal transport eliminates taste responses and taste buds. J. Neurosci. 3:117–123.

Smith, D. V., Van Buskirk, R. L., Travers, J. B., and Bieber, S. L. 1983. Coding of taste stimuli by hamster brain stem neurons. J. Neurophysiol. 50:541–558.

Stewart, W. B., Kauer, J. S., and Shepherd, G. M. 1979. Functional organization of rat olfactory bulb analysed by the 2-deoxyglucose method. J. Comp. Neurol. 185:715–734.

Trotier, D., and MacLeod, P. 1983. Intracellular recordings from salamander olfactory receptor cells. Brain Res. 268:225–237.

Motor Systems of the Brain: Reflex and Voluntary Control of Movement

VI

This section is concerned with what Charles Sherrington called the "integrative action" of the nervous system. To Sherrington, one of the most important features of nervous function was the regulation of motor output to achieve a *single purpose* even when an animal is presented with conflicting stimuli. He was therefore interested in the mechanisms responsible for bringing together the diverse parts of the nervous system to produce this highly focused and purposeful mode of action. Sherrington correctly recognized that reflexes intrinsic to the spinal cord provide the simplest expression of this integration, and he devoted much of his long career to analyzing their interactions and basic principles of operation.

As we saw in Part V, the spinal cord is an important sensory structure. Through its motor neurons and their associated interneuronal circuits, the spinal cord also provides the final output for voluntary as well as reflex actions. Thus, spinal mechanisms are critical for refined execution of all movements of the segmental musculature. The spinal cord can be seen as the first or lowest level in a four-level hierarchy of structures that control movement. The second level is the brain stem, the third the motor cortex, and the fourth the premotor cortex. Cellular studies on the motor and premotor cortices have revealed that other, nonmotor areas of cortex, such as the association cortices, can modulate the control of voluntary movements indirectly by exerting an influence on the motor cortex.

The cerebellum and basal ganglia also do not influence movements directly. Rather, both structures modulate the corticospinal and the rubrospinal systems that directly control the motor neurons and related spinal interneurons. Some functions of the basal ganglia and cerebellum and their disturbance by disease are now beginning to be understood in terms of transmitter pharmacology and biochemistry. In particular, information about the role of transmitters in the basal ganglia suggests that other neurological and psychiatric disorders may also result from altered functioning of specific chemical transmitter systems—transmitter synthesis, transport, release, and interaction with the postsynaptic receptor. Moreover, in the case of Huntington's disease, we now have the chance to learn how the mutation of a single gene can lead to premature cell death, which results in the symptoms of the disease.

Claude Ghez

Introduction to the Motor Systems

33

The skeletal muscles are the motor machinery for all the life of the animal which the older physiologists were wont to call the "life of external relation." Of the importance of that life of external relation the moralist has written that even in man the crown of life is an action, not a thought. Should we demur to this distinction, we can still endorse the old adage that to move things is all that mankind can do, and that for such the sole executant is muscle, whether in whispering a syllable or in felling a forest.

(Charles Sherrington, Linacre Lecture, Cambridge, England, 1924)

The motor systems allow us to move our body and limbs relative to the objects around us, and to maintain our posture—our attitude in space. Our entire behavioral repertoire is made up of movements and postural adjustments performed to achieve certain goals. It is up to the motor systems to initiate and coordinate all of the movements that contribute to realizing these goals. How do the motor systems achieve this action? In contrast to the sensory systems, which take physical energy and transform it into neural information, the motor systems act on the environment by transforming neural information into physical energy. Changes in external events or in our internal environment, signaled by our sensory systems, set up commands that are transmitted to our skeletal muscles by nerve impulses. The muscles translate this neural information into mechanical energy by generating a contractile force.

The control of movement and posture is achieved solely by adjusting the degree of contraction of skeletal muscles; however, this control requires that the motor systems be provided with a continuous flow of information about events in the periphery. Three types of afferent events are especially important. First, exteroceptors provide the motor systems with information about the spatial coordinates of the objects we encounter. Second, other receptors, called proprioceptors, relay information about the position of the body in space, the angles of the joints, and the length and tension of muscles. Through proprioceptors the motor systems gain access to information about the condition of the peripheral motor plant, the muscles and joints that have to be moved. Third, the motor systems need information about the consequences of their actions. Both exteroceptors and proprioceptors provide this information, which can then be used to calibrate the next series of motor commands. Thus, motor mechanisms are intimately related to and functionally dependent upon sensory information.

In this and subsequent chapters we shall not only consider the control of movement and posture and its regulation and updating by afferent information, but we shall also examine the constraints imposed on the motor system by the muscles and bones that must be moved. In particular, we shall consider how the motor systems are organized hierarchically to function effectively within these constraints. Finally, we shall discuss the components of the motor systems and the way in which afferent and sensory information acts on these components to influence both postural adjustments and skilled movements.

Motor Commands Are Tailored to the Physical Constraints of the Muscles, Bones, and Joints

Our motor systems may produce either a change in muscle length and a resultant change in joint angles, as when we reach for an object, or merely a change in tension, as when we tighten our grasp on an object already within our reach. To accomplish these different goals, the motor systems must take into account the limitations on movement imposed by the physical characteristics of the musculoskeletal system. Three constraints are especially important.

The first constraint results from the sluggish mechanical response of muscles to the neural signals that drive them. Muscles contract and relax slowly. As a result, changes in muscle tension do not represent a simple one-to-one transformation of the firing patterns of motor neurons. Rather, the muscles filter the information contained in the temporal pattern of the spike train produced by motor neurons. Because of this filtering action, muscles faithfully reproduce only those signals that vary slowly. When signals fluctuate rapidly, the ability of the muscle force to follow those fluctuations is greatly diminished. Thus, in order to produce rapid alternations in tension, it is necessary to alternate contraction in opposing muscles (see Chapter 34).

The second constraint results from the *springlike* properties of muscle. As is the case with a spring, the tension exerted by muscles varies in proportion to length. The effect of neural input is to change the muscles' resting length and stiffness (see Chapter 34). But, because muscles have springlike properties, actual changes in muscle length depend not only on the neural drive but also on the initial length of the muscle and on the external loads. *An important role of the mechanisms localized to spinal segments is to compensate for some of the more complex properties of muscle so as to simplify the accurate control of muscle contraction by the brain.* The complex properties of muscles and the loads to which they are ultimately attached also require that the motor systems calibrate their commands on the basis of previous experience. Skilled motor performance, therefore, depends crucially on learning.

The third and somewhat different constraint is that the motor systems typically need to control simultaneously many muscles acting at the same joint as well as muscles acting at different joints. Consider the task of reaching for an object while maintaining a standing position. A given trajectory of the hand can be achieved through several possible changes in angles at proximal and distal joints, and these changes involve the control of many muscles, some of which have more than one mechanical action. (The biceps, for instance, is both a flexor and a supinator of the forearm as well as a flexor of the shoulder.) Moreover, to bring a given limb segment to a desired position, it is not enough to contract a single group of muscles acting as prime movers (agonist muscles). Antagonist muscles, which oppose the actions of agonists, must also be controlled. For example, the antagonists may need to relax so that movement can take place with the least expenditure of energy, or they may need to contract late in the trajectory to decelerate the moving limb. In addition, postural muscles must also contract—some to fix the angle of proximal joints and others to prevent loss of balance. When we are in an upright position and lift an arm, the muscles of the legs contract before those of the arm; this prevents us from falling over when our center of gravity shifts suddenly. Finally, besides compensating for the inevitable changes in the center of gravity that occur when we move our limbs, or merely when we breathe, the motor systems also have to keep approximately 100 bones aligned end to end.

The motor systems and our muscles permit us a large number of adjustments in both posture and movement. As first pointed out by the Russian physiologist Nikolai Bernstein, the chief task of motor integration is to select one or more options from the large number of possibilities (or degrees of freedom) available. The motor systems of the brain and spinal cord reduce this wide array of choices to manageable proportions primarily by means of a hierarchy of several interconnected components. Let us now consider the components of this hierarchy.

The Four Major Components of the Motor Systems Are Hierarchically Organized

The idea that the motor systems are hierarchically organized was first appreciated in the nineteenth century by a British neurologist, Hughlings Jackson. Jackson recognized that different motor behaviors could be classified on a continuum that ranges from the most automatic behavior (such as reflexes) to the least automatic behavior (such as skilled voluntary movements). Jackson argued that the most automatic responses are organized at the level of the spinal cord, whereas the less automatic behaviors are organized by successively higher centers. Subsequent work has supported this idea and has indicated that the motor systems consist of separate neural circuits that are linked. These neural circuits are located in four distinct areas: (1) the spinal cord; (2) the brain stem and the reticular formation; (3) the motor cortex; and (4) the premotor cortical areas (Figure 33–1).

The Spinal Cord Is the First Level in the Motor Hierarchy

The first component in the motor hierarchy is the spinal cord. It is responsible for organizing the most automatic and stereotyped responses to stimuli. Even when disconnected from the brain stem by injury, the circuitry of the spinal cord is sufficient to generate a variety of automatic

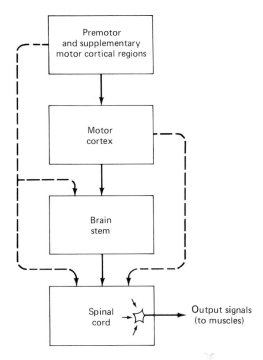

33–1 The motor systems consist of four hierarchical components. **Solid arrows** indicate hierarchical flow of commands. **Broken arrows** show parallel pathways.

behaviors. These automatic behaviors are known as reflex responses. They range from phasic behavioral responses such as the knee jerk or the withdrawal of the hand from a hot object to the alternating contraction of flexors and extensors that occurs during locomotion. In the spinal cord, sensory inputs are initially distributed either directly to the motor neurons innervating different muscles or indirectly to motor neurons through interneurons. Ultimately, whether directly or indirectly distributed, all motor processing is focused on a single target, the motor neurons, which constitute the "final common pathway" of the motor systems. As Sherrington stated,

The compounding together of reflexes is therefore a main problem in nervous co-ordination. For this problem it is important to recognize a feature in the architecture of the grey-centred (synaptic) nervous system which may be termed *the principle of the common path*. . . .

At the commencement of every reflex-arc is a receptive neurone extending from the receptive surface to the central nervous organ. This neurone forms the sole avenue which impulses generated at its receptive point can use whithersoever be their destination. This neurone is therefore a path exclusive to the impulses generated at its own receptive point, and other receptive points than its own cannot employ it. . . . its reflex-arcs spring from the one single shank or stem, i.e. from the one afferent neurone which conducts from the receptive point at the periphery into the central nervous organ.

But at the termination of every reflex-arc we find a final neurone, the ultimate conductive link to an effector organ (muscle or gland). This last link in the chain, e.g. the motor neurone, differs obviously in one important respect from the first link of the chain. It does not subserve exclusively impulses generated at one single receptive source, but receives impulses from many receptive sources . . . in many . . . regions of the body. It is the *sole* path which all impulses, no matter whence they come, must travel if they are to act on the muscle-fibres to which it leads.

(Charles Sherrington, Stillman Lecture, Yale University, 1904)

Although motor neurons are the final common pathway for motor actions, many of these actions are coordinated at the level of interneurons. For example, the reflex withdrawal from a noxious stimulus, or the alternating activity in flexors and extensors during locomotion, is organized by networks of spinal interneurons. Indeed, simple descending commands can produce surprisingly complex effects by acting on these interneurons.

Two examples illustrate this point. First, to produce movement of a limb in a desired direction, descending connections from the brain can activate the relevant motor neurons (see Chapter 38). However, a simple descending command acts simultaneously on motor neurons innervating the agonist muscles and on interneurons that inhibit the antagonists. Thus, the reciprocal control of two groups of muscles can be governed by a simple command signal, much as Ia afferents act both on the motor neurons to homonymous muscles and on the motor neurons to their antagonists.

Second, locomotion relies on networks of interneurons within the spinal cord that control alternating activity in flexor and extensor motor neurons. The existence of this circuitry at a low level in the motor hierarchy allows higher levels to control the complex sequences of muscle contraction necessary for locomotion by using simple commands.

Thus, a given descending pathway exerts control on the final motor response by acting either through interneurons or on motor neurons directly. Descending pathways can engage spinal interneurons to enhance or suppress specific reflex actions. These interneurons can act as gates that enable or prevent peripheral input from affecting motor output (Figure 33–2C). Gating can be achieved directly by descending fibers through presynaptic actions on the terminals of afferent fibers (Figure 33–2D). Indeed, the axons composing many descending pathways terminate as axo-axonic contacts with primary afferent fibers and can presynaptically inhibit the transmission of afferent information. Gating also allows higher centers to preselect which of several possible responses will follow a certain stimulus at a given moment. This capability decreases the information processing required and eliminates the need for decisions in the interval between stimulus and response.

The activity of both the spinal motor neurons and the interneurons reflects the sum of the several inputs impinging upon them: inputs from the periphery, from supraspinal regions, and from other interneurons or motor neurons (Figure 33–2B). The convergence of peripheral

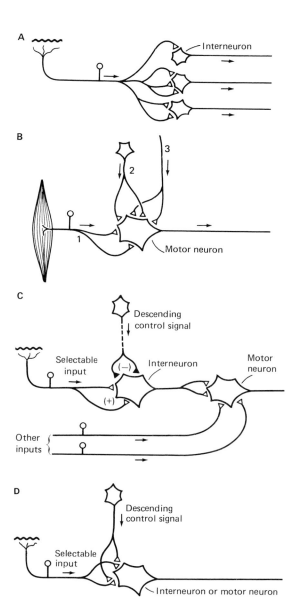

33–2 Several types and combinations of neuronal connections act on motor neurons. **A.** Divergence. Collaterals of a single neuron synapse on several target neurons. **B.** Convergence. The activity of a single neuron, such as the motor neuron shown here, depends upon the sum of inputs from afferent fibers (**1**), interneurons (**2**), and descending fibers from supraspinal regions (**3**). **C.** Gating by interneurons. An inhibitory command, direct or via an intercalated inhibitory interneuron (not shown), can prevent peripheral input from discharging an interneuron that acts on a motor neuron. **D.** Gating by presynaptic inhibition. A descending command can control afferent input by acting on presynaptic terminals of afferent fibers.

and descending synapses on spinal neurons allows for a great deal of flexibility in the way that the central nervous system can influence motor neuron activity. Subthreshold excitatory influences from descending pathways on a motor neuron (which depolarize the cell short of making it fire) can facilitate the action of a concurrent peripheral input. In this way the strength of a reflex can be increased. On the other hand, descending inhibitory influences on motor neurons can decrease reflex strength. In addition, interneurons and motor neurons give off branches, known as *collaterals*, that diverge and connect with other neurons, which allows individual motor neurons and interneurons to influence the activity of many other neurons (Figure 33–2A). Similarly, all motor neurons and interneurons receive converging inputs from many different sources, and a neuron's activity reflects the sum of excitatory and inhibitory influences (postsynaptic potentials) prevailing on it at the same time.

The Brain Stem Is the Second Level in the Motor Hierarchy

The brain stem contains neuronal systems that are necessary for integrating motor commands descending from higher levels as well as for processing information that ascends from the spinal cord and is conveyed from the special senses. The brain stem motor systems are crucial in processing selected categories of afferent input: those related to cranial nerve nuclei and those that are essential for postural adjustments. For example, the vestibular nuclei that receive information about the position of the head from organs of the inner ear relay this information to the spinal cord through the vestibulospinal tracts. This pathway allows the muscular adjustments needed to stabilize posture.

The importance of the brain stem motor systems is also illustrated by the fact that all descending motor pathways to the spinal cord originate in the brain stem with only one exception: the corticospinal tract.

The Motor and Premotor Cortices Are the Third and Fourth Levels in the Motor Hierarchy

The motor cortex (Brodmann's area 4), the third level in the motor hierarchy, is the node upon which the actions of the highest levels of cortical organization converge and from which certain descending motor commands requiring cortical processing are issued to the brain stem, to other subcortical structures, and to the spinal cord. These commands are mediated by the *corticospinal system*, which controls segmental neurons in the spinal cord, and by the *corticobulbar system*, which controls the motor nuclei in the brain stem.

The fourth and highest level of the hierarchy consists of premotor cortical regions in Brodmann's area 6. These areas are closely connected by corticocortical association fibers to the prefrontal and posterior parietal cortices. The premotor areas are responsible for identifying targets in space, for choosing a course of action, and for programming movement. These premotor areas act primarily on the motor cortex but also exert some influence on lower order brain stem and spinal systems (Figure 33–1).

There Are Three Important Aspects of the Hierarchical Organization

Three features of the hierarchy of motor structures are particularly important. First, with few exceptions, the different components of the motor systems contain somatotopic maps. In these maps, areas that influence adjacent body parts are adjacent to each other. This somatotopic organization is largely preserved in the interconnections of different levels. For example, the regions of motor cortex that control the arm receive input from premotor arm areas and, in turn, influence corresponding arm-control areas of the descending brain stem pathways. Second, each hierarchical level receives information from the periphery, so that sensory input can modify the action of descending commands (see Chapter 35). A third characteristic feature of the organization of the motor systems is the capacity of higher levels to control the information that reaches them, allowing or suppressing the transmission of the afferent volleys through sensory relays.

The Cerebellum and the Basal Ganglia Control the Components of the Motor Hierarchy

In addition to the four levels of the motor hierarchy, two other parts of the brain are important for motor function: the cerebellum and the basal ganglia. The *cerebellum* adjusts the actions of both the brain stem motor structures and the motor cortex by comparing descending control signals responsible for the intended motor response with sensory signals resulting from the consequences of motor action. On the basis of this comparison, the cerebellum is able to update and control movement when the movement deviates from its intended trajectory. The *basal ganglia* are not as well understood. They receive inputs from all cortical areas and focus their actions principally on premotor areas of the cerebral cortex. Diseases of the basal ganglia produce a unique set of motor abnormalities consisting of involuntary movements and disturbances in posture.

The Various Motor Control Levels Are Also Organized in Parallel

The brain stem and the motor and premotor cortical areas not only are organized hierarchically, so that each higher one influences the levels below it, but they also are organized in parallel, so that each can act *independently* on the final common pathway (Figure 33–1). For example, the corticospinal projection controls brain stem descending pathways, but it also controls spinal interneurons and even motor neurons. This parallel organization allows commands from higher levels either to modify or to supersede lower order reflex behavior. The combination of parallel and hierarchical control results in an overlap of different elements of the motor systems, similar to that which we encountered in the sensory sys-

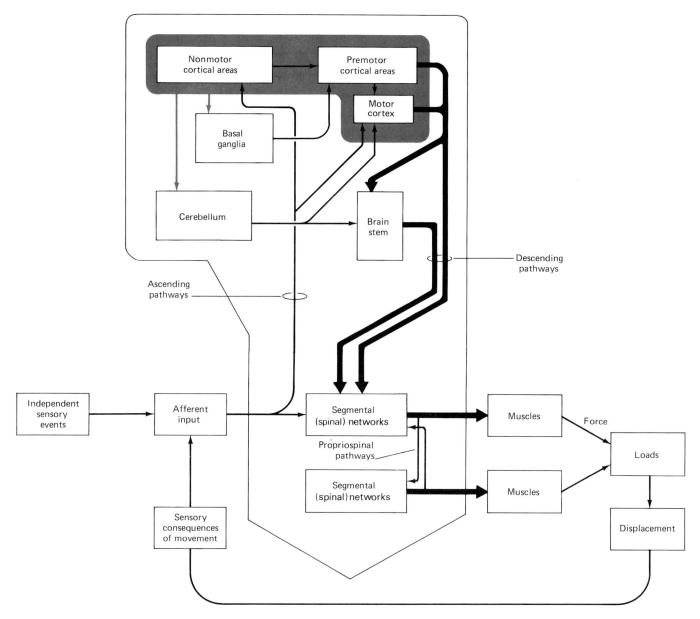

33–3 The major components of the motor systems are functionally interrelated. Note that **arrows** denote strong influences; they do not imply direct (monosynaptic) connections. Converging **arrows** do not necessarily imply convergence on the same individual neurons of the target structure. Crossing of pathways is not indicated nor are differences in connections of cortical areas. The thalamus has been omitted for clarity.

tems. This overlap allows motor commands to be divided into separate components, each making specific contributions to motor behavior; it is also important in the recovery of function after local lesions.

With these principles of hierarchical and parallel organization as a background, we can now survey the various components of the motor systems and review their functional interrelationships (Figure 33–3). Incoming volleys arising from the activation of sensory receptors are carried into the spinal cord by primary afferent fibers.

These axons act on segmental interneurons and motor neurons and thus generate reflex outputs mediated by the spinal cord. The neuronal networks of each segment connect to those of other segments through *propriospinal* neurons. Ascending pathways convey information to motor centers of the brain stem and, via the thalamic nuclei, to the cerebral cortex. Both the brain stem and cortical centers project back to the segmental networks and thereby are able to control reflex activity as well as produce skilled voluntary movements. The output of these supraspinal centers is influenced and ultimately integrated by the cerebellum and basal ganglia.

In addition, neural output can control muscle length indirectly: receptors in muscle (see Chapter 34) sense the displacement of muscles and limbs and can influence the output from spinal segments or higher levels. We shall now consider each of the main components of the motor systems in greater anatomical detail, emphasizing for each component its specific functional role.

In the Spinal Cord Motor Neurons Are Subject to Afferent Input and Descending Control

Afferent Fibers and Motor Neurons

On entering the spinal cord, the axons of the dorsal root ganglion cells send terminal branches to all laminae of the dorsal horn except lamina II. Some fibers continue within the intermediate zone, and a few of them reach the groups of motor neuron cell bodies in the ventral horn. In the ventral horn, the afferent fibers bifurcate and travel in rostral and caudal directions, sending off terminals at various segmental levels.

The motor neurons lie in the ventral horn. Those innervating a single muscle are collectively called a *motor neuron pool*. The motor neuron pools are segregated into *longitudinal columns* extending through two to four spinal segments (Figure 33–4A). The dendrites of the motor neurons are also oriented rostrocaudally within the respective cell columns. The longitudinal orientation of motor neurons and their dendrites matches that of primary afferent terminals in this zone. Thus, impulses in a given afferent axon tend to be distributed to motor neurons innervating the same muscle or muscles with similar function. (This set of connections gives rise to the stretch reflex discussed in Chapters 2 and 3.)

Two groups or divisions of motor neuron pools can be distinguished in the ventral horn. One group is located in the medial part of the ventral horn; the other, much larger group lies more laterally. These motor neurons connect to muscles according to a strict functional rule: *the motor neurons located medially project to axial muscles; those located more laterally project to limb muscles* (Figure 33–4A and B). Thus, the motor neurons of the medial division innervate the muscles of the neck and back. The motor neurons of the lateral division innervate the muscles of the arms and legs. The rule applies even within a group. Within the lateral group, the most medial motor neuron pools tend to innervate the muscles of the shoulder and pelvic girdles, while motor neurons located more laterally project to distal muscles of the extremities and digits. In addition to the proximal–distal rule, there is a flexor–extensor rule: *motor neurons innervating extensor muscles tend to lie ventral to those innervating flexors* (Figure 33–4B).

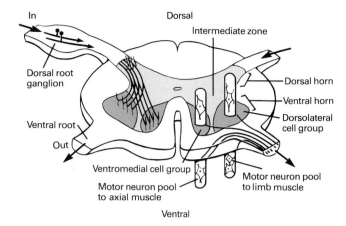

A Course of afferent fibers   Location of motor neuron pools

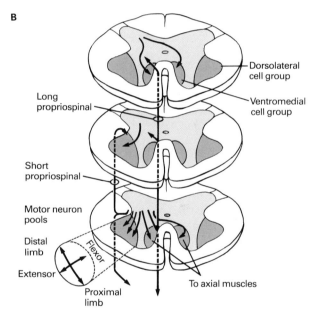

33–4 The spinal cord contains intrasegmental and intersegmental connections. **A.** Input–output organization of spinal segments and interconnections between segments. **B.** Direction of impulse traffic in interneurons and propriospinal neurons.

Interneurons and Propriospinal Neurons

Between the dorsal horn and the motor neuron pools lies the intermediate zone of the spinal cord. This zone contains interneurons that direct the impulse traffic according to their connections. The lateral parts of the intermediate zone project ipsilaterally to the dorsolateral motor neuron groups that innervate distal limb muscles. The medial regions of the intermediate zone project bilaterally to the medial motor neuron groups that innervate the axial muscles on both sides of the body. The areas in between the dorsolateral and the medial region project to the motor neurons innervating girdle muscles (Figure 33–4B).

Many of the interneurons in the intermediate zone have axons that course up and down the white matter of the spinal cord and terminate in homologous regions several segments away. These interconnecting interneurons, known as propriospinal neurons, send axons in the lateral columns that extend only a few segments (Figure 33–4B). Those in the ventral and ventromedial columns are longer and may extend the entire length of the spinal cord. This pattern of organization allows the axial muscles, which are innervated from many segments, to be activated in concert for appropriate postural adjustment. In contrast, distal limb muscles tend to be used independently.

In addition to an overall topographic organization, the interneurons also make precise connections. Specific populations of interneurons receive inputs from particular classes of afferent fibers (groups Ib, II, and joint receptors) and participate in specific reflexes. Many of these interneurons also receive characteristic connections from descending pathways (discussed in further detail in Chapters 35 and 38). These descending pathways terminate either on neurons in the dorsal horn and intermediate zone or directly on the motor neurons.

In considering the descending pathways, we shall begin by reviewing those that originate from brain stem nuclei. These pathways are thought to have developed first phylogenetically and to have persisted with little change in different mammalian species. We shall then consider the pathways originating from the cortex.

Two Groups of Descending Pathways from the Brain Stem Control Different Muscle Groups

The brain stem contains many groups of neurons whose axons form pathways projecting to the spinal gray matter. The Dutch anatomist H. G. J. M. Kuypers noted that these different pathways could be subdivided into *two distinct groups* according to the location of their terminations in the spinal cord. The first group, the *ventromedial pathways*, terminates in the ventromedial part of the spinal gray matter and thus *influences motor neurons innervating proximal muscles*. The second group, or *dorsolateral pathways*, terminates in the dorsolateral part of the spinal gray matter and *influences motor neurons controlling distal muscles of the extremities*. Kuypers drew the important conclusion that this difference in termination corresponds to a systematic difference in the functional roles of these two sets of descending systems. The ventromedial pathways (and the neuronal cell groups that give rise to them) are important in maintaining balance and in postural fixation, both of which rely especially on proximal muscles. The dorsolateral pathways play a crucial role in steering the extremities and in the fine control required for manipulating objects with the fingers and hand. The different uses to which we put proximal and distal muscles are reflected in differences in the fine organization of the connections of the ventromedial and dorsolateral systems, as we shall see below.

Ventromedial Pathways

The ventromedial group of pathways descends in the ipsilateral ventral columns of the spinal cord and terminates predominantly on medial motor neurons that innervate axial and girdle muscles. The pathways also end on interneurons, including long propriospinal neurons in the ventromedial part of the intermediate zone (Figure 33–5A).

The ventromedial pathways are characterized by the *divergent distribution of their terminals.* Many axons in the ventromedial pathways terminate bilaterally in the spinal cord. In addition, they send collaterals to different segmental levels. Thus, about one-half of the axons that reach the lumbar cord also have collaterals in the cervical gray matter. Moreover, the long propriospinal neurons controlled by this system also have many axons spreading widely up and down the spinal cord.

The ventromedial system has three major components: (1) The *lateral and medial vestibulospinal tracts* originate in the lateral and medial vestibular nuclei and carry information for the reflex control of equilibrium from the vestibular labyrinth. (2) The *tectospinal tract* originates in the tectum of the midbrain (superior colliculus), a structure that is important for the coordinated control of head and eye movements directed toward visual targets. (3) The *reticulospinal* tract originates in the reticular formation of the medulla and the pons. The reticular formation—the area of the medulla and pons composed mainly of interneurons and their processes—can best be considered as a rostral extension of the spinal intermediate zone into the brain stem. The other components of the ventromedial pathways send collaterals to the reticular formation. Three additional brain stem nuclei of lesser importance in motor function contribute to the ventromedial system: the interstitial nucleus of Cajal, the raphe nuclei (a serotonergic cell group), and the locus ceruleus (a noradrenergic cell group).

Dorsolateral Pathways

The dorsolateral group of pathways descends in the lateral quadrant of the spinal cord. It terminates in the lateral portion of the intermediate zone and among the dorsolateral groups of motor neurons innervating more distal limb muscles (Figure 33–5B). In contrast to the ventromedial pathways, in which individual fibers send off large numbers of collaterals at different levels, the dorsolateral pathways terminate on a small number of spinal segments.

The dorsolateral brain stem system is primarily composed of *rubrospinal fibers* that originate in the magnocellular portion of the red nucleus in the midbrain. Rubrospinal fibers cross the midline ventral to the red

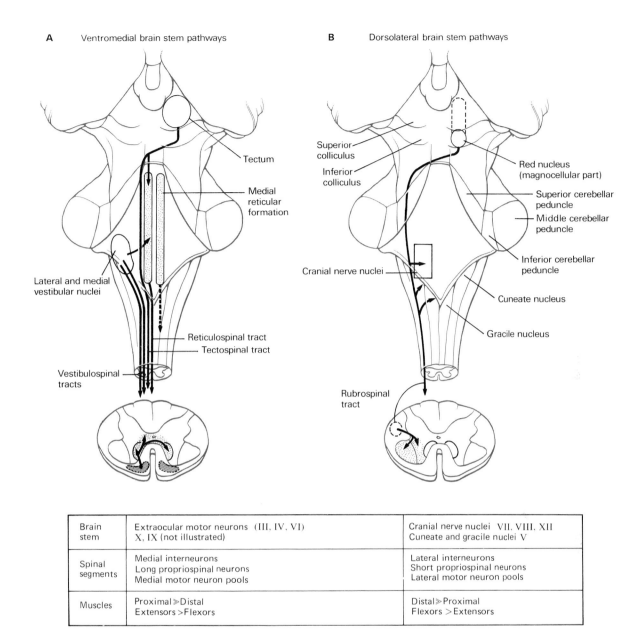

A Ventromedial brain stem pathways

Tectum

Medial
reticular
formation

Lateral and medial
vestibular nuclei

Reticulospinal tract
Tectospinal tract

Vestibulospinal
tracts

B Dorsolateral brain stem pathways

Superior
colliculus

Inferior
colliculus

Cranial nerve nuclei

Rubrospinal
tract

Red nucleus
(magnocellular part)

Superior cerebellar
peduncle

Middle cerebellar
peduncle

Inferior cerebellar
peduncle

Cuneate nucleus

Gracile nucleus

Brain stem	Extraocular motor neurons (III, IV, VI) X, IX (not illustrated)	Cranial nerve nuclei VII, VIII, XII Cuneate and gracile nuclei V
Spinal segments	Medial interneurons Long propriospinal neurons Medial motor neuron pools	Lateral interneurons Short propriospinal neurons Lateral motor neuron pools
Muscles	Proximal≫Distal Extensors >Flexors	Distal≫Proximal Flexors >Extensors

33–5 The two groups of descending brain stem pathways control different groups of neurons and different groups of muscles. **A.** Ventromedial pathways. The main components are the reticulospinal, the medial and lateral vestibulospinal, and the tectospinal tracts that descend in the ventral funiculus. These terminate in the **shaded portions** of the gray spinal matter. **B.** Dorsolateral pathways. The main pathway is the rubrospinal tract, which originates in the caudal, magnocellular portion of the red nucleus. The rubrospinal tract descends in the contralateral dorsolateral funiculus and terminates in the **shaded area** of the spinal gray matter. **Boxed insert:** Target neurons and muscle groups controlled by the two groups of pathways.

nucleus and descend in the ventrolateral quadrant of the medulla. The magnocellular portion of the red nucleus also gives rise to *rubrobulbar fibers,* which project both to the cranial nerve nuclei controlling facial muscles and to nuclei with a sensory function: the sensory trigeminal nucleus and the dorsal column nuclei (the cuneate and gracile nuclei).

The Motor Cortex Exercises Descending Motor Control via Corticospinal and Corticobulbar Tracts

We owe our repertory of discrete voluntary movements to the remarkable development of the cerebral cortex. Commands from the cerebral cortex are conveyed to the motor neurons by two main routes: the corticobulbar and corticospinal tracts. The *corticobulbar tract* controls the motor neurons innervating cranial nerve nuclei, and the *corticospinal tract* controls the motor neurons innervating the spinal segments. The two systems act directly on the motor neurons (or on the interneurons closely related to them). These two systems also act on the descending brain stem pathways, mainly the reticulospinal and rubrospinal tracts. Moreover, like the descending brain stem pathways, the corticospinal tract has both ventromedial and dorsolateral subdivisions that influence axial and distal muscles, respectively.

Some points of nomenclature need to be clarified. Strictly speaking, the term *corticobulbar* should refer only to fibers originating in the cortex and terminating in the medulla (the "bulb"). In practice, however, the term is often used to refer to cortical output fibers that terminate in nuclei (e.g. cranial nerve nuclei, reticular nuclei) of other parts of the brain stem as well. The *corticospinal fibers* originate in the cortex and terminate in the spinal cord. In the medulla, the corticospinal fibers form the medullary pyramids. The term *pyramidal tract* is therefore often used synonymously with corticospinal tract. However, because many fibers leave the medullary pyramids to innervate brain stem nuclei, the terms corticospinal and pyramidal are not strictly synonymous.

Origin, Course, and Terminations of the Corticospinal and Corticobulbar Tracts

In humans, approximately 30% of the corticospinal and corticobulbar fibers originate from a strip of cortex, the *precentral gyrus* of the frontal lobe (Brodmann's area 4), also known as the *motor cortex*. It is here that low-threshold electrical stimulation evokes movements of different body parts. Another 30% arise from area 6 (mainly the *premotor* cortex), a larger zone that lies in the frontal lobe anterior to area 4. The remaining 40% arise from the parietal lobe (especially the somatic sensory cortex, i.e., areas 3, 1, and 2). The corticospinal and corticobulbar fibers course through the *posterior limb of the internal capsule* to reach the ventral portion of the midbrain. Below the midbrain, in the pons, corticospinal fibers are no longer grouped together but form separate small bundles of fibers interspersed among the pontine nuclei. Lower still, in the ventral part of the medulla, corticospinal fibers again congregate to form the *medullary pyramids*. At the junction of the medulla and the spinal cord, most of the corticospinal fibers cross the midline in the *pyramidal decussation*. The crossed fibers descend in the dorsal part of the lateral columns (dorsolateral columns) of the spinal cord and form the *lateral corticospinal tract*, whereas the uncrossed fibers descend in the ventral columns and form the *ventral corticospinal tract*.

The lateral and ventral divisions of the corticospinal tract terminate in approximately the same regions of spinal gray matter as do the dorsolateral and ventromedial descending brain stem systems (Figure 33–6). In humans the lateral corticospinal tract projects to sensory neurons in the dorsal horn (laminae IV and V of Rexed),

to interneurons in the intermediate zone, and to motor neuron pools innervating distal limb muscles. The fibers that project to the dorsal horn originate in different areas of the cerebral cortex than do those that project to the intermediate zone and motor neurons (Figure 33–6B). The neurons that project to the dorsal horn (via the lateral corticospinal tract) are located in the somatic sensory cortex (areas 3, 1, and 2) of the postcentral gyrus. Those projecting contralaterally to the lateral parts of the intermediate zone and to the motor neurons that innervate distal limb muscles are located in the motor cortex (area 4) of the precentral gyrus, principally in regions controlling arm and leg muscles.

The ventral corticospinal tract projects bilaterally to the ventromedial motor neuron pools innervating axial and proximal muscles as well as to the adjoining portions of the intermediate zone. This projection derives mostly from that part of the precentral gyrus where stimulation causes contraction of proximal and axial muscles and from area 6, the region of cortex anterior to the precentral gyrus.

The corticobulbar fibers, which ultimately control muscles of the head and face, terminate in sensory and motor cranial nerve nuclei in the brain stem. In humans there are direct monosynaptic connections between corticobulbar fibers and motor neurons in the motor trigeminal, facial, and hypoglossal nuclei. The projections to the trigeminal motor nucleus are bilateral and approximately equal in size. Although the projection to the facial nucleus is also bilateral, *the motor neurons innervating muscles of the lower face receive predominantly contralateral fibers*. As a result, unilateral lesions that interrupt corticobulbar fibers on one side produce weakness only of the muscles of the contralateral lower part of the face.

Cortical Control of Movement Is Achieved Only Late in Phylogeny

Phylogenetically, the corticospinal and corticobulbar pathways first appear in mammals. In the most primitive species, the two pathways distribute their axons exclusively to sensory regions of the brain stem and spinal cord. In the hedgehog, a primitive mammal that has persisted essentially unchanged for millions of years, the corticospinal tracts are located in the dorsal columns and terminate exclusively in the dorsal horn. In this species the somatic sensory representations of the body surface in the cerebral cortex overlap precisely with that of the motor representation.

Phylogenetically higher mammals have distinct sensory and motor representations of the body in the cortex and have additional corticospinal terminations within the intermediate zone of the spinal cord. With still further phylogenetic development, there is a gradual increase in the number of corticospinal fibers distributed to more ventral regions of the spinal cord. Direct connections between corticospinal neurons and motor neurons appear first in lateral motor neuron cell groups (to

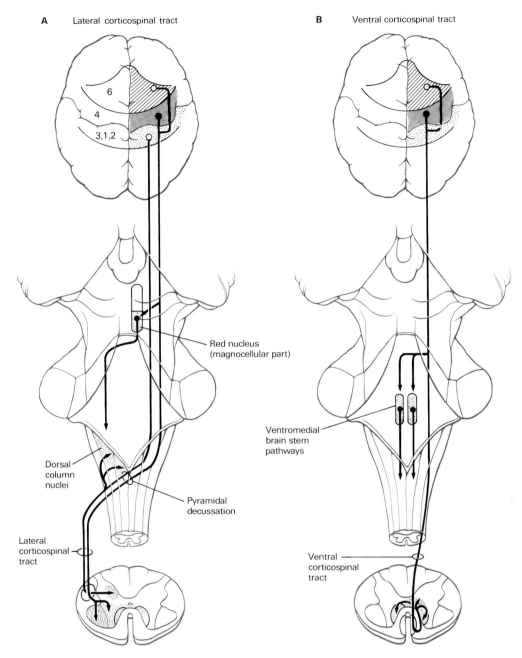

A Lateral corticospinal tract

B Ventral corticospinal tract

Red nucleus
(magnocellular part)

Ventromedial
brain stem
pathways

Dorsal
column
nuclei

Pyramidal
decussation

Lateral
corticospinal
tract

Ventral
corticospinal
tract

33–6 The descending cortical pathways to the spinal
segments constitute the corticospinal tracts.
A. Crossed pathways (lateral corticospinal tract) originate from
Brodmann's areas 4 and 6, cross at the pyramidal decussation,
descend in the dorsolateral funiculus, and terminate in the
shaded area of spinal gray matter. A few fibers cross the
midline. Collaterals reach rubrospinal neurons. The principal

area of termination of the corticospinal neurons originating
from the sensory cortex is the medial portion of the dorsal
horn. Collaterals project to dorsal column nuclei. **B.** Uncrossed
pathways (ventral corticospinal tract) originate principally in
Brodmann's area 6 and in zones controlling the neck and trunk
in area 4. Terminations are bilateral and collaterals project to
the ventromedial brain stem pathways.

distal limb muscles), then also in medial motor neuron
cell groups. Thus, in the phylogeny of primates, the
number of direct connections from the corticospinal
tract to the motor neurons increases progressively from
prosimians (e.g., lemurs such as the bushbaby) to monkeys (e.g., macaque), to apes (e.g., chimpanzee and gorilla), and finally to humans. In the more primitive primates, direct connections are seen only in the most

dorsolateral cell groups innervating the most distal muscles, whereas in monkeys the entire lateral division of
the motor neuron pool receives corticospinal input; in
higher apes and humans the medial motor neuron pools
also receive corticospinal input. In most carnivores corticospinal fibers terminate exclusively in the dorsal horn
and dorsolateral parts of the intermediate zone and do
not make any direct connections with motor neurons.

The Motor Cortex Is Itself Influenced by Both Cortical and Subcortical Inputs

All regions of the cortex are ultimately capable of influencing both the motor and premotor cortices through their *corticocortical connections*. These pathways take the form of bundles of axons in the white matter that link the different regions of cortex with each other.

An additional source of corticocortical inputs comes from the corpus callosum, which relays information from one hemisphere to the other. Callosal fibers interconnect homologous areas of both the sensory and motor cortices. There is only one exception to this rule: The regions that receive information from or project to the distal regions of the limbs do not receive callosal connections. These regions (the hand and foot areas of the somatic sensory and motor cortices of the two hemispheres) are thus functionally disconnected from one another.

The major subcortical input to area 6 and to the motor cortex comes from the thalamus, from the ventral anterior and the ventral lateral nuclei. In addition, the border zone between the ventral lateral and ventral posterior lateral nuclei relays important somatic sensory information to the precentral gyrus. The ventral anterior–ventral lateral complex receives most of its information from two important subcortical integrating centers: the basal ganglia and the cerebellum, which are important clinically because lesions within them produce serious motor disturbances.

The Several Levels of Motor Neuron Control Have Functional Consequences

The fact that ventromedial and dorsolateral pathways influence motor neurons innervating different classes of muscles and show different degrees of divergence has important functional implications. The dorsolateral brain stem and lateral corticospinal pathways control distal limb muscles. The presence of direct connections from the cortex to the motor neurons endows higher primates, including humans, with the ability to control individual muscles independently from one another. This important capacity is known as *fractionation of movement*. It is completely and irretrievably lost following lesions of the pyramidal tract. Monkeys whose pyramidal tracts have been interrupted are no longer able to grasp small objects between two fingers or to make isolated movements of the wrist or elbow. When attempting to grasp a small object, an animal with this lesion uses its hand as a shovel or, at best, contracts all the digits simultaneously around the object. However, these animals are not impaired in their ability to maintain balance or to control axial and girdle muscles; they can walk and climb without difficulty. In contrast, lesions interrupting the ventromedial brain stem pathways produce profound disorders in balance, and the animals become unable to sit or stand upright, walk, and climb.

The superimposition of several levels of control (corticospinal, brain stem, segmental interneurons, and mo-

tor neurons) contributes to the marked recovery of motor functions after lesions of one or another system. For example, ablation of the precentral gyrus is followed immediately by a profound paralysis of the muscles controlled by that area, but this paralysis is reversed to a remarkable extent. In different species, the extent and duration of the paralysis parallel the development of the direct corticospinal connections with motor neurons. The paralysis is briefer in the monkey than in humans and still briefer in the cat, which lacks cortical motor neuronal connections altogether. When the corticospinal tract is lesioned but the connections from the motor cortex to the red nucleus are spared, the brain is able to control distal limb muscles through the corticorubral pathway. In higher primates the rubrospinal pathway regresses somewhat relative to that of monkeys and other species, and the degree of functional recovery following cortical lesions is correspondingly smaller.

Lesions of the Corticospinal System Cause Characteristic Symptoms

Symptoms and signs resulting from lesions of the corticospinal system are especially common in neurological practice. This is easy to understand because corticospinal axons extend from the cerebral cortex through the brain stem to the spinal cord, and can be damaged by lesions at any of these locations. The most common cause of such lesions is vascular disease, especially occlusion of the middle cerebral artery (whose branches supply the lateral surface of the cortex and the internal capsule) or the vertebrobasilar artery (supplying the brain stem). Tumor, trauma, and demyelinating diseases are also common causes of damage to the corticospinal system.

Positive and Negative Signs

Hughlings Jackson recognized that lesions of the corticospinal system give rise to two kinds of abnormalities, or signs, which he referred to as negative and positive. *Negative signs* result from the loss of particular capacities normally controlled by the corticospinal system. *Positive signs* consist of abnormal responses to stimuli or of motor behaviors that emerge after the lesion. Also called *release phenomena*, these positive signs are attributable to the withdrawal of inhibitory influences acting on interneuronal networks that mediate the responses. One of the negative signs that accompanies corticospinal tract lesions is the loss of the ability to make independent movements of isolated muscle groups (loss of fractionation). This deficit results from the loss of the specific and direct connections made by corticospinal neurons onto motor neurons. Other important negative signs resulting from the withdrawal of facilitatory effects on spinal neurons are weakness and an inability to voluntarily contract muscles quite as rapidly as normal. The

A Normal plantar response

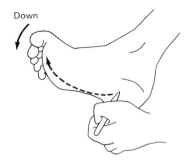

Down

B Extensor plantar response
(Babinski sign)

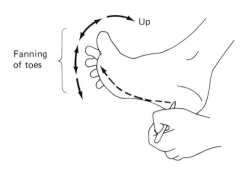

Up

Fanning
of toes

weakness may be profound immediately after the lesion, but it can diminish considerably with time.[1]

Among the release phenomena observed after injury to the corticospinal system, the *Babinski sign,* or *extensor plantar response,* is one of the most important and widely used in clinical neurology. The sign was discovered in 1896 by Joseph Babinski, a Polish neurologist in charge of a ward of syphilitic patients at the Pitié Hospital in Paris. A form of this disease, meningovascular syphilis, produces vascular lesions of the brain that often affect the corticospinal tract. Babinski noted that stroking the lateral aspect of the foot with a sharp object elicited a different reflex response in patients with corticospinal disease than it did in patients without this disorder. Normally, this stimulus produces flexion of all the toes, including the large one. In affected patients, however, there is a reflex extension of the big toe which may be accompanied by fanning of the others (Figure 33–7).

William Landau at Washington University and other researchers have now demonstrated that the extensor plantar response is actually an enhanced flexion reflex and is part of a larger family of withdrawal responses to noxious stimuli released by pyramidal lesions. (Extensors of the big toe represent physiological flexors because they do not oppose the action of gravity on the body.) The appearance under pathological conditions of a reflex response that is normally absent illustrates clearly that central lesions can lead to both negative and positive signs: to loss of some functions and to the release of others that are normally kept in check.

Upper and Lower Motor Neuron Lesions

Many lesions, both peripheral and central, can interfere with the normal balance of tonic inputs to the motor neurons and give rise to some features of the syndrome

[1]The recovery in muscle strength that often occurs with time is typically greater for younger patients than for older ones. It is generally believed that the amount of strength that the patient regains during the course of recovery results from a combination of factors, including the assumption by descending brain stem pathways of some of the functions of the corticospinal system and the sprouting of other axons to fill in the synaptic spaces vacated by the degenerating corticospinal axons.

33–7 The Babinski sign is diagnostic of a lesion of the corticospinal tract. When the sole of the foot is stroked firmly along the path indicated, the normal response (**A**) is flexion of the foot and toes. The Babinski sign (**B**) is extension of the big toe and fanning of the others.

of upper motor neuron lesion. As we saw in Chapter 18, the motor neurons of the ventral horn are often referred to as *lower motor neurons* in the clinical literature, whereas corticospinal neurons in the motor cortex as well as those giving rise to descending brain stem pathways are called *upper motor neurons.* The concept of upper and lower motor neurons continues to be used clinically to distinguish neurological disorders that result in muscular weakness. The clinician must first decide whether the underlying disease affects the motor neuron and its axon (lower motor neuron lesion) or whether it interferes with descending commands (upper motor neuron lesion).

Lesions of lower motor neurons often produce disturbances restricted to *single* muscles and are often associated with fasciculation (visible as twitches of muscle fascicles under the skin) and atrophy (loss of muscle volume). In addition, the affected muscles always show decreased tone, and tendon reflexes are reduced or absent (see Chapter 18). In contrast, upper motor neuron lesions affect groups of muscles, atrophy is rare, and there are no fasciculations.

In addition, a condition known as *spasticity* appears, in which muscle tone and deep tendon reflexes are both increased. Spasticity is detected by passively moving the limb segment about the joint and noting the resistance offered by the muscles. Under normal conditions, a mild amount of resistance is felt that derives in part from the stretch reflex and in part from the normal elastic properties of muscles. In spasticity, the limb opposes movement with increased resistance; frequently this is associated with the presence of a "clasp-knife" reflex, whereby the muscle tension abruptly melts away after an initial strong resistance. The increased muscle tone results from an increase in the excitability of alpha motor neurons produced by tonic descending activity from the brain stem as well as increased firing of gamma motor neurons (see Chapter 35). Both inputs tend to lower the threshold for the stretch reflex. As a result, the stretch reflex elicited by passive movement is much more powerful.

Although it was once believed that the heightened stretch reflexes and the clasp-knife reflex were produced by the withdrawal of an inhibitory action of the corticospinal neurons on segmental motor neurons and interneurons, it is now known that this is not so. Experiments in monkeys and other animals have shown that sectioning the corticospinal tract in the medullary pyramid always produces decreased muscle tone rather than spasticity. Spasticity arises not from damage to the corticospinal tract but from damage to corticobulbar or to descending brain stem pathways themselves.

Lesions affecting corticospinal and descending brain stem pathways can be understood in rather simple terms: they lead to a loss of facilitatory or inhibitory influences on segmental mechanisms. As a result, there is a decrease in strength and speed of muscle contraction, loss of fine muscle control, and impairment of muscle tone, causing disturbances in the ability to perform certain motor tasks. When the cerebellum and basal ganglia are damaged the motor deficits reflect interference with the processing mechanisms that ensure smoothly coordinated movements. The movements therefore become uncoordinated and clumsy, the spatial and temporal patterning of muscle contractions becomes abnormal, and involuntary movements may appear. These phenomena will be discussed further in Chapters 39 and 40.

Selected Readings

Bernstein, N. 1967. The Co-ordination and Regulation of Movements. Oxford: Pergamon Press.

Jackson, J. H. 1932. Selected Writings of John Hughlings Jackson, Vol. II. J. Taylor (ed.). London: Hodder and Stoughton.

Kuypers, H. G. J. M. 1981. Anatomy of the descending pathways. In V. B. Brooks (ed.), Handbook of Physiology, Section 1: The Nervous System, Vol. II, Motor Control. Bethesda, Md.: American Physiological Society, pp. 597–666.

Lundberg, A. 1979. Integration in a propriospinal motor centre controlling the forelimb in the cat. In H. Asanuma and V. J. Wilson (eds.), Integration in the Nervous System. Tokyo: Igaku-Shoin, pp. 47–64.

Sherrington, C. 1947. The Integrative Action of the Nervous System, 2nd ed. New Haven: Yale University Press.

Tower, S. S. 1940. Pyramidal lesion in the monkey. Brain 63:36–90.

References

Babinski, J. 1896. Sur le réflexe cutané plantaire dans certaines affections organiques du système nerveux central. C. R. Soc. Biol. (Paris) 48:207–208.

Landau, W. M., and Clare, M. H. 1959. The plantar reflex in man, with special reference to some conditions where the extensor response is unexpectedly absent. Brain 82:321–355.

Thomas J. Carew and Claude Ghez

Muscles and Muscle Receptors

34

As we saw in the last chapter, the central nervous system can act on the outside world only by means of muscle. In this chapter we shall first discuss how skeletal muscles produce the forces necessary to move our limbs. We shall then examine how specialized receptors within skeletal muscles convey information about both muscle length and muscle tension. Finally, we shall see that the central nervous system can control the flow of information it receives from skeletal muscles by adjusting the sensitivity of sensory receptors located in the muscles.

Skeletal Muscle Fibers and Motor Neurons Are Functionally Specialized

Skeletal muscle is composed of elongated multinucleated cells, the *muscle fibers.* These fibers contain the muscle's contractile machinery in the form of *myofilaments* composed of polymerized actin and myosin molecules as well as the proteins with which they are associated. Contraction occurs because the proteins of the myofilament slide relative to each other to produce tension or change in length. This process is dependent on energy supplied by the conversion of ATP to ADP. Although sliding filament mechanisms operate in all muscles, individual muscle fibers can be subdivided into two distinct classes—fast and slow—each of which has different physiological and biochemical properties.

Fast (or pale) muscle fibers contract and relax rapidly when stimulated (Figure 34–1). These fibers are capable of generating great force. They have a relatively low myoglobin content and are poorly vascularized, which gives them a pale color. They have few mitochondria and rely on glycolysis and

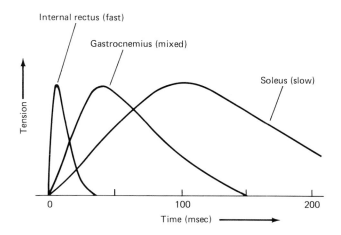

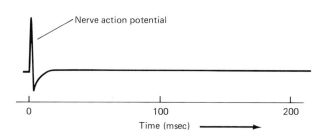

34–1 Fast and slow muscles differ in the time course of their twitch contractions in response to a single brief electrical stimulus to the muscle. For fast muscles such as extraocular muscles, maximum twitch tension develops in about 7.5 msec, whereas in a slow muscle such as the soleus, maximum twitch tension develops only after about 100 msec. The gastrocnemius contains both fast and slow fibers, and has an intermediate twitch contraction time. Notice also the difference in relaxation times. A nerve action potential is shown to indicate the difference in duration of spikes compared to muscle contraction. (Adapted from Henneman, 1980.)

glycogen for their energy requirements. As a result, fast muscle fibers typically fatigue rapidly and are best suited for intense activity of short duration.

Slow (or red) muscle fibers contract and relax slowly (Figure 34–1) and generate only low levels of force. Because these fibers have a high myoglobin content and are richly vascularized, they are red. They also have many mitochondria and utilize oxidative metabolism. They are therefore more resistant to fatigue and are specialized for sustained contraction. Individual muscles typically contain different proportions of these two principal fiber types. Muscles specialized for sustained activity contain predominantly slow fibers, and a few muscles, such as the soleus (an ankle extensor), contain only slow fibers.

In 1925 E. G. T. Liddell and Charles Sherrington introduced the term *motor unit* to describe the smallest functional unit that can be controlled by the nervous system. The motor unit consists of a single motor neuron, its axon, and all the muscle fibers that it innervates

(see Chapter 18). Because the muscle fibers of individual motor units are widely distributed and intermingle with fibers of other units (Figure 34–2), a more or less uniform tension results at the muscle tendon, even when very few motor units are active. Motor units vary considerably in the number of muscle fibers they contain. The number of muscle fibers in a motor unit is expressed as the innervation ratio of that motor unit: the fewer the muscle fibers innervated by a motor neuron, the lower the innervation ratio. Similarly, a muscle with a low innervation ratio has a large number of motor neurons relative to the number of its muscles fibers. As we shall see later, a low innervation ratio implies a potential for finer control of the total force that the muscle can generate, much as small receptive field sizes allow greater spatial resolution in the somatic sensory and visual systems.

Motor units also differ in physiological properties. Characteristically, the properties of the motor neuron are matched to the physiological and biochemical properties of the muscle fibers. Just as muscle types differ in their ability to contract rapidly, motor neurons differ in their ability to fire rapidly, and there is a close correspondence between the functional properties of the muscle and the motor neuron. Fast muscle fibers are innervated by motor neurons that can fire at high frequencies and have fast conduction velocities, whereas slow muscle fibers are innervated by motor neurons that fire at lower frequencies and have slower conduction velocities. Thus, motor units are also referred to as *fast* or *slow*. The properties of the muscle fibers depend to a large degree on the patterns of neural activation reaching them. The way in which the central nervous system brings about this match of functional properties will be discussed in Chapter 56.

The Nervous System Can Grade the Force of Muscle Contraction in Two Ways

Given the arrangement of motor units described above, how does the nervous system produce graded increases in muscular forces? The nervous system grades force in two principal ways: (1) Through *recruitment*, it increases the number of active motor units and thereby increases the force of contraction. (2) Through *rate coding*, it increases the frequency of activation of individual motor neurons; when the motor neurons fire faster, they increase muscle tension.

Recruitment: The Size Principle

Elwood Henneman and his colleagues at Harvard University discovered that when motor neurons are activated by a synaptic drive, they are recruited in an orderly fashion according to their size. Neurons with the smallest cell bodies have the lowest threshold for synaptic activation and are recruited by the weakest afferent input. As the afferent input increases in strength, it recruits progressively larger motor neurons. Because larger motor neurons innervate fast muscle fibers, which develop

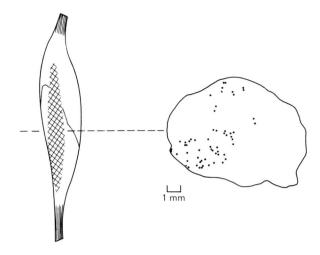

34-2 A single motor neuron can innervate many muscle fibers, and these muscle fibers are typically distributed quite widely, as shown by this example in the soleus muscle. The location of individual muscle fibers making up the motor unit was determined by stimulation of a single motor neuron for a prolonged period of time; this caused all the muscle fibers to which that motor neuron connected to contract and to deplete their stores of glycogen. The fibers were then identified histochemically with a stain selective for glycogen. On the **right** is an outline of a cross section taken from the muscle (**left**) at the level shown by the **broken line.** The **hatched area** is the approximate amount of motor unit territory projected onto the muscle surface. Each **dot** on the cross section represents a single muscle fiber. (Adapted from Burke et al., 1974.)

greater tension, each motor unit that is recruited adds a larger increment in force than the last one. This stereo-typed recruitment order is known as the *size principle*[1] and applies equally to reflex activation and to voluntary contraction.

Rate Coding

The second way the nervous system can command greater muscular force is by increasing the firing rate of motor neurons. When muscles are activated by succes-sive action potentials at intervals that are less than the time it takes for the muscle to contract and relax again (called the muscle's *twitch* time), the forces generated by each impulse summate until a plateau is reached. This state of maintained contraction is called *tetanus.*

The rate of stimulation of a muscle nerve affects the tension produced isometrically in the muscle (Figure 34-3A). At low and intermediate rates some relaxation can take place between impulses, and the tension record shows ripples corresponding to the peaks of each twitch; this is called *unfused tetanus.* At very high frequencies a smooth tension record is observed; this is called *fused tetanus.* Complete fusion, however, takes place only with the most rapid and forceful natural muscle contrac-tions. Movements requiring less than maximal contrac-

tion have smoother trajectories because motor units are always activated asynchronously: when one motor unit is at the peak of its twitch, others are relaxed.

The force developed by a motor unit also depends on the unit's pattern of activity. Robert Burke and his col-leagues have shown that insertion of one extra action

34-3 Muscle tension is affected by the firing rate of motor neurons through a process called rate coding.
A. Examples of unfused and fused tetanus. Stimulation of a muscle fiber at progressively higher frequencies (**dots below trace**) produces progressively more tension. (Adapted from Buchthal, 1942.) **B.** Effect of an initial doublet on tension produced by a train of stimuli. **Trace 1:** Unfused tetanus is produced by a train of stimuli (**dots below trace**). **Trace 2:** Much greater tension is produced when a single extra stimulus (**at arrow**) is added at the beginning of the stimulus train (**dots above trace**).

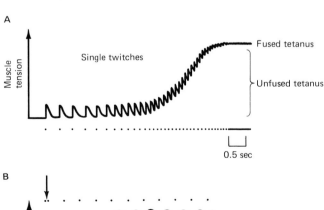

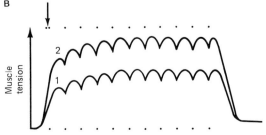

---

[1]The cellular mechanisms underlying the size principle derive from at least two factors. One important factor is the *input resistance* of the motor neuron. The size of an excitatory postsynaptic potential depends on the product of the synaptic current and the passive input resistance of the neuron. There is an inverse relationship between a neuron's sur-face area and its input resistance—the smaller the neuron, the larger its passive input resistance. Thus, the same synaptic current produces a larger excitatory postsynaptic potential in a small neuron than in a large neuron. Another important factor is the *density of presynaptic current.* In some systems there is evidence that small motor neurons may also receive greater synaptic input than large motor neurons; thus, the higher current density onto these small cells will bring them to threshold sooner than large motor neurons.

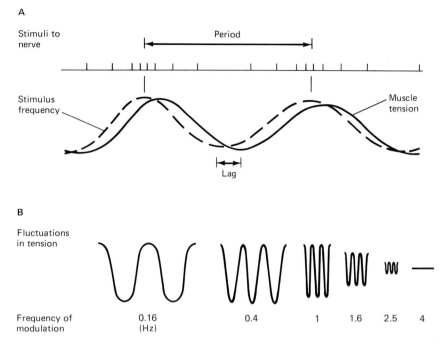

34–4 Muscle mechanics filter the information contained in the train of neural impulses. **A.** The stimuli are applied to the muscle nerve **(ticks on top trace)** with a sinusoidal frequency **(broken line in lower trace).** The oscillation in the muscle tension **(solid line in lower trace)** lags behind the changes in stimulus frequency. **B.** Changes in the frequency of the sinusoidal stimulation cause changes in the frequency and amplitude of muscle tension. At high rates, the tension no longer fluctuates. (Adapted from Partridge, 1966.)

potential at the onset of a relatively low-frequency stimulus train produces a remarkable enhancement of the tension output (Figure 34–3B). The tension produced when the pair of spikes occurs close together (called a *doublet*) is much greater and develops much more rapidly than the sum of the tensions that would be produced by either spike alone. Moreover, the effect of the second impulse can last many seconds. This mechanism for increasing both the tension in a muscle and the rate at which that tension increases is thought to be used for producing rapid movement.

Recruitment and rate coding are not mutually exclusive strategies for grading muscular force. In humans, successive single motor units are recruited and rate-modulated in an orderly fashion when the motor task involves a slowly increasing force. Under these conditions each motor unit is recruited at a specific force threshold. However, to produce rapid ballistic contractions all motor units must be mobilized quickly, almost at the same time. The number of motor units recruited is therefore also dependent on the rate at which the force develops; nonetheless, the recruitment order is preserved, and large motor units are activated only after all of the smaller ones are recruited.

Skeletal Muscles Filter the Information Contained in the Neural Spike Trains That Control Them

The control that the nervous system exerts over skeletal muscles does not occur through a simple one-to-one transformation of trains of action potentials in motor neurons to changes of muscle length or tension; rather, *the changes in muscle tension represent a filtered transformation of the changes in the frequency of neural im-*

pulses. This is best demonstrated by applying sinusoidally varying electrical inputs to nerve and examining how the signal is modified at the output by changes in muscle tension. This method has been used to characterize properties of sensory receptors and muscles as well as synaptic relays. Sinusoidally varying inputs allow one to determine how faithfully a signal reaching a processing element (such as a neuron-to-neuron synapse or a nerve-to-muscle synapse) is transmitted; conversely, sinusoidal inputs allow one to specify how such signals are distorted by intervening processes.

This method was first applied to muscle by Lloyd Partridge, who used it to examine changes in tension as the rate of nerve impulses delivered to the muscle was varied sinusoidally. He found that sinusoidal modulation of a stimulus train produces oscillations in muscle tension that slightly lag behind the fluctuations in impulse frequency of the stimuli (Figure 34–4A). As the frequency of the impulse train is varied, systematic changes develop in peak-to-peak tension of the muscle (Figure 34–4B). When the impulse frequency is oscillated more rapidly the changes in tension become smaller. In Figure 34–4B a 50% drop in tension has occurred from 0.16 Hz to 1.6 Hz; by 4 Hz, almost no fluctuation in muscle tension is present.

From records of this type Partridge concluded that the muscles exclude signals modulated at high frequencies and thus act as *low-pass filters.* This property is closely related to the fact that the muscle twitch produced by a single impulse is very long (10–100 msec) relative to the duration of the action potential itself (about 1 msec; see Figure 34–1). The low-pass filter properties in muscle have two important implications. First, muscles reproduce faithfully only slowly varying signals. Since mus-

A

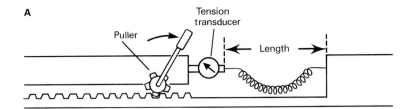

B

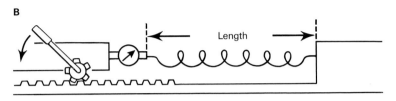

34–5 Changes in tension are produced by stretching a spring. **A.** When the length is less than the set point, the spring is slack. **B.** When the length is greater than the set point a restoring force is produced. **C.** As the length of the spring, L, increases beyond the set point, L_0, the tension, T, increases. The stiffness, K, is a ratio between the increases in both.

C

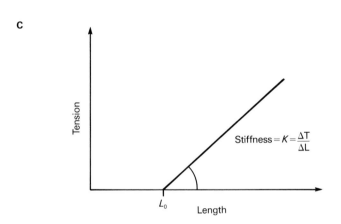

$$\text{Stiffness} = K = \frac{\Delta T}{\Delta L}$$

cles are activated by trains of action potentials in the muscle nerves, these trains must vary slowly if the changes in frequency are to be reflected with fidelity by changes in muscle tension. Second, rapid alternations in tension cannot be produced readily by one muscle acting alone. Since we can, in fact, produce alternating changes in tension at frequencies up to 8–10/sec, additional mechanisms must be available to compensate for this loss of force. One such mechanism operates by stimulating agonist and antagonist muscles in alternating bursts of activity.

Muscles Have Springlike Properties

The most common way our nervous system puts our muscles to use is to cause them to change their length; yet changes in muscle length are only an indirect consequence of neural activation. The degree to which a muscle can change in length (for example, in response to a given neural drive or train of spikes in a muscle nerve) depends on the *initial length* of the muscle and on the *forces opposing* changes in length. The dependence on initial length arises because muscles behave mechanically, like springs.

Alterations in Set Points

A spring is a mechanical device that responds to an increase in length by generating a restoring force that is proportional to the change in length. Moreover, in any spring (for example, a rubber band), this restoring force is developed only when the length exceeds a threshold known as the *set point* or resting length (L_0). Until L_0 is exceeded, the spring is slack (Figure 34–5A). In Figure 34–5B, as length is increased beyond L_0, the tension increases linearly. The slope of the line shown in Figure 34–5C—that is, the increment in tension (ΔT) divided by the increment in length (ΔL)—represents the spring constant K, also known as the *stiffness*:

$$K = \frac{\Delta T}{\Delta L}.$$

Thus, the tension or force produced by the spring can be described by the simple equation

$$T = K(L - L_0).$$

Measurements of muscle tension at different lengths indicate that muscles are like springs in that the tension

A

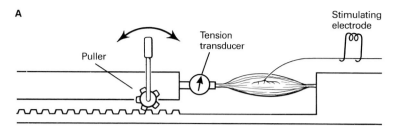

B

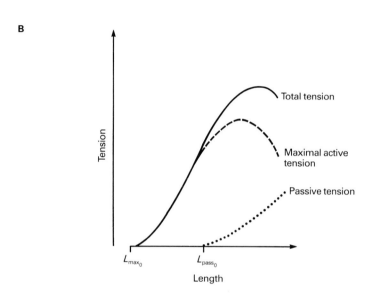

34–6 In normal muscle the amount of tension varies in proportion to length throughout most of the muscle's range. The **dotted line** shows the length–tension curve of a denervated muscle and represents the contribution of passive elastic elements (crossbridges in muscle fibers, connective tissue). The shape of the line is known as the passive stiffness of the muscle (K_{pass}). The **solid line** shows the length–tension curve for the same muscle when it is stimulated to produce maximal tetanic tension. The amount of tension developed by muscle increases as the muscle is stretched. **A.** The stretch of the muscle is depicted by a ratchet mechanism. **B.** For lengths greater than L_{pass_0}, the total tension (**solid line**) is the sum of active (**broken line**) and passive (**dotted line**) components.

exerted by muscle varies in proportion to the muscle's length (Figure 34–6). The muscle does not offer resistance until the set point is reached (i.e., the passive set point, L_{pass_0}). As the muscle is pulled beyond this point, a gradual increase in tension occurs. With maximal stimulation, as the muscle is stretched, it starts to develop tension at a much shorter length (its new set point, L_{max_0}) than it did in the passive state. This is equivalent to taking up the slack of a rubber band by excising a portion of it to shorten its initial length. In addition, when the muscle nerve is stimulated, the increase in tension produced by a given change in length (i.e., the slope of the length–tension relation) also increases. As a general rule, as the frequency of nerve impulses reaching the muscle increases, the set point length (L_0) decreases and the stiffness (K) increases. As we shall see in Chapter 35, however, stiffness is highly dependent on afferent signals acting on spinal motor neurons. Thus, it follows that the change in force produced by a given amount of neural activity is dependent on muscle length.

Let us now take a specific example and apply the physical principles we have just discussed in a physiological context. The biceps muscle can be represented as a spring acting to flex the elbow joint as shown in Figure 34–7A, and a change in set point (from L_1 to L_2 in Figure

34–7C) can be represented by a ratchet mechanism. An increase in neural activity (Figure 34–7B) is equivalent to clockwise rotation of the ratchet, and the increase in stiffness is equivalent to a thickening of the spring. The rotation of the ratchet pulls on the spring, which in turn moves the forearm to a specific point where the external forces (for example, the weight of the forearm) just balance the forces generated by the spring. The angle of the elbow joint where muscle tension precisely matches the external force is called the equilibrium point. The concept of equilibrium point is crucial for understanding how the nervous system controls limb position. Although the control of limb position will be discussed in detail when voluntary movements are considered in Chapter 38, it is worthwhile at least to consider some aspects of the principle of equilibrium point here, in the context of the springlike properties of muscle.

Equilibrium Points and the Control of Limb Position

The problem of accurately positioning a joint to the proper angle is simplified when an antagonist muscle can be controlled together with the agonist. The consequence of this dual control is that the central nervous

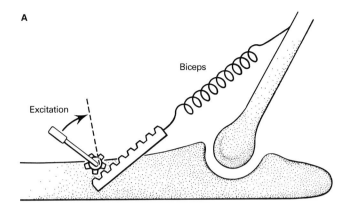

A

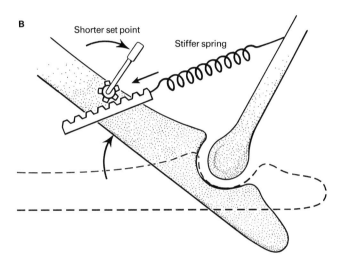

B

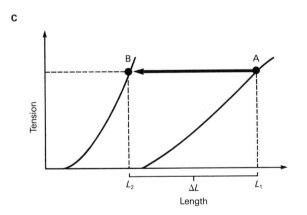

C

34–7 Changes in stiffness and set point of idealized elbow
flexor muscle (biceps) alter the limb position. **A.** The
ratchet mechanism represents a change in the set point of the
biceps, shown as a spring. **B.** Clockwise rotation of the ratchet
(lower set point resulting from increased neural activity) pulls
on the spring, which flexes the forearm. **C.** The graph
illustrates the change in length–tension relationships in
conditions **A** and **B.** In **A** the set point (L_1) is longer and the
stiffness (slope) is less than in **B.** The change in length, ΔL,
occurs because the opposing force (the mass of the arm)
remains the same in the two positions.

system can produce a given change in angular position
in several different ways. Two of these are illustrated
schematically in Figure 34–8A and B. Contractions of
muscles are shown as rotations of the ratchet mechanisms operating on a pair of springs representing biceps
(agonist) and triceps (antagonist). In Figure 34–8A the
contraction of the agonist is accompanied by *relaxation*
of the antagonist. This occurs through a mechanism
called *reciprocal innervation* (the neural mechanisms of
reciprocal innervation will be discussed in Chapter 35).
The activation (shortening) of the biceps increases its
stiffness and decreases its set point length (as shown in
Figure 34–7), whereas the relaxation of the triceps brings
about a decrease in stiffness and a corresponding increase
in set point length. These changes in both muscles result
in a new equilibrium position of the limb: the elbow is
flexed to the newly specified joint angle (Figure 34–8A
and B).

The same final joint position can be achieved in a different way by contracting both the agonist and the antagonist muscles, a process called *co-contraction*. Now,
however, the agonist must contract more than in reciprocal innervation because of the larger opposing forces
developed by the antagonist (Figure 34–8C). The increased contraction and stiffness of both muscles result
in an overall increase in the stiffness of the joint itself.
Thus, with the contraction of two opposing muscles, the
central nervous system can control both joint angle and
joint stiffness (Figure 34–8C).

Co-contraction is more costly in energy than is reciprocal innervation because two muscles are activated instead of one. Why, then, would the nervous system use
this second strategy? Co-contraction, although less efficient, provides a greater stability in response to unanticipated changes in external forces or loads. Because the
joint is stiffer with co-contraction, an unexpected change
in load will have less of a negative effect on achieving
the final desired angle of the joint than if reciprocal innervation were used.

Thus, there are two ways to achieve the same equilibrium point, each having a benefit and a cost: reciprocal
innervation is more energy efficient, but it requires that
the loads be accurately known; co-contraction uses more
energy but does not require that the loads be known precisely and decreases the effect of unexpected disturbances. One might expect, then, that as we learn to an-
ticipate loads during movements, we might switch from
one strategy to another. When we first practice a movement requiring accuracy, we typically use the co-contraction strategy. Only when we become familiar with
all external mechanical forces with practice, do we tend
to use the more energy-efficient solution of relaxing the
antagonist. As we shall see later, reflex actions also play
an important role in adjusting and regulating the stiffness of muscles and joints.

The idea that the central nervous system might control limb position (and posture in general) through the
specification of an equilibrium point was first docu-

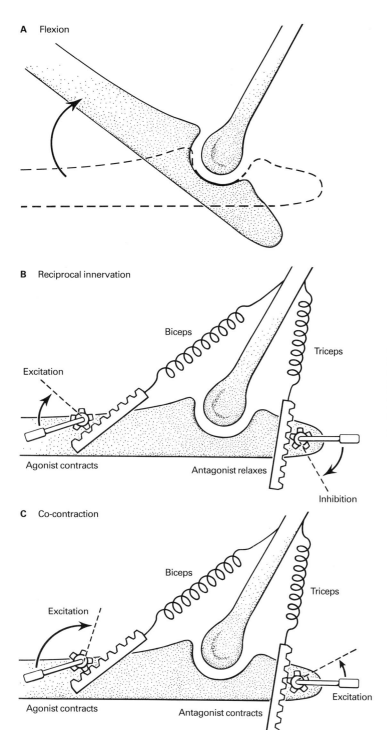

A Flexion

B Reciprocal innervation

Biceps

Triceps

Excitation

Agonist contracts

Antagonist relaxes

Inhibition

C Co-contraction

Biceps

Triceps

Excitation

Agonist contracts

Antagonist contracts

Excitation

34–8 The same change in equilibrium point, or joint angle (**A**), can be produced by reciprocal innervation (**B**) or co-contraction (**C**). Rotations of the ratchet mechanisms indicate changes in the set points of the muscles, represented by springs. **B.** The elbow is flexed by reciprocal innervation. The set point of the excited biceps is lowered and the muscle contracts while the inhibited triceps relaxes. **C.** The elbow is flexed by co-contraction. The agonist (biceps) must contract enough to overcome the force of the contracting antagonist (triceps).

mented experimentally by the Russian physiologist Anatol Feldman and later extended by Emilio Bizzi at the Massachusetts Institute of Technology. This concept is important because it led to one of the first attempts by motor physiologists to take into account the mechanical properties of muscles while considering how the brain could control limb position. This particular solution to the problem of controlling limb position allows the ner-

vous system to specify the angular position of the whole joint rather than control each individual muscle independently. Moreover, as emphasized by Feldman and by Bizzi, since the equilibrium point at the end of a movement specifies an intended final limb position, the central commands that control this end point need not be concerned with the position of the limb before movement.

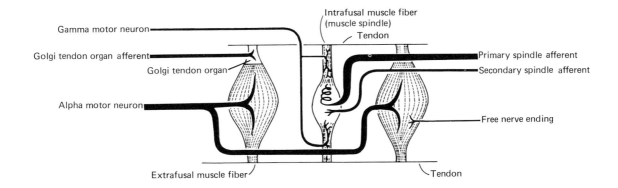

Muscles Have Specialized Receptors That Convey Information to the Central Nervous System

Muscles and joints contain a variety of receptors. Some inform the central nervous system about the length of the muscle, others detect its tension, and still others respond to pressure or to noxious stimuli. Among these different receptors, two have been most thoroughly studied and have important and specific actions on motor neurons. These are the *muscle spindles* and the *Golgi tendon organs.* Although both of these receptors discharge when the muscle is stretched, differences in their anatomical arrangement within the muscle are reflected in differences in the information they convey to the central nervous system. Muscle spindles, arranged in parallel with the muscle fibers, provide information about the length of the muscle. Golgi tendon organs are arranged in series with the muscle fibers and inform the nervous system of the tension exerted by the muscle on its tendinous insertion to the bone (Figure 34–9).

Muscle Spindles

Mammalian muscle spindles are receptors that are distributed throughout the fleshy parts of skeletal muscle. Each spindle, which consists of an encapsulated group of fine specialized muscle fibers, is tapered at each end and expanded at its center in a fluid-filled capsule. Within this capsule the muscular elements are entwined by the terminal branches of afferent fibers. The small muscle fibers within the spindle are called *intrafusal fibers;* they do not contribute to the overall tension of the muscle but regulate the excitability of the spindle afferents by mechanically deforming the receptors. Intrafusal fibers are innervated by small motor cells of the ventral horn called *gamma motor neurons* (Figure 34–9). The large skeletal muscle fibers that do develop substantial muscle tension are called *extrafusal fibers* and are innervated by the large *alpha motor neurons* in the ventral horn.

Muscle spindles contain two types of intrafusal muscle fibers called *nuclear bag fibers* and *nuclear chain fibers* after the arrangement of nuclei in their equatorial region (Figure 34–10). The bag fibers have nuclei clustered in twos or threes; the chain fibers have nuclei in

34–9 The muscle spindles (intrafusal fibers) are in parallel with the extrafusal fibers; the Golgi tendon organs are in series. The thicknesses of the afferent and efferent fibers represent their relative diameters. The intrafusal fibers do not actually attach to tendons; they attach directly to the extrafusal fibers, occupying only a small fraction of their length.

single file and are shorter and more slender than the bag fibers. The bag and chain fibers also differ in the kind of contraction they exhibit: bag fibers produce slow contractions, whereas chain fibers produce fast (or twitch) contractions.

There are two types of afferent terminals in muscle spindles: primary and secondary. The primary and secondary endings differ in several ways. The most important difference is their relationship to the two types of intrafusal fibers. *Primary endings innervate every single intrafusal fiber within a spindle,* however many there

34–10 Nuclear bag and nuclear chain intrafusal fibers within a muscle spindle each have their own efferent control (relative lengths of fibers not shown). Group I (primary) afferents innervate both the nuclear bag and the nuclear chain fibers, whereas group II (secondary) afferents usually innervate only the nuclear chain fibers; however, they occasionally can innervate bag fibers (indicated by the **thin branch**). (Adapted from Matthews, 1964.)

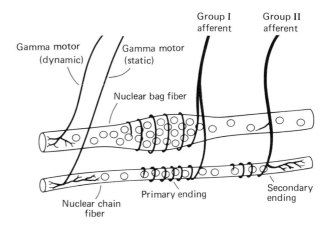

are, and irrespective of whether they are nuclear bag or nuclear chain fibers. *Secondary endings lie almost exclusively on nuclear chain fibers* (Figure 34–10). Because of differences in their morphology, the primary endings were once called annulospiral, and the secondary endings were referred to as *flower spray* endings.

Golgi Tendon Organs

The Golgi tendon organ is a slender capsule approximately 1 mm long and 0.1 mm in diameter. Each organ is in series with about 15–20 extrafusal skeletal muscle fibers that enter the capsule through a tight-fitting, funnellike collar. The muscle fibers terminate in musculotendinous junctions after entering the capsule and give rise to collagen fiber bundles that become braided and run the length of the capsule. An afferent fiber enters the capsule in the middle and branches many times, so that the axons of the afferent fiber become twisted within the braids of the collagen fiber bundles. When the skeletal muscle fibers contract they cause the collagen bundles to straighten; this, in turn, compresses the axons of the afferent fibers, causing them to fire. Thus, the braided arrangement of the collagen fiber bundles gives them a significant mechanical advantage in compressing the intertwined afferent axons, making those axons very sensitive to small changes in muscle tension. Moreover, because the afferent fiber is entwined in collagenous fibers that transmit force from many muscle fibers to the tendon proper, the afferent fiber responds to multiple motor units and can thus register the effects of recruitment.

Muscle Afferents

The standard classification of muscle afferents was introduced by David Lloyd and H.-T. Chang in 1948. Lloyd and Chang found that the myelinated afferent fibers from muscle fall into three main categories of diameters, which they classified as groups I, II, and III. (Lloyd and Chang's classification system, described in Chapter 23, includes another category—group IV, which are unmyelinated fibers.)

In 1954, Carlton Hunt studied the conduction velocity of fibers from different receptors. By inferring the fiber diameter from the conduction velocity,[2] he showed that the largest of the group I fibers (called Ia fibers) contain axons that innervate the muscle spindles; the smaller diameter subpopulation of group I fibers (called Ib fibers) are from Golgi tendon organs. However, the Ia and Ib populations overlap considerably. The group II fibers have smaller axons that innervate muscle spindles. The diameters of the two types of afferents from muscle spindles correspond to the function of these afferents: the large afferents make primary endings and the small afferents make secondary endings. These relationships are summarized in Figure 34–11. Much less is known about group III and the unmyelinated group IV fibers (not shown in Figure 34–11), but these fibers probably have free nerve endings. They are presumed to be responsible for sensations of muscle pressure and pain.

Muscle Stretch Receptors Convey Information About Muscle Length, Tension, and Velocity of Stretch

The relationship between muscle spindles and Golgi tendon organs was first analyzed by B. H. C. Matthews at Cambridge University in a classic series of studies carried out in 1933. Matthews found that, when he recorded from the axon afferent of a muscle spindle or a tendon organ and *stretched* the muscle, the afferent from either the tendon organ or the spindle would *increase* its rate of discharge. On the other hand, if the muscle was made to *contract actively* while still stretched (for example by stimulation of the motor neuron that supplies the muscle), the *tendon organ further increased its discharge but the spindle discharge decreased or ceased altogether* (Figure 34–12). The reason for this difference in response lies in the anatomical arrangement of the two types of receptors. The spindle organs are arranged in parallel with the extrafusal muscle fibers, whereas the Golgi tendon organs are arranged in series with the extrafusal fibers (Figure 34–9).

34–11 Relationship between receptor type, fiber diameter, and conduction velocity in muscle nerves. Note the bimodal distribution of afferents from muscle spindles (**solid line**) and the unimodal distribution of afferents from Golgi tendon organs (**broken line**). (Adapted from Hunt, 1954.)

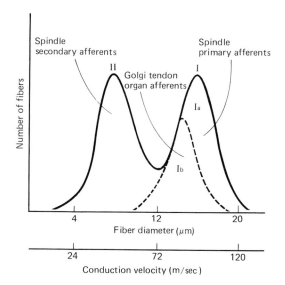

---

[2]Years before, J. B. Hursh had shown that conduction velocity (in meters per second) is roughly six times the fiber diameter (expressed in micrometers). This conversion factor (conduction velocity equals fiber diameter multiplied by 6) has subsequently been shown to be inexact for smaller diameter fibers, where the appropriate conversion factor has been estimated to be between 3 and 4. Thus, a 3-μm fiber, which would have been estimated to conduct at 18 m/sec using Hursh's factor, usually conducts at approximately 9–12 m/sec.

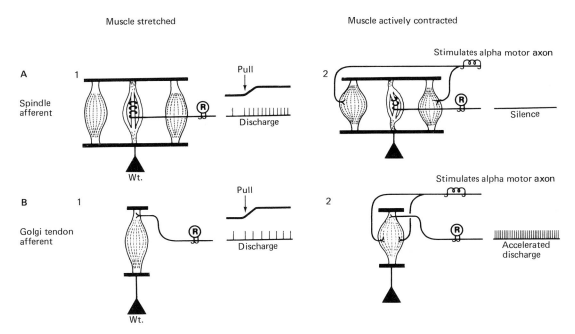

Muscle stretched   Muscle actively contracted

34–12 The two types of muscle stretch receptors give different responses to muscle stretch and, particularly, to muscle contraction. **A.** Muscle spindle responses. **B.** Golgi tendon organ responses. Both afferents discharge to stretch of the muscle (**A1, B1**), the Golgi tendon organ less than the spindle. However, when the muscle is made to contract actively by stimulation of its motor neuron, the spindle is unloaded (**A2**) and therefore goes silent, whereas the tendon organ output is further increased (**B2**). (Adapted from Patton, 1966.)

Passive stretching of the muscle distorts and thereby activates both the tendon organ and the muscle spindle receptors. (Stretching of the muscle spindle is called *loading*.) Contraction further stretches the tendon organ. (Tendon organs are much more sensitive to muscle contraction than to passive stretch, as will be discussed in Chapter 35.) However, active contraction of the extrafusal muscle fibers makes the intrafusal fibers go slack, *unloading* the spindle (Figure 34–12A, 2) so that it is no longer stretched. The discharge of tendon organs is increased and the discharge of spindle organs is decreased during muscle contraction. Thus, tendon organs, because they are in series with the extrafusal muscles, sense *muscle tension*, whereas the spindle organs, which are in parallel with the extrafusal fibers, sense *muscle length*.

When a muscle is stretched, the primary and secondary afferents in the muscle spindles respond quite differently. Both fiber types respond to static (steady-state) stretch, although secondary endings are a bit more sensitive; but the fibers respond differently to the dynamic phase of stretch (when the muscle is actually changing in length). Primary endings are very sensitive to the dynamic phase of stretch, whereas the secondary endings are not. *Thus the secondary endings are mainly sensitive to the length of the muscle, whereas the primary endings are sensitive both to the length of the muscle and to the rate of change in length.*

The dynamic sensitivity of the primary endings is largely due to the mechanical properties of the nuclear bag fibers. As early as 1933 B. H. C. Matthews had sug-

gested that the dynamic response of the primary afferents results from differences in viscoelastic properties between the receptor region and the polar region of the intrafusal muscle fibers. More recently, I. A. Boyd has clarified matters further by demonstrating an interesting mechanical property of the nuclear bag fiber that he called "intrafusal creep." Boyd found that, during prolonged passive stretch of the bag fiber, the fiber starts to creep back toward its unstretched length as its equatorial region (the region innervated by the primary afferent; Figure 34–10) begins to relax. This effect is exaggerated dramatically when the stretch is accompanied by stimulation of a dynamic gamma motor neuron innervating that bag fiber (see below). Thus, the dynamic sensitivity of the primary afferent reflects the mechanical properties of the bag fiber, whose equatorial region is maximally stretched as the length is increased, but begins to relax and shorten once the length remains steady.

The Central Nervous System Can Directly Control the Sensitivity of Muscle Spindles

As we saw earlier, contraction of extrafusal muscle fibers is produced by large alpha motor neurons; intrafusal muscle fibers are controlled by the smaller gamma motor neurons. The gamma motor neurons innervate the intrafusal muscle fibers at their polar regions, where the contractile elements of the fibers are located. The equatorial region of intrafusal fibers is almost devoid of contractile elements. Activation of a gamma efferent has the

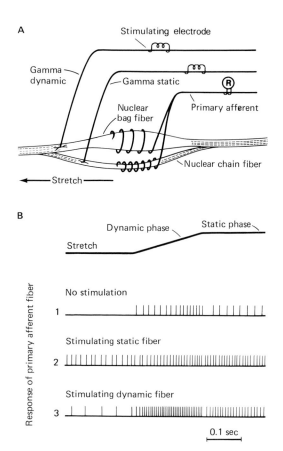

34–13 Crowe and Matthews demonstrated the difference between static and dynamic gamma motor neurons. **A.** Experimental setup. Extracellular electrodes can activate either gamma$_d$ or gamma$_s$ fibers before and during a ramp stretch applied to an extrafusal muscle, and the discharge response of the primary afferent (**R**) is measured. **B.** Differences in the primary afferent response are recorded when the stretch is superimposed on static or dynamic gamma activity. First, the extrafusal muscle is stretched and the primary afferent response is recorded (**1**). Next, a static gamma motor fiber is stimulated prior to and during the stretch (**2**). Then a dynamic gamma motor fiber is stimulated prior to and during the stretch (**3**). (Adapted from Crowe and Matthews, 1964.)

effect of contracting and shortening the intrafusal fiber at its ends, thereby stretching the equatorial region.

Dynamic and Static Gamma Motor Neurons

There are two types of gamma motor neurons. One type innervates nuclear bag fibers (*gamma dynamic* or γ_d); the other type innervates nuclear chain fibers (*gamma static* or γ_s). The reason for the names dynamic and static is that these gamma motor neurons regulate the sensitivity of the spindle afferents either to dynamic or to static phases of stretch. This distinction can be best appreciated through an experiment carried out by A. Crowe and P. B. C. Matthews about 20 years ago (Figure 34–13). These investigators recorded from a single primary afferent fiber while stretching a muscle (Figure 34–

13A). The primary afferent response typically showed a high rate of discharge initially (Figure 34–13B, 1) during the stretch (dynamic phase) and increased firing during the maintained stretch (static phase). They let the muscle relax and repeated the procedure, but this time they also activated a static gamma fiber before and during the stretch. This background static gamma activation enhanced the primary afferent response to static stretch (Figure 34–13B, 2). After allowing the muscle to relax they repeated the procedure again, this time stretching the muscle while stimulating a dynamic gamma fiber. This procedure enhanced the primary afferent response to the phasic, or dynamic, phase of stretch (Figure 34–13B, 3). The primary afferent response is influenced by both types of gamma fibers because the Ia afferent fiber innervates both the nuclear bag and the nuclear chain intrafusal fibers. As might be expected, because secondary endings are generally restricted to nuclear chain fibers group II afferents are influenced almost exclusively by static gamma motor neurons.

Functional Role of the Gamma System

An important role of the gamma system is to allow the spindle to maintain its high sensitivity over a wide range of muscle lengths during reflex and voluntary contractions. This function of the gamma system was first suggested by Carlton Hunt and Stephen Kuffler about 30 years ago. They reasoned that during large active contractions of extrafusal muscles the spindles become unloaded and would thus be unable to signal any further changes in muscle length (Figure 34–14A and B). Although they did not distinguish between static and dynamic efferents, they suggested that one role of the gamma system is to reload the spindle during active contractions, thereby keeping it responsive to further changes in length. Hunt and Kuffler's experiments confirmed this hypothesis, for they found that the characteristic pause in spindle discharge that occurs during a twitch contraction due to unloading of the spindle could be filled in by activation of a gamma efferent to the spindle during the contraction (Figure 34–14B and C). Stimulation of the gamma motor neuron during the extrafusal contraction prevents the spindle from being unloaded during the contraction, thereby keeping it responsive to further changes in length. Not surprisingly, this effect is due entirely to static gamma motor neurons.

Skeletofusimotor Innervation

Thus far we have considered how the central nervous system exerts relatively independent efferent control over (1) the intrafusal muscle fibers in the muscle spindles through gamma neurons and (2) the extrafusal muscle fibers through alpha motor neurons. However, it is now recognized that some muscle spindles are innervated by the same axon that innervates the extrafusal fibers. This is called *skeletofusimotor*, or *beta, innervation*. Skeletofusimotor innervation has been found in the cat, and it is likely that this kind of innervation exists in

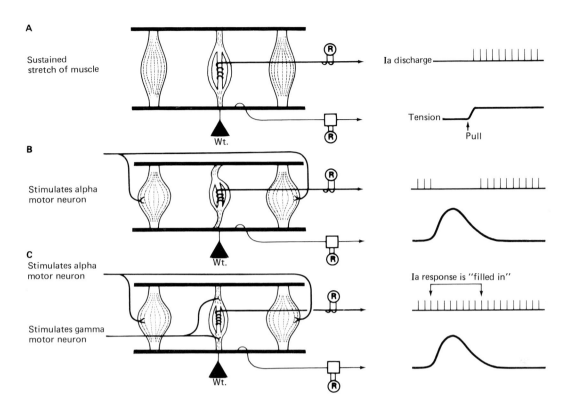

34–14 During active contractions, spindles can be reloaded by gamma activation. **A.** Sustained tension elicits steady firing of Ia afferent. **B.** Characteristic pause occurs in ongoing Ia discharge when the muscle is caused to contract by stimulation of its alpha motor neuron. The Ia fiber stops firing because the spindle is unloaded by the contraction. **C.** During a comparable contraction, a gamma motor neuron to the spindle is also stimulated, "filling in" the pause in Ia discharge by preventing unloading of the spindle during the contraction. (Adapted from Hunt and Kuffler, 1951.)

humans as well. The functional significance of beta innervation, compared with the dual alpha and gamma systems, remains an intriguing question for future research.

An Overall View

The function of the spindle afferents cannot be fully appreciated without understanding the modulation of those afferents by the gamma motor system. It is the integrated output of the two systems that is important for the successful operation of the motor system. To appreciate how the gamma system allows the spindle to maintain its high sensitivity over wide ranges of muscle length, we must consider how gamma motor neurons are controlled by descending influences. The gamma motor neurons for a particular muscle lie within the alpha motor neuron pool for the same muscle. Most descending systems that impinge upon alpha motor neurons (for example, those involved in postural adjustments or voluntary movements) also activate the smaller gamma motor neurons. Thus, alpha and gamma motor neurons are both activated by descending systems. Recent evidence suggests that dynamic and static gamma motor neurons can also be controlled independently by descending systems. In the next chapter we shall return to the process of co-activation. In addition, in our discussion of the cen-

tral actions of the muscle spindles and their role in the stretch reflex, we shall also consider other possible roles of the gamma system such as compensation for variations in the mechanical properties of muscle and compensation for changes in load during voluntary movement.

Selected Readings

Asatryan, D. G., and Feldman, A. G. 1965. Biophysics of complex systems and mathematical models. Functional tuning of the nervous system with control of movement or maintenance of a steady posture.—I. Mechanographic analysis of the work of the joint on execution of a postural task. Biophysics 10:925–935.

Bizzi, E., and Abend, W. 1983. Posture control and trajectory formation in single- and multi-joint arm movements. In J. E. Desmedt (ed.), Motor Control Mechanisms in Health and Disease. New York: Raven Press, pp. 31–45.

Brooks, V. B. (ed.). 1981. Handbook of Physiology, Section 1: The Nervous System, Vol. II, Motor Control. Bethesda, Md.: American Physiological Society.

Freund, H.-J. 1983. Motor unit and muscle activity in voluntary motor control. Physiol. Rev. 63:387–436.

Gurfinkel', V. S., Surguladze, T. D., Mirskii, M. L., and Tarko, A. M. 1970. Work of human motor units during rhythmic movements. Biophysics 15:1131–1137.

Harris, D. A., and Henneman, E. 1980. Feedback signals from muscle and their efferent control. In V. B. Mountcastle (ed.), Medical Physiology, 14th ed., Vol. 1. St. Louis: Mosby, pp. 703–717.

Henneman, E. 1980. Skeletal muscle: The servant of the nervous system. In V. B. Mountcastle (ed.), Medical Physiology, 14th ed., Vol. 1. St. Louis: Mosby, pp. 674–702.

Homma, S. (ed.). 1976. Understanding the stretch reflex. Prog. Brain Res. 44:1–507.

Jewett, D. L., and Rayner, M. D. 1984. Basic Concepts of Neuronal Function. Boston: Little, Brown, pp. 329–388.

Matthews, P. B. C. 1981. Muscle spindles: Their messages and their fusimotor supply. In V. B. Brooks (ed.), Handbook of Physiology, Section 1: The Nervous System, Vol. II, Motor Control. Bethesda, Md.: American Physiological Society, pp. 189–228.

Patton, H. D. 1965. Reflex regulation of movement and posture. In T. C. Ruch and H. D. Patton (eds.), Physiology and Biophysics, 19th ed. Philadelphia: Saunders, pp. 181–206.

Polit, A., and Bizzi, E. 1978. Processes controlling arm movements in monkeys. Science 201:1235–1237.

Stein, R. B. 1974. Peripheral control of movement. Physiol. Rev. 54:215–243.

References

Boyd, I. A. 1976. The response of fast and slow nuclear bag fibres and nuclear chain fibres in isolated cat muscle spindles to fusimotor stimulation, and the effect of intrafusal contraction on the sensory endings. Q. J. Exp. Physiol. 61:203–253.

Buchthal, F. 1942. The mechanical properties of the single striated muscle fibre at rest and during contraction and their structural interpretation. Dan. Biol. Med. 17:1.

Burke, R. E., Levine, D. N., Saloman, M., and Tsairis, P. 1974. Motor units in cat soleus muscle: physiological, histochemical and morphological characteristics. J. Physiol. (Lond.) 238:503–514.

Burke, R. E., Rudomin, P., and Zajac, F. E., III. 1976. The effect of activation history on tension production by individual muscle units. Brain Res. 109:515–529.

Crowe, A., and Matthews, P. B. C. 1964. The effects of stimulation of static and dynamic fusimotor fibres on the response to stretching of the primary endings of muscle spindles. J. Physiol. (Lond.) 174:109–131.

Henneman, E., Somjen, G., and Carpenter, D. O. 1965. Functional significance of cell size in spinal motoneurons. J. Neurophysiol. 28:560–580.

Hunt, C. C. 1954. Relation of function to diameter in afferent fibers of muscle nerves. J. Gen. Physiol. 38:117–131.

Hunt, C. C., and Kuffler, S. W. 1951. Stretch receptor discharges during muscle contraction. J. Physiol. (Lond.) 113:298–315.

Hursh, J. B. 1939. Conduction velocity and diameter of nerve fibers. Am. J. Physiol. 127:131–139.

Liddell, E. G. T., and Sherrington, C. S. 1925. Recruitment and some other features of reflex inhibition. Proc. R. Soc. Lond. [Biol.] 97:488–518.

Lloyd, D. P. C., and Chang, H.-T. 1948. Afferent fibers in muscle nerves. J. Neurophysiol. 11:199–207.

Matthews, B. H. C. 1933. Nerve endings in mammalian muscle. J. Physiol. (Lond.) 78:1–53.

Matthews, P. B. C. 1964. Muscle spindles and their motor control. Physiol. Rev. 44:219–288.

Partridge, L. D. 1966. Signal-handling characteristics of load-moving skeletal muscle. Am. J. Physiol. 210:1178–1191.

Thomas J. Carew

The Control of Reflex Action

35

In the previous chapter we considered muscles and receptors—the peripheral machinery involved in the production of movement. In this chapter we shall examine how this machinery is brought into action by the central nervous system to generate a wide variety of behavioral acts.

The simplest behavioral acts are reflexes, machinelike responses that are elicited by particular types of sensory stimuli. One of the best known is the knee-jerk reflex, in which the primary afferent fibers from muscle spindles act directly on the motor neurons innervating the quadriceps muscle and its synergists to produce a brisk extension of the knee. In other reflexes, one or more interneurons may be interposed between the primary afferent fibers and the motor neurons. Interneurons are present in all reflexes produced by stimulation of cutaneous mechanoreceptors. An example is the flexion reflex. Here noxious stimulation of the foot leads to withdrawal of the entire leg, a reflex that involves the coordination of many muscle groups. Interneurons distribute excitation and inhibition to many different motor neurons. In general, reflexes are characterized by a fixed spatial relationship between the locus of a stimulus and the particular muscles that contract. This specific topographic relationship is known as the *local sign*. Reflexes are also typically graded so that the intensity of the stimulation governs the intensity of the response.

The neuronal circuits that mediate reflexes are relatively simple. Moreover, descending influences from higher brain centers often use these same neuronal circuits to generate more complex behavior. Therefore, an understanding of the organizational principles of reflexes is essential for understanding more complex motor sequences. Reflexes also are valuable for clinical diagnosis. They can be used to assess the integrity of both afferent and motor connections as well as the general excitability of the spinal cord.

We shall begin by considering reflexes triggered by receptors in muscle because they are relatively simple and because a great deal is known about the muscle spindles and Golgi tendon organs. These reflexes are designed to correct motor output rapidly and automatically at the level of the spinal cord, providing the higher centers of the brain with the time needed to integrate other incoming information and to determine the appropriate motor output.

Ia Afferent Fibers Contribute to the Stretch Reflex

Basic Features of the Stretch Reflex

Charles Sherrington began the modern analysis of reflex physiology in the late nineteenth century. He developed an experimental preparation using cats whose brain stems had been transected surgically at the level of the midbrain between the superior and inferior colliculi. In this procedure, discussed in Chapter 37, the cerebrum is disconnected from the spinal cord, thus blocking pain sensation. Because decerebrate animals show heightened reflexes and a dramatic increase in muscle tone in the extensor muscles of their limbs, they have been used extensively to study postural control (see Chapter 37). In examining the reflexes in the hind limb of a decerebrate cat, Sherrington and Edward Liddell found that when they attempted to force the rigidly extended limb passively into a flexed position, the limb resisted the force by active muscular contraction. They called this the *stretch reflex* or *myotatic reflex* (*myotatic* from two Greek words meaning extended muscle). By 1925, Sherrington and Liddell had carefully characterized the stretch reflex in the knee extensor (quadriceps) and had concluded that the stretch reflex enhances the springlike properties of muscle and offers a graded resistance to change in length.

Stretch reflexes are seen in both flexor and extensor muscles, but they are most highly developed in muscles called *physiological extensors*, whose predominant action is to oppose gravity. Sherrington and Liddell found that the stretch reflex has two components: (1) a *phasic component*, which is short-lasting and relatively strong, and which is tested clinically by examining the tendon jerks, for example, by tapping the patellar tendon; and (2) a *tonic component*, which is weaker but lasts longer and is thought to be important for maintaining posture. The two components of the reflex are initiated by different aspects of the muscle's action. The phasic component is triggered by the *change in muscle length* that accompanies movement of the limb, whereas the tonic component is determined by the *steady stretch* of the muscles. In active muscles the tonic component predominates. For example, when a stretch is applied to actively contracting muscles in cats, there is little phasic response to

the stretch; the predominant response is a tonic increase in tension as the muscle is increasingly stretched.

The work on reflexes led Sherrington and Liddell to the discovery of a key principle of reflex organization: *reciprocal innervation* (see Figure 34–8A). Stretching the antagonist knee flexors (such as the biceps or the semitendinous muscle) causes neurons in the spinal cord to inhibit the extensor stretch reflex. In this reciprocal arrangement, the final efferent output of the spinal cord ensures an integrated motor response.

Central Connections of the Ia Afferent Fibers

What is the neuronal circuit for the stretch reflex? Specifically, which afferent fibers mediate this behavior? In the 1940s David Lloyd at the Rockefeller Institute worked out the synaptic connections made by the Ia afferents in the spinal cord and found that they beautifully accounted for the stretch reflex. To activate axons of a given diameter selectively, Lloyd applied carefully graded electrical stimuli to nerves of muscle origin. At the same time, he recorded the efferent (reflex) output of the spinal cord from the ventral roots. Remember that the threshold of an axon to extracellular current is inversely related to its diameter.[1] Thus, with the weakest stimulus strength, Lloyd could activate the largest fibers (the Ia afferents) selectively and examine the efferent volley (the reflex action) they produced. By increasing the stimulus he also activated the Ib afferents and was able to identify any new effects as a function of their contribution. By carefully measuring the latency of the efferent volley produced by (1) stretching of the gastrocnemius (ankle extensor) muscle and (2) electrical stimulation of the dorsal root, Lloyd estimated the number of synaptic delays that exist in the reflex pathway. Using this technique, he traced the path of the central connections of the Ia fibers in the spinal cord.

A few years later, with the advent of intracellular recording techniques, John Eccles and his colleagues confirmed and extended Lloyd's observations, and the following picture emerged (Figure 35–1):

1. The Ia fibers from both extensor and flexor muscles make direct monosynaptic excitatory connections with alpha motor neurons that innervate the same muscles *(homonymous muscles)*. In this arrangement, called *autogenetic excitation*, an afferent from a particular muscle either excites or inhibits a motor neuron that

---

[1]The fact that large-diameter fibers have low thresholds does not contradict the size principle described in the previous chapter, which states that, given the same synaptic current, small neurons are recruited into activity before large neurons. Large axons have a lower threshold than small axons when stimulated with extracellular current because of their geometry. When current flows extracellularly it has two paths: (1) through the extracellular space and (2) across the axon membranes. Cells with a large-diameter axon are affected by more of the extracellular current than cells with a small-diameter axon. The lower input resistance of large neurons, which raises their threshold to *synaptic* current, is more than offset by their increased axon diameter, which lowers their threshold to *extracellular* current.

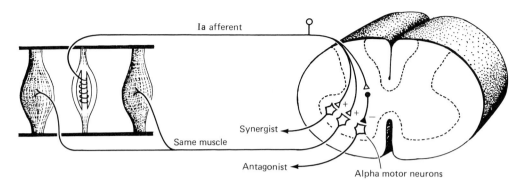

35–1 In the basic reflex circuitry for the myotatic reflex, Ia afferents monosynaptically excite motor neurons to the same (homonymous) muscle from which they arise and

motor neurons to synergist muscles; they also inhibit motor neurons to antagonist muscles through an inhibitory **(black)** interneuron.

produces contraction of the same muscle. Thus, the receptor has some degree of control over the muscle in which it resides. The distribution of Ia afferent fibers to alpha motor neurons supplying homonymous muscles is quite extensive. Using *spike-triggered averaging,*[2] in which a computer is triggered by the impulse in a single Ia afferent to detect the excitatory postsynaptic potentials produced by that afferent in the alpha motor neurons, Lorne Mendell and Elwood Henneman estimated that a single Ia afferent from the cat's medial gastrocnemius muscle sends synaptic terminals to *all* of the motor neurons innervating that muscle—approximately 300 motor neurons!

2. The Ia fibers also make direct monosynaptic excitatory connections on alpha motor neurons that innervate synergist muscles as well as the muscle from which the Ia fiber originated.

3. The Ia fibers provide direct excitatory synaptic input to *inhibitory* interneurons; these in turn connect directly to alpha motor neurons controlling muscles that are *antagonistic* to those from which the Ia fibers originated. Thus, the Ia fiber inhibits the antagonist motor neuron disynaptically by means of an intercalated inhibitory interneuron. This class of interneuron, called the Ia inhibitory interneuron (black in Figure 35–1), has been extensively studied (see Figure 35–2). Inhibition of antagonist motor neurons that occurs at the same time that

homonymous and synergist neurons are excited is called *reciprocal inhibition*. Reciprocal inhibition accounts for the reciprocal innervation described by Sherrington: as motor neurons to homonymous and synergist muscles are excited, motor neurons to antagonist muscles are inhibited.

Another important inhibitory spinal interneuron is the *Renshaw cell*, named after its discoverer, Birdsey Renshaw. This neuron receives direct excitation from collateral branches of spinal motor neurons, and in turn inhibits many motor neurons, including the one that gave rise to its input. This process is called *recurrent inhibition* (Figure 35–2). Recurrent inhibition can have several functional consequences. Perhaps the most obvious is that it tends to curtail the motor output from a particular collection of motor neurons, called a *motor pool*. Recurrent inhibition may also highlight the output

35–2 The elementary circuitry underlying recurrent inhibition involves the Renshaw cell, an inhibitory interneuron that is directly excited by collateral branches of spinal motor neurons; it inhibits many motor neurons, including the one that gave rise to its input. It disinhibits antagonist motor neurons by inhibiting Ia inhibitory interneurons.

[2]Spike-triggered averaging increases the signal-to-noise ratio of recorded voltage deflections in the postsynaptic cell produced by a given presynaptic spike. A computer is used to average all voltage deflections during a specified period after the occurrence of action potentials in a specific afferent axon (recorded by a second electrode). The signals examined with this method are thus *time-locked* to the spike. Since a monosynaptic excitatory postsynaptic potential from the Ia fiber will always occur at the exact same time after the spike, it will be constantly added into the average. On the other hand, randomly occurring events (for example, postsynaptic potentials from other cells or electrical noise) will sometimes add to the average and sometimes subtract from it. This method allows very small excitatory postsynaptic potentials that are triggered by a specific spike of interest to be detected, since the contribution of random fluctuations is progressively smaller with successive averages.

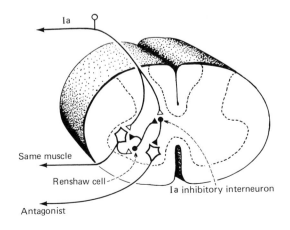

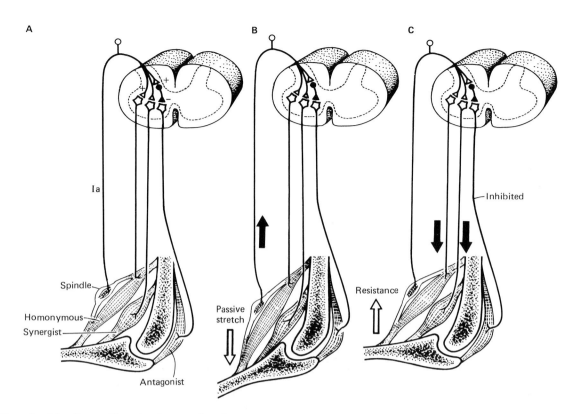

35-3 The role of Ia afferent fibers in the stretch reflex is exemplified by this reflex of flexor muscles. **A.** The connections of the Ia afferents excite the homonymous and synergist muscles and inhibit the antagonist muscles. **B.** Passive stretch of the limb **(open arrow)** gives rise to an increased Ia fiber discharge **(solid arrow). C.** The Ia fiber discharge causes homonymous and synergist alpha motor neurons to fire **(solid arrows)**, producing resistance to the stretch **(open arrow)**. (Figure adapted from Merton, 1972.)

of motor neurons that are strongly activated, because those motor neurons exert strong feedback inhibition (by means of the Renshaw cells) to other neighboring motor neurons, suppressing their output. Although the strongly activated motor neurons themselves also receive recurrent inhibition, their output, though diminished, can still be expressed because they are highly activated.

Among the many connections of the Renshaw cell, one of the most thoroughly studied is its direct connection to Ia inhibitory interneurons. Studies of the distribution of inhibition show that the Ia inhibitory interneurons receive their recurrent inhibition, via the Renshaw cells, from motor neurons to the same muscles that give rise to their Ia afferent input (Figure 35-2). Thus, alpha motor neurons and Ia inhibitory interneurons that receive the same Ia input also receive recurrent inhibition from the same set of Renshaw cells. An important functional consequence of this arrangement is that the Renshaw cell can limit the duration and magnitude of a Ia afferent-mediated reflex response, since Ia afferent activation of a homonymous motor neuron will in turn produce Renshaw inhibition of that motor neuron and, at the same time, disinhibition of the antagonist motor neuron by inhibiting the Ia inhibitory interneuron.

If we now consider the central connections of the Ia fibers discussed above, along with the reflex actions described by Liddell and Sherrington, we can see how the

Ia fibers contribute to the stretch reflex (Figure 35-3). In this example a stretch reflex of flexor muscles is illustrated. Passive extension of a partially flexed limb stretches the flexor muscles, thereby stretching (or loading) the muscle spindles of those muscles, which gives rise to a Ia fiber discharge from the spindles. The Ia fiber discharge excites both the homonymous and synergist flexor muscles monosynaptically, and disynaptically inhibits antagonist extensor muscles.

Although there is no question that the elementary circuits shown in Figures 35-1 to 35-3 do contribute to the stretch reflex, it is worth emphasizing that the patterns of Ia connectivity in the spinal cord are certainly more complex. In addition to the short-latency monosynaptic pathways shown in Figure 35-3, the Ia system also activates polysynaptic spinal pathways that contribute to the reflex. Moreover, Ia fibers can activate interneuronal systems that produce both excitatory and inhibitory effects on motor neurons.

Given that the Ia system has powerful monosynaptic and polysynaptic effects on motor neurons mediating the stretch reflex, the question arises whether the Ia system alone can account for the entire reflex. This question can be addressed directly by taking advantage of the fact that the *spindle primary afferent terminals are exceptionally sensitive to tendon vibration.* This sensitivity highlights a feature of the primary afferents that was discussed in the previous chapter, namely, that they are primarily sensitive to the *rate of change* of stretch. For example, a vibratory stimulus that displaces the soleus muscle by only 10 μm activates the Ia fibers selectively. Thus, vibration can be used as a tool to investigate the central actions of the Ia fibers in two ways: (1) if the amplitude and frequency of vibration are large enough, *all* Ia fibers are activated; and (2) vibration can be used to *saturate* the Ia fibers, virtually clamping them at the vibration frequency and thus making them unresponsive to other stimuli, such as muscle stretch.

These features allowed P.B.C. Matthews at Oxford University to use vibration to study the Ia contribution to the stretch reflex. By delivering a prolonged vibratory stimulus to the tendon, he elicited the *tonic vibration reflex.* Using this reflex, he showed that the spindle primaries provide a steady excitatory contribution to the stretch reflex that shows little central fatigue over time. He also found that the spindle primaries cannot account for the entire stretch reflex, and suggested that other afferent systems also make a contribution. We shall return to this point when we discuss the secondary (group II) spindle afferents.

Ib Afferent Fibers Contribute to the Inverse Myotatic Reflex

The success that Lloyd experienced in relating a specific identifiable class of afferent fibers to a specific reflex behavior has encouraged the search for other correlations between afferent fiber types such as the Ib afferents and behavioral responses. An appreciation of some of the functional properties of the Ib afferent system can be gained by examining the central connections of the Ib fibers. These connections were first studied by Yves Laporte and Lloyd, who increased the strength of an electrical stimulus to a nerve just above the threshold necessary to elicit the myotatic (Ia fiber-mediated) afferent response. They observed a reflex action that appeared to be the opposite of the myotatic reflex: the innervated muscle and its synergists were inhibited and its antagonists were excited. Laporte and Lloyd called this the *inverse myotatic reflex.*

The central connections of Ib fibers are shown in Figure 35–4. They have three features: (1) all connections to motor neurons are made through interneurons; (2) Ib afferents make weak connections to flexor muscles but connect powerfully to extensors; and (3) the connections of Ib afferents are much more widespread in the spinal cord and somatic muscles than those of Ia afferents. The reflex actions of the Ib afferent system are not simply the opposite of those of the Ia afferent system, but are qualitatively different. Because the central connections of the Ib afferents are more widespread than those of the Ia afferents, and the Golgi tendon system measures *tension* whereas the spindle system measures *length,* many investigators now believe that calling the reflex actions of the Ib system the inverse myotatic reflex is not appropriate.

What is the function of this Ib afferent-mediated reflex? Because the Golgi tendon organs were known to have a high threshold when activated by passive stretch, it was originally believed that the primary function of the Ib afferent system is protective, preventing the muscle from producing excessive tension by inhibiting homonymous and synergist motor neurons and exciting antagonists. However, by stimulating single large motor fibers to the soleus muscle and recording the Ib fiber discharge, James Houk and Henneman found that the Golgi tendon organs are very sensitive to active muscle contraction. These investigators therefore proposed that the Ib afferent system could act as a *tension feedback system.* Increases in muscle tension beyond a desired point would produce negative feedback from Golgi tendon organs that would inhibit the further development of tension. Decreases in muscle tension, as occurs when a muscle begins to fatigue, would have the opposite effect. As the tendon organ is less activated there would be less inhibition onto homonymous and synergist motor cells and more tension would develop, compensating for the fatigue.

Recently, Anders Lundberg and his colleagues provided further insight into how Ib afferent reflex pathways operate. They found that interneurons in these pathways receive convergent short-latency excitation from low-threshold cutaneous afferents and from joint afferents. The

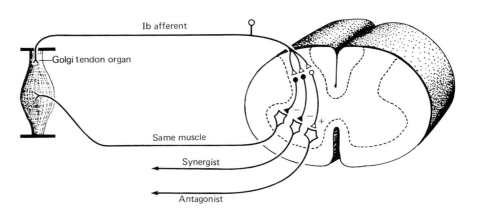

35–4 All connections of the Ib afferent fibers to motor neurons are through interneurons. In the reflex mediated by the Ib afferent system, inhibitory interneurons (**black**) inhibit motor neurons to the muscle of origin and its synergists, and excitatory interneurons excite the antagonists.

functional implication of this convergence is quite interesting. If a limb begins to move but suddenly meets a physical obstruction, low-threshold cutaneous and joint afferents would probably be activated. Their activity would facilitate Ib afferent inhibitory transmission, reducing muscle tension in the limb and thereby preventing further force against the obstacle.

There is another possible role for low-threshold joint afferent facilitation of Ib fiber transmission. If these afferents are activated at the end of a flexor or an extensor movement, their facilitation of Ib fiber inhibitory transmission might provide a mechanism to decrease force when a particular movement approaches the mechanical limit of the range over which the joint operates.

Group II Afferent Fibers Contribute to Stretch and Flexion Reflexes

Direct Actions on Homonymous Motor Neurons: Stretch Reflex

In 1969, Matthews first suggested that the secondary afferent terminals in muscle spindles contribute significantly to the stretch reflex in decerebrate animals. Using the tonic vibration reflex that we discussed earlier, Matthews showed that the reflex of a particular muscle to simple stretch is often greater than the reflex response of the same muscle to vibration, even though the vibratory stimulus excites the Ia fibers more powerfully. Since simple stretch also excites the group II afferents as well as the Ia fibers, this finding suggested that the group II afferents contribute to the reflex as well. Furthermore, if the Ia afferents were saturated by a tonic vibratory stimulus (thus making them unresponsive to stretch), a stretch reflex could *still* be elicited, providing further indirect support for a group II contribution. More recently, experiments conducted in several laboratories using the

spike-triggered averaging technique have shown conclusively that spindle secondary afferents produce monosynaptic excitation in homonymous motor neurons, although this action is now recognized to be relatively weak.

Polysynaptic Pathways: Flexion Reflexes

Eccles and Lundberg obtained intracellular recordings from different spinal motor neurons and found that electrical stimuli activating group II fibers in a variety of muscle nerves excite motor neurons to flexors and inhibit those to extensors. The postsynaptic potentials in the motor neurons produced by such stimulation occur with long latencies indicative of a polysynaptic pathway. These polysynaptic actions appear primarily in experimental animals with transected spinal cords, in which, as we shall see, flexion reflexes can be excited by stimulating very different types of afferents. Thus, the group II afferents have often been suggested to play a role in the flexion reflexes, which will be discussed later in this chapter.

The major problem in interpreting the actions of the group II afferents is that there are other afferent fibers in the group II diameter range that arise from *nonspindle afferents* (for example, from free nerve endings). These fibers exert powerful flexor activity in the spinal cord and thus, when activated by electrical stimulation, mask the myotatic reflex normally mediated by the group II spindle afferents. The modern view is that there are at least two functional classes of fibers falling in the group II range: those that arise from spindle secondaries that produce a myotatic reflex, and those that arise from nonspindle afferents whose predominant action is to produce a flexion reflex. The latter afferents fall into the general category of flexor reflex afferents, which will also be discussed later in this chapter.

Reflexes of Muscle Origin Are Functionally Significant

The Gamma Loop and the Length-Servo Hypothesis

The excitability of the stretch reflex depends critically upon tonic descending control from higher brain centers. The way in which higher centers influence the stretch

35–5 Alpha motor neurons can be activated indirectly via the gamma loop. The gamma motor neuron (**1**) is activated by input from higher centers, producing contraction of intrafusal muscle fibers (**2**) located on either side of the afferent ending. This stretches the afferent endings in the equatorial region of the spindle, increasing the discharge of the Ia fiber (**3**). This discharge is transmitted monosynaptically to the alpha motor neuron (**4**) leading to the contraction of extrafusal muscle fibers (**5**).

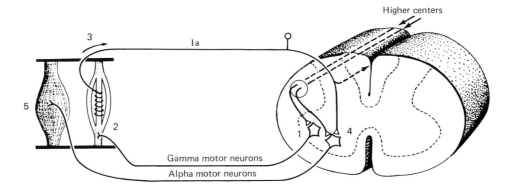

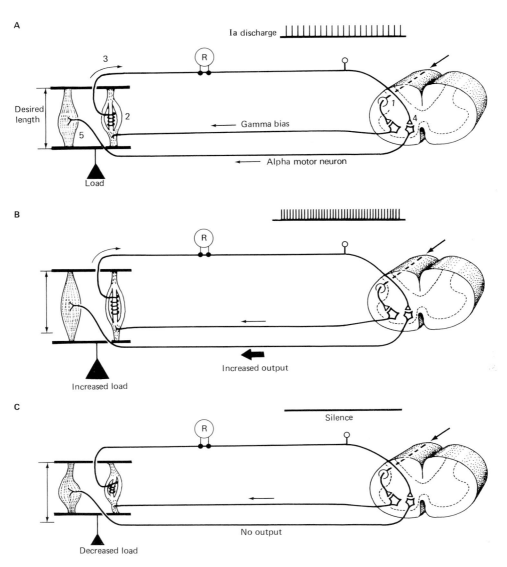

35–6 According to the length-servo hypothesis for the role of the gamma loop in the stretch reflex, the degree of contraction is determined by the gamma bias, which is controlled by higher centers. **A.** Higher centers activate alpha motor neurons via the gamma loop (**numbers** as in Figure 35–5). The firing of the gamma neurons (the gamma bias) increases the Ia fiber discharge (recorded at **R**) enough to drive alpha motor neurons, producing a reflex contraction of the muscle to a given desired length. **B.** Increasing the load on the muscle increases Ia fiber discharge and thereby increases alpha motor neuron output, counteracting the increased load and returning the muscle to the desired length. **C.** Decreasing the load unloads the spindle. With no Ia fiber input the alpha motor neuron output ceases and the muscle relaxes until the desired length is achieved, at which point the spindle is reloaded.

reflex has thus received a great deal of experimental and theoretical attention. Descending control could produce a movement directly by acting on alpha motor neurons or indirectly by acting on gamma motor neurons. Direct activation of alpha motor neurons from higher centers leads to contraction of extrafusal muscle fibers. Why, however, is there also descending control over gamma motor neurons? One attractive hypothesis is that activation of the somatic muscles can also be brought about indirectly by activation of gamma motor neurons from higher centers. This is called activation through the *gamma loop.* Activation of gamma motor neurons would load the intrafusal muscle spindles, provoking increased Ia fiber firing from the muscle, which in turn would ac-

tivate the homonymous and synergist motor neurons, thereby producing a contraction of the extrafusal fibers of this muscle (Figure 35–5).

Why would the nervous system use such an indirect route to activate alpha motor neurons, since it is slower and less precise than direct activation? Peter Merton recognized that spindle discharge can be modulated both by changes in gamma motor neuron activity and by changes in length of the extrafusal muscle fibers. He therefore proposed that the stretch reflex could be made to function as a *servomechanism* regulating muscle length. Although this idea has now been shown to be incorrect, it was historically important because it suggested a fruitful experimental approach. (Figure 35–6).

When contraction of somatic muscles is produced by the gamma route, the extrafusal muscle fibers contract at a given length (predetermined by the amount of gamma motor neuron discharge produced from higher centers; this discharge is called the *gamma bias*). If the extrafusal muscle fiber shortens any further—for example, because of a sudden decrease in load—the spindles in the muscle become unloaded, with the result that the Ia fiber discharge from those spindles ceases, thereby removing their excitation to motor neurons controlling the extrafusal muscle fiber (Figure 35–6C). The muscle then begins to relax until it lengthens to the point that the spindles are stretched (reloaded) and the muscle again contracts via the gamma loop. Thus, the extrafusal muscle fiber *follows automatically* the degree of contraction of the intrafusal fiber, which is determined by the gamma bias. Merton further suggested that this servo system could provide for load compensation, as any change in load (lengthening or shortening of the muscle) could be counteracted by an increase or decrease in Ia fiber discharge (Figure 35–6). Thus, a central concept in any form of servo hypothesis involving the gamma loop is the notion of *misalignment between intended muscle length and actual muscle length*, which reduces to the difference between spindle length and extrafusal fiber

length. When there is no difference between spindle and extrafusal fiber lengths, there is no misalignment.

A direct test of a major prediction of Merton's hypothesis, namely, that extrafusal contraction occurs as a result of central commands to the muscle spindle, was recently carried out by Å. B. Vallbo. Vallbo's results showed conclusively that movement is not initiated by activation of the gamma motor neurons but by co-activation of both alpha and gamma motor neurons. Vallbo recorded from the Ia afferents from muscle spindles in his own wrist and finger flexor muscles (by means of fine wires inserted into his muscle nerves) during both rapid and slow voluntary movements. A critical prediction from Merton's hypothesis is that the Ia fiber discharge should *precede* contraction of the muscle because, according to the hypothesis, gamma motor cells initiate the movement by contracting spindles, setting up a Ia discharge that then activates alpha motor cells and produces measurable movement. Vallbo actually found that the Ia discharge did not precede but actually *followed* electrical activity in the muscle (and the resultant muscle tension) after a short delay. This indicates that the movement was initiated by the direct alpha motor cells and not by the gamma motor cells. However, the fact that the Ia afferents fired at all showed that gamma motor neurons are also activated during normal movement. Had the gamma motor neurons not been activated, the spindles would have been unloaded by the contraction and the Ia discharge would have ceased. Vallbo concluded that the alpha and gamma motor neurons are essentially activated together. Co-activation of alpha and gamma motor neurons has subsequently also been observed in several other motor systems, including those involved in breathing, jaw contraction, human voluntary thumb movements, and (as we shall see in Chapter 37) locomotion.

The work of Vallbo and others led to the proposition that the gamma loop might function only to provide *servo assistance* in an auxilliary capacity: even though the gamma loop is not responsible for the initiation of a

35–7 The stretch reflex is a negative feedback mechanism.
   Descending control signals act upon the alpha motor neurons where their action sums (Σ) with feedback signals from the muscle spindle. This descending control is designed to maintain a set muscle length, the controlled variable. This, however, is achieved by controlling muscle tension, which interacts and sums (Σ) with external disturbances, such as load changes or muscle fatigue, to yield the actual length change. The difference between the actual and intended change in length is sensed by the spindle, which is informed about the intended length by the gamma drive. If the muscle shortens more than intended, the spindle output will drop, thus reducing the Ia excitatory input to the motor neuron, and it will fire less. This, in turn, will reduce muscle tension.

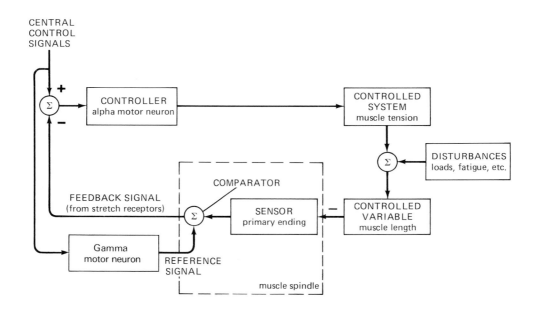

movement, it may still operate to assist in load compensation. However, the role of the gamma loop and the stretch reflex in load compensation is limited because the muscle spindles are primarily sensitive to very small changes in length. Moreover, the strength of the reflex connections between Ia fibers and motor neurons is modest. Because of these considerations, it is now believed that the stretch reflex compensates effectively only for small disturbances.

Although erroneous, Merton's idea drew attention to the role of negative feedback in the control of muscle length and tension. The essential feature of negative feedback is to provide stability by producing an action that opposes changes in the desired state (called the *regulated variable*). In Chapter 34 we examined the springlike properties of muscle. These properties provide a mechanical equivalent of negative feedback. A load applied to a springlike muscle produces an increase in length, which in turn increases the muscle's tension or restoring force. This process continues until the force exerted by the muscle equals the force exerted by the load. The stretch reflex is superimposed on this mechanical effect to provide a true form of negative feedback (Figure 35–7).

In a servo-controlled system, feedback information is provided by sensors reflecting the quantity that is being controlled. This information is compared with the signal reflecting the desired state, called a *reference signal*. The difference between these two signals is then used to counteract an external disturbance by acting on the controlled system through a control element. In the stretch reflex the muscle spindle acts both as sensor and comparator (since its sensitivity is controlled by the gamma fibers, which thus serve as a reference signal). A mismatch between an actual and intended length constitutes the error signal that is then delivered to the motor neurons that control the muscles.

Reflexes Mediated by Muscle May Regulate the Stiffness of Muscle

An important new perspective concerning the role of muscle receptors has recently emerged from the work of T. Richard Nichols and James Houk at Northwestern University Medical School. These investigations suggested that the major function of the reflexes mediated by muscle receptors is to compensate for undesirable irregularities in mechanical properties of muscle. Nichols and Houk compared the tensions produced by muscle stretch in cats whose feedback loop was intact with cats whose feedback was interrupted by a severed dorsal root. In the absence of feedback, a ramp stretch applied to the muscle produces an initial increase in tension that suddenly yields even though stretch is continuing (Figure 35–8).[3] However, when dorsal roots are intact and feed-

---

[3]This peculiar yielding of muscle is seen only when it is rapidly stretched and should not be confused with the usual length–tension relationships (discussed in Chapter 34) that are obtained with slow stretch. The transient yield with rapid stretch derives from the breaking of bonds at the cross bridges between actin and myosin molecules.

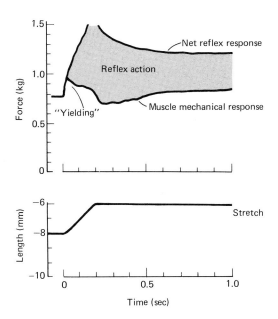

35–8 "Yielding" (abrupt failure in muscular stiffness) in response to a rapid and large stretch in the functionally isolated soleus muscle of the decerebrate cat is compensated for by the stretch reflex in the normal cat. (Adapted from Houk, 1979.)

back loops can operate, the muscle no longer yields. Instead, it continues to generate tension as a function of length and thus a more linear relationship between length and tension is maintained. These observations led Houk to suggest that length and tension feedback arise, respectively, from muscle spindles and from Golgi tendon organs that function in concert to regulate muscle stiffness.

To summarize, the reflexes mediated by Ia and Ib fibers *act together* to control muscle stiffness. The Ia reflex does not uniquely control length, nor does the Ib reflex uniquely control tension (Figure 35–9).

Descending Control of Muscle Set Point

We have seen earlier that muscle stiffness and set point are critical mechanical features of muscles. Which of these two is controlled by descending inputs to motor neurons? To address this question, A. G. Feldman and G. N. Orlovsky stimulated descending pathways (such as Deiters' nucleus in the vestibulospinal pathway) in cats and determined the effect of this stimulation on reflex force elicited by muscle stretch. They found that the set points of muscle were reduced while the stiffness was unaltered (Figure 35–10), illustrating a general principle in the study of motor control. The behavior of muscles is fundamentally springlike, and descending control signals act mainly by modifying the set point of the spring (the point beyond which a restoring force develops), while changes in the stiffness of the spring are small. However, as we saw in Chapter 34, the stiffness of the

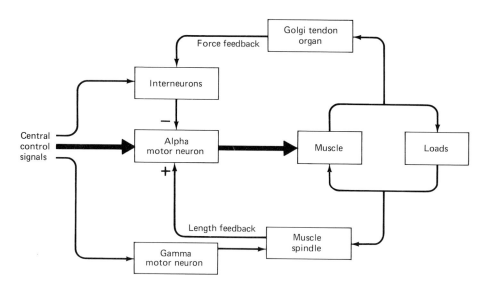

35–9 Length and force feedback act together to control muscle stiffness. Muscles act on loads to produce both changes in length and changes in tension. Changes in length are sensed by muscle spindles, whose afferents facilitate (indicated by + sign) the motor neurons innervating the same muscle. Changes in tension are signaled by Golgi tendon organs, which inhibit the motor neurons via an interneuron (indicated by − sign). Central control signals can influence both length and force feedback by acting on the spindle via gamma motor neurons or by acting on interneurons mediating force feedback.

joint as a whole can be controlled by co-contraction of both agonist and antagonist muscles—a strategy that is useful when loads cannot be anticipated. Thus, spinal reflex systems are capable of maintaining stiffness so that control of set point by descending commands can lead to predictable results in the face of unpredictable loads.

35–10 Descending control of muscle set point is demonstrated by gradually stretching the gastrocnemius muscle of the cat while applying various intensities of tonic stimulation to Deiters' nucleus to mimic a tonic descending command. The slope of these curves reflects the stiffness of the muscle, and the (extrapolated) intercept with the abscissa reflects the set point (the stretch reflex threshold). With increasing stimulation the curves are shifted progressively to the left (the set point is reduced) while the slope (stiffness) is relatively unaltered.

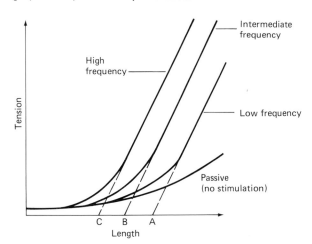

Afferent Fibers from Cutaneous and Deep Receptors Mediate a Reflex Consisting of Ipsilateral Flexion and Contralateral Extension

Group III and IV afferents arise from deep receptors in muscle and cutaneous receptors in skin. Most of the myelinated group III and the unmyelinated group IV fibers carry information about painful stimuli, such as extreme pressure, heat, or cold; thus the reflexes that they produce serve as protective or escape responses. These fiber groups give rise to ipsilateral flexion, usually accompanied by contralateral extension. This reflex response is mediated by polysynaptic connections in the spinal cord (Figure 35–11). The degree of flexion can vary from a flexor twitch, produced by relatively innocuous tactile stimulation, to complete withdrawal of the limb from a noxious stimulus. The crossed extensor part of the general reflex pattern makes sense because it provides a way for an animal to maintain balance, with the extended leg bearing the weight of the body while the opposite limb is withdrawn from the noxious stimulus.

Because group II and group III muscle afferents can produce flexion responses, they are often lumped together with afferents from skin and joints and collectively called *flexor reflex afferents.* In common practice this has become a term (albeit an imprecise one) for almost any afferents that produce a flexion response.

The general picture of ipsilateral flexion and contralateral extension produced by group III and IV afferents has several important exceptions. For example, Edward Perl has found that group II fibers can set into motion a bilateral flexion reflex. If group III fibers are also activated, however, the classic ipsilateral flexion and contra-

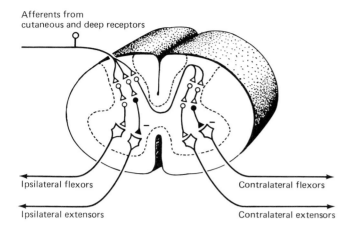

Afferents from
cutaneous and deep receptors

Ipsilateral flexors

Contralateral flexors

Ipsilateral extensors

Contralateral extensors

35–11 The basic circuitry for reflexes of cutaneous and deep receptor origin usually leads to ipsilateral flexion and contralateral extension via a network of excitatory and inhibitory interneurons.

lateral extension are seen. Thus, caution is necessary in interpreting studies that use only nerve stimulation because artificial stimulation of this sort can cause one class of reflex actions to be masked by another, more powerful, reflex pattern.

Another important exception to the general scheme described above is that special reflex effects can be obtained from cutaneous regions. For example, in a dog whose spinal cord has been transected at the cervical level, light tactile pressure applied to the footpads of the forepaw produces a reflex *extension* of the whole limb. This reflex has obvious utility when an animal is standing, for reflex tightening of the extensor muscles allows the animal to keep its leg straight automatically. However, another stimulus, such as a pinprick, to the same skin region of the footpad immediately produces a *flexion withdrawal* of the paw. Thus, *the quality of the stimulus as well as its location on the skin is an important determinant of the type of reflex action.*

Reflex Activity Is Subject to Supraspinal and Intraspinal Influences

One striking feature of the afferent fiber systems we have considered is that their influence on motor neurons is usually exerted by means of polysynaptic pathways. As a result, there are many sites within the spinal cord where modulation of reflex responses can occur. A dramatic illustration of reflex modulation is seen when all descending influences from supraspinal regions to spinal circuits are removed by cutting the cord. Immediately after spinal transection, all reflex activity is lost and a condition of areflexia, called *spinal shock*, results.

Sherrington showed that the loss of reflex activity after spinal transection is not due to the trauma of the transection per se. He cut the spinal cord and waited for recovery from spinal shock. He then performed a second transection just below the previous one, and little or no

spinal shock occurred, even though the surgical trauma of the second transection was comparable to that of the first. Sherrington concluded that the reflex depression is chiefly due to loss of facilitation from higher brain centers.

After some time, reflex activity gradually begins to return. In carnivores this may take only minutes to hours; in monkeys, days or weeks; and in humans it can take several months or even longer. The reflexes that return become progressively more abnormal and exaggerated, developing into a condition of hyperreflexia. This is particularly true of flexion reflexes, which can become so exaggerated that cutaneous input triggers a mass reflex involving generalized contraction of all flexor muscles. The hyperreflexia after spinal shock is not well understood. Many contributing factors have been suggested, including increased sensitivity of spinal interneurons and motor neurons to transmitter substances and removal of descending inhibitory influences from supraspinal centers onto reflex circuits.

Another interesting suggestion has been advanced by Gordon McCouch and his colleagues, who investigated the mechanism of late hyperreflexia that occurs in animals weeks or months after spinal injury, when tendon reflexes have returned and the flexor reflex becomes exaggerated. These investigations suggest that the hyperreflexia is due at least partly to the sprouting of afferent pathways below the spinal transection. It is thought that terminals from supraspinal tracts degenerate, leaving postsynaptic vacancies on interneurons and motor neurons that are then filled by sprouting branches of the still intact afferent systems, and new connections are formed. Therefore, the recovery of reflex function actually reflects the establishment of new abnormal reflex actions rather than the restoration of normal reflex function. There is compelling evidence that in other regions of the central nervous system (especially in the red nucleus, the septal nucleus, and the hippocampus) sprouting occurs after a lesion and the newly sprouted connections can be functional.

Spinal shock reveals the importance of descending influences on spinal reflex circuits. However, ascending influences are also exerted from lower spinal regions onto higher spinal regions. An interesting example of this is the *Shiff–Sherrington reflex.* As mentioned earlier, a decerebrate animal shows exaggerated extensor reflexes of the limbs and neck (*decerebrate rigidity*). If the spinal cord of a decerebrate animal is cut in the midthoracic region, below the level of the spinal output to the forelimbs, the degree of extensor rigidity in the forelimbs increases dramatically. This is thought to occur because lower regions of the spinal cord exert inhibitory influences over higher regions that mediate extensor reflexes of the forelimbs.

The key principle that emerges from studies on the relative influence of supraspinal and intraspinal regions on spinal reflexes is that the spinal cord contains within itself the basic neural machinery necessary to generate all reflex actions. These local spinal circuits, however, are constantly modulated (both facilitated and inhibited) by descending pathways from higher brain regions as well as by other regions within the spinal cord itself.

Selected Readings

Baldissera, F., Hultborn, H., and Illert, M. 1981. Integration in spinal neuronal systems. In V. B. Brooks (ed.), Handbook of Physiology, Section 1: The Nervous System, Vol. II, Motor Control. Bethesda, Md.: American Physiological Society, pp. 509–595.

Henneman, E. 1980. Organization of the spinal cord and its reflexes. In V. B. Mountcastle (ed.), Medical Physiology, 14th ed., Vol. 1. St. Louis: Mosby, pp. 762–786.

Houk, J. C., and Rymer, W. Z. 1981. Neural control of muscle length and tension. In V. B. Brooks (ed.), Handbook of Physiology, Section 1: The Nervous System, Vol. II, Motor Control. Bethesda, Md.: American Physiological Society, pp. 257–323.

Hunt, C. C., and Perl, E. R. 1960. Spinal reflex mechanisms concerned with skeletal muscle. Physiol. Rev. 40:538–579.

Jewett, D. L., and Rayner, M. D. 1984. Basic Concepts of Neuronal Function. Boston: Little, Brown.

Lundberg, A. 1975. Control of spinal mechanisms from the brain. In D. B. Tower (ed.), The Nervous System, Vol. 1: The Basic Neurosciences. New York: Raven Press, pp. 253–265.

Matthews, P. B. C. 1972. Mammalian Muscle Receptors and Their Central Actions. Baltimore: Williams & Wilkins.

Matthews, P. B. C. 1981. Muscle spindles: Their messages and their fusimotor supply. In V. B. Brooks (ed.), Handbook of Physiology, Section 1: The Nervous System, Vol. II, Motor Control. Bethesda, Md.: American Physiological Society, pp. 189–228.

Sherrington, C. S. 1947. The Integrative Action of the Nervous System, 2nd ed. New Haven: Yale University Press.

References

Chambers, W. W., Liu, C. N., and McCouch, G. P. 1973. Anatomical and physiological correlates of plasticity in the central nervous system. Brain Behav. Evol. 8:5–26.

Eccles, J. C. 1964. The Physiology of Synapses. Berlin: Springer.

Eccles, J. C., Fatt, P., and Koketsu, K. 1954. Cholinergic and inhibitory synapses in a pathway from motor-axon collaterals to motoneurones. J. Physiol. (Lond.) 126:524–562.

Eccles, R. M., and Lundberg, A. 1959. Synaptic actions in motoneurones by afferents which may evoke the flexion reflex. Arch. Ital. Biol. 97:199–221.

Feldman, A. G., and Orlovsky, G. N. 1972. The influence of different descending systems on the tonic stretch reflex in the cat. Exp. Neurol. 37:481–494.

Houk, J., and Henneman, E. 1967. Responses of Golgi tendon organs to active contractions of the soleus muscle of the cat. J. Neurophysiol. 30:466–481.

Houk, J. C. 1979. Motor control processes: New data concerning motoservo mechanisms and a tentative model for stimulus-response processing. In R. E. Talbott and D. R. Humphrey (eds.), Posture and Movement. New York: Raven Press, pp. 231–241.

Laporte, Y., and Lloyd, D. P. C. 1952. Nature and significance of the reflex connections established by large afferent fibers of muscular origin. Am. J. Physiol. 169:609–621.

Liddell, E. G. T., and Sherrington, C. 1924. Reflexes in response to stretch (myotatic reflexes). Proc. R. Soc. Lond. [Biol.] 96:212–242.

Liddell, E. G. T., and Sherrington, C. 1925. Further observations on myotatic reflexes. Proc. R. Soc. Lond. [Biol.] 97:267–283.

Lloyd, D. P. C. 1943. Conduction and synaptic transmission of the reflex response to stretch in spinal cats. J. Neurophysiol. 6:317–326.

Mendell, L. M., and Henneman, E. 1971. Terminals of single Ia fibers: Location, density, and distribution within a pool of 300 homonymous motoneurons. J. Neurophysiol. 34:171–187.

Merton, P. A. 1953. Speculations on the servo-control of movement. In G. E. W. Wolstenholme (ed.), The Spinal Cord. London: Churchill Livingstone, pp. 247–255.

Merton, P. A. 1972. How we control the contraction of our muscles. Sci. Am. 226(5):30–37.

Nichols, T. R., and Houk, J. C. 1973. Reflex compensation for variations in the mechanical properties of a muscle. Science 181:182–184.

Perl, E. R. 1958. Crossed reflex effects evoked by activity in myelinated afferent fibers of muscle. J. Neurophysiol. 21:101–112.

Vallbo, Å. B. 1970. Discharge patterns in human muscle spindle afferents during isometric voluntary contractions. Acta Physiol. Scand. 80:552–566.

Vallbo, Å. B. 1971. Muscle spindle response at the onset of isometric voluntary contractions in man. Time difference between fusimotor and skeletomotor effects. J. Physiol. (Lond.) 218:405–431.

Lewis P. Rowland

Clinical Syndromes of the Spinal Cord

36

Knowledge of the anatomy and physiology of the spinal cord helps clinicians to recognize spinal cord disease *(myelopathy)*, to localize the disease to a particular segment or region of the spinal cord, and often to identify the nature of the disorder. In this chapter we shall review the anatomy that is important for examining patients with neurological disorders of the spinal cord and consider the major diseases that affect it.

Clinically Important Anatomy

The only *descending* tracts of major clinical importance are the corticospinal tracts in the lateral columns of the spinal cord (Figure 36–1A). Other descending pathways, such as the rubrospinal tract, also function in the control of posture and movement, but only lesions of the corticospinal tracts have clinically evident effects.

In contrast, three *ascending* tracts are important clinically:

1. The dorsal column–medial lemniscal system carries sensations of discriminative touch, vibration, and joint position. The axons run ipsilateral to the roots of entry and cross to the other side above the spinal cord, in the medulla, after synapsing in the dorsal column nuclei (Figure 36–1B).
2. The lateral spinothalamic tracts convey sensations of pain, temperature, and crude touch from the contralateral side of the body (Figure 36–1C).
3. The spinocerebellar tracts provide information about the position of the body in space and about the position of body segments relative to one another (Figure 36–1D). These tracts are affected in some hereditary ataxias (Chapter 39) but are not the source of symptoms in other spinal cord diseases.

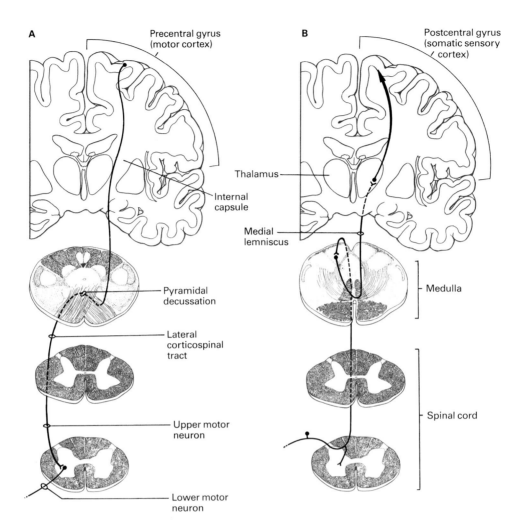

36–1 Clinically important ascending and descending tracts. **A.** The corticospinal tract is the only descending pathway in which lesions lead to clinically detectable changes.

B. The dorsal column–medial lemniscal system conveys sensations of light touch, vibration, and joint position.

Somatotopic Organization of the Spinothalamic Tract Is an Aid to Diagnosis

The fibers in the corticospinal tracts, posterior columns, and spinothalamic tracts are somatotopically organized. This organization is diagnostically important in two conditions, both of which affect the spinothalamic tracts: (1) lesions of the central parts of the cervical or thoracic cord, and (2) surgical procedures designed to relieve pain.

In the thoracic and cervical cord, fibers originating in the lowermost (sacral) region are pushed laterally by fibers entering from successively higher levels. Therefore, when lesions, such as tumors, arise in the innermost portion of the thoracic or cervical cord, a phenomenon called *sacral sparing* may result. As these lesions extend outward, they first compress the most medial fibers from higher segments but they may not affect the most lateral

sacral fibers. In such cases, all cutaneous sensation may be abolished below the level of the lesion but the sacral segments (perineum, scrotum, and saddle area) are spared (Figure 36–2F).

Neurosurgeons take advantage of the somatotopic organization of these tracts in the operation called *cordotomy*, which is sometimes performed to control intractable pain in the pelvis or legs. Because the spinal cord itself is insensitive to pain, it is possible to section the spinothalamic tracts selectively under local anesthesia. When the scalpel enters the outer aspect of the spinal cord and spinothalamic tract, it encounters the sacral fibers first. As the knife goes deeper, the level at which sensation is lost rises. Because the patient is awake and cooperative, the extent of sensory loss can be ascertained continuously during the procedure to ensure that only the desired level is attained.

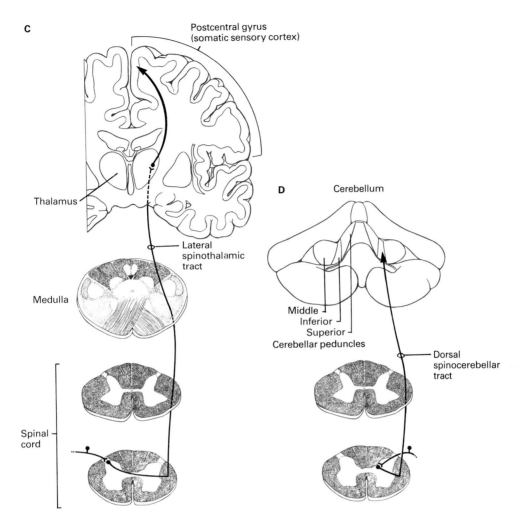

C. The lateral spinothalamic tracts carry sensations of pain, temperature, and crude touch from the other side of the body.

D. The spinocerebellar tracts convey unconscious proprioception.

Function Is Lost below a Transverse Spinal Lesion

Lesions of the spinal cord give rise to motor or sensory symptoms that are often related to a particular sensory or motor segmental level of the spinal cord. Identification of the appropriate level of the motor or sensory loss (called a *motor* or *sensory level*) is crucial for recognizing focal lesions within the spinal cord or external compressive lesions that interrupt functions below the lesion.

Motor Level

When motor roots are involved, or when motor neurons are affected focally, clinical findings may indicate the spinal level of the injury. This clinical evidence would include the typical lower motor neuron signs: weakness, wasting, fasciculation, and loss of tendon reflexes. The muscles and tendon reflexes that serve as landmarks for locating motor level lesions are listed in Table 36–1. However, because it is clinically difficult to relate the innervation of muscles of the trunk and thorax to specific spinal segments, the motor level may not be evident. For instance, a lesion anywhere above the first lumbar segment may cause signs of upper motor neuron disease in the legs. Under these circumstances sensory abnormalities are more valuable for localizing the lesion.

Sensory Level

The characteristic pattern of sensory loss after a transverse spinal cord lesion is loss of cutaneous sensation below the level of the lesion (Figure 36–2C), contralateral to the damaged spinothalamic tract if the lesion is unilateral (Figure 36–2B). The sensory level is often more evident

Table 36–1. Indicators of Motor Level Lesions

Root	Major muscles affected	Reflex loss
C3–5	Diaphragm	—
C5	Deltoid, biceps	Biceps
C7	Triceps, extensors of wrist and fingers	Triceps
C8	Interossei, abductor of fifth finger	—
L2–4	Quadriceps	Knee jerk
L5	Long extensor of great toe, anterior tibial	—
S1	Plantar flexors, gastrocnemius	Ankle jerk

36–2 The sensory level is correlated with the anatomical level of the lesion. (Adapted from Collins, 1962.)

than the motor level. However, sensory loss due to spinal lesions must be differentiated from the pattern of sensory loss caused by lesions of peripheral nerves or isolated nerve roots. In multiple symmetrical peripheral neuropathy *(polyneuropathy)*, there is a glove-and-stocking pattern of impaired perception of pain and temperature. This pattern, as we have seen in Chapter 18, is attributed to "dying-back" or impaired axonal transport; the parts of the axons most severely affected are those most distant from the sensory neuron cell bodies in the dorsal root ganglia. In injuries of *single peripheral nerves*, the distribution of sensory loss is more restricted and can be recognized by reference to sensory charts that were originally generated by studies of the long-term effects of traumatic nerve injuries incurred during war.

Nerve root or segmental sensory loss and spinal sensory levels can be identified by the dermatomes typically affected (Figure 36–3). The landmarks for the major sensory levels are listed in Table 36–2. The spinal cord ends at the base of the second lumbar (L2) vertebra. Below this level the spinal canal is occupied by the lower nerve roots (the cauda equina).

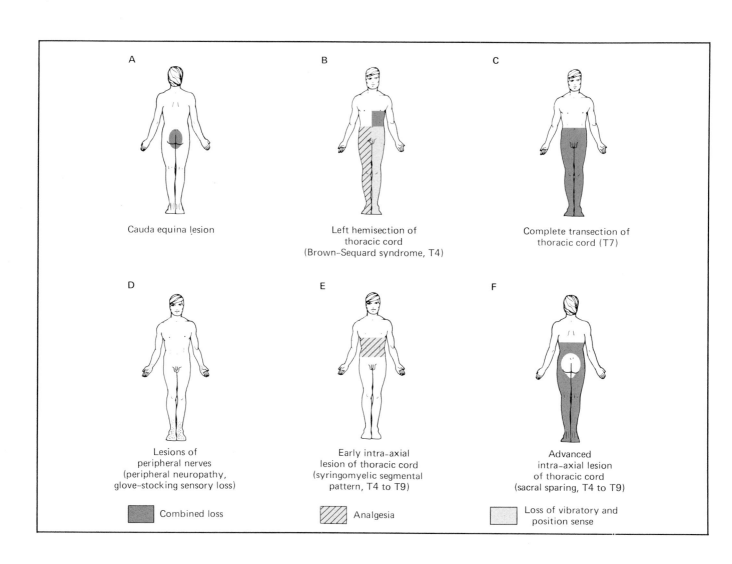

A Cauda equina lesion

B Left hemisection of thoracic cord (Brown-Sequard syndrome, T4)

C Complete transection of thoracic cord (T7)

D Lesions of peripheral nerves (peripheral neuropathy, glove-stocking sensory loss)

E Early intra-axial lesion of thoracic cord (syringomyelic segmental pattern, T4 to T9)

F Advanced intra-axial lesion of thoracic cord (sacral sparing, T4 to T9)

■ Combined loss   ▨ Analgesia   ▦ Loss of vibratory and position sense

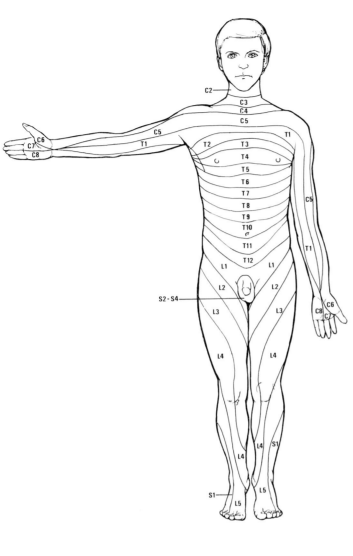

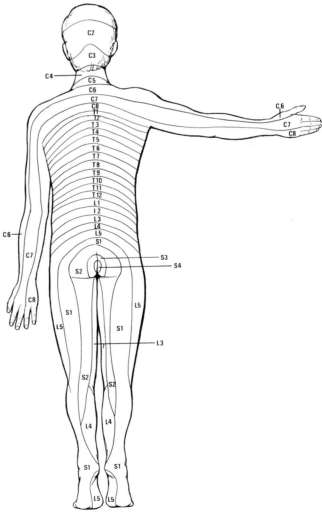

36–3 The segmental arrangement of dermatomes can be used as a map to determine the sacral (**S**), lumbar (**L**), thoracic (**T**), or cervical (**C**) level of a spinal lesion by the sensory loss.

Table 36–2. Indicators of Sensory Level Lesions

Root	Major sensory areas affected
C4	Clavicle
C8	Fifth finger
T4	Nipples
T10	Umbilicus
L1	Inguinal ligament
L3	Anterior surface of the thigh
L5	Great toe
S1	Lateral aspect of the foot
S3–5	Perineum

In examining patients, students are sometimes perplexed by abnormalities that patients report but that do not seem to fit the disorder suspected. It is important to realize that sensory testing may be difficult even in normal individuals and is especially difficult for anxious patients. Two general rules help: (1) If you find cutaneous sensory loss and the patient does not complain of paresthesias (tingling, pins and needles, lack of sensation, numbness), be wary of the sensory loss; it is probably an artifact of the examination. (2) Conversely, if the patient does complain of parethesias and you do not find any cutaneous sensory loss on examination, try again.

It Is Important to Distinguish Intra-axial from Extra-axial Disease

In practical terms, it is important to know whether a lesion arises within the spinal cord (intra-axial or intramedullary), or whether the spinal cord is being compressed by an external mass (extra-axial or extramedullary). Clinical evidence may give some clues that are helpful in making the distinction. For instance, pain is more common in extra-axial lesions because a compressive lesion (such as a tumor) may affect the dura, posterior nerve roots, or blood vessels that are innervated by sensory neurons mediating pain. In contrast, because there are no pain receptors within the spinal cord itself (or the brain), intra-axial lesions may be painless. Intra-axial lesions may be marked by sacral sparing of sensation (Figure 36–2F) or may cause a segmental pattern of sensory loss (Figure 36–2E), as in syringomyelia (described below). In addition, bladder function is affected earlier in intra-axial disorders than it is in extra-axial disease.

None of these characteristics is absolutely reliable, however; definite diagnosis depends on radiographic contrast procedures, the most important of which is now myelography. In this procedure a radiopaque material is introduced into the subarachnoid space to outline the spinal cord, the nerve roots, and the bony margins of the canal, permitting assessment of compressive lesions or those that distort the cord from within. Vascular lesions can be assessed by spinal angiography, in which spinal blood vessels are selectively catheterized and injected with radiopaque dyes.

To provide more detailed views of the contents of the spinal canal, computerized tomography is combined with injection of contrast material (metrizamide) into the subarachnoid space. As we saw in Chapter 22, magnetic resonance imaging may soon provide this information without the discomfort, expense, and hazards of injection into the subarachnoid space.

It is also possible to evaluate conduction in the human dorsal column–medial lemniscal system by measuring somatic sensory evoked potentials, a series of waves that are recorded at the scalp or over the spine in response to a sensory stimulus. (For further discussion of somatic sensory evoked potentials see Chapters 25 and 48.) These impulses are differentiated from random background electrical activity by computerized averaging of many stimulus-locked responses. To test the somatic sensory system, the median nerve is stimulated by cutaneous electrodes at the wrist, or the posterior tibial nerve is stimulated at the ankle. Recording electrodes are placed over the brachial plexus at Erb's point, the cervical spine, and the contralateral parasagittal scalp (corresponding to the primary somatic sensory cortex) to detect the afferent sensory volley from the arm as it travels from the periphery to the cortex. When the posterior tibial nerve is used, electrodes are placed over the lumbar spine and the contralateral scalp. In a typical somatic sensory evoked potential elicited by median nerve stimulation, the several peaks are attributed to sequential nerve activity in the brachial plexus (Erb's point), cervical spinal cord, medial lemniscus, and primary somatic sensory cortex. Although fibers entering both the spinothalamic and dorsal column pathways are activated when a peripheral nerve is stimulated, the somatic sensory evoked potential is derived almost exclusively from synchronous activity transmitted by the dorsal column–medial lemniscal system.

Evoked potentials are a measure of central conduction, and the test is of greatest use in evaluating patients with suspected multiple sclerosis or other demyelinating diseases in which conduction within myelinated fiber tracts may be slowed or blocked altogether. Because of the lesion, one or more peaks of the somatic sensory evoked potential may be absent or delayed. Evoked potentials are valuable because they may reveal lesions that are not detectable clinically, and they aid in interpreting a clinically equivocal symptom or sign. Somatic sensory evoked potentials may also be abnormal with compressive or infiltrative lesions, but the type of abnormality does not vary with etiology. In addition, these evoked potentials are used in the operating room to prevent spinal cord injury during surgical procedures on the spine or cord itself.

Lesions of the Spinal Cord Often Give Rise to Characteristic Syndromes

Spinal cord injuries are most often caused by trauma, especially automobile accidents. The resulting syndrome depends on the extent of direct injury of the cord or compression of the cord by displaced vertebrae or blood clots. In extreme cases trauma may lead to complete or partial transection of the spinal cord.

Complete Transection

The spinal cord may be completely severed acutely in fracture–dislocations of vertebrae or by knife or bullet wounds. Acute transection of the cord may also result from an inflammatory condition called transverse myelitis or from compression due to a tumor, especially metastatic tumors. In myelitis and tumors, symptoms evolve in days or weeks.

Immediately after traumatic section of the cord, however, there is loss of all sensation (Figure 36–2C) and all voluntary movement below the lesion. Bladder and bowel control are also lost. If the lesion is above C3, breathing may be affected. Although upper motor neuron signs might be expected, tendon reflexes are usually absent—a condition of *spinal shock* that persists for several weeks. After a while, reflex activity returns at levels below the lesion. Hyperactive reflexes, *clonus* (rapid and repeated contraction and relaxation of passively stretched muscle), and Babinski signs then appear as signs of damage to the corticospinal tract. The legs become spastic; this condition is often preceded by intermittent hypertonia and flexor spasms that occur spontaneously or may be provoked by cutaneous stimuli. Later, flexor and extensor spasms may alternate, and the ultimately fixed posture may be either flexion or extension of the knees and hips. Bladder and bowel function may become automatic, with emptying in response to moderate filling. Automatic bladder emptying may be retarded by severe distention of the bladder or infection in the acute stage, or by damage to lumbar or sacral cord segments.

Partial Transection

In partial transection of the spinal cord, some ascending or descending tracts may be spared. In slowly progressing lesions, as in compression by an extramedullary tumor, the same tracts may be affected but less severely. Partial function is retained, but specific motor and sensory signs can still be recognized.

Hemisection (Brown-Séquard Syndrome)

Because of spinal cord anatomy, hemisection of the right side of the cervical spinal cord (at C4, for example) has four main clinical consequences:

1. *Ipsilateral (right) signs of a lesion in the corticospinal tract.* There is weakness of the right arm and leg, with more active tendon reflexes in the right arm and leg. In addition, several abnormal reflexes appear. One is the Babinski sign—abnormal extension of the great toe, instead of the normal flexor (downward) plantar reflex in response to a moving stimulus on the lateral border of the sole of the foot (see Figure 33–7). This reflex abnormality reliably indicates a disorder of the corticospinal tract on that side of the spinal cord. Another abnormal reflex is the *Hoffmann sign*, an abnormal flexor reflex of the thumb and other fingers induced by stretching the flexors of the middle finger by flicking the distal phalanx of that finger. Finally, there may be clonus, which is best detected at the ankle when the examiner abruptly moves the patient's foot upward (stretching the gastrocnemius). Sometimes, clonus is so easily evoked that it occurs vigorously in response to a simple tap on the Achilles tendon or when the patient places the foot on the floor. The reaction can

be stopped promptly by passively moving the foot down or plantar-flexing the foot, relieving the stretched position of the gastrocnemius.
2. *Ipsilateral signs of a posterior column lesion* are indicated by a loss of position sense and vibratory sensation.
3. *Contralateral loss of pain and temperature perception* to the level of C4 follows interruption of the right spinothalamic tract.
4. *Loss of autonomic function* results in Horner's syndrome (miosis, ptosis) on the same side.

Multiple Sclerosis

The two most common nontraumatic disorders of the spinal cord are probably amyotrophic lateral sclerosis (described in Chapter 18) and multiple sclerosis. Upper motor neuron signs and proprioceptive sensory loss are almost always present in advanced cases of multiple sclerosis, although there may be no signs referable to a lesion of the spinal cord. Nonetheless, when patients who have had these signs come to autopsy, there are usually many small lesions throughout the spinal cord. Some combinations of signs are almost diagnostic of multiple sclerosis; for instance, the combination of proprioceptive sensory loss and signs of upper motor neuron disease together with evidence of either cerebellar dysfunction—ataxia, tremor of the arms, disorders of eye movement (nystagmus), difficulty in speaking (dysarthria)—or a history or signs of optic neuritis. In addition to signs of disorder elsewhere in the nervous system, there is often a clinical episode of transverse myelitis with corresponding motor and sensory levels.

Syringomyelia

Syringomyelia is a condition defined by the formation of cysts within the spinal cord. The cause is unknown, but the lesion affects the central portion of the cord first and then spreads peripherally. Intramedullary tumors may also cause the same clinical syndrome. The clinical picture of syringomyelia is characterized by two unusual patterns of segmental dysfunction (involving cutaneous sensation and motor neurons) as well as interruption of ascending or descending tracts. Because the lesion starts centrally, the first fibers to be affected are those carrying pain and temperature sensations as they cross in the anterior commissure (Figure 36–4). This usually causes bilateral loss of cutaneous sensation, restricted to the segments involved and resulting in a "shawl" or "cuirass" (French, breastplate) pattern, affecting a few cervical or thoracic segments and sparing sensation below (Figure 36–2E). Sometimes the segmental sensory loss is unilateral. The lesion is chronic and the loss of sensation may lead to painless injuries of the digits or painless burns. Because touch perception is conveyed in posterior columns as well as in spinothalamic tracts, there may be dissociated sensory loss, sparing touch as well as position and vibration sense (Figure 36–4). If motor neurons in the

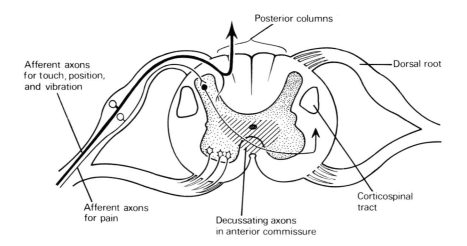

36–4 Syringomyelia disrupts pain sensation, not proprioception. The cavity (**shaded area**) within the spinal cord interrupts transmission of information about painful stimuli to the brain stem and thalamus. Sensory loss is seen only in the segments affected (as in Figure 36–2). In contrast, tactile sensation and limb proprioception remain undisturbed because the cavity does not encroach upon the posterior columns. Large cavities may extend into the anterior horn to disrupt motor neuron function in the affected segments. (Adapted from Collins, 1962.)

diseased segment are affected, there are lower motor neuron signs, such as weakness, wasting, and loss of reflexes, in the appropriate area. If the lesion extends laterally, the corticospinal tracts are affected and there may be upper motor neuron signs in the legs.

Subacute Combined Degeneration

Degeneration of the spinal cord that affects both the corticospinal tracts and the posterior columns (often called *subacute combined degeneration*) is usually the result of vitamin B_{12} deficiency. This disorder is most commonly due to loss of gastric intrinsic factor, resulting in macrocytic anemia *(pernicious anemia)*. As a consequence of the combined degeneration, there is a gait disorder, with upper motor neuron signs and loss of position and vibratory perception in the legs. The loss of position sense may be so severe that the patients are uncertain where their feet are. The unsteady gait is therefore due to sensory loss rather than motor incoordination, a disorder called *sensory ataxia*. Because the spinothalamic tracts are not involved primarily, loss of cutaneous sensation would not be expected but almost always occurs and is attributed to concomitant degeneration of peripheral nerves. The peripheral neuropathy may also abolish tendon reflexes, modifying or masking the expected upper motor neuron signs. Because this is a system degeneration rather than a focal cord lesion, there is no motor or sensory level.

Friedreich's Ataxia

Friedreich's ataxia is a genetic condition in which the distribution of spinal cord lesions is similar to that of combined system disease. In addition, spinocerebellar tracts are affected. As a result, the first symptoms, occurring in adolescence, are usually unsteadiness or ataxia in walking. There may be spastic weakness of the legs and loss of proprioception. The combination of lesions results in the incongruous appearance of Babinski signs although knee and ankle jerks are lost. Other signs of cerebellar disease (nystagmus and tremor of the arms, which we shall consider in Chapter 39) may appear later. (It is not clear why tendon reflexes are lost; there is no cutaneous sensory loss to imply peripheral neuropathy. Perhaps cerebellar influences on reflexes are important.)

An Overall View

The spinal cord may be affected by three types of diseases: traumatic, inherited, and acquired. The damage resulting in the spinal cord in each of these three types of disease may be segmental or longitudinal. The pattern of motor and sensory signs, and the severity of the resulting disorder, depend on the extent of the lesion.

Segmental lesions result most commonly from trauma or from tumors. There is characteristically a spinal level of disability below which motor or sensory functions are impaired. The pattern and severity of the resulting disorder depends on the extent of the lesion. For instance, traumatic transection of the cord may be complete or partial, and this difference is expressed in different patterns of neurological abnormality. Some segmental lesions pose diagnostic problems, however. For instance, syringomyelia and intramedullary tumors may be impossible to differentiate clinically because either lesion may cause segmental loss of cutaneous sensation or segmental loss of motor neuron function, with or without long tract signs. Another difficult distinction is that between intramedullary tumors and extramedullary compressive lesions. Myelography, angiography, computerized tomography, or magnetic resonance imaging are then necessary to determine the precise nature of the lesion.

"Longitudinal" disorders differ from segmental disorders in several ways. Longitudinal disorders are usually the result of hereditable or metabolic conditions that selectively affect particular sets of nerve cells and their axons in the spinal cord ("system degenerations"). For instance, the combination of lesions in descending corticospinal tracts and descending proprioceptive sensory tracts can be recognized clinically as indicating either combined system disease due to vitamin B_{12} deficiency or Friedreich's ataxia. Sometimes, as in multiple sclerosis, there are clinical signs of both segmental and longitudinal lesions.

The clinical syndromes that result from either segmental or longitudinal disorders are important diagnostically. They also provide insight into the organization of cells and tracts in the spinal cord.

Selected Readings

Collins, R. D. 1962. Illustrated Manual of Neurologic Diagnosis. Philadelphia: Lippincott.

DeJong, R. N. 1979. The Neurologic Examination, 4th ed. New York: Harper and Row.

Ischia, S., Luzzani, A., Ischia, A., and Maffezzoli, G. 1984. Bilateral percutaneous cervical cordotomy: Immediate and long-term results in 36 patients with neoplastic disease. J. Neurol. Neurosurg. Psychiatry 47:141–147.

Simpson, J. F., and Magee, K. R. 1973. Clinical Evaluation of the Nervous System, 1st ed. Boston: Little, Brown.

References

Chiappa, K. H., and Ropper, A. H. 1982. Evoked potentials in clinical medicine. N. Engl. J. Med. 306:1205–1211.

Thomas J. Carew

Posture and Locomotion

37

The motor neurons of the spinal cord are constantly bombarded by input from a variety of sources: from receptors in muscle and in skin and from neurons in several higher brain centers. These sources can act on the motor neurons directly or through spinal interneurons. In this chapter we shall consider how higher brain centers exert control on segmental motor neurons and interneurons. Specifically, we shall discuss the importance of descending control in the maintenance of posture and in the control of locomotion. To maintain posture, descending influences modulate motor output; this permits us to keep a set position in the face of changing external forces. In locomotion, descending influences permit spinal circuits to express a rhythmic motor output.

Descending Influences Play a Major Role in Postural Control

Decerebrate Rigidity Provides a Model for Studying Tonic Modulation

In 1898 Sherrington observed an exaggerated tonus of the limb extensors in cats that had been decerebrated by transection of the brain stem at midbrain level, a condition that he called *decerebrate rigidity*. In this condition, which persists indefinitely, the animals typically have great stiffness in both fore and hind legs with abnormally high activity in extensor muscles. Sherrington saw that the decerebrate cat might be useful for studying an important aspect of postural control: the maintenance of tone in gravity-opposing muscles (usually extensor muscles) that is required for standing upright. He therefore used decerebrate cats to analyze the role of spinal reflexes in the control of posture.

Sherrington discovered that decerebrate rigidity is maintained by reflex action. After dorsal spinal

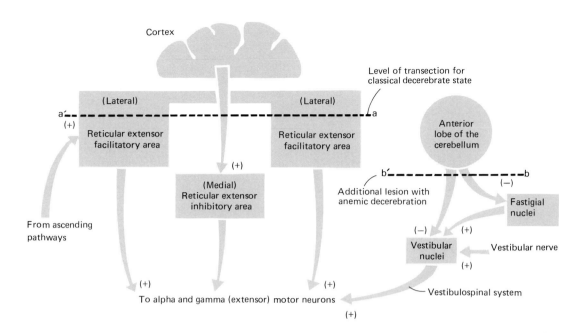

37–1 The major pathways involved in decerebrate and decerebellate rigidity are reticulospinal, vestibulospinal, and cerebellar. Both excitatory (+) and inhibitory (−) influences are involved. Mesencephalic transection at the level of a'–a produces decerebrate rigidity; additional disruption of inhibition from the cerebellum onto the fastigial and the vestibular (especially Deiters') nuclei at the level of b'–b produces decerebellate rigidity.

roots to a particular limb are sectioned, that limb becomes flaccid while the other limbs remain rigid. Thus, cutting the dorsal roots that carry afferent information from the limb abolishes the rigidity in that limb. This finding indicated that the extensor rigidity is reflex in origin, requiring afferent input for its maintenance. It later became clear, however, that several descending neural systems, especially the reticulospinal and vestibulospinal tracts and the cerebellum, are critically involved in the tonic modulation underlying decerebrate rigidity. We shall therefore examine the role that each of these systems plays in controlling posture.

Reticulospinal Influences. A significant advance in understanding decerebrate rigidity came in the mid-1940s from the work of Horace Magoun and Ruth Rhines. These investigators found that two different regions within the reticular formation of the brain stem profoundly influence the reflex activity of the spinal cord. When Magoun and Rhines stimulated a certain region in the medulla, extensor reflex activity was inhibited; they called this brain stem region the *medial reticular extensor inhibitory area.* Stimulation of another region, more rostral and lateral to the medullary region, facilitated extensor reflex activity; Magoun and Rhines called this region the *lateral reticular extensor facilitatory area*[1] (Fig-

ure 37–1). Both of these reticular areas influence alpha as well as gamma motor neurons to extensor muscles. Thus, when both reticular systems are intact, the normal state is a constant balance of descending facilitation and inhibition onto segmental alpha and gamma motor neurons.

How do these reticulospinal influences relate to decerebrate rigidity? The two reticular areas that influence the spinal cord receive excitatory input from several regions of the brain. In decerebrate rigidity the midbrain transection removes a major portion of excitatory input (mainly from the cortex) to the inhibitory region (Figure 37–1). Although some of the input to the facilitatory area is also removed, the facilitatory area still receives sufficient input, especially from ascending pathways, to exert its influence in the cord. This facilitation, however, is now largely unopposed by the inhibitory region, whose main excitatory input is missing, creating a severe imbalance that favors the facilitatory influence over extensor motor neurons.

Why is decerebrate rigidity reduced by cutting the dorsal roots? The reason is that most excitatory input to the extensor alpha motor neurons is contributed by the gamma loop. Here we see once again the operation of the size principle. Because the gamma motor neurons are smaller than the alpha motor neurons, an increase in descending facilitatory input onto the alpha and gamma (extensor) motor neuron pool activates the gamma motor

---

[1]There are two main reticulospinal tracts: the *medullary,* which gives rise to the lateral reticulospinal tract; and the *pontine,* which gives rise to the medial reticulospinal tract. The inhibitory area of Magoun and Rhines overlaps with the medullary (bulbar) region. Stimulation of this region not only inhibits extensors (as Magoun and Rhines showed), but also excites flexors. Functionally this makes sense. The congruence of the facilitatory area with the pontine reticular area is much less clear, since the facilitatory area is lateral and rostral to the pontine region. When Magoun and Rhines called the inhibitory area *medial,* they meant this *with respect to the more rostral and lateral facilitatory area.* This bulbar region gives rise to the *lateral* reticulospinal tract.

neurons more intensely. The large contribution of gamma motor neurons in decerebrate animals led Ragnar Granit to call this form of rigidity *gamma rigidity.*

Vestibulospinal Influences. Although the imbalance in the reticulospinal system plays the major role in decerebrate rigidity, the vestibulospinal system is also important. Unilateral destruction of the vestibular nuclei (especially the lateral or Deiters' nucleus) greatly reduces or even abolishes decerebrate rigidity on the side of the lesion. This occurs because Deiters' nucleus has powerful descending excitatory influence directly onto alpha and gamma (extensor) motor neurons. Without sufficient background excitation from Deiters' nucleus, the increased facilitation from reticulospinal neurons cannot by itself maintain the rigidity. By virtue of receiving positional information from the vestibular labyrinth, the vestibular nuclei also play a major role in the dynamic control of posture (see Chapter 44). Furthermore, many postural reflexes mediated by the vestibular nuclei can also be triggered by visual stimulation. Thus, the visual system can often compensate dramatically for lesions (or disease states) that involve the vestibular system.

Cerebellar Influences. The extensor rigidity is increased if the anterior lobe of the cerebellum of a decerebrate cat is lesioned. Surprisingly, however, cutting the dorsal roots in this cat no longer abolishes the rigidity. This was shown by Lewis Pollock and Loyal Davis, who were concerned about the surgical side effects of the midbrain transection used to produce decerebrate rigidity. They therefore devised a new kind of procedure to produce rigidity that they thought was less traumatic. They tied off both carotid arteries and the basilar artery to interrupt the blood supply to regions of the brain rostral to the mesencephalon, and thereby caused *anemic decerebration.* However, in this procedure the anterior cerebellum was also destroyed, and this proved to be the crucial difference from the decerebrate cat described by Sherrington.

Why would ablation of the cerebellum increase rigidity and stimulation of the cerebellum decrease it? The Purkinje cells of the anterior lobe of the cerebellum directly inhibit both Deiters' nucleus and a deep cerebellar nucleus called the *fastigial nucleus* (see Chapter 39). As mentioned earlier, Deiters' nucleus excites alpha and gamma (extensor) motor neurons, and the fastigial nucleus excites Deiters' nucleus. Thus, when the cerebellum is removed, Deiters' nucleus is relieved of the tonic cerebellar inhibition. Moreover, Deiters' nucleus now receives increased drive from the fastigial nucleus, which has also been relieved of cerebellar inhibition. These factors combine to allow the vestibulospinal pathway to overdrive extensor motor neurons (Figure 37–1). Cutting the dorsal roots does not abolish this rigidity because alpha motor neurons now receive so much excitation *directly* from Deiters' nucleus that the contribution of excitation from the gamma loop becomes relatively less

important. Thus, even when the dorsal roots are cut, depriving the alpha motor neurons of gamma loop input, the alpha motor neurons still receive sufficient excitation from the vestibulospinal system to maintain the rigidity. Because of the preponderant role of direct excitation of alpha motor neurons from Deiters' nucleus in decerebellate rigidity, this condition is sometimes called *alpha rigidity.*

Applicability of the Model to Clinical Syndromes of Spasticity and Rigidity. The main concept that has emerged from studying the decerebrate cat is that *static stretch reflex mechanisms act on posture to help an animal maintain a set position.* This concept is supported by the observation that animals that require significant flexor tone to maintain posture (such as sloths and opossums, which hang upside down from trees) show *flexor* rigidity after decerebration. These inverted animals illustrate a point about *physiological extensors,* a notion often encountered clinically that sometimes causes confusion. A muscle (or muscle group) is considered to be a physiological *extensor,* even though its anatomical action is *flexion,* if that muscle's normal action opposes gravity. For example, if, when standing upright, we flex our toes against the ground, this anatomical flex opposes gravity and is considered physiological extension. Thus, extension is a functional concept relating a muscle's action to the opposition of gravity.

Although the decerebrate cat has been useful for studying aspects of postural control mechanisms, a word of caution is necessary. The extensor rigidity exhibited by a decerebrate animal is, as Sherrington put it, at best, a "caricature of normal standing"—an extreme form that allows the study of some of the key factors in postural control. For example, when normal animals stand, they exhibit a distribution of muscle tone (with some coactivation of flexors and extensors), they show righting reflexes if placed on their sides, they can adjust to changes in the slope of the ground by adjusting the weight distribution on their limbs, and so forth. Decerebrate animals are severely impaired in most of these abilities.

An important question from a clinical perspective concerns the consequences of decerebration in humans compared with the decerebrate state in animals. When decerebrate rigidity occurs in humans, both the arms and legs are extended, the feet are flexed ventrally, the hands are pointed, and the back is arched with the head flexed dorsally. It is important to distinguish between this decerebrate state and the decorticate state that is sometimes also observed clinically and that can be produced in animals by transecting above, and thus sparing, diencephalic and mesencephalic structures. In animals the effects of decortication on posture are much less severe than those of decerebration: placing and hopping reactions are impaired, but decorticate animals show relatively normal tonic (postural) reflex activity. In humans, the decorticate state (such as that caused by oxygen deficiency to the brain) is characterized by flexor rigidity in the upper limbs and extension of the lower limbs. The reason for this configuration is not known, although flexor muscles may be antigravity muscles in the upper limbs of humans.

Interestingly, the flexor rigidity of decorticate patients interacts with tonic neck reflexes. Thus, if the head is rotated to the right, the flexor rigidity is predominantly expressed in the left arm, and vice versa. When the range and degree of postural impairment that accompany progressively greater amounts of decerebration are examined, a simplified overview of the clinical picture is that decortication produces exaggerated leg extension and arm flexion; decerebration (transection below Deiters' nucleus) produces exaggerated arm and leg extension; and spinal transection produces areflexia (spinal shock, discussed in Chapter 35). Thus, the more decerebration, the greater the impairment of tonic descending modulations.

Clinical Syndromes of Spasticity and Rigidity. It is important to distinguish between experimentally produced hypertonus, such as decerebrate or decerebellate rigidity, and clinically observed motor impairment, such as spasticity and rigidity. *Spasticity* is a hypertonic, hyperreflexive state characterized by increased resistance to passive movement. It has three distinguishing characteristics. One, it is unidirectional; the resistance is usually much greater in antigravity muscles. Therefore, extending the arm meets with more resistance than flexing it because of increased tone in the biceps. (The biceps is another example of a physiological extensor, as flexing the elbow normally opposes gravity.) Two, the resistance of the spastic muscle to passive extension largely depends on the velocity of the movement: the more rapid the extension, the greater the resistance to the movement. Finally, spastic patients show a hyperactive tendon jerk.

Rigidity is one of the major signs of Parkinson's disease (discussed in Chapter 40). In contrast to spasticity, rigidity has the following characteristics: (1) The increased resistance to passive movement is bidirectional: the resistance is seen more or less equally in flexors and extensors. (2) Rigidity is relatively independent of the velocity of movement. (3) Patients with Parkinson's disease do not have a hyperactive tendon jerk.

Considering our earlier discussion of decerebrate rigidity, some confusion can arise from the term *rigidity* used to describe decerebrate rigidity, because this form of experimentally produced hypertonus has some of the features of clinically observed *spasticity*: the resistance to passive movements is greater in extensors, it is velocity dependent, and hyperactive tendon jerks are present.

A final observation is that the clasp-knife reflex, which is commonly seen in spastic patients, is absent in decerebrate cats. However, following a lesion of a specific region of the pontine reticular formation, the clasp-knife reflex appears. Thus, the pontine region of the mesencephalon tonically inhibits the clasp-knife reflex in decerebrate cats. This, then, is a clear example of a reflex pathway that is normally closed in the decerebrate state, but is opened by removing a descending inhibitory influence from a higher brain center. As we shall see below, opening and closing of reflex pathways also occur in the normal control of posture and locomotion.

Descending Influences and Reflex Mechanisms Interact in Controlling Human Posture

Descending systems regulate posture not only by providing a tonic excitatory bias to extensor motor systems, but also by opening and closing spinal reflex circuits. An elegant series of recent studies by Lewis Nashner illustrates this point. Nashner investigated the stabilizing influences of *long-latency reflexes* triggered by rotation of the ankle joint of human subjects. Long-latency reflexes are thought to involve supraspinal as well as spinal circuits, and thus have considerably longer latencies (120 msec) than purely spinal reflexes such as the myotatic stretch reflex, which has a latency of 45–50 msec.

Using a servo-controlled movable platform, Nashner could produce body sway in two different ways: by sliding the platform backward, which would cause the subject to sway forward (Figure 37–2A), or by tilting the platform upward, which would cause the subject to sway backward (Figure 37–2B). In both examples, the gastrocnemius muscles are stretched by the movement, triggering a stretch-evoked response that extends the ankle joints. However, the consequences of ankle extension are quite different for the two movements. In induced forward swaying (Figure 37–2A), ankle extension *opposes* sway, whereas when the platform is tilted upward, ankle extension *increases* sway (Figure 37–2B). Thus, in one instance the reflex would be appropriate and in the other it would be inappropriate in maintaining normal posture. During these experiments, Nashner measured the electrical activity of the medial portion of the gastrocnemius muscles, the amount of ankle torque (torsional force exerted on the platform by the ankle muscles), and the amount of body sway (traces on right-hand side of Figure 37–2).

Nashner found that the reflex became progressively more facilitated with repeated trials when the reflex stabilized posture (Figure 37–2A), whereas it adapted and became progressively weaker when it destabilized posture. Thus, the same reflex was enhanced when triggered in one context and suppressed when triggered in another. Nashner used the term *postural set* to describe this context-specific tonic modulation of the reflex. Interestingly, the adaptation exhibited by normal subjects is severely impaired in patients with cerebellar disease, illustrating in a clinical context the critical role played by the cerebellum in a form of motor learning. Nashner's results illustrate an essential point: *descending influences* (in this case postural set) *can gate reflex loops, that is, they can open or close them.* We shall see in later sections that gating of reflexes occurs in other types of motor output as well.

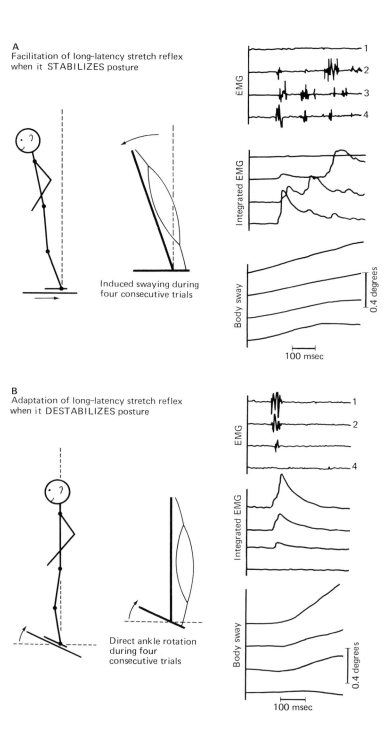

A
Facilitation of long-latency stretch reflex when it STABILIZES posture

Induced swaying during four consecutive trials

B
Adaptation of long-latency stretch reflex when it DESTABILIZES posture

Direct ankle rotation during four consecutive trials

37–2 The facilitation and adaptation of the long-latency stretch reflex of the human ankle can be studied with the use of a moving platform. **A.** Sway induced by unexpected backward movement of a platform triggers a long-latency stretch reflex that facilitates with repeated trials, because the reflex serves to stabilize posture. Notice reduction in body sway **(lower right-hand panel)** with four repeated trials as electromyogram **(EMG)** activity increases, i.e., as reflex facilitates. (**Numbers** opposite **EMG** traces refer to consecutive trials.) **B.** When the ankle is rotated as a direct consequence of the upward motion of the platform, a long-latency reflex is triggered that diminishes (adapts) with repeated trials because the reflex serves to destabilize posture. (Adapted from Nashner, 1976.)

Neural Control of Locomotion Involves Translation of a Tonic Descending Message into Rhythmic Locomotor Output

Descending control is involved in locomotion as well as in posture. In locomotion, a *tonic* descending message is translated into a *rhythmic* or *periodic locomotor output.* How the central nervous system achieves this has interested neural scientists for more than 100 years. Sherrington first observed that alternating movements of the hind limbs persisted in cats and dogs whose spinal cords had

been severed. With his colleague F. W. Mott, Sherrington cut the dorsal roots conveying sensory impulses from the ipsilateral fore and hind limbs of a monkey. This procedure produced a severe impairment of the monkey's motor ability: the monkey would not use the deafferented limbs at all during normal walking. These observations suggested that peripheral (afferent) feedback is required for normal movement. Sherrington and Mott thus advanced the notion that locomotion might be accomplished by a set of "chain reflexes" in which the sensory input resulting from a given part of a step cycle would

37–3 Spinal and supraspinal control of locomotion are demonstrated by limb movement of the decerebrate cat. **A.** The spinal cord and lower brain stem of the cat are isolated from cerebral hemispheres by transection at the level of **a'–a.** Locomotion can be produced in this preparation by electrical stimulation of the mesencephalic locomotor region (**filled circle**). Transection of the spinal cord at the level of **b'–b** isolates the hind limb segments of the cord. The hind limbs are still able to walk on a treadmill after recovery from surgery. **B.** Locomotion of a cat transected at **b'–b** (as in part **A**) on a treadmill. Reciprocal bursts of electrical activity can be recorded from flexors during the swing phase and from extensors during the stance phase of walking. (Adapted from Pearson, 1976.)

trigger the next part of the cycle by reflex action, giving rise to further afferent input that would trigger the next part, and so forth.

In 1911 this idea was shown to be incorrect by T. Graham Brown, who found that sectioning of the spinal cord triggered rhythmic walking movements that persisted for a minute or so following the transection, even in animals whose dorsal roots had been previously severed bilaterally. Thus, the rhythmic alternation between flexion and extension in walking is *not reflex in origin; it is generated by neurons located exclusively in the spinal cord.* Brown proposed that, although afferent input is not essential for the fundamental motor pattern, it is probably important "in grading the individual component movements to the temporary exigencies of the environment." After more than 70 years this viewpoint is still believed to be essentially correct.

In the mid-1960s, the Russian scientists M. L. Shik, F. V. Severin, and G. N. Orlovsky found that tonic electrical stimulation of the remaining brain stem of decerebrate cats causes the animals to walk normally when placed on a treadmill (walking was unrelated to the pattern of electrical stimulation). Furthermore, the gait of the animal depends on the strength of the stimulation and the speed of the treadmill. Weak stimulation produces walking, whereas progressively stronger stimulation produces trotting and finally galloping. The region of the brain stem that produces locomotion is a rather circumscribed area of the mesencephalon, called the *mesencephalic locomotor region* (Figure 37–3). The perfor-

mance of the decerebrate cats on the treadmill is useful for studying the neural mechanisms of locomotion, since nerve cells of interest can be recorded from or stimulated during locomotion in place, which is produced by stimulating the mesencephalic locomotor region. As a result, our understanding of locomotion has increased dramatically in the past 15 years.

The Central Program Controlling Locomotion Is Located in the Spinal Cord

The basic rhythmic pattern of neural activity underlying locomotion is generated by neurons intrinsic to the central nervous system. Thus, there is a *central program* (or pattern generator) for locomotion: there is a particular program of motor output that does not require afferent feedback for its pattern or maintenance. (This should not be taken to indicate that, in normal locomotion, afferent feedback is unimportant—on the contrary, it is critical, as we shall see in a later section.) To demonstrate that a central program exists for a behavior, it is necessary to show that a given behavioral output, such as the alternating contraction of flexors and extensors during walking, can be generated in the absence of peripheral (afferent) feedback. Central programs are also involved in many other types of motor acts, including voluntary movements (see Chapter 38) and complex sequences of innate behavior (see Chapter 60).

Direct evidence that locomotion is produced by a central program has come from Sten Grillner and his co-workers in Sweden, as well as from the Russian group mentioned previously. The evidence is based on two types of experiments: (1) locomotion was examined in animals whose dorsal roots to their limbs had been cut; and (2) alternating efferent outputs from ventral root filaments to flexors and extensors were examined in cats paralyzed with curare (this has been called *fictive*, or imitative locomotion). Both of these procedures eliminate afferent feedback to the spinal cord, the former by eliminating the afferent pathway, the latter by preventing movements that would in turn produce afferent feedback; in both, normal locomotor output is observed in motor neurons. Furthermore, by simultaneously recording electrical activity in several leg muscles, Grillner and P. Zangger have shown that the central program produces not just alternate flexor and extensor activation, but a much more delicate pattern that correctly times the contraction of appropriate muscles at just the right moment for normal walking. Thus, compelling evidence supports Brown's original observations that a central program exists for locomotion.

Grillner and his colleagues also have shown that cats with only the spinal cord connected to the limbs can be made to walk on a treadmill with a speed determined by the treadmill. Similar observations have been made on cats whose spinal cords were transected at 1–2 weeks of age. Thus, *the central program is located in the spinal cord.* Furthermore, Grillner has shown that there are individual pattern generators for each limb. For example, in animals with spinal transections that isolate the hind limb segment (Figure 37–3B), normal treadmill walking of the hind legs can be produced either by electrical stimulation of the dorsal roots or by intravenous injection of L-dihydroxyphenylalanine (L-DOPA; see below), and this walking does not require afferent feedback. Moreover, if one hind limb is prevented from walking, the other limb goes right on walking normally. By recording muscle activity in the restrained leg, it can be shown that the central program to that limb is frozen in midcycle, while the other limb's program continues to cycle rhythmically. Thus, the pattern generator for each limb does not require activity in the other generators. However, when all limbs are active, as in normal walking, the pattern generators from the limbs are coupled to one another.

In cats with the spinal cord cut in the cervical region, walking is accomplished by co-activation of alpha and gamma (both dynamic and static) motor neurons. Spindle discharge increases during the contractions of various limb muscles, indicative of co-activation. If gamma motor neurons were not co-active with alpha motor neurons, shortening of the muscle would unload the spindles, thereby reducing their discharge.

The Central Program Is Modulated by Descending Influences

Neurons giving rise to the rubrospinal tract, the vestibulospinal tract (especially from Deiters' nucleus), and the reticulospinal tract are rhythmically active in phase with locomotor movements. However, most attention has been focused on noradrenergic neurons located in the locus ceruleus and the lower brain stem that send their axons to the lumbosacral region of the spinal cord. These neurons are believed to mediate, at least in part, the actions of the mesencephalic locomotor region.

Grillner found that many of the effects of stimulating the mesencephalic locomotor region can be mimicked by intravenous injections of the adrenergic precursor L-DOPA into the spinal cat. It is believed that L-DOPA is taken up into the spinal cord and increases the amount of norepinephrine released from the terminals of noradrenergic fibers from the locus ceruleus. Thus, Grillner and Shik have suggested that the mesencephalic reticular formation gives rise to a command system for locomotion. (Command systems will be discussed further in Chapter 60.) Other descending systems are also important, since destruction of the noradrenergic system does not abolish locomotion.

Ascending Information from the Spinal Cord Is Sent to Higher Brain Centers During Locomotion

Yuri Arshavsky and his colleagues have studied the activity of neurons in the ventral and dorsal spinocerebellar tracts during locomotion. These tracts carry input to the cerebellum from muscle spindles, Golgi tendon organs, and joint afferents. The dorsal spinocerebellar tract neurons (in Clarke's column) receive specific synaptic input from the muscle afferents and are therefore easily influenced from the periphery, whereas the ventral spinocerebellar tract neurons are more difficult to influence because they receive weaker and more diffuse peripheral input. Both dorsal and ventral spinocerebellar tract neurons are phasically active during locomotion. After deafferentation, the dorsal neurons are no longer phasically activated during locomotion, indicating that they are modulated from the periphery. However, Arshavsky and co-workers found that after deafferentation the ventral cells still show phasic modulation during locomotion, in perfect phase with the step cycle. This indicates that the ventral neurons are involved in transmitting a *copy* of the central program for locomotion to the cerebellum. Thus, the dorsal and ventral spinocerebellar tracts transmit different information to the cerebellum: the dorsal tract informs the cerebellum about the *activity of muscles*, whereas the ventral tract informs it about the *active processes within the spinal cord* (in this case the pattern generator for locomotion).

Afferent Information Is Crucial for Locomotion

The importance of central programs for locomotion should not be taken to indicate that these programs are autonomous. Although the spinal networks possess the requisite oscillatory properties for pattern generation, locomotion requires afferent feedback. In the absence of feedback, the normal rhythm is greatly altered; it may be much slower than normal. Moreover, feedback from afferents plays an important role in modifying the timing and the details of the normal locomotor pattern. For example, changes in hip angle trigger changes in the direction of hip movement, whereas the afferents from knee and ankle joints alter the details of other aspects of the normal locomotor pattern. Thus, locomotion is not mediated primarily by a central program that is simply modulated by afferent input. Rather, it is now clear that *afferent input constitutes an essential element in the total program for locomotion.*

Two specific roles of afferent information have been elucidated recently by Grillner and his colleagues H. Forssberg and S. Rossignol. The first is in *switching the motor program from one phase to another.* During locomotion there are two phases in a step cycle: the *swing phase* (when the foot is off the ground and swinging forward) and the *stance phase* (when the foot is planted and the leg is moving backward relative to the body). The swing phase is mediated by flexors, the stance phase by extensors. Grillner and co-workers have found that preventing extension of one hind leg in a spinal cat inhibits the swing phase of that leg, and the limb displays maintained extensor muscle activity. When the limb is slowly extended, the extensor activity suddenly ceases at a certain critical point, and a prompt flexion occurs. Thus, the afferent feedback during a critical part of the stance phase allows the central motor program to switch to the swing phase. Preventing the occurrence of the afferent input can arrest the central program in midcycle.

The second role of afferent input is in *channeling information to different reflex pathways* in different parts of a step cycle. A typical reflex pattern exhibited by cats is a tactile placing reaction. If the top of a cat's foot is touched, the foot is rapidly placed in a more rostral position by a prompt flexion and subsequent extension of the limb. A weak electrical stimulus to the top of the foot produces exactly the same reflex. Grillner and colleagues examined this reflex in spinal cats during locomotion on a treadmill. They found that electrical stimulation of the top of the foot during the swing (flexion) phase enhances flexion of the limb and that identical stimulation during the stance (extension) phase enhances extension. The effect of the stimulus is channeled, through interneurons, to flexors during the flexion phase of walking and to extensors during the extensor phase; in other words, a *reflex reversal* occurs.

This is an elegant example of the basic phenomenon of *gating* in the spinal cord described in Chapter 33 and discussed earlier in this chapter in relation to Nashner's studies of stretch reflexes in human posture. This channeling of afferent input is important because a particular reflex may be appropriate only at certain times. For example, it would be adaptive for a tactile stimulus to the top of the foot to elicit flexion during the swing phase of locomotion because the reflex action is appropriate for stepping over something; but if the same flexion reflex were produced during the stance phase (when the animal's weight is being supported by the limb), the animal would collapse. Thus, afferent input during normal locomotion is not only critical for the expression of the total locomotion program but is also channeled to particular

reflex pathways in ways that are behaviorally appropriate during different phases of locomotion.

Arshavsky and his colleagues have investigated another form of modulation from higher brain centers—the scratch reflex in the cat. They have shown that this behavior shares many features with locomotion: (1) it is centrally programmed; (2) the pattern generator is located in the spinal cord, primarily in the fourth and fifth lumbar segments; (3) the reflex is modulated by afferent input (if the hind limb is moved out of the scratch position by extension of the hip, scratching immediately stops); and (4) the ventral spinocerebellar tract (and, in addition, the spinoreticulocerebellar pathway) sends a copy of the central program to higher centers. Another interesting suggestion from the work of the Arshavsky group is that locomotion and scratching might make use of at least some of the same spinal interneurons, which can operate in different modes depending on the source of the tonic descending input. Thus, there may be an economy of spinal circuitry that can produce different types of limb movements depending on two factors: the supraspinal centers that activate the circuitry and the type of afferent feedback that modulates the circuitry.

An Overall View

Our understanding of the neural mechanisms involved in locomotion has come almost exclusively from experimental animals. How relevant are these experiments to humans? They are quite likely of great importance. A large amount of experimental work in both vertebrate and invertebrate animals using such different types of locomotion as swimming, flying, and walking indicates that widely varying forms of locomotion rely on the same general principles of neuronal organization. It appears that evolution may have found an optimal solution to accomplish locomotion: a central program provides the requisite oscillatory network necessary for rhythmic output, and afferent input is essential for timing and shaping the locomotor pattern, as well as for reflex adjustment of the program to compensate for a changing environment.

Selected Readings

Brodal, A. 1981. Neurological Anatomy in Relation to Clinical Medicine, 3rd ed. New York: Oxford University Press.

Granit, R. 1955. Receptors and Sensory Perception. New Haven: Yale University Press.

Grillner, S. 1981. Control of locomotion in bipeds, tetrapods, and fish. In V. B. Brooks (ed.), Handbook of Physiology, Section 1: The Nervous System, Vol. II, Motor Control. Bethesda, Md.: American Physiological Society, pp. 1179–1236.

Henneman, E. 1980. Motor functions of the brain stem and basal ganglia. In V. B. Mountcastle (ed.), Medical Physiology, 14th ed., Vol. 1. St. Louis: Mosby, pp. 787–812.

Nashner, L. M. 1981. Analysis of stance posture in humans. In A. L. Towe and E. S. Luschei (eds.), Handbook of Behavioral Neurobiology, Vol. 5. New York: Plenum Press, pp. 527–565.

Pearson, K. 1976. The control of walking. Sci. Am. 235(6):72–86.

References

Arshavsky, Yu. I., Berkinblit, M. B., Fukson, O. I., Gelfand, I. M., and Orlovsky, G. N. 1972. Recordings of neurones of the dorsal spinocerebellar tract during evoked locomotion. Brain Res. 43:272–275.

Arshavsky, Yu. I., Berkinblit, M. B., Gel'fand, I. M., Orlovsky, G. N., and Fukson, O. I. 1972. Activity of the neurones of the ventral spino-cerebellar tract during locomotion. Biophysics 17:926–935.

Brown, T. G. 1911. The intrinsic factors in the act of progression in the mammal. Proc. R. Soc. Lond. [Biol.] 84:308–319.

Forssberg, H., Grillner, S., and Rossignol, S. 1975. Phase dependent reflex reversal during walking in chronic spinal cats. Brain Res. 85:103–107.

Grillner, S. 1973. Locomotion in the spinal cat. In R. B. Stein, K. G. Pearson, R. S. Smith, and J. B. Redford (eds.), Control of Posture and Locomotion. New York: Plenum Press, pp. 515–535.

Grillner, S. 1985. Neurobiological bases of rhythmic motor acts in vertebrates. Science 228:143–149.

Grillner, S., and Shik, M. L. 1973. On the descending control of the lumbosacral spinal cord from the "mesencephalic locomotor region." Acta Physiol. Scand. 87:320–333.

Grillner, S., and Zangger, P. 1975. How detailed is the central pattern generation for locomotion? Brain Res. 88:367–371.

Lindsley, D. B., Schreiner, L. H., and Magoun, H. W. 1949. An electromyographic study of spasticity. J. Neurophysiol. 12:197–205.

Magoun, H. W. 1963. Reticulo-spinal influences and postural regulation. In H. W. Magoun, The Waking Brain, 2nd ed. Springfield, Ill.: Thomas, pp. 23–38.

Magoun, H. W., and Rhines, R. 1946. An inhibitory mechanism in the bulbar reticular formation. J. Neurophysiol. 9:165–171.

Mott, F. W., and Sherrington, C. S. 1895. Experiments upon the influence of sensory nerves upon movement and nutrition of the limbs. Preliminary communication. Proc. R. Soc. Lond. 57:481–488.

Nashner, L. M. 1976. Adapting reflexes controlling the human posture. Exp. Brain Res. 26:59–72.

Pollock, L. J., and Davis, L. 1930. The reflex activities of a decerebrate animal. J. Comp. Neurol. 50:377–411.

Pollock, L. J., and Davis, L. 1931. Studies in decerebration. VI. The effect of deafferentation upon decerebrate rigidity. Am. J. Physiol. 98:47–49.

Sherrington, C. S. 1898. Decerebrate rigidity, and reflex coordination of movements. J. Physiol. (Lond.) 22:319–332.

Shik, M. L., Severin, F. V., and Orlovsky, G. N. 1966. Control of walking and running by means of electrical stimulation of the mid-brain. Biophysics 11:756–765.

Claude Ghez

Voluntary Movement

38

The neural events leading to purposeful movement involve several interrelated processes. Consider a thirsty person reaching for a glass of water on a table. This act can be divided into three phases. First, the object that the person wants to reach must be identified with the goal (reducing thirst), and the strategy for attaining it must be determined (moving the arm toward the glass). In this phase, attention is focused on the spatial coordinates of the object of interest.

Second, a plan of action must be developed. The sensory systems provide the brain with the spatial coordinates of the surrounding objects relative to each other (in this case, the glass in relation to the contours of the table). Now, however, a fundamental translation of this information is required. The spatial coordinates of the glass must be reinterpreted in terms of a corresponding set of body coordinates, such as the changes in joint angles that are necessary to bring the hand to the glass. The plan of action must also include the orientation of the wrist and digits so that the glass can be efficiently grasped when it is within reach. Furthermore, the plan must specify the direction of gaze and the position and orientation of the body.

Once the object has been identified in the context of a goal and a plan of action has been formulated, the third phase of the action follows: the motor systems must coordinate the activity of the different descending pathways that convey the commands to the motor neurons, the final common pathway. These commands specify the muscle groups to be used, the forces to be exerted by different muscles to move the limb, and the temporal sequence of their activation.

Although these three phases are closely related, they are largely governed by three distinct regions of the cerebral cortex: (1) the motor cortex, (2) the premotor cortex and supplementary motor areas of the frontal lobe, and (3) the posterior parietal cortex. In this chapter we shall see how these brain regions contribute to purposeful movement. We shall begin by considering the motor cortex.

The Motor Cortex Is Topographically Organized

Partly as an overreaction to the excesses of phrenology (a doctrine we considered in Chapter 1), established scientific opinion in the mid-nineteenth century held that the entire cerebral cortex functions as one indivisible unit. Later in that century, however, Hughlings Jackson proposed that motor functions might be localized to particular portions of the cortex. He observed that a common type of focal seizure, often associated with a small cortical lesion, characteristically started with convulsive contractions of the distal part of an extremity, for example, a finger. The contractions then spread proximally to involve the wrist, the forearm, arm, and shoulder (a sequence known as the *Jacksonian march*). Although Jackson did not have the benefit of modern neurophysiology, he correctly surmised that this series of symptoms resulted from the spread of discharges from a site in the cortex controlling distal extremity muscles to other cortical sites that control more proximal body parts. In 1870, the German neurologists Gustav Fritsch and Eduard Hitzig discovered that electrical stimulation of different parts of the cortex of the dog produces contractions of different contralateral muscles. This finding

provided the first direct evidence that distinct areas of the brain control movement in contralateral body parts.

The observations of Fritsch and Hitzig were soon extended to the monkey by the British physiologist David Ferrier, who elicited movements of contralateral limbs by stimulating the pre- and postcentral gyri, and movements of the eyes by stimulating the posterior parietal cortex. It remained for Charles Sherrington to discover that, in primates, motor effects are elicited most readily, and with the lowest stimulus intensities, from the precentral gyrus. This region is now referred to as the *motor cortex*; it corresponds to Brodmann's area 4.

These discoveries, together with those on speech by Broca and Wernicke, indicated that the cerebral cortex is functionally subdivided and that, within a subdivision, different areas are concerned with different functions or with different parts of the body. The significance of these observations was not lost on clinicians. The existence of a motor representation in the cerebral cortex immediately explained the weakness of face, arm, or leg that followed lesions of the contralateral frontal lobe. In addition, neurologists were struck by the similarity of the movements elicited by electrical stimulation of the cortex and those occurring during focal epileptic seizures. The early observations of Jackson and Ferrier allowed neurosurgeons to localize and to remove small tumors of the meninges, which, either through compression or by compromising the local vascular supply, irritated nearby areas of cortex and produced focal seizures.

Using modern stimulation techniques, Wilder Penfield, a neurosurgeon working in Canada, succeeded in 1950 in mapping the motor cortex in human patients

38–1 The body is somatotopically represented in the motor cortex. **A.** Map of body representation in a lateral view of the motor cortex of the chimpanzee. The **shaded** area indicates the precentral gyrus; electrical stimulation of the region indicated by **vertical lines** produces eye movements. (Adapted from Sherrington, 1906.) **B.** Body representation in the human motor cortex. (Adapted from Penfield and Rasmussen, 1950.)

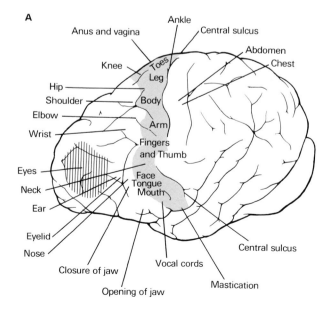

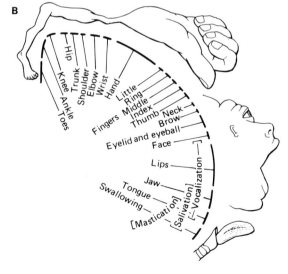

prior to neurosurgery (see Chapter 25). Penfield's work illustrates two important principles. First, the body representation in humans is arranged in an orderly fashion within the precentral gyrus, as was earlier found in primates. The head is represented close to the Sylvian fissure with the arms, trunk, and legs above it (Figure 38–1). Second, the muscle groups used in movements that require fine control—those of facial expression and of the hands—are given a disproportionately large representation.

The discovery of a systematic motor map in area 4 raised a new question. Do local areas in the motor cortex represent individual *muscles* or, rather, elementary *movements* involving the coordinated activity of several muscles? Early studies invariably stressed that cortical stimulation produces the simultaneous contraction of several related muscles and the relaxation of their antagonists. This led to the incorrect view that movements rather than muscles are represented in the motor cortex.

However, these studies had relied on stimulation of the surface of the cortex using high stimulus currents—a method that activates large populations of neurons underlying the electrode. In 1967 Hiroshi Asanuma, now at Rockefeller University, and H. Sakata reexamined this issue using a novel method that allowed them to stimulate within the depth of the motor cortex using microelectrodes. By inserting a stimulating microelectrode directly into the motor cortex they found that single muscles contracted in response to very low stimulus currents (a factor of 10 less than when stimulation was applied to the surface of the cortex). The sites where stimulation produced contraction of individual muscles were typically arranged in *radial arrays*, similar to the cortical columns of neurons found in the somatic sensory and visual cortices. Asanuma called these columnar arrays *cortical efferent zones*. Other discrete radial arrays produced inhibition of tonic activity in other muscles.

More recent work emphasizes that although the dominant projection from a local area of cortex may be to a single muscle, a single output neuron in the cortex often has many axon collaterals that may influence *several* muscles. Moreover, individual muscles, especially distal muscles, seem to be represented more than once in area 4. Thus, there is *convergence* from different cortical points into a single pool of motor neurons.

The Corticospinal Tract Originates from Pyramidal Neurons in the Cortex

In 1874, shortly after Fritsch and Hitzig's demonstration that stimulation of the precentral gyrus produces muscle contraction, Vladimir Betz discovered that the precentral gyrus contains a characteristic population of giant (50–80 μm in diameter) pyramid-shaped neurons now called the *Betz cells*. The axons of Betz cells run in the pyramidal (or corticospinal) tract. Initially the Betz cells were thought to be the *exclusive* origin of the pyramidal tract and to be solely responsible for the motor effects of cortical stimulation. This idea became untenable, however,

when it was discovered that the number of axons in the medullary pyramid (about 1 million) far exceeds the number of giant pyramidal neurons (about 30,000). More recent anatomical studies have shown that *the corticospinal tract originates from large, medium-sized, and small neurons, all located in layer V of the cortex.* Moreover, as we have seen in Chapter 33, only 30% of the axons in the pyramidal tract come from the motor cortex (Brodmann's area 4). Most of the remaining axons come from cells in area 6 (mainly the premotor cortex), which lies in front of area 4, and from the somatic sensory cortex (areas 3, 2, and 1) in the parietal lobe.

Corticospinal Neurons of the Motor Cortex Play a Preeminent Role in Controlling Distal Muscles

The effects produced by stimulation of the precentral gyrus are not all mediated by the *corticospinal tract*, the component of the pyramidal tract that projects to the spinal cord. Sectioning of the *medullary pyramid* (which contains all corticospinal as well as some corticobulbar fibers) abolishes only contraction of distal muscles. Proximal muscles can still be made to contract (though with higher stimulus currents), indicating that there must be alternative pathways to proximal muscles. Recent studies indicate that these alternative pathways originate in the brain stem as medial and lateral descending brain stem pathways that are driven by impulses in the corticobulbar system (see Chapter 33).

Although the motor cortex also regulates proximal muscles, it plays a special role in the control of distal muscles. Indeed, destruction of the precentral gyrus abolishes not only all effects on distal muscles that normally result from stimulation of the motor cortex, but also the distal effects produced by stimulation of other motor areas. Thus, both the *supplementary motor area* and the *premotor cortex*, which we shall consider later, act on distal muscles by projecting to the motor cortex in the precentral gyrus.

Corticospinal Neurons of the Motor Cortex Influence Motor Neurons Through Direct and Indirect Connections

James Preston at the State University of New York in Syracuse and Charles Phillips at Oxford and their colleagues demonstrated that corticospinal neurons make direct connections with alpha motor neurons in primates. They did this by recording excitatory postsynaptic potentials in motor neurons evoked at monosynaptic latencies following stimulation of the motor cortex. In addition, they found that the same regions of the motor cortex that excite the alpha motor neurons also excite gamma motor neurons, although through polysynaptic pathways. This co-activation of alpha and gamma motor neurons allows muscle spindles to remain sensitive to changes in muscle length even when limb movement shortens a muscle (see Chapter 34).

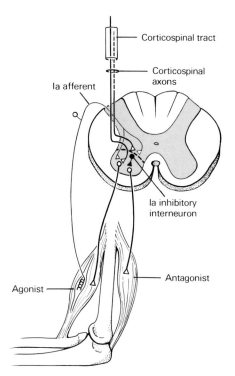

38–2 Corticospinal neurons exert inhibitory control on the Ia inhibitory interneuron.

Besides making direct connections with individual motor neurons, the corticospinal neurons produce and modify movement through their influence on spinal cord interneurons. These spinal interneurons form several classes distinguished by the patterns of peripheral and central inputs they receive. An important principle of interconnection discovered by Anders Lundberg and his coworkers in Goteborg, Sweden, is that *descending connections are typically made on the same interneurons that also mediate spinal reflexes. This allows the motor cortex to govern complex patterns of muscle activation (and thereby movements) through the control of automatic reflex behaviors organized at a lower level.* In this way, the corticospinal system combines its direct actions on motor neurons with interneuronal control over behavioral sequences. An example of coordination between direct actions on a given motor neuron pool and on an identified interneuron was discovered by Elsbieta Jankowska and her colleagues, also at Goteborg. They found that in addition to producing monosynaptic excitation in some motor neurons, corticospinal neurons produce disynaptic inhibition in motor neurons that innervate the antagonist muscle (Figure 38–2). This inhibition is mediated by the Ia inhibitory interneuron discussed in Chapter 35.

Local sectors of cortex also exert indirect control over spinal mechanisms through parallel projections to brain stem neurons. For example, rubrospinal neurons receive direct connections from the collaterals of small corticospinal neurons and from an independent set of "private" corticorubral neurons located mainly in Brodmann's area 6. Similarly, neurons in the motor and premotor cortices

terminate on reticulospinal, vestibular, and other brain stem neurons that project to the spinal cord. These connections allow the cortex to control a variety of automatic behavioral responses organized in the brain stem, including postural responses and synergistic actions of proximal muscles associated with limb movement.

Neurons of the Motor Cortex, Which Become Active before the Onset of Voluntary Movement, Encode the Force to Be Exerted

Anatomical studies and cortical stimulation experiments indicate how the motor cortex influences the final common pathway. These studies do not, however, provide direct information about the role played by neurons in the motor cortex in the performance of natural movements. In 1966 Edward Evarts at the National Institutes of Health introduced a method by which the activity of single cells in the brain could be recorded in awake animals that had been trained to perform specific motor tasks for a food reward. Eberhard Fetz and Paul Cheney in Seattle have recently refined this method by developing a cross-correlation technique that pinpoints the motor neurons that are monosynaptically activated by the cortical neurons being recorded. Using this technique they could establish the precise relationship between neuronal activity and the muscular force produced by muscles with which the neuron is connected. These methods made it possible for Evarts, Fetz, and others to correlate changes in the activity of neurons in the motor system with specific aspects of a motor behavior.

Evarts first examined the patterns of discharge of neurons in the precentral cortex projecting to the pyramidal tract in a monkey trained to flex and extend alternately its wrist (Figure 38–3A).[1] Evarts found that the activity of pyramidal tract neurons in the wrist area of the motor cortex changed in relation to the direction of the wrist movement. Some neurons increased their activity with flexion, others with extension. In addition, these neurons typically discharged before the onset of muscle contraction (Figure 38–3B).

Evarts next asked: What aspect of movement is encoded in the activity of individual pyramidal tract neurons? Is it the *movement of the limb* (change in position) or is it *force* exerted by the limb's muscles? If neurons encode an intended change in position, without regard to force, then the discharge of the neurons should remain the same if the animal makes the same movement against different loads. Conversely, if the cells encode the force exerted, neuronal activity should change in proportion to the load and remain independent of the change

---

[1]To ascertain that the neuron being recorded projected through the pyramidal tract, Evarts stimulated pyramidal fibers through a separate electrode implanted in the medullary pyramid to produce action potentials traveling antidromically. The antidromic activation of pyramidal tract neurons in the motor cortex can be recognized by the short and invariant latency of the evoked spike. In contrast, orthodromic activation, through pathways such as the medial lemniscus located nearby, occurs at longer and variable latency because of synaptic delays.

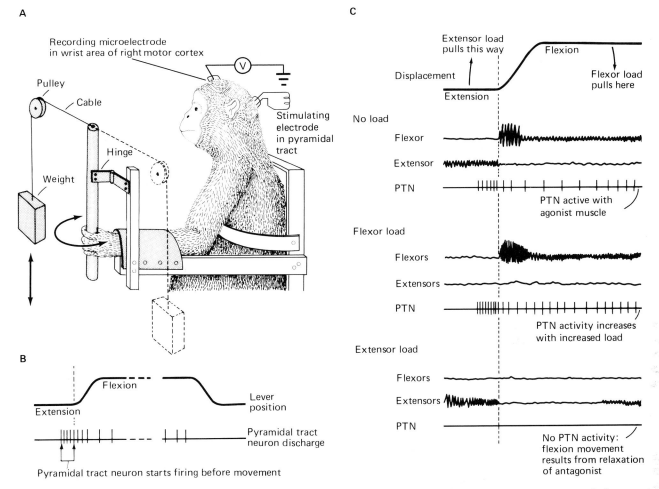

38–3 This experiment demonstrated that activity of motor cortical neurons reflects the direction of force exerted. **A.** Setup for recording discharge of specific pyramidal tract neurons in the motor cortex while awake monkey alternately flexes and extends its wrist. **B.** Pyramidal tract neuron starts firing before movement **(arrows). C.** Records of a pyramidal tract neuron **(PTN)** that increases its activity with flexion of the wrist. Flexor and extensor electromyograms and pyramidal tract neuron discharge records are shown under different load conditions. Absence of neuronal activity with extensor load indicates that the neuronal output codes for force rather than displacement. (Adapted from Evarts, 1968.)

in position. Evarts tested these alternatives by placing a weight on one or the other side of a pulley system attached to a handle that the monkey could move.

He discovered that the discharge frequency of pyramidal tract neurons encodes the force the animal uses to move the limb rather than the change in the position of the limb itself. This is illustrated in Figure 38–3C, which shows a neuron that is active during wrist flexion. This neuron increases its discharge when the flexor load is increased, but when the weight is shifted to assist flexion and oppose extension, the neuron no longer fires. Recordings taken from wrist flexor and extensor muscles show that flexion is accomplished solely by the relaxation of the antagonist (extensor) muscles. In contrast, when the load opposes flexion and the animal has to contract wrist flexor muscles to a greater degree, the cell discharges at a higher frequency than when no load is present.

Subgroups of Neurons in the Motor Cortex Encode Different Aspects of the Force Trajectory Required for Movement

The studies by Evarts indicated that pyramidal tract neurons are not uniquely related to change in position; rather, the neurons increase their activity as a function of the force the animal must exert. What aspects of force are then represented in the firing pattern of cells in the motor cortex: the rate of force or the steady-state level? To address this question, Alan Smith, Marie-Claude Hepp-Reymond, and U. R. Wyss in Zurich examined the discharge of neurons in the motor cortex of monkeys trained to squeeze a force transducer between the thumb and index finger. This task did not require shortening of muscles during contraction (thereby obviating changes in muscle tension resulting from mechanical properties of muscle) and allowed the researchers to distinguish three groups of neurons on the ba-

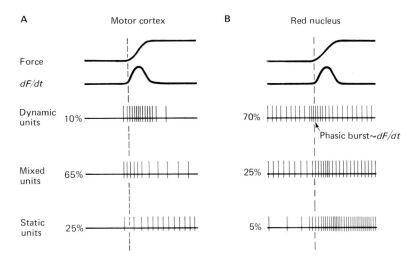

38–4 Dynamic, static, and mixed neurons are distinguished by their patterns of activity in the cat during voluntary isometric contraction. **A.** Recordings from the motor cortex. **B.** Recordings from rubrospinal neurons in the red nucleus. dF/dt = rate of change of force. Broken line denotes onset of movement. (Adapted from Ghez and Vicario, 1978; and Vicario, Martin, and Ghez, 1983.)

sis of their patterns of activity: dynamic, static, and mixed (Figure 38–4A). *Each of these groups encodes a different feature of the force trajectory.*

The *dynamic neurons* code for *the rate of force development.* These neurons changed their activity only briefly when the animal increased the level of force it was applying. Their activity returned to baseline even when the new force was maintained. *Static neurons* code for the *steady-state level of force.* These neurons discharged throughout the entire period during which higher forces were exerted. The third group, the *mixed neurons,* exhibit intermediate properties. The finding of these three types of cells shows that neurons in the corticospinal region not only control the steady-state level of force, but that a specialized subgroup of dynamic neurons also control the rate of force development and can therefore control the speed of movement.

As we saw in Chapter 33, the magnocellular division of the red nucleus also contributes to the lateral descending systems through the rubrospinal tract. Although this system acts in parallel with the corticospinal tract, it controls different features of movement. Recordings of single neurons in the red nucleus have shown that rubrospinal neurons code primarily for force development and speed of movement; they contribute much less to the control of the steady-state level of force (Figure 38–4B).

Neurons in the Motor Cortex Are Informed of the Consequences of Movement

Neurons in the motor cortex participate in the initiation of skilled voluntary movements. In addition, they are kept informed about the consequences of movement itself through sensory input. Neurons of the motor cortex have peripheral receptive fields that resemble those of neurons in the somatic sensory cortex. Some neurons in the motor cortex respond to tactile stimuli, others to joint rotation, and still others to stretch of individual muscles.

What is the relationship between the receptive fields of cortical neurons and the muscle groups controlled by local sectors of cortex? This issue was first examined by Asanuma and his colleagues. They found a specific relationship between the target muscle and the peripheral areas that excite the neurons (that is, their receptive field). The neurons in the motor cortex receive input either from the muscle to which they project (proprioceptive input) or from a region of skin related to the function of that muscle (tactile input). For example, neurons within cortical efferent zones that control flexor muscles of the digits are activated by stretching these muscles or by applying cutaneous stimuli to the ventral surface of the digits and palm (Figure 38–5). Although the pathways that transmit this sensory input are still not fully traced, both corticocortical fibers from the somatic sensory cortex and direct pathways from the thalamus are thought to be involved.

The specific topographic relationship between the input and output of local sectors of the cortex is similar to the organization of segmental connections between muscle afferents and motor neuron pools. Charles Phillips suggested that the input/output organization of the motor cortex might function in parallel with the stretch reflexes mediated in the spinal cord. Phillips envisioned a *transcortical reflex* whereby afferent information from muscle could control the contraction of a given muscle by a long "loop" circuit through the motor cortex (Figure 38–5). This feedback would provide servo assistance, supplementing the stretch reflex, when the moving limb encountered an unexpected obstacle. If the movement were appreciably slowed, misalignment would occur between the length of the muscle and its spindles (which, as discussed in Chapters 34 and 35, are also actively shortened because of co-activation of alpha and gamma motor neurons). This misalignment would then boost the output from the efferent zone. A similar process might be set in motion from cutaneous receptors. Skin contains activating receptors that can project to the efferent zone to control agonist muscles.

The skin of an arm or leg is a useful location for these receptors because obstacles are most likely to meet with the tip of an advancing limb.

The function of this transcortical pathway was studied directly by Vernon Brooks and his collaborators at the University of Western Ontario, and by Edward Evarts and J. Tanji at the National Institutes of Health. Brooks trained monkeys to move a handle between two target zones by flexing and extending the forearm. A motor attached to the handle was used to introduce loads opposing the movement at various times during the response. When, shortly after the onset of the movement, a sudden load was exerted that tended to extend the forearm, the monkey had to use more force to move the handle to the target zone. The presence of an unexpected load produced a marked change in the pattern of cortical discharge, consisting of an early burst of activity in response to the stimulus produced by the load and a later response during which the monkey repositioned the lever in the target zone (Figure 38–6). The presence of an early burst of cortical activity indicates that the motor cortex responds to muscle stretch in much the same way as the alpha motor neurons in the spinal cord, supporting Phillips' hypothesis. Although these early responses were at first thought to compensate for unexpected loads encountered during movement, the strength of this pathway is now known to be relatively modest, so that it can compensate only for very small disturbances. This is also compatible with the properties of muscle spindles, which are most sensitive to minute changes in length. When the disturbance is large, another voluntary response has to be triggered that embodies an updated or corrected estimate of the new loads opposing the movement. The late change in neural activity shown in Figure 38–6 is part of this updating process.

Not All Movements Are under the Control of the Motor Cortex

Whereas activity of motor cortex neurons precedes the onset of voluntary movement and varies with the level of force exerted, *not all movements are under cortical control*. The nervous system can activate the same set of muscles using different components of the central motor system. Evidence for the convergence of different motor systems on the same muscles was obtained by Donna Hoffmann and Eric Luschei, who recorded corticobulbar neurons controlling jaw muscles. They found that cortical neurons that were modulated during the performance of a conditioned biting response often did not change their activity when the animal contracted the same muscles during chewing. Similar evidence concerning the control of limb muscles was obtained by Eberhard Fetz. He discovered that when a monkey became agitated and used its arm to bang a lever from side to side rather than skillfully perform the task it was trained to do, many corticospinal neurons stopped firing altogether. Presumably, the inhibition of corticospinal neurons was compensated for by activity in another component of the motor system. This suggested that not all arm movements are produced by the same set of central neurons. These observations illustrate three points:

1. The central nervous system can shift control of a given set of muscles from one neural system to another.

2. The emotional context and the degree to which a motor act is automatic are critical in determining which of the central motor systems control a given set of muscles at any time.

38–5 Input–output organization of the neurons in the cortical efferent zone controlling a flexor of the digit. The neurons are activated by either stretch of the muscle or stimulation of the skin. A parallel pathway in the spinal cord is also shown. (Adapted from Asanuma, 1973.)

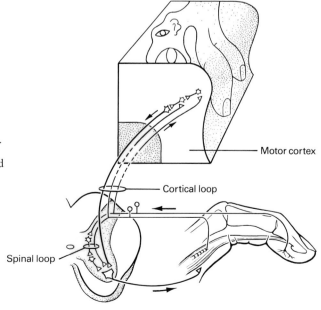

Motor cortex

Cortical loop

Spinal loop

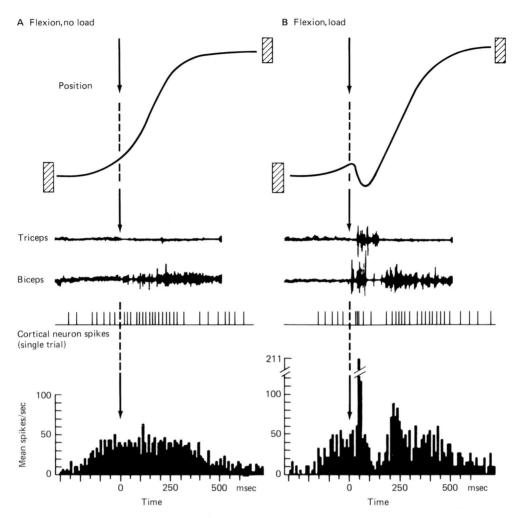

38–6 Unexpected load increases the activity of neurons in the motor cortex. From top to bottom, **traces** show position, triceps and biceps electromyograms, neuronal discharge during a single trial, and histograms of neuronal activity over 20 trials. **A.** Control movement between two target zones **(hatched rectangles). B.** Movement opposed by transient increase in opposing force **(at arrow).** The two transient periods of increased activity following the application of the load reflect, first, the activation of the neuron's receptive field (first period) and then the execution of a second motor command to overcome the load (second period). (Adapted from Conrad et al., 1974.)

3. Of these several neural systems, the motor cortex is more important in producing *skilled and accurate movements than in generating relatively automatic or rhythmic patterns of contraction.*

Voluntary Movement Requires a Plan of Action: The Central Motor Program

Before we reach out for an object, our nervous system must first select a motor program that specifies (1) the sequence of muscles needed to bring the hand to the desired point in space and (2) how much each muscle must contract. The major components of this motor program are believed to be developed not by the motor cortex it-self, but by three interconnected cortical regions: the supplementary motor area, the premotor cortex, and the posterior parietal cortices in the posterior portions of the parietal lobe. Together, these three regions specify the movement toward the item of interest (as opposed to other surrounding objects) and thus play a crucial role in generating a motor response that is appropriate to the intended goal. The locations and cytoarchitectonic boundaries of these regions are shown in Figure 38–7.

The supplementary motor area and the premotor cortex were discovered by Penfield and C. N. Woolsey, respectively, in the course of mapping the motor effects produced by cortical stimulation. They found that stimulation of two cortical areas rostral to area 4 produces muscle contractions and movements. Movements elic-

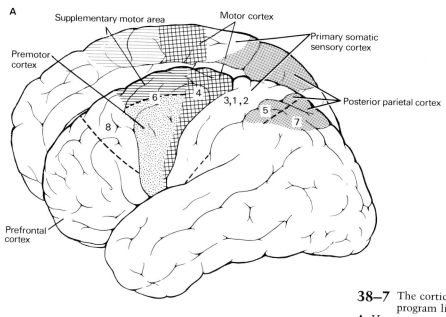

A

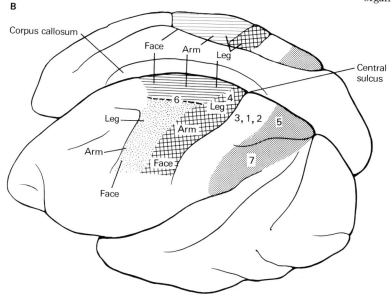

B

38–7 The cortical regions responsible for the central motor program lie near the motor cortex (Brodmann's area 4). **A.** Human cortex. **B.** Macaque monkey cortex. The somatotopic organization in the motor and premotor cortices is indicated.

ited from these areas are typically more complex than those elicited from the motor cortex and require larger stimulus currents. Each of the two areas is, however, somatotopically organized and receives cortical projections from *the posterior parietal areas 5 and 7*. These areas, in turn, receive major inputs from the somatic sensory and visual cortices, respectively. Both the supplementary motor area and premotor cortex project somatotopically to the motor cortex (Figure 38–8).

Gerald Schell and Peter Strick at the Veterans Administration Hospital in Syracuse, N.Y., have recently shown that although the premotor and supplementary motor

cortices both receive input from the posterior parietal areas (5 and 7) and both project to the motor cortex, they receive different subcortical inputs. The supplementary motor area receives a dominant input from portions of the ventral lateral nucleus of thalamus, which is influenced by output from the globus pallidus. In contrast, the premotor cortex is influenced primarily by cerebellar outflow through other portions of the ventral lateral nucleus. These differences in input suggest that the supplementary motor area and premotor cortex have somewhat different functions in the final specification of movement.

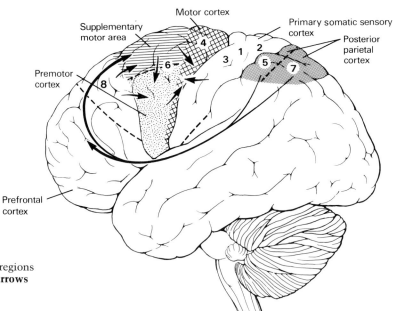

38–8 Corticocortical projections interconnect all the regions involved in the central program. Although the **arrows** are unidirectional, the interconnecting pathways are all reciprocal.

The role played by these regions is illustrated by a remarkable deficit discovered by L. Moll and H. G. J. M. Kuypers, who made frontal lesions involving both the supplementary motor area and the premotor cortex in the monkey. These lesions disrupted the animal's ability to orient its body properly and to reach for a morsel of food through a hole in a transparent plastic plate when the food was visible on the other side of the plate but not aligned with the hole. Whereas an intact animal readily reached around the barrier, the lesioned animal reached directly toward the food so that its hand hit the plastic barrier.

We shall now consider each of these cortical areas involved in the planning of movement.

The Supplementary Motor Area Is Important in Programming Motor Sequences

The supplementary motor area lies on the medial aspect of the hemisphere and plays an important role in the programming of complex sequences of movement. Movements elicited by stimulating the supplementary motor area require more intense and longer lasting trains of pulses. Although there is a crude somatotopic arrangement in the supplementary motor area, the responses evoked by stimulation include complex patterns of movement such as orienting the body or opening or closing the hand. The movements are frequently bilateral. Movements involving proximal muscles are mediated through direct projections from the supplementary motor area to the brain stem or spinal cord. Those involving distal muscles are mediated indirectly through connections to the motor cortex; they are abolished by lesions

of the motor cortex. Single-unit recordings in experimental animals also point to a more global role of this region in the control of movement. Although the neurons of the supplementary motor area discharge in association with arm movements, their activity is not related to *details* of the movement produced, and many neurons discharge during movements performed by either arm. Thus, the supplementary motor area plays a more indirect, preparatory role in motor function as compared with that of the motor cortex.

The most compelling demonstration of the role of the supplementary motor area in the programming of complex movement sequences has come from recent studies of regional cerebral blood flow in humans by Per Roland and his co-workers in Denmark. This method, which will be further described in Appendix IB, is based on the observation that local blood flow increases when neuronal activity increases. In order to assess the amount of cerebral blood flow in various cortical areas, Roland gave his subjects an intravenous injection of radioactive xenon dissolved in saline. Then, he measured the amount of radiation, using an array of detectors on the scalp. The subjects were then asked to perform several motor tasks that varied in complexity. In simple tasks, such as maintaining a spring compressed between the thumb and index finger, cerebral blood flow increased dramatically within the contralateral hand areas of both the motor and somatic sensory cortices (Figure 38–9A) but did not increase significantly over premotor areas. However, when the subjects performed a more complex sequence of movements involving all of the digits, the region of increased cerebral blood flow was no longer restricted to the motor and sensory hand areas; rather, blood flow also increased markedly in the supplementary motor area bilaterally (Figure

A Simple finger flexion (performance)

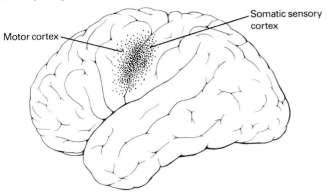

Motor cortex

Somatic sensory cortex

B Finger movement sequence (performance)

Supplementary motor area

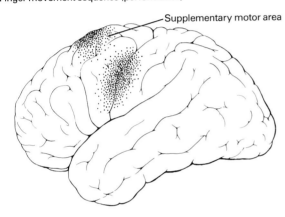

38–9 Changes in cerebral blood flow (increase indicated by **stippling**) during finger tasks indicate different roles played by the different cortical areas. **A.** Activity during simple finger flexion against a spring. **B.** Activity during a complex sequence of finger movements. **C.** Activity during mental rehearsal of sequence. (Adapted from Roland et al., 1980.)

C Finger movement sequence (mental rehearsal)

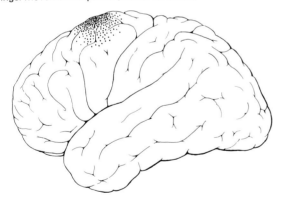

38–9B). An intriguing finding by Roland and his colleagues was that when subjects were told to rehearse mentally the sequence of finger movements but not to perform the sequence, the blood flow increased in the supplementary motor area (Figure 38–9C) but not in the motor cortex. This suggests that the supplementary motor area is involved in the programming rather than the execution of motor sequences.

The role of the supplementary motor area has recently been further analyzed in monkeys by Cobie Brinkman, at the Australian National University in Canberra. She pro-

duced lesions of the supplementary motor cortex and found two deficits. First, when reaching for a peanut in a small well, the monkey did not orient its hand and digits appropriately as the arm moved toward the nut; rather, the hand assumed awkward positions as it approached the target. Second, the monkey was severely impaired in its ability to use the two hands together. This deficit in bimanual coordination could be demonstrated by presenting the monkey with a morsel of food stuck into a hole drilled in a transparent plastic plate. A normal monkey gets the food out by pushing it with the index finger of

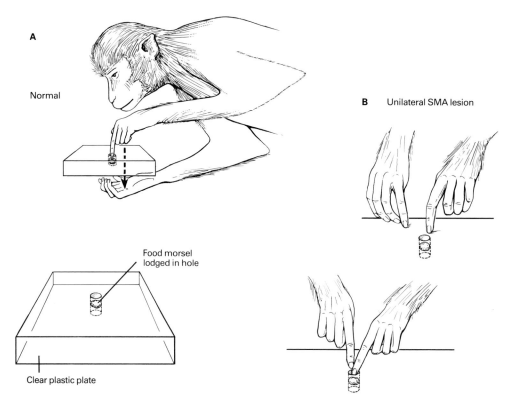

38–10 A deficit in bimanual coordination results from unilateral lesion of the supplementary motor area (**SMA**). **A.** A normal monkey pushes food through the hole with one hand and catches it with the other. **B.** The lesioned animal uses both hands to push the food, which falls out the bottom. (Adapted from Brinkman, 1984.)

one hand and catching it with the other (Figure 38–10A). After a unilateral lesion of the supplementary motor area, the monkey can no longer manage this coordinated bimanual strategy: it uses both hands to push the food through the hole, and the food drops to the ground (Figure 38–10B).

A major input to the supplementary motor area comes from the basal ganglia. This input may provide an important clue for both the functions of the basal ganglia and the programming of complex movement sequences.

The Premotor Cortex Is Important in Arm Projection and Sensory Guidance

The premotor cortex is located on the lateral surface of the hemisphere. It acts primarily on motor neurons innervating proximal muscles and is important in the sensory guidance of limb movements. Although the premotor cortex is the most poorly understood of the cortical regions that project to the motor cortex, some preliminary insights into its functions are starting to emerge from studies correlating anatomy, single-cell recording, and behavior.

The premotor cortex sends profuse output projections to regions of the brain stem that contribute to the medial descending systems (notably the reticulospinal system), as well as to the region of the spinal cord that controls proximal and axial muscles. In addition, the premotor cortex receives input from the posterior parietal cortex. This finding led Kuypers to suggest that the premotor cortex plays a primary role in the control of proximal and axial muscles and that it is necessary for the initial phases of orienting the body and arm toward a target.

Two lines of evidence support the idea that the premotor cortex is also concerned with controlling outputs governed by tactile and other peripheral stimuli. First, premotor lesions in humans and monkeys release a variety of involuntary tactile responses. Most commonly seen is the *grasp response*, in which grasping movements of fingers are evoked by tactile stimuli to the palmar surface of the hand (tactile grasp) or by stretching the extensor muscles of the fingers (proprioceptive grasp). Second, Kisou Kubota and I. Hamada, and more recently, Michael Weinrich and Steven Wise, have shown that neurons in the premotor cortex respond to sensory stimuli in a way that is contingent on the "intent" to use the information to direct movement. Thus, when an arm is moved toward a suddenly illuminated target, some neurons in the premotor cortex become active in close temporal association with the presentation of the target stimulus, whereas others become active with the movement.

Weinrich and Wise also found other neurons in the premotor cortex whose properties suggest a specific role in *response preparation.* They recorded from neurons while a monkey performed a complex task that required reaching for one of several targets when a lamp located beneath the target was illuminated. Before this "go" signal, the monkey was given a cue as to which target it should reach for. Under these conditions, a distinct class of neurons is active only in the interval between the initial stimulus presentation and the "go" signal. These neurons are called *set related* to indicate that their activity is altered in relation to what the animal is set to do when the "go" signal is given.

The Posterior Parietal Cortex Plays a Critical Role in Providing the Spatial Information for Targeted Movements

In monkeys, lesions of the *posterior portion of the parietal lobe* give rise to effects similar to those produced by damage to the premotor cortex. In both cases the animal is unable to use complex sensory information about its surroundings to produce a correct strategy for movement. These symptoms are similar to the deficits, known as *apraxias*, that occur in humans with lesions of the *frontal association* or *posterior parietal cortices*. Patients with these lesions lose the ability to execute learned sequences of movements in the appropriate spatiotemporal context but otherwise show no weakness, ataxia, or other disruption in their ability to control limb or axial muscles. They are unable to execute simple acts, such as eating with a knife and fork or opening a door, and cannot perform complex motor acts either on command or by imitating the examiner. In one form of this condition seen with both parietal and frontal lesions *(kinesthetic apraxia)*, patients are unable to generate movements that accord with the spatial coordinates of nearby objects. These patients cannot orient their hands to an object of interest; they will reach for an object but will miss, and will have to grope around to find it.

The finding of features common to lesions of the premotor cortex and those of the posterior parietal lobe fits well with the fact that these two areas are interconnected anatomically (Figure 38–8).

Both clinical and experimental evidence now indicate that the posterior parietal lobe is crucial for processing sensory stimuli leading to purposeful movement. Patients with lesions in this cortex exhibit a syndrome of "neglect" and an inability to respond to stimuli on the contralateral side of the body or in the contralateral visual field. Neglect is especially pronounced with lesions of the nondominant hemisphere. Although sensation may be entirely normal, these patients are unable to recognize complex objects placed in the hand or to draw three-dimensional objects. They typically do not assimilate any information from either the contralateral side of the body or the contralateral visual field into their percept of their body or of the space around them. Thus, they appear to synthesize the spatial coordinates of objects in abnormal ways and behave as if their movements are not in accord with the coordinates of the object in space. For example, when drawing a clock, a patient with a posterior parietal

lesion puts all the numbers on one side and does not notice that the drawing is inaccurate (see Chapter 51).

Vernon Mountcastle and his co-workers have characterized the properties of neurons in areas 5 and 7 of the posterior parietal cortex of monkeys. Two classes of neurons are especially interesting for their possible role in the initiation of movement. The first, called *arm projection neurons*, fire only when the monkey reaches for a desired object within its immediate surroundings (for instance, food or reward-related stimuli). These neurons are otherwise unresponsive to any form of passive sensory stimulation and do not fire when the animal moves its limb to the same region of space when the object of interest is absent. The second class of neurons, in area 5, called *hand manipulation neurons*, becomes active only when the animal manually explores objects of interest.

Neurons with similar movement-dependent properties have been found in area 7, but this area also includes neurons that are related specifically to visual stimuli and eye movements. For example, some neurons begin to fire before and during a rapid eye movement toward a target of interest, but not during spontaneous eye movements or in the dark. All *hand–eye coordination neurons* discharge at highest rates when the animal simultaneously fixes the eyes on the target and reaches for it. Thus, neurons in the posterior parietal cortex can be driven by sensory stimuli, but only in the context of very specific behavioral motor responses. Even so, the discharge of these neurons is in no way related to the fine details of the movement. It is unclear whether these neurons function as the earliest components of a command system ultimately impinging on premotor areas or whether the neural process is one of selective attention to particular objects of interest. Nevertheless, the parietal lobe is important in decoding sensory stimuli that are ultimately used to direct and to guide limb movement.

An Overall View

Although knowledge of how different cortical regions participate in directing voluntary movements is still sketchy, there recently have been several important conceptual advances. First, the motor system has been found to have a *modular arrangement* similar to the one that exists in sensory systems. Until recently it was thought that the motor cortex, as well as other brain regions, is composed of "centers" where a particular function is encoded. According to this view, a movement is evoked when a suitable trigger activates the region. This conception has been shown to be wrong; rather, local areas of cortex function as modules that transform the complex information they receive and direct their output to other modules according to specific rules. Moreover, specific cooperative arrangements exist between widely separate areas of cortex and between the cortex and subcortical structures, an arrangement Mountcastle referred to as *distributed processing.*

Second, the characterization of processes as being sensory, motor, or emotional obscures the underlying interdependence of these processes. Even the concept of "motor program" is misleading because of the interactions between sensory and motor events. Third, as is clear from the first two considerations, it is unlikely that a specific set of instructions for producing any motor act is restricted to any one structure. Rather, movement emerges from a complex interplay of series and parallel processes whereby the means for achieving a goal (for example, quenching one's thirst) are specified. The appropriate movement can be achieved only on the basis of prior knowledge of the properties of the effector system, of the objects around us, and of the expected consequences of our actions.

Selected Readings

Asanuma, H. 1981. The pyramidal tract. In V. B. Brooks (ed.), Handbook of Physiology, Section 1: The Nervous System, Vol. II, Motor Control. Bethesda, Md.: American Physiological Society, pp. 703–733.

Evarts, E. V. 1981. Role of motor cortex in voluntary movements in primates. In V. B. Brooks (ed.), Handbook of Physiology, Section 1: The Nervous System, Vol. II, Motor Control. Bethesda, Md.: American Physiological Society, pp. 1083–1120.

Humphrey, D. R. 1979. On the cortical control of visually directed reaching: Contributions by nonprecentral motor areas. In R. E. Talbott and D. R. Humphrey (eds.), Posture and Movement. New York: Raven Press, pp. 51–112.

Phillips, C. G., and Porter, R. 1977. Corticospinal Neurones: Their Role in Movement. London: Academic Press.

References

Asanuma, H. 1973. Cerebral cortical control of movement. Physiologist 16:143–166.

Asanuma, H., and Sakata, H. 1967. Functional organization of a cortical efferent system examined with focal depth stimulation in cats. J. Neurophysiol. 30:35–54.

Bernstein, N. 1967. The Co-ordination and Regulation of Movements. Oxford: Pergamon Press.

Betz, V. 1874. Anatomischer Nachweis zweier Gehirncentra. Centralbl. Med. Wiss. 12:578–580, 595–599.

Brinkman, C. 1984. Supplementary motor area of the monkey's cerebral cortex: Short- and long-term deficits after unilateral ablation and the effects of subsequent callosal section. J. Neurosci. 4:918–929.

Cheney, P. D., and Fetz, E. E. 1980. Functional classes of primate corticomotoneuronal cells and their relation to active force. J. Neurophysiol. 44:773–791.

Conrad, B., Matsunami, K., Meyer-Lohmann, J., Wiesendanger, M., and Brooks, V. B. 1974. Cortical load compensation during voluntary elbow movements. Brain Res. 71:507–514.

Evarts, E. V. 1966. Pyramidal tract activity associated with a conditioned hand movement in the monkey. J. Neurophysiol. 29:1011–1027.

Evarts, E. V. 1968. Relation of pyramidal tract activity to force exerted during voluntary movement. J. Neurophysiol. 31:14–27.

Evarts, E. V., and Tanji, J. 1976. Reflex and intended responses in motor cortex pyramidal tract neurons of monkey. J. Neurophysiol. 39:1069–1080.

Ferrier, D. 1875. Experiments on the brain of monkeys. No. I. Proc. R. Soc. Lond. 23:409–430.

Fetz, E. E., Cheney, P. D., and German, D. C. 1976. Corticomotoneuronal connections of precentral cells detected by postspike averages of EMG activity in behaving monkeys. Brain Res. 114:505–510.

Fritsch, G., and Hitzig, E. 1870. Ueber die elektrische Erregbarkeit des Grosshirns. Arch. Anat. Physiol. Wiss. Med., pp. 300–332.

Fulton, J. F., and Keller, A. D. 1932. The Sign of Babinski. A Study of the Evolution of Cortical Dominance in Primates. Springfield, Ill.: Thomas.

Ghez, C., and Vicario, D. 1978. Discharge of red nucleus neurons during voluntary muscle contraction: Activity patterns and correlations with isometric force. J. Physiol. (Paris) 74:283–285.

Hoffman, D. S., and Luschei, E. S. 1980. Responses of monkey precentral cortical cells during a controlled jaw bite task. J. Neurophysiol. 44:333–348.

Jackson, J. H. 1931. Selected Writings of John Hughlings Jackson, Vol. I. J. Taylor (ed.). London: Hodder and Stoughton.

Jane, J. A., Yashon, D., DeMyer, W., and Bucy, P. C. 1967. The contribution of the precentral gyrus to the pyramidal tract of man. J. Neurosurg. 26:244–248.

Jankowska, E., Padel, Y., and Tanaka, R. 1976. Disynaptic inhibition of spinal motoneurones from the motor cortex in the monkey. J. Physiol. (Lond.) 258:467–487.

Kohlerman, N. J., Gibson, A. R., and Houk, J. C. 1982. Velocity signals related to hand movements recorded from red nucleus neurons in monkeys. Science 217:857–860.

Kubota, K., and Hamada, I. 1978. Visual tracking and neuron activity in the post-arcuate area in monkeys. J. Physiol. (Paris) 74:297–312.

Leyton, A. S. F., and Sherrington, C. S. 1917. Observations on the excitable cortex of the chimpanzee, orang-utan, and gorilla. Q. J. Exp. Physiol. 11:135–222.

Lloyd, D. P. C. 1941. The spinal mechanism of the pyramidal system in cats. J. Neurophysiol. 4:525–546.

Lundberg, A. 1979. Integration in a propriospinal motor centre controlling the forelimb in the cat. In H. Asanuma and V. J. Wilson (eds.), Integration in the Nervous System. Tokyo: Igaku-Shoin, pp. 47–64.

Lynch, J. C., Mountcastle, V. B., Talbot, W. H., and Yin, T. C. T. 1977. Parietal lobe mechanisms for directed visual attention. J. Neurophysiol. 40:362–389.

Moll, L., and Kuypers, H. G. J. M. 1977. Premotor cortical ablations in monkeys: Contralateral changes in visually guided reaching behavior. Science 198:317–319.

Mountcastle, V. B. 1978. An organizing principle for cerebral function: The unit module and the distributed system. In G. M. Edelman and V. B. Mountcastle (eds.), The Mindful Brain. Cambridge, Mass.: MIT Press, pp. 7–50.

Mountcastle, V. B., Lynch, J. C., Georgopoulos, A., Sakata, H., and Acuna, C. 1975. Posterior parietal association cortex of the monkey: Command functions for operations within extrapersonal space. J. Neurophysiol. 38:871–908.

Penfield, W., and Rasmussen, T. 1950. The Cerebral Cortex of Man. A Clinical Study of Localization of Function. New York: Macmillan.

Preston, J. B., and Whitlock, D. G. 1961. Intracellular potentials recorded from motoneurons following precentral gyrus stimulation in primate. J. Neurophysiol. 24:91–100.

Roland, P. E., Larsen, B., Lassen, N. A., and Skinhøj, E. 1980. Supplementary motor area and other cortical areas in organization of voluntary movements in man. J. Neurophysiol. 43:118–136.

Schell, G. R., and Strick, P. L. 1984. The origin of thalamic inputs to the arcuate premotor and supplementary motor areas. J. Neurosci. 4:539–560.

Sherrington, C. 1906. The Integrative Action of the Nervous System. 2nd ed. New Haven: Yale University Press, 1947.

Smith, A. M., Hepp-Reymond, M.-C., and Wyss, U. R. 1975. Relation of activity in precentral cortical neurons to force and rate of force change during isometric contractions of finger muscles. Exp. Brain Res. 23:315–332.

Vicario, D. S., Martin, J. H., and Ghez, C. 1983. Specialized subregions in the cat motor cortex: A single unit analysis in the behaving animal. Exp. Brain Res. 51:351–367.

Weinrich, M., and Wise, S. P. 1982. The premotor cortex of the monkey. J. Neurosci. 2:1329–1345.

Woolsey, C. N. 1958. Organization of somatic sensory and motor areas of the cerebral cortex. In H. F. Harlow and C. N. Woolsey (eds.), Biological and Biochemical Bases of Behavior. Madison: University of Wisconsin Press, pp. 63–81.

Claude Ghez and Stanley Fahn

The Cerebellum

39

The cerebellum (Latin, little brain) is one of the most interesting structures in the central nervous system. First, by weight it constitutes only 10% of the total brain, yet it contains more than half of all the neurons in the brain! Second, it has a highly regular structure. The cerebellar cortex has an almost crystalline organization, a regularity that results from a repetition of the same elementary circuit modules. This regular organization suggests that all areas of the cerebellum perform a set of similar functions but that each area performs that function on a different set of inputs. Third, the cerebellum is not necessary for basic perception or for the movement of muscle. Although both the sensory systems and the motor systems are mapped onto the cerebellum, complete destruction of the cerebellum produces no sensory impairment, and muscle strength typically remains intact. Rather, the cerebellum plays a crucial role in movement and posture indirectly, by adjusting the output of the major descending motor systems of the brain. Lesions of the cerebellum disrupt coordination of limb and eye movements, impair balance, and decrease muscle tone. The signs of cerebellar damage thus differ dramatically from those of damage to the motor cortex (upper motor neuron disease), which reduces the strength and speed of movement and causes the patient to lose the ability to contract individual muscles. The cerebellum also regulates visceral output, but this function is less well understood and will not be discussed here.

How does the cerebellum adjust the output of the motor systems? The most attractive idea is that the cerebellum acts as a *comparator*, a device that compensates for errors by *comparing intention with performance*. The cerebellum compares the central commands for movement with the actual movements themselves. Three features of its organization are important to this function:

1. The cerebellum receives information about plans for movement from brain structures concerned with the programming and execution of movement. This type of information is often called *corollary discharge* or *internal feedback*.

2. The cerebellum receives information about motor performance from sensory feedback arising in the periphery during the course of movement. This type of information is often called *reafference* or *external feedback*. These internal or external feedback signals allow the cerebellum to compare central information (corresponding either to the intended goal or to the desired trajectory) with the actual motor response.

3. The cerebellum projects to the descending motor systems of the brain.

Through comparisons of external and internal feedback signals, the cerebellum is able to correct ongoing movements when they deviate from their intended

course as well as to modify central motor programs so that subsequent movements can fulfill their goal. How are these corrections made? Recent work indicates that the corrections depend in part on the capacity of certain classes of inputs to modify cerebellar circuits for long periods of time. Thus, the function of the cerebellum is modified by experience; indeed, the cerebellum plays an important role in the learning of motor tasks.

In this chapter we shall first consider the organization of the cerebellum—its several regions and the functional role of each. We shall next examine the "wiring diagram" of the cerebellum to see how this structure functions on the cellular level. Finally, we shall review disorders of cerebellar function.

The Regional Organization of the Cerebellum Reflects Its Functions

The cerebellum occupies most of the posterior cranial fossa. It is composed of an outer mantle of gray matter (the *cerebellar cortex*), internal white matter, and three pairs of *deep nuclei*: the *fastigial* nucleus, the *interposed* nucleus (itself composed of two nuclei, the *globose* and the *emboliform*), and the *dentate* nucleus (Figure 39–1A).

The cerebellum receives input from three sources: the periphery, the brain stem, and the cerebral cortex. The input pathways to the cerebellum synapse on neurons in both the deep nuclei and the cerebellar cortex. Most of the outflow from the cortex projects back to the deep nuclei (rather than out of the cerebellum). As a result, neurons in the deep nuclei can compare afferent input reaching them directly with the same information after it has been processed by the cerebellar cortex. In addition to the outflow to the deep nuclei, some portions of the cerebellar cortex project directly to the vestibular nuclei in the brain stem. Together, *the deep cerebellar nuclei and the vestibular nuclei transmit the entire output of the cerebellum.* This cerebellar output in turn is focused primarily upon motor regions of the cerebral cortex and the brain stem.

The input and output connections of the cerebellum course through three symmetrical pairs of tracts that connect the cerebellum to the brain stem. These tracts, called the *cerebellar peduncles*, consist of the *inferior cerebellar peduncle* (or *restiform body*), the *middle cerebellar peduncle* (or *brachium pontis*), and the *superior cerebellar peduncle* (or *brachium conjunctivum*) (Figure 39–1A and B).

The Cerebellum Is Divided into Three Lobes by Two Deep Transverse Fissures

A striking feature of the cerebellar surface is the many parallel transverse convolutions that run from one side to the other. Two deep transverse fissures divide the cerebellum into three major lobes. The *primary fissure*, lo-

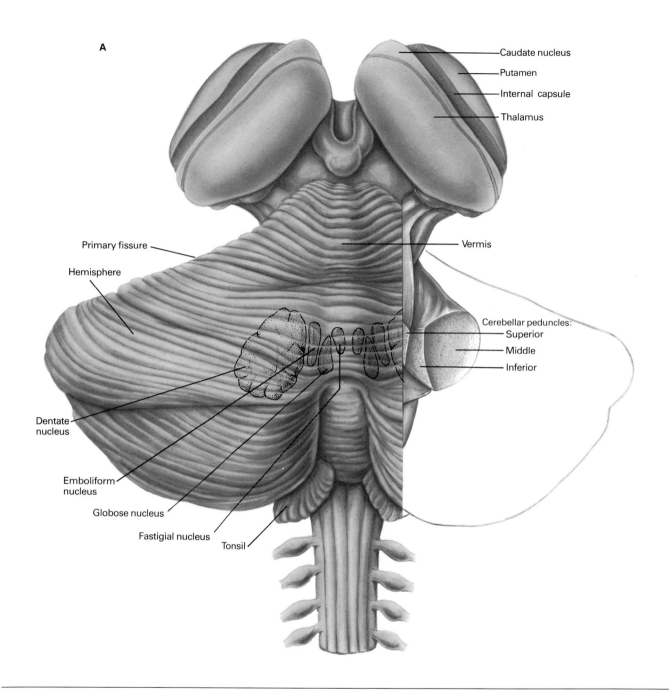

cated on the upper surface of the cerebellum, divides the cerebellum into an *anterior* and a *posterior lobe.* The *posterolateral fissure* on the underside of the cerebellum separates the large posterior lobe from the small *flocculonodular lobe.* Shallower fissures subdivide each lobe into several lobules. The fissures are best seen in a midsagittal section (Figure 39–1C), which shows the lobes and lobules arranged as branches of a tree on a common trunk of white matter. On the surface of each branch are also innumerable offshoots, called *folia* (Latin, leaves), that run from side to side. Anatomists have identified 10

different lobules (denoted by different names and Roman numerals, Figure 39–2). Although the names of most of these lobules need not be learned, one set of them, called the *cerebellar tonsils,* located on the undersurface of the cerebellum (Figures 39–1A and 39–2B), is of clinical importance. The cerebellar tonsils are prone to injury when a mass (for example, a tumor or hemorrhage) in a cerebral hemisphere displaces the brain stem and cerebellum downward. The cerebellar tonsils may then be squeezed out of the skull at the *foramen magnum*—a condition known as tonsillar herniation.

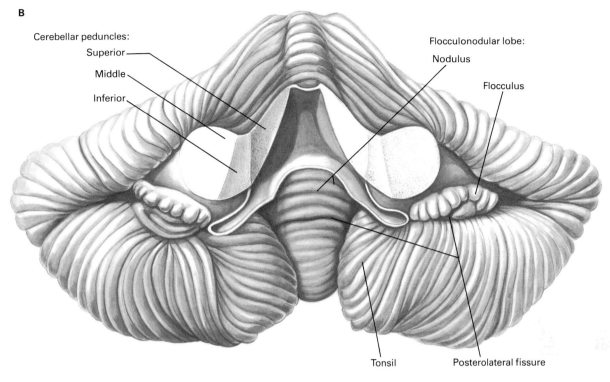

B

Cerebellar peduncles:
Superior
Middle
Inferior

Flocculonodular lobe:
Nodulus
Flocculus

Tonsil   Posterolateral fissure

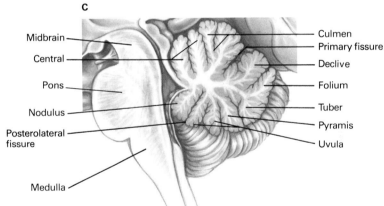

C

Midbrain
Central
Pons
Nodulus
Posterolateral fissure
Medulla

Culmen
Primary fissure
Declive
Folium
Tuber
Pyramis
Uvula

39–1 Gross features of the cerebellum are evident in three views. **A.** Dorsal view of the cerebellum. A notch on the right side has been cut out to show the underlying cerebellar peduncles. **B.** Ventral view of the cerebellum detached from the brain stem. **C.** Midsagittal section through the brain stem and cerebellum. (Adapted from Nieuwenhuys, Voogd, and van Huijzen, 1981.)

Two Longitudinal Furrows Divide the Cerebellum into Medial and Lateral Regions

The surface of the cerebellum also has two longitudinal furrows that are most prominent on the undersurface of the posterior lobe. These furrows separate three sagittal areas from one another: a thin longitudinal strip in the midline, known as the *vermis* (Latin, worm), is separated from the left and right *cerebellar hemispheres* on either side (Figures 39–1 and 39–2). Each hemisphere in turn is composed of an *intermediate* and a *lateral* zone (Figure 39–2B). These zones are not separated by any surface landmarks but represent distinct functional subdivisions by virtue of their different connections.

Jan Jansen and Alf Brodal in Norway made the important discovery that the vermis and the two zones of each hemisphere are connected to different deep cerebellar nuclei. The vermis projects to the fastigial nucleus, the intermediate zone of the hemisphere to the interposed nucleus, and the lateral zone to the dentate nucleus. These three longitudinal areas project differentially to the medial and lateral descending systems. The vermis projects

A

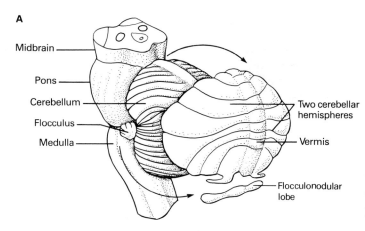

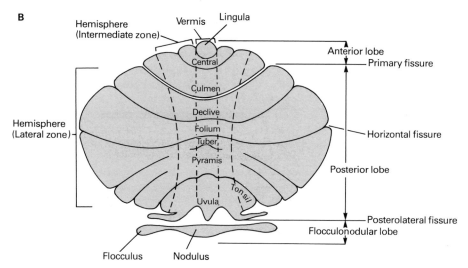

39–2 Schematic views show the divisions of the cerebellar surface. **A.** The cerebellum is unfolded to reveal the different lobes and lobules normally hidden from view. **B.** The symmetrical arrangement is evident in the lobes and lobules of the cerebellum.

to cortical and brain stem regions that give rise to the ventromedial descending systems, and thus controls proximal muscles (see Chapter 33). The intermediate zone projects to the cortical and brain stem regions that give rise to the dorsolateral descending systems through which distal limb muscles are controlled. The lateral zone connects primarily with motor and premotor regions of the cerebral cortex, regions involved in the planning of voluntary movements.

We shall see later how these divisions contribute differently to motor function through their different inputs and through their action on different parts of the motor system.

The Cellular Organization of the Cerebellum Is Highly Regular

The Cerebellar Cortex Is Divided into Distinct Molecular, Purkinje, and Granular Layers

The cerebellar cortex is a simple and uniform structure consisting of three layers that contain only five types of neurons: stellate, basket, Purkinje, Golgi, and granule cells (Figure 39–3).

The *molecular layer* is outermost and is composed primarily of granule cell axons, known as *parallel fibers*, that run parallel to the long axis of the folium. It also contains scattered local interneurons, the stellate and basket cells, as well as the dendrites of neurons lying in deeper layers.

The *Purkinje cell layer* consists of the large (50–80 μm) cell bodies of Purkinje neurons. These neurons send their dendrites up into the molecular layer, where they branch extensively. Their extensive dendritic arbor is confined to a single plane that is perpendicular to the main axis of the folium. The Purkinje neurons send their axons down through the third layer of the cortex into the underlying white matter. *They provide the sole output of the cerebellar cortex.* Masao Ito in Japan made the crucial discovery that Purkinje neurons are inhibitory.

The *granular layer* is the innermost and contains a vast number of densely packed small neurons (about 10^{11}, a number that exceeds the total in the cerebral cortex). Most of the neurons in the granular layer are small granule cells; a few larger Golgi cells are found at the outer border. Light microscopy reveals small, clear spaces called *cerebellar glomeruli* within the granular layer. These spaces are actually the bulbous expansions of afferent (mossy) fibers forming complex synaptic contacts with cells in the granular layer (Figure 39–3B).

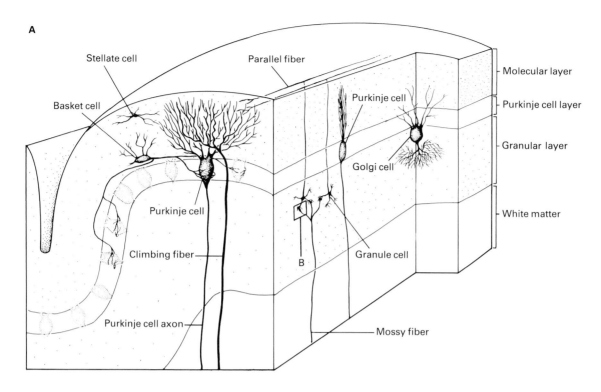

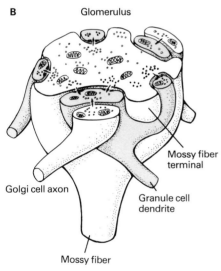

39–3 Five types of neurons are organized into three layers in the cerebellar cortex. **A.** A single cerebellar folium is sectioned vertically, in both longitudinal and transverse planes, to illustrate the general organization of the cerebellar cortex. **B.** An area (**B**) of part **A** is blown up to show the structure of a cerebellar glomerulus.

Input Reaches the Cerebellum via Two Excitatory Fiber Systems: Mossy and Climbing Fibers

Two excitatory inputs, the mossy fibers and the climbing fibers, determine the activity of the only cortical output system, the Purkinje neurons. The mossy and climbing fibers arise from different sources (as we shall see below), terminate in different ways in the cerebellum, and have different functional roles. However, both afferent systems send collateral axon branches to the deep cerebellar nuclei; *these collateral pathways, given off by the mossy and climbing fibers to activate neurons in deep nuclei, constitute the primary cerebellar circuit.* This primary circuit is then modulated by the inhibitory action of the cerebellar cortex (mediated by the Purkinje neurons), which is driven by the same inputs.

The *mossy fibers* constitute the largest contingent of cerebellar afferents. They originate from a variety of brain stem nuclei, including nuclei receiving input from the cerebral cortex, as well as ones receiving input from the spinal cord. These fibers influence Purkinje neurons indirectly through synapses within the cerebellar glomeruli on granule cells, which are excitatory interneurons (Figure 39–3B). Peripheral stimuli typically activate local clusters of granule cells. The granule cell axons ascend into the molecular layer, where they make synaptic contact with several overlying Purkinje cells. These axons then bifurcate and give rise to *parallel fibers* that

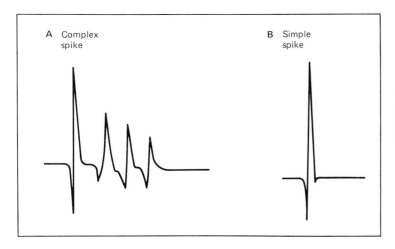

39–4 The excitatory input from a climbing fiber produces a much greater response in Purkinje neurons than input from a mossy fiber. **A.** Action potential in Purkinje neurons evoked by climbing fiber activation (complex spike). **B.** Action potential in Purkinje neurons evoked by mossy fiber activity (simple spike).

produce action potentials in a long row of Purkinje neurons. This occurs because the parallel fibers, which extend several millimeters along the long axis of the cerebellar folia, intersect the dendrites of several thousand Purkinje cells that are oriented perpendicular to the parallel fibers. Thus, individual mossy fiber inputs indirectly influence a large number of Purkinje cells. Individual mossy fibers also send collaterals to adjacent cerebellar folia. Moreover, each Purkinje cell receives converging input from approximately 200,000 parallel fibers from granule cells that collect input from many mossy fibers.

The *climbing fibers* originate in a single site in the medulla, the inferior olivary nucleus. The name climbing fiber derives from the morphology of the terminations of olivary neurons upon the Purkinje neurons. Their axons enter the cortex and wrap around the soma and dendrites of Purkinje neurons, where they make numerous synaptic contacts. Climbing fiber synapses are all excitatory. Individual climbing fibers contact only 1–10 Purkinje neurons, and *each Purkinje neuron receives synaptic connections from only a single climbing fiber.* This synaptic connection is one of the most powerful in the nervous system. A single action potential in a climbing fiber invariably elicits a gigantic excitatory postsynaptic potential, which produces a high-frequency burst of action potentials in the Purkinje cells; this burst is called a *complex spike* (Figure 39–4A). In contrast, the mossy fiber input transmitted by parallel fibers results in smaller excitatory postsynaptic potentials. Spatial and temporal summation of these smaller postsynaptic potentials is required for the Purkinje cell to produce a single action potential, called a *simple spike* (Figure 39–4B).

The mossy and climbing fiber inputs are modulated quite differently during natural behaviors. Mossy fibers fire spontaneously at high rates, producing 50–100 simple spikes per second in Purkinje neurons. Sensory stimuli or voluntary movements enhance this firing even further. These mossy fiber inputs are essential for controlling the firing of the Purkinje cell. In contrast, the

neurons in the inferior olive that give rise to the climbing fibers fire at low irregular rates and, on average, produce only one complex spike per second. Sensory stimuli or movement elicit only one or two complex spikes, suggesting that the climbing fibers do not function directly in controlling motor behavior. Recent experiments by Ito and his co-workers suggest that, instead, climbing fibers modulate the responsiveness of Purkinje neurons to mossy fiber inputs and that this action is crucial to the role of the cerebellum in learning.

Inhibitory Side Loops Modulate Purkinje Cell Activity

The activity of Purkinje neurons is modulated by three types of inhibitory interneurons: stellate, basket, and Golgi cells. Stellate and basket cells are located in the molecular layer (Figure 39–3) and receive excitatory connections from the parallel fibers. The axons of these two inhibitory neurons remain in the molecular layer but are perpendicular to the parallel fibers. As a result, when a row of Purkinje neurons is excited by a beam of parallel fibers, the stellate and basket cells inhibit the Purkinje neurons on either side of the beam (Figure 39–5). This action resembles the function of surround inhibition in sensory cortical areas and relay nuclei.

The third inhibitory interneuron, the Golgi cell, also receives its principal input from the parallel fibers in the molecular layer, where it has an elaborate dendritic tree, but the Golgi cell distributes its terminals on the granule cells in the form of axodendritic synapses within the glomeruli (Figure 39–3B). Thus, the Golgi neurons act to suppress the excitation of the granule cells in response to mossy fiber input. The overall function of this elaborate inhibitory network is still not known. By analogy to the surround inhibition in sensory systems, the stellate and basket cell inhibition is thought to sharpen the boundaries between active clusters of Purkinje neurons, whereas Golgi inhibition provides temporal focusing of the excitation.

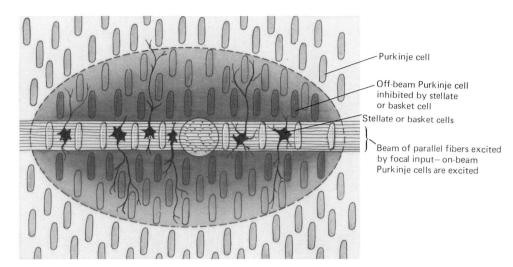

39–5 Excitation of a beam of parallel fibers by focal mossy fiber input leads to excitation of on-beam Purkinje cells and inhibition of off-beam Purkinje cells (via excitation of inhibitory stellate or basket cells). In this schematic view of the surface of the cerebellar folium, the **light area** through the center indicates excitatory effects and the **dark areas** indicate inhibitory effects. (Adapted from Eccles, Ito, and Szentágothai, 1967.)

As first conceived by Ito, information flowing through the cerebellum acts initially on the deep nuclei, which also provide the output from the cerebellum. The circuit is modulated by the inhibitory action of the Purkinje neurons in the cerebellar cortex. The Purkinje neuron itself receives two excitatory inputs. The actions of these excitatory lines is further modified by inhibitory side loops mediated by local interneurons (Figure 39–6).

Aminergic Systems Project from Brain Stem Nuclei

In addition to the specific connections made by climbing and mossy fibers, the cerebellar cortex also receives more diffuse afferents from two groups of brain stem nuclei, the *raphe* and the *locus ceruleus*. The projection from the raphe nuclei is serotonergic and terminates in both the granular and the molecular layers. The projection from the locus ceruleus is noradrenergic and terminates as a plexus in all three layers of the cerebellar cortex. Both systems are thought to have a widespread modulatory action.

39–6 The input–output organization of the cerebellum incorporates inhibitory modulation of an excitatory input. (Excitatory interneurons omitted for clarity.)

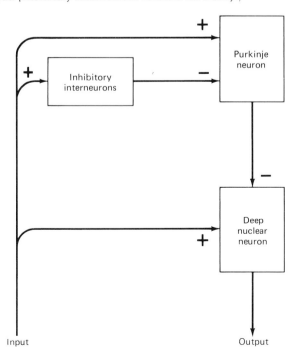

The Three Functional Divisions of the Cerebellum Have Different Connections and Different Phylogenetic Origins

We saw earlier that the cerebellar surface has conspicuous landmarks such as fissures, lobes, and lobules. From a functional perspective, however, the cerebellum is divided into separate sagittal regions with distinctive anatomical connections. These divisions form three functionally distinct parts of the cerebellum: the vestibulocerebellum, the spinocerebellum, and the cerebrocerebellum. Lesions in these three regions give rise to characteristic clinical syndromes. Moreover, the three regions correspond roughly to subdivisions based on comparative studies, suggesting that these regions have developed successively in the course of vertebrate phylogeny. The locations of these regions of the cerebel-

39—7 The functional subdivisions of the cerebellum project to different structures to subserve different functions.

Spinocerebellum

To medial descending systems

To lateral descending systems

Motor execution

To motor and premotor cortices

Motor planning

Cerebrocerebellum

To vestibular nuclei

Balance and eye movements

Vestibulocerebellum

lum and their projections are depicted in Figure 39–7; the afferent inputs reaching the different zones of the cerebellum are indicated in Figure 39–8.

The *vestibulocerebellum* occupies the flocculonodular lobe. This region receives its input from the vestibular nuclei in the medulla and projects directly back to them, hence its name. This part of the cerebellum appeared first in vertebrate evolution; it is therefore also called the *archicerebellum*. In primitive vertebrates such as bony fish, the vestibulocerebellum still constitutes the largest component of the cerebellum. It has retained its functional connections with the vestibular apparatus throughout phylogeny. Through its afferent and efferent connections with the vestibular nuclei, the vestibulocerebellum of humans governs eye movements and body equilibrium during stance and gait.

The *spinocerebellum* extends rostrocaudally through the central part of both the anterior and posterior lobes

39—8 Different regions of the cerebellar cortex receive afferent input from different sources.

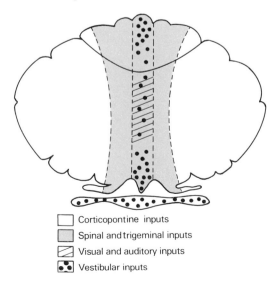

☐ Corticopontine inputs

▨ Spinal and trigeminal inputs

▧ Visual and auditory inputs

⬚ Vestibular inputs

and *includes two longitudinal regions:* the *vermis* at the midline and the *intermediate zone* of the hemispheres. These two regions are the areas of the cerebellum that receive sensory information from the periphery. The spinocerebellum is so named because a major source of its input arises in the spinal cord. The output of the spinocerebellum is through the fastigial nuclei, to which the vermis projects, and through the interposed nuclei, to which the intermediate zone projects. Through these two deep nuclei the spinocerebellum controls the medial and lateral components of the descending motor systems, respectively. The spinocerebellum thus plays a major role in controlling limb movement. It developed later in vertebrate phylogeny than did the vestibulocerebellum and emerged in conjunction with the need for more precise control of limb muscles. The spinocerebellum is therefore also called the *paleocerebellum*.

The *cerebrocerebellum* is the lateral zone of the cerebellum. Its inputs originate exclusively in pontine nuclei that relay information from the cerebral cortex, and its output is conveyed by the dentate nucleus to the thalamus and then to the motor and premotor cortices. In conjunction with the motor and premotor regions of the cerebral cortex with which it is connected, the cerebrocerebellum is thought to have a special function in the planning and initiation of movement. Phylogenetically, the cerebrocerebellum increases in size with the progressive development of the cerebral cortex and is largest in humans, in whom the contribution of cortical mechanisms to the control of movement is greatest. Because it is the most recent zone to have developed, it is often referred to as the *neocerebellum*.

Let us now consider each of these divisions in detail.

The Vestibulocerebellum Controls Balance and Eye Movements

The dominant input to the vestibulocerebellum comes from primary vestibular afferents originating both in the semicircular canals, which signal changes in head position, and in the otoliths, which signal the orientation of the head with respect to gravity, and secondary afferents arising from the vestibular nuclei (Figure 39–9). (Among the multiple sources of input to reach the cerebellar cortex, primary vestibular afferents are the only afferents that can do so directly from ganglion cells in the periphery without an intervening relay.) The vestibulocerebellum also receives visual information from the lateral geniculate nucleus, superior colliculi, and striate cortex, most of which is relayed through the pontine nuclei. The output of the vestibulocerebellum is reflected back onto the vestibular nuclei.

By its action on the vestibular nuclei the vestibulocerebellum plays a critical role in equilibrium and in the control of the axial muscles that are used to maintain balance. In addition, the vestibulocerebellum functions to control eye movement and to coordinate movements of the head with those of the eyes.

The Spinocerebellum Contains Topographical Maps of the Body That Receive Sensory Information from the Spinal Cord

The principal input to the spinocerebellum comes from the spinal cord through the *spinocerebellar tracts* and conveys information about somatic sensibility. However, the spinocerebellum also receives information from the auditory, visual, and vestibular systems. As was first shown in the 1940s by Edgar Adrian in England and by Ray Snider in the United States, all of these afferent projections are organized somatotopically. *The entire body is mapped in two different areas of the spinocerebellar cortex* (Figure 39–10). One map lies mainly in the anterior lobe and the other lies in the posterior lobe. These two maps are inverted relative to one another: the body map in the anterior lobe has its feet oriented forward while the face extends backward into the first lobule of the posterior lobe. The other body map is oriented head forward and is located in the intermediate zone of the posterior lobe on either side of the vermis. Auditory and visual stimuli elicit maximal activity in the posterior lobe vermis.

The earliest studies of afferent processing by the cerebellar cortex were based on the recording of surface potentials evoked in a population of neurons by peripheral stimuli. Although two apparently continuous somatotopic maps of the body were revealed by this technique, more refined studies using single-cell recordings have complicated this simple view. First, mossy fiber input from restricted peripheral sites diverges to influence several independent patches of granule cells that excite small arrays of Purkinje neurons. This is dramatically seen in the detailed maps of mossy fiber inputs to granule cells obtained in the rat by G. Shambes and his colleagues (Figure 39–11). Even though input from a given site activates a small, sharply demarcated area, adjacent regions may receive information from distant body parts—an arrangement that has been called a *fractured somatotopy*. The apparent conflict with earlier observations based on recordings of surface potentials can be re-

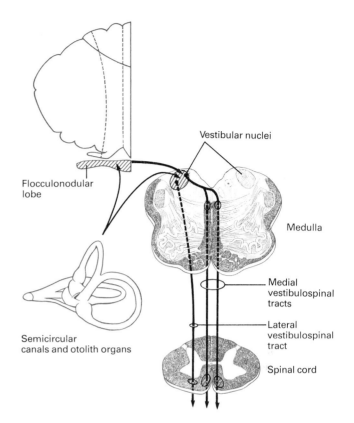

39–9 The flocculonodular lobe forms the vestibulocerebellum. It receives input from the labyrinth and projects directly to the vestibular nuclei. (Oculomotor connections of the vestibular nuclei are omitted for clarity.)

solved because the peripheral area giving rise to the largest potential represents only the predominant input to a particular region of the cerebellar cortex.

In addition to receiving sensory information directly from the periphery, the spinocerebellum also receives information from the somatic sensory and motor cortices, and this information is mapped to correspond with the peripheral body representations. Similarly, information

39–10 Two regions of the cerebellar surface each contain somatotopic maps of the entire body.

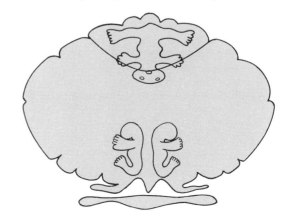

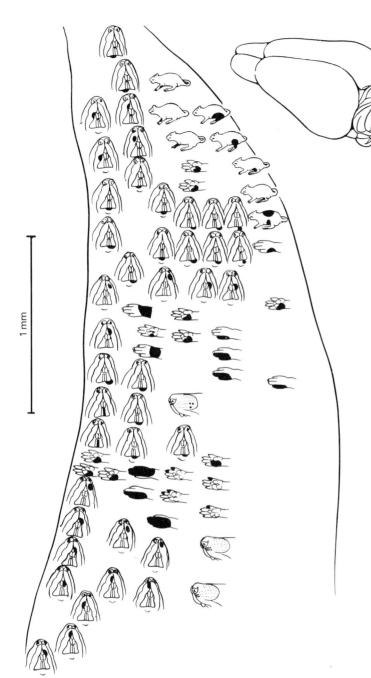

1 mm

39–11 The receptive fields of granule cells recorded in the rat cerebellum reveal that there are multiple representations of the same body parts in different locations. In the expanded portion of the cerebellum **(left)**, the receptive fields of individual granule cells are depicted as **shaded** areas on body parts. (Adapted from Shambes, Gibson, and Welker, 1978.)

from visual and auditory cortical regions reaches the visual and auditory receiving areas in the posterior vermis. The entire vermis also receives input from primary and secondary vestibular axons (Figure 39–8).

Somatic Sensory Information Reaches the Cerebellum Through Direct and Indirect Mossy Fiber Pathways

Information from spinal levels is conveyed to the cerebellum by numerous pathways terminating in the vermis and the intermediate zone. Four pathways carry somatic sensory information to the cerebellar cortex directly

from the spinal cord and are termed direct pathways. The *dorsal* and *ventral spinocerebellar tracts* are the direct pathways that convey information from the lower part of the body (trunk and legs), and the *cuneo-* and *rostral spinocerebellar tracts* are the corresponding pathways from the upper body (arms and neck).

The *dorsal spinocerebellar tract* originates from neurons in Clarke's nucleus, which lies in the spinal intermediate zone between the levels of T1 and L2. Individual neurons within this nucleus receive information either from *muscle* or from *cutaneous* receptors and relay this information to small, discrete areas of the cerebellum. The dorsal spinocerebellar tract ascends ipsilaterally in

Table 39–1. Principal Input and Output Pathways of the Cerebellum

Functional region	Anatomical region	Principal afferent input	Deep nucleus	Principal destination	Function
Vestibulocerebellum	Flocculonodular lobe	Vestibular labyrinth	Lateral vestibular	Medial systems: Axial motor neurons	Axial control; vestibular reflexes
Spinocerebellum	Vermis	Vestibular labyrinth, proximal body parts; face, visual, and auditory to posterior lobe only	Fastigial	Medial systems: Medial brain stem system Axial regions of motor cortex	Axial and proximal motor control; ongoing execution
Spinocerebellum	Intermediate part of hemisphere	Spinal afferents (distal body parts)	Interposed	Lateral systems: Red nucleus (magnocellular part) Distal regions of motor cortex	Distal motor control; ongoing execution
Cerebrocerebellum	Lateral part of hemisphere	Cortical afferents	Dentate	Motor integration areas: Red nucleus (parvocellular part) Motor cortex (area 4, distal limb areas) Premotor cortex (area 6)	Initiation; planning; timing

the lateral quadrants of the spinal cord and enters the cerebellum through the inferior cerebellar peduncle.

The *ventral spinocerebellar tract* originates primarily from the *spinal border cells*, a group of neurons located at the lateral edge of the spinal gray matter. These cells receive *convergent* inputs from both cutaneous and muscle receptors, especially Golgi tendon organs, as well as from descending pathways and spinal interneurons. Their axons ascend in the ventral quadrants of the spinal cord (some crossed, some uncrossed) to enter the cerebellum through the superior cerebellar peduncle.

Work by Anders Lundberg, Olov Oscarsson, and their co-workers in Sweden suggests that whereas the information carried by the dorsal spinocerebellar tract faithfully reflects sensory events arising in the periphery, the information carried by the ventral spinocerebellar tract is different in character and represents an internal feedback that monitors the final commands reaching motor neurons. This final command integrates both descending and peripheral information. This important idea was confirmed by Yuri Arshavsky and co-workers in Moscow, who recorded the activity of dorsal and ventral spinocerebellar tract neurons during locomotion both in intact cats and in deafferented cats whose dorsal roots had been cut. Dorsal spinocerebellar tract neurons in Clarke's column were modulated during locomotion only when the dorsal roots were intact, whereas ventral spinocerebellar tract neurons continued to be modulated even in the absence of peripheral input after section of the dorsal roots (see Chapter 37). This experiment showed that, although dorsal spinocerebellar tract neurons provide the cerebellum with information about evolving movements, the ventral spinocerebellar neurons are principally driven by central commands that determine the locomotor cycle.

The cerebellum also receives information from cranial nerve nuclei that mediate input from the face and from special senses. The principal pathways carrying this information are listed in Table 39–1.

In addition to the direct dorsal and ventral spinocerebellar pathways, the cerebellum receives information from the periphery indirectly through relays in different brain stem nuclei. Two of these nuclei, the *lateral reticular nucleus* and the *inferior olivary nucleus*, both located in the medulla, are particularly important. The lateral reticular nucleus receives input from the spinal cord, cranial nerve nuclei, and the cerebral cortex. The peripheral receptive fields of lateral reticular neurons are typically larger than those of either dorsal or ventral spinocerebellar tract neurons, and the discharge evoked in them by sensory stimuli is longer lasting. These neurons project to widespread areas of the ipsilateral cerebellar cortex through the inferior cerebellar peduncle. The inferior olivary nucleus is the only source of the climbing fibers; we shall therefore consider its contribution later in this chapter in the context of the cerebellum's role in learning.

Efferent Spinocerebellar Projections Control the Medial and Lateral Descending Systems

As we saw earlier, the Purkinje neurons in the cerebellar vermis and the adjacent intermediate part of the hemisphere project to different deep nuclei. These nuclei in turn control different components of the descending motor pathways.

514

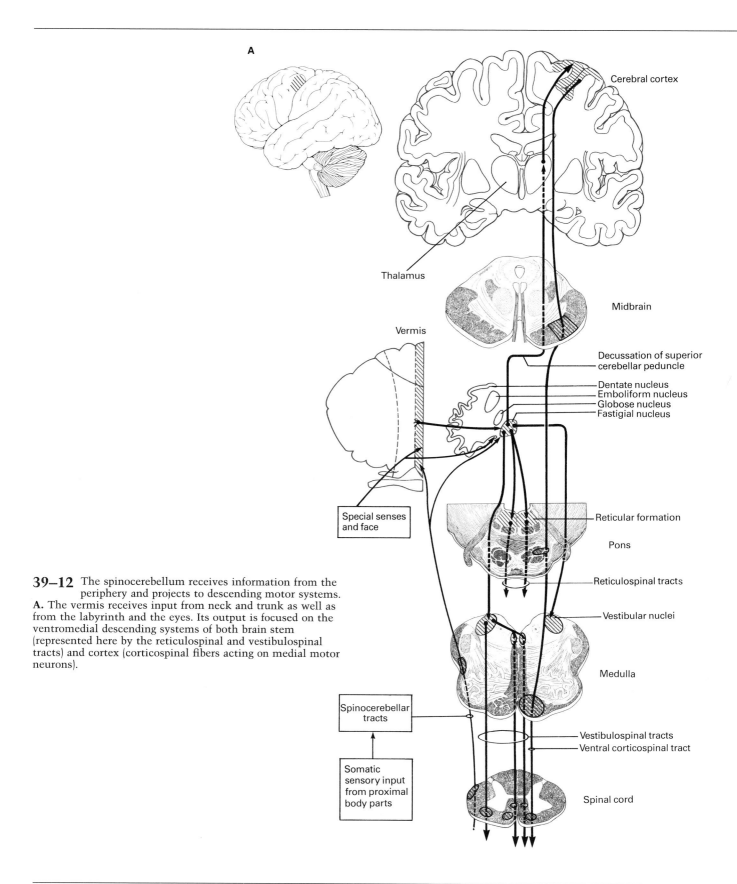

A

Cerebral cortex

Thalamus

Midbrain

Vermis

Decussation of superior
cerebellar peduncle

Dentate nucleus
Emboliform nucleus
Globose nucleus
Fastigial nucleus

Special senses
and face

Reticular formation

Pons

Reticulospinal tracts

39–12 The spinocerebellum receives information from the
periphery and projects to descending motor systems.
A. The vermis receives input from neck and trunk as well as
from the labyrinth and the eyes. Its output is focused on the
ventromedial descending systems of both brain stem
(represented here by the reticulospinal and vestibulospinal
tracts) and cortex (corticospinal fibers acting on medial motor
neurons).

Vestibular nuclei

Medulla

Spinocerebellar
tracts

Vestibulospinal tracts
Ventral corticospinal tract

Somatic
sensory input
from proximal
body parts

Spinal cord

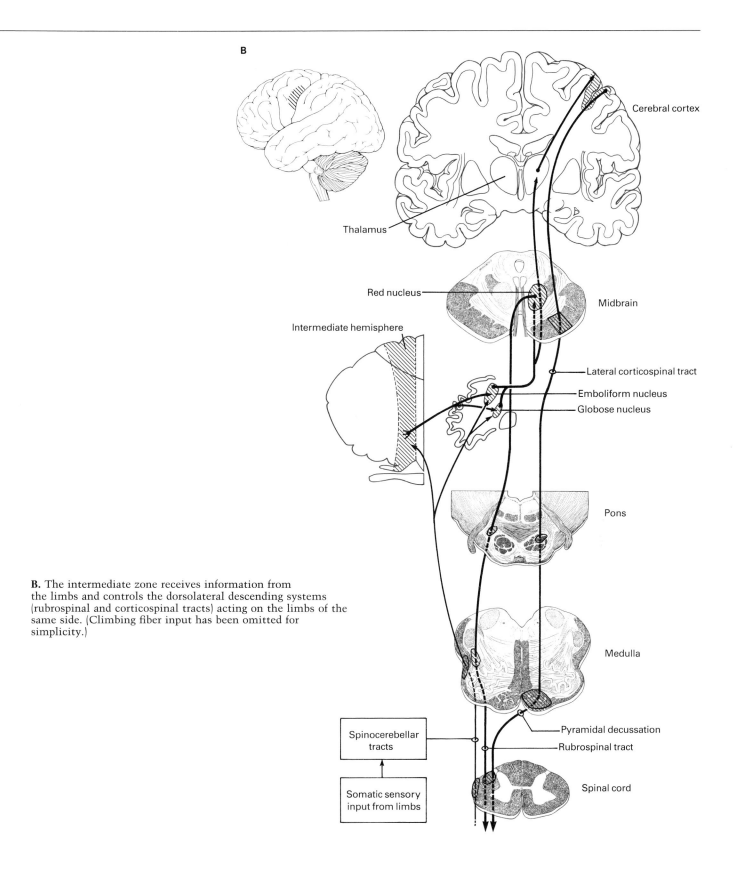

B

Cerebral cortex

Thalamus

Red nucleus

Midbrain

Intermediate hemisphere

Lateral corticospinal tract

Emboliform nucleus

Globose nucleus

Pons

B. The intermediate zone receives information from the limbs and controls the dorsolateral descending systems (rubrospinal and corticospinal tracts) acting on the limbs of the same side. (Climbing fiber input has been omitted for simplicity.)

Medulla

Pyramidal decussation

Rubrospinal tract

Spinal cord

Spinocerebellar tracts

Somatic sensory input from limbs

The fastigial nuclei receive topographically organized projections from the anterior and posterior lobe vermis and project bilaterally to the *brain stem reticular formation* and to the *lateral vestibular nuclei*. Both the vestibular nuclei and the reticular formation give rise to fibers that descend to the spinal cord. The fastigial nuclei also have crossed ascending projections that reach the motor cortex after relaying in the ventrolateral nucleus of the thalamus. Through both its ascending and descending projections, the *medial region of the cerebellum controls the cortical and brain stem components of the medial descending systems*. This region of the cerebellum controls axial and proximal musculature (Figure 39–12A).

The intermediate zones of the cerebellar cortex projects to the interposed nuclei. The interposed nuclei also influence movement through their connections to the brain stem and cortical components of the lateral descending systems: the rubrospinal and lateral corticospinal tracts. The interposed nuclei project to the contralateral magnocellular portion of the red nucleus (Figure 39–12B) in the brain stem via the superior cerebellar peduncle. Many of these fibers continue rostrally to the ventral lateral nucleus of the thalamus, where they terminate on neurons projecting to the limb areas of the motor cortex. (Although the ventral lateral nucleus also receives projections from the globus pallidus, the pallidal and cerebellar projections terminate on separate neuronal populations.) By controlling the rubrospinal and corticospinal components of the dorsolateral descending systems, the intermediate zone and the interposed nuclei focus their action on distal limb muscles. Because the cerebellar connections (in the superior cerebellar peduncle) with the rubrospinal and corticospinal systems are crossed, and because these two pathways cross again before terminating in the spinal cord, *the deficits produced by lesions of the intermediate zone affect limbs on the same side as the lesion* (Figure 39–12B).

The Spinocerebellum Uses Sensory Feedback to Control Muscle Tone and the Execution of Movement

The spinocerebellum has two principal functions: (1) to control the execution of movement, and (2) to regulate muscle tone. The spinocerebellum carries out these functions by regulating the peripheral muscular apparatus so as to compensate for small variations in loads encountered during movement and to smooth out small oscillations (physiological tremor). This control is thought to be dependent both on information that the spinocerebellum receives from cortical motor areas about the intended motor command and on feedback from the spinal cord and periphery, which provides details about the evolving movement. These inputs allow the spinocerebellum to correct for deviations from the intended movement. This view is supported by the finding that although neurons in interposed nuclei are well modulated during movement, their change in activity occurs only after neurons in the motor cortex have started firing.

Lesions of the spinocerebellum produce an abnormality in the sequence of muscle contractions during rapid movement. Normally, rapid movements directed to a target are accomplished by the brief and transient contraction of agonist muscles with concurrent relaxation of the antagonist. At the midpoint of the movement, the antagonist contracts to terminate movement accurately. With cerebellar lesions this normal pattern is altered. The initial contraction of the agonist is prolonged, while the antagonist does not initially relax as it normally does but may actually contract. Moreover, the phasic contraction of the antagonist, which serves to decelerate the limb, neither occurs when it should nor is sufficient to stop the movement in time. Studies carried out by John Soechting and his collaborators at the University of Minnesota have shown that the neural commands required to decelerate the limb at its terminal point depend on proprioceptive feedback information from the moving limb. Patients as well as experimental animals with lesions of the spinocerebellum are unable to use this information effectively. Slow movements also become disrupted. The movements become clumsy and inaccurate (*ataxia* and *dysmetria*; see below) and a tremor appears. This tremor typically is greatest at the end point of a movement and under conditions in which precise control is necessary.

Lesions of the cerebellum that interrupt the projections to either the brain stem or the cortical motor areas from the interposed or dentate nuclei also lead to decreased muscle tone, or *hypotonia*. Neurons in the deep cerebellar nuclei show a high rate of spontaneous activity even in the absence of movement. A lesion of these nuclei therefore removes the tonic drive originating from them and inactivates the ipsilateral corticospinal and rubrospinal neurons. Sid Gilman, now at the University of Michigan, discovered that a major factor contributing to decreased muscle tone is a systematic decrease in the drive of gamma motor neurons innervating the muscle spindles. Because of the resulting decrease in steady background of spindle afferent activity, the firing threshold of motor neurons is elevated and the resistance to muscle stretch during passive motion is decreased.

The Cerebrocerebellum Coordinates the Planning of Limb Movements

Input from the Cerebral Cortex Is Conveyed to the Cerebellum Through the Pontine Nuclei

The cerebrocerebellum receives its input from wide areas of the cerebral cortex and does not receive peripheral sensory input. Most of its input originates from sensory and motor cortices and from the premotor and posterior parietal cortices (Figure 39–13). These regions do not project directly to the cerebellum but rather to the pontine nuclei, which then distribute cortical information to the contralateral cerebellar hemisphere through the middle cerebellar peduncle.

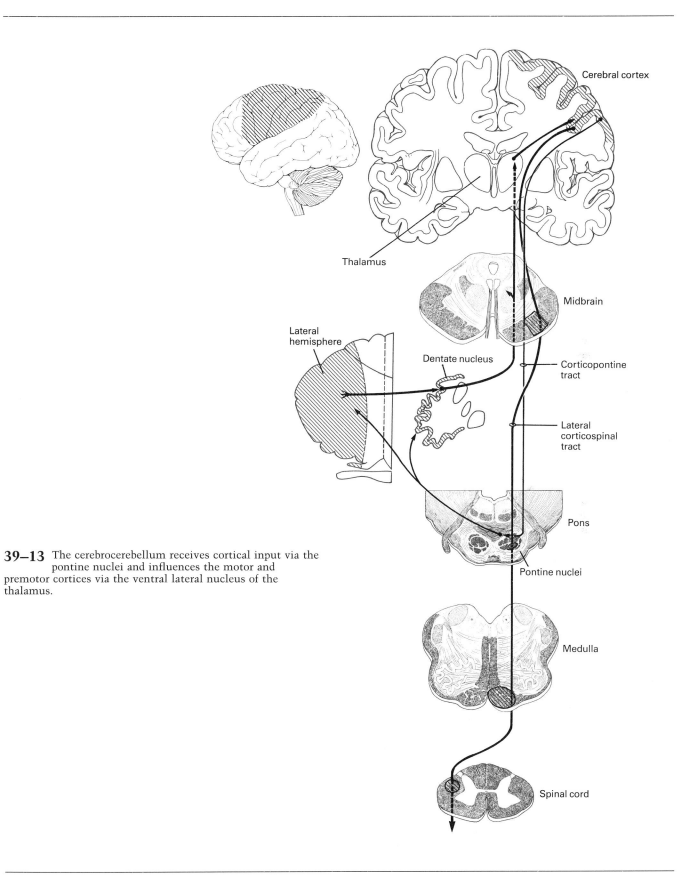

Cerebral cortex

Thalamus

Midbrain

Lateral hemisphere

Dentate nucleus

Corticopontine tract

Lateral corticospinal tract

Pons

Pontine nuclei

Medulla

Spinal cord

39–13 The cerebrocerebellum receives cortical input via the pontine nuclei and influences the motor and premotor cortices via the ventral lateral nucleus of the thalamus.

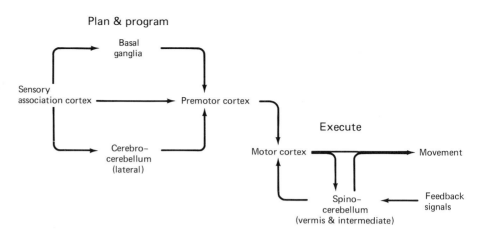

39–14 This hypothetical flow diagram shows the likely role of the cerebellum in the initiation of voluntary movement. The thalamic relay for basal ganglia, cerebellar, and somatic sensory input is omitted for simplicity. (Adapted from Allen and Tsukahara, 1974.)

The Output of the Cerebrocerebellum Is Mediated by the Dentate Nuclei, Which Control Motor and Premotor Areas of the Cortex

The lateral zone of the cerebellar cortex projects to the dentate nucleus, which sends fibers through the superior cerebellar peduncle to terminate in the ventral lateral nucleus of the thalamus. From the ventral lateral nucleus, the dentate nucleus influences motor and premotor regions of the cerebral cortex. The dentate nucleus also projects to the parvocellular component of the red nucleus. This portion of the red nucleus does not contribute to the rubrospinal tract; rather, it is part of a complex feedback circuit that sends information back to the cerebellum primarily through the ipsilateral inferior olivary nucleus. The function of this circuit is poorly understood.

Lesions of the Cerebrocerebellum Produce Delays in Movement Initiation and in Coordination of Limb Movement

The effects of lesions of the lateral parts of the cerebellum are largely restricted to the control of distal limb muscles and consist of three disturbances: (1) delays in the initiation of movement, (2) decreased muscle tone (hypotonia), and (3) distortion of muscular coordination (ataxia).

Two mechanisms have been proposed to account for the delay in the initiation of movement. First, the dentate nucleus might provide background facilitation to either cortical or subcortical neurons so that, after dentate lesions, commands to initiate movement could bring the motor neurons to fire only after an increased period of summation. Alternatively, the dentate nucleus might participate in, or indeed convey, the commands initiating movement.

This question was addressed by Vernon Brooks and his collaborators at the University of Western Ontario. They recorded the patterns of activity of neurons in the motor cortex of monkeys while the animals performed prompt movements to a visual cue, and then compared these patterns before and after the dentate nucleus was reversibly inactivated. This was achieved by using a cooling probe inserted through a cannula into the deep cerebellar nuclei. Had the dentate merely provided background excitation to subcortical structures, the change in activity of neurons in the motor cortex should have occurred at the normal time, but more time would have elapsed before the onset of movement. This, however, was not the case. When the dentate nucleus was cooled, both the discharge of motor cortex neurons associated with the movement and the onset of the movement itself were delayed.

Although the results may be interpreted to suggest that the dentate nucleus provides the signal that directly triggers activity in the motor cortex, another possibility is that the dentate participates with the premotor cortex in the programming of movement. The initiation of movement would then involve complex comparisons between different signals reaching the lateral cerebellum while its output would contribute to an earlier "decision" to move. This scheme is more compatible with the finding by Meyer-Lohmann, Hore, and Brooks that when the dentate nucleus is reversibly inactivated by cooling, the occurrence of movement is not prevented; under these conditions the patterns of cortical activity are (as the movement itself) only delayed by a few hundred milliseconds at most and are not otherwise abnormal. Thus, it is generally believed that whereas the execution of movements is controlled by the spinocerebellum, the lateral cerebellum plays a role in the preparation to move (Figure 39–14).

Does the Cerebellum Have a Role in Motor Learning?

In 1970, David Marr and later James Albus suggested that the cerebellum is crucial in the learning of motor skills on the basis of mathematical models they developed to simulate the operation of cerebellar circuitry. Both investigators proposed that the function of the climbing fiber input is to modify, for prolonged periods of time, the response of Purkinje neurons to mossy fiber inputs. Ito had already suggested that the cerebellum consists of an excitatory loop circuit in which specific information is processed in the deep nuclei, and that this process is regulated by changing Purkinje inhibition. In the context of Ito's ideas, Marr suggested that the climbing fiber input on specific Purkinje cells would act to increase the effectiveness of mossy fiber synapses on any one Purkinje neuron. In turn, Albus suggested that the climbing fiber decreases the effectiveness of the mossy fibers.

Many experimental studies now support the idea that cerebellar circuits are modified by experience and that these changes are important for motor learning. Much of this work has focused on the control of eye movement when the visual world is experimentally altered. A. Gonshor and G. Melvill Jones in Canada and David Robinson at Johns Hopkins studied the vestibulo-ocular reflex, which maintains the eyes on a fixed target if the head is rotated. In this reflex, motion of the head in a given direction (sensed by the vestibular labyrinth; see Chapter 43) produces eye movements in the opposite direction. When humans and animals wear prismatic lenses that reverse the left and right visual fields, the direction of the vestibulo-ocular reflex becomes reversed over a period of time. This learning is prevented by lesions of the cerebellum.

Concurrently Ito and his colleagues have shown that climbing fiber activity modifies the response of Purkinje neurons to mossy fiber inputs for a long period of time and that this modification is responsible for learned changes in the vestibulo-ocular reflex (see Chapter 43).

P. F. C. Gilbert and W. T. Thach in St. Louis have provided fascinating insights into the role of the cerebellum, and climbing fiber inputs in particular, in the learning of skilled movements. Gilbert and Thach trained monkeys to hold a handle in a fixed position and to return the handle when it was deflected by an external force. They then recorded the activity of Purkinje neurons in the arm area of the anterior lobe. As long as the signal remained constant—and thus predictable—each movement made by the monkey was accompanied by the same change in simple spikes from mossy fiber excitation, with only an occasional complex spike indicating climbing fiber activity. When the external force was abruptly changed, however, the animal at first was unable to return the handle to the original position. Gradually, however, as the monkey became familiar with the new pattern, it learned to respond correctly, and rapidly brought the handle back to the appropriate position.

This behavioral adaptation was accompanied by two concomitant changes at the cellular level (Figure 39–15).

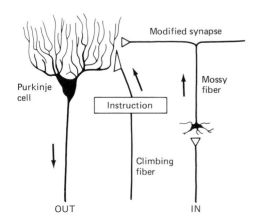

A Normal movement

Wrist position

Purkinje neuron

Flexion

Simple spike

Complex spike

B Increased load

C Adapted

D

Modified synapse

Purkinje cell

Instruction

Mossy fiber

Climbing fiber

OUT   IN

39–15 Changes in simple and complex spike activity take place as a monkey learns to move a novel load.
A. A control trial prior to load presentation produces only occasional complex spikes. **B.** The trial immediately following the application of a novel load exhibits numerous complex spikes. **C.** The trial after practice with the new load shows a return to preload level of complex spikes and a decrease in simple spikes. **D.** Simplified neural circuit showing the convergence of the two major inputs onto the cerebellum, the mossy fibers and the climbing fibers. The changes that occur in the cerebellum following the learning of a novel motor task result from the ability of the climbing fibers to depress the actions of the mossy fibers on the Purkinje cells. According to this view, the climbing fibers *instruct* or *modulate* the action of the mossy fibers.

First, when the new load was introduced, bursts of complex spikes characteristic of climbing fiber activity accompanying the response increased dramatically in frequency and then gradually decreased as performance returned to normal. The second change was that simple spikes characteristic of mossy fiber activity gradually decreased and remained diminished, even after the complex spikes again reached normal levels, until the force was again changed. This result agrees with Albus' hypothesis and suggests that, during the learning of a new task, climbing fibers of olivary neurons detect a mismatch between the intended role of the motor program and the result achieved. The message sent to the cerebellar cortex through the climbing fibers serves to depress Purkinje neuron responses to mossy fiber inputs.

Richard Thompson and his colleagues at Stanford University have shown that the role of the cerebellum in motor adaptation may be the expression of a more general role in certain forms of classical or Pavlovian conditioning. In the rabbit, lesions of the cerebellum both prevent the acquisition and selectively disrupt the retention of a conditioned eyeblink reflex. This finding suggests that the cerebellum plays a crucial role in learning this response. Thus, *the cerebellum appears to have functions that go beyond its contribution to the control of movement.* Its role in motor learning is crucial to movement because even normal motor behavior requires constant adaptation as circumstances change.

Cerebellar Diseases Can Be Localized by Their Clinical Features

Disorders of the cerebellum result in distinctive symptoms and signs that were comprehensively and elegantly described by Gordon Holmes in 1939. These symptoms often help localize a disease process to specific portions of the cerebellum. One of the features of movement disturbed by cerebellar disease is *synergy*, the coordinated contractions of agonist and antagonist muscles to produce a smooth, well-controlled movement. The normal cerebellum provides this control. *Asynergia* is the lack of synergy manifested in a combination of abnormally coordinated movements, including inaccurate range and direction *(dysmetria)*, amplitude, and force, as well as delays in the initiation of movement (Figure 39–16A and B). Instead of smooth movement, there is *decomposition of movement*, in which the various components of an act are not executed in a smooth sequence (Figure 39–16B). *Hypermetria* is an excessive extent of movement, as when a limb overshoots the desired point; and *hypometria* is a deficient extent of movement so that the limb stops before reaching the goal. *Dysdiadochokinesia* is an irregular pattern of movement seen when a patient performs rapid alternating movements, such as patting the thighs with palms up (back of the hand) followed by palms down in a rapidly alternating pattern (Figure 39–16C). The clinician commonly uses the term *limb ataxia* for asynergia. *Ataxia* of gait is characterized by a wide

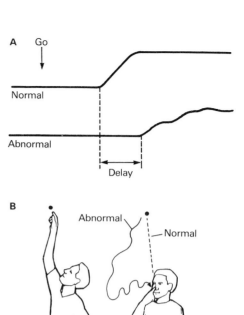

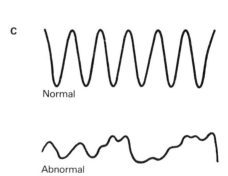

39–16 Typical defects observed in cerebellar diseases. **A.** Here, a patient with a lesion in the right cerebellar hemisphere shows a delay in the initiation of movement. The patient is told to flex both arms at the same time at a "go" signal. The left arm is flexed later than the right, as evident in the recordings of elbow position. **B.** A patient moving his arm from a raised position to touch the tip of his nose exhibits dysmetria (inaccuracy in range and direction) and decomposed (unsmooth) movement. **C.** Dysdiadochokinesia, an irregular pattern of alternating movements, can be seen in the position trace on the bottom.

stance and unsteady walking with a tendency to fall. The "drunken sailor's" gait is a characteristic ataxic gait.

Muscle tone is the degree of resistance to passive manipulation of the limbs. *Normal tone* can be defined as a slight constant tension of healthy muscles, so that when the limbs are handled or moved passively, they offer only modest resistance to displacement. *Hypotonia* is a cerebellar sign denoting diminished resistance to passive movement. *Lack of check* is the inability of a rapidly moving limb to stop rapidly and sharply; the limb overshoots and then may rebound excessively. *Tremor* is an oscillatory movement about a joint due to alternating contractions of agonists and antagonists. The characteristic tremor seen in cerebellar disease occurs with movement of a limb and is most marked at the end of the movement; this is known as *terminal tremor* and more commonly as *intention tremor*. Intention tremor is a common consequence of lesions in the superior cerebellar peduncle. *Titubation* is a truncal tremor and may be present when the patient is standing or sitting.

Disorders in the articulation of speech (dysarthria) are also seen in cerebellar disease. Word use is normal (aphasia is absent), but the mechanical aspects of speech are impaired. Speech is slurred and somewhat slow, and syllables are prolonged. This characteristic has been referred to as *scanning speech*, because of its sing-song quality. *Nystagmus*, or oscillatory movements of the eyes, is a sign of vestibular dysfunction and is often present with lesions involving the flocculonodular lobe.

It is possible to relate localization within the cerebellum to specific disorders by means of four principles:

1. Lesions in the cerebellum produce disturbances in the ipsilateral limbs.
2. Because of the somatotopic organization of the cerebellum, lesions in the lateral part of the cerebellum produce limb asynergia, whereas lesions in the vermis produce disorders of the trunk, such as titubation or gait ataxia.
3. Lesions of the deep cerebellar nuclei produce symptoms much more severe than those seen with disorders restricted to the cortex. The symptoms and signs produced by lesions involving the superior cerebellar peduncle are also intense.
4. The symptoms of cerebellar disease tend to improve gradually with time (if the underlying disease process does not itself progress), especially when the lesion occurs in childhood.

Disease of the Vestibulocerebellum Causes Disturbances of Equilibrium

Because of the connections of the *flocculonodular lobe* with the vestibular system, disease that affects this lobe causes prominent disturbances of equilibrium, including ataxic gait and a compensatory wide-based stance.

These patients lack the ability to use vestibular information to coordinate movements of either body or eyes; thus, the patient moves normally when lying down. Nystagmus is also seen. The most common lesion involving the vestibulocerebellum is the medulloblastoma, a tumor usually occurring in childhood.

Disease of the Spinocerebellum Usually Affects the Anterior Lobe and Causes Disorders of Stance and Gait

A common disease involving the *anterior lobes* (vermis and leg areas) is a restricted form of cerebellar cortical degeneration occurring in alcoholic patients. The cardi-

nal features of disease in this part of the cerebellum are involvement of the legs and impaired gait, with relative sparing of the arms. The heel–shin test, which consists of sliding the heel of one foot slowly down the shin of the opposite leg, shows abnormal movement (asynergia). Gait is wide-based and ataxic. In contrast to the ataxia of gait following lesions of the flocculonodular lobe, the ataxia that accompanies disease of the anterior lobe vermis is not improved when the patient is physically supported. Thus, it is a more general deficit than an inability to control leg movements according to gravity.

Diseases of the Cerebrocerebellum Cause Disorders of Speech and Coordinated Movement

Lesions in the *lateral parts of the posterior lobe* result in asynergia of the ipsilateral limbs. Abnormalities of the finger-to-nose and heel–shin tests, with dysmetria, dysdiadochokinesia, lack of check, and hypotonia may all be present. Bilateral lesions are common in degenerative diseases of the cerebellum. Dysarthric speech may be present with bilateral involvement.

When considering cerebellar function, it is instructive to consider a comment made by a patient of Gordon Holmes who had a lesion of his right cerebellar hemisphere: "The movements of my left arm are done subconsciously, but I have to think out each movement of the right [affected] arm. I come to a dead stop in turning and have to think before I start again." Eccles has proposed that the cerebellum spares us this mental task: a general command can be given by higher brain centers that leaves the specific details of the execution of movement to be carried out by subcortical, notably cerebellar, mechanisms.

Selected Readings

Adams, R. D., and Victor, M. 1981. Principles of Neurology, 2nd ed. New York: McGraw-Hill, pp. 60–68.

Brooks, V. B., and Thach, W. T. 1981. Cerebellar control of posture and movement. In V. B. Brooks (ed.), Handbook of Physiology, Section 1: The Nervous System, Vol. II, Motor Control. Bethesda, Md.: American Physiological Society, pp. 877–946.

Ito, M. 1984. The Cerebellum and Neural Control. New York: Raven Press.

References

Adrian, E. D. 1943. Afferent areas in the cerebellum connected with the limbs. Brain 66:289–315.

Albus, J. S. 1971. A theory of cerebellar function. Math. Biosci. 10:25–61.

Allen, G. I., and Tsukahara, N. 1974. Cerebrocerebellar communication systems. Physiol. Rev. 54:957–1006.

Arshavsky, Y. I., Berkenglit, M. B., Fukson, O. I. Gel'fand, I. M., and Orlovsky, G. N. 1972. Recordings of neurones of the dorsal spinocerebellar tract during evoked locomotion. Brain Res. 43:272–275.

Arshavsky, Y. I., Berkenglit, M. B., Fukson, O. I., Gel'fand, I. M., and Orlovsky, G. N. 1972. Origin of modulation in neurones of the ventral spinocerebellar tract during locomotion. Brain Res. 43:276–279.

Eccles, J. C., Ito, M., and Szentágothai, J. 1967. The Cerebellum as a Neuronal Machine. New York: Springer.

Gilman, S. 1969. The mechanism of cerebellar hypotonia. An experimental study in the monkey. Brain 92:621–638.

Holmes, G. 1939. The cerebellum of man. Brain 62:1–30.

Jansen, J., and Brodal, A. (eds.). 1954. Aspects of Cerebellar Anatomy. Oslo: Grundt Tanum.

McCormick, D. A., and Thompson, R. F. 1984. Cerebellum: Essential involvement in the classically conditioned eyelid response. Science 223:296–299.

Marr, D. 1969. A theory of cerebellar cortex. J. Physiol. (Lond.) 202:437–470.

Meyer-Lohmann, J., Hore, J., and Brooks, V. B. 1977. Cerebellar participation in generation of prompt arm movements. J. Neurophysiol. 40:1038–1050.

Nieuwenhuys, R., Voogd, J., and van Huijzen, Chr. 1981. The Human Central Nervous System: A Synopsis and Atlas, 2nd rev. ed. Berlin: Springer.

Oscarsson, O. 1973. Functional organization of spinocerebellar paths. In A. Iggo (ed.), Handbook of Sensory Physiology, Vol. 2: The Somatosensory System. New York: Springer, pp. 339–380.

Robinson, D. A. 1976. Adaptive gain control of vestibuloocular reflex by the cerebellum. J. Neurophysiol. 39:954–969.

Shambes, G. M., Gibson, J. M., and Welker, W. 1978. Fractured somatotopy in granule cell tactile areas of rat cerebellar hemispheres revealed by micromapping. Brain Behav. Evol. 15:94–140.

Snider, R. S., and Stowell, A. 1944. Receiving areas of the tactile, auditory, and visual systems in the cerebellum. J. Neurophysiol. 7:331–357.

Soechting, J. F., Ranish, N. A., Palminteri, R., and Terzuolo, C. A. 1976. Changes in a motor pattern following cerebellar and olivary lesions in the squirrel monkey. Brain Res. 105:21–44.

Thach, W. T. 1978. Correlation of neural discharge with pattern and force of muscular activity, joint position, and direction of intended next movement in motor cortex and cerebellum. J. Neurophysiol. 41:654–676.

Lucien Côté and Michael D. Crutcher

Motor Functions of the Basal Ganglia and Diseases of Transmitter Metabolism

40

The basal ganglia were once believed to be the major components of the *extrapyramidal motor system*, which was thought to control movement in parallel with and independently of the *pyramidal motor system*. The division of the motor systems into pyramidal and extrapyramidal was used clinically to distinguish between two motor syndromes: one characterized by spasticity and paralysis, the other by involuntary movements, rigidity, and immobility without paralysis. As we have seen in the preceding chapters, there are several reasons why this simple dichotomy is not a satisfactory description of the motor systems. First, in addition to the basal ganglia and pyramidal motor system, several other brain structures are now known to mediate voluntary movement: the red nucleus, the motor nuclei of the brain stem, and the cerebellum. Second, the extrapyramidal system (the basal ganglia) and pyramidal system are not independent; rather, they are interconnected extensively and cooperate in the control of movement. Indeed, the motor actions of the basal ganglia are mediated in part by the pyramidal system. Third, the concept of an extrapyramidal system can prove misleading clinically. The category of "extrapyramidal diseases" includes different syndromes of diverse etiologies, often without evidence of pathology in the basal ganglia, the brain stem, or the cerebellum. For these reasons, the concept of the extrapyramidal motor system, while historically important, is no longer considered to be useful.

The main components of the *basal ganglia* are three large subcortical nuclei: the *caudate*, the *putamen*, and the *globus pallidus* (pallidum). They, in turn, are interconnected with and functionally related to two other subcortical nuclei: the *subthalamic nucleus* and the *substantia nigra*. These five nuclei participate in the control of movement together with the cerebellum, the corticospinal system, and the brain stem motor nuclei. Unlike most other components of the motor systems, however, the basal ganglia do not have direct afferent or efferent connections with the spinal cord; instead, their primary input is from widespread areas of the neocortex and their output is directed back to the prefrontal and premotor cortices of the frontal lobes by way of the thalamus. The motor functions of the basal ganglia are therefore mediated by the frontal cortex.

The insight that the basal ganglia are involved in the control of movement initially came from clinical observations. Postmortem examination revealed pathological changes in the basal ganglia in patients who died with Parkinson's disease, Huntington's disease, and hemiballismus. These diseases produce three characteristic types of motor disturbances: (1) involuntary movements, including tremor; (2) poverty and slowness of movement without paralysis; and (3) changes in posture and muscle tone.

An important feature of several of these diseases is that they involve deficiencies in chemical transmitters. In fact, Parkinson's disease was the first disease of the central nervous system in which a defect in transmitter metabolism was shown to have a causal role. Study of diseased basal ganglia has therefore been instructive in two ways: it has provided important basic and clinical information about the motor functions of the basal ganglia, and it has suggested paradigms for studying the relationship of transmitters to disorders of mood and of thought (see Chapters 53 and 54).

Nuclei of the Basal Ganglia

The caudate nucleus and putamen develop from the same telencephalic structure. As a result, these two nuclei are composed of identical cell types and are fused anteriorly. Together, they are referred to as the *striatum*, and they serve as the input component of the basal ganglia. The globus pallidus derives from the diencephalon.[1] It has two segments, the internal and the external. The internal segment of the globus pallidus is a major output nucleus of the basal ganglia. The globus pallidus lies medial to the putamen and lateral to the internal capsule (Figure 40–1). Together, the putamen and globus pallidus form a lens-shaped structure that is sometimes referred to as the lenticular nucleus. As we saw in Chapter 21, the caudate nucleus is C-shaped and lies lateral to the lateral ventricle and medial to the internal capsule.

---

[1]Since the caudate and putamen are phylogenetically the most recent nuclei of the basal ganglia, they have been collectively called the *neostriatum*. The terms neostriatum and striatum are used synonymously. The globus pallidus, phylogenetically older, is sometimes referred to as the *paleostriatum*. The term *corpus striatum* includes both neostriatum and paleostriatum. The amygdaloid nucleus, which is embryologically related to the basal ganglia but belongs functionally to the limbic system, is older than the globus pallidus and is called the *archistriatum*.

Because the subthalamic nucleus and the substantia nigra are closely linked to these nuclei both anatomically and functionally, they are often considered to be part of the basal ganglia. The subthalamic nucleus (of Luys) lies in the basal portion of the diencephalon, at the junction with the mesencephalon (Figure 40–1). The substantia nigra is the largest nuclear mass of the mesencephalon. It has two zones: a ventral pale zone *(pars reticulata)* that resembles the globus pallidus cytologically; and a dorsal, darkly pigmented zone *(pars compacta)* whose nerve cell bodies contain *neuromelanin* with its end-stage lysosomes. This dark pigment, which appears to be a polymer of dopamine or its metabolites, gives the substantia nigra its name because this part of the brain appears black in cut sections. The neurons of the pars compacta use dopamine as a neurotransmitter, and the degree of their pigmentation is correlated with the concentration of dopamine they contain, but the function of the pigment is uncertain.

Basal Ganglia Receive Input from the Cortex, Thalamus, and Substantia Nigra and Project Mainly Back to the Cortex via the Thalamus

The basal ganglia have separate input and output components. All of the afferent inputs to the basal ganglia terminate in the striatum. The internal segment of the globus pallidus and the substantia nigra (pars reticulata) generate all of its major efferent systems (Figure 40–2).

Afferent Connections

The striatum receives afferent input from three major sources: the cerebral cortex, the intralaminar nuclei of the thalamus, and the substantia nigra (Figure 40–2A).

The most important input is from the cortex by means of the *corticostriate projection*. The entire cerebral cortex, including the motor, the sensory, and the association cortices, projects to the striatum. This projection is topographically organized: specific areas of the neocortex project to different parts of the striatum. In general, the rostral areas of the cortex project to the rostral striatum and more posterior cortical areas project to progressively more posterior parts of the striatum. However, there is considerable overlap in the terminations of corticostriatal projections that originate from functionally related and interconnected cortical areas, suggesting that the striatum integrates related cortical inputs. The extensive input from diverse regions of the cortex also suggests that the basal ganglia are involved in other functions besides motor control.

A second input to the striatum is the projection from the intralaminar nuclei of the thalamus. This projection arises mainly from the centromedian nucleus and terminates in the putamen. Because the centromedian nucleus receives input from the motor cortex, this pathway provides an additional means by which the motor cortex can influence the basal ganglia. A third major input to the

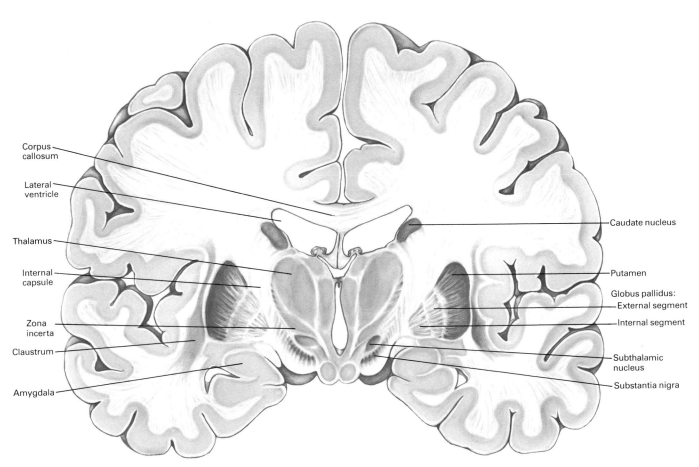

40–1 This coronal section shows the basal ganglia in relation to surrounding structures. (Adapted from Nieuwenhuys, Voogd, and van Huijzen, 1981.)

striatum is the dopaminergic projection from the pars compacta of the substantia nigra. This important projection to the striatum is also topographically organized.

Internuclear Connections

Cells in both the caudate and the putamen project to both segments of the globus pallidus and to the pars reticulata of the substantia nigra (Figure 40–2B). These striatal efferent projections are topographically organized so that each part of the striatum projects to circumscribed parts of the globus pallidus and substantia nigra. Because the corticostriatal pathway and the striatopallidal and striatonigral pathways are topographically organized, specific parts of the cortex act on specific parts of the globus pallidus and substantia nigra via the striatum.

The globus pallidus and substantia nigra are intimately connected to the subthalamic nucleus. The entire output of the external segment of the globus pallidus is directed to the subthalamic nucleus, which in turn has topographic projections to both segments of the globus pallidus and to the substantia nigra pars reticulata. The subthalamic nucleus also receives direct, topographically

organized inputs from the motor and premotor cortices. Thus, the motor cortex has another means for modulating the output of the basal ganglia through the subthalamic nucleus.

Efferent Connections

The internal segment of the globus pallidus and the pars reticulata of the substantia nigra give rise to the major efferents from the basal ganglia, which project to parts of the *ventral lateral* and the *ventral anterior thalamic nuclei*. The internal segment of the globus pallidus has an additional projection to the centromedian nucleus of the thalamus. The projections to the thalamus from the globus pallidus are conveyed by two fiber bundles, the *ansa lenticularis* and the *lenticular fasciculus;* these two bundles later fuse and reach the thalamus in the *thalamic fasciculus*. The portions of the ventral anterior and ventral lateral nuclei of the thalamus that receive input from the basal ganglia project to the prefrontal and premotor cortices. This projection is by far the major outflow of the basal ganglia. Through it the basal ganglia can influence other descending systems such as the corticospinal and the corticobulbar systems. In addition to these major efferent projections, projections have recently been described from the globus pallidus to the brain stem and the habenula and from the pars reticulata of the substantia nigra to the superior colliculus.

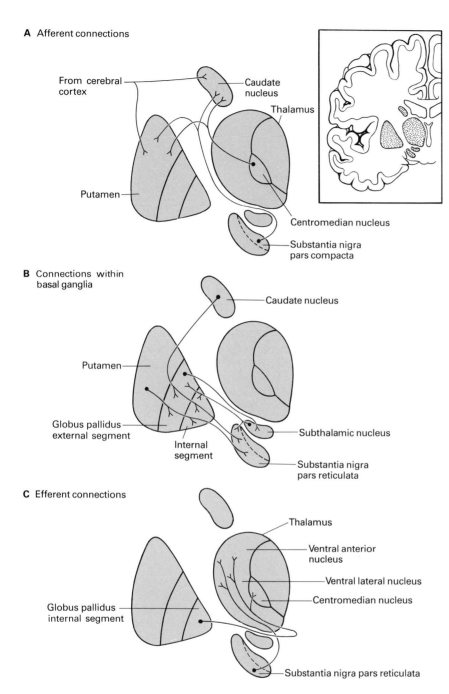

A Afferent connections

From cerebral cortex

Caudate nucleus

Thalamus

Putamen

Centromedian nucleus

Substantia nigra pars compacta

B Connections within basal ganglia

Caudate nucleus

Putamen

Globus pallidus external segment

Internal segment

Subthalamic nucleus

Substantia nigra pars reticulata

C Efferent connections

Thalamus

Ventral anterior nucleus

Ventral lateral nucleus

Centromedian nucleus

Globus pallidus internal segment

Substantia nigra pars reticulata

40–2 Major anatomical connections of the basal ganglia. **A.** The caudate nucleus and putamen receive all afferent input. **B.** The internuclear connections include topographically organized connections between all of the nuclei of the basal ganglia. **C.** The principal target of efferent connections from the basal ganglia is the thalamus.

The complex connections of the basal ganglia can be viewed simply as four interconnected loops (Figure 40–3). The first loop, and the most important, runs from the neocortex to the basal ganglia and thalamus and then back to the frontal neocortex. The second loop runs from the external segment of the globus pallidus to the sub-thalamic nucleus and back to both segments of the globus pallidus. The third loop runs from the striatum to the substantia nigra and then back to the striatum. The fourth loop runs from the striatum through the globus pallidus and centromedian nucleus of the thalamus back to the striatum.

The basal ganglia and the cerebellum constitute major subcortical reentrant loops of the motor system (Figure 40–4): they both receive inputs from the cerebral cortex and both project back to the cortex via the thalamus. However, there are important differences between the connections of the basal ganglia and cerebellum. First, the basal ganglia receive inputs from the entire cerebral cortex, whereas most of the cortical inputs to the cerebellum arise from those areas of the cortex most closely related to sensorimotor functions. Second, a major output of the cerebellum is back to the motor cortex (area 4) by means of the thalamus, whereas the basal ganglia project via the thalamus to the prefrontal and premotor cortices, not to the motor cortex. Finally, unlike the basal ganglia, the cerebellum receives somatic sensory information directly from the spinal cord and has impor-

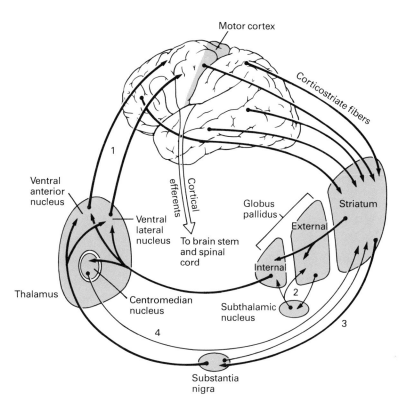

40–3 The anatomical connections of the basal ganglia comprise four interconnected loops (see text). Note the major afferent and efferent connections with the neocortex. (Adapted from DeLong, 1974.)

40–4 The basal ganglia and cerebellum both participate in major subcortical reentrant loops, but there are differences in their anatomical connections that suggest their differing functions. **A.** Connections of the basal ganglia. **B.** Cerebellar connections.

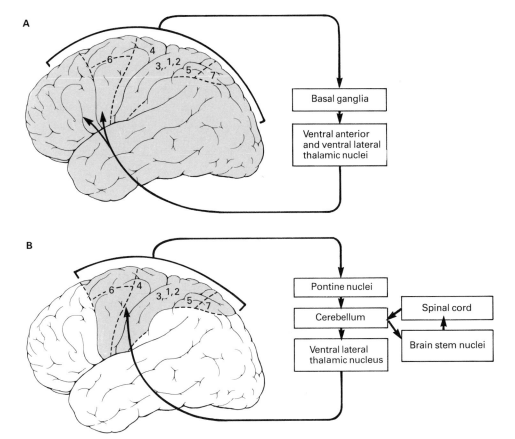

tant projections to brain stem nuclei that generate descending motor projections. These differences suggest that the cerebellum is more directly involved than the basal ganglia in the on-line control of movement, movement that requires feedback from the periphery for rapid correction of errors. In contrast, the basal ganglia seem to be involved in more complex aspects of motor control than is the cerebellum. Indeed, there is now evidence that the basal ganglia participate in cognitive functions as well (see below).

Modular and Somatotopic Organization

For many years the striatum was considered to be a relatively homogeneous structure. However, with the application of new anatomical and physiological techniques it has become apparent that the striatum is divided into anatomically and functionally distinct modules similar to those we previously encountered in the cerebral cortex. Tracer techniques have shown that the corticostriate and thalamostriate projections end in discontinuous patches of terminals in the striatum. During early stages of development, the dopaminergic nigrostriatal projection is also patchy. Recently, areas 200–600 μm in diameter containing clusters of cells that share common neurotransmitters have also been described.

Electrophysiological studies of the activity of single cells during movement have shown that the striatum is also organized into clusters of neurons with similar functional properties. For example, all of the cells in a given cluster might be active only during movements of the elbow, and microstimulation at that site would result in elbow movement. These clusters probably represent the basic functional units of the striatum, much like the functional columns of the neocortex. In addition to providing information about the cellular organization of the basal ganglia, these single-cell recordings have revealed a somatotopic organization. Neurons related to movements of a single body part are segregated from neurons related to other body parts. This somatotopic organization of the basal ganglia reflects the topographic nature of their afferent and efferent connections. For example, the arm areas of the motor and sensory cortices project to the arm area of the putamen, which then projects to the arm area of both segments of the globus pallidus. Similarly, the arm area of the subthalamic nucleus is interconnected with the arm areas of the globus pallidus and receives an additional input from the arm area of the motor cortex. These precise topographic interconnections provide the anatomical basis for processing information about a single body part in discrete areas of each nucleus of the basal ganglia.

Basal Ganglia May Contribute to Cognition

In addition to the segregation of neurons related to movement of different body parts, the basal ganglia also show a segregation of motor from nonmotor functions. Parts of these nuclei participate in cognitive aspects of behavior, a role consistent with the finding that the striatum receives inputs from the entire neocortex. Whereas the motor functions of the basal ganglia are carried out predominantly by the putamen, the cognitive functions are thought to be carried out by the caudate nucleus. This general pattern of segregation of functions is also seen within the caudate nucleus, where different cognitive functions are subserved by different regions. For example, in primates, circumscribed bilateral lesions in the dorsolateral prefrontal neocortex produce deficits in performance of delayed alternation tasks, tasks thought to measure the capability for spatial memory. Lesions in the orbitofrontal neocortex result in impaired performance in object reversal tasks.[2] These two areas of neocortex have distinct and separate projections to the head of the caudate nucleus. Similarly, bilateral lesions in the caudate restricted to either of these projection areas cause the expected behavioral deficit. The segregation of motor functions of the basal ganglia in the putamen and of cognitive functions in the caudate is maintained in all of the sequential projections through the globus pallidus and thalamus to the cortex. The output of the putamen is thought to be directed primarily to the premotor cortex and supplementary motor area, and the output of the caudate to the prefrontal cortex.

Diseases of the Basal Ganglia Cause Characteristic Symptoms

Diseases of the basal ganglia characteristically produce involuntary movements (dyskinesias), poverty and slowness of movement, and disorders of muscle tone and postural reflexes. These abnormal movements include the following: *tremor* (rhythmic, involuntary, oscillatory movements of a body part); *athetosis* (slow, writhing movements of the fingers and hands, and sometimes of the toes and feet, which can also involve the proximal part of the limb); *chorea* (rapid, flick-like movements of the limbs and facial muscles that may resemble normal restlessness or fidgeting); and *ballism* (violent, flailing movements primarily involving proximal parts of the limb).

As we saw in Chapter 33, Hughlings Jackson first pointed out that all motor disorders fall into two classes of deficits: *primary functional deficits* (negative signs), which can be attributed to the loss of function subserved by specific neurons; and *secondary deficits* (positive signs or *release phenomena*), which may be caused by the malfunction of neurons or the emergence of an abnormal pattern of action in neurons when part of their controlling input (usually their inhibitory input) is destroyed or dys-

---

[2]In delayed alternation tasks the monkey is required to alternate responses on successive trials to two identical foodwells placed on the right or left. Trials are separated by a delay, so the monkey must remember which choice he made on the preceding trial. In object reversal tasks the monkey must discriminate between two different objects and respond only to one of the objects. After a block of trials, the reward contingencies are reversed.

Table 40–1. Disorders of the Basal Ganglia

Disorder	Pathophysiology	Chemical changes	Clinical manifestations	Treatment
Parkinson's disease	Degeneration of the nigrostriatal pathway, raphe nuclei, locus ceruleus, and motor nucleus of vagus	Reduction in dopamine, serotonin, and norepinephrine	Slowly progressive disease, third most common neurological disease (affects 500,000 Americans); about 15% of patients have a first degree relative with the disease; mean age of onset is 58 years; findings are tremor at rest (3–6 beats/sec), cogwheel rigidity, bradykinesia, and postural reflex impairment	L-DOPA with or without peripheral DOPA decarboxylase inhibitor Anticholinergic agents: trihexyphenidyl (Artane) or benztropine (Cogentin), and others
Huntington's disease	Degeneration of intrastriatal and cortical cholinergic neurons and GABA-ergic neurons	Reduction in choline acetyltransferase and glutamic acid decarboxylase activities and GABA	Progressive disease with associated dementia and death within 15–20 years; incidence about 10,000 cases in the United States; autosomal dominant; onset at any age, but usually in adulthood; findings are chorea, decreased tone (may occur), and dementia	No specific therapy; dopamine antagonists (phenothiazines, butyrophenones) useful to control chorea; so far, GABA agonists not effective
Ballism	Damage to one subthalamic nucleus, often due to acute vascular accident	No data	Most severe form of involuntary movement disorder known; tends to clear up slowly	Neuroleptics (butyrophenones)
Tardive dyskinesia	Alteration in dopaminergic receptors causing hypersensitivity to dopamine and its agonists	Normal cerebrospinal fluid and homovanillic acid (acid metabolite of dopamine) levels	Iatrogenic disorder due to long-term treatment with phenothiazines or butyrophenones; abnormal involuntary movements, especially of the face and tongue; usually temporary but can be permanent	Stop offending drug; reserpine

functional because of disease. The abnormal movements that occur in basal ganglia disease are thought to fall into the second category. These movements apparently result from abnormal activity in neurons of the basal ganglia caused by removal of inhibitory influences on them. Indeed, some of the symptoms of the various forms of movement disorders have been alleviated by surgically lesioning the globus pallidus or the ventral anterior and ventral lateral nuclei of the thalamus and thereby abolishing the abnormal neural activity. Some of the major disorders of movement are summarized in Table 40–1.

Parkinson's Disease

In 1817 James Parkinson, a physician working in London, described in the following terms the motor disorder that now bears his name: "involuntary tremulous motion, with lessened muscular power, in parts not in action and even when supported; with a propensity to bend the trunk forwards, and to pass from a walking to a running pace, the senses and intellects being uninjured."

Parkinson's disease (paralysis agitans), one of the best characterized diseases of the basal ganglia, is accompanied by (1) a rhythmic tremor at rest, (2) a unique kind of increased muscle tone or rigidity that often has a cogwheellike characteristic, and (3) a slowness in the initiation of movement (akinesia) as well as in the execution of movement (bradykinesia). This slowness is often evident in the way the patient gets up from a bed or chair and in a shuffling gait. The presumptive site of the lesion in Parkinson's disease is the dopaminergic projection from the substantia nigra to the striatum.

The tremor and rigidity of Parkinson's disease have been attributed to a loss of an inhibitory influence within the basal ganglia, leading to an abnormal outflow from the internal segment of the globus pallidus to the ventral anterior and ventral lateral nuclei of the thalamus, and finally to the cortex. Surgical interruption of the outflow from the basal ganglia, either in the globus pallidus or in the ventral lateral nucleus of the thalamus, decreases the abnormal neural activity and thus alleviates the positive symptoms of tremor and rigidity. Unfortunately, the slowness in the initiation and execution of movement does not change, perhaps because they are primary deficit symptoms. Although surgical intervention is sometimes remarkably successful in alleviating tremor and rigidity, many patients do not improve significantly in their daily activities because the bradykinesia and impaired postural reflexes remain unchanged and are so disabling. Moreover, tremor and rigidity often recur within 1–3 years after surgery. Because of the success of drug therapy (see below), surgery for Parkinson's disease is now rarely performed.

Several major breakthroughs in our understanding of diseases of the basal ganglia were made in the late 1950s. Arvid Carlsson and, independently, two Swedish pharmacologists, A. Bertler and E. Rosengren, observed that dopamine constitutes about one-half of the catecholamine in the brain, 80% of which is localized in the basal ganglia (an area that makes up less than 0.5% of the total weight of the brain). Soon afterward, Oleh Hornykiewicz, studying human brains obtained at postmortem examination at the University of Vienna, found that some brains had low amounts of dopamine, norepinephrine, and serotonin. In reviewing the medical histories of these patients, Hornykiewicz discovered that all of the patients with low brain levels of biogenic amines had Parkinson's disease at the time of death. He next observed that, of the three biogenic amines, dopamine was most drastically reduced. Parkinson's disease therefore became the first documented example of a disease of the brain consistently correlated with a deficiency in a specific neurotransmitter. This discovery has provided the impetus for a thorough search for neurotransmitter changes in other disorders of the brain, including depression, schizophrenia, and dementia.

Patients with Parkinson's disease also show loss of nerve cells and depigmentation in the pigmented nuclei of the brain stem—the substantia nigra and the locus ceruleus. The severity of changes in the substantia nigra parallels the reduction of dopamine in the striatum. Because the pars compacta of the substantia nigra contains most of the dopaminergic nerve cell bodies in the brain, these observations first suggested that the nigrostriatal dopaminergic pathway is involved in Parkinson's disease. Later, iontophoretic application of dopamine onto neurons of the basal ganglia suggested that the predominant effect of dopamine on striatal neurons is inhibition. At that time it was hypothesized that the reduction in the release of the inhibitory transmitter dopamine in the striatum could lead to disinhibition and abnormal discharge of the cells in the striatum and in the globus pallidus (Figure 40-5). This could explain the positive symptoms of Parkinson's disease. However, at present, there is still debate about whether dopamine is inhibitory or excitatory. If dopamine is excitatory, as some believe, then the loss of this excitatory input into the striatum

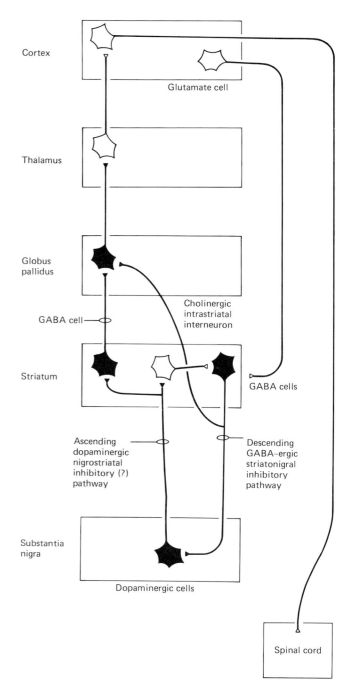

40–5 Interaction of neurons that use GABA, acetylcholine, and dopamine in the striatum and substantia nigra. There is still debate about whether the nigrostriatal projection is excitatory or inhibitory. (**Black** neurons are inhibitory; **white** neurons are excitatory.)

could result in the primary deficits of akinesia and bradykinesia. In either case, some of the symptoms of Parkinson's disease can be explained by the loss of dopamine in nigrostriatal neurons.

With these ideas in mind, Walther Birkmayer and Hornykiewicz reasoned that patients with Parkinson's disease might improve if the amount of dopamine in the brain could be restored to normal. They therefore gave 3,4-dihydroxyphenylalanine (DOPA) intravenously to patients with Parkinson's disease. This amino acid is a precursor of dopamine but, unlike dopamine, it crosses the blood–brain barrier (which normally excludes many substances). Birkmayer and Hornykiewicz observed a remarkable, albeit brief, remission in their patients' symptoms and thus provided a dramatic new approach to the treatment of Parkinson's disease.

Although L-DOPA therapy has been hailed as the most significant breakthrough in the treatment of Parkinson's disease, it is not the panacea hoped for when it was first introduced. At that time, cautious optimism was expressed that L-DOPA might not only ameliorate the symptoms of Parkinson's disease, but also arrest the disease and even reverse some of the degenerative changes seen in the substantia nigra. Experience gained in the past few years with L-DOPA therapy, however, has shown that this does not happen: L-DOPA does not alter the course of the disease; it only controls some of the symptoms.

It is still unclear how L-DOPA ameliorates the symptoms of Parkinson's disease. Dopamine normally is synthesized in the striatum, in the nerve endings of dopaminergic neurons whose cell bodies lie in the substantia nigra; at these nerve endings the transmitter is taken up into vesicles and released in the synaptic cleft when the cell fires. In Parkinson's disease, as many as 90% of the dopaminergic neurons have degenerated or are in the process of doing so. What, then, is the fate of L-DOPA in patients with Parkinson's disease? Presumably the L-DOPA is taken up and converted into dopamine (see Chapter 13) by the remaining dopaminergic nerve cells. The few remaining healthy dopaminergic neurons and those that have partially degenerated may be able to compensate by carrying out the entire function of the nigrostriatal system once the rate-limiting enzyme for the synthesis of dopamine (tyrosine hydroxylase) is bypassed with the large amounts of L-DOPA. Another possibility is that DOPA decarboxylase, which is not specific to dopaminergic neurons and which is abundant and ubiquitous in the brain, can synthesize dopamine from the orally administered L-DOPA in nondopaminergic cells—for example, in serotonergic neurons, in other neurons, and perhaps even in glial cells. This newly formed dopamine might then be released or secreted in amounts large enough to act on appropriate target cells.

Although the primary pathology in Parkinson's disease is the degeneration of the dopaminergic projection to the striatum, not all the symptoms of these patients are exclusively attributable to the loss of nigrostriatal dopamine. For example, there are losses of noradrenergic neurons in the locus ceruleus and serotonergic neurons in the raphe nuclei. Both of these areas have very widespread projections throughout the brain, including the cerebellum and neocortex. In addition to the dopaminergic projection to the striatum, there are also dopaminergic projections to parts of the limbic system (nucleus accumbens, olfactory tubercle, and amygdala) and the

frontal neocortex. There is some experimental evidence that the akinesia seen in parkinsonian patients may be due partly to dopamine depletion in the nucleus accumbens. Some of the symptoms of patients with Parkinson's disease may also be due to loss of dopamine from nerve endings in the cortex. In primates, regional depletion of dopamine in the prefrontal cortex leads to specific cognitive deficits. Because of the degenerative changes in these aminergic systems with widespread projections, it is difficult to be certain of the specific loci and synaptic mechanisms that account for all of the parkinsonian symptoms in patients.

Huntington's Disease and the Dopaminergic–Cholinergic–GABA-ergic Loop

In 1872 George Huntington, a graduate of the College of Physicians and Surgeons of Columbia University, described a disease that he, his father, and his grandfather had observed during several generations of practice. The disease occurred in a cluster of families and was characterized by four features: (1) heritability, (2) chorea, (3) dementia, and (4) death after 15 or 20 years. This disease, later called Huntington's disease, has now been shown to affect men and women with equal frequency, about 5 per 100,000 population. In most cases the onset of the disease occurs in the fourth to fifth decade of life. Thus, the disease strikes after most individuals have married and had children. Each child of an affected parent has a 50% chance of inheriting the disease. One of the tragic aspects of the disease is that no test has been available that makes the diagnosis before the symptoms become apparent. As a result, the children of an affected individual live for decades in the fear that they, too, have inherited the gene for the disease.

The first signs of the disorder are subtle and may consist of absentmindedness, irritability, and depression, accompanied by fidgeting, clumsiness, or sudden falls. Uncontrolled (choreiform) movements, a prominent feature of the disease, gradually increase, until the patient becomes confined to bed or to a wheelchair. Speech is at first slurred, then incomprehensible, and finally it ceases altogether as facial expressions become distorted and grotesque. Mental functions undergo similar deterioration, and eventually the ability to reason disappears. There is no treatment available to slow the course of the disease, much less to cure it. Once the disease has begun its inexorable course, the afflicted person faces years of gradually decreasing capacity, followed by total disability and certain death.

Huntington's disease results from the loss of specific sets of cholinergic neurons and neurons that synthesize gamma-aminobutyric acid (GABA-ergic neurons) in the striatum (Figure 40–5). The nerve cell death (up to 90%) in these nuclear groups is thought to cause the choreic movements. The impaired cognitive functions and eventual dementia may be due to the concomitant loss of cortical neurons. It has recently become possible to demonstrate the selective loss of neurons in Huntington's

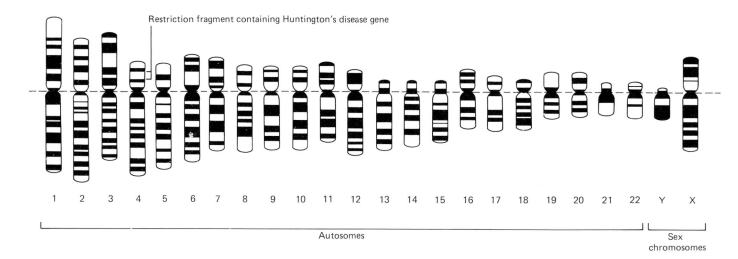

Restriction fragment containing Huntington's disease gene

1 2 3 4 5 6 7 8 9 10 11 12 13 14 15 16 17 18 19 20 21 22 Y X

Autosomes

Sex chromosomes

40–6 The general location of the Huntington's disease gene on the short arm of chromosome 4 is indicated on this map of human chromosomes at metaphase. (Adapted from Watson, Tooze, and Kurtz, 1983.)

disease while individuals are still alive by the use of computerized tomography, positron emission tomography, and magnetic resonance imaging.

Normally a balance is maintained among the activities of three biochemically distinct but functionally interrelated systems: (1) the nigrostriatal dopaminergic system; (2) the intrastriatal cholinergic neurons; and (3) the GABA-ergic system, which projects from the striatum to the globus pallidus and substantia nigra (Figure 40–5). As we have seen in Parkinson's disease, reduction of the dopaminergic system causes an imbalance in the output of the globus pallidus to the thalamus, leading to tremor, rigidity, and bradykinesia. In Huntington's disease, on the other hand, there is profound destruction of small intrastriatal cholinergic neurons and of striatopallidal and striatonigral GABA-ergic neurons. It is postulated that dopaminergic cells in the substantia nigra then become disinhibited because their GABA-mediated inhibition is missing. If dopamine is excitatory to striatal neurons, then this disinhibition would produce excessive excitation of the remaining striatal neurons, with resulting abnormal pallidal output to the thalamus. This could produce the choreic movements of Huntington's disease.

In line with the pathological changes, there is a marked decrease in the striatum of both choline acetyltransferase, the enzyme required for the formation of acetylcholine, and glutamic acid decarboxylase, the biosynthetic enzyme required for GABA. These biochemical findings are consistent with the clinical observation that if a patient with Huntington's disease is given L-DOPA, the choreic movements are substantially worsened. Similarly, a parkinsonian patient given too much L-DOPA develops involuntary movements such as chorea, athetosis, and dystonia. Thus, an imbalance anywhere in the dopaminergic–cholinergic–GABA-ergic loop can cause involuntary movements. This is a fundamental principle

in the pharmacology of the brain. As defects in one transmitter have widespread consequences that are both direct and indirect, so may therapeutic intervention have serious secondary consequences. Sometimes they are as serious as the disease itself!

The Genetic Marker for Huntington's Disease

The genetic transmission of Huntington's disease became evident when it was discovered that practically all patients with this disease who lived on the East Coast of the United States were descendants of two ancestors who were born in Suffolk, England, and who emigrated to Salem, Massachusetts, in 1630. In all likelihood, several of the unfortunate and apparently deranged individuals in Salem who were executed for being witches were actually exhibiting symptoms of Huntington's disease. The familial pattern is impressive; traced through 12 generations (over 300 years), the disease was expressed in each generation.

Huntington's disease is inherited as an autosomal dominant disorder. The normal human complement of chromosomes consists of 22 pairs of autosomes (nonsex chromosomes) and one pair of sex chromosomes (Figure 40–6). Using recombinant DNA procedures, James Gusella and his colleagues at Massachusetts General Hospital have been able to narrow the locus of the gene responsible for Huntington's disease to a portion of the short arm of chromosome 4 and to detect a marker linked with this gene.

How was this accomplished? By definition, a genetic defect such as that found in Huntington's disease must reflect an alteration in the nucleotide sequence of DNA. The techniques of molecular genetics now allow the comparison of DNA sequences between the DNA of normal people and of those who have genetic diseases. Where the defective gene product is known, as, for example, in the case of the defective hemoglobin molecule of sickle cell anemia, the mutation can be identified directly by determining how the abnormal DNA sequence of the gene differs from normal (wild type).

However, in Huntington's disease, the abnormal gene product and the gene itself have not yet been identified. Therefore, the less direct approach was attempted of finding a marker in the DNA so close to the gene that it is almost always inherited with it. If two genes are located very near one another, they are likely to be inherited together. For example, if one gene produces a disease and a nearby gene codes for a phenotypic marker that is readily recognized (such as hair or eye color), or it codes for a readily detectable gene product (such as a protein present in the blood), it might be possible to establish that people who express the marker also express the disease—even though the marker may have nothing to do with the disease. These markers represent *genetic polymorphisms:* the trait or gene product, such as eye color, represents the expression of a particular genetic locus, and both trait and locus vary in the normal population. Genetic markers have proved very useful in the analysis of some neurological diseases, such as myotonic muscular dystrophy; a blood group protein allowed this disease to be localized to chromosome 19. This approach did not work for Huntington's disease, however, because no known protein markers are near the gene.

With recombinant DNA technology, it has been possible to develop a novel approach to genetic markers based on the finding that there are variations in DNA sequences that are inherited, even though they may not be expressed as proteins. These presumably neutral variations in the DNA are called *DNA polymorphisms* or *restriction fragment length polymorphisms.* Bacterial restriction enzymes cut DNA only at a specific nucleotide sequence. Restriction fragment length polymorphisms are the result of differences in DNA sequence that are detected because they produce or eliminate a cutting site for a particular restriction enzyme. Consequently, different lengths are produced by a given restriction enzyme from the two alleles on the paired chromosomes. Chromosomal DNA can be "fingerprinted." The fragments that differ in length can be separated by electrophoresis in agarose gel and distinguished by specific DNA probes in a Southern hybridization (Figure 40–7). When such a polymorphic region of the DNA is closely linked to a particular gene, the inheritance of the gene can be traced by following the inheritance of a particular pattern of restriction fragments (Figure 40–8). The method can be applied to the analysis of polymorphisms in any population of subjects; like fingerprints, which are also genetic polymorphisms, the polymorphism need not be related to the genetic defect with which it happens to be linked.

Gusella and his colleagues used this method to search for a correlation between a particular pattern of restriction enzyme polymorphism and the Huntington's disease gene. To follow the inheritance of the gene and correlate it with the restriction fragment marker, they relied on a previously identified population in Venezuela that carries the gene for Huntington's disease. This population was descended from a Venezuelan woman who lived near Lake Maracaibo at the beginning of the nineteenth century. The woman developed Huntington's disease, most

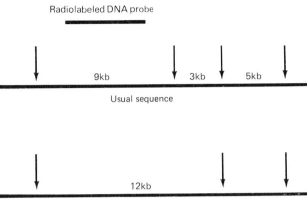

40–7 A hypothetical restriction fragment length polymorphism. Two alleles of an arbitrary genetic marker are shown. **Arrows** indicate the cleavage recognition sites in the DNA sequence for a particular restriction endonuclease. The normal sequence contains four recognition sites for this enzyme. In the variant DNA sequence, a change has occurred in one segment that alters one recognition site and reduces the number of recognition sites in this stretch to three. As illustrated, the sets of fragments resulting from the digestion of the two segments with the restriction enzyme will therefore differ significantly in size. To detect the size differences, the DNA fragments are first separated according to size by means of electrophoresis through gel slabs. Next, using a procedure developed by E. M. Southern, the DNA fragments are denatured and fixed on the gel and then transferred to nitrocellulose paper, where they are fixed in place. On the nitrocellulose paper the fragments are exposed to a radiolabeled DNA probe made from a clone of the critical region. This probe will then hybridize to the critical fragments and, because the labeled fragments from the two sources differ in size, they can be distinguished by their different positions on the gel. (Adapted from Houseman and Gusella, 1982.)

40–8 The inheritance of the gene responsible for Huntington's disease can be traced by following the inheritance of restriction fragment polymorphisms for chromosome 4.

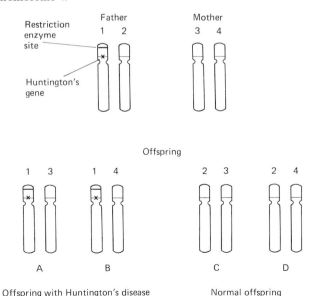

Offspring with Huntington's disease   Normal offspring

likely because her father, a sailor from Europe, carried the gene. Most of the woman's offspring have stayed near Lake Maracaibo, and she now has more than 3000 living descendants; 100 of them have Huntington's disease. In addition, there are 1100 children, with a 25%–50% chance of inheriting the disease. Gusella and his colleagues examined this population and found a consistent correlation between Huntington's disease and a restriction enzyme DNA fragment cut on the short arm of chromosome 4. By this means the Huntington's disease gene has now been localized to an area of the chromosome several million base pairs in length, an area large enough to hold about 50 genes.

Although the exact locus of the Huntington's disease gene is not known, even the degree of localization that has been obtained will lead to two important consequences. First, it will allow the disease to be diagnosed presymptomatically or even prenatally. Second, this localization should allow the defective gene to be cloned, a prerequisite for identifying the gene product and ultimately determining how a mutation of this gene causes the disease.

Tardive Dyskinesia

Tardive dyskinesia is another clinical disorder that may involve the basal ganglia; it is manifested by involuntary movements, especially of the face and tongue. It is a medically induced disorder caused by long-term treatment with antipsychotic agents—the phenothiazines (e.g., chlorpromazine, perphenazine) and the butyrophenones (e.g., haloperidol)—that decrease the function of dopaminergic cells. It is not understood how these drugs affect the dopaminergic system, but they appear to block dopaminergic cells. In the long run this blockage makes the receptors hypersensitive to dopamine. The balance between the dopaminergic, intrastriatal cholinergic, and GABA-ergic systems is altered, and involuntary movements appear as a consequence.

Experimental Manipulation of Transmitter Systems

Although clinicopathological studies in humans indicate that the basal ganglia are involved in the control of movement, attempts to reproduce clinical symptoms in experimental animals by lesioning the basal ganglia have not been particularly successful. In contrast, manipulation of specific transmitter systems in experimental animals has been quite effective in simulating disease states. For example, akinesia (lack of movement)—often associated with rigidity, postural abnormalities, and tremor—results from destruction of the ascending dopamine pathways, or from application of drugs that block dopamine receptors or inhibit the synthesis or storage of dopamine in experimental animals. Because these symptoms, which resemble those of Parkinson's disease, can be more easily reproduced in experimental animals by manipulating specific transmitter systems than by anatomical lesions, it is likely that the underlying pathology in human disorders of the basal ganglia disrupts transmitter metabolism, causing an *abnormal output* from the basal ganglia rather than *eliminating* the output.

A possible exception is hemiballismus, which commonly develops suddenly as a result of a vascular occlusion that destroys the subthalamic nucleus. Indeed, experimental lesions of the subthalamic nucleus in primates produce involuntary movements of the contralateral limbs similar to those seen in patients with hemiballismus. However, these involuntary movements are abolished if subsequent lesions are made to the output pathways of the basal ganglia (the globus pallidus or thalamus), or the motor cortex, or the corticospinal pathway. This suggests that the output of the basal ganglia is mediated, at least in part, by the corticospinal system.

An Overall View

In 1949, Linus Pauling revolutionized medical thinking by introducing the concept of a "molecular disease." He and his collaborators had observed a change in the electrophoretic mobility of hemoglobin S and reasoned that sickle cell anemia, a disease known to be genetic, could be explained by a mutation governing a specific protein. A decade later, Vernon Ingram showed that this alteration in charge occurs in the β polypeptide chain of hemoglobin S where a glutamic acid residue is replaced by a valine. This change from a single negatively charged residue in normal hemoglobin to a neutral one explains the altered molecular properties of hemoglobin S, and these, in turn, account for the intermolecular and cellular differences observed in sickled red cells. Thus, the molecular change is fundamental to understanding the patients' pathology, symptoms, and prognosis.

While the explanation for other diseases may not be as simple, it is a fundamental principle of modern medicine that each disorder has a molecular basis. With myasthenia gravis, the molecular target involved has been identified as the acetylcholine receptor. With the disorders of the basal ganglia, it appears that the metabolism of biogenic amine transmitters is the system affected: some components involved in the synthesis, packaging, or turnover of dopamine and serotinin is altered in these diseases. Parkinson's disease and myasthenia gravis are disorders that historically have made the medical community realize that specific molecular components of chemical synapses are likely to be loci for disease. What causes the pathological alterations at these loci, whether genetic, infectious, toxic or degenerative, is not yet known. With Huntington's disease, we are in a position to identify the mutant gene, but as yet have no idea about the molecule affected by the disorder. For each neurological disease, rational treatment demands a good understanding of the various steps involved in synaptic transmission. Conversely, these diseases prove to be a powerful motivation for expanding our insight into synaptic physiology, brain function, and motor behavior.

Selected Readings

Barden, H. 1981. The biology and chemistry of neuromelanin. In R. S. Sohal (ed.), Age Pigments. Amsterdam: Elsevier North-Holland Biomedical Press, pp. 155–166.

Botstein, D., White, R. L., Skolnick, M., and Davis, R. W. 1980. Construction of a genetic linkage map in man using restriction fragment length polymorphisms. Am. J. Hum. Genet. 32:314–331.

Curzon, G. 1977. The biochemistry of the basal ganglia and Parkinson's disease. Postgrad. Med. J. 53:719–725.

DeLong, M. R., and Georgopoulos, A. P. 1981. Motor functions of the basal ganglia. In V. B. Brooks (ed.), Handbook of Physiology, Section 1: The Nervous System, Vol. II, Motor Control. Bethesda, Md.: American Physiological Society, pp. 1017–1061.

Harper, P. S. 1984. Localization of the gene for Huntington's chorea. Trends Neurosci. 7:1–2.

Marks, J. 1977. Physiology of abnormal movements. Postgrad. Med. J. 53:713–718.

Martin, J. B. 1984. Huntington's Disease: New approaches to an old problem. Neurology 34:1059–1072.

References

Bertler, Å., and Rosengren, E. 1959. Occurrence and distribution of dopamine in brain and other tissues. Experientia 15:10–11.

Birkmayer, W., and Hornykiewicz, O. (eds.). 1976. Advances in Parkinsonism: Biochemistry, Physiology, Treatment. Fifth International Symposium on Parkinson's Disease, Vienna. Basel: Roche.

Carlsson, A. 1959. The occurrence, distribution and physiological role of catecholamines in the nervous system. Pharmacol. Rev. 11:490–493.

Cotzias, G. C., Van Woert, M. H., and Schiffer, L. M. 1967. Aromatic amino acids and modification of parkinsonism. N. Engl. J. Med. 276:374–379.

Crutcher, M. D., and DeLong, M. R. 1984. Single cell studies of the primate putamen. I. Functional organization. Exp. Brain Res. 53:233–243.

DeLong, M. R. 1974. Motor functions of the basal ganglia: Single-unit activity during movement. In F. O. Schmitt and F. G. Worden (eds.), The Neurosciences, Third Study Program. Cambridge, Mass.: MIT Press, pp. 319–325.

Evarts, E. V. 1976. Neurophysiological mechanisms in Parkinson's disease. In W. Birkmayer and O. Hornykiewicz (eds.), Advances in Parkinsonism: Biochemistry, Physiology, Treatment. Fifth International Symposium on Parkinson's Disease, Vienna. Basel: Roche, pp. 37–54.

Goldman, P. S., and Nauta, W. J. H. 1977. An intricately patterned prefronto-caudate projection in the rhesus monkey. J. Comp. Neurol. 171:369–385.

Grabiel, A. M. 1984. Neurochemically specified subsystems in the basal ganglia. In D. Evered and M. O'Connor (eds.), Functions of the Basal Ganglia. Ciba Foundation Symposium 107. London: Pitman, pp. 114–149.

Gusella, J. F., Wexler, N. S., Conneally, P. M., Naylor, S. L., Anderson, M. A., Tanzi, R. E., Watkins, P. C., Ottina, K., Wallace, M. R., Sakaguchi, A. Y., Young, A. B., Shoulson, I., Bonilla, E., and Martin, J. B. 1983. A polymorphic DNA marker genetically linked to Huntington's disease. Nature 306:234–238.

Hornykiewicz, O. 1966. Metabolism of brain dopamine in human parkinsonism: Neurochemical and clinical aspects. In E. Costa, L. J. Côté, and M. D. Yahr (eds.), Biochemistry and Pharmacology of the Basal Ganglia. New York: Raven Press, pp. 171–185.

Houseman, D., and Gusella, J. 1982. Molecular Genetic Approaches to Neural Degenerative Disorders. In F. O. Schmitt, S. J. Bird, and F. E. Bloom (eds.), Molecular Genetic Neuroscience. New York: Raven Press.

Ingram, V. 1963. The Hemoglobins in Genetics and Evolution. New York: Columbia University Press.

Johnson, T. N., and Rosvold, H. E. 1971. Topographic projections on the globus pallidus and the substantia nigra of selectively placed lesions in the precommissural caudate nucleus and putamen in the monkey. Exp. Neurol. 33:584–596.

Lee, T., Seeman, P., Rajput, A., Farley, I. J., and Hornykiewicz, O. 1978. Receptor basis for dopaminergic supersensitivity in Parkinson's disease. Nature 273:59–61.

Nieuwenhuys, R., Voogd, J., and van Huijzen, Chr. 1981. The Human Central Nervous System: A Synopsis and Atlas, 2nd rev. ed. Berlin: Springer.

Parkinson, J. 1817. An Essay on the Shaking Palsy. London.

Pauling, L., Itano, H. A., Singer, S. J., and Wells, I. C. 1949. Sickle Cell Anemia: A molecular disease. Science 110:543–548.

Ungerstedt, U., Ljungberg, T., Hoffer, B., and Siggins, G. 1975. Dopaminergic supersensitivity in the striatum. In D. Calne, T. N. Chase, and A. Barbeau (eds.), Advances in Neurology, Vol. 9: Dopaminergic Mechanisms. New York: Raven Press, pp. 57–65.

Watson, J. D., Tooze, J., and Kurtz, D. 1983. Recombinant DNA: A Short Course. New York: Freeman.

The Brain Stem and Reticular Core: Integration of Sensory and Motor Systems

VII

The brain stem is the region of the central nervous system situated between the spinal cord and the diencephalon. It is composed of many nuclei, long tracts (both motor and sensory), and the various components of the reticular formation, all contained in a relatively small volume. Its clinical significance is far out of proportion to its size, however. Damage to the brain stem often has profound effects not only on motor and sensory processes but also on consciousness.

Since most of the cranial nerves arise from the brain stem, we shall discuss their organization here. The cranial nerves innervate the structures of the head and neck, and the general principles underlying their organization are similar to those already encountered earlier in the chapters on spinal nerves. However, the head is more complicated than the trunk and limbs, and the nerves innervating the head reflect this complexity anatomically. In addition, many of the cranial nerves are concerned with special senses—sight, hearing, taste, and smell.

The brain stem also contains neurons that govern several key reflex behaviors, in particular those involving eye movements; as we shall see, these reflexes illustrate nicely how several independent neural systems can regulate a single set of motor behaviors.

Finally, we shall consider the clinical consequences of damage to the brain stem. The resulting neurological syndromes often consist of many symptoms that may seem unrelated. These complex syndromes occur because in the brain stem long tracts and nuclei are concerned with very different functions. Thus, long ascending and descending tracts course near different nuclear groups, and one vascular accident can affect neurons that mediate completely different aspects of sensation or motor function. The organization of the brain stem is so well understood that knowing the location of even a small lesion in the brain stem makes it possible to predict the clinical consequences of the lesion. Conversely, the clinical symptoms can indicate the precise location of a brain stem lesion.

James P. Kelly

Cranial Nerve Nuclei, the Reticular Formation, and Biogenic Amine-Containing Neurons

41

The brain stem lies between the spinal cord and the diencephalon. It is divided into three major regions: the medulla, the pons, and the midbrain. As the rostral continuation of the spinal cord, the brain stem innervates the head and neck and shares with the spinal cord common principles of organization. As in the spinal cord, there are somatic and visceral afferent and motor fibers in the brain stem. In addition, the brain stem is concerned with a variety of special senses mediated by the cranial nerves, and these senses introduce a new complexity not found in the spinal cord. Furthermore, lying outside the major tracts and nuclei of the brain stem are nerve cells that seem less discretely organized at first glance, yet they have an important modulatory effect on the brain stem as a whole, as well as on the spinal cord and the cerebral cortex. These neurons collectively are called the *reticular formation* because they are usually enmeshed in a network, or reticulum, of fine fibers. Originally the reticular formation was thought to be diffuse in its organization, but as we shall see, recent studies with modern neuroanatomical tracing methods have shown that the neurons of the reticular formation make rather precise connections with other parts of the brain: functional groups of neurons can be identified in the reticular formation by their neurotransmitter biochemistry.

In this chapter we shall first consider the location of the cranial nerves in relation to the major landmarks that characterize each of the three regions of the brain stem. We shall then discuss these nerves and associated nuclei and follow the peripheral course of certain nerves to illustrate principles that govern their distribution. Finally, we shall examine the reticular core along with the trajectories of the major brain stem tracts to gain insight into the functions and organization of the reticular formation.

Most Cranial Nerves Originate in the Brain Stem and Innervate the Head, Neck, and Special Sense Organs

The cranial nerves are concerned with three main functions: (1) the motor and sensory innervation of the head and neck, (2) the innervation of special sense organs, and (3) the parasympathetic innervation of autonomic ganglia that control important visceral functions such as breathing, heart rate, blood pressure, coughing, and swallowing.

The twelve pairs of cranial nerves are numbered in the rostrocaudal sequence in which they pierce the dura mater during their course. Some of them are purely motor, others are sensory, and the rest are mixed, mediating both motor and sensory innervation. The cranial nerves and their functions are summarized in Table 41–1.

An assessment of the functioning of these nerves is an extremely important part of a clinical neurological examination because disease states in the brain are often

Table 41–1. Functions of the Cranial Nerves

	Cranial nerve	Type of nerve	Functions
I	Olfactory	Sensory	Smell
II.	Optic	Sensory	Vision
III.	Oculomotor	Motor	Eye movements: innervates all extraocular muscles except the superior oblique and lateral rectus muscles (see N. IV and VI)
			Innervates the striated muscle of the eyelid
			Contains autonomic fibers that mediate pupillary constriction and accommodation of lens for near vision
IV.	Trochlear	Motor	Eye movements: innervates superior oblique muscle
V.	Trigeminal	Mixed	Sensory: mediates cutaneous and proprioceptive sensations from skin, muscles, and joints in the face and mouth, and sensory innervation of the teeth
			Motor: innervates muscles of mastication
VI.	Abducens	Motor	Eye movements: innervates lateral rectus muscle
VII.	Facial	Mixed	Motor: innervates muscles of facial expression
			Sensory: mediates taste sensation from the anterior $2/3$ of the tongue

reflected in functional abnormalities of one or more of the cranial nerves. Since the cranial nerves originate from different regions in the brain stem, disorder in the function of one or more nerves can provide valuable information about the site of a lesion.

The origins of most cranial nerves can best be illustrated by examining several views of the brain stem with the cerebral hemispheres and cerebellum removed. Let us begin with a ventral view (Figure 41–1). Here, three purely motor nerves (nerves III, VI, and XII) exit from the brain stem close to the midline. Ontogenetically and phylogenetically, these three cranial nerves belong to a common class (see below), and the motor neurons that give rise to them are always found adjacent to the midline of the brain stem. Let us consider each of the cranial nerves in turn. The oculomotor nerve (III) emerges at the caudal border of the midbrain, the abducens nerve (VI) emerges at the caudal border of the pons, and the hypoglossal nerve (XII) emerges from the medulla just lateral to the medullary pyramids. The oculomotor and abducens nerves innervate extraocular muscles. The hypoglossal nerve innervates the intrinsic muscles of the tongue.

Only one cranial nerve, the trochlear (IV), exits from the dorsal aspect of the brain stem. The trochlear nerve is also a purely motor nerve and, like nerves III and VI, it innervates extraocular muscles. The trochlear nerve exits from the midbrain just caudal to the inferior colliculus near the midline to innervate the superior oblique muscle of the eye (Figure 41–2). (Recall that the superior

and inferior colliculi are two symmetrical pairs of swellings on the dorsal surface of the midbrain, and that they are related to the visual and auditory systems, respectively; Figure 41–2.)

A lateral view of the brain stem (Figure 41–3) illustrates seven of the remaining eight cranial nerves. The trigeminal nerve (V) enters the pons. This mixed sensory–motor nerve mediates sensation from facial skin and innervates the muscles of mastication. The facial (VII) and vestibulocochlear (VIII) nerves originate at the junction between the pons and the medulla. The lateral view also shows that the glossopharyngeal (IX), vagus (X), and accessory (XI) nerves arise in the medulla as a series of fine rootlets just dorsal to the inferior olive. We shall discuss the functional classes of fibers found in these nerves later in this chapter. The optic (II) and olfactory (I) nerves terminate not in the brain stem but in the lateral geniculate nucleus of the thalamus and in the olfactory bulb, respectively. We shall, therefore, not consider them here.

To understand the organization of the cranial nerves, let us consider the ontogenetic development of the spinal cord and the spinal nerves. The principles governing the organization of the cranial nerves are quite similar to those governing the organization of the spinal nerves; however, the existence of special sense organs in the head and the complicated embryology of this region make the anatomy of the cranial nerves more intricate than the anatomy of the spinal nerves.

Table 41–1. *(continued)*

	Cranial nerve	Type of nerve	Functions
VIII.	Vestibulocochlear	Sensory	Audition
			Equilibrium, postural reflexes, orientation of the head in space
IX.	Glossopharyngeal	Mixed	Contains autonomic axons that innervate the parotid gland
			Swallowing: mediates visceral sensations from the palate and posterior third of the tongue
			Innervates the carotid body
			Innervates taste buds in posterior third of the tongue
X.	Vagus	Mixed	Contains autonomic fibers that innervate smooth muscle in heart, blood vessels, trachea, bronchi, esophagus, stomach, and intestine
			Innervates striated muscles in the larynx and pharynx and controls speech
			Mediates visceral sensation from the pharynx, larynx, thorax, and abdomen
			Innervates taste buds in the epiglottis
XI.	Spinal accessory	Motor	Motor innervation of trapezius and sternocleidomastoid muscles
XII.	Hypoglossal	Motor	Motor innervation of intrinsic muscles of the tongue

542

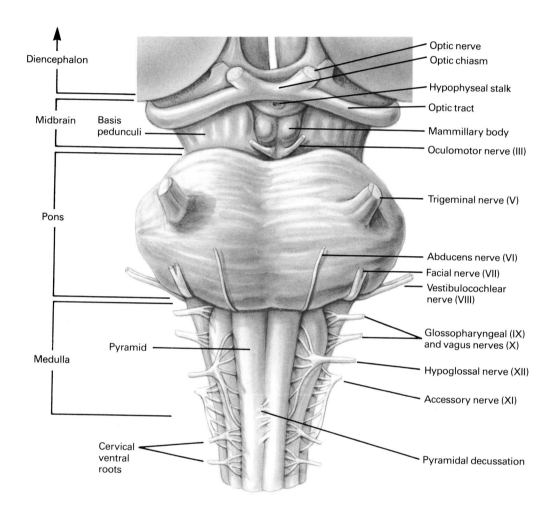

Diencephalon

Midbrain

Basis
pedunculi

Pons

Medulla

Pyramid

Cervical
ventral
roots

Optic nerve

Optic chiasm

Hypophyseal stalk

Optic tract

Mammillary body

Oculomotor nerve (III)

Trigeminal nerve (V)

Abducens nerve (VI)

Facial nerve (VII)

Vestibulocochlear
nerve (VIII)

Glossopharyngeal (IX)
and vagus nerves (X)

Hypoglossal nerve (XII)

Accessory nerve (XI)

Pyramidal decussation

41–1 The origins of most of the cranial nerves are evident in
a ventral view of the brain stem.

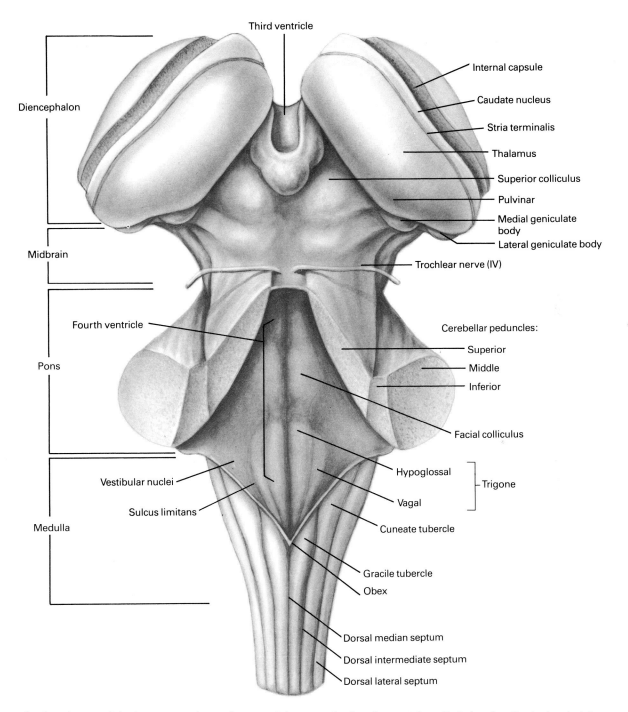

41–2 The dorsal view of the brain stem shows the exit of the trochlear nerve (IV). The dorsal surface of the pons is made up of the floor of the fourth ventricle medially and the three cerebellar peduncles more laterally. The caudal border of the fourth ventricle, called the *obex* (Latin, barrier), is an important surgical landmark in the medulla. Lying lateral to the obex are the dorsal column nuclei and their associated tracts.

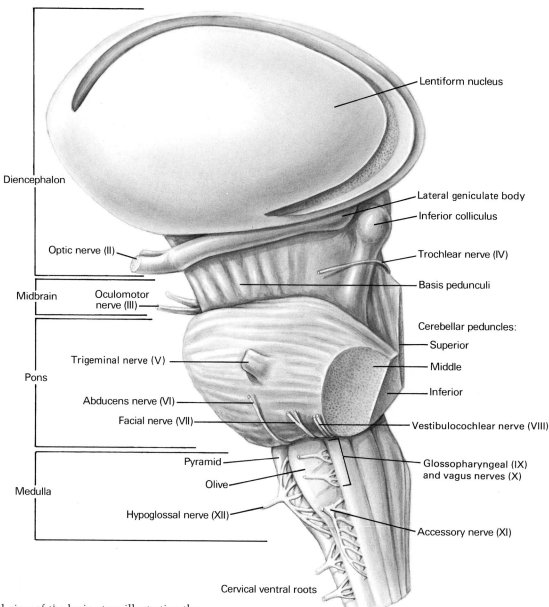

41–3 Lateral view of the brain stem illustrating the emergence of the cranial nerves in a rostrocaudal sequence. The origins of the facial (VII) and vestibulocochlear (VIII) nerves can best be seen in this view of the brain stem.

Cranial Nerves Contain Visceral and Somatic Afferent and Efferent Fibers

As we saw in Chapter 21, after the neural tube closes, the developing spinal cord is roughly cylindrical in outline, with a diamond-shaped central canal (Figure 41–4). The dorsal region of the cord is called the *alar plate*, and the ventral region is called the *basal plate*. The cleft indicating the division between the alar and basal plates is termed the *sulcus limitans*. The division into alar and basal regions is significant because the sensory neurons that receive input from the dorsal roots are derived from

the alar plate, whereas motor neurons that send their axons out in the ventral roots are derived from proliferating cells in the neuroepithelium of the basal plate.

There are two classes of *motor neurons* in the spinal cord: *somatic motor neurons*, which innervate the skin and muscle of the trunk and limbs, and *visceral (autonomic) motor neurons*, which are preganglionic neurons belonging to the autonomic nervous system, that innervate blood vessels, glands, and the viscera of the body cavity. There are also two classes of *afferent neurons* that have their cell bodies in the dorsal root ganglia: *somatic afferent neurons* and *visceral (autonomic) afferent*

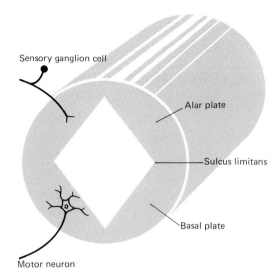

41–4 The sensory neurons of the spinal dorsal roots and the motor neurons of the spinal ventral roots are derived from the alar and basal plates of the primitive neural tube.

neurons. The types of afferent and efferent fibers in a spinal nerve that originate from these neurons are summarized in Table 41–2.

The organization of the cranial nerve nuclei is similar to that of the spinal nerves. As in the spinal cord, the cell bodies of motor and sensory (or afferent) neurons differ in location from one another. The cell bodies of motor neurons that send their axons into the cranial nerves are located within the brain stem, whereas the cell bodies of the afferent fibers in the cranial nerves lie outside the brain stem, either in ganglia analogous to the dorsal root ganglia or in specialized end-organs such as the eye. However, both the somatic and visceral afferent and motor neurons can be subdivided into further functional subclasses.

There Are Three Types of Motor Neurons in the Brain Stem: Somatic, Special Visceral, and General Visceral

Whereas the spinal cord contains only two classes of motor neurons, the brain stem contains three: one type of *somatic motor neuron*, and two types of *visceral motor neurons*—*special visceral motor neurons* and *general visceral motor neurons.*

The *somatic motor neurons* and the *special visceral motor neurons* innervate the skeletal muscles of the head and neck. But the two classes of motor neurons innervate two different categories of muscles because the striated muscles in the head and neck arise from two sources during development: (1) from myotomes and (2) from the primitive branchial arches.

Striated muscle fibers that arise from the *myotomes* give rise to the extraocular muscles and the intrinsic muscles of the tongue. These muscles are similar in their development to other striated muscles in the body and

Table 41–2. Types of Fibers in Spinal Nerves

Fiber type	Structures innervated
Somatic motor	Striated muscle
Visceral motor	Smooth muscle, glands, blood vessels
Somatic afferent	Sensory receptors in skin, muscles, and joints
Visceral afferent	Viscera of the body cavity

are innervated by *somatic motor neurons* (located in nuclei III, IV, VI, and XII). These motor neurons resemble the large motor neurons of the ventral horn of the spinal cord in both appearance and function.

The striated muscles that arise from the *primitive branchial arches* control chewing, facial expression, the larynx, and the pharynx. These branchiomeric muscles are innervated by *special visceral motor neurons* (located in nuclei V, VII, IX, X, and XI). In appearance they are similar to somatic motor neurons, but, as we shall see, their location in the brain stem is different.

The *general visceral motor neurons* are preganglionic parasympathetic neurons that regulate the activity of glands, blood vessels, and smooth muscle. The parasympathetic neurons have their cell bodies in brain stem nuclei, and their axons exit as part of nerves III, VII, IX, and X. These preganglionic axons synapse upon neurons in the autonomic ganglia of the head. The axons of the postganglionic parasympathetic neurons in these ganglia innervate the target organs. Sympathetic neurons that innervate structures in the head have their cell bodies outside the brain stem in the superior cervical ganglion, the most rostral part of the sympathetic chain. Axons of sympathetic neurons run along the internal carotid artery for part of their course and eventually join one of the cranial nerve branches to reach the appropriate end-organ. The organization of motor neurons contributing to the cranial nerves is summarized in Table 41–3.

All three types of motor neurons (somatic, general visceral, and special visceral) are located in the cranial motor nuclei of the brain stem. As is the case with their

Table 41–3. Classification of Motor Neuron Fiber Types in Cranial Nerves

Fiber type	Structures innervated	Cranial nerves containing these fibers
Somatic	Muscles derived from the myotomes	III, IV, VI, XII
Special visceral (branchial)	Muscles derived from the branchial arches	V, VII, IX, X, XI
General visceral	Smooth muscle, glands, and blood vessels	III, VII, IX, X

Table 41–4. Classification of Afferent Fiber Types in Cranial Nerves

Fiber type	Structures innervated	Cranial nerves containing these fibers
General somatic	Skin of the face and mucous membrane of the mouth	V, VII, IX, X
Special somatic	Sensory organs of the inner ear	VIII
General visceral	Internal organs	IX, X
Special visceral	Taste buds	VII, IX, X

counterparts in the spinal cord, these cranial motor neurons are called *lower motor neurons.* In contrast, the cell bodies of the afferent fibers in the cranial nerves lie outside the brain stem, as do the dorsal root ganglion cells. The sensory nuclei in the brain stem therefore are composed of second-order neurons that receive input from the primary afferent neurons.

There Are Four Types of Afferent Neurons: General Somatic, Special Somatic, General Visceral, and Special Visceral

Because of the presence of *special* sensory organs in the head as well as the mixed embryological origin of muscle in the facial region *specialized* types of afferent fibers that are not present in spinal nerves are found in the cra-

nial nerves. As a result, the two types of afferent neurons (somatic and visceral) in the cranial nerves may be further subdivided to include these specialized fiber types. There are *general somatic afferent* fibers innervating the skin of the face and the mucous membranes of the mouth as well as *special somatic afferent* fibers from the cochlea and vestibular apparatus, the sensory organs in the inner ear. The *general visceral afferent* fibers provide sensory innervation to internal structures such as the larynx and pharynx, as well as to internal organs. The *special visceral afferents* innervate the taste buds and mediate the sense of taste. These classes of afferent fibers and the cranial nerves that contain them are summarized in Table 41–4.

Cranial Nerve Nuclei Are Grouped into Seven Columns

The cranial nerve nuclei are organized into seven longitudinal columns according to function. Neurons belonging to particular functional classes are always in the same place with respect to other functional classes, and each class of neurons forms a column that is oriented rostrocaudally in the brain stem. Each column is found in a relatively constant position, but it may be interrupted at points along its length. The general principles underlying the organization of these columns are illustrated in Figure 41–5.

Neurons innervating somatic muscles in the head derived from the myotomes are situated adjacent to the midline, immediately ventral to the floor of the fourth ventricle (Figures 41–5 and 41–6). These neurons consti-

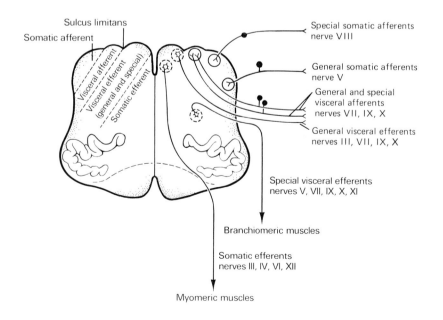

41–5 The cranial nerve nuclei, shown in a cross section of the brain stem, are organized into columns according to function.

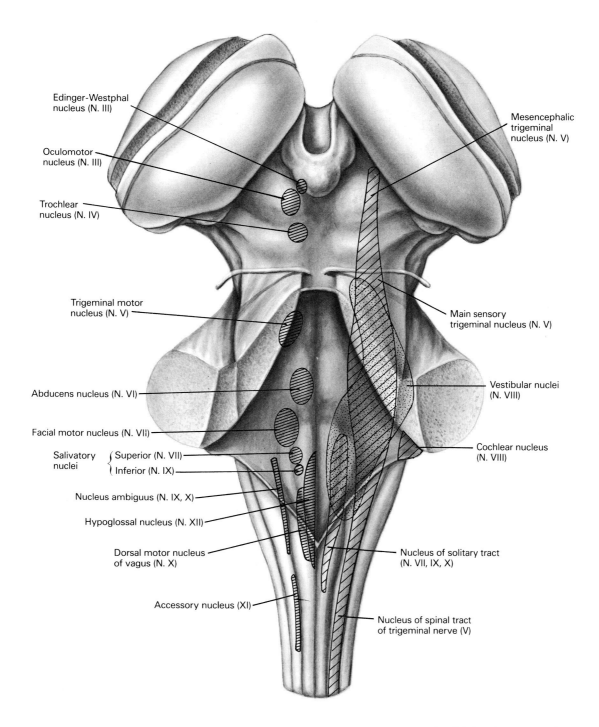

Edinger-Westphal nucleus (N. III)

Oculomotor nucleus (N. III)

Trochlear nucleus (N. IV)

Trigeminal motor nucleus (N. V)

Abducens nucleus (N. VI)

Facial motor nucleus (N. VII)

Salivatory nuclei { Superior (N. VII) / Inferior (N. IX) }

Nucleus ambiguus (N. IX, X)

Hypoglossal nucleus (N. XII)

Dorsal motor nucleus of vagus (N. X)

Accessory nucleus (XI)

Mesencephalic trigeminal nucleus (N. V)

Main sensory trigeminal nucleus (N. V)

Vestibular nuclei (N. VIII)

Cochlear nucleus (N. VIII)

Nucleus of solitary tract (N. VII, IX, X)

Nucleus of spinal tract of trigeminal nerve (V)

41–6 The motor nuclei (**left-hand side**) and afferent nuclei (**right-hand side**) of the cranial nerves can be viewed from the dorsal aspect of the brain stem. (See transverse sections in Figures 41–7 to 41–13.)

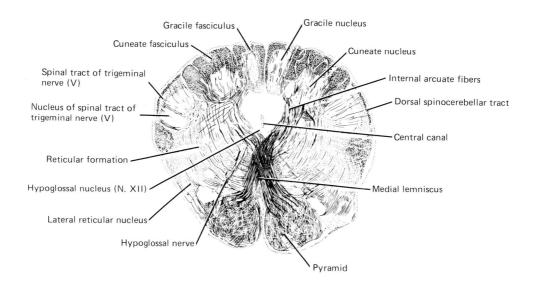

41–7 Cranial nerve nuclei viewed from the level of the lower medulla. (Adapted from Ranson and Clark, 1953.)

tute the *somatic motor column*. Motor neurons innervating the branchiomeric muscles are displaced ventrally and laterally from the somatic motor column (Figures 41–5 and 41–6). These branchiomeric motor neurons constitute the *special visceral motor column*. The parasympathetic neurons of the *general visceral motor column* are found immediately lateral to the somatic motor column (Figure 41–5).

41–8 Cranial nerve nuclei viewed from the level of the upper medulla. (Adapted from Ranson and Clark, 1953.)

The Somatic Motor Column Contains Motor Neurons That Innervate the Extraocular Muscles and the Tongue

The somatic motor column of neurons consists of four nuclear groups: the oculomotor (III), trochlear (IV), abducens (VI), and hypoglossal (XII) nuclei. This column of neurons is not continuous along its rostrocaudal extent. Each of the nuclei is found in the same relative position, just below the floor of the ventricular system near the midline, but at different rostrocaudal levels of the brain stem. The locations of cranial nerve nuclei in the longitudinal axis of the brain stem are shown schematically in Figure 41–6 and in the subsequent series of transverse sections stained for myelin (Figures 41–7 to 41–13), which are arranged in sequence from the medulla to the midbrain. The oculomotor nucleus lies in the rostral part of the midbrain (Figure 41–13) at the level of the superior

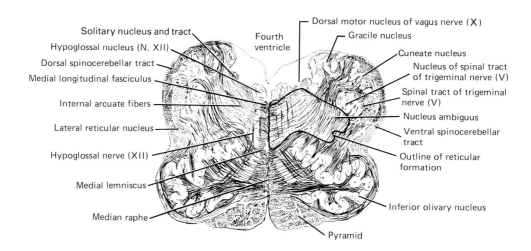

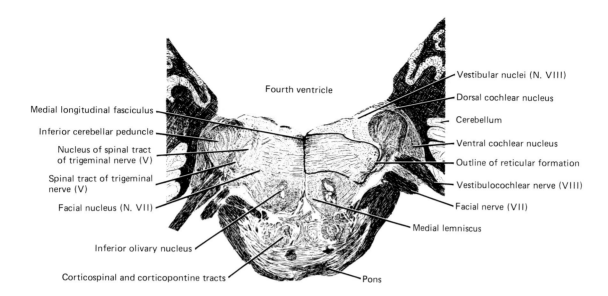

41–9 Cranial nerve nuclei viewed from the level of the lower pons. (Adapted from Ranson and Clark, 1953.)

colliculus. The trochlear nucleus lies more caudally in the midbrain, at the level of the inferior colliculus (Figure 41–12). Both of these nuclei lie ventral to the cerebral aqueduct. The abducens nucleus is in the pons (Figure 41–10), and the hypoglossal nucleus is in the medulla (Figure 41–8). Both of these nuclei lie ventral to the floor of the fourth ventricle.

The Special Visceral Motor Column Contains Motor Neurons That Innervate the Branchiomeric Muscles of the Larynx, Pharynx, Face, and Jaw

The motor neurons of the special visceral motor column are also clustered in four distinct nuclei that occupy the same relative position in the brain stem (Figure 41–5).

They are displaced ventrally and laterally from the somatic motor column. The motor nucleus of the trigeminal nerve (V) lies in the pons (Figure 41–6). It is the most rostral component of the special visceral motor column and contains the motor neurons that innervate the muscles of mastication. The motor nucleus of the facial nerve (VII) lies caudal to the motor nucleus of the tri-

41–10 Cranial nerve nuclei viewed from the level of the midpons. (Adapted from Ranson and Clark, 1953.)

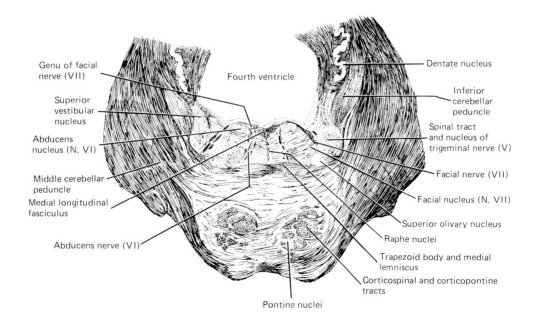

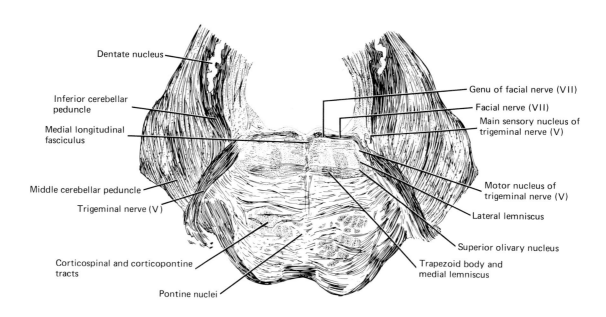

41–11 Cranial nerve nuclei viewed from the level of the upper pons. (Adapted from Ranson and Clark, 1953.)

geminal nerve in the pons (Figures 41–6 and 41–10) and contains motor neurons that innervate the muscles of facial expression. The special visceral motor neurons contributing to the glossopharyngeal (IX), vagus (X), and accessory (XI) nerves lie most caudally in the medulla.

The cell bodies of the branchiomeric motor neurons of the glossopharyngeal (IX) and vagus (X) nerves are clustered in a single group that is called the *nucleus ambiguus* because it is penetrated by fibers running from

41–12 Cranial nerve nuclei viewed from the level of the inferior colliculus. (Adapted from Ranson and Clark, 1953.)

the inferior olive to the cerebellum and is consequently difficult to identify in sections stained for cell bodies (Figure 41–6). Neurons in the nucleus ambiguus innervate striated muscles in the larynx and pharynx and are therefore critical for both speech and swallowing (Figure 41–8). The nucleus of the spinal accessory nerve (XI) is the most caudal member of this column. The motor neurons of this nucleus stretch into the cervical regions of the spinal cord; they innervate the sternocleidomastoid and trapezius muscles.

The General Visceral Motor Column Contains Preganglionic Parasympathetic Neurons

The general visceral motor column, which is just lateral to the somatic motor column, is divided into four principal nuclei (Figure 41–5). The most rostral of these is

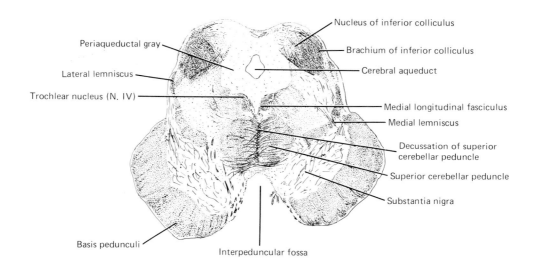

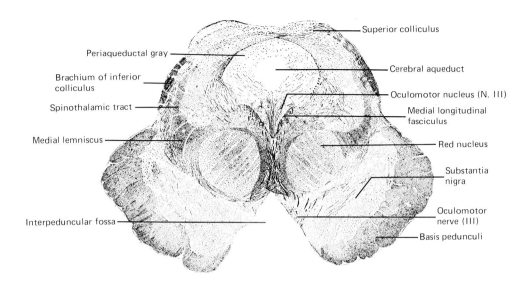

Periaqueductal gray

Brachium of inferior colliculus

Spinothalamic tract

Medial lemniscus

Interpeduncular fossa

Superior colliculus

Cerebral aqueduct

Oculomotor nucleus (N. III)

Medial longitudinal fasciculus

Red nucleus

Substantia nigra

Oculomotor nerve (III)

Basis pedunculi

the Edinger–Westphal nucleus (Figure 41–6). It lies adjacent to the third nerve motor nucleus and contains some, but not all, of the preganglionic parasympathetic neurons that send their axons out of the midbrain with the third nerve. These axons terminate in the ciliary ganglion. The postganglionic fibers innervate the pupillary constrictor and the ciliary muscle of the eye. The sympathetic axons that innervate the eye arise from the superior cervical ganglion. These postganglionic axons innervate three smooth muscles in the orbit: the smooth muscle of the eyelid, the pupillary dilator, and Mueller's muscle, which holds the eye forward in the orbit by opposing the force of the extraocular muscles, which tend to pull the eye deeper into the orbit.

It is useful to compare what happens to the eye when the oculomotor nerve is severed with what happens when the sympathetic innervation of the eye is severed. Damage to the third nerve causes a paralysis of the eye on the affected side. The eye looks downward and outward because of the unopposed action of the remaining extraocular muscles (the superior oblique and the lateral rectus). Since the striated muscle of the eyelid is denervated, the eyelid droops. This condition is called *ptosis*. The pupil is dilated *(mydriasis)* because the pupillary constrictor is denervated, and the eye is drawn forward in the orbit *(exophthalmos)* due to the unopposed action of Mueller's muscle. Interrupting the sympathetic innervation also produces ptosis because the smooth muscle of the eyelid is denervated. In contrast to a nerve III lesion, however, sympathetic damage produces a *miosis*, a constriction of the pupil, because the pupillary dilator is denervated; the eye also recedes into the orbit, a condition termed *enophthalmos*, because Mueller's muscle is denervated. These three symptoms—ptosis, miosis, and enophthalmos—are collectively called *Horner's syndrome* along with anhidrosis, a loss of sweating, and are important indicators of damage to the sympathetic divi-

41–13 Cranial nerve nuclei viewed from the level of the superior colliculus. (Adapted from Ranson and Clark, 1953.)

sion of the autonomic nervous system. This damage may occur in pre- or postganglionic axons, or in descending axons that run from the hypothalamus through the lateral aspect of the brain stem to the intermediolateral cell column of the spinal cord.

The superior and inferior salivatory nuclei are components of the general visceral motor column in the rostral part of the medulla, but the borders of these nuclei are difficult to delineate. The neurons of the superior salivatory nucleus send their axons into the root of the facial nerve (VII). The axons of neurons in the inferior salivatory nucleus run in the glossopharyngeal nerve (IX). The visceral motor axons in both of these nerves synapse in autonomic ganglia in the head; the postganglionic axons innervate salivary glands, mucous glands, and blood vessels. The inferior salivatory nucleus innervates, for example, the parotid gland via the optic ganglion. Neurons in the superior salivatory nucleus innervate the sublingual and submandibular glands via the submandibular ganglion, and the lacrimal glands via the sphenopalatine ganglion.

The last component of the general visceral motor column is the dorsal motor nucleus of the vagus (X), which lies adjacent to the hypoglossal nucleus (XII) in the medulla (Figure 41–8). Neurons in the dorsal motor nucleus of the vagus give rise to the preganglionic parasympathetic axons that run in the various branches of the vagus nerve to innervate the viscera of the body: the heart, the lungs, and the gut. Vagal stimulation causes a decrease in heart rate, whereas sympathetic stimulation causes an increase. In the gut, the vagus nerve promotes peristalsis, while sympathetic fibers slow gut motility.

Just lateral to the general visceral motor column there is a slight indentation in the ventricular wall, the *sulcus limitans*. This cleft marks the division between sensory and motor regions of the developing neural tube, and in the adult brain stem it marks the division between the afferent and efferent cell columns. The motor neurons described above are medial to the sulcus limitans. The afferent cell columns, to be described next, lie lateral to it.

The General and Special Visceral Afferent Columns Contain Neurons That Provide the Sensory Innervation for the Taste Buds, Larynx, Pharynx, Blood Vessels, and Viscera

Neurons in the visceral afferent column (Figure 41–5) lie adjacent to the general visceral motor column in the medulla and receive fibers conveying the sense of taste, fibers carrying input from the carotid body, afferent fibers innervating the larynx and pharynx, and afferent fibers innervating the heart, lungs, and gut. This column of cells exists only in the medulla and is called the *solitary nucleus* (Figure 41–8). The nucleus has two parts. The rostral part of the solitary nucleus is a relay for taste and for visceral afferents from the gastrointestinal tract. The caudal part of the nucleus receives input from the carotid body, which monitors carbon dioxide tension in the blood and is important for cardiovascular control. Other neurons in the caudal part of the solitary nucleus receive afferent input from the lungs and bronchi.

The neurons conveying sensory input to the solitary nucleus have their cell bodies in ganglia that lie outside the brain stem in association with cranial nerves VII (facial), IX (glossopharyngeal), and X (vagus). The centrally directed processes of the sensory neurons in these ganglia run into the brain stem and join the *solitary tract* (Figure 41–8), which terminates in the solitary nucleus. The axons of cells in the solitary nucleus that mediate taste sensation synapse in the thalamus. Thalamic neurons, in turn, relay information about taste to the cerebral cortex. The other regions of the nucleus that deal with cardiovascular function have local connections with the reticular formation, and indirect connections with the limbic system of the forebrain, which has an important role in autonomic regulation.

The Special Somatic Afferent Column Contains Neurons That Innervate the Cochlear and the Vestibular Sensory Organs

The somatic afferent columns (Figure 41–5) lie lateral to the visceral afferent column. The special somatic afferent nuclei in the caudal part of the pons and the rostral part of the medulla receive the fibers of the vestibulocochlear nerve (VIII). The cochlear nuclei (Figures 41–6 and 41–9) receive the centrally directed branches of neurons in the spiral ganglion running in the cochlear division of the eighth nerve. The vestibular nuclei (Figures 41–6 and 41–9) receive input from the vestibular division of the eighth nerve; this nerve is concerned with detecting the motion and position of the body in space. Both of these nuclei lie in the floor of the lateral recess of the fourth ventricle.

The General Somatic Afferent Column Contains Neurons That Innervate the Face and the Mucous Membranes of the Mouth

The general somatic afferent column is displaced ventrolaterally (Figure 41–5). It is composed of the three separate divisions of the sensory trigeminal nucleus (V), which are arranged in rostrocaudal sequence. The mesencephalic nucleus of the trigeminal nerve (Figure 41–6) lies in the mesencephalon and modulates proprioception from the muscles and joints of the face. The main sensory nucleus of the trigeminal nerve lies in the pons. The spinal nucleus of the trigeminal nerve runs the entire length of the medulla and extends into the spinal cord. These nuclei receive afferent input from the muscles, skin, and joints of the face and the mucous membranes of the mouth, mostly via the trigeminal nerve. This sensory input is conveyed to the thalamus and then to the cerebral cortex. The organization of the trigeminal nuclei will be discussed in greater detail in Chapter 42.

Principles of Organization Governing the Cranial Nerves

Three principles underlie the organization of the cranial nerves: First, *most of the motor nuclei in the brain stem are associated with individual cranial nerves.* For example, the oculomotor nerve has its own motor nucleus, as do the trochlear nerve and the trigeminal nerve. These neurons are analogous to the lower motor neurons in the spinal cord. They receive input from the motor area of the cerebral cortex and send their axons to muscles in the periphery.

Afferent nuclei in the brain stem, on the other hand, often receive fibers from several cranial nerves. The solitary nucleus, for example, collects fibers carrying information about taste from the facial, glossopharyngeal, and vagus nerves. As we shall see in Chapter 42, the nucleus of the spinal tract of the trigeminal nerve also receives sensory input from several cranial nerves. The interesting point is that sensory information of a particular type, such as taste, is forwarded to a single nucleus no matter which cranial nerve pathway this information takes. This principle, considered before, appears again and again in discussions of sensory systems: *afferent fibers bearing similar modalities of input usually terminate within similar sites in the brain.*

The third principle is related to location: *neurons with different functional properties occupy consistently different positions in the brain stem.* Specificity of localization arises during development. Neurons destined for different functions arise from distinctive parts of the neuroepithelium lining the neural tube, differentiate at characteristic times in development, and migrate to specific positions within the brain stem. The eventual functional role of a neuron can therefore be correlated with early events in its developmental history.

Specific Sensory and Motor Tracts Traverse the Brain Stem

The paths through the brain stem of four major tracts— the corticospinal, corticobulbar, medial lemniscal, and spinothalamic—are shown in Figure 41–14. The corticospinal tract descends on the ventral aspect of the brain stem within the pyramids to the caudal border of the medulla, where it crosses to form the lateral corticospinal tract (Figure 41–14A). Corticobulbar fibers also run in the pyramids, but they peel off at various levels to reach the motor nuclei of the cranial nerves (Figure 41–14B). The neurons that give rise to corticobulbar axons are upper motor neurons whose effects are similar to those exerted by corticospinal axons upon spinal motor neurons. Medial lemniscal axons ascend initially near the midline after their origin in the dorsal column nuclei, but they fan out laterally before reaching the thalamus (Figure 41–14C). The spinothalamic tract runs near the medial lemniscus after ascending from its origin in the spinal cord and gives off collaterals to the reticular formation (Figure 41–14D). Aside from these tracts and a few others (e.g., the rubrospinal tract), the major cranial nerve nuclei, and nuclei related to cerebellar function (e.g., the inferior olive), the rest of the brain stem is composed of reticular neurons and their processes.

It will become apparent in Chapter 45 that a knowledge of these tracts and of the cranial nerves is essential in clinical neurology. Vascular lesions often affect adjacent tracts and nuclei in the brain stem, and the symptoms that result from such lesions can be understood only if the regional anatomy is known in detail.

Cranial Nerve Fiber Types Mix in the Periphery

The motor neurons of the cranial nerves and their associated sensory nuclei lie in distinct regions of the brain. In the periphery, however, there is considerable mixing of different fiber types. As an example of this phenomenon let us examine the peripheral course of the facial nerve (VII).

The motor neurons of the facial nerve lie ventrolaterally in the pons (Figure 41–10). The axons of these cells run dorsomedially, curve sharply around the abducens nucleus (genu of the facial nerve; Figure 41–10), and then run ventrolaterally toward their point of exit at the lower border of the pons. The facial nerve exits from the brain stem medial to the vestibulocochlear nerve. The region immediately outside the brain stem, where both nerves

are found, is called the *cerebellopontine angle* (see Chapter 45 for the clinical significance of this region). As these two nerves run toward the internal auditory meatus, they are joined by the small intermediate nerve. This nerve carries sensory fibers and visceral efferent fibers (arising from the superior salivatory nucleus) associated with the facial nerve.

After they leave the internal auditory meatus, the facial and intermediate nerves run in the facial canal (Figure 41–15). The facial canal at first runs directly laterally, but then takes a sharp turn posteriorly. The geniculate ganglion, containing the cell bodies of sensory fibers associated with the facial nerve, is found in the region of this turn. The facial canal then takes a second bend, directly ventrally, to reach the stylomastoid foramen, where the facial nerve exits from the cranium. Before it reaches the foramen, branchiomeric motor axons leave the main trunk of the nerve to form the small stapedius nerve, which innervates the stapedius muscle of the middle ear (Figure 41–15). The stapedius muscle acts to dampen the motion of the ear ossicles in response to loud sounds. The remaining branchiomeric motor fibers of the facial nerve leave through the stylomastoid foramen and branch widely in the periphery to innervate the muscles of facial expression (the frontalis, orbicularis oculi, orbicularis oris, and buccinator, for example).

The fibers of the intermediate nerve leave the facial nerve during its course through the facial canal. The greater superficial petrosal nerve leaves near the geniculate ganglion (Figure 41–15) and then runs back into the cranial cavity. This nerve passes just lateral to the internal carotid artery (Figure 41–15) and eventually exits from the cranium via the foramen lacerum. There the nerve is joined by the deep petrosal nerve, which is composed of sympathetic axons arising from the sympathetic chain. These two nerves form the nerve of the pterygoid canal, which eventually reaches the sphenopalatine ganglion. The visceral motor (parasympathetic) axons synapse here, and the postganglionic fibers course further in the periphery to innervate the lacrimal glands. These fibers actually reach the gland by joining a branch of the trigeminal nerve (V). The frequent association of autonomic axons and branches of the trigeminal nerve will be considered in Chapter 42.

The chorda tympani leaves the facial nerve near the stylomastoid foramen (Figure 41–15). It runs through the tympanic cavity to join the lingual nerve, a branch of the trigeminal nerve, which carries the preganglionic visceral motor fibers of the chorda tympani to their termination in the submaxillary ganglion. Postganglionic fibers from this ganglion innervate the submaxillary and sublingual glands.

The chorda tympani also contains sensory fibers mediating taste from the anterior two-thirds of the tongue. These fibers are distributed to the tongue in the lingual nerve (a branch of the trigeminal nerve) and have their cell bodies in the geniculate ganglion. The centrally directed branches of these cells run in the intermediate

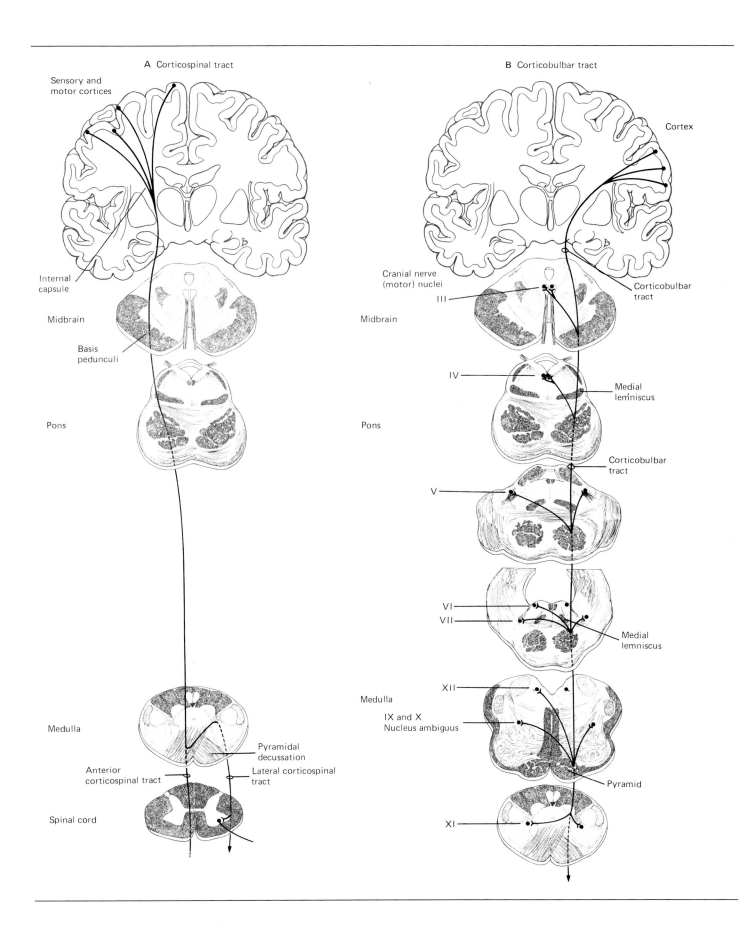

A Corticospinal tract

Sensory and motor cortices

Internal capsule

Midbrain

Basis pedunculi

Pons

Medulla

Anterior corticospinal tract

Pyramidal decussation

Lateral corticospinal tract

Spinal cord

B Corticobulbar tract

Cortex

Cranial nerve (motor) nuclei

III

Corticobulbar tract

Midbrain

IV

Medial lemniscus

Pons

Corticobulbar tract

V

VI

VII

Medial lemniscus

Medulla

XII

IX and X Nucleus ambiguus

Pyramid

XI

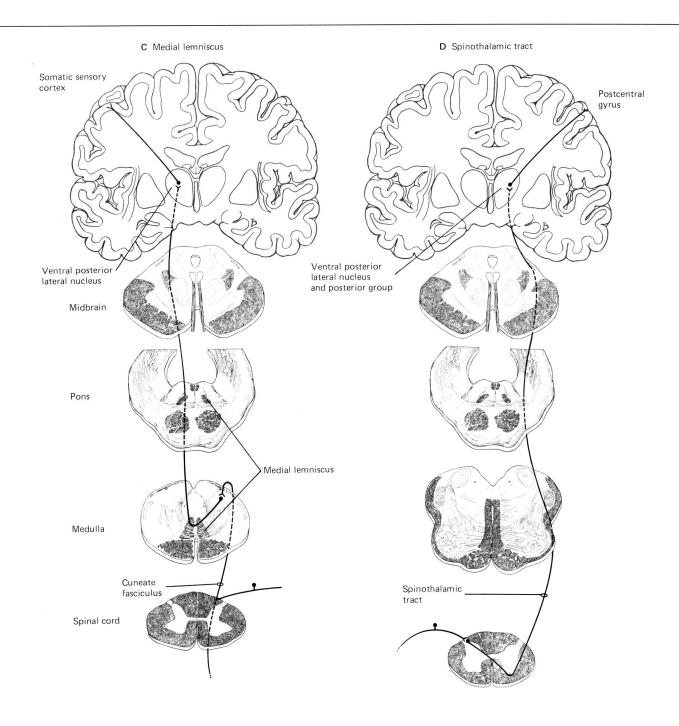

C Medial lemniscus

Somatic sensory cortex

Ventral posterior lateral nucleus

Midbrain

Pons

Medial lemniscus

Medulla

Cuneate fasciculus

Spinal cord

D Spinothalamic tract

Postcentral gyrus

Ventral posterior lateral nucleus and posterior group

Spinothalamic tract

41–14 Four major pathways course through the brain stem.
A. Corticospinal tract. **B.** Corticobulbar tract.
C. Medial lemniscal tract. **D.** Spinothalamic tract.

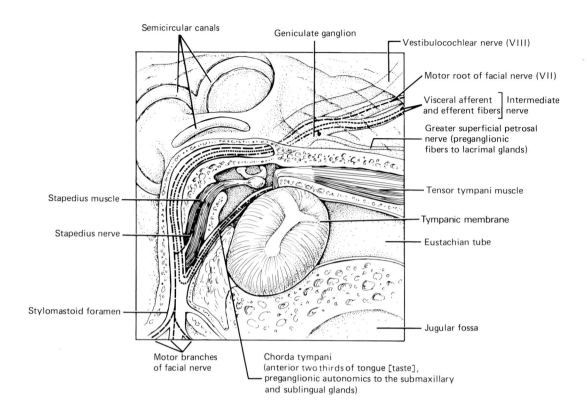

Semicircular canals

Geniculate ganglion

Vestibulocochlear nerve (VIII)

Motor root of facial nerve (VII)

Visceral afferent and efferent fibers] Intermediate nerve

Greater superficial petrosal nerve (preganglionic fibers to lacrimal glands)

Stapedius muscle

Tensor tympani muscle

Stapedius nerve

Tympanic membrane

Eustachian tube

Stylomastoid foramen

Jugular fossa

Motor branches of facial nerve

Chorda tympani (anterior two thirds of tongue [taste], preganglionic autonomics to the submaxillary and sublingual glands)

41–15 Fiber types mix along the peripheral course of the facial nerve.

nerve to reach the brain stem, where they synapse in the anterior one-third of the nucleus of the solitary tract.

On the basis of the anatomy we have just considered, it should now be possible to explain why a lesion in the facial nerve, as it exits from the brain stem in association with the intermediate nerve, would cause disturbances in the secretion of saliva and tears, an exceptionally acute sense of hearing, and a paralysis of the muscles of facial expression on the affected side, accompanied by a severe diminution in taste sensation from the anterior two-thirds of the tongue.

Reticular Neurons Form Widespread Networks

The reticular formation is composed of neurons that are outside the major nuclear groups of the brain stem. The reticular formation represents the rostral extension of the interneuronal network found in the spinal cord. In the brain stem, however, this network of neurons is more extensive than in the cord. We shall first examine the general distribution of reticular neurons and then consider their morphology and transmitter biochemistry. We shall end by considering some aspects of their function and their topological relationship to the major tracts of the brain stem.

The reticular formation is distributed throughout the medulla, pons, and midbrain and is most conveniently divided along a medial-to-lateral axis. Lying in the midline are the *raphe nuclei*, so named because of their proximity to the midline seam or raphe. Adjacent to the raphe is the *large-cell region* of the reticular formation; more laterally is the *small-cell region.* Two examples of discrete nuclear groups that can be identified in these broad subdivisions of the reticular formation at the level of the medulla are the *nucleus raphe magnus* and the *gigantocellular reticular nucleus* (Figure 41–16). We shall discuss the functions of these nuclei later in the chapter.

Although some reticular neurons such as those of the raphe nuclei are grouped in circumscribed clusters, most are not. Nearly all reticular neurons have an inordinately widespread network of connections. Thus, the unique feature of reticular neurons, irrespective of the nuclear group to which they belong, is the far-flung distribution of their axons, often in both rostral and caudal directions along the brain stem. An example of the axonal plexus established by a single gigantocellular reticular neuron is shown in Figure 41–17. The axon not only branches to reach the dorsal column nuclei and the spinal cord, but also ascends to terminate in the thalamus and hypothalamus. Reticular neurons thus can exert an extensive influence on the brain. However, not all reticular neurons branch in this manner. Some local regions of the reticular formation contain cells that send their axons either rostrally, to higher regions of the brain, or caudally to the spinal cord.

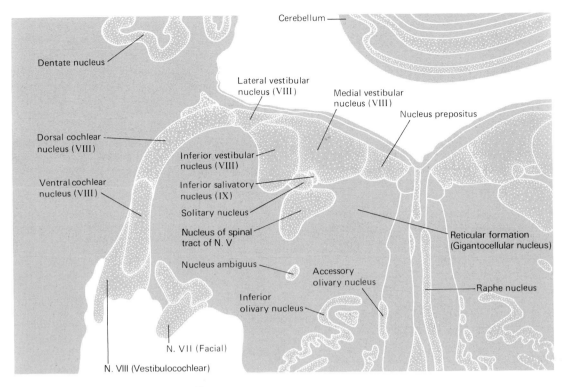

41–16 The location of some major reticular cell groups is shown through a section of the medulla. (Adapted from DeArmond, Fusco, and Dewey, 1976.)

41–17 The axonal plexus established by an individual gigantocellular neuron of the reticular formation is widespread, as shown by this example in a 2-day-old rat. It emits an axon that bifurcates into an ascending and a descending branch. The latter gives off collaterals to the adjacent gigantocellular reticular nucleus, the gracile nucleus, and the ventral horn in the spinal cord. The ascending branch gives off collaterals to the reticular formation and the periaqueductal gray matter and then appears to supply several thalamic nuclei (the parafascicular, paracentral, and others), the hypothalamus, and the zona incerta. (Adapted from Scheibel and Scheibel, 1958.)

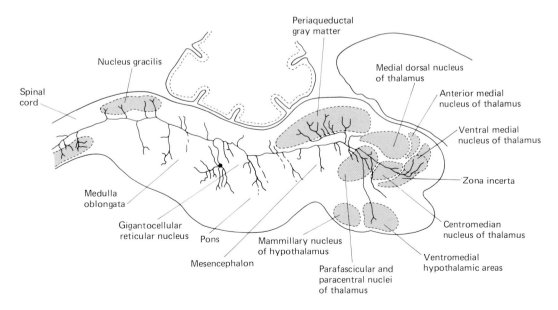

Some Reticular Neurons Are Grouped According to Their Chemical Messengers

Studies of the brain using histochemical techniques have shown that many reticular neurons contain biogenic amines and neuroactive peptides that presumably are used as chemical messengers. The three most prominent groups of reticular neurons are those that contain norepinephrine, dopamine, or serotonin. In sections of a brain that has been exposed to radiolabeled transmitter substances or treated with appropriate histochemical reagents, it is possible to identify the distinctive fluorescence emitted by each of these biogenic amines. In addition, the localization of specific peptide sequences can be determined immunocytochemically. The distribution of neurons containing monoamines and peptides can therefore be mapped throughout the extent of the reticular formation.

Noradrenergic System

The *locus ceruleus* (Latin, blue place), which lies in the caudal midbrain and upper pons at the lateral margin of the periaqueductal gray matter, is made up of noradrenergic neurons that have extensive axonal connections with the entire forebrain. At least five noradrenergic tracts, including the central tegmental tract, run rostrally from the locus ceruleus to the diencephalon and telencephalon; among their terminations are the hippocampus and cerebral cortex (Figure 41–18). Fibers from this nucleus also run through the superior cerebellar peduncle to reach the cerebellar cortex. Recent physiological studies by Roger Nicoll and his colleagues at the University of California in San Francisco have demonstrated that the axons of these neurons mediate an excitatory modu-

lation in the regions where they terminate. This excitatory modulation is due to the closure of a K$^+$ channel by means of cyclic AMP-dependent protein phosphorylation.

Dopaminergic System

The distribution of dopaminergic neurons in the brain stem was first mapped in 1964 by Annica Dahlström and Kjell Fuxe, two pioneers in the application of fluorescence microscopy to the brain. They found that the dopaminergic cells are grouped into small clusters at several loci in the brain stem. They identified these clusters with the letter *A* followed by a number (serotonin cell groups were labeled with a *B*). The distribution of axons arising from several dopaminergic cell groups is shown in Figure 41–19. Many dopaminergic neurons are found in the ventral tegmentum of the midbrain and in the adjacent substantia nigra. The axons of these cells are directed toward the basal ganglia (see Chapter 40), the hypothalamus and the limbic system (see Chapters 46 and 47), and the neocortex.

Serotonergic System

The clusters of serotonergic neurons, designated as groups B1–B9 by Dahlström and Fuxe, are found along the raphe. The connections established by some of these cell groups are illustrated in Figure 41–20. Immunocytochemical studies have revealed that most of the raphe neurons contain a neuroactive peptide as well as serotonin. This was first demonstrated by Tomas Hökfelt and his collaborators at the Karolinska Institute and by Victoria Chan-Palay at the Harvard Medical School, who showed that *individual* raphe cells and processes contain both substance P and serotonin. Coexistence in raphe

41–18 Connections established by the neurons of the locus ceruleus, which are noradrenergic (viewed in the sagittal plane). **AON,** anterior olfactory nucleus. **AP-VAB,** ansa peduncularis–ventral amygdaloid bundle system. **BS,** brain stem nuclei. **C,** cingulum. **CC,** corpus callosum. **CER,** cerebellum. **CTT,** central tegmental tract. **CTX,** cerebral neocortex. **DPS,** dorsal periventricular system. **DTB,** dorsal catecholamine bundle. **EC,** external capsule. **F,** fornix. **H,** hypothalamus. **HF,** hippocampal formation. **LC,** locus ceruleus. **ML,** medial lemniscus. **MT,** mamillothalamic tract. **OB,** olfactory bulb. **PC,** posterior commissure. **PT,** pretectal area. **RF,** reticular formation. **S,** septal area. **SC,** spinal cord. **ST,** stria terminalis. **T,** tectum. **TH,** thalamus. (Adapted from Cooper, Bloom, and Roth, 1982.)

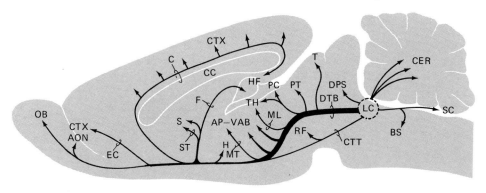

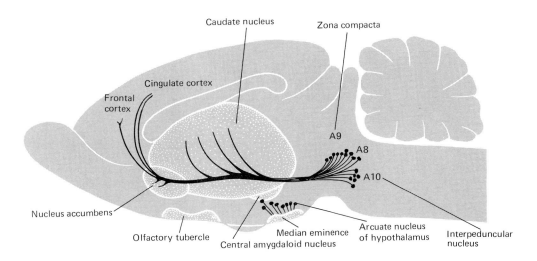

41–19 Connections of certain dopaminergic cell groups in the brain stem of the rat.

neurons was next shown for Leu-enkephalin, Met-enkephalin, and thyrotropin-releasing hormone. In a recent quantitative study making use of specific antibodies to serotonin and the peptides combined with neuroanatomical tracing using horseradish peroxidase, Joe Dan Coulter and his co-workers in Galveston have shown that a large majority of the raphe neurons that project to the spinal cord are serotonergic and that about half of them contain substance P immunoreactivity. The rest of the serotonergic raphe neurons were stained with antibodies either for the enkephalins or for thyrotropin-releasing hormone. Only a few of the neurons appeared to contain serotonin alone.

It therefore seems likely that the neurons that make up the raphe–spinal system consist of distinct sets of cells: some cells contain only serotonin, and others contain serotonin and a neuroactive peptide. The action of the nucleus raphe magnus on the dorsal horn of the spinal cord appears to be mediated by serotonin. Electrical stimulation of this nucleus inhibits the cells that give rise to the spinothalamic tract, and serotonin released iontophoretically onto spinothalamic neurons inhibits them. What then is the purpose of coexistence of a neu-

rotransmitter and a neuroactive peptide in the same terminal? Each population of raphe neurons with its different complement of chemical messengers could have different actions on spinal cord target cells. Raphe neurons with different chemical messengers might each project to different cells in the spinal cord; alternatively, different raphe neurons could control the activity of the same spinal cells, each in a different fashion.

Multiple chemical messengers could produce their different postsynaptic actions in several ways. For example, serotonin could act on a postsynaptic spinal neuron, and the peptide could act on adjacent spinal cells. The peptide could influence another neuron in the cord presyn-

41–20 Distribution of the main serotonin-containing pathways in the rat central nervous system. (Adapted from Cooper, Bloom, and Roth, 1982.)

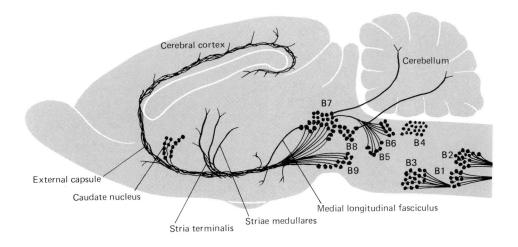

aptic to the serotonoceptive spinal cell or even modulate the transmission from the raphe neuron itself by acting on autoreceptors on the raphe neuron's terminal in the spinal cord. Enormous complexity in function can thus be coded by raphe neurons with quite specific properties.

Reticular neurons can influence the processing of sensory information not only at higher centers through connections to the thalamus, but also at lower levels—even at the initial level of input to the spinal cord. Despite the diversity of their targets, these neurons seem to make connections that are quite specific. Their connections, rather than being diffuse, therefore, are better described as being widespread. Presumably, the anatomical arrangement of the neurons of the reticular core, with projections to many distant parts of the central nervous system, and the diverse but nonetheless characteristic biochemical organization of their chemical messengers, endow these neurons with the capacity to regulate behavioral arousal and to control levels of mental awareness.

Reticular Neurons Have Several Functions

Because the reticular formation is composed of so many isolated cell clusters, it is difficult to study physiologically, although significant advances are being made in examining reticular control of motor events and sensory processing in the spinal cord. Originally the reticular core was thought to be a diffuse "activating" system that regulated general levels of activity in the brain. This view came from the work of Giuseppe Moruzzi and Horace Magoun, who stimulated the reticular formation of deeply anesthetized animals and produced changes in the overall electrical activity of the brain (as measured by the electroencephalogram). This stimulation transformed the electroencephalogram into a pattern resembling the awake state. However, as we have seen, recent anatomical studies have shown that the reticular formation is not diffusely organized at all, but instead is composed of many groups of neurons that are well defined morphologically and biochemically.

The "activation" of the brain for behavioral arousal and for controlling levels of awareness is evidently only one physiological role of the reticular core. At least three other functions, some of which have already been noted, are associated with the reticular formation:

First, it influences the modulation of segmental stretch reflexes and muscle tone by the medullary and pontine reticulospinal tracts. The reticulospinal axons principally originate in the medial regions of the pons and medulla, where large reticular neurons are found. The medullary reticulospinal tract arises from the gigantocellular reticular nucleus and terminates widely in the intermediate zone of the ventral horn from cervical to lumbar levels of the spinal cord. This tract exerts an inhibitory influence on extensor muscle tone. The pontine reticulospinal tract terminates near the motor nuclei of the anterior horn and it facilitates extensor muscle tone. The antagonistic activity of these two tracts is important for the control of motor function (discussed in Chapter 37).

Second, the reticular formation is involved in the control of breathing movements and cardiac function. Many reticular neurons that regulate respiration send their axons to the spinal cord, where they control the activity of motor neurons innervating the muscles for inhalation and exhalation. Reticular neurons important for cardiovascular functions receive input from a wide variety of peripheral receptors, including the carotid body, through a relay in the solitary tract. The activity of these neurons is also influenced from higher areas in the hypothalamus and prefrontal association cortex. The cardiovascular neurons regulate the output of preganglionic neurons associated with the vagus nerve and of preganglionic sympathetic neurons in the intermediolateral cell column of the spinal cord, and they can therefore accelerate or depress the heart rate in response to an appropriate stimulus.

Finally, reticulospinal pathways modulate the sense of pain by influencing the flow of information through the dorsal horn of the spinal cord (see Chapter 24).

Thus, the principal functions of the reticular formation (behavioral arousal, regulation of muscle reflexes, coordination of autonomic functions, and modulation of pain sensation) are carried out by neurons with widespread sets of connections unlike those found in the major sensory and motor systems. Even though many of its neurons are not grouped into distinct nuclei, the reticular formation is organized quite precisely to accomplish its functional role.

Selected Readings

Brodal, A. 1981. Neurological Anatomy in Relation to Clinical Medicine, 3rd ed. New York: Oxford University Press, Chapter 7.

Cooper, J. R., Bloom, F. E., and Roth, R. H. 1982. The Biochemical Basis of Neuropharmacology, 4th ed. New York: Oxford University Press.

Dahlström, A., and Fuxe, K. 1964. Evidence for the existence of monoamine-containing neurons in the central nervous system. Acta Physiol. Scand. Suppl. 232:1–55.

References

Bowker, R. M., Westlund, K. N., Sullivan, M. C., Wilber, J. F., and Coulter, J. D. 1983. Descending serotonergic, peptidergic and cholinergic pathways from the raphe nuclei: A multiple transmitter complex. Brain Res. 288:33–48.

Chan-Palay, V. 1979. Combined immunocytochemistry and autoradiography after in vivo injections of monoclonal antibody to substance P and ³H-serotonin: Coexistence of two putative transmitters in single raphe cells and fiber plexuses. Anat. Embryol. 156:241–254.

Clark, R. G. 1975. Manter and Gatz's Essentials of Clinical Neuroanatomy and Neurophysiology, 5th ed. Philadelphia: Davis.

DeArmond, S. J., Fusco, M. M., and Dewey, M. M. 1976. Structure of the Human Brain: A Photographic Atlas, 2nd ed. New York: Oxford University Press.

Hökfelt, T., Lundberg, J. M., Schultzberg, M., Johansson, O., Ljungdahl, Å., and Rehfeld, J. 1980. Coexistence of peptides and putative transmitters in neurons. In E. Costa and M. Trabucchi (eds.), Neural Peptides and Neuronal Communication. New York: Raven Press, pp. 1–23.

Molliver, M. E., Grzanna, R., Lidov, H. G. W., Morrison, J. H., and Olschowka, J. A. 1982. Monoamine systems in the cerebral cortex. In V. Chan-Palay and S. L. Palay, (eds.), Neurology and Neurobiology, Vol. 1: Cytochemical Methods in Neuroanatomy. New York: Liss, pp. 255–277.

Moruzzi, G., and Magoun, H. W. 1949. Brain stem reticular formation and activation of the EEG. Electroencephalogr. Clin. Neurophysiol. 1:455–473.

Nicoll, R. A. 1982. Neurotransmitters can say more than just "yes" or "no." Trends Neurosci. 5:369–374.

Ranson, S. W., and Clark, S. L. 1953. The Anatomy of the Nervous System: Its Development and Function, 9th ed. Philadelphia: Saunders.

Scheibel, M. E., and Scheibel, A. B. 1958. Structural substrates for integrative patterns in the brain stem reticular core. In H. H. Jasper, L. D. Proctor, et al. (eds.), Reticular Formation of the Brain (Henry Ford Hospital International Symposium). Boston: Little, Brown, pp. 31–55.

James P. Kelly

Trigeminal System

42

In this chapter we shall consider the structure, connections, and functions of neurons associated with the fifth cranial nerve. This nerve carries most of the sensory innervation to the face and the mucous membrane of the oral cavity and the motor innervation to the muscles of mastication. The most important principle that emerges from study of the trigeminal system is that *even when different modalities of sensation are carried from the periphery to the central nervous system by a single cranial nerve, they still are relayed to different sites in the brain.* This anatomical principle, which is evident in the projection of the dorsal roots to the spinal cord, is also essential for understanding the central trigeminal nuclei. As we shall see, information about pain and temperature, proprioception, and touch and pressure carried by the fifth nerve is relayed to distinct central sites. Each of these central trigeminal nuclei, in turn, has special connections with other parts of the brain, so that a separation of afferent connections according to modality is maintained at higher levels of the nervous system.

The Fifth Nerve Has Three Major
Peripheral Branches

The fifth cranial nerve is called *trigeminal* because it branches into three major peripheral nerves—the ophthalmic, the maxillary, and the mandibular—that exit from the skull through three separate openings: the superior orbital fissure, the foramen rotundum, and the foramen ovale, respectively. We shall first consider the sensory fibers of the nerve.

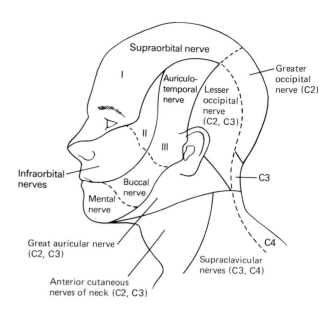

42–1 Different areas of the skin are innervated by the three branches of the trigeminal nerve: the ophthalmic (**I**), maxillary (**II**), and mandibular (**III**). (Adapted from Brodal, 1981.)

All Three Major Branches Contain Sensory Fibers

Sensory fibers with cell bodies in the trigeminal ganglion run in all three branches of the trigeminal nerve. The area of skin innervated by each branch is shown in Figure 42-1. The overlap in the areas is much smaller than the overlap in the spinal dermatomes of the trunk, but the overlap between the areas supplied by the fifth nerve and those supplied by the cervical dorsal roots is more extensive. In the perioral region there is bilateral overlap of innervation, so that unilateral destruction of the fifth nerve does not completely deprive this region of sensation on the affected side.

In the skin of the face, three physiological classes of receptors have been found: (1) mechanoreceptors, both rapidly adapting and slowly adapting; (2) thermoreceptors, sensitive to changes in skin temperature; and (3) nociceptors, sensitive to stimuli that damage the skin. Certain animals, most notably rodents, have whiskers, called *mystacial vibrissae*, on the hairy skin of the face. These whiskers are used to explore the physical environment around the animal's head and, as we shall see later, they have a unique pattern of representation in the somatic sensory part of the central nervous system.

The peripheral receptive fields of trigeminal touch fibers vary considerably in size, but they are smallest near the mouth. Nearly all these cells rapidly adapt to mechanical stimuli. Slowly adapting touch units rarely are present in hairy facial skin.

The trigeminal nerve provides sensory innervation to most of the oral mucosa, to the anterior two-thirds of the tongue, and to the dura mater of the anterior and middle cranial fossae. Sensory cells associated with the vagus nerve innervate the dura mater in the posterior cranial fossa. (As we saw in Chapter 41, taste is mediated by cranial nerves VII, IX, and X.) The trigeminal nerve also mediates the sensory innervation of tooth pulp as well as that of the surrounding gingiva and the periodontal membrane.

Autonomic Fibers Run with Branches of the Fifth Nerve

In the periphery, efferent autonomic fibers often join branches of the trigeminal nerve before they reach their final targets. An example is the autonomic and general sensory innervation of the eye (Figure 42–2). The *nasociliary nerve*, a branch of the ophthalmic division, innervates the sclera, the conjunctiva, and the cornea of the eye, and a portion of the nasal cavity. The several branches of the nasociliary nerve that innervate the eyeball are called *long ciliary nerves*. The ciliary ganglion is physically attached to one of the branches of the nasociliary nerve. This ganglion receives its input from a branch of the oculomotor nerve. Postganglionic axons leave the ganglion via the *short ciliary nerves* to reach the pupillary constrictor and the ciliary muscle of the eye. The sympathetic fibers innervating the pupillary dilator muscle have their cell bodies in the superior cervical ganglion. The axons of these cells course for a while in the internal carotid plexus, but they eventually leave to join the nasociliary nerve. The sympathetic axons may reach their final target by running in either the long or the short ciliary nerves. Unlike the roots of other cranial nerves that mediate autonomic functions, the root of the trigeminal does not contain autonomic axons; however, these axons are commonly associated with branches of the nerve in the periphery. There may be some special developmental affinity between trigeminal and autonomic axons, or, alternatively, the wide peripheral spread of the trigeminal nerve may simply make it a convenient pathway for autonomic fibers to reach peripheral targets.

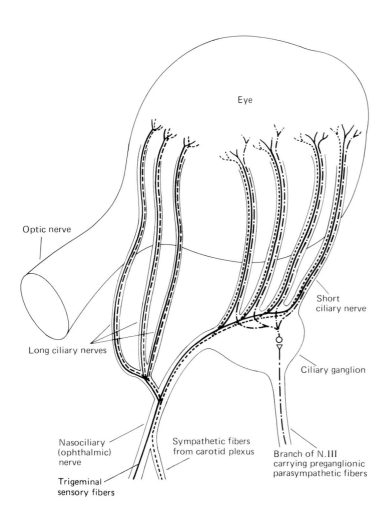

42–2 Efferent autonomic fibers join the sensory fibers of the nasociliary nerve to innervate the eye.

Fifth Nerve Fibers Ascend to the Main Sensory Nucleus and Descend to the Spinal Nucleus

The central branches of the afferent neurons in the trigeminal ganglion enter the pontine region of the brain stem. There are relatively few unmyelinated fibers in the fifth nerve. The numbers of myelinated and unmyelinated fibers entering the brain stem in the trigeminal nerve root are about equal. This contrasts with most spinal nerves, for which this ratio is nearly 1:4. Like dorsal root fibers, the majority of entering nerve fibers bifurcate into ascending and descending branches (Figure 42–3). The ascending branch terminates in the main sensory nucleus of the trigeminal nerve located in the pons. The descending branch runs in the descending or spinal tract of the trigeminal nerve to terminate in the descending or spinal nucleus of the trigeminal nerve. A few fibers do not branch but go directly to either the main sensory nucleus or the spinal tract of nerve V. The similarity between the connections of the trigeminal fibers and the connections of dorsal root fibers is quite striking. The main sensory nucleus of nerve V corresponds to the dorsal column nuclei. The spinal tract and nucleus of nerve V correspond to the tract of Lissauer and to the substantia gelatinosa of the dorsal horn, respectively. In fact, the descending

tract and nucleus of the trigeminal complex become continuous with their spinal homologues in the upper cervical region of the cord.

The Mesencephalic Nucleus of the Fifth Nerve Mediates Proprioception from the Muscles of the Jaws

The mesencephalic nucleus (Figure 42–3) of the trigeminal nerve extends from the rostral end of the main sensory nucleus to the superior colliculus. It consists of a column of monopolar primary sensory neurons. This is the only instance in which the cell bodies of primary sensory neurons lie within the adult vertebrate central nervous system. The peripheral branches of the mesencephalic neurons innervate stretch receptors in the jaw muscles and mechanoreceptors in the periodontal membrane. A collateral branch from the mesencephalic nucleus goes directly to the motor nucleus of the trigeminal nerve (Figure 42–3), providing a monosynaptic reflex arc to the motor neurons similar to the stretch reflex mediated by the Ia spindle afferents in the spinal cord. For example, depressing the lower jaw by pressing on the mandibular teeth causes a reflex contraction of the mus-

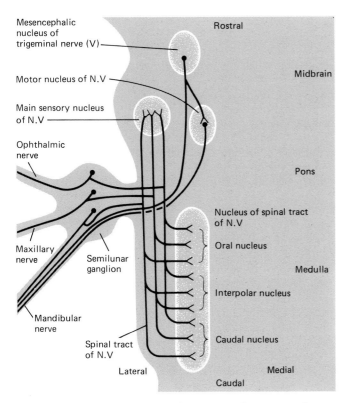

Mesencephalic nucleus of trigeminal nerve (V)

Motor nucleus of N.V

Main sensory nucleus of N.V

Ophthalmic nerve

Maxillary nerve

Semilunar ganglion

Mandibular nerve

Spinal tract of N.V

Rostral

Midbrain

Pons

Nucleus of spinal tract of N.V

Oral nucleus

Medulla

Interpolar nucleus

Caudal nucleus

Lateral   Medial

Caudal

42–3 Central connections of the trigeminal nerve are shown schematically in the horizontal plane.

cles of mastication (the jaw reflex) that is mediated by this set of connections. The trigeminal motor neurons send their axons into the mandibular nerve to supply the masseter, temporalis, and pterygoid muscles. The motor nucleus of nerve V, which lies in the pons near the main sensory nucleus (see Figure 42–6), also innervates the anterior belly of the digastric muscle, the mylohyoid, and the tensor tympani.

The Spinal Tract and Nucleus of the Fifth Nerve Mediate Pain and Temperature Sensation

Let us now consider the anatomy of the sensory nuclei within the trigeminal complex in greater detail. Primary trigeminal fibers, descending in the spinal tract of nerve V, are organized somatotopically. The location of this tract and its associated nucleus is shown in Figure 42–4.

Sensory fibers from the ophthalmic division of the nerve are found ventrolaterally in the tract, fibers from the mandibular division are found dorsomedially, and fibers from the maxillary division lie in between. Thus, there is an inverted representation of the ipsilateral face in the spinal tract of nerve V. Primary sensory fibers from other cranial nerves (VII, IX, and X) also enter the descending tract of nerve V. These fibers carry input from a portion of the skin of the external ear, the larynx, and the pharynx.

Most of the superficial fibers in the spinal tract of the fifth nerve are myelinated and tend to be larger (2–8 μm in diameter) than the fibers located at the internal aspect of the tract. Most of the internal fibers are unmyelinated and small (less than 1 μm in diameter). If the root of the trigeminal nerve is severed at its point of entry into the brain stem, the superficial fibers of the spinal tract degenerate but the deep fibers do not, indicating that the fine internal fibers are of local origin.

Near their point of termination, fibers in the descending tract turn abruptly inward and ramify in the underlying *spinal nucleus* of the fifth nerve. This nucleus is continuous with the main sensory nucleus of the fifth nerve rostrally and descends caudally to the level of C2 in the spinal cord.

42–4 The location of the spinal tract and nucleus of the fifth nerve is shown in a cross section through the medulla stained for myelin. (Adapted from Ranson and Clark, 1953.)

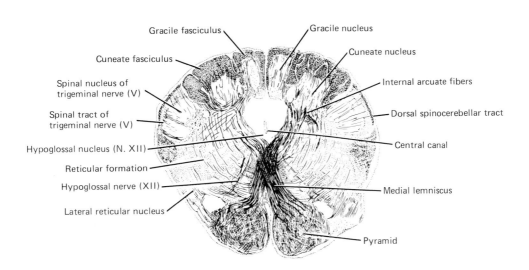

Gracile fasciculus

Cuneate fasciculus

Spinal nucleus of trigeminal nerve (V)

Spinal tract of trigeminal nerve (V)

Hypoglossal nucleus (N. XII)

Reticular formation

Hypoglossal nerve (XII)

Lateral reticular nucleus

Gracile nucleus

Cuneate nucleus

Internal arcuate fibers

Dorsal spinocerebellar tract

Central canal

Medial lemniscus

Pyramid

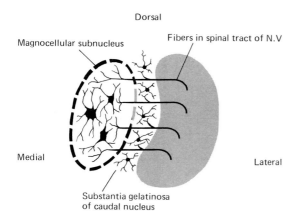

Dorsal

Magnocellular subnucleus

Fibers in spinal tract of N.V

Medial

Lateral

Substantia gelatinosa
of caudal nucleus

42–5 A cross section through the caudal nucleus of the fifth nerve shows the external part (substantia gelatinosa) and the internal part (magnocellular subnucleus) of the nucleus.

The spinal nucleus has three clear subdivisions along its rostrocaudal extent. The caudal part of the spinal nucleus is called the *caudal nucleus* (Figure 42–3). It is organized just like the dorsal horn of the spinal cord (Figure 42–5). The external part of the caudal nucleus underlying the spinal tract is called the *substantia gelatinosa.* The internal part of the nucleus is composed of large cells and is called the *magnocellular subnucleus.* The large cells are similar to those seen in the deeper laminae of the dorsal horn in the spinal cord. More rostrally near the obex, a change occurs in the structure of the spinal nucleus of the trigeminal nerve. It becomes filled with scattered small cells and is called the *interpolar nucleus* (Figure 42–3). More rostral still (just caudal to the main sensory nucleus), the cells of the spinal nucleus become tightly packed; this segment of the spinal nucleus of nerve V is termed the *oral nucleus* (Figure 42–3). The subdivisions of the nucleus of the spinal tract of the trigeminal nerve have different functional roles, and we shall consider these in the following sections of this chapter.

Caudal Nucleus. Trigeminal neuralgia is a very distressing condition of unknown etiology that is characterized by severe paroxysmal pain in the face without any local damage to the skin or skull. One treatment for this ailment is to sever the nerve V root, thereby depriving the face of its sensory innervation. This operation offers relief in most patients, but it has several deleterious side effects. Cutting the fifth nerve interrupts the afferent limb of the blinking reflex by making the cornea anesthetic, so that *keratitis* (a drying out and thickening of the cornea) tends to develop.

During the 1930s the neurosurgeon Olof Sjöqvist found that the fine fibers of the trigeminal root terminate selectively in the caudal nucleus. He therefore suggested that cutting the spinal tract of nerve V just before it enters the caudal nucleus might remove the pain fibers selectively, leaving the other aspects of facial sensation intact. The operation is anatomically possible because the

spinal tract and nucleus of nerve V bulge out of the lateral aspect of the medulla, forming the *tuberculum cinereum,* a structure that can be visualized directly. This operation, called the *medullary or trigeminal tractotomy of Sjöqvist,* often alleviates trigeminal neuralgia without totally eliminating facial sensation.

Because of the success of Sjöqvist's neurosurgical procedure, Patrick Wall and Arthur Taub suggested in 1962 that the caudal nucleus would be a good site to study the properties of specific nociceptors. They examined the responses of cells in the caudal nucleus of anesthetized cats while mechanical stimuli were delivered to the face. Unexpectedly, they could find no neurons that were selectively responsive to noxious stimuli in the awake animal. These physiological observations made the success of the Sjöqvist procedure seem puzzling. However, further experiments done in 1973 by Lawrence Kruger and his colleagues on the caudal nucleus of the trigeminal nerve provided the explanation: most cells in the magnocellular subnucleus (which is equivalent to the nucleus proprius of the dorsal horn) are sensitive to light mechanical stimuli delivered to the skin of the face; other cells are selectively responsive to vibratory stimuli; and still others respond to light touch of the cornea. In the substantia gelatinosa of the caudal nucleus (Figure 42–5), however, many cells respond only to strong mechanical stimuli that are painful in the awake cat. Specific nociceptors are most probably confined to this subdivision of the caudal nucleus, and because these cells are small and it is difficult to record from them, they could have been missed by Wall and Taub. Specific thermoreceptors also appear to be confined to the substantia gelatinosa of the caudal nucleus. As we shall see in the next section, the caudal nucleus also mediates the innervation of the tooth pulp.

Interpolar Nucleus. The interpolar nucleus, which is adjacent to the caudal nucleus, plays an important role in mediating dental pain. It has been known for some time that sectioning the peripheral branches of the fifth-nerve ganglion cells does not lead to complete degeneration of their central processes. In fact, this is true of all sensory ganglion cells associated with the cranial nerves, and of dorsal root ganglion cells as well. However, Lesnick Westrum, Stephen Gobel, and their colleagues found that the central branches of the trigeminal ganglion cells degenerate completely if peripheral fifth-nerve axons are cut and then prevented from reforming connections with their original terminals. This shows clearly that trophic interactions between axons and target organs are important biologically, and that blocking these interactions can have a widespread effect on the neurons in a given pathway. This example has direct clinical relevance as well, since tooth pulp removal, accompanied by filling of the pulp chamber and root canal, is a routine practice used to halt the spread of carious infection. Westrum and Gobel removed the pulp from all the mandibular teeth on one side of the jaw in rats. When the pulp is removed, the receptors connected with fifth-nerve axons innervating the pulp are destroyed and the axons

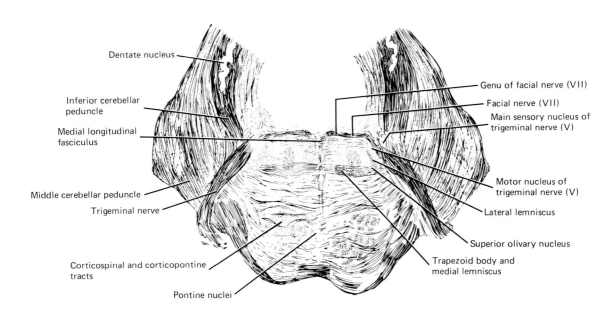

Dentate nucleus

Inferior cerebellar
peduncle

Medial longitudinal
fasciculus

Middle cerebellar peduncle

Trigeminal nerve

Corticospinal and corticopontine
tracts

Pontine nuclei

Genu of facial nerve (VII)

Facial nerve (VII)

Main sensory nucleus of
trigeminal nerve (V)

Motor nucleus of
trigeminal nerve (V)

Lateral lemniscus

Superior olivary nucleus

Trapezoid body and
medial lemniscus

42–6 The location of the main sensory nucleus of the fifth nerve is shown in a section through the pons stained for myelin. (Adapted from Ranson and Clark, 1953.)

themselves are cut. When the pulp chamber and the root canal are filled with dental cement, the pulp afferents are prevented from reaching receptors in their original terminal site. Deprived of their connections with the periphery, the trigeminal neurons innervating the pulp degenerate.

With the neuroanatomical tracing method described in Chapter 4, the degenerating central terminals of these neurons can be found principally in the interpolar nucleus, an important locus in the mediation of pain from the tooth pulp. There is in this nucleus a bilateral sensory representation of the pulp from an individual tooth. Electron microscopy or silver staining by the Nauta method demonstrates that there are degenerating terminals in this nucleus that occur on *both* sides of the brain in the rat. In addition, some degenerating terminals are also found in the substantia gelatinosa of the caudal nucleus. Finally, about a month after removal of the pulp, transneuronal degeneration occurs in the central sites where tooth pulp afferents terminate. When the pulp afferents degenerate, neurons receiving synapses from them are deprived of their normal input and undergo a transneuronal atrophy characterized by severe shrinkage of the cell body and dendrites.

Oral Nucleus. The oral nucleus, which lies immediately rostral to the interpolar nucleus, appears to contain a portion of the representation of tactile sense from mucous membranes in the mouth.

The Main Sensory Nucleus Mediates Touch Sensation from the Face

The receptive fields of the cells in the main sensory nucleus are confined largely to the ipsilateral side of the face. Most of these cells have small receptive fields (about 5 mm in diameter) and respond to light mechanical stimuli. Tactile sensation from the teeth is repre-

sented in a distinct dorsomedial segment of the nucleus. The location of the main sensory nucleus is illustrated in the tissue section stained for myelin in Figure 42–6.

Ascending Information from the Trigeminal Complex Reaches the Cortex via the Thalamus

Cells in the caudal nucleus send their rostrally directed axons to the other parts of the spinal nucleus as well as to the intralaminar nuclei and the posterior group of thalamic nuclei on both sides of the brain. The intralaminar nuclei lie in the medullary lamina, or fiber bundle, that separates the major thalamic nuclei. The posterior group of nuclei is a poorly defined collection of cells lying just behind the ventral posterior nucleus of the thalamus. The terminal sites of the caudal nucleus are similar to those of the anterolateral system, a pathway also concerned with the mediation of pain. As in the anterolateral system, the ascending efferents from the caudal nucleus also have collateral branches that terminate in the reticular formation of the brain stem.

Most of the cells in the main sensory nucleus of nerve V, along with the cells in the oral nucleus and the interpolar nucleus, send their axons to the contralateral side of the brain, where they join with the medial lemniscus and terminate in the *medial* part of the *ventral posterior* nucleus of the thalamus. There is a small *ipsilateral* projection to the ventral posterior medial nucleus from the main sensory nucleus of the trigeminal nerve; the tract carrying these fibers is the *dorsal trigeminal tract*. In monkeys and humans, a curved, cell-free band separates the medial part of the ventral posterior nucleus (also

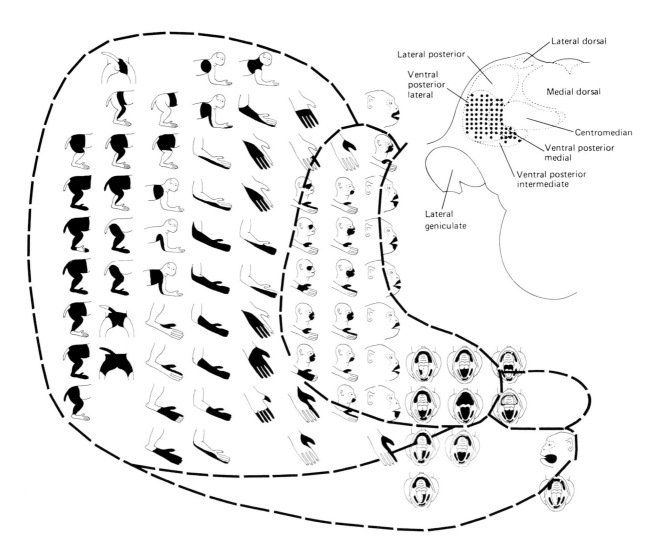

42–7 The somatotopic organization in the ventral posterior lateral and medial nuclei of the thalamus in the monkey has been determined by the evoked potential technique. The drawing of the thalamus was prepared from a frontal section of the brain in the plane of electrode penetrations; **dots** indicate positive points, and each figurine drawing is arranged accordingly. Tactile stimulation of the skin of the areas marked on the figurines evoked responses at the points indicated. With the exception of ipsilateral intraoral and perioral regions, all responses were obtained only from stimulation of the contralateral side of the body and head. (Adapted from Mountcastle and Henneman, 1952.)

called the *arcuate nucleus*) from the lateral part, which is devoted to the somatic sensory representation of the rest of the body. In the ventral posterior medial nucleus, there is a somatotopic representation of the contralateral half of the face. The lower jaw is represented most ventrally and the mouth is represented closest to the midline, as shown in Figure 42–7.

From the ventral posterior medial nucleus of the thalamus, axons run to the face region in the primary somatic sensory cortex, which occupies most of the postcentral gyrus, where there is a complete representation of the contralateral face and a bilateral representation of the perioral region (Figure 42–7). The receptive fields of neurons in the face region of the somatic sensory cortex tend to be about two times larger than those seen at lower levels of the trigeminal system, and they have more pronounced inhibitory surrounds. The representation of the face lies in the ventrolateral part of the postcentral gyrus. The area of the cortex devoted to the mouth, perioral region, and tongue is disproportionately large with respect to the representation of other parts of the face because the peripheral innervation density is greatest in the region of the mouth.

Ventral and posterior to the primary somatic sensory cortex is the secondary somatic sensory cortex, which is smaller than the primary cortex but contains a complete representation of the entire body surface. The projection from the ventral posterior medial nucleus to the cortex terminates principally in the primary somatic sensory cortex. The secondary somatic sensory cortex receives a substantial part of its thalamic input from the sites where the spinothalamic tract and the caudal nucleus of the spinal tract of nerve V terminate most heavily, particularly the posterior group of nuclei; but fibers from the

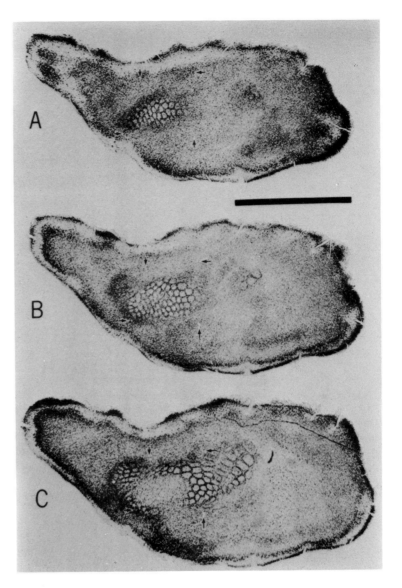

42–8 Neurons are arranged in discrete units, or barrels, in layer IV of the somatic sensory cortex of the mouse as shown in photomicrographs of three serial tangential sections. Orientation: anterior, **left;** posterior, **right;** medial, **up;** lateral, **down. Arrows** point to some of the vessels that, appearing in subsequent sections, are commonly used to spatially relate serially cut sections to one another. Formalin fixation, methylene blue-Cl, 50-μm thick sections. **Bar:** 2 mm. **A.** Most superficial of the three sections. **B.** Next section. **C.** Deepest of the three. (Adapted from Woolsey and Van der Loos, 1970.)

ventral posterior medial nucleus also terminate in this cortex. Some cells in the posterior group have branching axons that terminate in both the primary and secondary somatic sensory cortices. The receptive fields of neurons in the posterior group are large and often include the face. Many cells in this part of the thalamus are *polysensory:* an individual neuron may respond both to stroking of the facial skin and to auditory stimuli. Further work on the anatomy and physiology of the posterior group is required to define its functional role unequivocally.

Whiskers in Rodents Have a Unique Functional Representation in the Cerebral Cortex

As Thomas Woolsey and Hendrik Van der Loos showed in 1970, animals with mystacial vibrissae have a unique arrangement of cells in the portion of the somatic sensory cortex representing the face. The whiskers of the rodent are important tactile receptors, and their pattern

is quite regular and similar from animal to animal. At the base or follicle of an individual vibrissa, specialized receptors transduce the bending of the hairs into electrical activity in afferent fibers of the trigeminal nerve. Each whisker is innervated by a separate vibrissal nerve containing about 100 myelinated fibers. Recordings from these fibers show them to be sensitive to movements of the whiskers. The fibers have their cell bodies in the trigeminal ganglion and their central terminals in the main sensory nucleus and the oral nucleus of the descending trigeminal complex. As we have seen, these nuclei project to the ventral posterior medial nucleus of the thalamus, which in turn projects to the primary somatic sensory cortex.

In layer IV of the somatic sensory cortex, where the fibers from the ventral posterior medial nucleus terminate, the neurons are arranged in discrete functional units called *barrels* (Figure 42–8). This organization of the central representation of whisker stimuli is similar

Table 42–1. Functions of Trigeminal Nuclei

Nucleus	Function
Main sensory	Cutaneous sensation from skin of the face and from the oral mucosa; tactile sensation from the teeth
Spinal tract	
Oral	Cutaneous sensation from the oral mucosa
Interpolar	Sensation of pain from the tooth pulp
Caudal	Pain, temperature, and light touch from the skin of the face; sensation of pain from the tooth pulp
Mesencephalic	Proprioception from the muscles of the face and the extraocular muscles; jaw reflex arc
Motor	Motor innervation to muscles of mastication (masseter, temporalis, and pterygoid muscles), to the tensor tympani and tensor palati, and to the anterior belly of the digastric muscle

in principle to the columnar organization described in Chapter 25 for the somatic sensory system and in Chapter 28 for the visual system. A single barrel contains about 2500 neurons arranged in a cylindrical array around a hollow center. Each barrel processes tactile input derived from a single whisker. The number of barrels is the same as the number of whiskers on the contralateral face, and the barrels are arranged in a regular pattern that corresponds to the topography of the whiskers.

An Overall View

The functional role of each of the central trigeminal nuclei is summarized in Table 42–1. Underlying the organization of the trigeminal nerve is the general principle that the motor output and the different modalities of sensation are processed by separate nuclei in the brain stem. The caudal nucleus of the spinal tract of nerve V, for example, is concerned with pain and temperature sensation in the head, but not only from regions innervated by the fifth nerve. Both the seventh and tenth nerves innervate a small patch of skin in the concha of the ear, and the tenth nerve innervates the dura mater in the posterior cranial fossa. The cell bodies that give rise to the sensory axons lie in the geniculate and jugular ganglia associated with nerves VII and X. The central branches of the sensory neurons terminate in the nucleus of the spinal tract of nerve V, along with trigeminal fibers. Thus, even though sensory information from the head reaches the brain by different paths, this information converges in a single locus for further processing. As a result, the skin of the face, the oral mucosa, and the dura mater are represented by a continuous map in the spinal nucleus of the trigeminal system, even though these regions are innervated by several different cranial nerves.

Selected Readings

Brodal, A. 1981. Neurological Anatomy in Relation to Clinical Medicine, 3rd ed. New York: Oxford University Press, pp. 508–532.

Gobel, S., and Binck, J. M. 1977. Degenerative changes in primary trigeminal axons and in neurons in nucleus caudalis following tooth pulp extirpations in the cat. Brain Res. 132:347–354.

Mosso, J. A., and Kruger, L. 1973. Receptor categories represented in spinal trigeminal nucleus caudalis. J. Neurophysiol. 36:472–488.

Sjöqvist, O. 1938. Studies on pain conduction in the trigeminal nerve. Acta Psychiatr. Neurol. [Suppl.] 17:1–139.

Wall, P. D., and Taub, A. 1962. Four aspects of trigeminal nucleus and a paradox. J. Neurophysiol. 25:110–126.

Woolsey, T. A., and Van der Loos, H. 1970. The structural organization of layer IV in the somatosensory region (S I) of mouse cerebral cortex. The description of a cortical field composed of discrete cytoarchitectonic units. Brain Res. 17:205–242.

References

Mountcastle, V. B., and Henneman, E. 1952. The representation of tactile sensibility in the thalamus of the monkey. J. Comp. Neurol. 97:409–439.

Ranson, S. W., and Clark, S. L. 1953. The Anatomy of the Nervous System: Its Development and Function, 9th ed. Philadelphia: Saunders.

Westrum, L. E., Canfield, R. C., and Black, R. G. 1976. Transganglionic degeneration in the spinal trigeminal nucleus following removal of tooth pulps in adult cats. Brain Res. 101:137–140.

Peter Gouras

Oculomotor System

43

We move our eyes to locate, see, and track objects in visual space. The parts of the brain that control eye movement are collectively called the *oculomotor system*. Because the eyeball is a constant load, the repertoire of eye movements produced by this motor system is more predictable than is the repertoire of limb movements. There are five principal movements; these movements and the conditions that elicit them can be defined and analyzed quantitatively. We shall first examine the five movements and then consider how they are controlled by motor neurons and premotor cells in the brain.

Three Pairs of Muscles Move the Eyeball along Three Axes

The eyes can be rotated around any axis, but for descriptive purposes it is helpful to use a three-dimensional model based on three imaginary axes that intersect in the center of the eyeball: vertical, horizontal, and torsional axes (Figure 43–1). Around the vertical axis the eyeball rotates from side to side in *adducting* (toward) or *abducting* (away from) movements. Rotation around the horizontal axis leads to eye movements that are directed upward *(elevation)* or downward *(depression)*. Torsional movements occur around an anterior–posterior axis and are either clockwise or counterclockwise. When the upper cornea moves in a circular arc in the nasal direction, the movement is called *intorsion;* when it moves in the temporal direction, the movement is called *extorsion.*

Eye movements are controlled by three antagonistic pairs of muscles: the lateral and medial recti, the superior and inferior oblique, and the superior and inferior recti (Figure 43–2). Although all of the

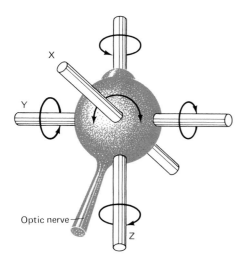

43–1 The three principal axes of rotation (shown for the right eye) are the vertical axis (**X**), which is also the center of motion, the transverse axis (**Y**), and the anterior–posterior axis (**Z**).

In most eye movements both eyes move together in the same direction. These movements are called *conjugate*. In convergence or divergence, however, the eyes move in opposite directions; these movements are called *disjunctive.* Two muscles that are excited together in a movement are called a *yoked pair*—for example, the lateral and medial recti of opposite eyes in horizontal conjugate movements. Muscles that oppose each other are called *antagonistic*—for example, the lateral recti of both eyes in horizontal movements. Antagonistic pairs for conjugate eye movements share the same nuclei on opposite sides of the brain stem. Since eye movements involving pairs of antagonistic muscles are common, strong inhibitory interactions are important in governing the activity of the motor nuclei for these muscles.

The movements of some eye muscles are among the fastest in the body. In contrast to other striated muscles, the extraocular muscles do not pull against gravity, and they carry the same mechanical load throughout life. The relatively few muscle spindles that do exist in extraocular muscles undoubtedly play a more general role in proprioception, possibly in muscle coordination or spatial orientation via the cerebellum.

Extraocular muscles are innervated by three cranial nerves. The medial, inferior, and superior recti, and the inferior oblique muscles are innervated by motor neurons of the oculomotor nerves, the nuclei of which are located in the midbrain at the level of the superior colliculus. The superior oblique muscle is innervated by the trochlear nerve. Like the oculomotor nucleus, the trochlear nucleus is located in the midbrain but at the level of the inferior colliculus. The lateral rectus muscle is innervated by the abducens nerve. The abducens nucleus

extraocular muscles contribute to some degree to all eye movement by either contracting or relaxing, each movement is determined by only two muscles in any one plane. Thus, the lateral and medial recti are chiefly responsible for moving the eyes horizontally. Both the superior and inferior oblique and the superior and inferior recti can move the eye vertically as well as torsionally; their exact contribution to vertical or torsional movement depends upon the position of the eye in the orbit (Figure 43–3 and Table 43–1).

43–2 The origins and insertions of the three pairs of extraocular muscles.

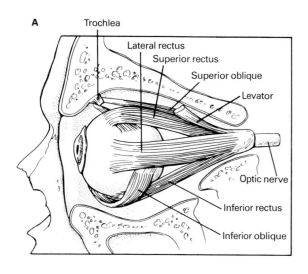

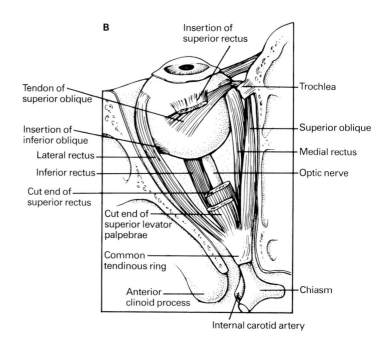

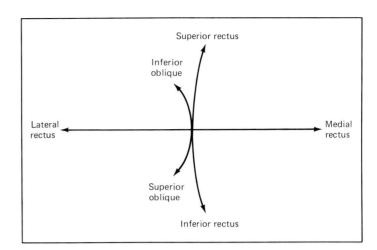

43–3 This scheme, devised by Ewald Hering, shows how each individual extraocular muscle operating alone would move the right eye as you looked at it. (Adapted from Hering, 1879.)

can be seen as a small bump in the floor of the fourth ventricle. This bump is actually called the *facial colliculus* because it is formed by the facial nerve wrapping around and over the abducens nucleus.

These motor neuron complexes in the brain stem that give rise to the three oculomotor nerves that move the eyeball are called the *oculomotor nuclei* (Figure 43–4). Neural signals coordinating the oculomotor nuclei with each other and with the vestibular system are carried in part in the medial longitudinal fasciculus. This pathway is a paired structure that runs just beneath the floor of the ventricle on both sides of the midline. Lesions of one side of the medial longitudinal fasciculus cause a specific clinical syndrome in humans. The deficits in horizontal conjugate gaze caused by this lesion have been pinned down to the interruption of the axons of one specific cell type, the axons of abducens internuclear neurons.

One of the major purposes of the oculomotor system is to keep images centered on the retinal region of greatest visual acuity. Although we can detect objects over a large visual angle (about 200°), we see them best within a relatively small arc in our visual field, the central 5°. This central area of high visual acuity corresponds to the fovea, a discrete retinal structure about 1 mm in diameter that we considered in Chapter 27 (Figure 43–5). Optimal examination of objects in our visual environment requires that images be kept on the fovea for seconds or even minutes. If an object tends to wander off the fovea the motor system can correct the slippage by moving the head, body, or eyes.

Five Neural Control Systems Keep the Fovea on Target

The oculomotor system puts the fovea on target and keeps it there by means of five separate neural control systems, each sharing the same effector pathway—the motor neurons of the oculomotor nuclei in the brain stem. The five systems are saccadic eye movement, smooth pursuit movement, optokinetic movement, vestibulo-oculomotor reflex, and vergence movement.

Table 43–1. Innervation and Actions of the Extraocular Muscles

Cranial nerve	Muscle	Main action	Subsidiary action
III	Superior rectus	Elevator, maximal on lateral gaze	Adduction, intorsion
III	Inferior oblique	Elevator, maximal on medial gaze	Abduction, extorsion
III	Inferior rectus	Depressor, maximal on lateral gaze	Adduction, extorsion
IV	Superior oblique	Depressor, maximal on medial gaze	Abduction, intorsion
VI	Lateral rectus	Abductor	None
III	Medial rectus	Adductor	None

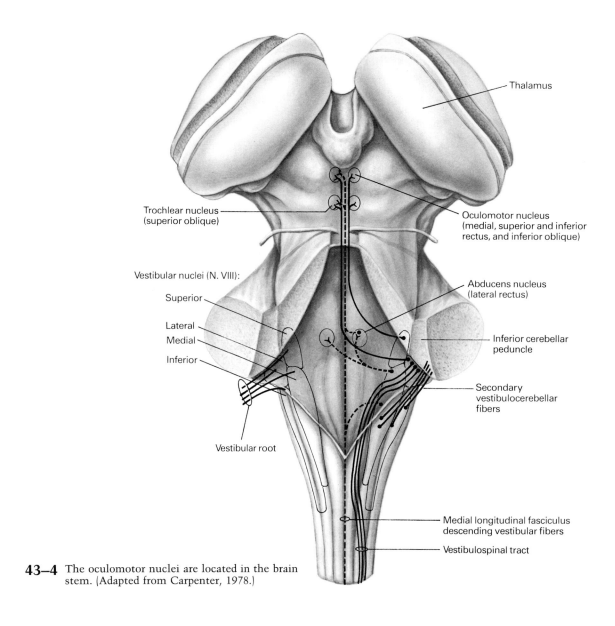

Thalamus

Trochlear nucleus
(superior oblique)

Oculomotor nucleus
(medial, superior and inferior
rectus, and inferior oblique)

Vestibular nuclei (N. VIII):

Superior

Abducens nucleus
(lateral rectus)

Lateral

Medial

Inferior

Inferior cerebellar
peduncle

Secondary
vestibulocerebellar
fibers

Vestibular root

Medial longitudinal fasciculus
descending vestibular fibers

Vestibulospinal tract

43–4 The oculomotor nuclei are located in the brain
stem. (Adapted from Carpenter, 1978.)

Saccadic Eye Movement System

The saccadic eye movement system is responsible for
rapidly directing the fovea to a target of interest in visual
space. This system generates a conjugate, ballistic movement of the eyes, called a *saccade*, that brings the fovea
on a target. Saccades are extremely fast, taking place
within a fraction of a second, at speeds of up to 600°–
700°/sec. There is a distinct advantage in this speed because vision becomes blurred during an eye movement.
A saccadic eye movement is called ballistic because once
initiated, it is extremely difficult to correct in flight.
There is a delay of about 0.2 sec between spotting the
target and initiating the saccade. After this latent period,
it takes about 0.05 sec for the movement to be completed. Once the saccadic process has been initiated, the
system is unable to make another saccade until 0.2 sec

later, regardless of target behavior. For example, if a target is moved during that fraction of a second when the
eye is making a saccade toward it, the fovea will always
end up at the position where the target was at the beginning of the saccade. The ballistic nature of the saccade
appears to be alterable only by a simultaneous vestibular
input, such as occurs when the head moves during a saccade. Despite their ballistic nature, saccades may be under continuous feedback control, as the model of Figure
43–14 implies.

The speed with which a monkey can make horizontal
saccades is shown in Figure 43–6. Eye movements that
monkeys make are about twice as fast as those of humans. The saccadic eye movement system depends on
both retinal position and eye position. The movement
requires that the retina first sense the location of a target
in visual space (retinal position); the movement also de-

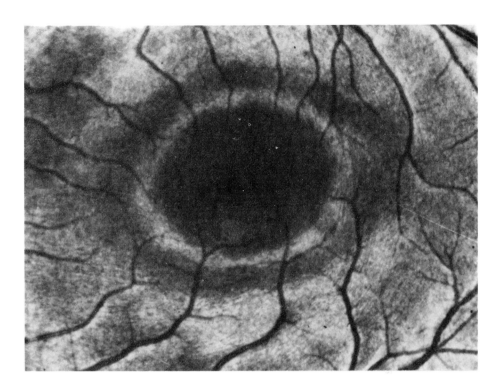

43–5 The human fovea is approximately 1 mm in diameter. The oculomotor systems keep images centered on this area of high visual acuity.

pends upon the initial position of the eyes in the orbit when the object is sighted (eye position). Both retinal position and eye position are taken into account before the command for a saccade is initiated. The brain must continuously monitor the position of the eye in the orbit so that it can deliver an appropriate command for a saccade. This command then includes information about the direction and amplitude of the saccade. The direction of the saccade is coded by exciting the appropriate group of motor neurons, and its amplitude is coded by the duration (pulse-width control) of their discharge frequency.

Saccades are also under voluntary control and can be made in the dark or with closed eyes. Part of the command center appears to be located in the cerebral cortex, which sends signals to the brain stem that are thought to initiate each saccade, although this has not been proved experimentally. Saccades to the left are initiated in the right cerebral hemisphere and those to the right in the left hemisphere. It is possible to induce a conjugate eye movement by stimulating the frontal cortex.

Smooth Pursuit Movement System

The smooth pursuit eye movement system is concerned with keeping the fovea on a target once that target has been located. This system operates for stationary as well as moving objects and uses different processes for each kind of target. If both eyes and the target are stationary, fixation *(foveation)* can be maintained by conscious effort, presumably by suppressing any conscious saccades.

43–6 A monkey can make horizontal saccadic eye movements of up to 40° within 50 msec; these superimposed tracings of movements in steps between 5° and 40° were selected as representative from one monkey. All the responses to a target step were averaged with regard to magnitude, duration, and maximum velocity. (Adapted from Fuchs, 1967.)

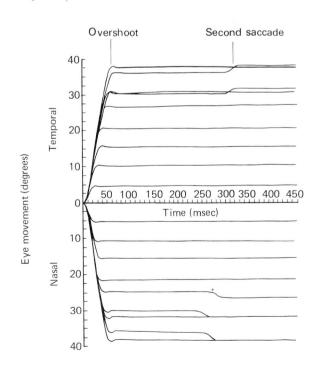

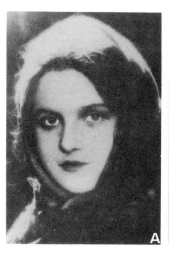
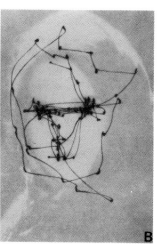

43–7 The eyes are constantly moving during continued fixation on an object. As a subject examined the photograph in part **A** with both eyes for 1 min, the record of eye movements (in part **B**) was obtained by using contact lenses with light-reflecting mirrors attached to them. (From Yarbus, 1967.)

Nevertheless, during steady fixation on a target, there are continuous, unconscious small movements of the eyes, characterized as slow drifts and quick flicks (10–15 min of arc). The *drifts* move the fovea over a target of interest; the *flicks* are small saccades that return the fovea to a target after a drift carries it too far away. Because of the flicks, there is no net displacement of the target. The drifts appear to be essential for continuous vision. Objects that are totally stabilized on the retina, such as retinal blood vessels, disappear. We are able to continue seeing objects only if their edges are continuously moving on the retina. Take a thin flashlight and rub it gently along your lid on the lateral side of your eye and see your

43–8 Smooth pursuit responses to 10°, 15°, and 20°/sec target ramps in the macaque monkey. The dotted lines show the path of the target the monkey must follow; the continuous lines show the eye movements of the monkey; note the initial "catch up" saccades. (Adapted from Fuchs, 1967.)

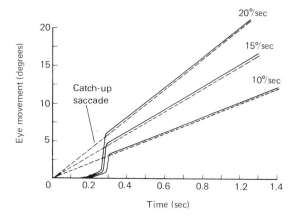

retinal blood vessels appear, as the shadows they produce are made to move on your retina. Remember that cells in the visual cortex are best excited by *moving* contours of appropriate orientation. The Russian physiologist Alfred Yarbus has cleverly demonstrated how our eyes move during continued fixation on an object of interest (Figure 43–7).

If a target moves and the viewer remains stationary, the eyes pursue the image so that it remains continuously on the fovea. For this smooth pursuit movement to occur, the brain must calculate the direction and velocity of the image on the retina. These operations appear to be carried out under the control of the occipital cortex, where, as we saw in Chapter 29, perception of form occurs. The smooth pursuit system can operate only with a target on the retina; it does not operate in the dark.

Smooth pursuit movements of a monkey following a target moving at designated velocities are illustrated in Figure 43–8; note the quick saccade necessary to catch up with the target initially. The differences in properties of the smooth pursuit and saccadic eye movements are summarized in Table 43–2.

Vestibulo-Oculomotor Reflex System

The vestibular eye movement system is concerned with stabilizing the eye against changes in head position. If the position of the head is altered, this reflex system keeps the eye looking in the same direction as it did before the movement. The signal initiating this reflex does not arise within the visual system but, rather, in the membranous labyrinth of the inner ear (Figure 43–9), which detects movements of the head along the three axes of space (Figure 43–1).

Each of the three semicircular canals senses the angular acceleration of the head around a different axis and transmits corresponding signals to neurons in the vestibular nuclei. Higher acceleration (i.e., greater head velocities) produces greater discharge rates along the nerves innervating any one canal. Because of the viscosity of the fluid surrounding the hair cells in the semicircular canals, these discharge rates are proportional to head velocity, not acceleration, for most normal head movements. Neurons in the vestibular nuclei assess the change in head position by integrating information about velocity coming from each canal, and a suitable correction signal is sent to the oculomotor nuclei to stabilize the eyes. At the end of a brief acceleration, these signals *persist* because the *velocity* is constant. As acceleration becomes zero, the velocity signals fade away in 10–20 sec, but that is much longer than the duration of most head movements. Therefore, when the head moves, information about the velocity and direction of the movement is always available to enable the brain to determine head position and consequently to initiate appropriate compensatory eye movements. The gain of the vestibulo-oculomotor reflex can be altered by environmental changes: changes in the relationship between corresponding hand, eye, or retinal movements, revealing

Table 43–2. Properties of Saccadic Versus Smooth Pursuit Movements of the Eye

Property	Saccadic	Smooth pursuit
Visual acuity during movement	Poor	Excellent
Target required	No	Yes
Maximum velocity	700°/sec	100°/sec
Velocity under voluntary control	No	No, a function of target velocity
Stimulus to elicit a movement	Target displacement	Target velocity
Latency	0.2 sec	0.13 sec
Barbiturate sensitivity	Least	Most
Control system	Discrete	Continuous

Source: Adapted from Fuchs, A. F. 1967. Saccadic and smooth pursuit eye movements in the monkey. J. Physiol. (Lond.) 191:609–631.

plasticity in the synaptic circuitry of the oculomotor system. The vestibulo-oculomotor reflex can be tested by gently irrigating the external auditory canal with warm (42°–47°C) or cold (20°C) water. A thermal gradient is established across the canal that induces flow of the endolymph in one direction or the other and thus influences the cupula (see Chapter 44). This procedure simulates head movement, which in turn produces compensatory eye movements via the vestibular system.

Optokinetic Movement System

When an animal moves through an object-filled space with its eyes open, a reflex compulsion to track these objects, especially large ones, is powerfully induced. This kind of oculomotor behavior is especially well developed in birds but also occurs in any moving animal with vision.

The optokinetic reflex is a backup system for the vestibulo-oculomotor reflex. For head movements that last about 0.5 sec, the vestibulo-oculomotor reflex stabilizes retinal images well and needs no assistance. When a unidirectional head movement is prolonged to 20–30 sec, however, the vestibulo-oculomotor reflex adapts and can no longer compensate for the head movement. The optokinetic reflex then comes into play. This reflex uses a continuous retinal signal rather than a phasic signal from the labyrinth to sense head movement. To keep the image on the retina stationary, the eye automatically begins to track a target as the head moves. This tracking move-

43–9 The membranous labyrinth of the inner ear (shown for the left ear) is where the vestibulo-oculomotor reflex is initiated. (Adapted from Brödel, in Hardy, 1934.)

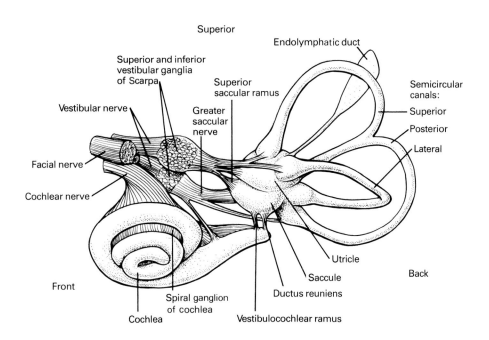

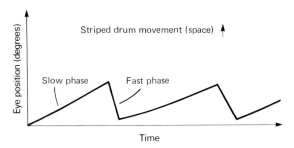

43–10 Optokinetic nystagmus is induced by having a subject observe a rotating striped drum. The eyes move slowly in the direction of drum movement (**slow phase**) and then rapidly in the opposite direction (**fast phase**).

ment keeps the relative velocity of the retinal image at zero; that is, it keeps eye velocity equal and opposite to head velocity. When the object that is being tracked moves out of the visual field, the eye makes a rapid saccade toward a new target, which it then proceeds to track.

This reflex can be induced by placing a subject within a rotating striped drum that completely surrounds him. The rotating drum will induce a rhythmic oscillatory movement of the eyes called *optokinetic nystagmus* (from the Greek *nystagmos*, nod), which has a slow phase as the head drops and a fast phase as the head snaps back to an erect position (Figure 43–10). The eyes automatically begin to track one stripe on the drum (slow phase), until it becomes impossible to do so without turning the head or body. Before this occurs, the eyes rapidly make a saccade in the direction opposite to that of the motion of the drum to allow a new stripe to be fixated (fast phase). This generates a rhythmic train of saw-tooth, conjugate eye movements, one slowly in the direction of drum movement followed by one rapidly in the opposite direction. Eye movements in different directions can be examined clinically with this device. If stripe size is progressively reduced, visual acuity can also be examined, especially in young children or uncooperative adults. If optokinetic movements do not occur, the stripe width is below visual acuity. Similar nystagmoid movements occur when one looks out of the window of a moving vehicle *(railroad nystagmus)*.

Vergence Movement System

The optokinetic, vestibulo-oculomotor, smooth pursuit, and saccadic systems generate conjugate eye movements. Whenever your eyes view an object moving toward or away from you, each eye must move differently (disjunctively) to keep the image of the object precisely aligned on both foveas. If the object moves closer, the eyes must converge; if it moves away, they must diverge. This operation is performed by the *vergence system*. The stimulus for this reflex leads to *stereopsis*, or the fusion of a single image in depth (see Appendix II). The vergence

system works together with the pupil- and lens-controlling systems in the so-called accommodation reflex (see Appendix II). The control center for vergence appears to be located in the occipital cortex, especially the prestriate cortex, where, as we have seen, the perception of depth (stereopsis) is mediated.

Misalignment

All five oculomotor control systems must move the eyes together precisely to maintain binocular vision. If the eyes are misaligned by abnormalities of muscle or nerve, double vision *(diplopia)* occurs. Merely displacing the position of one eye relative to the other with one's finger is sufficient to cause diplopia. Inappropriate alignment of the eyes at rest is called *heterotropia*. In heterotropia, one or several eye muscles must be contracted to prevent diplopia, even for a distant target. Often, muscular effort is no longer successful in aligning the two eyes, and the visual axes do not fix on the same point in space. This condition, called *strabismus*, or squint, would lead to diplopia were it not for the tendency to suppress the image from the weaker eye, the eye whose axis of vision cannot be aligned by muscular effort. Unfortunately, suppression in turn leads to reduction in visual acuity in the weaker eye.

Oculomotor Neurons Fire at Very High Rates

All the motor neurons that drive eye muscles (in cranial nerves III, IV, and VI) have similar properties. The features of these motor neurons can be illustrated by considering a lateral rectus motor neuron that causes a lateral horizontal eye movement (Figure 43–11). To produce a saccade, this motor neuron discharges briskly before each contraction (lateral abduction); the discharge then persists throughout the saccade. The duration of the saccade is determined by the duration of the burst. The larger the saccade, the longer the duration of the burst. While the lateral rectus muscle is contracting, motor neurons innervating the antagonist muscle, the medial rectus, are inhibited from firing.

Oculomotor neurons differ from spinal motor neurons in several ways. Spinal motor neurons tend to fire slowly at 50–100 impulses/sec, but oculomotor neurons fire at much higher rates of 100–600 impulses/sec. The ability to fire at higher rates results from intrinsic properties of the motor neurons and from the absence of recurrent inhibition, which is a prominent feature of the organization of spinal motor nuclei. The higher rates of discharge in oculomotor neurons probably serve to endow eye movements with a wider linear range and finer gradation of controls. Although there are many muscle spindles in the eye muscle, there is no stretch reflex. Each motor neuron has its own threshold for steady firing. Therefore, muscle tension is increased by the recruitment of motor neurons of different thresholds as well as by acceleration in the firing rate of each motor neuron.

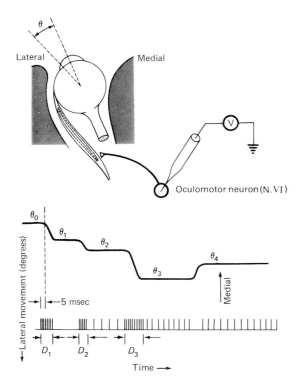

43–11 A saccade to the left (indicated by a movement of the eye through angle θ) is associated with a burst of impulses (**D**) in the lateral rectus motor neuron that lasts the duration of the saccade. Fixation in the new position is associated with steady firing that is increased in proportion to the eccentricity of the fixation. Medial saccades cause an inhibition in the firing pattern of the lateral rectus motor neuron. (Adapted from Fuchs and Luschei, 1970.)

Premotor Centers Act Directly and Indirectly on Oculomotor Neurons

Three major premotor regions of the brain impinge either directly or indirectly on the oculomotor neurons and participate in the control of gaze: the pontine gaze center of the reticular formation, the vestibular nuclei, and the superior colliculus. The pontine gaze center and the vestibular nuclei project directly to oculomotor neurons. In contrast, the superior colliculus appears to influence the oculomotor neurons only indirectly, through the pontine gaze center. We shall consider each of these three premotor centers in turn.

The Vestibular Nuclei Are Important for Many Types of Eye Movement

The vestibular nuclei bring signals about head movement from the semicircular canals directly to oculomotor neurons. In addition, the cells of the vestibular nuclei are a major source of all commands for eye movements *except* saccades. Saccadic eye movements are largely controlled by the pontine gaze center.

Neurons in the Pontine Gaze Center Are Heavily Involved in Programmed Eye Movements Such as Horizontal Saccades

There is clinical evidence that the pontine gaze center, an area in the reticular formation of the pons, plays an important role in eye movement, especially horizontal movements. Lesions in this part of the pons cause an enduring conjugate paralysis of horizontal gaze. In this type of paralysis, the eyes cannot move into the hemifield on the same side as the lesion but remain in the contralateral visual fields. Moreover, minor lesions cause an absence or slowing of saccades toward the side of the lesion. Stimulation of the gaze center in the pontine reticular formation causes short-latency eye movement, and gross recordings in this area reveal large potentials that are generated 10–15 msec before a saccade. Figure 43–12 illustrates how the synaptic circuitry of the pontine gaze center is organized to mediate horizontal saccades (in this example to the right). In these horizontal saccades the abducens nucleus plays a pivotal role.

A similar disturbance of horizontal gaze can be produced by lesions in two other brain areas: lesions of the abducens nucleus (nerve VI) and a combined lesion of the frontal cortex and superior colliculus.

There are four types of neurons in the reticular formation of the pons that discharge in relation to horizontal eye movements: burst cells, tonic cells, burst–tonic cells, and pause cells. We shall consider each of these to illustrate how a saccadic eye movement to a target of interest can arise (Figure 43–13).

Burst Cells. The burst cells are thought to initiate the saccade. They discharge at a high frequency just before and during voluntary saccades, and usually are silent at all other times (Figure 43–13). The burst precedes the saccade by 12 msec, and the number of spikes is proportional to the size of the saccade. Typically, these cells continue to fire at the beginning of any saccade and stop discharging just before the eye reaches the new position. The burst cells can be excited through vestibular, visual, and voluntary pathways to create saccades voluntarily as well as during the fast phases of vestibular and optokinetic nystagmus. Lesions in the pontine reticular formation that affect the burst cells selectively abolish the fast phase of vestibular nystagmus, suggesting that the locus for both saccades and the quick phase of vestibular and optokinetic nystagmus resides in the reticular formation.

Tonic Cells. These premotor neurons are thought to be involved in initial slow pursuit and fixation movements. The tonic cells are active in all eye movements because they carry the eye position signal. Any change in the position of the eye is associated with a concomitant change in the discharge pattern of the entire population of tonic neurons, some increasing and some decreasing depending on eye position. This pattern of activity provides the brain with a continuous signal for the position of the eye in the orbit. The tonic cells fire

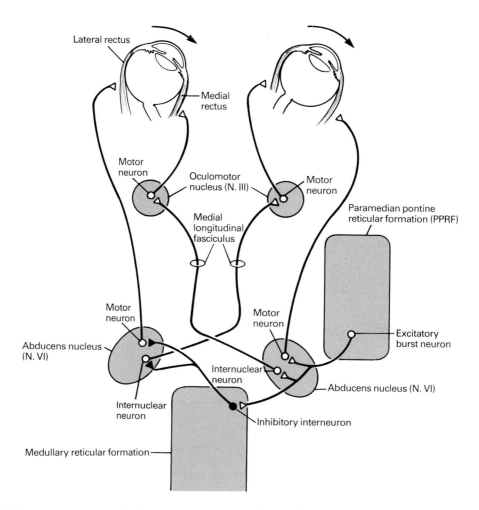

43–12 This simplified synaptic circuitry for the pontine gaze center shows how a horizontal saccade to the right is programmed. An excitatory burst neuron in the paramedian pontine reticular formation initiates a saccade by exciting several neurons in the abducens nucleus and an inhibitory neuron in the medullary reticular formation. One of the neurons in the abducens nucleus is a motor neuron that excites the lateral rectus muscle of the right eye; the other neuron is an interneuron that crosses the midline to excite a motor neuron in the oculomotor nucleus, which in turn excites the medial rectus of the left eye. The inhibitory interneuron in the medullary reticular formation also crosses the midline to inhibit the corresponding neurons in the abducens nucleus of the left side that are responsible for saccades to the left.

at a steady rate with eye fixation, and the firing rate increases linearly with increasing lateral rotation of the eye. In saccades their activity changes from the steady pre- to the faster postsaccadic level (Figure 43–13), suggesting that the burst and the late steady-state firing of a motor neuron during a saccadic movement are produced independently by different premotor cells.

Burst–Tonic Cells. These cells exhibit a burst of activity for lateral saccades and fire steadily during fixation, increasing their firing frequency with lateral eye rotation. The burst–tonic cells, which may be interneurons, have been found in several brain stem nuclei (the prepositus nucleus and the interstitial nucleus of Cajal) and in the pontine gaze center.

Pause Cells. In addition to the premotor neurons that discharge during different phases of eye (or head) movement, there are cells that fire at fairly constant rates but pause during rapid eye movements (Figure 43–13). These cells are located in the reticular formation in the gigantocellular tegmental field just behind and below the abducens nucleus. They are exclusively contralateral in their axonal projection fields. They are also involved in saccadic eye movements. Their firing is thought to inhibit burst cells: by pausing, they allow burst cells to initiate a saccade (Figure 43–13).

Interconnection of Cell Types. A schematic diagram (Figure 43–14) shows how these various cells may be interconnected. Burst neurons and tonic neurons are

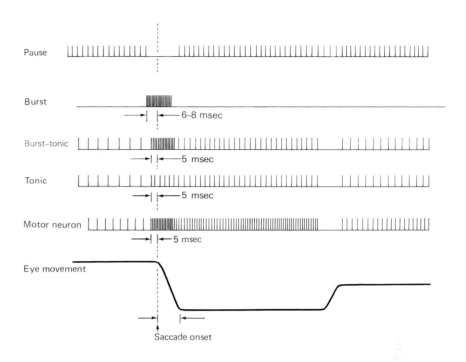

43–13 The various prototype neurons (pause, burst, burst–tonic, and tonic premotor cells in the pontine gaze center, and oculomotor neurons) in the oculomotor system change their frequency of firing during an eye movement. The burst neuron appears to initiate the saccade, since it begins firing before the other premotor cells. The burst–tonic and the tonic neurons begin firing from 1 to 3 msec afterward. The eye movements begin with a large saccade, then the eye remains stationary before returning part of the way to its initial position.

43–14 This schematic circuit shows how various classes of neurons (pause, burst, tonic, and motor neurons) can be synaptically connected to produce a saccade to a desired position in space. The model shows tonic and burst cells feeding the motor neuron directly. However, an intermediary burst–tonic cell may also contribute to the final output of the motor neuron. (Adapted from Robinson, 1981.)

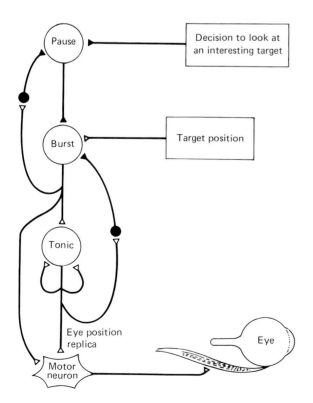

thought to provide the input that produces the burst–tonic discharge of the motor neurons. When the eye is not making a saccade, pause neurons prevent the burst neurons from firing. The appearance of an interesting target can lead to a decision in the brain to look at the target. This in turn leads to a brief trigger stimulus that inhibits the pause neurons, allowing burst neurons to respond to the excitatory input stimulated by the target. The burst neurons now fire at a high rate, and the eye begins to move. One hypothesis as to how the brain might control saccadic movement is that a neural replica of the eye position (called a *corollary discharge*) is fed back and inhibits the burst neuron. When the eye is on target the burst neuron stops firing and the inhibitory connection from the burst neuron to the pause neuron is turned off, reactivating the pause neuron and deactivating the burst neuron.

The Superior Colliculus Coordinates Visual Input with Eye Movements

The superior colliculus is thought to translate visual input to oculomotor commands. Neurons coding for the spatial location of visual stimuli as well as for the amplitude and direction of saccades are arranged topographically in an orderly fashion. In the dorsal layer, cells respond selectively to visual stimuli. Some respond vigorously to movement in any direction. These cells are called *event detectors*. The dorsal layer of the superior colliculus receives input from the entire visual field through direct retinal projections as well as from a cortical projection. In the ventral layer, oculomotor cells predominate that discharge before saccadic eye movements. The ventral layer of the superior colliculus in turn gives off fibers that travel in the tectal spinal, tectal pontine, and tectoreticular tracts to the brain stem. The superior colliculus is thought to be exclusively involved in saccadic performance, having nothing to do with pursuit, fixation, or optokinetic nystagmus.

Two Cortical Eye Fields Act on the Premotor Cells

Two regions in each hemisphere, the frontal and occipital eye fields, are particularly important for eye movement. These functionally distinct eye fields are essential for pursuit and saccadic movements and for visual reflexes that depend on these basic movements.

43–15 This scheme shows all the neural centers currently known to affect the common motor neuron output to the ocular muscles. The frontal cortex eye fields (Brodmann's area 8) direct saccades; areas 17 and 18 of the occipital cortex direct fixation and smooth pursuit; area 19 directs vergence and stereopsis; the semicircular canals and the vestibular nuclei stabilize the eye in the head; and the cerebellum, superior colliculus, and pretectal nuclei coordinate those movements in ways we have yet to discover. (Adapted from Robinson, 1968.)

Frontal Eye Fields

The frontal eye fields are located opposite the motor cortex in the region corresponding to Brodmann's area 8. These fields contribute to the initiation of voluntary gaze although they are not absolutely essential for initiation. Efferent fibers leaving this region pass through the posterior limb of the internal capsule and continue caudally within the cerebral peduncle, which contains the corticospinal and corticobulbar fibers. Arriving at the midbrain, the tract deviates away from the main bundle of peduncular fibers and travels a short distance to terminate in the general area of pontine gaze center interneurons. The frontal eye fields also project to the colliculus.

Electrical stimulation of frontal eye fields on one side produces conjugate eye movements to the opposite side. A lesion in the frontal eye fields produces a sustained, conjugate deviation of the eyes to the side of the lesion and an inability to move the eyes voluntarily to the opposite direction (although rapid improvement usually occurs as a result of the compensatory effect of uncrossed fibers from the contralateral eye field). If there is bilateral destruction of frontal eye fields, the patient loses the ability to gaze laterally in either direction, as well as the ability to direct visual attention to an object introduced suddenly into the peripheral vision. The patient cannot initiate voluntary saccades and consequently is unable to initiate the visual fixation reflex. Patients may look

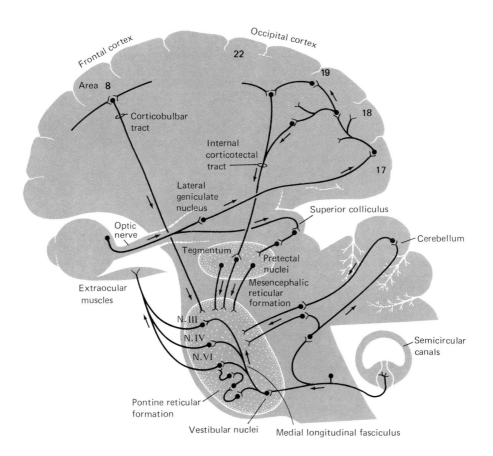

compulsively at objects that appear abruptly in the periphery, even when told not to do so. It is thought that this behavior is caused by a superior collicular response that has been released from higher control by the lesion. This deficit may only be transient; voluntary saccades are permanently lost only when both the frontal eye fields and the superior colliculus are destroyed.

Occipital Eye Fields

The occipital cortex is also involved in oculomotor activity and reflexes. Without it there is no conscious visual perception, and visual pursuit movements become impossible. Ablation studies suggest that the occipital fields are involved in smooth pursuit tracking movements and in optokinetic nystagmus, including both the slow component (smooth pursuit movements) and the fast component (reflex saccades). In lower animals, the optokinetic system is located mainly in the brain stem, but in primates it has come to depend significantly on the geniculostriate system. It is thought that a cortical area anterior to the visual areas gathers information about the pursuit and optokinetic movement and transmits this information to the brain stem. The occipital eye fields also play some role in supporting the visual fixation reflex.

In neurological diseases in which certain areas of the frontal cortex are destroyed, this fixation reflex can no longer be broken without blocking the visual input to the eyes. Patients whose posterior cortical eye fields have been impaired and whose frontal areas are still intact may still be able voluntarily to direct their gaze with little impairment. Nevertheless, attempts to fixate on a target are undermined by severe instability and wandering of the eyes, with considerable deterioration of perception. Since the lesions also directly interfere with the visual pathway, diagnosis of the causes of the visual and ocular impairments may be difficult.

An Overall View

The oculomotor system is another example of the modular design of the brain. Specific groups of neurons perform specific operations: some compute head velocity, others eye velocity in space; some groups of neurons compute the differences between the two, and still others relate these variables to retinal targets. Although each operation is performed by separate groups of cells, most of the modules influence and control the computations made by the others through synaptic interactions. Many modules also share computational circuits, and all share the final common pathway of the system, the pool of oculomotor neurons. All of the neural centers known to affect this pool are shown in Figure 43–15. In addition to the flexibility inherent in this kind of system, modular design enables the neurologist to pinpoint the area where something has gone wrong in the diseased nervous system.

Selected Readings

Cohen, B. (ed.). 1981. Vestibular and oculomotor physiology. Ann. N.Y. Acad. Sci. 374:1–892.

Fuchs, A. F. 1967. Saccadic and smooth pursuit eye movements in the monkey. J. Physiol. (Lond.) 191:609–631.

Fuchs, A. F., and Kaneko, C. R. S. 1981. A brain stem generator for saccadic eye movements. Trends Neurosci. 4:283–286.

Leigh, R. J., and Zee, D. S. 1983. The Neurology of Eye Movements. Contemporary Neurology Series. Philadelphia: Davis.

Raphan, T., and Cohen, B. 1978. Brainstem mechanisms for rapid and slow eye movements. Annu. Rev. Physiol. 40:527–552.

Robinson, D. A. 1981. The use of control systems analysis in the neurophysiology of eye movements. Annu. Rev. Neurosci. 4:463–503.

Westheimer, G. 1954. Mechanism of saccadic eye movements. A.M.A. Arch. Ophthalmol. 52:710–724.

References

Carpenter, M. B. 1978. Core Text of Neuroanatomy, 2nd ed. Baltimore: Williams & Wilkins.

Fuchs, A. F., and Luschei, E. S. 1970. Firing patterns of abducens neurons of alert monkeys in relationship to horizontal eye movement. J. Neurophysiol. 33:382–392.

Hardy, M. 1934. Observations on the innervation of the macula sacculi in man. Anat. Rec. 59:403–418.

Hering, E. 1879. Der Raumsinn und die Bewegungen des Auges. In L. Hermann (ed.), Handbuch der Physiologie, Band III, Teil I. Leipzig: F. C. W. Vogel, pp. 343–601.

Mays, L. E., and Sparks, D. L. 1980. Saccades are spatially, not retinocentrically coded. Science 208:1163–1165.

Robinson , D. A. 1968. Eye movement control in primates. Science 161:1219–1224.

Schiller, P. H., True, S. D., and Conway, J. L. 1979. Effects of frontal eye field and superior colliculus ablations on eye movements. Science 206:590–592.

Wurtz, R. H., and Albano, J. E. 1980. Visual-motor function of the primate superior colliculus. Annu. Rev. Neurosci. 3:189–226.

Yarbus, A. L. 1967. Eye Movements and Vision. Basil Haigh (trans.). New York: Plenum Press.

James P. Kelly

Vestibular System

44

The vestibular system detects the position and the motion of the head in space by integrating information from peripheral receptors located in the inner ear on either side of the head. Unlike taste, smell, vision, audition, and somesthesis—the sensations we have considered earlier—the vestibular sense is not prominent in our consciousness. Although we normally are not aware of the vestibular dimension of our sensory experience, this dimension is essential for the coordination of motor responses, eye movement, and posture. Moreover, malfunctioning of the vestibular system leads to dizziness and nausea—sensations that all too quickly impinge upon our consciousness.

The inner ear, or labyrinth, is made up of two parts: the bony labyrinth and the membranous labyrinth. The *bony labyrinth,* which houses the vestibular as well as the auditory sense organs, consists of a series of cavities in the petrous portion of the temporal bone. Within these cavities is the *membranous labyrinth,* so called because it consists of fine membranes made up of a simple epithelium. In specialized regions, the epithelium becomes elaborated into a sensory epithelium that serves as a transducing structure for both audition and balance. The membranous labyrinth is separated from the bony labyrinth by a fluid called *perilymph* (Figure 44–1).

In the bony labyrinth, the vestibular division of the membranous labyrinth is closely associated with the cochlea, the auditory end-organ. We have considered the auditory portion of the membranous labyrinth in Chapter 31. The adjacent vestibular division of the membranous labyrinth is filled with a fluid called *endolymph;* one portion of the vestibular apparatus, the saccule, communicates freely with the cochlea. On the outside, the *perilymph*

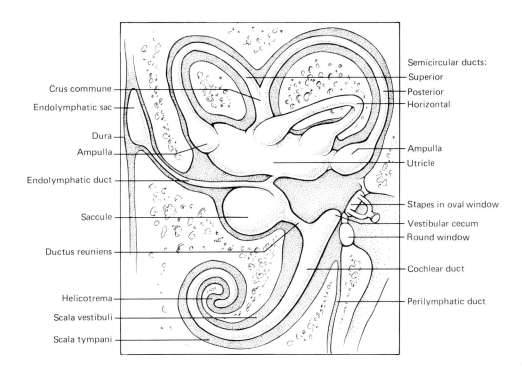

Crus commune
Endolymphatic sac
Dura
Ampulla
Endolymphatic duct
Saccule
Ductus reuniens
Helicotrema
Scala vestibuli
Scala tympani

Semicircular ducts:
Superior
Posterior
Horizontal
Ampulla
Utricle
Stapes in oval window
Vestibular cecum
Round window
Cochlear duct
Perilymphatic duct

44–1 The membranous labyrinth contains auditory structures (cochlear duct) and vestibular structures (utricle, saccule, and semicircular ducts). (Adapted from Iurato, 1967.)

that bathes the vestibular portion of the membranous labyrinth also is continuous with and bathes the outside of the cochlear duct, the auditory portion of the membranous labyrinth.

The vestibular labyrinth consists of two principal sets of structures: (1) a pair of saclike swellings—*the otolith organs*—called the *utricle* and the *saccule;* and (2) three directionally sensitive, more or less orthogonal, *semicircular ducts.* The sensory receptor cells in each of these structures respond to accelerated movement of the head, or to changes in acceleration resulting from an altered position of the head. Different segments of the end-organ respond to different aspects of acceleration. The three semicircular ducts lie in three different planes that are mutually perpendicular to one another. As a consequence of their arrangement in three-dimensional space, they detect angular acceleration of the head in any of these three directions. The otolith organs detect linear acceleration when the head moves and they are also important for determining the position of the head with respect to the vertically oriented gravity vector.

Information from both components of the peripheral end-organ is relayed by the vestibular portion of the eighth nerve to the vestibular nuclei in the brain stem and to the vestibular portion of the cerebellum (the flocculonodular lobe). Different subdivisions of the vestibular nuclear complex, in turn, connect in a highly specific manner with the motor nuclei of the extraocular muscles and with the spinal cord. The whole apparatus functions to keep the body balanced, to coordinate head and body movements, and most remarkably to enable the eyes to remain fixed on a point in space even when the head is moving.

In this chapter we shall first consider the structure of the two principal segments of the vestibular labyrinth: the semicircular ducts and the otolith organs. Located in the two segments of the vestibular labyrinth are specialized receptor cells sensitive to mechanical displacement—the vestibular hair cells; we shall examine the mechanisms of transduction used by the hair cells. Finally, we shall discuss the central connections of the vestibular system and the role of this system in eye, head, and body coordination.

The Vestibular Labyrinth Is Part of the Membranous Labyrinth

The organization of the membranous labyrinth is depicted in Figure 44–1. The vestibular labyrinth is directly connected to the cochlear duct by the *ductus reuniens.* The saccule and the utricle, the two otolith organs, lie in the vestibule of the inner ear. The other portion of the vestibular apparatus, the membranous *semicircular ducts,* lie in the bony *semicircular canals* and are separated from them by narrow sheaths of connective tissue. There are three ducts on each side of the head: the anterior, posterior, and horizontal. These ducts are paired with functional counterparts on the opposite side of the head so that at least one pair is affected by any given angular acceleration.

Endolymph Fills the Vestibular Labyrinth and Perilymph Surrounds It

The membranous labyrinth is filled with endolymph. This extracellular fluid is peculiar because its ion composition is very similar to that of intracellular fluid: the endolymph has a high potassium concentration ($\approx$ 150 meq/liter) and a low sodium concentration ($\approx$ 20 meq/liter). These ion concentrations vary somewhat in different portions of the labyrinth, but they never approach the normal ion balance found in other extracellular fluids. The unusual ion concentration of endolymph may partly explain why there is a net potential difference between the membranous labyrinth and the surrounding perilymph. The utricular endolymph is about 4 mV positive with respect to ground, while the fluid within the cochlear duct is about 70 mV positive. This is largely due to the active pumping of positive ions from the cochlear duct. The significance of these potentials is still not understood, but they may play a role in the transduction processes occurring in the hair cells.

The endolymph of the vestibular labyrinth is probably produced by secretory cells in the transitional epithelium surrounding the sensory epithelia, and by the *stria vascularis*, the epithelium lining the upper part of the cochlear duct. It drains into the venous sinuses of the dura mater through the endolymphatic duct. Perilymph is thought to be secreted by arterioles lying in the periosteum surrounding the labyrinth. It drains into the subarachnoid space through the perilymphatic duct. If normal production or drainage of either fluid is disturbed, the function of the entire labyrinth is impaired. For example, the overproduction of endolymph may lead to a condition called Ménière's syndrome, in which both auditory and vestibular functions are disturbed. Given the continuity between the cochlear duct and the vestibular labyrinth, it is not surprising that both functions are affected by the excessive production of endolymph. The disease is characterized by transient attacks of dizziness or vertigo that are so severe that the afflicted individual cannot stand or walk. Nausea, vomiting, abnormal eye movements (nystagmus), and a sensorineural hearing loss also occur. These symptoms may be consequences of fluid imbalance in the labyrinth.

Specialized Regions of the Vestibular Labyrinth Contain Receptors

Both ends of each fluid-filled semicircular duct terminate in the utricle (Figure 44–1), although one limb of the superior duct fuses with the posterior duct before joining the utricle. Each duct has an enlargement called the *ampulla*, where it joins the utricle. In part of the ampulla, the epithelium of the duct is thickened and contains specialized receptor cells, the *vestibular hair cells*. The thickened zone containing the hair cells is termed the *ampullary crest* (Figure 44–2A). Peripherally directed processes of bipolar sensory neurons in the vestibular

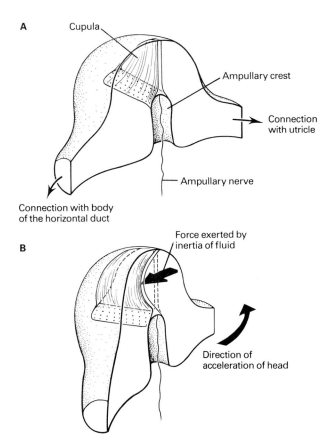

44–2 The ampullae of the semicircular ducts contain a receptor system. **A.** The ampullary crest of the horizontal duct. **B.** Displacement of the cupula by flow of endolymph caused by head movement.

ganglion innervate the hair cells in the crest. The crest is covered with a gelatinous mass called the *cupula* (Latin, small inverted cup) that stretches from the crest to the roof of the ampulla. When the head is rotated, the inertia of the fluid in the semicircular ducts causes the fluid to push against the cupula, producing an angular displacement of the sensory hairs on the receptor cells. As we shall see, the resulting distortion of the cupula elicits a receptor potential in the hair cells of the crest and eventually alters the level of activity in the eighth-nerve fibers innervating them.

The receptor system of the vestibular apparatus is so sensitive that it can respond to angular accelerations or decelerations as small as $0.5°/\text{sec}^2$. The displacement of the cupular system at the threshold of sensitivity is less than 10 nm, which is somewhat greater than the physical displacement produced by low-amplitude sounds in the auditory system. This sensitivity is made possible by the arrangement of the cupula, which forms a diaphragmlike partition across the ampullary lumen (Figure 44–2B). The displacement of the base of the cupula is greatest near the center of the ampullary crest, and therefore receptor cells near the center of the crest have the greatest sensitivity to this displacement. Increasing acceleration recruits more and more receptor cells toward the periphery of the crest, since these cells are located near the edge of the diaphragm. This anatomical relationship therefore leads to a graded response in the population of hair cells.

As is the case with the ampullae of the semicircular ducts described above, a portion of the floor of the utricle is also thickened and contains hair cells along with the distal branches of vestibular ganglion cells. This zone of the utricle, termed the *macula* (Latin, spot), is the receptor region of the utricle. The macula is covered with a gelatinous substance in which crystals of calcium carbonate, called *otoliths* (Greek, *lithos*, stone), are embedded. The macula of the utricle lies roughly in the horizontal plane when the head is held horizontally, so that the otoliths rest directly upon it. If the head is tilted or if the head undergoes linear acceleration, the otoliths deform the gelatinous mass, which in turn bends the hairs of the receptor cells. A receptor-rich macula is also found in the saccule. In contrast to the macula of the utricle, the macula of the saccule is oriented vertically when the head is in its normal position. The macula of the saccule also detects the position of the head in space, but it responds selectively to vertically directed linear forces.

The Arrangement of Vestibular Hair Cells Is Integral to Their Function as Receptors

Hair Cells Are Polarized Structurally and Functionally

Vestibular hair cells are restricted to the ampullary crests of the semicircular ducts and the maculae of the saccule and utricle. Hair cells are separated from one another by supporting cells, to which they are joined at their apical surfaces by tight junctions (Figure 44–3). The free surface of each hair cell is differentiated into 40–70 stereocilia per cell and a single *kinocilium* (Figure 44–3). The stereocilia increase in length with increasing proximity to the kinocilium (Figure 44–4A). In the semicircular ducts, these "hairs" project into the overlying cupula. The kinocilium is always found on one side of the hair bundle. This gives each hair cell a *morphological axis of polarity*. We can define the axis as running from the smallest stereocilium to the kinocilium. This structural arrangement is important because hair cells respond to bending of the apical hairs in a directional manner. Bending of the hair bundle toward the kinocilium leads to depolarization of the hair cell and an increase in the firing of afferent fibers

44–3 The hair cells of the vestibular sensory epithelium are surrounded by supporting cells, to which they are joined at their apical surfaces by tight junctions. The surfaces of the supporting cells are covered with microvilli. The hair cell is innervated at its base by the afferent process of vestibular ganglion cells, and by efferent terminals that arise from cells in the brain stem; these efferent processes provide a pathway for the brain to regulate the activity of vestibular receptor cells directly. The apical surface of the hair cell displays several rows of stereocilia that are packed with actin filaments and a single kinocilium. At the base of each stereocilium is an anchoring rootlet that extends into the underlying cuticular plate. The kinocilium arises from the cytoplasmic surface of the hair cell and is longer than the stereocilia. In the ampullae of the semicircular ducts, the hair bundle extends into the overlying cupula. In the maculae of the utricle and saccule, the hair bundle extends into the overlying otolithic membrane.

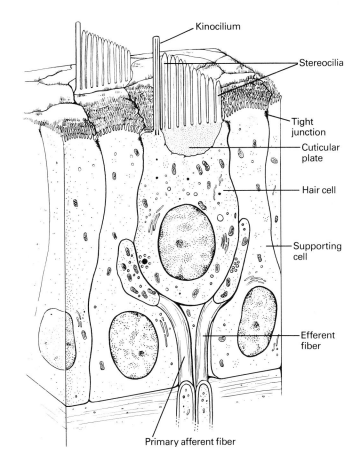

Kinocilium

Stereocilia

Tight junction

Cuticular plate

Hair cell

Supporting cell

Efferent fiber

Primary afferent fiber

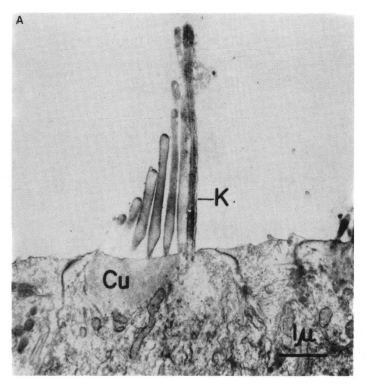

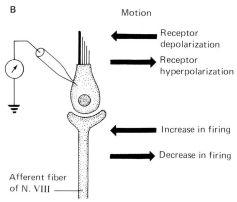

44–4 The arrangement of the apical hairs determines changes in the polarization of the hair cell. **A.** A transmission electron micrograph of the hair cell apical surface shows that the stereocilia increase in length toward the kinocilium (**K**). The cuticular plate (**Cu**) occupies the top of the sensory cell except for an area around the basal body of the kinocilium. Osmium tetroxide fixation, uranyl acetate stain. x11,000. (Adapted from Flock, 1964.) **B.** The direction in which the apical hairs bend (toward or away from the kinocilium) affects the polarization of the hair cell and the firing rate of eighth-nerve afferent fibers.

in the eighth nerve; conversely, bending away from the kinocilium leads to hyperpolarization of the hair cell and decreased firing in the vestibular fibers of the eighth nerve (Figure 44–4B).

The hair cells in the ampullae of the semicircular ducts are arranged in an orderly pattern. In the vertical ducts, the kinocilia face away from the utricle. In the horizontal ducts, the kinocilia all face the utricle (Figure 44–5), and therefore bending of the hairs in the direction of the utricle is excitatory. The outcome of this morphological polarity can be demonstrated by extracellular single-unit recordings from the afferent fibers innervating the hair cells. At rest, the vestibular nerve fibers discharge spontaneously at a rate of about 100 spikes/sec. If the sensory hairs are bent in one direction, this rate is increased, and if they are bent in the other, the rate is decreased (Figure 44–6). Therefore, the vestibular nerve fibers to each duct respond to rotation in one direction with an increase in activity and, since there is a resting discharge, with a decrease in activity to rotation in the opposite direction.

Semicircular Ducts Work in Pairs

To examine the way that paired ducts on either side of the head work together, imagine that we are looking down on top of the two horizontal ducts (Figure 44–7).

44–5 The kinocilia of hair cells in the ampullary crest of the horizontal duct all face the utricle.

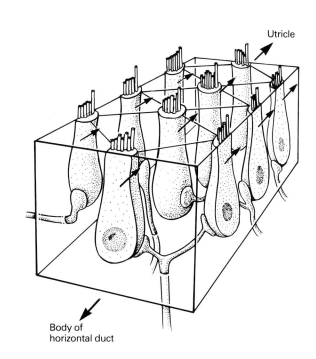

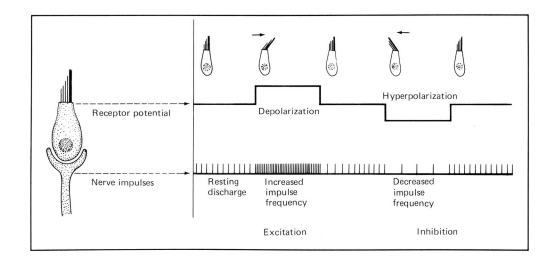

44–6 The firing of vestibular nerve fibers depends upon the direction in which the hairs are bent. (Adapted from Flock, 1965.)

Remember that the horizontal ducts are connected to the utricle at both ends (Figure 44–1). Furthermore, the morphological axis of polarity of each hair cell in both horizontal ampullae points toward the nearest juncture between the ducts and the utricle. As the head turns to the left, the fluid in the ducts lags behind the turning motion because of inertia. As a consequence, the fluid in the left duct deflects the hair bundles in the direction of their axes of polarity, while the fluid in the right duct deflects the hair bundles against their axes. The hair cells of the left ampulla therefore depolarize and release transmitter substance to excite the afferent fibers innervating them. The hair cells of the right ampulla hyperpolarize, and the firing rate of the afferent fibers innervating them decreases. The brain then receives two indications of this turning motion: an increase in the firing of eighth-nerve fibers on one side, and a decrease on the other.

The horizontal ducts lie in approximately the same plane on each side, and they work together to detect motion. The situation is not so simple for the other ducts because of their orientation in the head (Figure 44–8). The *anterior duct* on one side lies approximately in the same plane as the *posterior duct* on the opposite side, so the anterior and posterior ducts of either side are functional pairs. The component of motion in the plane of these ducts causes excitation of hair cells in one ampulla and inhibition in the other, and thus provides a bilateral indication of head movement.

Hair Cells in the Utricle Are Polarized toward the Striola

Hair cells in the macula of the utricle are also arranged in an orderly pattern but their kinocilia do not face in a single direction. Because the cells are not polarized in a

uniform pattern in the utricular macula, this structure can respond to tilt or to linear acceleration in any one of several directions. This works as follows: The hair cells of the utricle are in a specialized epithelium much like the crests of the ampullae. Their sensory hairs project

44–7 View of the horizontal ducts from above shows how paired canals work together to provide a bilateral indication of head movement.

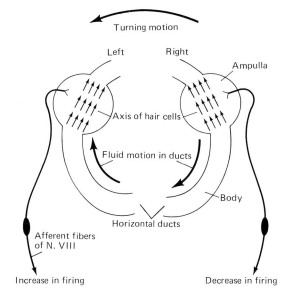

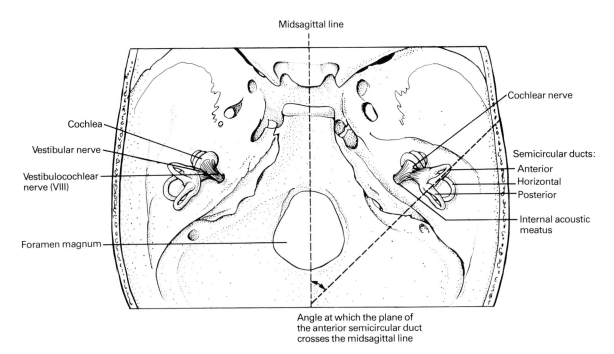

Midsagittal line

Cochlear nerve

Cochlea

Vestibular nerve

Vestibulocochlear
nerve (VIII)

Semicircular ducts:
Anterior
Horizontal
Posterior

Internal acoustic
meatus

Foramen magnum

Angle at which the plane of
the anterior semicircular duct
crosses the midsagittal line

44–8 The orientation of the semicircular ducts. The
horizontal ducts on both sides lie on the same plane. In
contrast, the anterior duct on either side lies on the same plane
as the posterior duct on the opposite side.

44–9 The apical hairs of hair cells in the utricular macula
project into the otolithic membrane, in which the
otoliths are embedded. (Adapted from Iurato, 1967.)

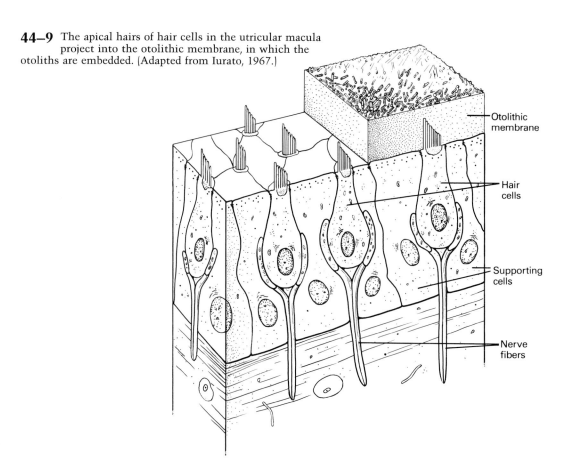

Otolithic
membrane

Hair
cells

Supporting
cells

Nerve
fibers

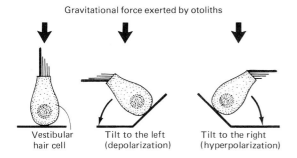

Gravitational force exerted by otoliths

Vestibular hair cell | Tilt to the left (depolarization) | Tilt to the right (hyperpolarization)

44–10 The response of an individual macular hair cell to a tilt of the head depends upon the direction in which its hairs are bent by the gravitational force of the otoliths.

into an overlying gelatinous matrix in which the otoliths are embedded (Figure 44–9). The macular hair cells are also polarized, with their kinocilia located toward one side of the cells' apical surface.

The response of an individual macular hair cell to the gravitational force exerted by the otoliths and otolithic membrane is shown in Figure 44–10. When the head is held in the horizontal plane, gravitational force is directed downward upon the hair bundle. When the head is tilted to the left, the hair bundle of the cell is displaced along the axis of polarization, causing it to depolarize and excite its afferent fiber. A tilt to the right has the opposite effect. Therefore, the afferent fiber innervating an individual macular hair cell is either excited or inhibited by a given tilt of the head. The intriguing structural feature of the macula is that the axes of the hair cells all point toward a single curving landmark called the *striola* (Figure 44–11, arrows). Tilt in any direction depolarizes some macular hair cells and hyperpolarizes others. This dual signal most probably aids in providing the brain with an accurate measure of head position.

44–11 The axes of all hair cells in the macula of the utricle point toward the striola (**arrows**). (Adapted from Spoendlin, 1966.)

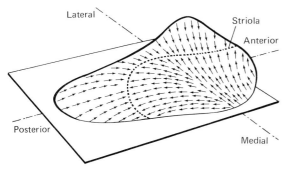

Lateral | Striola | Anterior | Posterior | Medial

The Central Connections of the Vestibular Labyrinth Reflect Its Dynamic and Static Functions

The vestibular labyrinth has two interrelated functions. The *dynamic* function, mediated principally by the semicircular ducts, enables us to detect the rotation of the head in space, and, as we shall see, is important for the reflex control of eye movements. The *static* function, mediated principally by the utricle and saccule, enables us to monitor the absolute position of the head in space and plays a pivotal role in the control of posture. We shall now consider the central connections established by ganglion cells innervating the ampullae of the ducts and the maculae of the utricle and saccule. As might be expected, the central connections of these two sets of ganglion cells are different—a reflection of their distinctive physiological roles.

The Central Axons of the Neurons of the Vestibular Ganglion Run in the Eighth Cranial Nerve to the Brain Stem

The afferent fibers of the vestibular system have their cell bodies in the vestibular ganglion (Scarpa's ganglion) lying near the internal auditory meatus. There are about 20,000 cells in each vestibular ganglion. These cells are bipolar: The peripheral axon innervates the hair cells and the central axon runs into the vestibular division of the vestibulocochlear nerve (VIII) to terminate in the brain stem. Both the axons and the cell body are myelinated.

The vestibular ganglion is divided into two portions. The *superior division* innervates the macula of the utricle, the anterior part of the macula of the saccule, and the cristae of the horizontal and anterior semicircular ducts. The *inferior division* innervates the posterior part of the macula of the saccule and the crista of the posterior duct. The centrally directed axons of cells in Scarpa's ganglion join with axons from the spiral ganglion in the cochlea to constitute the eighth cranial nerve. The nerve runs through the internal auditory meatus, along with the facial nerve (VII). After exiting from the meatus, the eighth nerve runs through the cerebellopontine angle to reach the lateral aspect of the pons, where the axons enter the brain.

Each Nucleus of the Vestibular Nuclear Complex Has Distinctive Connections

The vestibular nuclear complex occupies a substantial portion of the medulla beneath the floor of the fourth ventricle (Figure 44–12). In this complex there are four distinct nuclei: the lateral vestibular nucleus, or Deiters' nucleus; the medial vestibular nucleus; the superior vestibular nucleus; and the inferior, or descending, vestibular nucleus. Each of the nuclei can be distinguished on the basis of its architecture, but more important, each nucleus has a distinctive set of connections with the ves-

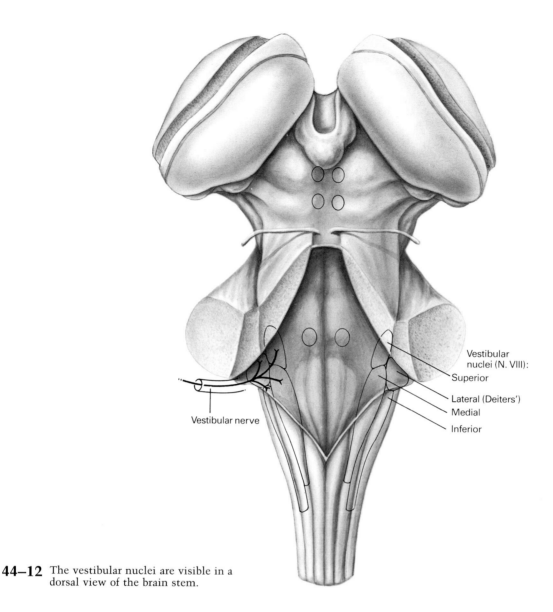

44–12 The vestibular nuclei are visible in a dorsal view of the brain stem.

Vestibular nerve

Vestibular nuclei (N. VIII):
Superior
Lateral (Deiters')
Medial
Inferior

tibular periphery and with certain regions in the central nervous system—notably, the spinal cord, the oculomotor nuclei (III, IV, and VI) of the brain stem, and the cerebellum.

Lateral Vestibular Nucleus. Deiters' nucleus is diamond shaped when viewed from the side. The rostroventral portion of the nucleus receives primary vestibular fibers innervating the macula of the utricle. The dorsocaudal portion of the nucleus receives input from the cerebellum and the spinal cord. Deiters' nucleus is easily recognized because it contains large nerve cells (about 50–100 μm in diameter) along with smaller neurons. All of these cells send their axons into the lateral vestibulospinal tract, which terminates ipsilaterally in the ventral horn of the spinal cord at cervical, thoracic, and lumbar levels. The lateral vestibulospinal tract, along with descending reticulospinal fibers, has a pro-

nounced facilitatory effect on both alpha and gamma motor neurons that innervate antigravity muscles in the limbs. This tonic excitation of antigravity muscles (the extensors of the leg and the flexors of the arm) enables us to maintain an upright body posture.

The neurons in Deiters' nucleus respond selectively to tilting of the head. These neurons have a resting discharge that increases in response to tilt in one direction and decreases in response to tilt in the opposite direction. The magnitude of the response increases with increasing angle of tilt. A smaller number of neurons respond whenever the angle of the head is changed. Both types of cells receive input from the macula of the utricle. The dorsocaudal part of Deiters' nucleus receives direct inhibitory input from the cerebellum. Electrical stimulation of Purkinje cell axons emanating from the vermis of the cerebellum produces monosynaptic inhibitory postsynaptic potentials in the large cells of Deiters' nucleus.

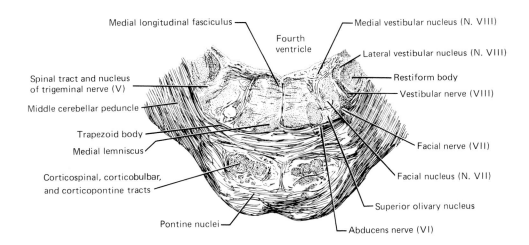

Medial longitudinal fasciculus

Fourth ventricle

Medial vestibular nucleus (N. VIII)

Lateral vestibular nucleus (N. VIII)

Spinal tract and nucleus of trigeminal nerve (V)

Restiform body

Middle cerebellar peduncle

Vestibular nerve (VIII)

Trapezoid body

Medial lemniscus

Facial nerve (VII)

Corticospinal, corticobulbar, and corticopontine tracts

Facial nucleus (N. VII)

Superior olivary nucleus

Pontine nuclei

Abducens nerve (VI)

44–13 This section of the lower pons stained for myelin illustrates the relationship of the medial longitudinal fasciculus to the medial vestibular nucleus.

As we saw in Chapter 37, the input from the vermis is important for understanding the factors that modify decerebrate rigidity. This rigidity is characterized by increased reflex tone in the antigravity muscles, and it appears when the brain stem is transected above the level of the vestibular nuclei. If the transection occurs caudal to the vestibular nuclei, the rigidity does not occur. Decerebrate rigidity is undoubtedly due to the unopposed excitatory effect of the lateral vestibulospinal tract upon motor neurons supplying the antigravity muscles. If the portion of the cerebellum connected to Deiters' nucleus is removed, this condition is greatly exacerbated because the inhibitory actions of the Purkinje cells on the giant cells of Deiters' nucleus are eliminated. Conversely, electrical stimulation of the anterior part of the cerebellar vermis alleviates the rigidity.

Medial and Superior Vestibular Nuclei. These nuclei receive input principally from the ampullae of the semicircular ducts. The medial vestibular nucleus gives rise to the medial vestibulospinal tract, which terminates bilaterally in the cervical region of the cord. The axons in this tract make monosynaptic connections with motor neurons innervating the neck muscles. This tract participates in the reflex control of neck movements so that the position of the head can be maintained accurately and correlated with eye movements.

Cells in both the medial and the superior vestibular nuclei participate in vestibulo-oculomotor reflexes. They send their axons into the *medial longitudinal fasciculus,* a tract running to rostral parts of the brain stem just beneath the midline of the fourth ventricle. The locations of these structures are indicated in Figure 44–13. The function of the medial and superior vestibular nuclei can be illustrated by examining an elementary vestibulo-oculomotor reflex arc. If the head is tilted to one side, for example, the eyes rotate in the opposite direction, and this helps to maintain the visual field in the horizontal plane. The precise central pathways that mediate this reflex have not been completely mapped out, but it is dependent upon tonic input from the utricle.

To understand vestibulo-oculomotor reflexes that are mediated by inputs from the semicircular ducts, imagine that a person seated on a stool is being spun to the left around a vertical axis. When the acceleration to the left first begins, the eyes undergo a slow conjugate deviation to the right, in a direction opposite the motion of the head. This tends to keep the eyes fixed on a single point in space. The eyes do not remain in this position; when they have reached the limit of their excursion, they move rapidly to the left, in the direction of the angular acceleration. These slow and fast movements are termed the *slow and fast phases of vestibular nystagmus.* Note that the fast phase of nystagmus is in the direction of the angular acceleration. When the movement to the left is stopped abruptly, it is equivalent to producing a rapid acceleration to the right due to the inertia of the fluid in the horizontal semicircular ducts. The eyes now undergo repeated slow movements to the left, accompanied by rapid return movements to the right until the vestibular stimulus subsides. This *postrotatory nystagmus* is used clinically to evaluate the functional state of the vestibular system.

A highly simplified circuit diagram for the initial phase of this vestibulo-oculomotor reflex is shown in Figure 44–14. As the head accelerates to the left, there is increased firing in the nerve fibers innervating the ampulla of the horizontal duct of the left side. This increase in activity is carried through several synaptic relays and leads to contraction of the muscles that turn both eyes to the right. At the same time the activity of nerve fibers innervating the crista of the right horizontal duct diminishes, and this causes a relaxation of antagonist muscles. These coordinated effects are achieved by specific sets of connections between the medial and superior vestibular nuclei and the motor nuclei of the extraocular muscles.

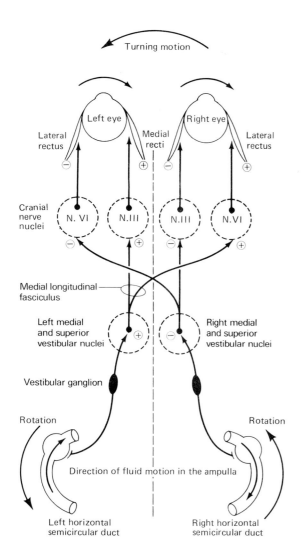

44–14 This circuit diagram for the initial phase of the vestibulo-oculomotor reflex arc shows how excitation of fibers in the ampulla of the left horizontal duct leads to contraction of the muscles that turn both eyes to the right. Increase (+) or decrease (−) in rate of firing along a particular pathway is limited.

For motion in planes other than the horizontal, the other ducts work together in pairs just as do the horizontal ducts.

The coordinated regulation characteristic of the vestibulo-oculomotor reflex was examined experimentally in the 1950s by Janos Szentágothai. He sealed a cannula in the left horizontal semicircular duct of an experimental animal and alternately pushed and pulled the endolymph while recording the tension in each of the extraocular muscles. When the endolymph was pushed, simulating a rotational movement to the left, the medial rectus of the left eye and the lateral rectus of the right eye contracted, while the lateral rectus of the left eye and the medial rectus of the right eye showed reduced tension.

As we saw in Chapter 43, the *voluntary* control of eye movements is independent of the vestibular system. The most important regions of the cerebral cortex involved in voluntary movements of the eyes are the frontal eye fields, located in the frontal lobes. When the frontal eye fields are stimulated electrically on one side of the brain, there is a conjugate deviation of the eyes to the opposite side. Patients with lesions in the frontal fields are unable to make voluntary eye movements to the side opposite the lesion, but other reflex movements of the eyes, mediated by the vestibular system, remain intact.

Inferior Vestibular Nucleus. The descending vestibular nucleus appears to receive primary vestibular fibers from the semicircular ducts and from the utricle and saccule. Like Deiters' nucleus, this nucleus also receives afferents from the vermis of the cerebellum. The majority of efferent fibers contribute to the vestibulospinal and vestibuloreticular pathways, and they exert a major influence on the cerebellum. This nucleus, therefore, is structured to integrate input from the peripheral vestibular apparatus and the cerebellum, and to affect the activity of centers at higher levels in the brain stem, perhaps even in the thalamus.

Some primary vestibular fibers terminate directly in the flocculonodular lobe of the cerebellum. These axons terminate as mossy fibers in the granular layer. They are important for the cerebellar control of posture. Some neurons in the vestibular complex itself (the medial, superior, and inferior nuclei) also send their axons to the cerebellum and are similarly important for postural control.

Movements of the Head and Neck Can Produce Tonic Neck and Labyrinthine Reflexes

In experimental animals, reflex alterations in the tone of limb muscles may be produced by movements of the head that cause activity in joint receptors in the neck. By keeping the angle of the neck constant while moving the head, or by bending the neck and maintaining the head in a constant position in relation to gravitational force, it is possible to separate the effects of *tonic neck reflexes* from those of *tonic labyrinthine reflexes* arising in the vestibular system. In the cat, for example, tonic neck reflexes cause the forelimb to extend and the hind limb to flex when the neck is bent backward or dorsiflexed. This has the net effect of destabilizing the animal's posture. Tonic labyrinthine reflexes counterbalance the neck reflexes so that appropriate postural adjustments are made in response to changes in head position to allow the nervous system to maintain global control of body posture.

An Overall View

The central connections of the vestibular nuclei are summarized in Figure 44–15. This vestibular system receives input from a complex peripheral receptor, the vestibular

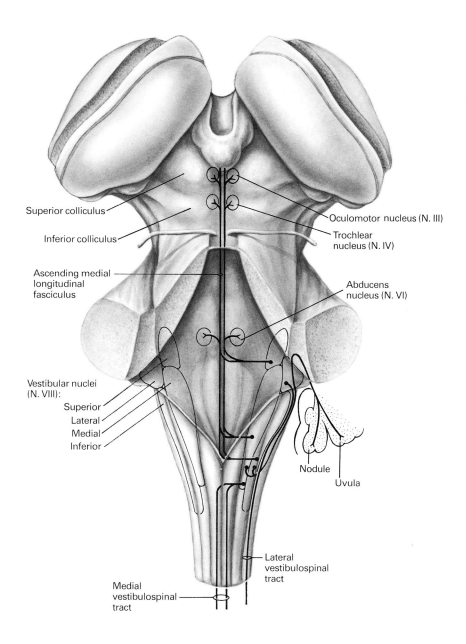

Superior colliculus

Inferior colliculus

Ascending medial
longitudinal
fasciculus

Vestibular nuclei
(N. VIII):

Superior
Lateral
Medial
Inferior

Oculomotor nucleus (N. III)

Trochlear
nucleus (N. IV)

Abducens
nucleus (N. VI)

Nodule

Uvula

Lateral
vestibulospinal
tract

Medial
vestibulospinal
tract

44–15 The central connections of the vestibular nuclei are summarized in this dorsal view of the brain stem.

hair cell, whose physiological properties determine several aspects of vestibular function. Many peripheral receptors, for example the Pacinian corpuscle, depolarize in response to an appropriate stimulus. Others, such as vertebrate photoreceptors, hyperpolarize. The vestibular hair cell, however, may either depolarize or hyperpolarize depending upon the direction of head movement or tilt. Furthermore, any motion of the head affects both sides, so there must be extensive interaction in the central nervous system between the inputs arising from both labyrinths. The bidirectional nature of the hair cell response, along with the bilateral interaction of the labyrinth, provides multiple indications of head movement and position.

An analysis of vestibular function also shows clearly the important difference between *sensory* and *afferent*

information reaching the brain. A large percentage of dorsal root fibers relay sensory information to the spinal cord. This information—about the size, intensity, or temperature of stimuli impinging upon the skin—is then relayed to higher centers in the brain and eventually reaches consciousness. Much of the input carried centrally via the vestibular division is purely *afferent* in nature: the input is used to mediate a variety of reflexes but much of it never reaches consciousness. Even though we are usually unaware of the functions of the vestibular system, its normal operation is essential for the performance of most motor behaviors.

Selected Readings

Brodal, A. 1981. Neurological Anatomy in Relation to Clinical Medicine, 3rd ed. New York: Oxford University Press, pp. 470–495.

Corey, D. P., and Hudspeth, A. J. 1979. Ionic basis of the receptor potential in a vertebrate hair cell. Nature 281:675–677.

Flock, Å. 1964. Structure of the macula utriculi with special reference to directional interplay of sensory responses as revealed by morphological polarization. J. Cell Biol. 22:413–431.

Hudspeth, A. J., and Corey, D. P. 1977. Sensitivity, polarity, and conductance change in the response of vertebrate hair cells to controlled mechanical stimuli. Proc. Natl. Acad. Sci. U.S.A. 74:2407–2411.

Ohmori, H. 1984. Mechanoelectrical transducer has discrete conductances in the chick vestibular hair cell. Proc. Natl. Acad. Sci. U.S.A. 81:1888–1891.

Wilson, V. J., and Melvill Jones, G. 1979. Mammalian Vestibular Physiology. New York: Plenum Press.

References

Flock, Å. 1965. Transducing mechanisms in the lateral line canal organ receptors. Cold Spring Harbor Symp. Quant. Biol. 30:133–145.

Iurato, S. 1967. Submicroscopic Structure of the Inner Ear. Oxford: Pergamon Press.

Spoendlin, H. 1966. Ultrastructure of the vestibular sense organ. In R. J. Wolfson (ed.), The Vestibular System and Its Diseases. Philadelphia: University of Pennsylvania Press, pp. 39–68.

Szentágothai, J. 1950. The elementary vestibulo-ocular reflex arc. J. Neurophysiol. 13:395–407.

Wersäll, J., and Flock, Å. 1965. Functional anatomy of the vestibular and lateral line organs. In W. D. Neff (ed.), Contributions to Sensory Physiology, Vol. 1. New York: Academic Press, pp. 39–61.

Lewis P. Rowland

Clinical Syndromes of the Brain Stem

45

Crowded into the small space of the brain stem are the nuclear groups and nerve fibers of the cranial nerves, the long sensory tracts ascending from the spinal cord to the thalamus and cortex, and the motor pathways descending from the cortex and the subcortical nuclei to the brain stem and spinal cord. In addition, the brain stem contains the reticular formation, with autonomic centers that control respiration, blood pressure, and gastrointestinal functions as well as centers that mediate arousal and wakefulness. Finally, the brain stem surrounds a narrow passage for the circulation of cerebrospinal fluid; that channel, the aqueduct of Sylvius, is susceptible to occlusion. No other region of the central nervous system is as densely packed with vital structures; it is therefore not surprising that a small lesion in the brain stem can have disastrous results.

Knowledge of the anatomy of the cranial nerves and of the ascending and descending tracts is essential for accurate diagnosis of disorders of the brain stem. Abnormalities in the function of specific cranial nerves can localize a lesion to particular levels of the brain stem, for example, to the medulla or to the pons (Figure 45–1). At that horizontal level, the signs caused by lesions of the long tracts—such as the corticospinal tract medially or the spinothalamic tract laterally—can localize the lesion to the medial or lateral segment of that level. The combined information provided by disorders of tracts and cranial nerves can therefore indicate that the lesion affects a specific site in the brain stem.

In this chapter, we shall consider the structures of the brain stem from a clinical perspective. Rather than examining all possible abnormalities, we shall concentrate on illustrative vascular lesions at four critical levels because they cause

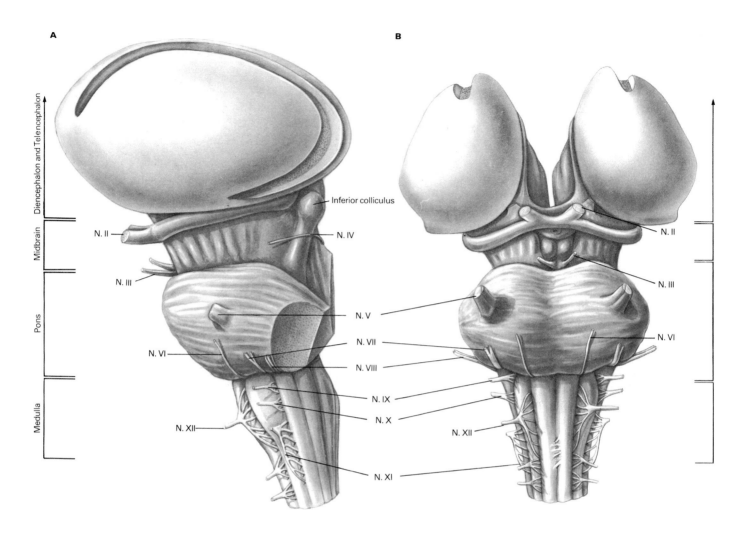

45–1 Two views of the brain stem show the location of the cranial nerves. **A.** Lateral view. **B.** Ventral view.

characteristic symptoms that can readily be inferred from the anatomy. Other conditions also affect the brain stem, but we cannot consider them here; for instance, lesions in the brain stem are common in multiple sclerosis and in brain tumors of the posterior fossa.

Familiarity with Anatomy Is Necessary to Locate Lesions in the Brain Stem

To localize lesions within the brain stem, it is useful to delineate structures along two planes, the longitudinal and the cross-sectional. Along the longitudinal plane, areas of the brain stem that lie in the direction of the cerebral hemispheres are called *upper*, *superior*, or *rostral*; areas that lie in the direction of the spinal cord are called *lower*, *inferior*, or *caudal* (Figure 45–1). In cross section, the lowermost structures are called *ventral*; the upper structures are called *dorsal* or *tegmental*.

As is the case in spinal cord disease (see Chapter 36), it is critical in clinical practice to determine whether the site of a lesion lies within or outside the brain stem proper. A lesion that directly affects the tissue of the brain stem is called *intra-axial*, *intramedullary*, or *parenchymal*. A lesion outside the brain stem—such as one affecting the peripheral course of a cranial nerve—is called *extra-axial*.

Because of the anatomical arrangement, unilateral lesions within the brain stem tend to cause crossed syndromes, in which some signs are ipsilateral and others are contralateral to the lesion. Extra-axial lesions may affect only specific groups of cranial nerves, but extra-axial tumors may also compress the brain stem so that ascending and descending tracts are compromised, making it difficult to distinguish between intra- and extra-axial lesions on clinical grounds.

Extra-axial Lesions Are Illustrated by Tumors of the Cerebellopontine Angle

Small extra-axial lesions affecting the brain stem often begin by compressing and interfering with the function of individual cranial nerves. Neighboring structures within the brain stem may then be affected, causing long tract signs. Isolated cranial nerve disorders, however, are more likely to be due to peripheral lesions, affecting the nerves as they exit through the foramina of the skull. Intracranial tumors outside the brain stem may also begin by compressing cranial nerves.

As an example of a common extra-axial lesion we shall consider the *acoustic neuroma*. This extramedullary tumor originates from Schwann cells of the sheath of the acoustic nerve (VIII) within the acoustic canal and grows in the angle between the cerebellum and the pons (the cerebellopontine angle). The acoustic neuroma first compresses the cochlear nerve, causing ringing in the ear (tinnitus), loss of hearing, and ultimately deafness. The distance from the internal auditory meatus to neighboring nerves and the brain stem is short (Figure 45–2). As the tumor grows into the angle between the cerebellum and the pons, the corneal reflex may be lost, signifying compression of afferent fibers of the trigeminal nerve (V). Later, other trigeminal motor and sensory functions may also be lost. The next signs may involve the facial nerve (VII) or the ipsilateral cerebellar hemisphere. When the facial nerve is affected, there is a lower motor neuron type of paralysis on the same side of the face. If the cerebellar hemisphere is compressed, there is ipsilateral limb *ataxia* and *intention tremor* (a tremor that is intensified by voluntary movement) or *nystagmus* (rhythmical oscillation of the eyes, with a fast movement in one direction and a slow movement in the other) (Figure 45–3). The brain stem ultimately becomes compressed, causing corticospinal tract signs or narrowing the aqueduct to cause hydrocephalus and symptoms of increased intracranial pressure (as explained in Appendix IA). The tumor is now usually detected by computerized tomogra-

phy or magnetic resonance imaging before the condition progresses to hydrocephalus. Acoustic neuromas are benign and accessible tumors that can be removed surgically.

Intra-axial Lesions Often Cause Gaze Palsies and Internuclear Ophthalmoplegia

Gaze Palsies

Many lesions of the brain stem cause abnormalities of gaze (conjugate movements of both eyes) or nystagmus. It is therefore useful to review the relationship between two of the centers controlling eye movements that we considered in Chapter 43—the occipital and frontal eyefields and the pontine gaze center (Figure 45–3).

Discharging epileptic foci or electrical stimulation of frontal or occipital eye fields on one side causes both eyes to move conjugately to the opposite side (Figure 45–4A). Conversely, destructive lesions of the cortical frontal area may result in impaired gaze toward the side opposite the lesion. A patient with a lesion in the right frontal lobe, for example, cannot move the eyes conjugately to the left, and they tend to drift to the right (Figure 45–4B). If a lesion in the right hemisphere also causes a left hemiplegia, the eyes therefore seem to look *away* from the hemiplegia.

45–2 The acoustic neuroma grows in the cerebellopontine angle and causes a characteristic syndrome. **A.** A view of the inner surface of the cranium with the brain stem and cerebellum removed showing the normal cerebellopontine angle. **B.** Changes caused by an acoustic neuroma. (Adapted from Patten, 1977.)

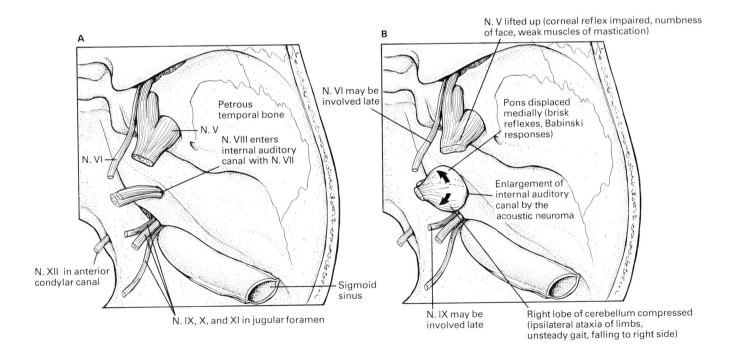

A

N. VI may be involved late

Petrous temporal bone

N. V

N. VIII enters internal auditory canal with N. VII

N. VI

N. XII in anterior condylar canal

Sigmoid sinus

N. IX, X, and XI in jugular foramen

B

N. V lifted up (corneal reflex impaired, numbness of face, weak muscles of mastication)

Pons displaced medially (brisk reflexes, Babinski responses)

Enlargement of internal auditory canal by the acoustic neuroma

N. IX may be involved late

Right lobe of cerebellum compressed (ipsilateral ataxia of limbs, unsteady gait, falling to right side)

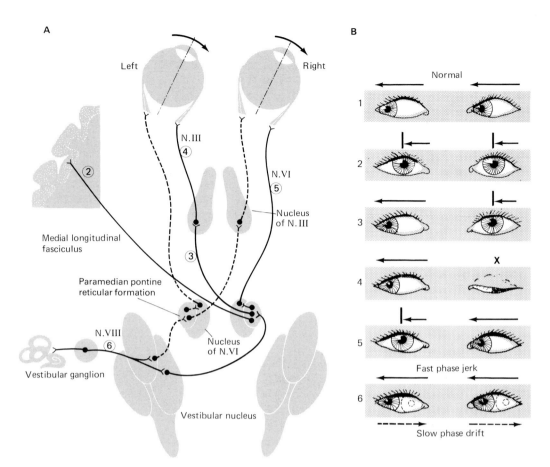

45–3 Lesions of the neural pathways subtending horizontal gaze lead to specific deficits. **A.** Pathways for horizontal gaze. **Numbers** indicate sites of lesions. **B.** Abnormalities of eye movements on attempted gaze to the right correspond to the numbered lesions in the horizontal gaze system shown in part **A. 1:** Normal right gaze. **2:** Left cortical lesion (gaze to the right is impaired). **3:** Left medial longitudinal fasciculus lesion (impaired adduction of the left eye; nystagmus of abducting right eye). **4:** Left oculomotor nerve lesion (impaired adduction of left eye plus other manifestations of third-nerve palsy, including the ptosis illustrated). **5:** Right abducens nerve lesion, with isolated paralysis of lateral rectus. **6:** Left vestibular nerve lesion (jerk nystagmus). (Adapted from Sears and Franklin, 1980.)

The fibers descending from the cortical eye fields cross the midline to the contralateral pontine gaze center in the reticular formation, near the sixth-nerve nucleus (Figure 45–3A). Lesions in or near the pontine gaze centers impair gaze toward the side of the lesion. For instance, a destructive lesion on the right side of the pons impairs gaze to the right, and the eyes tend to drift to the left. If corticospinal fibers are also involved, the right-sided lesion is above the decussation of the descending fibers. Therefore, a left hemiplegia results, and the eyes look *toward* the hemiplegia (Figure 45–4C).

Syndrome of the Medial Longitudinal Fasciculus: Internuclear Ophthalmoplegia

Gaze to the right requires coordinated activity of the right lateral rectus muscle (innervated by the sixth nerve) and the left medial rectus (innervated by the third nerve). This integration depends upon functions of the pontine gaze center or *paramedian pontine reticular formation.* The paramedian pontine reticular formation sends fibers to the ipsilateral abducens nucleus and the contralateral oculomotor nucleus (Figure 45–3A). These fibers travel with vestibular and other fibers in the medial longitudinal fasciculus. Lesions in the medial longitudinal fasciculus cause a characteristic combination of signs called *internuclear ophthalmoplegia* (Figure 45–3B, 3). In young adults the most common cause of internuclear ophthalmoplegia is multiple sclerosis. In later life, the syndrome is most often caused by occlusion of the basilar artery (described below) or paramedian branches of that artery.

If the lesion is unilateral, adduction of the eye on that side is impaired or paralyzed (Figure 45–3B,3). By convention, lesions within the medial longitudinal fasciculus—as opposed to those in the paramedian pontine reticular formation—are named for the side of the affected medial rectus. The supranuclear nature of the impaired adduction on attempted gaze can be deduced because the function of the medial rectus in the reflex responses of convergence for near vision is preserved. (If rostral lesions involve the third-nerve nucleus, convergence may also be lost.)

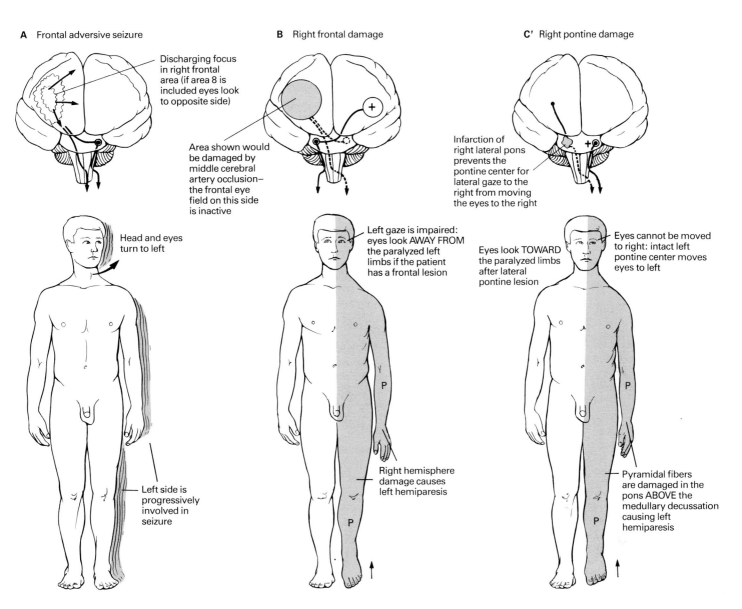

A Frontal adversive seizure

Discharging focus in right frontal area (if area 8 is included eyes look to opposite side)

Head and eyes turn to left

Left side is progressively involved in seizure

B Right frontal damage

Area shown would be damaged by middle cerebral artery occlusion—the frontal eye field on this side is inactive

Left gaze is impaired: eyes look AWAY FROM the paralyzed left limbs if the patient has a frontal lesion

Right hemisphere damage causes left hemiparesis

C' Right pontine damage

Infarction of right lateral pons prevents the pontine center for lateral gaze to the right from moving the eyes to the right

Eyes look TOWARD the paralyzed limbs after lateral pontine lesion

Eyes cannot be moved to right: intact left pontine center moves eyes to left

Pyramidal fibers are damaged in the pons ABOVE the medullary decussation causing left hemiparesis

45–4 Disorders of gaze in relation to other impairments can indicate the nature of the lesion. Direction of gaze (see **eyes**), functioning gaze center (**+**), paretic limbs (**P**), and the presence of the Babinski sign (↑) are indicated. **A.** Frontal adversive seizure. **B.** Right frontal damage. **C.** Right pontine damage. (Adapted from Patten, 1977.)

In internuclear ophthalmoplegia, there is often nystagmus of the abducting eye. The cause of this nystagmus is not known. Formerly attributed to an interruption of vestibular fibers, it is now regarded as evidence of persistent convergence; that is, the patient uses the only possible eye movement mechanism (convergence) remaining to adduct the paretic medial rectus. Convergence, however, involves both eyes, and the abducting eye also adducts momentarily. To resume its position, the abducting eye makes a quick movement to refixate on the laterally placed target, and this appears as nystagmus.

Vascular Lesions of the Brain Stem and Midbrain May Cause Characteristic Syndromes

The medulla is supplied by branches of the vertebral artery, including the posterior inferior cerebellar artery (Figure 45–5). The two vertebral arteries of each side join to form the *basilar artery*, which runs along the base of

the pons and produces three sets of branches: (1) *paramedian branches*, which supply midline structures of the pons; (2) *short circumferential branches*, which supply the lateral aspect of the pons and the middle and superior cerebellar peduncles; and (3) *long circumferential arteries*, the *inferior* and *superior cerebellar arteries*, which also supply lateral portions of the brain stem and run around the pons to reach the cerebellar hemispheres. (The basilar artery terminates by dividing into the two posterior cerebral arteries. These vessels are then linked to the corresponding carotid arteries by the posterior communicating arteries to complete the posterior portion of the circle of Willis.)

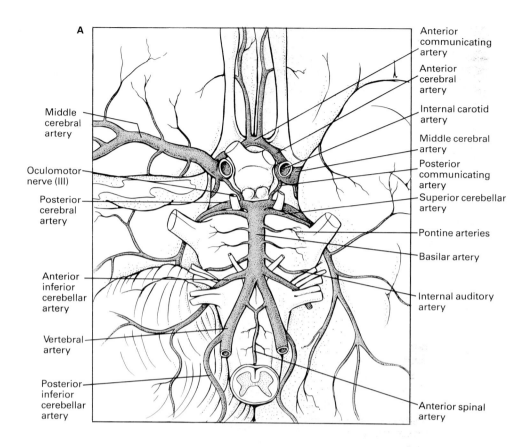

A

Anterior communicating artery

Anterior cerebral artery

Internal carotid artery

Middle cerebral artery

Posterior communicating artery

Superior cerebellar artery

Pontine arteries

Basilar artery

Internal auditory artery

Anterior spinal artery

Middle cerebral artery

Oculomotor nerve (III)

Posterior cerebral artery

Anterior inferior cerebellar artery

Vertebral artery

Posterior inferior cerebellar artery

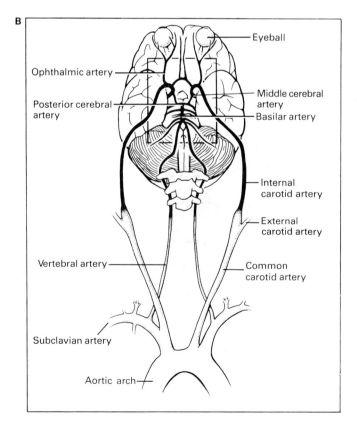

B

Eyeball

Ophthalmic artery

Posterior cerebral artery

Middle cerebral artery

Basilar artery

Internal carotid artery

External carotid artery

Vertebral artery

Common carotid artery

Subclavian artery

Aortic arch

45–5 Branches of the vertebral arteries carry the blood supply to the brain stem. **A.** Dorsal view. (Adapted from Patten, 1977.) **B.** Three-dimensional view along the longitudinal axis of the brain stem. Details of area indicated by **box** are illustrated in part **A.** (Adapted from Martinez Martinez, 1982.)

Table 45–1. Features Common to Syndromes at Any Level of the Medulla or Pons

Syndromes	Structure involved	Signs
Medial	Corticospinal tract	Hemiparesis (contralateral)
	Medial lemniscus	Loss of position and vibration sense (contralateral)
	Cerebellar connections (pons)	Limb ataxia or nystagmus (ipsilateral)
Lateral	Cerebellar connections	Limb ataxia (ipsilateral)
	Sensory nucleus or descending sensory tract of trigeminal nerve	Loss of cutaneous sensation on face (ipsilateral)
	Descending autonomic fibers	Horner's syndrome: miosis, ptosis, impaired sweating (ipsilateral)
	Spinothalamic tract	Loss of pain and temperature sensation (contralateral)
	Vestibular nuclei and connections	Nystagmus, nausea, vomiting
	Uncertain	Hiccup

Sometimes only a branch of the basilar artery is occluded selectively, resulting in a restricted lesion in the brain and often a characteristic syndrome. More often, either the vertebral or the basilar artery itself is occluded, giving rise to a more extensive lesion, which may be unilateral or bilateral and causes signs of more than one of the characteristic syndromes that occur when only a single branch is occluded. Here we shall consider the simple case of a single occluded branch vessel giving rise to a single syndrome. In actual clinical situations, however, the occlusion often leads to mixtures of the individual syndromes.

The longitudinal continuity of ascending and descending pathways places the different tracts in relatively constant medial or lateral positions that are maintained in cross sections at different levels. Because the locations of tracts and cranial nerve nuclei are fixed, specific combinations of signs reliably indicate the site of the lesion. Analysis of disorders of the brain stem is therefore greatly simplified by principles that help answer two questions:

1. *Is the lesion medial or lateral?* Below the midbrain, manifestations of lesions in long ascending and descending tracts indicate whether the lesion is medial or lateral (Table 45–1).

2. *What is the level of the lesion?* Specific cranial nerve signs delineate the actual level of the lesion (Table 45–2).

Table 45–2. Specific Syndromes Produced by Vascular Lesions of the Brain Stem

Syndrome	Artery affected	Structure involved	Specific manifestations
Medullary			
Medial	Paramedian branches	Emerging fibers of nerve XII	Ipsilateral hemiparalysis of tongue
Lateral	Posterior inferior cerebellar	Emerging fibers of nerves IX and X	Dysphagia, hoarseness, ipsilateral paralysis of vocal cord; ipsilateral loss of pharyngeal reflex
		Solitary nucleus and tract	Loss of taste on ipsilateral half of tongue
Inferior pontine			
Medial	Paramedian branches	Pontine gaze center, near nucleus of nerve XI	Paralysis of gaze to side of lesion
		Vestibular nucleus or connections, or medial longitudinal fasciculus	Gaze-evoked nystagmus
		Nucleus or emerging fibers of nerve VI	Paralysis of ipsilateral lateral rectus
Lateral	Anterior inferior cerebellar	Emerging fibers of nerve VII	Ipsilateral facial paralysis
		Pontine gaze center	Paralysis of gaze to side of lesion
		Nerve VIII or cochlear nucleus	Deafness, tinnitus
Superior pontine			
Medial	Paramedian branches	Medial longitudinal fasciculus	Internuclear ophthalmoplegia
		Uncertain	Palatal myoclonus

These signs, which localize the lesion in both the longitudinal and horizontal extent of the brain stem, can be best understood by referring to the figures that accompany the following descriptions of the lesions.

Medial Syndromes of the Medulla and Pons

Medial lesions arise from occlusion of the paramedian branches of the basilar artery. A unilateral medial lesion in the pons or upper medulla affects the corticospinal tract and medial lemniscus, with corresponding signs on the other side of the body: (1) contralateral hemiparesis and (2) contralateral loss of position and vibratory sensation (Table 45–1 and Figure 45–6). Cutaneous sensation, which is mediated by the spinothalamic tracts, is spared.

If the lesion is in the medulla, it will not affect the corticobulbar fibers to the facial nerve nucleus (which lies in the pons), so there will be no facial paralysis. Similarly, the connections to the cerebellum are spared, and there may be no ipsilateral limb ataxia or nystagmus. Ataxia does occur in medial pontine lesions, however, because of damage to the crossing cerebellar connections of the middle cerebellar peduncle.

The cranial nerve signs serve to identify the actual level of a medial lesion, differentiating medial syndromes of the medulla from those of the pons (Table 45–2 and Figure 45–6).

In the *medial syndrome of the medulla* (Figure 45–6A), the emerging fibers of the hypoglossal nerve (XII) are involved, causing ipsilateral weakness and later wasting of that half of the tongue. In the *medial syndrome of the pons* (Figure 45–6B), the lateral rectus muscle may be paralyzed if the lesion is rostral and extends dorsally to affect the nucleus of the abducens nerve (VI) or the emerging fibers of the nerve. Lesions involving the nucleus of the sixth nerve are likely to cause ipsilateral gaze palsy rather than isolated paralysis of the abducens. Nystagmus may also be present if the lesion involves vestibular or cerebellar connections or the medial longitudinal fasciculus.

Lateral Syndromes of the Medulla and Pons

Lateral lesions arise from occlusion of the posterior inferior cerebellar artery or the anterior inferior cerebellar artery. The resulting lesions affect lateral structures (not those affected in medial lesions). Lateral lesions involve the spinothalamic tract, descending autonomic fibers, the nucleus or descending sensory tract of the trigeminal nerve, vestibular nuclei, and cerebellar connections.

All lateral lesions involve a set of six common manifestations that may appear together or in different combinations (Table 45–1): (1) contralateral loss of pain and temperature sensation of the limbs and trunk due to damage in the spinothalamic tract; (2) ipsilateral Horner syndrome with miosis (small pupil with normal reaction

to light), ptosis of the eyelid, and decreased sweating on the ipsilateral side of the face due to interruption of descending autonomic fibers; (3) ipsilateral loss of cutaneous sensation on the face from involvement of the sensory trigeminal nucleus or descending tract; (4) nystagmus and nausea attributed to involvement of vestibular connections; (5) ataxia of the ipsilateral limbs due to interruption of cerebellar connections—the restiform body in the medulla, and the middle and superior peduncles in the pons; and (6) hiccup for reasons not known. Lateral lesions do not cause hemiparesis or loss of proprioception.

Vascular lesions can affect the brain stem at several levels to produce a variety of syndromes. Involvement of specific cranial nerves distinguishes the actual level of the syndrome.

The *lateral medullary syndrome* (Wallenberg syndrome) is caused by occlusion of the posterior inferior cerebellar artery or the vertebral artery (Figure 45–6A). This damages the dorsal portion of the lateral medulla, the lateral medullary tegmentum. In addition to the six common characteristics listed above, glossopharyngeal (IX) and vagal (X) cranial nerves may be involved, causing difficulty swallowing (dysphagia), hoarseness of the voice because of paralysis of the ipsilateral vocal cord, and loss of the ipsilateral pharyngeal reflex (Table 45–2). The solitary nucleus may also be destroyed, leading to loss of taste on the ipsilateral half of the tongue.

The *lateral syndrome of the lower pons* results from occlusion of the anterior inferior cerebellar artery (Figure 45–6B). It includes the six common lateral manifestations and three additional specific signs that arise from damage of the facial (VII) and auditory (VIII) nuclei (Table 45–2): (1) ipsilateral facial paralysis of the lower motor neuron type because the lesion involves either the facial nucleus or the emerging fibers of the seventh nerve; (2) deafness and tinnitus; and (3) ipsilateral gaze paralysis if the lesion extends medially to affect the pontine gaze center.

Lateral lesions of the midpons due to occlusion of a short circumferential artery cause a syndrome identical to that of the lower pons except that nerves VII and VIII are spared and there is no abnormality of facial movement or hearing. Instead, trigeminal motor functions are implicated. In *lateral lesions of the superior pons* (Figure 45–6C), which arise from occlusion of the superior cerebellar artery, there are no specific cranial signs. In other words, facial paralysis and hearing loss imply a lateral lesion of the lower pons; impaired trigeminal functions imply a lesion of the midpons; and none of these cranial nerves is affected by lesions of the upper pons.

45–6 Structures involved (**shaded areas**) in syndromes of brain stem vascular lesions. **A.** Medulla. **B.** Lower pons. **C.** Upper pons. (Adapted from Adams and Victor, 1977.)

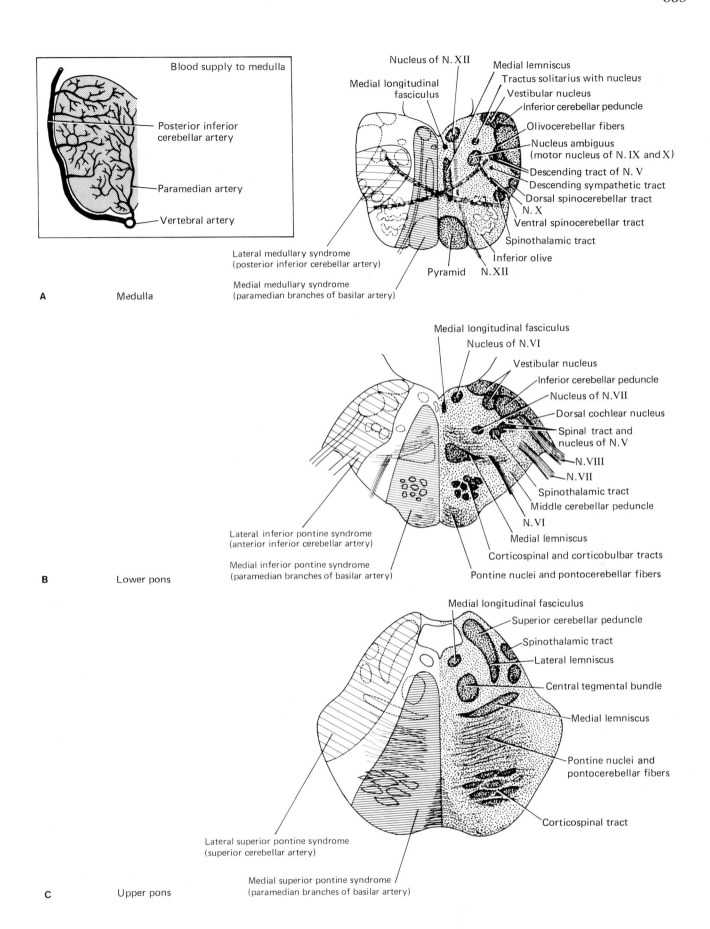

Blood supply to medulla

Posterior inferior cerebellar artery

Paramedian artery

Vertebral artery

Nucleus of N. XII

Medial longitudinal fasciculus

Medial lemniscus

Tractus solitarius with nucleus

Vestibular nucleus

Inferior cerebellar peduncle

Olivocerebellar fibers

Nucleus ambiguus (motor nucleus of N. IX and X)

Descending tract of N. V

Descending sympathetic tract

Dorsal spinocerebellar tract

N. X

Ventral spinocerebellar tract

Spinothalamic tract

Inferior olive

Pyramid

N. XII

Lateral medullary syndrome (posterior inferior cerebellar artery)

Medial medullary syndrome (paramedian branches of basilar artery)

A   Medulla

Medial longitudinal fasciculus

Nucleus of N.VI

Vestibular nucleus

Inferior cerebellar peduncle

Nucleus of N.VII

Dorsal cochlear nucleus

Spinal tract and nucleus of N. V

N.VIII

N.VII

Spinothalamic tract

Middle cerebellar peduncle

N. VI

Medial lemniscus

Corticospinal and corticobulbar tracts

Pontine nuclei and pontocerebellar fibers

Lateral inferior pontine syndrome (anterior inferior cerebellar artery)

Medial inferior pontine syndrome (paramedian branches of basilar artery)

B   Lower pons

Medial longitudinal fasciculus

Superior cerebellar peduncle

Spinothalamic tract

Lateral lemniscus

Central tegmental bundle

Medial lemniscus

Pontine nuclei and pontocerebellar fibers

Corticospinal tract

Lateral superior pontine syndrome (superior cerebellar artery)

Medial superior pontine syndrome (paramedian branches of basilar artery)

C   Upper pons

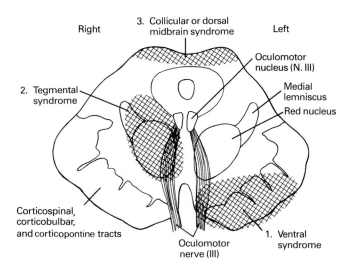

45–7 Areas affected (**cross-hatched areas**) in the three midbrain syndromes. (Adapted from Gatz, 1966.)

Midbrain Syndromes

The clinical anatomy of the mesencephalon is less complicated than that of the medulla and pons, but even in this small area three separate syndromes are recognized (Figure 45–7). In the *ventral syndrome* (Weber syndrome) a lesion of the cerebral peduncle causes (1) contralateral hemiparesis, including supranuclear facial paresis due to damage of the corticospinal and corticobulbar tracts, and (2) ipsilateral oculomotor nerve palsy from damage of the emerging third-nerve fibers.

In the *central or tegmental syndrome* oculomotor nerve palsy is again seen because of a lesion in either a nucleus or emerging fibers, but there is also a tremor or involuntary movement of the contralateral limbs. This condition, called *hemichorea*, is attributed to a lesion in the red nucleus. In addition, there is contralateral hemianesthesia that includes both primary forms of sensation: cutaneous sensation (carried by the spinothalamic tract) and proprioception (carried in the medial lemniscus). The corticospinal tract is spared if the lesion is limited, as in Figure 45–7.

The *dorsal midbrain or collicular syndrome* (Parinaud syndrome) is usually caused by an extra-axial lesion, most often a tumor of the pineal gland (pinealoma) that compresses the superior colliculi and pretectal structures. This compression causes paralysis of upward gaze but does not affect other eye movements.

Coma and the Locked-in Syndrome

Because brain stem mechanisms are normally so important in maintaining alertness, lesions in this area often cause coma. It is therefore important to recognize brain stem signs in the examination of a comatose patient (see Chapter 50) or patients with massive lesions that are likely to cause brain stem signs due to downward tentorial herniation or herniation of the cerebellum through the foramen magnum.

Bilateral lesions of the ventral pons, usually due to occlusion of the basilar artery, may interrupt the corticobulbar and corticospinal tracts on both sides. As a result, the patient is quadriplegic, unable to speak, and incapable of facial movement. This state may resemble coma, but the eyes are open and move, and the patient is fully conscious and able to communicate by movement of the eyelids or eyes, although otherwise completely immobile or "locked in."

An Overall View

There are many brain stem syndromes and the analysis of these syndromes is of more than diagnostic importance; it tells us something about how the brain is organized and how it functions.

Selected Readings

Adams, R. D., and Victor, M. 1977. Principles of Neurology. New York: McGraw-Hill.

Ash, P. R., and Keltner, J. L. 1979. Neuro-ophthalmic signs in pontine lesions. Medicine (Baltimore) 58:304–320.

Bauer, G., Gerstenbrand, F., and Rumpl, E. 1979. Varieties of the locked-in syndrome. J. Neurol. 221:77–91.

Bilaniuk, L. T., Zimmerman, R. A., Littman, P., Gallo, E., Rorke, L. B., Bruce, D. A., and Schut, L. 1980. Computed tomography of brain stem gliomas in children. Radiology 134:89–95.

Britt, R. H., Herrick, M. K., and Hamilton, R. D. 1977. Traumatic locked-in syndrome. Ann. Neurol. 1:590–592.

Caplan, L. R. 1980. "Top of the basilar" syndrome. Neurology 30:72–79.

Daniels, D. L., Williams, A. L., and Haughton, V. M. 1982. Computed tomography of the medulla. Radiology 145:63–69.

Glaser, J. S. 1978. Neuro-ophthalmology. Hagerstown, Md.: Harper & Row.

Harner, S. G., and Laws, E. R., Jr. 1981. Diagnosis of acoustic neurinoma. Neurosurgery 9:373–379.

Ho, K.-L., and Meyer, K. R. 1981. The medial medullary syndrome. Arch. Neurol. 38:385–387.

Levin, B. E., and Margolis, G. 1977. Acute failure of automatic respirations secondary to a unilateral brainstem infarct. Ann. Neurol. 1:583–586.

Plum, F., and Posner, J. B. 1980. The Diagnosis of Stupor and Coma, 3rd ed. Philadelphia: Davis.

Seales, D. M., Torkelson, R. D., Shuman, R. M., Rossiter, V. S., and Spencer, J. D. 1981. Abnormal brainstem auditory evoked potentials and neuropathology in "locked-in" syndrome. Neurology 31:893–896.

References

Baloh, R. W., Furman, J. M., and Yee, R. D. 1985. Dorsal midbrain syndrome: Clinical and oculographic findings. Neurology 35:54–60.

Bydder, G. M., Steiner, R. E., Thomas, D. J., Marshall, J., Gilderdale, D. J., and Young, I. R. 1983. Nuclear magnetic resonance imaging of the posterior fossa: 50 cases. Clin. Radiol. 34:173–188.

Collins, R. D. 1962. Illustrated Manual of Neurologic Diagnosis. Philadelphia: Lippincott.

Curtis, B. A., Jacobson, S., and Marcus, E. M. 1972. An Introduction to the Neurosciences. Philadelphia: Saunders.

Flannigan, B. D., Bradley, W. G., Jr., Mazziota, J. C., Rauschning, W., Bentson, J. R., Lufkin, R. B., and Hieshima, G. B. 1985. Magnetic resonance imaging of the brain stem: normal structure and basic functional anatomy. Radiology 154:375–383.

Gatz, A. J. 1966. Manter's Essentials of Clinical Neuroanatomy and Neurophysiology, 3rd ed. Philadelphia: Davis.

Kalovidouris, A., Mancuso, A. A., and Dillon, W. 1984. A CT-clinical approach to patients with symptoms related to the V, VII, IX-XII cranial nerves and cervical sympathetics. Radiology 151:671–676.

Martinez Martinez, P. F. A. 1982. Neuroanatomy, Development and Structure of the Central Nervous System. Philadelphia: Saunders, p. 101.

Mawad, M. E., Silver, A. J., Hilal, S. K., and Ganti, S. R. 1983. Computed tomography of the brain stem with intrathecal metrizamide. Part I: The normal brain stem. Am. J. Neuroradiol. 4:1–11.

Patten, J. 1977. Neurological Differential Diagnosis. London: Starke. New York: Springer.

Reznik, M. 1983. Neuropathology in seven cases of locked-in syndrome. J. Neurol. Sci. 60:67–78.

Sears, E. S., and Franklin, G. M. 1980. Diseases of the cranial nerves. In R. N. Rosenberg (ed.), The Science and Practice of Clinical Medicine, Vol. 5: Neurology. New York: Grune & Stratton, pp. 471–494.

Hypothalamus, Limbic System, and Cerebral Cortex: Homeostasis and Arousal

VIII

A major function of the nervous system is to maintain the constancy of the internal environment. Homeostatic, regulatory processes that maintain the internal environment have intrigued many of the founders of modern physiology, among them Claude Bernard, Walter B. Cannon, and Walter Hess. Although virtually the whole brain is involved in homeostasis, neurons controlling the internal environment are concentrated in the hypothalamus, a small area of the diencephalon that comprises less than 1% of the total volume of the brain.

The hypothalamus and closely linked structures in the limbic system keep the internal environment constant by regulating three related functions: endocrine secretion, the autonomic nervous system, and emotions and drives. By controlling the endocrine system and autonomic nervous system, the hypothalamus maintains homeostasis by acting *directly* on the internal environment. By controlling emotions and motivated behavior, the hypothalamus maintains homeostasis *indirectly* by acting through the external environment. Because it acts on the external environment by regulating emotional expression, the hypothalamus functions in conjunction with higher control systems located in the limbic system and in the neocortex.

In addition to regulating specific motivated behaviors, the hypothalamus and the cerebral cortex are involved in arousal—the maintenance of a general state of awareness that affects many behaviors simultaneously. The level of arousal varies from states of excitement on the one hand to drowsiness, sleep, and coma on the other. Because the electrical activity of the cortex is an index of wakefulness, studies of arousal and sleep provide insights into the collective behavior of neurons. The electrical activity of the cortex also is important diagnostically for analyzing abnormalities of consciousness, particularly those due to epilepsy.

Irving Kupfermann

Hypothalamus and Limbic System I: Peptidergic Neurons, Homeostasis, and Emotional Behavior

46

In 1878, Claude Bernard, then professor at the Collège de France, first pointed out that human beings and other higher animals live in two environments:

a *milieu extérieur* in which the organism is situated, and a *milieu intérieur* in which the tissue element lives. The living organism does not really exist in the *milieu extérieur*—the atmosphere it breathes, salt or fresh water if that is its element—but in the liquid *milieu intérieur* formed by the circulatory organic liquid which surrounds and bathes all the tissue elements; this is the lymph and the plasma . . . . The *milieu intérieur* surrounding the organs, the tissue and their element never varies . . . . Here we have an organism which has enclosed itself in a kind of hot house. The peripheral changes of external conditions cannot reach it; it is not subject to them, but is free and independent . . . . All the vital mechanisms, however varied they may be, have only one object, that of preserving constant the conditions of life in the internal environment.

The vital mechanisms referred to by Bernard are centered in the hypothalamus and limbic system. Moreover, as Walter B. Cannon, Professor of Physiology at Harvard Medical School, later pointed out, the mechanisms within the hypothalamus ensure not so much constancy as, rather, limited variability. The process by which this limited variability is achieved Cannon called *homeostasis*. The hypothalamus is so important because it is critically responsible for the homeostatic mechanisms that provide, to paraphrase Bernard, the necessary conditions for free and independent life.

The hypothalamus constitutes less than 1% of the total volume of the brain, yet it contains a large number of neuronal circuits concerned with vital functions. These circuits control the regulation of temperature, heart rate, blood pressure, blood osmolarity, and water and food intake. The hypothalamus and related structures in the limbic system are not the only structures in the brain involved in homeostasis. However, they participate in the regulation of homeostasis by receiving information directly from the internal environment and by operating directly on the internal environment, whereas other parts of the brain regulate the internal environment largely indirectly, through action on the external environment. These alternative means of regulating the internal environment often function in parallel. If a room is cold, one can maintain a constant body temperature by peripheral vasoconstriction—a primarily hypothalamic mechanism involving actions on the internal environment. In addition, one can utilize primarily thalamic and cortical mechanisms to operate on the external environment—by, for example, closing the window or writing a note to the landlord asking for more heat.

The hypothalamus exerts its influence on both the internal and external environments through three major systems: the endocrine system; the autonomic nervous system; and an ill-defined neural system concerned with motivation and drive. In this chapter we shall briefly examine the anatomy of the hypothalamus and limbic system and then consider how these structures regulate homeostasis, with an emphasis on endocrine and auto-

nomic control; in Chapter 47 we shall focus on the motivational mechanisms of homeostatic regulation. In addition to homeostatic functions, hypothalamic and limbic structures are important in the regulation of emotional and sexual behavior. In this chapter we shall consider aspects of emotion. Chapter 58 will deal with sexual behavior.

The Anatomy of the Limbic System and Hypothalamus Is Related to Their Functions

The hypothalamus is extensively interconnected with a ring of cortical structures that is part of the limbic system. This area is often referred to as the *visceral brain* because, in conjunction with the hypothalamus, it is concerned with the maintenance of basic autonomic and homeostatic function. An understanding of the anatomy of the hypothalamus can be facilitated by first considering the structure and interconnections of the components of the limbic system.

Higher Cortical Centers Communicate with the Hypothalamus via the Limbic System

The concept of the limbic system derives from the idea of a *limbic lobe* (Latin, *limbus*, border) a term introduced by Pierre Paul Broca to characterize the phylogenetically primitive cortical gyri that form a ring around the brain stem (Figure 46–1A). The limbic lobe includes the parahippocampal gyrus, the cingulate gyrus, and the subcallosal gyrus, which is the anterior and inferior continuation of the cingulate gyrus. It also includes the underlying cortex of the hippocampal formation, which is morphologically even more primitive. The hippocampal formation includes the hippocampus proper, the dentate gyrus, and the subiculum.

In 1937 James Papez, at Cornell University Medical School, suggested that the limbic lobe forms a neural circuit that provides the anatomical substratum for emotions (Figure 46–2). He was influenced by experiments suggesting that the hypothalamus has a critical role in the expression of emotion. (We shall consider these findings later in the chapter.) Papez tried to answer the following question: How do higher cortical centers communicate with the hypothalamus? A cortical connection must exist, Papez argued, since emotions reach consciousness; likewise, thought and other higher cognitive functions affect emotions. Papez therefore proposed that

46–1 The limbic system consists of the limbic lobe and deep-lying structures. **A.** This medial view of the brain shows the limbic lobe, which consists of primitive cortical tissue (**dots**) that encircles the upper brain stem. Also included in the limbic lobe are the underlying cortical structures (hippocampus and dentate gyrus). **B.** This view schematically illustrates the interconnections of deep-lying structures included as part of the limbic system. The most prominent directions of flow of neural activity are indicated by **arrows**, but the designated tracts typically have bidirectional activity. (Adapted from Nieuwenhuys, Voogd, and van Huijzen, 1981.)

A

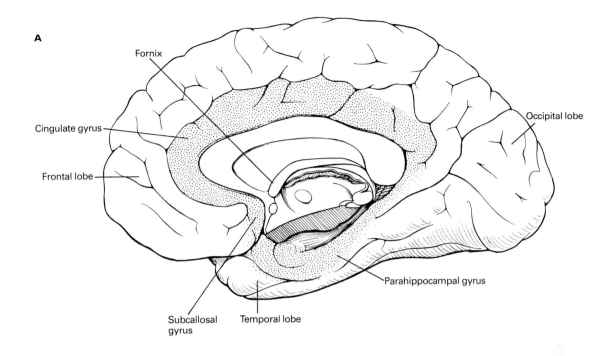

Fornix

Cingulate gyrus

Frontal lobe

Occipital lobe

Parahippocampal gyrus

Subcallosal gyrus

Temporal lobe

B

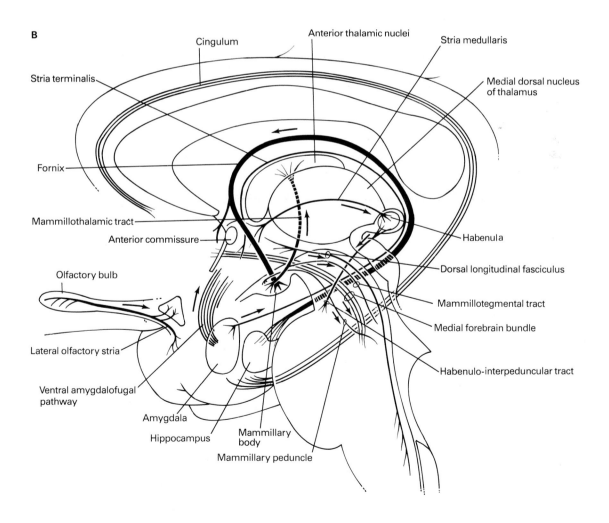

Cingulum

Anterior thalamic nuclei

Stria medullaris

Medial dorsal nucleus of thalamus

Stria terminalis

Fornix

Mammillothalamic tract

Anterior commissure

Olfactory bulb

Lateral olfactory stria

Ventral amygdalofugal pathway

Amygdala

Hippocampus

Mammillary body

Mammillary peduncle

Habenula

Dorsal longitudinal fasciculus

Mammillotegmental tract

Medial forebrain bundle

Habenulo-interpeduncular tract

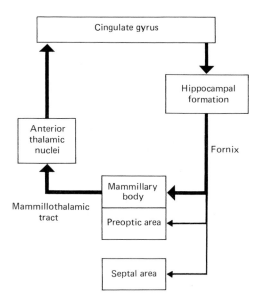

46–2 This is a modified version of the neural circuit for emotion (**thick arrows**) proposed by Papez; known projections of the fornix to the septal area and hypothalamic regions (mammillary bodies and preoptic anterior hypothalamic area) are also indicated (**fine arrows**). The septal area of animals corresponds to a region near the anterior commissure of the human brain just ventral to the septum pellucidum.

cortical influences are funneled to the hypothalamus through connections of the cingulate gyrus to the hippocampal formation. The hippocampal formation would, according to this scheme, process this information and project it, by way of the fornix, to the mammillary bodies of the hypothalamus (Figures 46–1 and 46–2). The hypothalamus would in turn provide information to the cingulate gyrus by a pathway from the mammillary bodies to the anterior thalamic nuclei (through the mammillothalamic tract) and from the anterior thalamic nuclei to the cingulate gyrus (Figures 46–1 and 46–2).

In the same year that Papez outlined this circuit, Heinrich Klüver and Paul Bucy at the University of Chicago reported their extraordinary finding (which we shall also consider later) that bilateral destruction of the temporal lobe, a lobe that includes a number of limbic structures, produces dramatic changes in the emotional behavior of the monkey. The papers by Papez and by Klüver and Bucy provided the background for many of the subsequent theoretical and experimental approaches to the neurobiology of emotions.

The concept of the limbic system was later expanded by Paul MacLean at the National Institute of Mental Health to include other structures functionally and anatomically related to those outlined by Papez. MacLean included in the limbic system parts of the hypothalamus, the septal area, the nucleus accumbens (a part of the striatum), and, finally, neocortical areas such as the orbitofrontal cortex. Also included in MacLean's definition of the limbic system is the amygdala, a subcortical structure located at the dorsomedial tip of the temporal lobe

and continuous with the uncus of the parahippocampal gyrus.

The *amygdala* is composed of numerous nuclei that are reciprocally connected to the hypothalamus, hippocampal formation, and thalamus. The amygdala gives rise to two major efferent projections: the stria terminalis and the ventral amygdalofugal pathway. The *stria terminalis* innervates the bed nucleus of the stria terminalis, the septal area, the nucleus accumbens, and the hypothalamus. The second efferent projection, the *ventral amygdalofugal pathway*, provides input to the hypothalamus, dorsomedial nucleus of the thalamus, and rostral cingulate gyrus. The amygdala in turn receives an important afferent input from the olfactory system and lesser inputs from other afferent systems. Despite extensive olfactory input, the amygdala is not essential for olfactory discrimination. Lesions and stimulation of the amygdala have produced effects similar to those found for the lateral or medial regions of the hypothalamus; these effects (as we shall see below and in Chapter 47) include alterations of autonomic responses, emotional behavior, and feeding.

Modern anatomical studies have greatly expanded our knowledge of the connections of the limbic system and have demonstrated extensive and direct connections between the hippocampal formation, amygdala, and neocortical areas. The input connections to the hippocampus arise by way of the entorhinal cortex and the fornix. The entorhinal cortex receives input from areas of the association cortex and thereby provides a neocortical–limbic link. Some of the fibers from the entorhinal cortex on the way to the hippocampus (the *perforant path*) pass through the *subiculum*, a gray matter structure that is interposed between the primitive cortex of the hippocampus proper and the neocortical tissue of the temporal cortex. The subiculum receives a major output from the hippocampus and has extensive reciprocal connections with many areas of the brain, including several areas of the neocortex. It is of interest that the relative size of the subiculum increases in phylogeny and is greatest in humans. The subiculum is now known to be the origin of those fibers in the fornix that innervate the hypothalamus. The fornix also contains axons of hippocampal pyramidal cells that innervate nonhypothalamic structures.

The Structure of the Hypothalamus Reflects Its Diverse Functions

One of the primary functions of the hypothalamus, its control of the pituitary gland, can be inferred by its position dorsal to the pituitary, to which it is attached by a stalk called the *infundibulum* (Figure 46–3). The posterior extent of the hypothalamus is delimited by the mammillary bodies. The anterior extent is delimited by the optic chiasm, preoptic area, and lamina terminalis.

The hypothalamus can be grossly divided into periventricular, lateral, and medial regions. The *periventricular region* consists of that part of the hypothalamus immediately bordering the third ventricle. The *lateral region* has extensive short-fiber, multisynaptic ascending

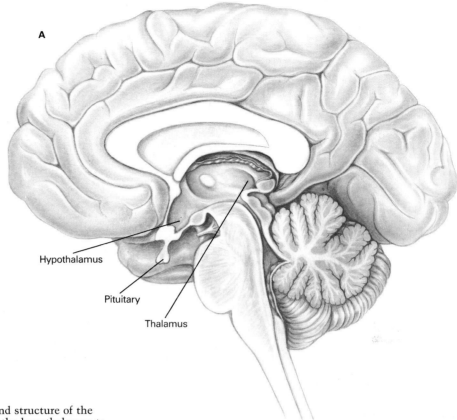

46–3 Medial views show the location and structure of the
hypothalamus. **A.** Relationship of the hypothalamus to
the pituitary and thalamus. **B.** Positions of the main
hypothalamic nuclear groups. (Adapted from Nieuwenhuys,
Voogd, and van Huijzen, 1981.)

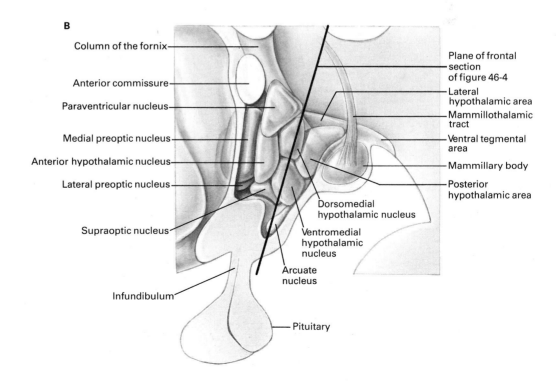

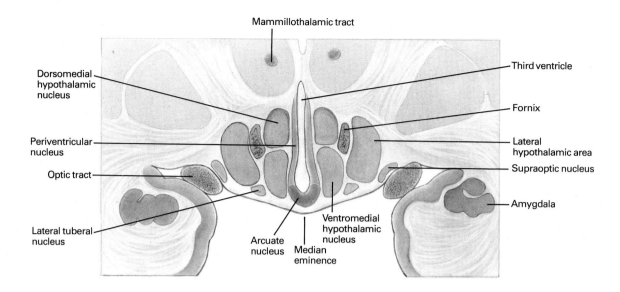

and descending pathways. Most prominent of these is the *medial forebrain bundle,* a major fiber tract that runs through the lateral hypothalamus and continues rostrally to end on the various regions of the forebrain. Many aminergic neurons originating in the brain stem course to neocortical regions through fibers in the medial forebrain bundle and its rostral continuation in the *cingulum bundle.* The *medial region* is separated from the lateral region by the descending columns of the fornix (Figure 46–4). The medial region contains most of the well-delineated nuclear groups of the hypothalamus. The basal portion of this medial region contains many of the hypothalamic neurons that secrete the peptide-releasing factors (which we shall consider later). Within the basal region are the tuberal nucleus, found in the primate brain, as well as the arcuate nucleus and other nuclei found in lower animals.

Most fiber systems of the hypothalamus are bidirectional. One exception is the *hypothalamohypophyseal tract;* this tract contains the axons of the paraventricular and supraoptic neurons, which terminate primarily in the posterior pituitary. The hypothalamus also receives one-way afferent connections directly from the retina. These fibers terminate primarily in the suprachiasmatic nucleus.

Projections to and from areas caudal to the hypothalamus are carried in the medial forebrain bundle, the mammillotegmental tract, and the dorsal longitudinal fasciculus. Other rostral structures are interconnected to the hypothalamus by means of the mammillothalamic tract, fornix, and stria terminalis.

The Hypothalamus Contains Various Classes of Peptidergic Neuroendocrine Cells

Recent studies of the hypothalamus reveal that several cell groups in this region secrete peptides. Some peptides are released into the local or systemic circulation and

46–4 Frontal view of the hypothalamus (section along plane shown in Figure 46–3).

serve as hormones acting on specific receptors located on distant cells. Others are released into a synaptic cleft and act in a manner analogous to transmitter substances. The actions of neuroactive peptides, no matter where they are released, tend to be enduring and to serve a so-called modulating function, controlling neuron excitability and synaptic effectiveness (see Chapter 13). These long-lasting actions are thought to be important for a variety of behavioral functions including the modulation of mood, motivational state, and learning.

Many of the peptidergic neurons of the hypothalamus that project to other regions of the nervous system innervate, in particular, structures of the limbic system and structures related to the autonomic nervous system. For example, the paraventricular nucleus, in addition to its classical peptidergic projections to the posterior pituitary, sends oxytocin- or vasopressin-containing axons to the amygdala, to the locus ceruleus, to the solitary nucleus, to the dorsal vagal complex, and to the intermediolateral cell column of the spinal cord. In addition, neurons in the arcuate nucleus containing adrenocorticotropin, β-endorphin, and related peptides project to the thalamus, periaqueductal gray matter, limbic structures (nucleus accumbens, bed nucleus of the stria terminalis, and amygdala), and the major catecholamine-containing nuclei of the brain. These extrahypothalamic peptidergic projections are well suited to coordinate neuroendocrine and autonomic responses, but their exact function is largely unknown.

The Hypothalamus Controls Endocrine Function by Means of Peptidergic Neurons

One of the main functions of the hypothalamus is the control of the endocrine system. This is accomplished in

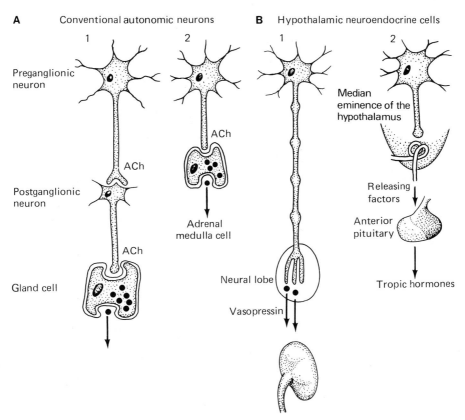

A Conventional autonomic neurons **B** Hypothalamic neuroendocrine cells

46–5 In contrast to conventional autonomic neurons, hypothalamic neuroendocrine cells release secretory products into the blood stream. **A.** Conventional autonomic neurons. **1:** Exocrine glands are innervated by postganglionic neurons that stimulate secretion through direct action of acetylcholine **(ACh)** on membrane receptors. **2:** The adrenal medulla is innervated by preganglionic sympathetic neurons of the nervous system that end on cell receptors. **B.** Hypothalamic neuroendocrine cells. **1:** In the neurohypophyseal system, the secretions (vasopressin or oxytocin) are formed in the cell body of the neuron and transported by axoplasmic flow to the nerve terminals in the neural lobe of the pituitary. Activity of the neuron leads to the release of the hormone into the general circulation. **2:** In the adenohypophyseal system, the secretions (hormone-releasing factors) are also formed in the cell body of the neuron and are transported by axoplasmic flow to nerve terminals in the median eminence (and in some species, the pituitary stalk). Activity of these neurons leads to secretion of the releasing factors into the hypophyseal–portal circulation, and the release of hormones from the anterior pituitary. (Adapted from Reichlin, 1978.)

two ways: (1) directly, by secretion of neuroendocrine products into the general circulation via the vasculature of the posterior pituitary (neural lobe or neurohypophysis); and (2) indirectly, by secretion of regulating hormones (releasing and inhibiting hormones) into the local portal plexus (within the median eminence), which drains into the blood vessels of the anterior pituitary (adenohypophysis). The hypothalamic regulating hormones, in turn, control the synthesis and release of anterior pituitary hormones into the general circulation.

The current understanding of the hypothalamus derives from the analysis of these two types of control by Ernst and Berta Scharrer, then at Case Western Reserve University, and by Geoffrey Harris at the Maudsley Hospital in London. Scharrer and Scharrer developed the concept of *neurosecretion*, the idea that certain neurons function in two roles: as nerve cells that receive and

transmit electrical information, and as endocrine cells that release their secretory products into the blood stream (Figure 46–5). They serve as "neuroendocrine transducers" to convert neural information into hormonal information. Harris recognized the importance of the blood supply that connects the pituitary to the hypothalamus (the pituitary–hypophyseal–portal system) and showed that this vascular link carries hormonal information from the hypothalamus to the pituitary (Figure 46–6). These concepts form the basis of modern neuroendocrinology and our current understanding of the hypothalamic control of endocrine activity.

The two types of endocrine control (direct and indirect) are mediated by two classes of peptidergic neuroendocrine cells. In both classes of neurons the various neurohormones or precursor peptides are synthesized in the cell bodies and packaged in neurosecretory vesicles that

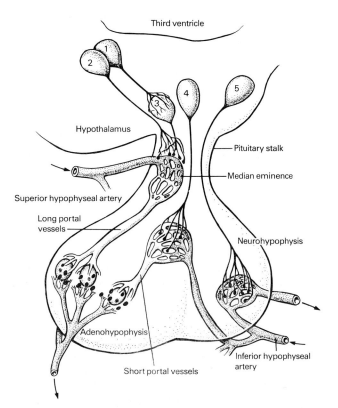

46–6 Various functional elements participate in the control of the pituitary by the hypothalamus. Peptidergic neurons (**5**) that produce oxytocin or vasopressin release their secretions into the general circulation via the posterior pituitary. Two general types of neurons are involved in anterior pituitary regulation. Peptidergic neurons (**3, 4**) form the releasing hormones that enter the capillary plexus of the hypophyseal–portal vessels. The second type of neuron (**1, 2**) is the link between the rest of the brain and the peptidergic neuron. These neurons, some of which are monoaminergic, are believed to end on the cell body of the peptidergic neuron in a conventional manner (**1**), or to end on the axon terminal of the peptidergic neuron (**2**) by means of axo-axonic synapses. (Adapted from Reichlin, 1978; Gay, 1972.)

eral hypothalamic regions: in the medial basal region, in the arcuate and tuberal nuclei, the periventricular region, and also in the preoptic, paraventricular, and suprachiasmatic nuclei. The parvicellular neurons release their secretions into the portal vasculature to stimulate or inhibit secretions from the anterior pituitary. The capillaries of the posterior pituitary and median eminence are highly fenestrated (i.e., contain perforations or openings), facilitating the entry of the released magnocellular hormones into the general circulation (via the posterior pituitary) or of parvicellular hormones into the portal plexus (from the median eminence).

Magnocellular Neurons Release Oxytocin and Vasopressin

In 1950 Vincent du Vigneaud, at Cornell University Medical School, determined the amino acid sequence of oxytocin. Four years later he worked out the sequence of vasopressin, thereby proving that hormonal functions of the brain are mediated by peptides. Vasopressin and oxytocin contain nine amino acid residues each (Table 46–1). As with most peptide hormones, both vasopressin and oxytocin are cleaved from a larger precursor, called the *prohormone*. The prohormones for vasopressin and oxytocin are synthesized in the cell bodies of the magnocellular neurons, and cleavage occurs within vesicles during transport along the axons of the neurons. Neurophysin is produced as a cleavage product in both vasopressin and oxytocin neurons; however, the neurophysin formed in one type of neuron differs somewhat from that produced in the other. Each neurophysin is released along with its hormone at terminals in the posterior pituitary.

Parvicellular Neurons Release Inhibiting and Releasing Hormones

The discovery of the structure of oxytocin and vasopressin and the work of Harris on the neural control of the anterior pituitary gland stimulated Roger Guillemin and Andrew Schally and their colleagues to isolate and characterize the structure of hormones that regulate the anterior pituitary. After 12 years of intense work on several tons of hypothalamic fragments, the laboratories of Guillemin and Schally independently characterized the structure of thyrotropin-releasing hormone (Figure 46–7). In 1971 Schally characterized luteinizing hormone–releasing hormone, and in 1973 Guillemin characterized somatostatin (Figure 46–7). Recently, corticotropin-releasing

are transported rapidly down axons to axon terminals, where they are stored for secretion when the neuron is stimulated. The *magnocellular* (large) neuroendocrine neurons are located in the paraventricular and supraoptic nuclei, and release their secretion (the neurohypophyseal hormones, oxytocin and vasopressin) into the general circulation by way of the posterior pituitary. The *parvicellular* (small) neurosecretory neurons are located in sev-

Table 46–1. Neurohypophyseal Hormones

Name	Structure	Function
Vasopressin	H-Cys-Tyr-Phe-Gln-Asn-Cys-Pro-Arg-Gly-NH₂ $\quad$ S-S	Vasoconstriction, water resorption by the kidney
Oxytocin	H-Cys-Tyr-Ile-Gln-Asn-Cys-Pro-Leu-Gly-NH₂ $\quad$ S-S	Uterine contraction and milk ejection

46–7 Structures of the first fully characterized hypothalamic releasing and inhibiting hormones.

pyro Glu — His — Pro — NH₂
Thyrotropin-releasing hormone

pyro Glu — His — Trp — Ser — Tyr — Gly — Leu — Arg — Pro — Gly — NH₂
Luteinizing hormone—releasing hormone

H — Ala — Gly — Cys — Lys — Asn — Phe — Phe — Trp — Lys — Thr — Phe — Thr — Ser — Cys — OH
S———————————S
Somatostatin

factor (CRF) and growth hormone–releasing factor have been sequenced in the laboratories of both Wylie Vale and Guillemin. Utilizing immunohistochemical techniques, P. E. Sawchenko, L. W. Swanson, and a number of other investigators have found that, similar to the other hypophyseotropic hormones, CRF is contained in neurons outside of the hypothalamus-adenohypophyseal system, and in fact it is one of the most widely distributed of those that have been described to date. Within the hypothalamus, CRF is found in a number of regions. It is present in magnocellular neurons of the paraventricular nucleus and of the supraoptic nucleus, where it exists together with oxytocin in some neurons and, like oxytocin, may be released into general circulation via the posterior pituitary. The CRF that is released in the median eminence to act on the pituitary appears to originate in parvicellular neurons in the paraventricular nucleus, and some of these same neurons also contain vasopressin.

It is now clear that most hormones of the anterior pituitary are controlled by peptide neurohormones synthesized by parvicellular neurons that release their product into the capillaries of the median eminence. The release of most of the hormones of the anterior pituitary is regulated by both enhancing and inhibiting substances. For example, growth hormone is inhibited by somatostatin and stimulated by growth hormone–releasing factor (a *factor* is a chemically uncharacterized substance). There is evidence that at least one inhibiting hormone is not a peptide: the inhibition of prolactin release is controlled by dopamine. In many instances, a single releasing hormone affects more than one pituitary hormone. The known hypothalamic releasing and inhibiting hormones are listed in Table 46–2 along with their most common abbreviations and the anterior pituitary hormones they affect. The releasing hormones are not the only peptides of neurobiological interest found in neurons of the hypothalamus: the morphinelike peptides, β-endorphin and the enkephalins (see Chapter 26), are also found here, as are angiotensin II, substance P, neurotensin, and several other peptides.

Systematic electrical recordings from identified groups of neurons secreting releasing factors have not been made, but there is reason to believe that, as with magnocellular neurons, many of the parvicellular neurons discharge in bursts. This inference is based on the obser-

Table 46–2. Hypothalamic Substances That Release or Inhibit the Release of Anterior Pituitary Hormones

Hypothalamic substance	Anterior pituitary hormone
RELEASING	
Thyrotropin-releasing hormone (TRH)	Thyrotropin, prolactin
Corticotropin-releasing hormone (CRH)	Adrenocorticotropin, β-lipotropin
Luteinizing hormone (follicle-stimulating hormone)–releasing hormone (LH/FSH-RH, LRH, or GnRH)	LH, FSH
Growth hormone–releasing hormone (GHRH or GRH)	GH
Prolactin-releasing factor (PRF)	Prolactin
Melanocyte-stimulating hormone–releasing factor (MRF)	MSH, β-endorphin
INHIBITING	
Prolactin release–inhibiting hormone (PIH), dopamine	Prolactin
Growth hormone release–inhibiting hormone (GIH or GHRIH; somatostatin)	GH, thyrotropin
Melanocyte-stimulating hormone release–inhibiting factor (MIF)	MSH

vation that hormonal secretion is typically pulsatile: blood concentrations of hormones show periodic surges throughout the day. This pattern is seen even for hormones, such as growth hormone, that regulate non-episodic physiological functions. Episodic release may have evolved because the continuous exposure of a receptor in a cell membrane to its hormone often leads to inactivation of the receptor *(down regulation)*. Down regulation occurs much more slowly in the case of periodic exposure.

Hypothalamic Neurons Participate in Four Classes of Reflexes

The hypothalamus has both neural and humoral outputs and inputs. The hypothalamus can therefore participate in four classes of reflexes: (1) conventional reflexes involving neural input and neural output; (2) reflexes in which the input to the hypothalamus is neural and the output is humoral; (3) reflexes in which the input is humoral and the output is neural; and (4) reflexes in which both the input and output are humoral. In this and the next two sections we shall consider simple examples of these four types of reflexes, but any normal physiological function typically involves more than one of these hypothalamic reflex modes.

Milk Ejection and Uterine Contraction Are Regulated by a Neural Input and a Humoral Output

The paraventricular and supraoptic nuclei contain neurons that release oxytocin, which induces contraction of the myoepithelial cells of the mammary gland. Oxytocin also increases the amplitude of uterine smooth muscle contraction (only if the muscle is appropriately primed by estrogens). This action of the hormone facilitates expulsion of the baby during delivery. In 1964 Eric Kandel, then at Harvard Medical School, recorded intracellularly from magnocellular neurons in the goldfish and found them to resemble conventional neurons in many respects. They have resting potentials, fire action potentials, and receive excitatory and inhibitory synaptic input. Electrical stimulation of the posterior pituitary results in antidromic action potentials in many of these neurons, demonstrating that they send axons to the posterior pituitary.

B. A. Cross and J. D. Green, in 1959, and C. Brooks and co-workers, in 1966, were the first to record extracellularly from mammalian neurons in the supraoptic and paraventricular nuclei while animals were exposed to various sensory stimuli. In 1974, D. W. Lincoln and J. B. Wakerley succeeded in recording from identified neuroendocrine cells in the female rat while the rat was presented with a natural stimulus for oxytocin release—suckling of rat pups. Milk ejection was simultaneously measured by recording intramammary pressure. Lincoln and Wakerley found that a continuous suckling stimulus produced periodic bursts of action potentials in many of the identified neuroendocrine cells. Approximately 13

sec after the burst, there was an increase in intramammary pressure, indicating the arrival of a pulse of oxytocin to the mammary glands (Figure 46–8). Thus, the oxytocin cells participate in a relatively simple reflex in which the afferent limb is neural and the efferent limb is humoral. As appears to be true for all the hypothalamic neurosecretory products, the release of oxytocin can be affected by higher brain structures. For example, in a lactating mother, the sight or sound of her child may trigger milk ejection. Presumably, excitatory cortical influences project to oxytocin-containing cells in the hypothalamus. Because anxiety and worry can inhibit the milk ejection reflex, inhibitory cortical influences may also affect these cells.

Urine Flow Is Regulated by a Humoral Input and a Humoral Output

The paraventricular and supraoptic nuclei also contain neurons that release the hormone arginine vasopressin (also called antidiuretic hormone). Vasopressin alters the membrane permeability of the collecting ducts and convoluted tubules of the kidneys so that their membranes are more permeable to water. As a result, the recovery of water after filtration is facilitated, urinary volume is decreased, and body water is conserved.

In contrast to the neurons that release oxytocin, which tend to be triggered into a single burst of activity, the neurons that release vasopressin are spontaneously active and provide a constant basal concentration of the hormone in the blood. This concentration is decreased or increased according to physiological demand. Vasopressin-releasing neurons fire more rapidly when the animal is deprived of water, and less rapidly when the animal is loaded with water. The functioning of the vasopressin system is therefore analogous to that of graded neural reflexes and the oxytocin system to that of fixed action pattern responses (to be considered in Chapter 60).

The hypothalamic neurons that release vasopressin respond directly to the state of the *milieu intérieur* (specifically, the blood), although they can also be influenced through afferent neuronal pathways. Direct response to humoral factors, first suggested by E. B. Verney in 1947, is strongly supported by the observation made by John Sundsten and Charles Sawyer in 1961 that animals can regulate release of vasopressin even when the hypothalamus is disconnected from all structures except the pituitary. Evidence is accumulating that vasopressin-producing cells as well as other hypothalamic cells respond directly to osmotic stimuli or to changes in the blood concentration of Na^+. Other humorally mediated stimuli can affect vasopressin release directly or indirectly. For example, anesthetic agents increase the release of vasopressin, and ethanol decreases its release.

The release of vasopressin is also controlled by neural inputs from blood volume receptors in blood vessels: decreased blood volume enhances vasopressin release, and increased blood volume inhibits vasopressin release. Afferent input probably also comes from temp-

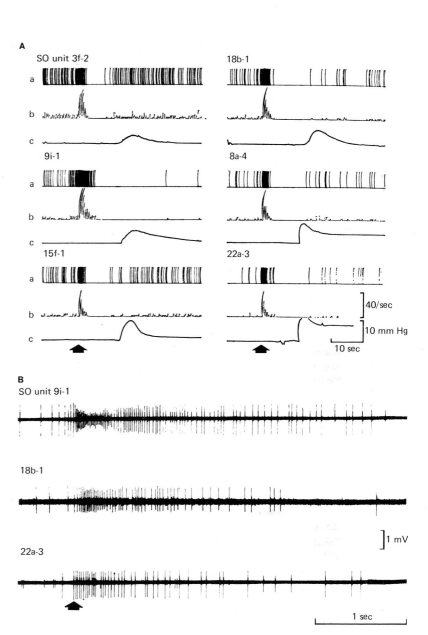

46–8 Recordings from oxytocin-releasing neuroendocrine cells in the female rat during suckling of pups illustrate the correlation of spike activity with milk ejection. **Arrows** indicate onset of neurosecretory response. **A.** Polygraph records of six responsive supraoptic neurons. Approximately 40 sec of spike activity, spanning one milk ejection, is shown for each unit. **Trace a,** unit activity, in which each vertical deflection corresponds to a single action potential. **Trace b,** an integration of the unit recording in which the height of the trace is proportional to frequency. **Trace c,** recording of intramammary pressure. Note the difference in the background activity of the six units, the dramatic and stereotyped acceleration in spike activity about 13 sec before milk ejection, the peak rates of spike discharge (30–50 spikes/sec), the duration of the response, and the period of afterinhibition. **B.** Photographs on a greatly expanded time scale of the spike trains in three of the units illustrated in part **A.** (Adapted from Lincoln and Wakerley, 1974.)

erature receptors in the skin: cold inhibits the release of vasopressin, while warmth enhances its release.

Some vasopressin-releasing cells in the paraventricular nucleus send axons to the external zone of the median eminence to terminate on the primary portal plexus. Furthermore, in 1973 Earl Zimmerman and colleagues at Columbia University showed that the portal blood contains high concentrations of vasopressin. Some of these vasopressin-containing neurons also contain corticotropin-releasing hormone and control the release of adrenocorticotropin. Interestingly, the action of corticotropin-releasing hormone is greatly potentiated in the presence of vasopressin, indicating that these substances act synergistically. Stress, pain, and anxiety, which increase vasopressin release, also increase the release of adrenocorticotropin. The absence of adrenal steroid hormones following adrenalectomy results in an increase of both CRF and vasopressin in paraventricular neurons.

In every instance studied, the releasing hormones are found not only in the median eminence, but also in other regions of the brain, where their release presumably affects neural systems that control various behavioral functions. Releasing hormones are particularly prominent in the limbic system.

The Brain Itself Is a Target for Hormone Action

Feedback Loops Involve a Humoral Input and a Humoral Output

Neurons in limbic as well as hypothalamic structures possess receptors that bind a variety of hormones. These receptors provide the substrate for *long feedback loops* in which the hormone of a peripheral endocrine gland (typically steroid hormones that readily cross the blood–

brain barrier) can modulate its own production by directly inhibiting the brain or the anterior pituitary. In turn, the regulatory hormones of the pituitary also can have feedback effects (*short feedback loops*) on the brain that modulate release of the hormones. These effects are examples of reflexes in which both input and output are humoral.

Central Effects of Hormones on Behavior Involve a Humoral Input and a Neural Output

Although certain hormones circulate widely through the brain, only a small subset of neurons possess receptors to a specific hormone. Therefore, the action of circulating hormones can be quite specific, and a given hormone that can cross the blood–brain barrier or is released into the extracellular space or cerebrospinal fluid will activate or inhibit only a restricted population of neurons. Hormonal effects on these nerve cells (sometimes referred to as *modulatory effects*) are slow and are suited to long-term regulation of excitability or synaptic effectiveness. These hormonal actions are thought to be involved in modifying mood and behavioral states, or in providing a triggering signal for the generation of a complex motor pattern in which the details are dependent upon conventional transmitter actions.

Releasing factors may modulate behavior by peripheral actions or by actions on the brain independent of their effects on the release of pituitary hormones. For example, R. L. Moss and S. M. McCann, and independently, Donald Pfaff, have found that subcutaneous injection of luteinizing hormone–releasing hormone into estrogen-treated female rats increases mating behavior as measured by the display of a stereotyped female sexual behavior (lordosis). Similar effects are obtained after injection of luteinizing hormone–releasing hormone into the medial preoptic area and arcuate nucleus of the hypothalamus. The action of this releasing hormone does not appear to be mediated through the ovaries, since the effect is not abolished by hypophysectomy or ovariectomy as long as estrogen is provided. A final example of a peptide that is involved in both peripheral and central actions is corticotropin-releasing factor, which acts on the pituitary in response to stress, but when injected intraventricularly also evokes many of the behavioral and autonomic reactions normally seen in response to stress.

Hormones May Be Important for Learning

In animals, adrenocorticotropin (and melanocyte-stimulating hormone, which has peptide sequences in common with adrenocorticotropin), as well as vasopressin, has been shown by D. de Wied and others to facilitate the learning (or to delay extinction) of tasks involving stress or aversive stimuli. These actions of adrenocorticotropin are not mediated by the adrenal glands, since the facilitation is also seen in adrenalectomized animals. Furthermore, fragments of the adrenocorticotropin mol-

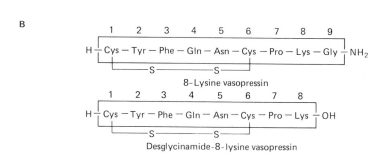

46–9 Fragments of certain peptide hormones affect memory retention although they lack the endocrine effects of the whole molecule. **A.** Amino acid sequences of complete α-melanocyte-stimulating hormone (α-MSH) and adrenocorticotropin (ACTH). **Shaded area** covers peptide sequences 4–10 in α-MSH and in ACTH, which have been found to restore deficient learning behavior in hypophysectomized rats. **B.** Amino acid sequence of complete vasopressin molecule and the fragment desglycinamide-8-lysine vasopressin, which has been found to have a positive effect on memory retention.

ecule with no corticotropic activity are also effective. The amino acid sequence of the fourth through seventh positions of adrenocorticotropin is sufficient to produce the behavioral effects on learning (Figure 46–9A). Similarly, analogues of vasopressin that have no antidiuretic properties are effective in facilitating memory (Figure 46–9B). It is unclear whether the effects of hormones on memory are due to a direct action on the learning process or whether they indirectly alter learning by, for example, altering the arousal state of the animal.

Evidence that hormones or peptides may regulate a variety of behavioral processes suggests an exciting new pharmacological approach to the effective treatment of behavioral disorders.

The Hypothalamus Helps Regulate the Autonomic Nervous System

Although the hypothalamus has important hormonal inputs and outputs, it also mediates conventional reflexes involving simple neural inputs and outputs. The hypothalamus functions in this manner in its role as the so-called head ganglion of the autonomic nervous system. Much of what we know about the autonomic function of the hypothalamus stems from a long series of experiments started in the early 1930s by Stephen W. Ranson at Northwestern University and Walter R. Hess in Switzerland. Ranson took advantage of the stereotaxic method developed by Horsley and Clarke in England, which permitted the precise and reproducible placement of electrodes in the deep structures of the brains of experimental animals by means of a triple-coordinate system that located each subcortical nucleus uniquely according to its position in the brain. (This technique was later refined to permit neurosurgeons to make therapeutic lesions deep within the brain.) In previous attempts to stimulate the hypothalamus, investigators had utilized drastic surgical procedures to visualize the appropriate structures. Using the stereotaxic technique, Ranson systematically stimulated different regions of the hypothalamus and evoked almost every conceivable autonomic reaction, including alterations in heart rate, blood pressure, gastrointestinal motility, piloerection, and bladder contraction. The most prominent responses involved the sympathetic nervous system, and these effects tended to occur with stimulation of the lateral and posterior hypothalamus.

Most of Ranson's experiments were done on anesthetized animals. Hess extended Ranson's approach by implanting electrodes and permanently fixing them to the skull of the animal. By attaching a long flexible cable to the implanted electrode he could observe the effects of brain stimulation in awake and completely unrestrained animals. In a brilliant series of investigations that ultimately earned him the Nobel Prize in 1949, Hess found that responses evoked by hypothalamic stimulation did not occur in isolation but in characteristic constellations that gave the appearance of being organized behaviors. For example, electrical stimulation of the lateral hypothalamus in cats elicited autonomic and somatic re-

sponses characteristic of anger: increased blood pressure, raising of the body hair, pupillary constriction, arching of the back, and raising of the tail. These observations indicated that the hypothalamus is not simply a motor nucleus for the autonomic nervous system: it is a coordinating center that integrates various inputs to ensure a well-organized, coherent, and appropriate set of autonomic and somatic responses.

The Hypothalamus Is Involved in Emotional Behavior

The evidence provided by Ranson, Hess, and others that stimulation of the hypothalamus produces autonomic, endocrine, and motor effects resembling those seen during various types of emotional behaviors suggests that the hypothalamus integrates and coordinates the behavioral expression of emotional states. This idea is supported by lesion studies indicating that different hypothalamic structures can be associated with a wide range of emotional states. Whereas stimulation of the lateral hypothalamus elicits anger, lesions of the lateral hypothalamus result in placidity. On the other hand, animals with lesions of the medial hypothalamus become highly excitable and are easily triggered into aggressive responses.

Similar irritability is also produced by decortication. The responses seen in decorticated cats include lashing of the tail, vigorous arching of the back, jerking of the limbs, clawing, attempts to bite, and autonomic responses such as erection of the tail hairs, sweating (of the toe pads), micturition, defecation, and increased blood pressure. There is also an increase in epinephrine and corticosteroid secretion into the blood. In 1925 Cannon and Britton termed this constellation of responses *sham rage* because it appeared to lack elements of conscious experience that are characteristic of naturally occurring rage. Sham rage reactions also differed from genuine rage in that the anger could occur spontaneously or could be triggered by very mild tactile and other stimuli. Even when elicited by strong stimuli, the sham rage responses subsided very quickly when the stimulus was removed. Finally, the aggressive responses were undirected, and the animal sometimes bit itself. In 1928, Philip Bard further analyzed sham rage by means of progressive transections down the neuraxis. He found that sham rage disappeared when the hypothalamus was included in the ablation (Figure 46–10). Nevertheless, a fragmented expression of emotional responses could still be obtained in animals in which the hypothalamus and all rostral forebrain structures had been removed. These responses (first described by Robert Woodworth and Charles Sherrington in 1904, who called them *pseudoaffective reflexes*), were, however, much less coordinated than those seen with the hypothalamus left intact, and very strong stimuli were required to elicit them.

Which forebrain structures account for the suppression of sham rage responses in normal animals? Bard and Vernon Mountcastle found that large portions of the neo-

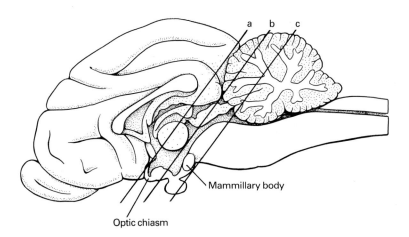

Optic chiasm

Mammillary body

46–10 This midsagittal section of the cat brain shows the levels of brain transections used to study sham rage. Transection of the forebrain (at level **a**) causes an animal to exhibit sham rage. Transection at the level of the hypothalamus (**b**) also produces sham rage unless the posterior hypothalamus is included (**c**), in which case only isolated elements of a rage response can be elicited.

cortex could be removed without producing sham rage. Sham rage phenomena were seen when the lesion included structures of the limbic system (for example, the cingulate cortex).

As mentioned earlier, in 1937 Klüver and Bucy reported that bilateral removal of the temporal lobe in the monkey—which included the amygdala and the hippocampal formation as well as the nonlimbic temporal cortex—produced a dramatic behavioral syndrome. The animals, formerly quite wild, became tame, showed a flattening of emotions, and exhibited remarkable oral tendencies (they put all manner of objects they encountered into their mouths). They also became hypersexual: they exhibited an enormous increase in sexual behavior, including a mounting of inappropriate objects and species. Finally, the animals showed *hypermetamorphosis*—a compulsive tendency to take note of and react to every visual stimulus, while failing to recognize familiar objects. Some of the features of the Klüver-Bucy syndrome tend to be the opposite of those encountered in patients with temporal lobe epilepsy, who show decreased sexuality and heightened emotionality (see Chapter 1).

What structures account for the individual symptoms of the Klüver-Bucy syndrome? Damage to the amygdala is particularly important in producing the oral tendencies, hypersexuality, and tameness; and damage to the visual association areas of the temporal cortex contributes to the visual deficits.

The current model of the neural basis of emotional behavior is not far from the ideas that Papez proposed more than 40 years ago. We think of the hypothalamus as functioning to integrate the motor and endocrine responses that produce appropriate emotional behavior. The forebrain suppresses emotional responses to trivial and inconsequential stimuli. Thus, the forebrain connects the hypothalamus with the outer world in such a manner that appropriate autonomic and endocrine concomitants of emotions are expressed in response to external conditions. Forebrain structures also provide the neural mechanisms needed to direct skeletomotor re-

sponses to external events, so that, for example, an object is appropriately approached or avoided. Finally, the forebrain seems to be crucial for the conscious experience of emotions.

An Overall View

The interplay between the neural activity of the hypothalamus and the neural activity of higher centers results in an emotional experience to which we can attach words such as fear, anger, pleasure, and contentment. The behavior of patients in whom the prefrontal cortex (parts of which appear to be related to the limbic system) has been removed or who have lesions of the cingulate gyrus supports this idea. These patients are no longer bothered by chronic pain. They sometimes perceive pain and exhibit appropriate autonomic reactions, but the perception is no longer associated with a powerful emotional experience (see Chapters 26 and 51).

Thus, noxious or pleasurable stimuli seem to have dual effects. These stimuli trigger a set of events that are integrated by the hypothalamus and result in an alteration of internal state that prepares the organism for appropriate action (attack, flight, sexual experience). These preparatory autonomic reactions are relatively simple in execution and require no conscious control. However, in executing complex actions such as attack, the organism must interact with its external environment; forebrain mechanisms come into play in these interactions and modulate the behavioral repertoire much as proprioceptive sensory feedback from an uneven terrain modulates the central program for locomotion. Perhaps consciousness evolved as a result of the enormous complexity involved in dealing with the external environment. Compared with our internal environment, the external environment is far less predictable and provides a much richer variety of stimuli. Furthermore, in dealing with the external environment we often have the luxury of delaying our responses, thus permitting actions to be guided by plans and strategy.

Selected Readings

Brownstein, M. J., Russell, J. T., and Gainer, H. 1980. Synthesis, transport, and release of posterior pituitary hormones. Science 207:373–378.

Gellhorn, E. (ed.). 1968. Biological Foundations of Emotion: Research and Commentary. Glenview, Ill.: Scott, Foresman.

Guillemin, R. 1978. Control of adenohypophyseal functions by peptides of the central nervous system. Harvey Lect. 71:71–131.

Hess, W. R. 1954. Diencephalon: Autonomic and Extrapyramidal Functions. New York: Grune & Stratton.

Krieger, D. T. 1983. Brain peptides: What, where and why? Science 222:975–985.

Leng, G., Mason, W. T., and Dyer, R. G. 1982. The supraoptic nucleus as an osmoreceptor. Neuroendocrinol. 34:75–82.

Mauk, M. D., Olson, G. A., Kastin, A. J., and Olson, R. D. 1980. Behavioral effects of LH-RH. Neurosci. Biobehav. Rev. 4:1–8.

Meyerson, B. J. 1979. Hypothalamic hormones and behaviour. Med. Biol. (Helsinki) 57:69–83.

Ranson, S. W. 1934. The hypothalamus: Its significance for visceral innervation and emotional expression. Trans. Coll. Physicians Phila. [Ser. 4] 2:222–242.

Renaud, L. P. 1981. A neurophysiological approach to the identification, connections and pharmacology of the hypothalamic tuberoinfundibular system. Neuroendocrinol. 33:186–191.

Silverman, A.-J., and Zimmerman, E. A. 1983. Magnocellular neurosecretory system. Annu. Rev. Neurosci. 6:357–380.

Swanson, L. W., and Sawchenko, P. E. 1983. Hypothalamic integration: Organization of the paraventricular and supraoptic nuclei. Annu. Rev. Neurosci. 6:269–324.

References

Bard, P. 1928. A diencephalic mechanism for the expression of rage with special reference to the sympathetic nervous system. Am. J. Physiol. 84:490–515.

Bard, P., and Mountcastle, V. B. 1948. Some forebrain mechanisms involved in expression of rage with special reference to suppression of angry behavior. Res. Publ. Assoc. Res. Nerv. Ment. Dis. 27:362–404.

Bernard, C. 1878–1879. Leçons sur les phénomènes de la vie communs aux animaux et aux végétaux, 2 Vols. Paris: Baillière.

Brooks, C. McC., Ishikawa, T., Koizumi, K., and Lu, H.-H. 1966. Activity of neurones in the paraventricular nucleus of the hypothalamus and its control. J. Physiol. (Lond.) 182:217–231.

Cannon, W. B., and Britton, S. W. 1925. Studies on the conditions of activity in endocrine glands. XV. Pseudaffective medulliadrenal secretion. Am. J. Physiol. 72:283–294.

Cross, B. A., and Green, J. D. 1959. Activity of single neurones in the hypothalamus: Effect of osmotic and other stimuli. J. Physiol. (Lond.) 148:554–569.

De Wied, D., and Gispen, W. H., 1977. Behavioral effects of peptides. In H. Gainer (ed.), Peptides in Neurobiology. New York: Plenum Press, pp. 397–448.

Du Vigneaud, V. 1956. Hormones of the posterior pituitary gland: Oxytocin and vasopressin. Harvey Lect. 50:1–26.

Gay, V. L. 1972. The hypothalamus: Physiology and clinical use of releasing factors. Fertil. Steril. 23:50–63.

Harris, G. W. 1955. Neural Control of the Pituitary Gland. Monograph No. 3 of The Physiology Society. London: Arnold.

Kandel, E. R. 1964. Electrical properties of hypothalamic neuroendocrine cells. J. Gen. Physiol. 47:691–717.

Klüver, H., and Bucy, P. C. 1937. "Psychic blindness" and other symptoms following bilateral temporal lobectomy in Rhesus monkeys. Am. J. Physiol. 119:352–353.

Klüver, H., and Bucy, P. C. 1939. Preliminary analysis of functions of the temporal lobes in monkeys. Arch. Neurol. Psychiatry 42:979–1000.

Lincoln, D. W., and Wakerley, J. B. 1974. Electrophysiological evidence for the activation of supraoptic neurones during the release of oxytocin. J. Physiol. (Lond.) 242:533–554.

MacLean, P. D. 1955. The limbic system ("visceral brain") and emotional behavior. Arch. Neurol. Psychiatry 73:130–134.

Moss, R. L., and McCann, S. M. 1973. Induction of mating behavior in rats by luteinizing hormone–releasing factor. Science 181:177–179.

Nieuwenhuys, R., Voogd, J., and van Huijzen, Chr. 1981. The Human Central Nervous System: A Synopsis and Atlas, 2nd rev. ed. Berlin: Springer.

Papez, J. W. 1937. A proposed mechanism of emotion. Arch. Neurol. Psychiatry 38:725–743.

Pfaff, D. W. 1973. Luteinizing hormone–releasing factor potentiates lordosis behavior in hypophysectomized ovariectomized female rats. Science 182:1148–1149.

Reichlin, S. 1978. Introduction. In S. Reichlin, R. J. Baldessarini, and J. B. Martin (eds.), The Hypothalamus. Res. Publ. Assoc. Res. Nerv. Ment. Dis. 56:1–14.

Sawchenko, P. E., and Swanson, L. W. 1985. Localization, colocalization, and plasticity of corticotropin-releasing factor immunoreactivity in rat brain. Fed. Proc. 44:221–227.

Schally, A. V. 1978. Aspects of hypothalamic regulation of the pituitary gland. Its implications for the control of reproductive processes. Science 202:18–28.

Scharrer, E., and Scharrer, B. 1954. Hormones produced by neurosecretory cells. Recent Prog. Horm. Res. 10:183–232.

Sundsten, J. W., and Sawyer, C. H. 1961. Osmotic activation of neurohypophyseal hormone release in rabbits with hypothalamic islands. Exp. Neurol. 4:548–561.

Vale, W., Spiess, J., Rivier, C., and Rivier, J. 1981. Characterization of a 41-residue ovine hypothalamic peptide that stimulates secretion of corticotropin and β-endorphin. Science 213:1394–1397.

Verney, E. B. 1947. The antidiuretic hormone and the factors which determine its release. Proc. R. Soc. Lond. [Biol.] 135:25–106.

Woodworth, R. S., and Sherrington, C. S. 1904. A pseudaffective reflex and its spinal path. J. Physiol. (Lond.) 31:234–243.

Zimmerman, E. A., Carmel, P. W., Husain, M. K., Ferin, M., Tannenbaum, M., Frantz, A. G., and Robinson, A. G. 1973. Vasopressin and neurophysin: High concentrations in monkey hypophyseal portal blood. Science 182:925–927.

Irving Kupfermann

Hypothalamus and Limbic System II: Motivation

47

In Chapter 46 we examined the role of the limbic system and the hypothalamus in the neuroendocrine and autonomic regulation of homeostasis. In this chapter we shall consider the control of homeostasis by the motivated behavior of the organism. These behavioral responses typically occur in parallel to the autonomic and neuroendocrine responses. We shall first consider the concept of motivational state and how control systems analysis can be used to study motivation. Temperature regulation, feeding, and drinking will serve as examples for the application of control systems analysis. We shall next examine the regulation of motivated behaviors by factors other than simple tissue deficits. Finally, we shall discuss systems of the brain concerned with reward or reinforcement.

Motivational or Drive States Are Thought to Intervene between Stimuli and Complex Responses

Psychologists refer to the internal conditions that arouse and direct voluntary behavior as *motivational states*. Specific motivational states are referred to as *drives*. Drives represent urges or impulses based upon bodily needs that impel humans and other animals into action. Thus, for example, behavioral regulation of body temperature, such as shivering or rubbing the hands together, is said to be due to a temperature-regulating drive. Other conditions that control behaviors such as curiosity and sex are also spoken of as drives because, in common with classical homeostatic drives, these behaviors also involve arousal and satiation; however, for the latter behaviors there do not appear to be any well-defined underlying states of physiological deprivation as there are for classical drives, such as thirst and hunger.

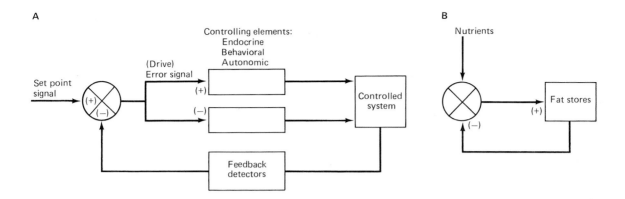

47–1 Control systems analysis can be applied to homeostatic processes. **A.** A system using a set point to turn behavior on or off is used for regulating body weight, temperature, etc. When the feedback signal indicating the level of the controlled variable is below or above the set point, an error signal is generated; this signal serves to turn on or to facilitate appropriate behaviors and physiological responses, and to turn off or to suppress incompatible responses. **B.** A negative feedback system without a set point controls fat stores. (Adapted from data of Di Girolamo and Rudman, 1968.)

Drives or motivational states are hypothetical mechanisms that are thought to determine the intensity and direction of a variety of complex behaviors such as temperature regulation, feeding, thirst, and sex. Behavioral scientists posit these internal states because observable features of the external environment are not sufficient to predict all aspects of these behaviors. In simple reflexes—for example, the pupillary response—the properties of the stimulus appear to account in large part for the properties of the behavior. On the other hand, the features of highly complex activities are not precisely correlated with external stimulus conditions. For example, when a long time has passed since the last meal, a food stimulus might produce vigorous feeding responses in an animal; but at other times, the same stimulus might produce no behavior or even rejection. In this example, the motivational state of hunger is inferred to explain the loose correlation between the food stimulus and the feeding response.

Neurobiologists are now beginning to define the actual physiological states that correspond to the hypothetical states inferred by psychologists. In some instances it has been possible to approach motivational states as examples of the interactions between external and internal stimuli. The problem of motivation thus can be reduced to that of a complex reflex under the excitatory and inhibitory control of multiple stimuli, some of them internal. This approach has worked well with temperature regulation. The relevant internal stimuli for hunger, thirst, and sexual behavior have been exceedingly difficult to identify or to manipulate. Therefore, for these behaviors the concept of drive state remains useful for behavioral scientists. As more is learned about the actual physiology of hypothetical drive states, the need for invoking these states to explain behavior may disappear, to be replaced by more precise concepts derived from physiology and systems theory.

Homeostatic Processes Can Be Analyzed in Terms of Control Systems

Temperature regulation as well as other homeostatic regulatory mechanisms can be understood in terms of the types of control systems—*servomechanisms*—that regulate machines. While the existence of a specific physiological control system has never been proved, this approach has provided a convenient and precise language to describe concepts and experimental results. It permits us to organize our thinking about highly complex systems. Furthermore, the servomechanism analogy defines the nature of the problem of physiological control in terms of experimentally approachable elements that can be analyzed one by one. As we shall see, analysis in terms of servocontrol systems has been most successfully applied to temperature regulation. Application to more complex regulatory behaviors such as feeding and thirst has been less successful, but this is probably still the best approach to the analysis of these poorly understood, multidetermined functions.

Control systems regulate a *controlled variable* (e.g., temperature) that is maintained within a certain range. One way of regulating the controlled variable is to measure it by means of a *feedback detector* and to compare it with a desired value or *set point*. This is accomplished by an *integrator* or *error detector* that generates an *error signal* when the measurement of the controlled variable does not match the set point signal. The error signal then drives *controlling elements* that adjust the controlled system in the desired direction. In Figure 47–1, two sets of controlling elements are indicated, since all examples of physiological control seem to involve dual effects, inhibitory and excitatory, which function together to adjust the control system. The control system used to heat a home provides a good example of a familiar servomechanism that illustrates these principles. The furnace system is the controlling element. The room temperature is

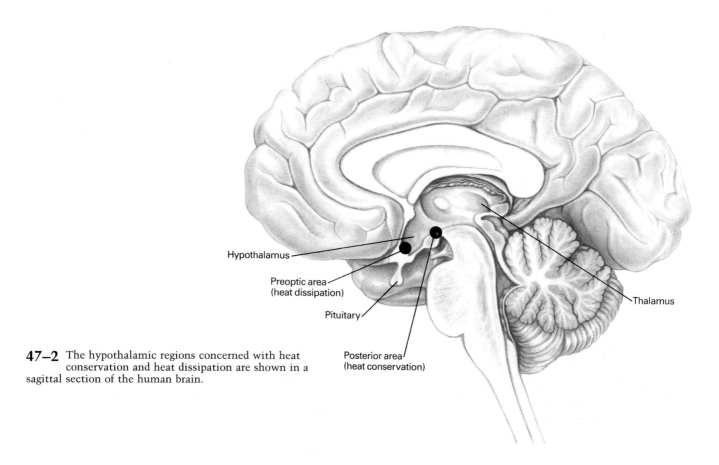

47–2 The hypothalamic regions concerned with heat conservation and heat dissipation are shown in a sagittal section of the human brain.

Labels in figure: Hypothalamus; Preoptic area (heat dissipation); Pituitary; Posterior area (heat conservation); Thalamus

the controlled variable. The home thermostat is the error detector. The setting on the thermostat is the set point. Finally, the output of the thermostat that turns the controlling element on or off is the error signal.

Temperature Is Regulated in Response to Peripheral and Central Input

In the system of temperature regulation, the integrator and many controlling elements appear to be located in the hypothalamus. Temperature regulation nicely fits a model of a servocontrol system (or several systems) in which normal body temperature is the set point. The feedback detector appears to collect information about body temperature from two main sources: peripheral temperature receptors located throughout the body (in the skin, spinal cord, and viscera), and central temperature receptors concentrated in the anterior hypothalamus. Although both anterior and posterior hypothalamic areas are involved in temperature regulation, detectors of temperature, both low and high, are located only in the anterior hypothalamus. The hypothalamic receptors are probably hypothalamic neurons whose firing rate is highly dependent on local temperature, which in turn is determined primarily by the temperature of the blood.

Because temperature regulation requires integrated autonomic, endocrine, and skeletomotor responses, the anatomical connections of the hypothalamus make this structure well suited for this task. Electrical stimulation of the hypothalamus indicates that it is organized anatomically in terms of dual mechanisms that control, respectively, increases and decreases in body temperature (Figure 47–2). Electrical stimulation of the *anterior hypothalamus* in unanesthetized animals causes dilation of blood vessels in the skin and a suppression of shivering—responses that result in a drop in body temperature. Electrical stimulation of the *posterior hypothalamus* produces a set of opposite responses that function to generate or conserve heat. As with hypothalamically evoked fear responses (see Chapter 46), electrically induced temperature regulation also includes appropriate responses involving the skeletomotor system. For example, rostral hypothalamic stimulation produces panting, while posterior stimulation produces shivering.

The results of ablation experiments corroborate the critical role of the hypothalamus in regulating temperature. Lesions of the anterior hypothalamus lead to chronic hyperthermia and eliminate the major responses that normally dissipate excess heat. Lesions in the posterior hypothalamus have relatively little effect if the animal is maintained at room temperature (approximately 22°C). If the animal is exposed to cold, however, it quickly becomes hypothermic because of failure of the homeostatic mechanisms that generate and conserve heat.

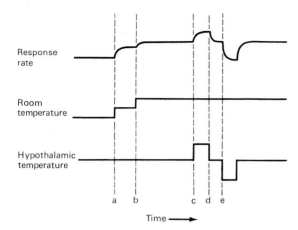

47–3 Changes in room temperature (**points a** and **b**) and in hypothalamic temperature (**points c, d,** and **e**) alter the response rate of rats trained to respond for the reward of a brief burst of cool air. (Adapted from data of Corbit, 1973, and Satinoff, 1964.)

The hypothalamus also controls endocrine responses to temperature challenges. Thus, long-term exposure to cold can enhance an animal's release of thyroxine and thereby increase body heat by increasing tissue metabolism.

The error signal of the temperature control system, in addition to driving appropriate autonomic, endocrine, and nonvoluntary skeletal responses, can also provide a signal to drive voluntary behavior that moves the controlled system in the direction that minimizes the error signal. For example, a rat can be taught to press a button to receive a puff of cool air in a hot environment. If the rat is placed in a room at normal temperature it will not press the cool-air button. If we now place a hollow probe into the anterior hypothalamus and locally warm this area by perfusing warm water through the probe, the rat will run to the cool-air button and press it. In the same rat we can demonstrate the summation of peripheral and central input to the hypothalamus by heating the environment and concurrently cooling or heating the hypothalamus (Figure 47–3). When both the environment and hypothalamus are heated, the rat presses faster than when either one is heated alone. Button pressing for cool air in a hot environment can be suppressed completely by directly cooling the hypothalamus.

Recordings from neurons in the preoptic area and from those in the anterior hypothalamus support the idea that the hypothalamus integrates peripheral and central information relevant to appropriate temperature regulation. Units in this region, called *warm-sensitive neurons,* increase their firing when the local hypothalamic tissue is warmed. Other neurons, called *cold-sensitive neurons,* respond to local cooling. The warm-sensitive neurons, in addition to responding to local brain warming, are generally excited by warming of the skin or spinal cord and are inhibited by cooling of the skin or spinal cord. The cold-sensitive neurons exhibit the opposite behavior. Thus, these neurons could serve to integrate thermal information from the periphery with that from the brain.

The control of body temperature is a clear example of the integrative function of the hypothalamus in autonomic, endocrine, and drive-state control, and illustrates how the hypothalamus operates directly on the internal environment or provides signals (derived from the internal environment) to control higher neural systems.

Feeding Behavior Is Regulated by a Variety of Signals

Feeding behavior also can be approached in terms of a control system in much the same fashion as temperature regulation, although at every level of analysis the understanding of feeding is less complete.

Set Point

One reason it appears that control theory can be applied to feeding behavior is that body weight seems to be controlled by some type of set point system. Humans often maintain body weight over a period of many years. Since even a small daily excess or deficit of caloric intake could result in a profound change of body weight over a period of years, in some way the body must provide feedback signals that control nutrient intake and metabolism. Control of nutrient intake can be clearly seen in animal studies in which body weight can be altered from the set point either by food deprivation or by force-feeding. In both cases, animals adjust their subsequent food intake (either up or down) until they regain a body weight appropriate for their age (Figure 47–4). Animals are said to "defend" their body weight against perturbations.

47–4 The tendency of animals to adjust their food intake to achieve a normal body weight is demonstrated by this schematized growth curve for a group of rats. At **arrow 1,** one-third of the animals were maintained on their normal diet (**curve b**), one-third were force-fed (**curve a**), and one-third were placed on a restricted diet (**curve c**). At **arrow 2,** all rats were placed on a normal (ad libitum) diet. The force-fed animals lost weight and the starved animals gained weight until the mean weight of the two groups approached that of the normal growth curve (**b**). (Adapted from Keesey et al., 1976.)

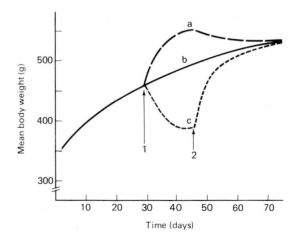

Regulation of body weight, however, is different from regulation of body temperature. Whereas body temperature is remarkably similar from individual to individual, body weight has an equally remarkable dissimilarity from individual to individual. Furthermore, the *apparent* set point of an individual can vary as a function of stress, palatability of the food, exercise, and numerous other factors. One possible explanation for these observations is that the set point itself can change on the basis of different factors. Another possibility is that feeding behavior utilizes some control systems in which there are no formal, fixed set point mechanisms, but the systems function as if there were set points. Feedback systems of this type do exist in the body. In Figure 47–1B a negative feedback system for the regulation of fat stores in cells is shown. Apparently, the more fat stored in the cell, the less conversion there is of nutrients to fat. Thus, fat stores may directly or indirectly exert a negative feedback that is proportional to the level of fat. Because of this feedback mechanism, fat stores tend to be stable in the face of varying nutrient input. If, however, nutrient input is increased, the system will seek a new set point that is above the former value. In this system, the fat stores cannot increase the negative feedback signal (to meet the demands of higher nutrient input) unless the fat stores first increase somewhat. Automatic physiological feedback systems of this type may play an important role in regulating body weight.

Controlling Elements

Food intake has been thought to be under the control of two centers in the hypothalamus. In 1942, A. W. Hetherington and S. W. Ranson reported that destruction in the region of the ventromedial hypothalamic nuclei (see Figure 46–4) and surrounding tissue produces hyperphagia, which results in severe obesity. In contrast, B. K. Anand and J. R. Brobeck found in 1951 that bilateral lesions of the lateral hypothalamus produce the opposite effect—a severe aphagia in which the animal dies unless force-fed and hydrated. Electrical stimulation of the hypothalamus produces the opposite effects: lateral stimulation elicits feeding, whereas medial stimulation suppresses feeding. These observations suggested that the lateral hypothalamus contains a feeding center, and the medial hypothalamus, a satiety center; however, this conceptually attractive conclusion is faulty. The brain is not organized into discrete centers that control specific functions; rather, individual functions are performed by neural circuits distributed among several structures in the brain.

Attempts to define precisely the normal function of the lateral or medial centers have not provided clear results. Even a small lesion in the hypothalamus affects many systems and produces complex effects. The observed results of hypothalamic lesions on feeding are now thought to be due to many different factors, including (1) effects on fibers of passage that influence the development of arousal, (2) alteration of sensory information, (3) alteration of set point, and (4) alteration of hormonal balance. One or more of these effects may be seen in patients who have sustained damage to the hypothalamus from vascular disease or a tumor.

Hypothalamic Lesions and Fibers of Passage. Lesions of the lateral hypothalamus have been found to damage dopamine-containing fibers coursing from the substantia nigra to the striatum. If these fibers are sectioned outside of the hypothalamus, animals exhibit a hypoarousal state and aphagia similar to that observed following lateral hypothalamic lesions. The hypothalamic aphagia, however, can be more profound and differs in detail.

The data suggesting that the effects of lateral hypothalamic lesions may be due to interruption of fibers of passage have led investigators to question whether the hypothalamus itself has *any* role in feeding behavior. Recent studies of the lateral hypothalamus have utilized local injection of *kainic acid*, a substance that produces a chemical lesion that primarily destroys cell bodies by an unknown mechanism that is thought to involve prolonged depolarization but does not severely damage fibers of passage (for a review of this type of approach see G. Jonsson, 1980). Chemical lesions were found to produce aphagia and certain other aspects of a lateral hypothalamic syndrome. Furthermore, Edmund T. Rolls and his collaborators have found that the hypothalamus contains many neurons that respond to the sight or taste of food and that the cells respond only when the animal is hungry.

Sensory and Motor Deficits. In some instances, lateral hypothalamic lesions may sever fibers of the trigeminal system, and the resultant sensory loss can contribute to the aphagia. Sectioning of peripheral trigeminal input can also disturb feeding behavior. Sensory or motor deficits might contribute to the phenomenon of *sensory neglect* seen after lateral hypothalamic lesions. Sensory neglect is most easily seen following *unilateral* lesions of the lateral hypothalamus. Animals with these lesions show greatly reduced orienting responses to visual, olfactory, and somatic sensory stimuli presented contralateral to the lesion. They also exhibit diminished feeding responses to food presented contralaterally. It is not clear whether this phenomenon is due to disruption of sensory systems or to interference with motor systems directing responses contralateral to the lesion.

Altered sensory responses are also seen in hyperphagic animals with lesions in the region of the ventromedial hypothalamic nucleus. These animals show heightened responsiveness to the noxious or attractive properties of food and other stimuli (Figure 47–5). Thus, on a normal diet they eat more than nonlesioned animals, but if the food is adulterated with a bitter substance they eat less than normal animals. This effect is similar to that seen in nonlesioned animals that are made obese. Therefore, the altered sensory responsiveness to food seen in ani-

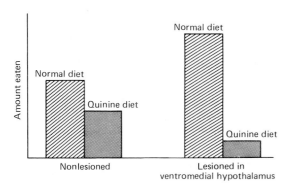

47–5 Rats with a lesion of the ventromedial hypothalamus exhibit extreme feeding responses on a normal diet or a diet adulterated with a bitter substance (quinine). In comparison to control animals, rats with ventromedial hypothalamic lesions, fed the quinine diet, decreased their food intake, whereas lesioned rats fed the normal diet overate.

mals with ventromedial hypothalamic lesions probably is, at least in part, a consequence rather than a cause of the obesity. This interpretation is supported by the work of Stanley Schachter at Columbia University, who found that obese humans with no evidence of damage to the ventromedial hypothalamus are also highly responsive to the taste of food.

47–6 Lateral hypothalamic lesions seem to alter the set point for body weight. Three groups of rats were used in this experiment. The control group was maintained on a normal diet. On day zero the animals of the other two groups received small lesions of the lateral hypothalamus. One of these groups had been maintained on a normal diet; the other group had been starved before the lesion and consequently had lost body weight. Following the lesion, all animals were given free access to food. The lesioned animals that had not been prestarved initially decreased food intake and lost body weight. The food intake of the lesioned animals that were prestarved was not inhibited, and they rapidly gained weight until they reached the level of the other lesioned animals. (Adapted from Keesey et al., 1976.)

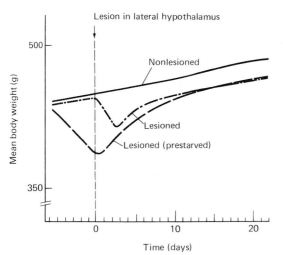

Alterations of Set Point. The results of several experiments have indicated that hypothalamic lesions may alter the set point for regulating body weight. In these experiments the animal's weight is changed by force-feeding or starvation before the lesion. An example of the results of this type of experiment is shown in Figure 47–6. After a relatively small lateral hypothalamic lesion is made, animals eventually resume eating, although ordinarily at a reduced level of intake. If the weight of the animals is reduced before the lateral hypothalamic lesion, the animals eat and gain weight immediately after the lesion, instead of losing weight as the control (non-prestarved) animals do. The prestarvation apparently brings their weight below the set point level determined by the lateral lesion. Analogous but converse results are obtained when animals are force-fed and then given hypothalamic lesions that ordinarily result in overeating.

Hormonal Effects. Feeding behavior is affected by many hormones including sex steroids, glucagon, insulin, and growth hormone. Large lesions of the hypothalamus invariably affect many hormonal control systems. For example, lesions of the medial hypothalamus result in a greatly increased release of insulin when animals are exposed to food. This response may explain, at least in part, the hyperphagia and weight gain seen after medial lesions, since a large amount of insulin in the blood can elicit feeding responses and also promotes the conversion of nutrients into fat. Interestingly, animals with medial hypothalamic lesions show a relative increase in body fat even when their overeating is controlled by limiting their caloric intake to normal levels.

Nonhypothalamic Elements

Although the role of the hypothalamus in a variety of regulatory mechanisms has been emphasized in this and the preceding chapter, it is very important to realize that other structures in the nervous system also contribute to regulation. Indeed, a limited degree of homeostatic regulation continues even in the complete absence of the hypothalamus and structures rostral to it. For example, a rat with this type of lesion will eat if food is placed in its mouth and will reject food (satiate) after an appropriate amount of food has been ingested.

Signals Regulating Feeding

A great deal of research has been devoted to analyzing the cues the organism uses to regulate feeding. There are two main sets of regulatory cues for hunger: *short-term cues* regulate the size of individual meals, and *long-term cues* regulate overall body weight. Short-term cues consist primarily of chemical properties of the food acting in the mouth to stimulate feeding behavior and in the gastrointestinal system and liver to inhibit feeding. The short-term satiety signals apparently impinge on the hypothalamus through afferent autonomic pathways communicating primarily with lateral hypothalamic regions. The effectiveness of short-term cues is modulated by some long-term signal reflecting body weight (perhaps related to total fat stores). By this means, body weight is kept reasonably constant over a broad range of activity and diet.

Several humoral signals are thought to be important for the regulation of feeding behavior. The hypothalamus has glucoreceptors that respond to blood glucose levels. This system, however, probably controls feeding behavior (in contrast to autonomic responses related to blood glucose) only in pathological "emergency" states in which blood glucose levels fall drastically. Other humoral signals that may suppress feeding include gut hormones that are released during a meal. The best evidence, although far from conclusive, is for a role of the peptide *cholecystokinin* in satiety. Cholecystokinin is released from the duodenum and upper intestine when amino acids are present in the tract. The systemic injection of cholecystokinin can inhibit feeding behavior.

Cholecystokinin also appears to be one of the peptide neurotransmitters in neurons of the brain (see Chapter 13), and the injection of small quantities of it into the ventricles of animals also inhibits feeding. Therefore, cholecystokinin released in the brain may inhibit feeding independently of cholecystokinin released from the gut. This is an example of a hormone or neuromodulator that appears to have independent central and peripheral actions that are functionally related. Other examples include luteinizing hormone–releasing hormone (sexual behavior), adrenocorticotropin (stress and avoidance behavior), and angiotensin (responses to hemorrhage; see the section on thirst).

It is possible that separate peripheral and central neurons, utilizing the same neuromodulator to control related behaviors, may have developed during evolution from precursor cells that performed multiple functions in more primitive forebears. Support for this idea is provided by studies by Klaude Weiss, Irving Kupfermann and their colleagues at Columbia University on serotonergic neurons that modulate feeding behavior in *Aplysia*. One of these neurons exerts modulatory hormone-like actions directly on the muscles that mediate biting, as well as on central neurons that control these muscles. Similar neurons have been described in other invertebrates. Both the central and peripheral actions serve an arousal function and improve the efficiency of the behavior. It is also possible that certain similar actions of peripheral and central substances may be a reflection of the fact that peripherally acting hormones have access to the brain. For example, R. M. Bergland and R. B. Page have shown that substances released from the anterior pituitary may enter the brain by means of retrograde blood flow in pituitary portal blood vessels. Blood-borne hormones may find their way into the brain through regions where the blood–brain barrier is weak. Similar peripheral and central actions would ensure that the responses in different parts of the organism work toward the same behavioral goal.

Thirst Is Regulated by Tissue Osmolality and Vascular Volume

As discussed in Chapter 46, the hypothalamus regulates water balance by direct physiological actions. The hypothalamus also regulates behavioral aspects of drinking. Unlike the ingestion of food, as long as a sufficient amount of water is ingested, the precise amount of water taken in is relatively unimportant. Within broad limits, excess intake is readily eliminated. Nevertheless, a set point or ideal level of water intake appears to exist, since either too much or too little drinking results in an inefficient partitioning of the organism's limited time (which can be spent either on drinking behavior or on other necessary activities). If an animal takes in too little liquid at one time, it must soon interrupt other activities and resume its liquid intake to avoid underhydration. Drinking a large amount at one time results in unneeded time spent drinking, as well as urinating in order to eliminate the excess fluid.

Drinking is controlled by two main physiological variables: *tissue osmolality* and *vascular (fluid) volume.* These variables appear to be handled by separate but interrelated mechanisms. Drinking also can be controlled by dryness of the tongue, and by hyperthermia, detected at least in part by thermosensitive neurons in the anterior hypothalamus.

The feedback signals for water regulation derive from many sources. Osmotic stimuli can act directly on osmoreceptor (or sodium-level receptor) cells (probably neurons) in the hypothalamus. Osmotic or sodium stimuli acting on the tongue also can regulate drinking behavior.

The feedback signals for vascular volume are located in the low-pressure side of the circulation—the right atrium and adjacent walls of the great veins. Large volume changes may also affect arterial baroreceptors in the aortic arch and carotid sinus, and signals from these sources can initiate drinking. Low blood volume (as well as other conditions that decrease body sodium) also leads to increased renin secretion from the kidney. Renin, a proteolytic enzyme, cleaves plasma angiotensinogen into angiotensin I, which is then hydrolyzed to the highly active octapeptide angiotensin II. *Angiotensin II* elicits drinking as well as three other physiological actions designed to compensate for water loss: (1) vasoconstriction, (2) increased release of aldosterone, and (3) increased release of vasopressin.

The signals that terminate drinking are less well understood than the signals that initiate drinking. It is clear, however, that the termination signal is not always merely the absence of the initiating signal. This principle holds for many examples of physiological and behavioral regulation, including feeding. Thus, for example, drinking initiated by low vascular fluid volume (e.g., after severe hemorrhage) terminates well before the deficit is rectified. This is highly adaptive since it prevents water intoxication due to excessive dilution of extracellular fluids. It also seems to prevent overhydration that could result because fluid from the alimentary system is absorbed after a relatively long delay.

Motivated Behaviors Can Be Regulated by Factors Other Than Tissue Needs

In this chapter we have dealt with the role of tissue needs in signaling the nervous system to initiate appropriate behavioral and physiological responses to minimize or eliminate deficits. A thorough understanding of motivated behaviors, however, requires knowledge of a number of factors not related to tissue deficit. For example, sexual responses and curiosity appear not to be controlled by the lack of specific substances in the body. Even homeostatic responses such as drinking and feeding are regulated by innate and learned mechanisms that modulate the effects of the feedback signals that indicate tissue deficits. In humans in particular, learned habits and subjective feelings of pleasure can override interoceptive feedback signals. For example, people often choose to go hungry rather than eat food that they have learned to avoid. In addition to hedonic factors, or pleasure, there are two other non-deficit factors that regulate motivated behaviors: the particular ecological requirements of the organism, and anticipatory mechanisms.

Ecological Constraints

The details of particular behavior patterns have been determined by evolutionary selection processes that have shaped responses so that they are appropriate for the ecology of the particular animal. One means of analyzing motivated behaviors in an ecological context is to do cost–benefit analyses similar to those done by economists. In feeding behavior, costs include the time and effort to search for and procure food. The benefit consists of nutrient intake that will ultimately support a given level of reproductive success. The spacing and duration of meals can be considered to reflect the operation of brain mechanisms that have evolved to maximize gain and minimize costs. According to this type of analysis, carnivores may eat very rapidly not because they have exceptionally powerful feedback signals indicating severe deprivation, but because they have evolved mechanisms that help ensure that their kill will not have to be shared with other animals. Ecological considerations need not preclude consideration of homeostatic mechanisms, since homeostatic mechanisms also have evolved to assist the organism in adapting to its particular environmental conditions.

Anticipatory Mechanisms

Homeostatic regulation often is anticipatory and can be initiated before any physiological deficit occurs. Clock mechanisms turn physiological behavioral responses on and off before the occurrence of tissue deficit or need. One such common mechanism is a daily rhythm with a

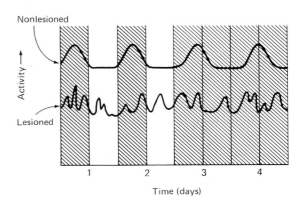

47–7 Lesions of the suprachiasmatic nucleus affect the daily activity rhythm of the rat. Normal animals exhibit 24-hr rhythms during periods of light (**white areas**) and dark (**hatched areas**) and approximately 24-hr rhythms in constant dark. Animals with lesions of the suprachiasmatic nucleus completely lose the 24-hr rhythm.

free-running period typically close to 24 hr, called a *circadian rhythm* (Latin *circa*, about, and *dies*, a day). In the presence of a repeated 24-hr signal (typically light–dark cycles), or *Zeitgeber*, the circadian rhythm runs exactly 24 hr. Circadian rhythms are autogenous, and under constant dark the rhythms continue, although in periods of somewhat more or less than 24 hr. Circadian rhythms exist for virtually every homeostatic function of the body. Since many of the rhythms are coordinated, the hypothalamus would seem to be the ideal location for a major clock mechanism that would drive them, or at least coordinate independent clock mechanisms located throughout the brain. The results of lesions of the suprachiasmatic nucleus in the hypothalamus of the rat and other animals support this suggestion (Figure 47–7). Animals with these lesions lose 24-hr rhythmicity of corticosteroid release, feeding, drinking, locomotor activity, and several other responses.

In primates, including humans, there appear to be two primary oscillators that are linked during normal light–dark cycles but that run free with independent cycles under conditions of constant light. One oscillator appears to be driven by the suprachiasmatic nucleus and controls functions such as slow-wave sleep, plasma growth hormone, skin temperature, and calcium excretion. The second oscillator controls rapid eye movement (REM) sleep, plasma corticosteroids, body core temperature, and potassium excretion.

Consistent with a role of the suprachiasmatic nucleus in circadian rhythmicity is the finding by Robert Moore and Nicholas Lenn that this nucleus receives direct retinal projections. The presence of a circadian mechanism in the suprachiasmatic nucleus provides a means of affecting many different systems with a minimal amount of wiring, and it illustrates the advantage of clustering related functions into an anatomically discrete structure.

Hedonic Factors

In humans an unquestionable factor in the control of motivated behaviors is pleasure. Humans sometimes even subject themselves to deprivation in order to heighten the pleasure obtained when the deprivation is relieved (e.g., skipping lunch in order to enjoy dinner more), or to obtain pleasure by satisfying some competing need (e.g., dieting to look attractive). Since pleasure is subjective, it is difficult to study in animals, but there are reasons to believe that a similar variable may control motivated animal behavior. For example, in 1976 Anthony Sclafani found that rats given a very palatable diet containing a variety of junk foods (chocolate chip cookies, salami, etc.) eat much more than when they are given a bland and comparably nutritious diet of rat chow. The neural bases of pleasure are poorly understood, but it seems reasonable to hypothesize that these mechanisms overlap or even coincide with brain mechanisms (including those in the hypothalamus) that are concerned with reward and the reinforcement of learned behavior.

Intracranial Self-Stimulation Can Reinforce Behavior

One of the most influential discoveries related to mechanisms of drive was the finding by James Olds and Peter Milner in 1954 that intracranial electrical stimulation of the hypothalamus and associated structures could act as a reward or reinforcement for operant conditioning of animals (see Chapter 61 for the definition of operant conditioning). In many respects, brain stimulation appears to act as an ordinary reinforcement such as food, but there is one important difference. Ordinary reinforcement is effective only if the animal is in a particular drive state. For example, food reinforces only a hungry animal. Brain stimulation seems to work regardless of the drive state of the animal. In 1963 these considerations led J. Anthony Deutsch and C. I. Howarth to postulate that reinforcing brain stimulation does two things: (1) it evokes a drive state, and (2) it activates systems that are normally activated by a reinforcing stimulus. Support for this idea has come from subsequent observations that many of the points in the brain that are effective in producing reward also stimulate complex behavioral patterns such as feeding and drinking. Brain stimulation at many different sites in the brain has been found to be reinforcing, but hypothalamic sites are particularly effective. Very effective sites are found along the medial forebrain bundle and the structures it innervates.

There have been many attempts to relate reinforcing brain stimulation to pathways utilizing specific neurotransmitters—usually one or another biogenic amine. The available evidence indicates that pathways utilizing dopamine may be involved in some way, although a complex behavioral phenomenon such as reinforcement is exceedingly unlikely to involve only a single transmitter.

An Overall View

In addition to the hypothalamus, other structures in the nervous system contribute to regulatory functions. Nevertheless, because of its intimate relationship with both the autonomic system and the endocrine system, the hypothalamus appears to play a central role in the physiological and behavioral regulatory mechanisms that are essential to the complex functioning of higher organisms.

Selected Readings

Bligh, J. 1973. Temperature Regulation in Mammals and Other Vertebrates. Amsterdam: North-Holland Pub. Co.

Booth, D. A., Toates, F. M., and Platt, S. V. 1976. Control system for hunger and its implications in animals and man. In D. Novin, W. Wyrwicka, and G. A. Bray (eds.), Hunger: Basic Mechanisms and Clinical Implications. New York: Raven Press, pp. 127–143.

Boulant, J. A. 1981. Hypothalamic mechanisms in thermoregulation. Fed. Proc. 40:2843–2850.

Friedman, M. I., and Stricker, E. M. 1976. The physiological psychology of hunger: A physiological perspective. Psychol. Rev. 83:409–431.

Kissileff, H. R., and Van Itallie, T. B. 1982. Physiology of the control of food intake. Annu. Rev. Nutr. 2:371–418.

Moore-Ede, M. C. 1983. The circadian timing system in mammals: Two pacemakers preside over many secondary oscillators. Fed. Proc. 42:2802–2808.

Rolls, B. J., and Rolls, E. T. 1982. Thirst. Cambridge, England: Cambridge University Press.

Rolls, E. T. 1981. Central nervous mechanisms related to feeding and appetite. Br. Med. Bull. 37:131–134.

Schoener, T. W. 1971. Theory of feeding strategies. Annu. Rev. Ecol. Syst. 2:369–404.

References

Anand, B. K., and Brobeck J. R. 1951. Localization of a "feeding center" in the hypothalamus of the rat. Proc. Soc. Exp. Biol. Med. 77:323–324.

Bergland, R. M., and Page, R. B. 1979. Pituitary–brain vascular relations: A new paradigm. Science 204:18–24.

Corbit, J. D. 1973. Voluntary control of hypothalamic temperature. J. Comp. Physiol. Psychol. 83:394–411.

Deutsch, J. A., and Howarth, C. I. 1963. Some tests of a theory of intracranial self-stimulation. Psychol. Rev. 70:444–460.

Di Girolamo, M., and Rudman, D. 1968. Variations in glucose metabolism and sensitivity to insulin of the rat's adipose tissue, in relation to age and body weight. Endocrinology 82:1133–1141.

Hetherington, A. W., and Ranson, S. W. 1942. The spontaneous activity and food intake of rats with hypothalamic lesions. Am. J. Physiol. 136:609–617.

Jonsson, G. 1980. Chemical neurotoxins as denervation tools in neurobiology. Annu. Rev. Neurosci. 3:169–187.

Keesey, R. E., Boyle, P. C., Kemnitz, J. W., and Mitchel, J. S. 1976. The role of the lateral hypothalamus in determining the body weight set point. In D. Novin, W. Wyrwicka, and G. A. Bray (eds.), Hunger: Basic Mechanisms and Clinical Implications. New York: Raven Press, pp. 243–255.

Moore, R. Y., and Lenn, N. J. 1972. A retinohypothalamic projection in the rat. J. Comp. Neurol. 146:1–14.

Olds, J., and Milner, P. 1954. Positive reinforcement produced by electrical stimulation of septal area and other regions of rat brain. J. Comp. Physiol. Psychol. 47:419–427.

Rolls, E. T., Sanghera, M. K., and Roper-Hall, A. 1979. The latency of activation of neurones in the lateral hypothalamus and substantia innominata during feeding in the monkey. Brain Res. 164:121–135.

Satinoff, E. 1964. Behavioral thermoregulation in response to local cooling of the rat brain. Am. J. Physiol. 206:1389–1394.

Schachter, S. 1971. Some extraordinary facts about obese humans and rats. Am. Psychol. 26:129–144.

Sclafani, A. 1976. Appetite and hunger in experimental obesity syndromes. In D. Novin, W. Wyrwicka, and G. A. Bray (eds.), Hunger: Basic Mechanisms and Clinical Implications. New York: Raven Press, pp. 281–295.

Stellar, J. R. and Stellar, E. 1985. The Neurobiology of Motivation and Reward. New York: Springer Verlag.

Weiss, K. R., Koch, U. T., Koester, J., Rosen, S. C., and Kupfermann, I. 1982. The role of arousal in modulating feeding behavior of Aplysia: Neural and behavioral studies. In B. G. Hoebel and D. Novin (eds.), The Neural Basis of Feeding and Reward. Brunswick, Maine: Haer Institute, pp. 25–57.

John H. Martin

Cortical Neurons, the EEG, and the Mechanisms of Epilepsy

48

What distinguishes the human brain most dramatically from those of other vertebrates is the enormous expanse of the cerebral cortex. One of the challenges for neurobiology is to understand how the cerebral cortex is organized and how this organization relates to the special perceptual, motor, and linguistic competence of human beings. This challenge is central to understanding the role of the brain in the higher cognitive functioning of humans.

As we have seen in previous chapters, functional differences in the various regions of the cortex derive more from their patterns of connections—from the input–output organization—than from differences in cellular properties or even intrinsic circuitry. In fact, studies of the intrinsic organization of the primary somatic sensory cortex (see Chapter 25) by Vernon Mountcastle, and of the primary visual cortex (see Chapter 29) by David Hubel and Torsten Wiesel, indicate that the two primary sensory cortices are quite similar and share a common organization. For example, in both the visual and somatic sensory cortices, neurons are organized in vertical columns that run from the pial surface to the white matter. In addition, in both cortices, cells in a given column have similar properties, which include a similar receptive field position and similar responses to an effective stimulus.

Thus, even though the different functional subdivisions of the cerebral cortex have characteristic morphologies, common principles govern many aspects of the intrinsic organization of the cortex. Furthermore, there are even common principles that govern the patterns of connections. For exam-

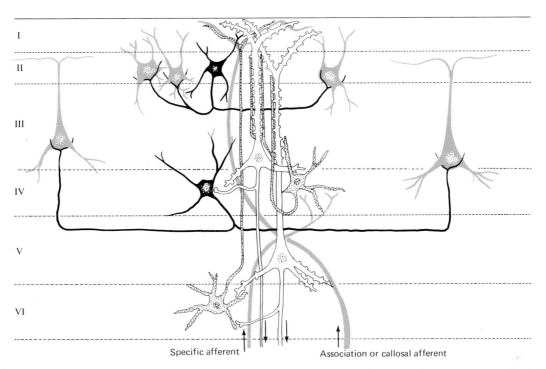

Specific afferent   Association or callosal afferent

48–1 The principal neuron types and their interconnections are similar in the various regions of the cerebral cortex. Note that the two large pyramidal cells (**white**) in layers III and V receive multiple synaptic contacts from the star-shaped interneuron (stellate cell, **stippled**) in layer IV. Basket cell (**black**) inhibition is directed to the somata of cortical neurons.

Major input to the cortex derives from specific thalamic nuclei (specific afferents) and is directed mostly to layer IV; association and callosal input (association and callosal afferents) is in large part directed to more superficial layers. (Adapted from Szentágothai, 1969.)

ple, the major input to the different primary sensory cortices invariably comes from specific nuclei in the lateral thalamus and the input is distributed predominantly to layer IV (Figure 48–1). The neurons of layer IV in turn distribute the information within a given column to neurons located more superficially as well as to those in deeper layers. In contrast to input from the thalamus, information from other cortical regions projects to neurons that lie superficial to layer IV, in layers II and III. The output functions of the cortex are served by neurons in layers II, III, V, and VI. These common organizational features led Mountcastle to suggest that the columns function as modular processing units in all parts of the cerebral cortex.

In this chapter, we shall examine the structure and electrophysiological properties of neurons and glia of the cerebral cortex and briefly consider some key aspects of the transmitter biochemistry of cortical neurons. Next we shall discuss two methods for determining the collective electrical activity of cortical neurons that are useful clinically for examining the function of the cerebral cortex: (1) the electroencephalogram (EEG), and (2) sensory evoked potentials. Finally, we shall consider epilepsy—a major disease of the cerebral cortex. In particular, we shall explore the connection between epilepsy and the electrophysiological properties of cortical neurons.

Cortical Neurons Have Properties That Are Specially Suited to Their Function

As we saw in Chapter 20, the nerve cells of the cerebral cortex are distributed in layers. On the basis of the number of layers and their developmental origin, anatomists have subdivided the cortex into three regions: archicortex, paleocortex, and neocortex. The phylogenetically older *archicortex* (hippocampus) and *paleocortex* (portions of the medial temporal lobe) contain only three cell layers. They are simpler than the six-layered *neocortex*, which emerged late in phylogeny and caps most of the cerebrum. Here we shall focus on the cellular organization of the neocortex. Because so much of the cortex is neocortex, we use the two terms interchangeably.

The Cerebral Cortex Contains Two Major Classes of Neurons

The cerebral cortex contains several different types of nerve cells that fall into two major classes, pyramidal and stellate (Figure 48–1). The *pyramidal cells*, so called because their cell bodies are shaped like pyramids, project their axons to other areas of the brain and spinal cord; they are excitatory neurons and are the major projection neurons of the cerebral cortex. For example, in the motor cortex the pyramidal cells of layer V (the largest of which are the Betz cells) project to the brain stem and spinal cord. The smaller pyramidal cells of layers II and III project to other cortical regions.

Pyramidal cells have a characteristic dendritic organization that facilitates the integration of a variety of inputs. Their apical dendrites often cross several layers and are always oriented perpendicular to the surface of the brain. This anatomical organization of pyramidal cells allows input from different sources to impinge at different points along the dendritic tree. In addition, the dendrites contain booster zones that amplify synaptic currents, thereby enabling distant synaptic sites to be effective (see below). Pharmacological experiments suggest that an amino acid (either glutamate or aspartate) is the neurotransmitter of pyramidal cells.

Stellate cells are neurons with rounded, or oval-shaped, cell bodies. In contrast to pyramidal cells, the axons of stellate cells typically do not leave the cortex but terminate on nearby neurons; thus, the stellate cells are interneurons and serve to establish the appropriate connections within cortical columns. One important class of stellate cells has axons that are oriented *vertically* in the plane of the cortical columns. These cells receive information directly from thalamic neurons, which they convey to other interneurons or pyramidal cells. An example of this kind of stellate interneuron is the spiny stellate cell of the visual cortex, so called because its dendrites are covered with small spines.

Stellate interneurons are quite heterogeneous and use various transmitters. One class, with vertically oriented axons, contains either vasoactive intestinal polypeptide or cholecystokinin. When administered to cortical neurons, both of these peptides are excitatory, and this suggests that the interneurons that contain them are excitatory.

Some stellate cells have axons that are oriented *horizontally*, in the plane of the cortical layers. An important cell with this axonal configuration is the *basket*

cell, which forms dense synaptic connections that envelop the soma of the postsynaptic neuron (hence the name "basket"). The terminals of basket cells contain large amounts of the enzyme glutamic acid decarboxylase, which catalyzes the synthesis of the inhibitory neurotransmitter γ-aminobutyric acid (GABA). For this reason, this cell is likely to be an inhibitory interneuron. The basket cell is thought to produce surround or pericolumnar inhibition, which enables neurons in a given cortical column to function in relative isolation from neighboring columns.

Powerful Inhibitory Synapses Are Located Close to the Cell Body

In 1959 E. G. Gray, at University College London, classified synapses in the cerebral cortex into two types (type I and type II) based on the morphological criteria considered in Chapter 12. Most *type I synapses* end on dendritic spines and are excitatory. *Type II synapses* end both on the dendrites and on cell bodies, and usually are inhibitory. In the cerebellum, the synapses on spines of the Purkinje cell dendrites are type I and excitatory; the basket cell synapses on the Purkinje cell body are type II and inhibitory.

Inhibitory synapses generally are located closer to the cell body than are excitatory synapses, and this is important for information processing. For example, basket cells synapse on the cell bodies of pyramidal cells in the neocortex; they therefore can exert an inhibitory veto on whether or not an impulse is generated at the initial segment of the pyramidal cell (Figure 48–1).

Not only are inhibitory synapses in cortical neurons strategically placed for decision-making, they are also very strong. Cortical inhibitory actions are much larger and last 10 to 20 times longer than the inhibitory actions exerted on spinal motor neurons (Figure 48–2). Rather than simply neutralizing the actions of an excitatory pathway, large cortical inhibitory postsynaptic potentials have a powerful influence on the activity of cells in a particular population.

Pyramidal Cells Are Capable of High-Frequency Firing

Like most neurons in the central nervous system, pyramidal cells have resting potentials of −50 to −70 mV and action potentials of about 100 mV. Pyramidal neurons differ from spinal motor neurons in the configuration of their afterpotentials, however. Motor neurons display a prominent hyperpolarizing afterpotential that limits the firing frequency to a low and stable rate; this biophysical feature presumably matches the mechanical properties of the muscle innervated. In contrast, neocortical pyramidal cells project onto other neurons and are not subject to the same temporal constraints on firing as are motor neurons. Such cells exhibit only a small hyperpolarizing afterpotential and can fire at frequencies up to

48–2 The inhibitory postsynaptic potential (**IPSP**) recorded from a hippocampal pyramidal cell is much greater than that recorded from a spinal motor neuron. (Adapted from Spencer and Kandel, 1968.)

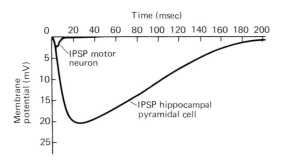

100/sec. Certain pyramidal cells of the hippocampus actually have depolarizing afterpotentials and fire brief high-frequency bursts.

Dendritic Trigger Zones Boost Remote Input

Spinal motor neurons have a single trigger zone located at the initial segment of the axon. In addition to a trigger zone in the initial segment, cortical cells have one or more trigger zones in the dendritic tree. In 1961 Alden Spencer and Eric Kandel, working at the National Institutes of Health, recorded intracellularly from the somata of hippocampal pyramidal cells. They observed small unitary potentials, which they called *fast prepotentials*, that appeared to be active responses occurring in dendrites that are detectable remotely in the soma. Later, Rodolfo Llinás and Charles Nicholson at New York University recorded intracellularly from the dendrites of the cerebellar Purkinje cells and found that these cells also have several trigger zones located in the dendrites. The intradendritic recordings revealed a complex action potential that has many notches on the rising and falling phases. These notches represent dendritic spikes; their variable shapes and sizes reflect different spatial relationships between the site of the recording microelectrode and the site of initiation of the dendritic spike (Figure 48–3). Because of their long duration, the dendritic action potentials in the Purkinje cell summate to produce large potentials.

Until recently, the pyramidal cells of the motor cortex and of the hippocampus were the only types of cortical neurons that had been studied in detail because their large cell bodies were the easiest to impale with intracellular microelectrodes. A recent technical advance in cellular physiological studies of cortical neurons has been the development of the *tissue slice preparation*, which allows in vitro experiments with sections of brain regions, especially the neocortex and hippocampus. Transverse slices of tissue are removed from the animal and perfused and aerated in an experimental chamber. Isolated from the rest of the brain in this manner, the neurons can be visualized and intracellular recordings can be obtained for several hours so that cellular mechanisms can be studied effectively. Moreover, the microenvironment of the neurons can be manipulated. David Prince and his colleagues at Stanford University have recorded directly from the dendrites of hippocampal pyramidal cells and observed both small fast spikes (fast prepotentials) and slow large spikes. The fast prepotentials are blocked by tetrodotoxin (a Na^+ channel inhibitor), which indicates that they are Na^+ spikes. In contrast, the larger spikes, which are insensitive to tetrodotoxin, are inhibited by Mg^{++}, which blocks Ca^{++} channels.

The dendritic trigger zones in cortical neurons serve to boost remote excitatory inputs because they allow the signal to be *actively* conducted toward the final common trigger zone in the axon. Thus, remote excitatory input may have an effect on the activity of neurons that is greater than predicted by the size of the postsynaptic po-

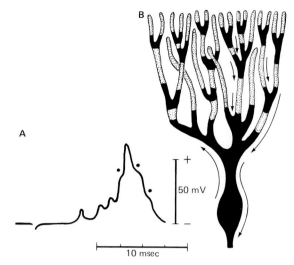

48–3 Dendritic spikes are produced by the dendritic trigger zones of cortical neurons. **A.** Sample intradendritic recording from a cerebellar Purkinje cell. Three all-or-none dendritic spikes precede the larger depolarization. **Dots** adjacent to the large depolarization correspond to inflection points and are presumably also dendritic spikes. **B.** Schematic representation of the probable set of events following orthodromic Purkinje cell activation of dendrites. **Black areas** on the dendrites correspond to sites capable of triggering dendritic spikes. In response to parallel fiber stimulation, active responses are initiated in the dendrites that summate, presumably at dendritic branch points (**downward arrows**). When an impulse is initiated at an axonal locus, it is antidromically conducted only to proximal dendrites (**upward arrow**). (Adapted from Llinás and Nicholson, 1971.)

tential. In the spinal motor neuron, the single spike-initiating zone summates synaptic inputs of various signs and magnitudes impinging on the soma and dendritic membranes. Inputs located farther out on the dendrites have a comparatively weaker influence on spike generation than do synapses near the soma. This situation poses a problem for neurons such as the pyramidal cell, which possesses long apical dendrites of 1 mm or more. Dendritic trigger zones enable synapses located on distal portions of the dendrites to be effective.

Glial Cells May Buffer the Extracellular K^+ Concentration

As in other regions of the brain, the cerebral cortex contains 10 times more glial cells than neurons. Of the major types of glia in the central nervous system (see Chapter 2), three are present in the cortex: astrocytes, oligodendrocytes, and microglia.

Intracellular recordings made by Stephen Kuffler and his colleagues have shown that glial cells cannot develop action potentials. Their membrane responds only passively to imposed electrical changes, and they are believed not to have a role in signaling. The glial cell mem-

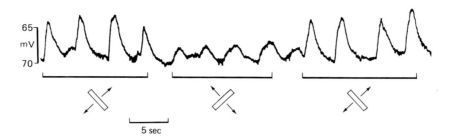

48–4 A glial cell in the visual cortex is depolarized by a visual stimulus with preferred orientation of nearby neurons. **Bars** below intracellular recording indicate the orientation of visual stimuli, each of which is presented for period indicated by **bracket.** (Adapted from Kelly and Van Essen, 1974.)

brane is extremely sensitive to changes in extracellular K^+ concentrations; however, unlike nerve cells, the glial membrane acts as an ideal electrode for K^+ (see Chapter 5). During neuronal activity, the efflux of K^+ from neurons increases, thereby increasing the concentration of K^+ in the extracellular space and, consequently, the depolarization of glial membranes (Figure 48–4). Glial cells are thought to take up this extra K^+ and thereby to buffer the K^+ concentration in the extracellular space. Glial cells are also believed to take up neurotransmitter and toxic substances from the intercellular space.

The Collective Behavior of Neurons Can Be Studied Noninvasively in Humans by Using Macroelectrodes

The function of the cerebral cortex depends on the actions of many neurons. An index of the behavior of neuronal ensembles can be obtained by reconstructing the responses of neuronal populations based on the responses of individual cells probed with microelectrodes. This approach is time-consuming, however, and can be applied only in experimental animals. Another approach is to use macroelectrodes (similar to those used by Wade Marshall, Clinton Woolsey, and Philip Bard to map responses in the somatic sensory cortex) to record the summated activity of large groups of neurons. Recordings of electrical responses of neuronal ensembles may be obtained in humans when the cortical surface is exposed during surgery (electrocorticogram, ECoG), or even from the surface of the scalp (electroencephalogram, EEG). These measurements of collective function are important for studying wakefulness, sleep, and dreaming, as well as for diagnosing epilepsy.

Macroelectrode recording from the cortex is similar in principle to electrocardiography: the electrical responses of a population of cells are recorded at sites distant from the source of the electrical activity. Both types of recordings are based on a theory called *volume conduction,* which describes the flow of ionic current generated by nerve cells through the extracellular space under various conditions of cellular activity.

Potential changes recorded from the scalp, as with the EEG, are generated by the summed ionic currents of the many thousands of neurons located under the recording electrode. The net ionic current can be recorded as a voltage across the resistance of the extracellular space. To elucidate the EEG, we shall first examine intracellular recordings of the response of a single neuron in an active population of neurons. Next we shall examine that neuron's response and those of its neighbors detected with a microelectrode positioned just outside the cell. Finally, we shall examine the summed responses of the neurons of the entire ensemble recorded by a macroelectrode located on the scalp.

Let us first consider the flow of current produced by an excitatory postsynaptic potential on the apical dendrite of a cortical pyramidal cell (Figure 48–5A). The excitatory postsynaptic potential is produced by a current, I_{EPSP}, flowing inward through the synaptic membrane and outward along the large expanse of the extrasynaptic membrane. The intracellular record is the measured voltage, V_m, across both the membrane resistance, R_m, and extracellular resistance, R_{ex} (Figure 48–5B, 1). Because the extracellular resistance is so small compared with the large resistance of the membrane, the voltage is effectively equal to the current multiplied by the membrane resistance ($I_{EPSP} \times R_m$).

To understand extracellular potentials, we must now focus on this small extracellular resistance. With the extracellular recording configuration shown in Figure 48–5B, 2, a recording is made across only the extracellular resistance. A given current (I_{EPSP}) flowing across the transmembrane resistance (R_m) causes a much greater potential change across the membrane, ΔV_m, than does the same current (I_{EPSP}) flowing across the extracellular resistance (R_{ex}). This is one reason that intracellular potentials are large (in the range of millivolts) and extracellular potentials small (in the range of microvolts). As a first approximation, we can calculate the voltage difference between intracellularly and extracellularly recorded potentials using Ohm's law. The current set up by the excitatory postsynaptic potential is the same throughout the circuit, encountering the membrane resistance (R_m) and the extracellular resistance (R_{ex}). From this it follows

A

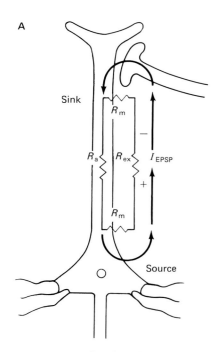

Sink

R_m

R_a R_{ex} I_{EPSP}

$-$

$+$

R_m

Source

B

Membrane

Intracellular   Extracellular

1

R_m R_{ex}

$\Delta V_m = I_{EPSP}(R_m + R_{ex})$
$R_m \gg R_{ex}$
$\Delta V_m = I_{EPSP}(R_m)$

2

R_m R_{ex}

$\Delta V_m = I_{EPSP}(R_{ex})$

48–5 A. Current flow (I_{EPSP}) in and around a cortical pyramidal cell. R_{ex}, extracellular resistance; R_m, membrane resistance; R_a, axoplasmic resistance. **B.** Comparison of intracellular (**1**) and extracellular (**2**) recording configurations. Whereas intracellular recordings measure the voltage drop principally across R_m, extracellular recordings are measurements across R_{ex}. Because R_m is much greater than R_{ex}, an intracellularly recorded electrical event is larger than such an event recorded extracellularly.

that if we assume an intracellularly recorded excitatory postsynaptic potential of 5 mV, the extracellular signal measured just outside the cell would be about 2.5 μV:

$$\frac{\Delta V_{in}}{R_m} = \frac{\Delta V_{ex}}{R_{ex}} = \frac{5 \times 10^{-3}\, V}{1 \times 10^5\, \Omega} = \frac{\Delta V_{ex}}{5 \times 10^1\, \Omega}$$

Therefore,

$$\Delta V_{ex} = \frac{(5 \times 10^{-3})\, V}{(1 \times 10^5)\, \Omega} (5 \times 10^1)\, \Omega = 2.5\ \mu V.$$

It is important to distinguish the sites of inward and outward current in order to interpret the polarity of the recorded potential. The site of inward current is called the *sink* because this is where the current flows into the cell. The site of outward current is called the *source*. (For simplicity, only one path of inward and outward current is shown in Figure 48–5A.) As illustrated in Figure 48–5A, the sink is on the negative side of the extracellular potential; the source is on the positive side.

This example can be taken one step further by considering the recorded polarity of such responses. As shown in Figure 48–6, when we examine the extracellular recording of the excitatory postsynaptic potential, we see that it is a signal of negative polarity. To understand why this recording differs from the intracellular recording, we must know the spatial relations between the tip of the recording electrode and the location of inward and outward currents. The electrode tip in Figure 48–6 (extracellular record, top right) is close to the site of inward cur-

48–6 The polarities of extracellular, not intracellular, recordings change with position. An intracellular recording is shown on the left. Two extracellular recordings are shown on the right. The top extracellular recording is near the site of inward current flow (sink) and the one below is near the site of outward current flow (source).

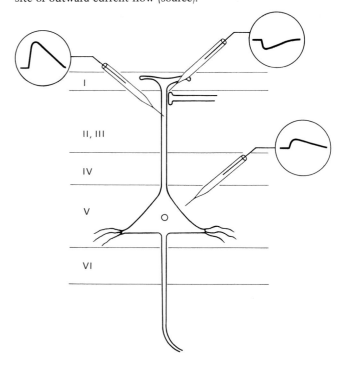

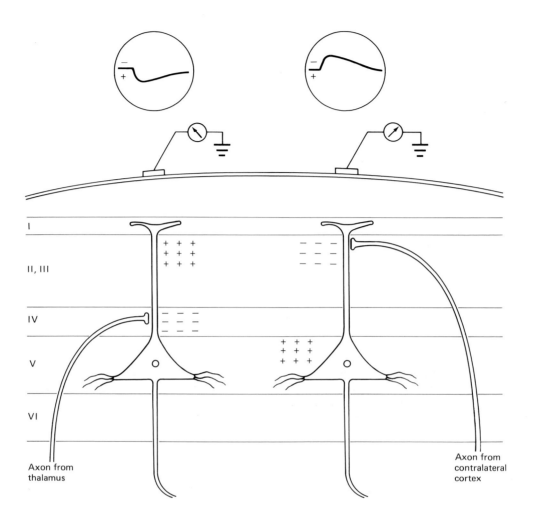

48–7 Scalp recordings and underlying synaptic mechanisms.
On the **left** is a potential recorded from a scalp electrode following activation of thalamic inputs. The terminals of thalamocortical neurons make excitatory connections on cortical neurons predominantly in layer IV. Thus, the site of inward current flow (sink) is in layer IV and the site of outward current flow (source) is in the superficial cortical layers. Since the recording electrode is located on the scalp, it is closer to the site of outward current flow than inward current flow and therefore records a positive potential. By convention, and unlike intracellular recordings, a positive extracellularly recorded potential is a downward deflection. On the **right** is a potential recorded from an excitatory input from a callosal neuron in the contralateral cortex. The axons of callosal neurons terminate in the superficial cortical layers. A negative potential (upward deflection) is recorded because the electrode is closer to the site of inward current flow than that of the outward flow.

cellular record) produced by the influx of positively charged ions. Intracellular recordings, therefore, have a similar polarity irrespective of the recording site.

These extracellular recordings have been illustrated with a signal from one cell, but an extracellular electrode records from many cells. The recorded signal comes principally from neurons near the electrode and only to a small extent from more distant neurons. As the electrode is moved from the site of generation of activity, the recorded amplitude decreases rapidly by the square root of the distance. In addition to the small value of the extracellular resistance, the rapid drop of potential with distance also contributes to the small size of the recorded extracellular potentials.

The small size of these potentials poses a serious problem when the electrode is far from the active neurons, as is the case when we record from the scalp with a macroelectrode. The small size of the potential precludes recording of the activity of single neurons. Fortunately, the scalp recording is the algebraically summed activity of large numbers of neurons. Thalamic input synchronously activates thousands of cortical neurons. Initially, this situation is associated with a sink in deeper layers (where the excitatory synapses are located) and a source in superficial layers (Figure 48–7, left). The source

rent (the sink). This represents the negative side of the voltage drop across the resistance and is therefore a negative potential. In contrast, when the tip of the electrode is close to the site of outward current (Figure 48–6, extracellular record, bottom right), a positive potential is recorded. Intracellularly recorded excitatory postsynaptic potentials are depolarizing potentials (Figure 48–6, intra-

Table 48–1. Directions of Deflection in Recordings of Excitatory and Inhibitory Potentials

Postsynaptic potential	Intracellular recording	Extracellular surface recording	
		Synapse in superficial layer	Synapse in deeper layer
Excitatory	Upward	Upward	Downward
Inhibitory	Downward	Downward	Upward

is therefore closer to a recording electrode located on the surface of the scalp than is the sink, which is located in a deeper cortical layer. Later, the configuration of sinks and sources may change because of further intracortical processing (not shown in figure). The convention adopted for the polarity of extracellular recording is that a positive potential is shown as a downward deflection. Therefore, excitatory postsynaptic potentials in deeper cortical layers are observed as downward deflections on an EEG recording device. (In contrast, in intracellular recordings, positive potentials are recorded as upward deflections.) The sign of the electrical signal will be different when the excitatory synapse is located in the superficial layers of the cortex. The right half of Figure 48–7 shows the scalp-recorded potential as a consequence of activation by a callosal neuron whose axon terminates in layers II and III. There, the sink is closer to the recording electrode and the recording is an upward deflection. Because the polarity of the recording depends on the sign of synaptic action, the relationship between synapse location and recording polarity is reversed during inhibition. Moreover, from surface recording alone, the cortical synaptic events that contribute to the scalp potential cannot be unambiguously determined. For example, a positive wave recorded from the surface of the scalp may correspond to either superficial excitation or deep inhibition. Additional information about the anatomical organization of cortical synapses is needed to define the synaptic mechanisms underlying surface-recorded potentials. The directions of deflection of recorded potentials in response to excitation and inhibition are summarized in Table 48–1.

Electroencephalograms Reflect Summated Postsynaptic Potentials in Cortical Neurons

An EEG is a record of fluctuations of electrical activity in the brain recorded from the surface of the scalp (Figure 48–8). The EEG is used chiefly for distinguishing the various stages of sleep (as we shall see in Chapters 49 and 50) and for diagnosing cerebral dysfunction (such as epilepsy). To record the EEG, two electrodes are used: an *active electrode* is placed over the presumed site of neuronal activity (i.e., the recording area), and an *indifferent electrode* is placed at some distance from this site. Numerous active electrodes situated over different parts of the head are used in clinical EEG recordings. (All recordings measure the potential difference between two electrodes: either between the active and indifferent electrode or between two active electrodes.) The recording

electrodes are usually placed on the scalp over the frontal, parietal, occipital, and temporal lobes according to a conventional scheme. In special circumstances, placement of nasopharyngeal or sphenoidal electrodes enhances detection of activity in the medial temporal lobes. This is particularly important in patients suspected of having seizures originating in limbic structures.

The frequencies of the potentials recorded from the surface of the scalp of a normal human vary from 1 to 50 Hz (usually 1–30 Hz), and the amplitudes typically range from 20 to 100 μV. The amplitude of the EEG is attenuated by the skull and scalp. Although the frequency characteristics of the EEG potential are extremely complex and the amplitude may vary considerably even within a relatively short time interval, a few dominant frequencies and amplitudes are typically observed. They are called alpha (8–13 Hz), beta (13–30 Hz), delta (0.5–4 Hz), and theta (4–7 Hz).

Alpha waves (sometimes called *Berger rhythm* after Hans Berger, who studied EEG extensively in disease states) are generally associated with a state of relaxed wakefulness; they are recorded best over the parietal and occipital lobes (Figure 48–8). *Beta waves* are normally seen over the frontal regions and more diffusely during intense mental activity. Beta waves have the smallest amplitudes of recorded EEG activity. *Delta* and *theta waves*, which are associated with stages of sleep in

48–8 An EEG recorded from the scalp surface at various points over the left and right hemispheres.

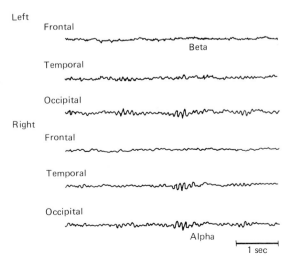

Left

Frontal

Beta

Temporal

Occipital

Right

Frontal

Temporal

Occipital

Alpha

1 sec

the normal adult, have the largest amplitudes of EEG activity.

The EEG is a record of the extracellular current flow associated with the summed activity of the individual cells underlying the electrode. Although it might seem that the most obvious source for these extracellular potentials is the action potential—the largest signal generated by neurons—action potentials actually contribute little to gross surface potentials except possibly when there is synchronous activity in large groups of neurons. The bulk of the gross potentials recorded from the scalp results from extracellular current flow associated with summated postsynaptic potentials in synchronously activated, vertically oriented pyramidal cells. As we saw above, the exact configuration of the gross potential is related in a complex way to the site and the sign of postsynaptic potentials. Knowledge of both extracellular current flow and anatomical pathways is essential for an understanding of the cellular basis of gross potentials.

Pyramidal cells are oriented parallel to one another, and their dendrites run perpendicular toward the surface of the cortex. Therefore, a synaptic potential generated on the dendrites is picked up with little attenuation due to geometrical factors because the sources and sinks are also oriented perpendicular to the cortical surface. In contrast, glial cells are not oriented in any particular fashion relative to one another or to the pyramidal cells; their contribution to the EEG is probably insignificant.

Stimulation of Sensory Pathways Can Be Recorded as Evoked Potentials

As we saw in Chapter 25, another type of clinically interesting potential recorded from the scalp is the *sensory evoked potential*. This potential is a specific change in the ongoing EEG resulting from stimulation of a sensory pathway. Sensory evoked potentials are time-locked to the stimulus and are specific for the sensory system that evokes them. The evoked potentials recorded from the scalp are not readily apparent in the background EEG, and special computerized averaging programs are necessary to detect them (Figure 48–9). For example, the sensory evoked potential recorded over the postcentral gyrus in response to an electrical stimulus or a tap to the skin has a short latency; its first phase is positive and is followed by a negative wave. The initial positive response reflects excitation of neurons in layer IV of the cortex produced by input from the ventral posterior nucleus of the thalamus. The later negative response is a result of the elaboration of excitatory input in superficial cortical layers and inhibition in deeper layers.

By using computers, it has also become possible to record the contribution of noncortical structures to the evoked potential and thereby to learn something about the role of these regions in processing stimuli. For example, in the auditory system one can assess the contribution of each relay in the auditory pathway in terms of its contribution to the recording from the scalp (Figure 48–10). This is possible because the tissue between a brain stem nucleus and the scalp electrode behaves as a volume conductor. Although the scalp electrode best records local activity in the immediate environment of the electrode, with appropriate averaging of repeated trials, unwanted signals are rejected and the stimulus-dependent activity of each relay becomes readily apparent in what is called the *far field potential*. In Figure 48–10, both far field potentials and cortical sensory evoked potentials are shown. Recording the far field potential is important clinically in assessing the function of subcortical sensory relays as well as in evaluating demyelinat-

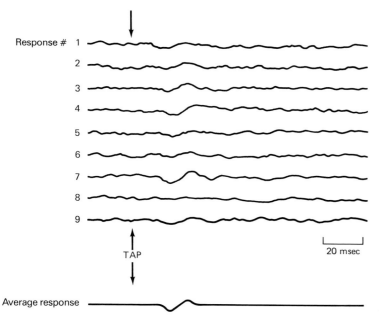

48–9 Signal averaging of sensory evoked potentials increases the signal-to-noise ratio. Sensory evoked potentials recorded over the postcentral gyrus (primary somatic sensory cortex) occur at a fixed latency following the mechanical stimulus; however, the size of these responses is small in relation to the amplitude of the fluctuations of the EEG. This schematic figure shows 9 separate EEG records made during 9 stimulus presentations (**tap**). With a computer, these 9 records are averaged. In this procedure, the randomly occurring fluctuations in the EEG cancel each other out, leaving a record of an average sensory evoked potential that clearly illustrates the time course and waveform of the electrical events involved with processing the sensory information.

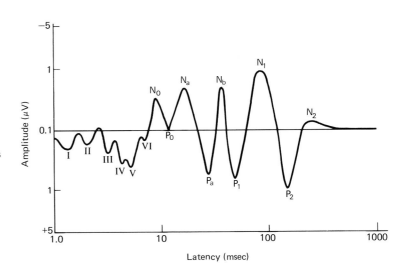

48–10 The contribution of each relay in the auditory pathway can be assessed by examining the auditory evoked potential components (plotted on a logarithmic scale). Available evidence suggests that components **I** to **VI** are generated by the succession of structures in the auditory pathway from the auditory nerve to the medial geniculate nucleus. These potentials are called *far field potentials*. Sources for later components (N_0–N_2 and P_0–P_2) probably include nonspecific thalamic nuclei, the auditory cortex, and association cortices. (Adapted from Picton et al., 1974.)

ing diseases, such as multiple sclerosis. Destruction of the myelin sheath causes a decrease in conduction velocity; as a result, in demyelinating diseases the latencies (i.e., the time that elapses between onset of stimulation and onset of response) of the far field potentials are longer than normal.

Epilepsy Is a Disease of Cerebral Neuron Dysfunction

About 1% of the population suffers from epilepsy, one of the most common neurological diseases. Epileptic seizures result when a large collection of neurons discharge in abnormal synchrony. This synchronous discharge produces stereotyped and involuntary paroxysmal alterations in behavior that profoundly alter the life of epileptic patients. Abnormal cellular discharge may be associated with a variety of specific causative factors: trauma, oxygen deprivation, tumors, infection, and metabolic derangements. However, no specific causative factors are found in about half the patients. Epileptic seizures can be either partial or generalized.

Partial and Generalized Seizures Have Different Clinical and EEG Features

Partial (or *focal*) *epilepsy* is a form of seizure that begins in a specific brain region. The clinical manifestations of a partial seizure reflect the region of the brain involved (Figure 48–11A). An epileptic focus located in the precentral gyrus (motor cortex) results in involuntary twitching of the striated muscles of the body, most commonly those of the contralateral fingers and face. Typically, there is sequential activation of different muscle groups as the abnormal electrical activity spreads from the focus to neighboring cortical tissue. Thus, the motor activity may involve first the fingers, followed by the wrist, elbow, shoulder, and eventually the face and leg. As we

have seen in Chapter 38, Hughlings Jackson first described the somatotopic organization of the motor cortex from observations made in patients with this type of seizure. These attacks are therefore called *Jacksonian motor seizures*. A patient experiencing a Jacksonian seizure remains conscious if the abnormal activity is restricted to one hemisphere. When the epileptic activity spreads to the other hemisphere, consciousness is lost. *Complex partial seizures*, sometimes referred to as *psychomotor epilepsy*, are characterized by complicated illusory phenomena and semipurposeful complicated motor acts that result from the involvement of structures within the temporal lobe.

The electrophysiological consequences of focal seizures can be recorded in a noninvasive manner with scalp electrodes. The signature of a focal seizure is a sharp spike of electrical activity, often called an *EEG spike* (Figure 48–11A). As we shall see below, this signal corresponds to the synchronous discharge of cortical neurons beneath the electrode.

Generalized (or *nonfocal*) *epilepsy* involves large parts of the brain from the outset (Figure 48–11B). These generalized seizures are subdivided into *petit mal* and *grand mal*: petit mal seizures are characterized by transient loss of consciousness; grand mal seizures are characterized by loss of consciousness associated with tonic-clonic movements (i.e., tonic periods of increased muscle tone alternating with clonic periods consisting of jerky movements). The difference in the spatial distribution of abnormal electrical activity recorded during generalized and focal seizures is remarkable (Figure 48–11). Generalized seizures also result in EEG spikes, but unlike focal seizures, seizure activity is present on EEG traces all over the skull simultaneously.

Epileptic Seizures Can Be Produced in Experimental Animals

Focal epilepsy has been studied most widely because it is quite prevalent in patients and is easy to produce in ex-

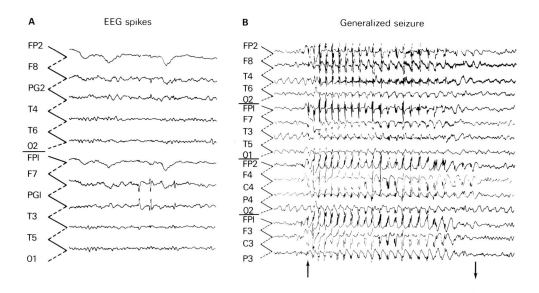

48–11 Scalp recordings during a focal epileptic seizure **(A)** and a generalized seizure **(B)**. In each part, various scalp electrodes record ongoing electrical activity over different cortical regions. The location and nomenclature of the electrodes conform to an international convention. For example, those overlying the parietal lobe are indicated by the letter P and a number to specify position further. Electrodes placed in the pharyngeal region, indicated by PG, preferentially record activity from the medial portions of the temporal lobes. **A.** Focal seizure. EEG spikes can be seen as sharp deflections recorded between electrodes F7 and PG1, and PG1 and T3. **B.** Generalized seizure. The beginning and end of the seizure are indicated by the **arrows.** During a generalized seizure, abnormal electrical activity is present from seizure onset on all recording electrodes. In contrast, focal seizures are characterized by abnormal electrical activity from only a subset of electrodes. (Adapted from Merritt, 1979, courtesy of Dr. Eli S. Goldensohn.)

perimental animals. An epileptic focus can be established by applying a convulsant agent to the surface of the cortex in an experimental animal. An effective method is the direct application of the antibiotic penicillin. The electrical activity recorded from the surface of the brain with macroelectrodes in an experimentally induced seizure is similar to that recorded from epileptic foci in humans.

The first abnormal electrical event after the experimental initiation of a focal seizure is the appearance of intermittent high-voltage negative waves on the EEG (Figure 48–12). These are called *interictal spikes* because they resemble the spikes seen in the EEG of humans between actual seizures. As the interictal spikes become more frequent, they become associated with a negative wave of slower time course. Collectively, the fast (spike-like) and slow components are referred to as the *interictal EEG paroxysm*. The slow negative component may also be associated with low-voltage fast waves riding on the crest. When a full-blown seizure occurs, it typically arises from these low-voltage components.

The interictal EEG paroxysm provides a convenient model for elucidating the electrophysiological mechanisms of epilepsy. Intracellular recordings from neurons in an experimental epileptic focus show cellular discharges during the interictal spike that are driven by a large depolarization (followed by a hyperpolarization). The origin of the paroxysmal depolarization is not completely understood but is believed to result from active membrane responses intrinsic to a cell. For example, pen-

48–12 Relationship between surface-recorded EEG discharges and intracellular and extracellular activity in a cortical epileptic focus in an experimental animal. (Adapted from Ayala et al., 1973.)

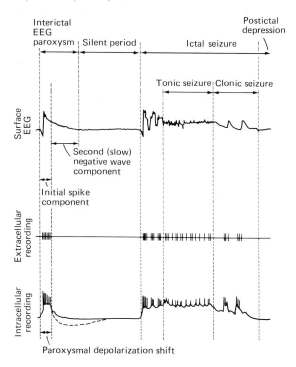

icillin, which blocks synaptic inhibition mediated by γ-aminobutyric acid, is thought to release and amplify the dendritic spike-generating mechanism that involves Ca^{++}. The afterhyperpolarization that follows the paroxysmal depolarization is thought to be due to the activation of the Ca^{++}-dependent K^+ channel by the influx of Ca^{++} into the dendrites. Synaptic inputs trigger and synchronize this process throughout a population of cells.

An Overall View

Basic research in epilepsy provides a good example of the application of cellular techniques to the investigation of cortical disease. One of the goals of research in neurobiology is to use similar approaches for other neurological and psychiatric diseases. In later chapters on sleep disorders, instinctive behavior, psychoses, and learning, we shall see that a cellular approach is becoming fruitful in the study of other human diseases.

Selected Readings

Ayala, G. F., Dichter, M., Gumnit, R. J., Matsumoto, H., and Spencer, W. A. 1973. Genesis of epileptic interictal spikes. New knowledge of cortical feedback systems suggests a neurophysiological explanation of brief paroxysms. Brain Res. 52:1–17.

Hubel, D. H., and Wiesel, T. N. 1977. Ferrier Lecture: Functional architecture of macaque monkey visual cortex. Proc. R. Soc. Lond. [Biol.] 198:1–59.

Mountcastle, V. B. 1978. An organizing principle for cerebral function: The unit module and the distributed system. In G. M. Edelman and V. B. Mountcastle, The Mindful Brain. Cambridge, Mass.: MIT Press, pp. 7–50.

Orkand, R. K. 1977. Glial cells. In E. R. Kandel (ed.), Handbook of Physiology, Section 1: The Nervous System, Vol. I, Cellular Biology of Neurons. Bethesda, Md.: American Physiological Society, pp. 855–875.

Prince, D. A. 1978. Neurophysiology of epilepsy. Annu. Rev. Neurosci. 1:395–415.

Schwartzkroin, P. A., and Wyler, A. R. 1980. Mechanisms underlying epileptiform burst discharge. Ann. Neurol. 7:95–107.

References

Glaser, G. H. 1979. Convulsive disorders (epilepsy). In H. H. Merritt, A Textbook of Neurology, 6th ed. Philadelphia: Lea & Febiger, pp. 843–883.

Gray, E. G. 1959. Axo-somatic and axo-dendritic synapses of the cerebral cortex: An electron microscope study. J. Anat. 93:420–433.

Kelly, J. P., and Van Essen, D. C. 1974. Cell structure and function in the visual cortex of the cat. J. Physiol. (Lond.) 238:515–547.

Kuffler, S. W. 1967. Neuroglial cells: Physiological properties and a potassium mediated effect of neuronal activity on the glial membrane potential. Proc. R. Soc. Lond. [Biol.] 168:1–21.

Llinás, R., and Nicholson, C. 1971. Electrophysiological properties of dendrites and somata in alligator Purkinje cells. J. Neurophysiol. 34:532–551.

Marshall, W. H., Woolsey, C. N., and Bard, P. 1941. Observations on cortical somatic sensory mechanisms of cat and monkey. J. Neurophysiol. 4:1–24.

Merritt, H. H. 1979. A Textbook of Neurology, 6th ed. Philadelphia: Lea & Febiger.

Picton, T. W., Hillyard, S. A., Krausz, H. I., and Galambos, R. 1974. Human auditory evoked potentials. I: Evaluation of components. Electroencephalogr. Clin. Neurophysiol. 36:179–190.

Spencer, W. A., and Kandel, E. R. 1961. Electrophysiology of hippocampal neurons. IV. Fast prepotentials. J. Neurophysiol. 24:272–285.

Spencer, W. A., and Kandel, E. R. 1968. Cellular and integrative properties of the hippocampal pyramidal cell and the comparative electrophysiology of cortical neurons. Int. J. Neurol. 6:266–296.

Szentágothai, J. 1969. Architecture of the cerebral cortex. In H. H. Jasper, A. A. Ward, Jr., and A. Pope (eds.), Basic Mechanisms of the Epilepsies. Boston: Little, Brown, pp. 13–28.

Spencer, W. A. 1977. The physiology of supraspinal neurons in mammals. In E. R. Kandel (ed.), Handbook of Physiology, Section 1: The Nervous System, Vol. I, Cellular Biology of Neurons. Bethesda, Md.: American Physiological Society, pp. 969–1021.

Stockard, J. J., and Rossiter, V. S. 1977. Clinical and pathologic correlates of brain stem auditory response abnormalities. Neurology 27:316–325.

Dennis D. Kelly

Sleep and Dreaming

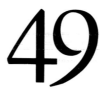

Ideas about sleep and dreaming have always been critical to man's concept of mind and consciousness. Thinking about sleep has followed one of two lines. One line of thought has characterized sleep as an analog of death during which mental function ceases, while another has held that sleep, like wakefulness, is a special form of mental activity. Thus, almost eight centuries before Christ, Hesiod called sleep "the brother of death." However, there have been many who, like Shakespeare's Hamlet, have viewed sleep less as a suspension of life than as a chance to dream, a chance to engage in a special form of mental activity. In 1900 Sigmund Freud significantly expanded the latter view. In *The Interpretation of Dreams*, Freud first recognized that the mental activity that occurs during sleep represents a unique avenue by which unconscious motivation might be explored. For as Freud pointed out, when waking consciousness is periodically interrupted by sleep, mental activity is not simply laid to rest; rather, the mental experience of waking is replaced with the even more intense mental experience of dreaming.

In a book published in 1913 that was to influence sleep research for several decades, Henri Piéron defined sleep as a state that has three features: (1) it is periodically necessary, (2) it has a rhythm relatively independent of external conditions, and (3) it is characterized by complete interruptions of the sensory and motor functions that link the brain with the environment. We now know that the third part of Piéron's definition is not completely correct. The isolation from the environment is far from complete even in the deepest stages of sleep. Sensory impulses from the periphery penetrate cortical areas even during sleep, and, conversely, cortical motor commands reach alpha motor neurons in the spinal cord, although the output of the motor neurons is actively inhibited.

Nevertheless, Piéron's definition remains interesting today, for it focuses our attention on two unsolved questions: How and why does the brain regularly undergo such a profound change in its activity?

Sleep Is an Active and Rhythmic Neural Process

There is a strict periodicity to sleep throughout the life cycle: from the polyphasic sleep–wake cycle of the newborn, to the biphasic pattern of the child who naps in the afternoon, and to the monophasic, circadian cycle of the adult. The sleep–wake cycle is one of the endogenous rhythms of the body that become entrained to the day–night cycle. If a person is completely isolated from the diurnal changes of light and temperature, from social cues, and especially from the knowledge of time, his sleep–wake rhythm will gradually drift from a strict 24-hr cycle to one of approximately 25 hr. This represents the length of the normal sleep–wake rhythm for three-quarters of the adult population. In the remainder, the period between successive awakenings under free-running conditions is longer.

A striking example of a person whose free-running sleep–wake cycle lengthened to 33 hr is shown in Figure

49–1 Body rhythms that are synchronized under normal conditions can become desynchronized under isolated, free-running conditions. In this subject the free-running sleep–wake cycle lengthened to 33.2 hr, as evidenced by the drift to the right in the **bars** showing cycles of activity (**black**) and rest (**white**). The drift in the activity–rest plot is caused by the subject awakening (the beginning of the line) several hours later each day. Rectal temperature (**triangles** plotted separately to the left) maintained a 24.8-hr rhythm. Thus, when superimposed upon the activity–rest plot, temperature shows more than one maximum or minimum per 33-hr cycle. (Adapted from Aschoff, 1969.)

49–1. These data illustrate that there is no single biological clock that regulates all of the body's circadian rhythms. Under free-running conditions the various rhythmic functions, such as maintenance of temperature, formation of urine, and secretion of cortisol, may become desynchronized with each other and with the sleep–wake cycle. Body temperature, for example, normally varies in a circadian pattern from a high in the late afternoon to a low in the early morning hours during sleep. Under normal conditions the sleep–wake and body temperature rhythms are linked. However, under free-running conditions, as in Figure 49–1, most vegetative functions cannot follow cycles longer than 25 hr. Therefore, when the sleep–wake cycle lengthens beyond this value, the rhythms become desynchronized and free-run with different periodicities.

In the 1950s sleep research was dominated by a passive theory of sleep, which held that the brain lapses into sleep when there is insufficient sensory stimulation to keep it awake. Because sleep was viewed simply as the end of the waking state, the central problem for neurophysiology was reduced to specifying those neural systems that maintained wakefulness—the primary, active state.

Compared with the simple notion of sleep as an idling state somewhere near the low end of a continuum of vigilance (a theory to which we shall return in Chapter 50 in relation to the study of coma), the concept of sleep that emerged during the 1950s and 1960s was revolutionary. Sleep became recognized as an active process characterized by a cyclic succession of different psychophysiological phenomena. The stages of sleep are programmed in a relatively predictable time sequence each night, and they appear to be controlled by different, but linked, neurochemical systems. Let us therefore consider the work that has led to the current understanding of sleep.

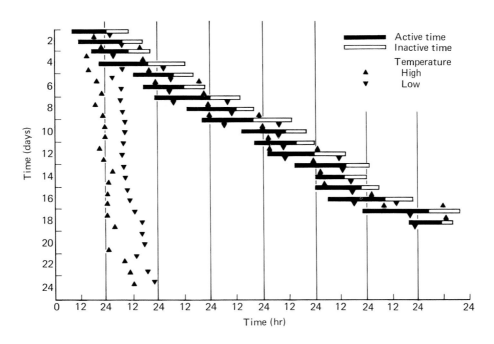

Normal Sleep Cycles Through Identifiable Stages within a Single Sleep Period

Slow-Wave Sleep without Rapid Eye Movements

The primary method for monitoring the stages of human sleep is the EEG, which we considered in Chapter 48. Stages 1–4 of slow-wave sleep are characterized by progressively slower frequencies and higher voltage activities and are correspondingly related to the depth of sleep (Figure 49–2A). As a person initially cycles into sleep, the EEG progresses over a 30–45 min span through stages 1–4 of slow-wave sleep, and then the EEG retraces the same stages in reverse order over a similar time span (Figure 49–2B). During slow-wave sleep, the muscles are relaxed, but somatic activity is not absent. The normal sleeper makes a major postural adjustment on the average of once every 20 min, and some sleepers do so every 5 min. During slow-wave sleep parasympathetic activity seems to predominate. Heart rate and blood pressure decline; gastrointestinal motility is increased. The threshold for arousal in slow-wave sleep varies inversely with EEG frequency, with stage 4 delta-wave sleep the most difficult to interrupt.

Sleep with Rapid Eye Movements

About 90 min after the onset of sleep, several abrupt physiological changes occur. The EEG suddenly becomes desynchronized (low-voltage, fast activity, characteristic of stage 1) and body temperature rises slightly. This active brain pattern (Figure 49–2A) is coupled with broad sympathetic activation. Heart rate and blood pressure increase; respiration becomes more rapid and irregular; and gastrointestinal movements cease. There is a profound loss of muscle tonus except for eye and middle ear muscles. As a result, snoring, if present, abates. The sleeper also becomes unable to regulate body temperature, which begins to change in the direction of the ambient temperature.

In 1957, William Dement and Nathaniel Kleitman, then both at the University of Chicago, described the rapid eye movements (REM) that are characteristic of this phase, which is also called *REM sleep*. Actually, most of the eye movements during REM sleep are slow and rolling; discrete episodes of rapid eye movements are superimposed upon this background of slow eye movements. Middle ear muscles are also phasically active, and both rapid eye movement and middle ear muscles appear to be driven by phasic bursts of electrical activity that can be recorded in animals from a variety of structures in the brain stem (the pons and the oculomotor nuclei), the thalamus (lateral geniculate nuclei), and the visual cortex. These monophasic electrical bursts (referred to as pontine–geniculate–occipital spikes) represent a primary triggering process for phasic ocular movements, a conclusion supported by the finding that the first derivative of the electrooculogram during episodes of rapid eye movement in the cat are perfectly correlated with the pontine–geniculate–occipital spikes.

During REM sleep the arousal threshold in animals is increased. Thus, by this criterion, the REM stage is the deepest stage of sleep. On the other hand, a human sleeper is also more likely to awaken spontaneously from

49–2 Stages of sleep form a cyclical pattern. **A.** EEG recordings during different stages of wakefulness and sleep. Each line represents 30 sec. The top recording of low-voltage, fast activity is that of an awake brain; the next four represent successively deeper stages of non-REM slow-wave sleep. Note that the stage 2 sample contains several characteristic bursts of waxing and waning waves (sleep spindles) of 1–2 sec duration. Stage 1 REM sleep can be distinguished from stage 1 non-REM sleep only by additional electrooculographic and electromyographic criteria. **B.** A typical night's pattern of sleep staging in a young adult. The time spent in REM sleep is represented by a **black bar.** The first REM period is usually short (5–10 min), but it tends to lengthen in successive cycles. Conversely, stages 3 and 4, which together are often referred to as "delta sleep," dominate the non-REM periods in the first third of the night, but are often completely absent during the later, early morning cycles. The amount of stage 2 non-REM sleep increases progressively until it completely occupies the non-REM periods toward the end of the night. Note that in this example, because the morning awakening interrupted the last REM period, the likelihood of a dream recall is good. If, instead, the REM period had been completed and the sleeper had been awakened by an alarm clock from the next stage 2 non-REM sleep, the chance of a dream recall would have been greatly reduced.

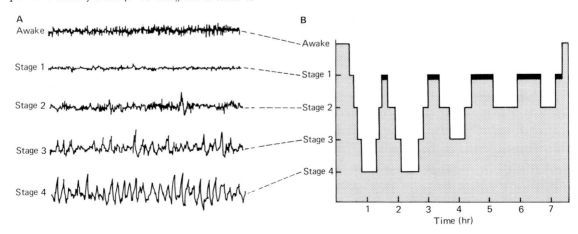

REM sleep than from any other stage of sleep. By this criterion, then, REM sleep is the lightest stage of sleep.

Finally, if the sleeper is awakened and asked, "Were you dreaming?," many more people will recall dreams during REM sleep (74%–95%) than during periods of non-REM sleep (0%–51%).[1]

Architecture of a Night's Sleep

During a typical night's sleep, outlined in Figure 49–2B, the normal person alternates between periods of REM and non-REM sleep, with stage REM recurring at regular intervals five to seven times each night. After the first REM period, the intervals between successive REM periods decrease throughout the night, while the length of each REM episode tends to increase. In all, REM sleep occupies approximately 20%–25% of the sleep time of young adults. Stage 2 non-REM sleep occupies about one-half of total sleep time, and stage 3 and stage 4 non-REM sleep about 15%.

In addition to the cyclic occurrence of REM sleep, another feature characterizes human sleep: stage 4 non-REM (deep) sleep appears primarily in the first half of the sleep period. Thus, the early morning hours with less stage 3 and 4 non-REM sleep and with longer REM periods are characterized by more frequent awakenings even in the normal sleeper.

Stage 4 non-REM sleep and REM sleep have distinctive characteristics. As we shall see in the next section, they show markedly different developmental patterns within the life span of the individual. Stage 4 non-REM sleep is highly responsive to the amount of prior wakefulness, whereas stage REM is much less so. REM and stage 4 non-REM sleep are also differentially affected by certain drugs. A broad spectrum of psychoactive agents, particularly alcohol and the barbiturates, suppress REM sleep, whereas stage 4 non-REM sleep is somewhat less responsive to these drugs but does respond to others. For instance, stage 4 non-REM sleep is reduced by the benzodiazepines to a much greater extent than REM sleep. We shall return to this important point in Chapter 50 when we consider the treatment of insomnia.

The Daily Sleep Requirement Varies with Age

Thus far we have considered only the nightly sleep pattern of the mature human brain. There are also dramatic ontogenetic and phylogenetic differences in the sleep process. The amount of sleep required declines steadily throughout childhood and adolescence, levels off through the middle years, and then further declines with the onset of old age (Figure 49–3).

---

[1]The range in these values depends principally on the definition of dreaming adopted by different investigators, and hence on their method of questioning the subject. REM sleep has also been called *paradoxical sleep* (because its EEG pattern resembles that recorded on an awake person), or *D-sleep* (which refers to dreaming coupled with a desynchronized EEG). In the latter terminology, non-REM sleep is referred to as *S-sleep* in reference to its characteristic slow-wave, synchronized, and spindling EEG patterns.

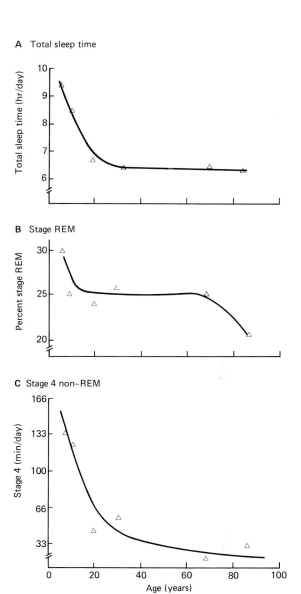

49–3 The human sleep pattern changes as a function of age. Each plot shows data points for the ages of 6, 10, 21, 30, 69, and 84 years (Δ). **A.** Total sleep time per day. (Adapted from Feinberg, 1969.) **B.** Percentage of sleep time spent in stage REM. **C.** Minutes per day spent in stage 4 non-REM sleep.

The most striking maturational changes in the architecture of human sleep involve the amounts of stage REM and stage 4 non-REM sleep (Figure 49–3B and C). The need for REM sleep begins in utero. REM sleep fills approximately 80% of the total sleep time of 10-week premature infants, and 60%–65% of the sleep time of infants born 2–4 weeks prematurely. In full-term neonates REM sleep fills one-half of the normal 16-hr total daily sleep time. REM sleep declines sharply to 30%–35% of sleep time by age 2 and stabilizes at about 25% by 10 years of age, after which it shows little change until the seventh or eighth decade. Thus, the absolute amount of REM sleep time per day declines sharply from about 8 hr at birth to 1.5–1.75 hr by the onset of puberty. Stage 4 non-REM sleep, on the other hand, declines exponentially throughout the developing and middle years, and often disappears after 60 years of age. This decline in stage 4 non-REM sleep in the elderly is correlated with an increase in the number of normal spontaneous awakenings and ultimately with a return to a biphasic circadian pattern of sleep (that is, a nap in the afternoon).

What is the importance of the development of these striking and systematic changes in REM sleep? Because the ontogenetic pattern of REM sleep roughly parallels cerebral myelinization, in 1966 Howard Roffwarg, then at the College of Physicians and Surgeons of Columbia University, suggested that REM sleep plays a role in the developing nervous system analogous to that of physical exercise in the development of muscles. This early theory took into account the fact that REM sleep causes intense activation of neuronal circuits; indeed, the consumption of oxygen by the brain is even greater during REM sleep than during either intense physical or mental exercise in the waking state. Thus, REM sleep was postulated to be a potential source of internal stimulation necessary for proper maturation of the brain. However, this theory does not explain why dreaming continues after the brain has fully developed.

The Phylogeny of Sleep May Provide a Clue to the Function of REM Sleep

Throughout phylogeny the pattern of sleep, like that of dietary habits, is partly determined by ecological adaptation. A lion sleeps by day and hunts at night, while the giraffe takes short daytime naps and then spends the night relaxed, but awake and vigilant. Dement, now at Stanford University, has suggested that the human pattern of a single, extended period of sleep through the night may have evolved as a protective measure because it is safer to sleep at night huddled in a cave than to hunt or graze when nocturnal carnivores are searching for prey.

In the early 1970s, Michel Jouvet of Lyons, France, developed a theory to account for REM sleep. EEG recordings show that sleep stages in nonhuman primates are similar to those of humans. However, the sleep of rodents, smaller mammals, and birds is characterized by only two distinct stages: slow-wave sleep, similar to human stage 4 non-REM sleep; and activated sleep, equivalent to REM sleep in humans. On the other hand, sleep associated with EEG desynchronization has not been clearly established in reptiles or amphibians, although EEG criteria may be useless for establishing the homology of sleep patterns in species that possess no neocortex. Because REM sleep is recognizable in mammals and birds but not in snakes or other reptiles, Jouvet suggested that REM may be a later phylogenetic process related to warm-blooded animals.

Jouvet also discovered that bilateral destruction of the medial portion of the locus ceruleus or of its descending pathway interrupts the strong motor inhibition of the REM state and allows observation of the unparalyzed behavior of cats during REM sleep. By analogy with the human REM state, these animals appear to be acting out their dreams. The behaviors most often exhibited when the other signs of REM sleep are present are those of predatory attack, rage, flight, grooming, exploration, and various other well-integrated, species-typical behavior patterns. These dream-related movement patterns are strongly linked to pontine–geniculate–occipital spikes.

Jouvet suggests that the stage REM "dreams" of lower mammals may be a way of programming species-specific behaviors—of practicing vital behavioral responses before the actual eliciting situation is encountered in the waking state. This is why, Jouvet argues, instinctive acts are nearly perfect the first time they are executed by individual members of the species: they have been rehearsed in dreams. By extension, dreams of all animals may be considered to be genetically preprogrammed. The control of instinctive behavioral sequences is added to the repertoire of the maturing brain during REM sleep when the necessary neuronal circuits are organized according to a genetic blueprint. In cold-blooded animals, Jouvet suggests, this genetic readout may be completed in ovo before birth; hence, there is no need for the REM state.

The Psychophysiology of Dream Content

The discovery by Dement of the strong correlation between REM sleep and visual dreaming in humans has reversed many commonly held notions about dreams. Although it was previously believed that dreaming is rare, modern physiological studies have proved that everyone dreams in regular REM cycles several times every night. The reason that dreams have been thought to be infrequent is that their memory traces are evanescent. The probability of dream recall falls to non-REM levels within 8 min after REM sleep. As a result, we usually remember only morning dreams, which also turn out to be those with the oldest and most emotional psychological content.

Intensity Gradient of Dreams within a Night's Sleep

Successive REM periods during a single night's sleep are characterized by increasing physiological intensity as measured by the frequency of phasic events (pontine–geniculate–occipital spikes, rapid eye movements, middle ear muscle contractions, cardiorespiratory irregularities, or muscular twitching). There is also a parallel increase through successive REM periods in the intensity of emotional tone and the activity of visual imagery in the content of the recalled dream. In this limited sense, eye movements appear to be related to dream imagery: eventful dreams are associated with more frequent rapid eye movements than inactive dreams. It is a matter of current dispute, however, whether any closer correspondence exists, as if the eye were scanning or looking at the dream. While some investigators find occasional cor-

Table 49–1. Reported Characteristics of REM and Non-REM Mentation

Characteristic	Sleep stage		
	Non-REM 3 and 4	Non-REM 2 (ascending)	REM
Features present (percent positive responses)			
Dreaming content	51	51	82
Thinking content	19	23	5
Emotion felt by self	28	29	50
Visual	73	62	90
Physical movement of self	33	38	67
Only one other character	62	50	34
Shift in scene	28	38	63
Recall makes sense to dreamer in terms of recent experience[a]	69	75	48
Median judged duration of reported mental experience	5 (min)	5 (min)	5 (min)
Subject mean ratings of dream characteristics[b]			
Anxiety	0.71	1.00	1.19
Violence/hostility	0.12	0.59	0.71
Distortion	1.12	0.41	1.68

Source: Adapted from Foulkes, D. 1966. The Psychology of Sleep. New York: Scribner's.
[a]Question asked on postsleep questionnaire rather than during nocturnal interview.
[b]Scale runs from 0 (low) to 5 (high).

relations between specific eye movements and shifts of gaze in dream imagery, others find that eye movements are driven in a locked frequency pattern along with other phasic phenomena and seem not to be guided by subjective dream content.

The Content of Dreams

Throughout history, dreams have been experienced as being portentous and important. In ancient times they were believed to provide insight into the future. Because of their presumed predictive value, dreams were extensively catalogued in antiquity. The most famous dream book was written by Artemidorus of Daldis. The dreams recorded in the second century A.D. are remarkably similar to contemporary ones.

Many normal dreams are unpleasant. Calvin Hall catalogued over 10,000 dreams from normal people and found that approximately 64% were associated with sadness, apprehension, or anger. Only 18% were happy or exciting. Hostile acts by or against the dreamer, such as murder, attack, or denunciation, outnumbered friendly acts by more than two to one. Only 1% of dreams involve sexual feelings or acts, and few of these involve sexual intercourse.

Dreams are primarily visual, although the congenitally blind have auditory dreams. Those who lose their sight gradually lose their visual dreams.

Erection Cycles during Sleep

Penile erection is a common physiological correlate of REM sleep. Erections slightly precede, then accompany, virtually every REM epoch in males. They usually bear little relationship to dream content, and they rarely correlate with overtly sensual dreaming, although tumescence may modulate, and ejaculation may occur at appropriate moments in a dream story. The ability to attain a normal erection during REM sleep has been used by some sex therapists to distinguish between physical and psychogenic causes of impotence.

Passage of Time in Dreams

Despite many popular anecdotes to the contrary, the passage of time in dreams is apparently not compressed. On the assumption that it would take more words to describe a long dream than a short one, Dement counted the number of words in dream reports and compared them to the length of the REM episodes. The length of dream narratives showed a highly positive correlation with the duration of REM sleep. In another experiment in the same series, Dement awakened subjects either 5 or 15 min after the onset of REM sleep and asked them to select the correct interval on the basis of the apparent duration of whatever dream material they recalled. A correct choice was made in 83% of instances.

REM Versus Non-REM Mentation

Although dreaming often occurs in REM sleep, mental activity also occurs during non-REM sleep. In general, non-REM mentation is more poorly recalled, less vivid and visual, more conceptual and plausible, under greater volitional control, less emotional, and more pleasant (Table 49–1). An important exception is that most nightmares occur during stages 3 and 4 non-REM sleep, a point to which we shall return in Chapter 50. The essential symptoms of true nightmares are respiratory oppression, paralysis, and anxiety. However, as is typical of non-REM mental activity, such episodes are not accompanied by full dream narratives: rather, a single oppressive situation is recalled, such as being locked up in a tomb.

Selective Deprivation of REM Sleep Results in a REM Rebound

By arousing subjects as they pass into REM sleep, an investigator can reduce REM sleep time drastically without curtailing non-REM sleep. The initial interest in selective REM deprivation was in its possible consequences for subsequent waking behavior. However, total REM deprivation does not lead to psychosis, bizarre behavior, anxiety, or irritability. Subjects deprived of REM sleep for as long as 16 days show no signs of serious psychological disturbance.

The most important effect of REM deprivation is a dramatic shift in subsequent sleep patterns when the subject is allowed to sleep uninterruptedly. Subjects denied REM sleep try to compensate for what was missed. Curtailment of REM sleep for several nights is followed by marked lengthening and increased frequency of REM periods; the more prolonged the deprivation, the larger and longer the REM rebound. This indicates that REM sleep is physiologically necessary and confirms the common belief that dreaming serves some important need. In 1900 Freud proposed that dreams may permit the sleeper to discharge psychologically upsetting stimuli that might arise from the environment during sleep, from concerns of the previous day, and from unsatisfied repressed impulses that otherwise might disturb the sleep: "The dream-process allows the result of such a combination to discharge itself through the channel of a harmless hallucinatory experience, and thus insures the continuity of sleep." Because the content of dreams has been believed often to represent thoughts that are more repressed and hence unavailable to consciousness, psychoanalysts have made use of the interpretation of dreams in therapy.

The mechanism and purpose of sleep and dreaming are still unexplained in neurobiological terms, but several hypotheses have been proposed. Among the more recent, Francis Crick and Graeme Mitchison have suggested that the functioning of neural circuits in the brain inevitably entails the build-up of informational errors. During the waking state, these errors accumulate. Sleep is necessary to erase these errors, and dreaming is a reflection of this process. One property of this theory is that it would explain why newborn infants have more REM sleep than adults. They need to unlearn the many accidental or meaningless connections that accrue as part of the early learning process. "We dream in order to forget," write Crick and Mitchison. In an opposing view, Bernard D. Davis has proposed that dreaming serves to reinforce weakened neural circuits so as to strengthen the important memories of the day.

Several Neural Mechanisms May Be Responsible for the Sleep–Wake Cycle

In 1913 Henri Piéron suggested that physical or mental activity during the day probably produces some chemical that induces sleep and that during sleep the chemical is destroyed. Piéron siphoned cerebrospinal fluid from dogs kept awake for several days and injected it into the ventricular system of recipient dogs, who subsequently slept for 2–6 hr.

In recent years improved biochemical techniques have led to the discovery and characterization of at least three potential sleep-promoting factors: one found in cerebral venous blood, another in cerebrospinal fluid, and a third in brain stem nervous tissue. In 1977 G. A. Schoenenberger and M. Monnier isolated a nonapeptide from the blood of rabbits in which the thalamus had been electrically stimulated to induce sleep. Because administration of this peptide (Trp-Ala-Gly-Gly-Asp-Ala-Ser-Gly-Glu) into the cerebral ventricles enhanced EEG delta waves typical of non-REM sleep and reduced general locomotor activity, it has been named *delta sleep-inducing peptide*. However, in most studies this peptide has proven to be a mild hypnotic and, like other peptides, its normal passage across the blood–brain barrier is difficult and slow.

Another peptide sleep-promoting substance with a molecular weight of less than 500 was concentrated by means of selective filtration from the cerebrospinal fluid of sleep-deprived goats. This factor, which was purified by John R. Pappenheimer and M. Karnofsky, acts by increasing the duration of slow-wave sleep (but not REM sleep) and by decreasing locomotor activity in recipient subjects. Chemical analysis showed this factor to be a peptidoglycan with a muramic acid residue. This type of compound had previously been thought to occur only in bacteria, but Pappenheimer and Karnofsky have shown that it is also synthesized by mammalian cells. How this cerebrospinal fluid factor acts in sleep is still unknown.

Early Concept of the Reticular Activating System

Whether or not these sleep factors function physiologically, it is now certain that on a neural level the onset of sleep is an actively induced process. This has been widely accepted only in the past 25 years, largely through the efforts of Giuseppe Moruzzi. The earlier theory that sleep might be a passive function of the brain took root in the mid-1930s because of the experiments of the Belgian neurophysiologist Frederic Bremer.

Bremer was interested in whether the isolated forebrain, disconnected from the caudal brain stem and thus deprived of almost all sensory input, would continue to cycle between sleep and wakefulness. Bremer completely transected the midbrain of a cat at a level between the superior and inferior colliculi (a *cerveau isolé* preparation), and found that the isolated forebrain displayed a continuous EEG pattern typical of sleep. There were only high-voltage slow-wave activity and permanently constricted pupils. When the transection was made lower in the brain stem, between the caudal medulla and the spinal cord (an *encéphale isolé preparation*), the forebrain showed normal cycles of sleep and waking. Bremer reasoned that the isolated forebrain of the cerveau isolé preparation slept permanently because there was insufficient sensory input to arouse it. The bulbospinal transection of the encéphale isolé cat preserved the sensory input of the cranial nerves, particularly the fifth (trigeminal) and eighth (vestibulocochlear), and this input in turn preserved normal sleep–wake cycling. To support this interpretation, Bremer showed that if the brain stem cranial sensory nerves were cut in an encéphale isolé preparation, a state of continuous forebrain sleep resulted similar to that with the cerveau isolé.

Bremer's assumption was that the stimulation that normally aroused the forebrain is carried rostrally by means of the specific sensory systems. However, in 1949 Moruzzi and Horace W. Magoun significantly qualified Bremer's theory by making partial lesions rather than complete brain stem transections at the midbrain level of the cat. They found that lateral tegmental lesions, which severed the classical ascending sensory pathways, did not significantly alter the balance between sleep and wakefulness. However, midline lesions that cut the rostral projections of the reticular formation resulted in a behavioral stupor and a continuous EEG delta pattern that resembled sleep. They concluded that the ascending projections of a tonically active reticular formation (fed by collaterals from the specific sensory systems) activated the cortex and kept the forebrain awake, and that reduction in this activity resulted in sleep. This passive view of sleep as a functional deafferentation regulated by an ascending reticular activating system dominated sleep research for many years.

Evidence for a Sleep-Inducing Area in the Brain Stem

In the late 1950s Moruzzi and his colleagues began to question the unitary view of the nonspecific reticular activating system. They found that when brain stem transections were performed at the midpontine level, only a few millimeters caudal to the midbrain cuts of Bremer, cats could not sleep. This suggested that the rostral reticular formation contains a population of neurons whose activity is required for wakefulness and, conversely, that the caudal brain stem contains neurons that are necessary for sleep. These neurons are part of the reticular formation, as demonstrated in 1959 in Moruzzi's laboratory and described in Chapter 41. Because these experiments are relevant to understanding coma that follows lower brain stem lesions, they will be more fully discussed in Chapter 50 (see Figure 50–5). In brief, Moruzzi showed that when injections of thiopental, a barbiturate anesthetic, were restricted to the rostral pons and cerebrum (by selectively tying off various cerebral arteries), awake cats were put to sleep, as might be expected. However,

when only the caudal brain stem was anesthetized, the cat woke up if it had been sleeping, and synchronous EEG activity was replaced by desynchronous EEG activity. Thus, these experiments demonstrate that somewhere in the caudal brain stem is an area whose *activity* is needed to induce sleep.

Raphe Nuclei. Later studies have suggested that this sleep-inducing area is the collection of cells that lie in the midline of the medulla known as the *raphe nuclei* (a collection of serotonergic nerve cells). Jouvet found that destruction of 80%–90% of the raphe nuclei produced complete insomnia in cats for 3–4 days. Non-REM sleep, but not REM sleep, gradually returned but never exceeded 2 hr/day. (Cats normally sleep 14.5 hr/day.) Smaller lesions resulted in more recovery, but REM sleep never reappeared until non-REM sleep totaled at least 3.5 hr/day.

Nucleus of the Solitary Tract. A secondary medullary system, located in the vicinity of the nucleus of the solitary tract, may also be involved in inducing sleep. Since activation of this area promotes sleep but damaging it does not result in insomnia, it may produce its effects on sleep by modulating the arousal properties of the reticular formation (see Chapter 41). Electrical stimulation of the nucleus of the solitary tract has a synchronizing effect upon forebrain EEG activity that long outlasts the stimulation. This portion of the medulla receives taste and visceral afferent input principally from the vagus nerve (X). Stimulation of afferent fibers in the vagus nerve also produces EEG synchrony, as does mild, low-frequency (3–8 Hz) stimulation of certain cutaneous nerves. Perhaps this frequency-sensitive mechanism calms the gently rocked baby.

The Suprachiasmatic Nucleus and the Biological Clock for the Sleep–Wake Cycle

At least two areas in the hypothalamus and adjacent basal forebrain are also essential for the induction of normal sleep: the preoptic area and the suprachiasmatic nucleus.

Direct application of serotonin to the *preoptic area* can induce non-REM sleep, as can certain patterns of electrical stimulation. Both effects can be attenuated by prior treatment with parachlorophenylalanine, an inhibitor of serotonin synthesis. Destruction of the preoptic area results in abrupt insomnia in rats.

As we saw in an earlier section and with reference to Figure 49–1, the sleep–wake cycle is one of the endogenous rhythms of the body that normally become entrained to the day–night cycle. Light serves as a *Zeitgeber*, literally a "time giver"—a stimulus that entrains an endogenous rhythm to the circadian clock. However, when both the primary optic tracts and the accessory optic system are severed caudal to the optic chiasm, light continues to entrain the sleep–wake cycle of animals.

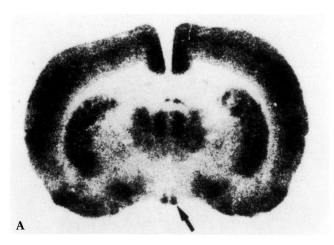

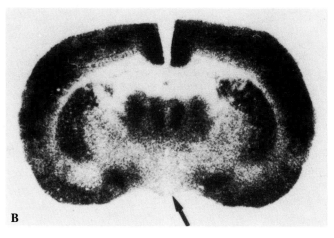

49–4 The metabolic activity of the suprachiasmatic nucleus changes during light/dark circadian cycles. Both autoradiographic micrographs of transverse sections through the rat brain were made after injections of radioactive 2-deoxyglucose. **A.** The **arrow** indicates the increased metabolic activity in the suprachiasmatic nucleus when the injections took place during the day. **B.** Control injections during the night did not produce evidence of metabolic activity at this site. (From Schwartz and Gainer, 1977.)

This unexpected result prompted the hypothesis that a direct retinohypothalamic pathway conveyed information about light to the internal circadian pacemaker. There is now evidence that, at least in nonhuman animals, the primary biological clock is located in the *suprachiasmatic nucleus.*

This hypothalamic nucleus receives direct input from retinal fibers. (In some species there are also retinal fibers that terminate in the preoptic area.) The suprachiasmatic nucleus is also remarkable for the density of dendrodendritic synapses that link its cells together and thus bias them toward synchronous activity. In 1972 Robert Y. Moore and Irving Zucker independently discovered that destruction of the suprachiasmatic nucleus not only prevents entrainment of rhythms by light, but also abolishes various endogenous behavioral and hormonal circadian rhythms, including the sleep–wake cycle. It appears, therefore, that the suprachiasmatic nucleus may house self-contained circadian oscillators and that the retinohypothalamic pathway may serve to couple the mammalian circadian system to the external light–dark cycle.

A remarkable demonstration of the circadian activity of the suprachiasmatic nucleus is shown in Figure 49–4. The rat is a nocturnal animal, active at night. William Schwartz and Harold Gainer injected rats with radioactive 2-deoxyglucose. As we have seen earlier, 2-deoxyglucose is taken up by cells and terminals in proportion to their metabolic activity, and phosphorylated by hexokinase within the functioning cell, where it accumulates and can be detected autoradiographically. The animals were prepared and observed during the day. As seen in Figure 49–4A, the suprachiasmatic nucleus, indicated by the arrow at the base of the brain, was heavily labeled, a consequence of the high metabolic activity in this nucleus resulting from activation of the retinohypothalamic pathway. The nucleus in animals prepared and observed during the night was not labeled.

Distinct Regions of the Brain Stem May Also Trigger REM Sleep

In addition to the postulated involvement in non-REM sleep of such brain stem populations as the raphe nuclei and the nucleus of the solitary tract, there is thought to be a special subset of anatomically and biochemically distinct regions that may trigger REM sleep. Most serotonergic neurons in the dorsal raphe nucleus in the midbrain periaqueductal gray matter fire maximally during waking and drastically reduce their firing rate during REM sleep. This pattern fits with the suggestion that they may normally suppress pontine–geniculate-occipital waves. Some raphe neurons cease firing specifically during pontine–geniculate–occipital spikes, while others remain silent throughout REM episodes. Jouvet suggested that these neurons inhibit more tonic REM events and that their silence during REM sleep indicates a termination of this inhibition.

A Perspective on Neurotransmitters and Sleep

There have also been several attempts to relate three specific chemical transmitters—serotonin, norepinephrine, and acetylcholine—to the various phases of sleep. The role of serotonin in inducing sleep has been explored by Jouvet. He found that lesions involving the raphe nuclei in the medulla depress the levels of serotonin in the cerebral cortex and cause insomnia, whereas cerebral injections of serotonin induce sleep. A difficulty with the hypothesis that serotonin controls sleep, however, is revealed by experiments with parachlorophenylalanine, which inhibits the synthesis of serotonin. When parachlorophenylalanine is administered chronically it leads initially to insomnia, as expected. But, after only one week of repeated daily injections, both REM and non-

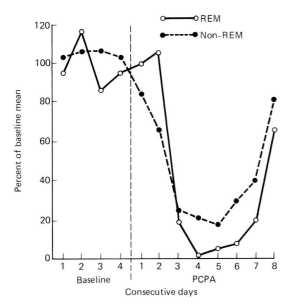

49–5 Although parachlorophenylalanine (PCPA) inhibits the synthesis of serotonin, it produces only a short-term effect on REM and non-REM sleep. In this experiment, parachlorophenylalanine was administered to a cat for 8 consecutive days and its effects on REM and non-REM sleep were compared with the cat's normal sleep as measured for 4 days before treatment (baseline). Shortly after treatment began, both types of sleep diminished sharply, but by the eighth day they were returning to their normal levels. In contrast, serotonin levels remained at approximately zero during the entire course of treatment, suggesting that serotonin is not the crucial factor for the normal production of either REM or non-REM sleep. (Adapted from Dement, 1965.)

REM sleep return to within 70% of normal, despite continued and complete suppression of brain serotonin levels (Figure 49–5).

J. Allan Hobson and Robert McCarley at Harvard have called attention to the possible importance of acetylcholine in REM sleep and norepinephrine in non-REM sleep. They have found two reciprocally interconnected populations of neurons that either fire or are inhibited during REM sleep. One population, cholinergic cells in the gigantocellular tegmental field, fires rapidly and in a phasic manner throughout REM sleep and is correlated with pontine–geniculate–occipital spikes, rapid eye movements, and muscle twitches (see Figure 41-17). The second population, noradrenergic cells in the locus ceruleus, are slowed down in their firing during REM sleep. This led Hobson and McCarley to propose that an intrinsic pattern of alternating activity between cholinergic and noradrenergic cells might account for the cyclicity of REM and non-REM sleep, respectively. Unfortunately for this hypothesis, Jerome Siegel and Dennis McGinty showed that the discharge of giant cholinergic tegmental cells is most highly correlated with movements in alert, awake animals, and thus appears not to be selective for REM sleep but for motor activation per se.

In light of these recent discouraging findings regarding the aminergic and cholinergic models of sleep, it may

now seem as if we actually know less about the neurochemistry of sleep than was presumed only 20 years ago, when the biogenic amine hypothesis was first framed by Jouvet and before the experiments that challenged it were carried out. Since Piéron and before, each generation has sought the presumed hypnogenic substance in the brain and experienced a common disappointment. But science is a self-correcting process, and in this context the exchange of one chemical hypothesis for another reflects the application of the scientific method. Perhaps the neurochemical model itself requires reexamination. For sleep, like other functions of the brain, probably makes use of more than one biochemical key.

Selected Readings

Borbély, A., and Valatx, J.-L. (eds.). 1984. Sleep Mechanisms. Exp. Brain Res. Suppl. 8. Berlin: Springer.

Drucker-Colín, R., Shkurovich, M., and Sterman, N. B. (eds.). 1979. The Functions of Sleep. New York: Academic Press.

Hobson, J. A. 1983. Neurophysiology of dreaming. In M. Monnier and M. Meulders (eds.), Functions of the Nervous System, Vol. 4: Psycho-Neurobiology. Amsterdam: Elsevier, pp. 249–274.

Jouvet, M. 1983. Neurobiology of dream. In M. Monnier and M. Meulders (eds.), Functions of the Nervous System, Vol. 4: Psycho-Neurobiology. Amsterdam: Elsevier, pp. 227–248.

Pappenheimer, J. R. 1976. The sleep factor. Sci. Am. 235(2):24–29.

Steriade, M., and Hobson, J. A. 1976. Neuronal activity during the sleep-waking cycle. Prog. Neurobiol. 6:155–376.

Takahashi, J. S., and Zatz, M. 1982. Regulation of circadian rhythmicity. Science 217:1104–1111.

Wyatt, R. J., and Gillin, J. C. 1976. Biochemistry and human sleep. In R. L. Williams and I. Karacan (eds.), Pharmacology of Sleep. New York: Wiley, pp. 239–274.

References

Artemidorus Daldianus. ca. 140–180 A.D. The Interpretation of Dreams (Oneirocritica). R. J. White (trans.). Park Ridge, N.J.: Noyes Press, 1975.

Aschoff, J. 1969. Desynchronization and resynchronization of human circadian rhythms. Aerosp. Med. 40:844–849.

Batini, C., Moruzzi, G., Palestini, M., Rossi, G. F., and Zanchetti, A. 1958. Persistent patterns of wakefulness in the pretrigeminal midpontine preparation. Science 128:30–32.

Bremer, F. 1936. Nouvelles recherches sur le mécanisme du sommeil. C. R. Séances Soc. Biol. Fil. (Paris) 122:460–464.

Crick, F., and Mitchison, G. 1983. The function of dream sleep. Nature 304:111–114.

Davis, B. D. 1985. Perspectives in Biology. Chicago: The University of Chicago.

Dement, W., and Kleitman, N. 1957. Cyclic variations in EEG during sleep and their relation to eye movements, body motility, and dreaming. Electroencephalogr. Clin. Neurophysiol. 9:673–690.

Dement, W. C. 1965. An essay on dreams: The role of physiology in understanding their nature. In New Directions in Psychology II. New York: Holt, Rinehart and Winston, pp. 135–257.

Feinberg, I. 1969. Effects of age on human sleep patterns. In A. Kales (ed.), Sleep: Physiology & Pathology. Philadelphia: Lippincott, pp. 39–52.

Foulkes, D. 1966. The Psychology of Sleep. New York: Scribner's.

Freud, S. 1900–1901. The Interpretation of Dreams, Vols. IV and V. J. Strachey (trans.). London: Hogarth Press and The Institute of Psycho-Analysis, 1953.

Freud, S. 1933. New Introductory Lectures on Psycho-Analysis. W. J. H. Sprott (trans.). London: Hogarth Press and The Institute of Psycho-Analysis, 1949.

Hall, C. S., and Van de Castle, R. L. 1966. The Content Analysis of Dreams. New York: Appleton-Century-Crofts.

Hobson, J. A., McCarley, R. W., and Wyzinski, P. W. 1975. Sleep cycle oscillation: Reciprocal discharge by two brainstem neuronal groups. Science 189:55–58.

Moore, R. Y., and Eichler, V. B. 1972. Loss of a circadian adrenal corticosterone rhythm following suprachiasmatic lesions in the rat. Brain Res. 42:201–206.

Moruzzi, G., and Magoun, H. W. 1949. Brain stem reticular formation and activation of the EEG. Electroencephalogr. Clin. Neurophysiol. 1:455–473.

Nagasaki, H., Kitahama, K., Valatx, J.-L., and Jouvet, M. 1980. Sleep-promoting effect of the sleep-promoting substance (SPS) and delta sleep-inducing peptide (DSIP) in the mouse. Brain Res. 192:276–280.

Pappenheimer, J. R., Miller, T. B., and Goodrich, C. A. 1967. Sleep-promoting effects of cerebrospinal fluid from sleep-deprived goats. Proc. Natl. Acad. Sci. U.S.A. 58:513–517.

Piéron, H. 1913. Le Problème Physiologique du Sommeil. Paris: Masson.

Roffwarg, H. P., Muzio, J. N., and Dement, W. C. 1966. Ontogenetic development of the human sleep-dream cycle. Science 152:604–619.

Sastre, J.-P., and Jouvet, M. 1979. Le comportement onirique du chat. Physiol. Behav. 22:979–989.

Schoenenberger, G. A., and Monnier, M. 1977. Characterization of a delta-electroencephalogram(-sleep)-inducing peptide. Proc. Natl. Acad. Sci. U.S.A. 74:1282–1286.

Schwartz, W. J., and Gainer, H. 1977. Suprachiasmatic nucleus: Use of ^{14}C-labeled deoxyglucose uptake as a functional marker. Science 197:1089–1091.

Siegel, J. M., and McGinty, D. J. 1977. Pontine reticular formation neurons: Relationship of discharge to motor activity. Science 196:678–680.

Stephan, F. K., and Zucker, I. 1972. Circadian rhythms in drinking behavior and locomotor activity of rats are eliminated by hypothalamic lesions. Proc. Natl. Acad. Sci. U.S.A. 69:1583–1586.

Dennis D. Kelly

Disorders of Sleep and Consciousness

50

Disorders of sleep can disrupt a life with extraordinary thoroughness. Sleep disorders can alter a person's mood and behavior and may exert far-reaching effects on one's life. By a conservative estimate, between 12% and 15% of people living in industrialized countries have serious or *chronic* sleep problems. An additional 20% complain of *occasional* insomnia. Among certain populations, such as institutionalized mental patients, the incidence is much higher still: in a survey of 700 patients at St. Elizabeth's Hospital in Washington, D.C., 70% of those interviewed identified a sleep complaint as that which first prompted them to seek medical help.

In this chapter, we shall consider the most important sleep disorders within the context of the neural mechanisms of normal sleep outlined in Chapter 49. A consideration of sleep disorders not only should enlighten our speculations about normal sleep but should also establish that sleep is not an isolated behavioral event.

Insomnia Is a Symptom, Not a Unitary Disease

Insomnia is the chronic inability to obtain the necessary amount or quality of sleep to maintain adequate daytime behavior. Because of the emphasis upon the complaints and self-evaluation of the patient, this widely accepted definition is independent of the actual number of hours the patient sleeps. As we shall see, insomnia encompasses many disorders, many of which are still poorly understood.

Necessary for the diagnosis of insomnia is some understanding of the range of normal sleep habits.

Few people adhere literally to Alfred the Great's formula of "eight hours for work, eight hours for play, and eight hours for sleep." Young adults do sleep, on the average, 7–8 hr each day, yet the normal range extends from 4–10 hr. Brief sleepers spend proportionately less time than do others in the lighter stages (1) and (2) of non-REM sleep, and more time in REM and in the deepest stage (4) of non-REM sleep.

A complaint of insomnia may not be enough to conclude that something is wrong with the physiology of a patient's sleep. When available, independent verification from a sleep partner is advisable, particularly in the absence of an EEG examination in a sleep laboratory. When tested in the laboratory, many self-professed insomniacs have been found to sleep, dream, and even snore normally. When awakened, however, these sleepers may deny they have been asleep, particularly if aroused from REM sleep. In an early laboratory study, William Dement examined 127 self-professed "insomniacs" and observed an average sleep onset time of 15 min and a mean sleep duration of 7 hr. He concluded that one cannot assume that "insomniacs" cannot sleep. One possibility is that these patients may dream that they are awake.

Two Normal Sources of Insomnia Are Disrupted Rhythms and Aging

Of those who actually cannot sleep, there is an identifiable cause in approximately one-third. The two most common causes are (1) disruptions of normal circadian rhythms or of their entrainment, and (2) the inevitable consequence of aging.

Normal circadian rhythms can be disrupted not only by travel ("jet lag") but also by other behavioral changes such as late-afternoon naps during vacations, altered meal times, and so on. As we saw in Chapter 49, the body's endogenous sleep–wake rhythm is entrained to the diurnal cycle; the stimuli that entrain the internal circadian rhythm to the 24-hr day are called *Zeitgebers*, or indicators of time. Besides the sun, these can be clocks, regular work or meal habits, rhythmic noise or silence (e.g., traffic), or even regularly occurring behavioral interactions imposed by another person's activity–rest cycle. Changes in any of these can result in a phase shift of the circadian cycle and, in turn, in a disturbance of sleep.

In the same way that they can be disrupted as a by-product of behavioral change, circadian rhythms can also be deliberately manipulated. For example, phase shifts to a more appropriate sleep cycle can be established by forcing persistent arousal at a specified time each day. Similarly, people who stay in bed too long on one day may have insomnia the next night. "Sunday night insomnia" after long weekend mornings in bed is common.

As we saw in Chapter 49, the single most powerful determinant of a person's normal sleep pattern is age. Furthermore, for reasons not wholly understood, the older one grows the more difficult it is to reset one's biological clock rapidly. Thus, travel across time zones more seriously upsets the normal sleep patterns of the elderly. Even under stable conditions, most people over 60 sleep no more than 5.5 hr/day. Elderly people worry about this normal change in their sleep pattern. In addition, as we saw in Figure 49–3, the amount of stage 4 non-REM sleep also declines with age. In fact, in many people it is virtually eliminated by the seventh decade. As a natural consequence, older people spend proportionately more time in the lighter stages of non-REM sleep, from which they awaken more often. Noise that will awaken an older sleeper may produce only a temporary shift toward lighter sleep in an EEG of a young adult.

Psychopathology Is Often Mirrored in Disturbed Sleep

Perhaps the most common cause of insomnia is emotional disturbance. At times the underlying psychological problem can be hidden, so that the sleep disturbance appears to be the primary complaint. What is more, psychopathology and poor sleep can potentiate each other; and drugs that affect one usually affect the other, although not always in the desired manner. In a study of patients with insomnia at the Hershey Medical Center in Pennsylvania, an emotional problem was the likely cause in 70%, with depression heading the list. However, most of these depressed patients had initially been treated with sleeping pills because their presenting complaint was lack of sleep, not depression.

Insomnia aside, however, there are some consistent quantitative differences in the sleep of depressed patients. They obtain less delta sleep (combined stages 3 and 4 non-REM). Although total REM sleep is not curtailed, D. J. Kupfer and F. G. Foster at the University of Pittsburgh found that seriously depressed persons consistently show very short REM latencies: depressed patients have been observed to enter REM sleep within 5–15 min after sleep onset. Compared with depressed, or even with severely anxious persons, schizophrenic patients sleep well, and show only subtle sleep abnormalities.

Medication May Initially Help, Then Harm Sleep

Many of the hypnotic drugs used to treat insomnia, although initially helpful, lose effectiveness within 2 weeks. Most patients also show rebound insomnia when withdrawn from hypnotics. Thus, the repeated administration of barbiturates, such as pentobarbital or phenobarbital, gradually leads to an increase in the liver enzymes responsible for degrading these drugs. The result is that their pharmacological action progressively diminishes with prolonged use (Figure 50–1). Moreover, since these enzymes tend to be relatively nonspecific, a broad cross-tolerance to other hypnotics tends to develop at the same time. Most hypnotics, especially barbiturates, severely suppress REM sleep, and drug withdrawal is associated with a profound REM rebound (Figure 50–2). Because of these properties, the administration of barbiturates beyond several days may actually aggravate insomnia.

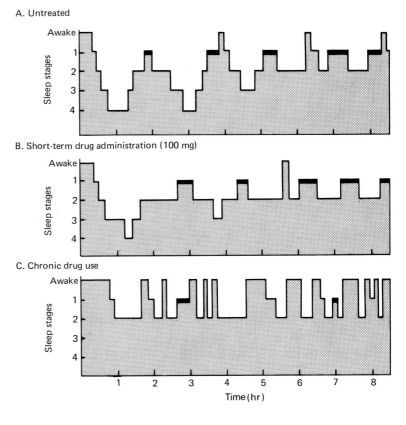

A. Untreated

B. Short-term drug administration (100 mg)

C. Chronic drug use

Time (hr)

50–1 Effect of pentobarbital treatment on sleep staging in a young adult. Time spent in REM sleep is indicated by **black bar. A.** Untreated patient complained of early morning awakenings. **B.** Initially 100 mg pentobarbital lengthened the latency to the first REM period and decreased spontaneous awakenings. **C.** However, with chronic nightly use and an increased dose reflecting tolerance, it took the patient almost 1 hr to fall asleep and there were 12 awakenings during the night. Note also the suppression of both REM sleep and stages 3 and 4 non-REM sleep. (Adapted from Kales and Kales, 1973.)

For these reasons there has been a notable shift away from the use of barbiturates as sleeping pills and toward the use of benzodiazepines. Interest in flurazepam, which currently accounts for more than one-half of all prescriptions for hypnotics, was initially sparked by preliminary reports that it remained effective for at least 28 consecutive nights. A recent and thorough clinical trial of this drug was performed at the National Institutes of Health by Wallace B. Mendelson and colleagues. Nightly use of flurazepam for 28 days by chronic insomniac patients resulted in a modest but overall significant increase in EEG measures of total sleep time, largely due to an increase in stage 2 non-REM sleep. (The benzodiazepines have

been known for a long time virtually to eliminate stage 4 non-REM sleep, a property that makes them effective in treating certain delta sleep disorders, as we shall see later.) Subjective reports of improved sleep were also modest and limited to the first few days of drug therapy. Both barbiturates and benzodiazepines are addictive.

There is some recent evidence that the mechanism of flurazepam's sleep-inducing properties may involve the neuronal benzodiazepine receptor, which may be involved in the physiological regulation of normal sleep (see Chapter 14). Mendelson and his colleagues found that in rats a benzodiazepine receptor antagonist (3-hydroxymethyl-β-carboline) induces a dose-dependent in-

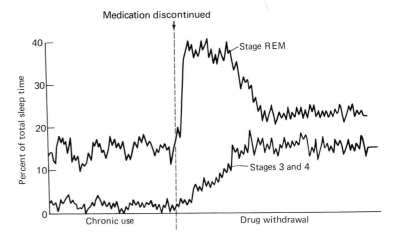

Medication discontinued

Stage REM

Stages 3 and 4

Chronic use   Drug withdrawal

50–2 Abrupt withdrawal of hypnotic drugs causes a marked increase in previously suppressed REM sleep, which is coupled with an increase in both the frequency and intensity of dreaming. Stages 3 and 4 non-REM sleep also recover to normal levels, but they do so gradually, displaying no overshoot or rebound phenomena. (Adapted from Kales and Kales, 1973.)

crease in sleep latency, a reduction in non-REM (but not REM) sleep, and a state of persistent wakefulness unaccompanied by changes in motor activity. Furthermore, at a low dose that by itself did not affect sleep, the same drug blocked sleep induction by large doses of flurazepam. Because this β-carboline drug also antagonizes the anxiolytic actions of the benzodiazepines, the previously noted relation between insomnia and anxiety states may also be traced in the future to alterations in a common neuronal receptor.

Most drugs that are used to prevent or reduce sleep, such as amphetamine, also cause profound alterations in motor activity and other behaviors. If a compound like β-carboline were found to act more directly upon a normal sleep mechanism and thus to reduce sleep without eliciting other major changes in motor behavior, it could be defined as a "somnolytic," a drug class that sleep researchers have long sought to develop. Such compounds might be useful in the treatment of sleep disorders that are characterized by excessive somnolence. We shall encounter these disorders later in the chapter.

Nocturnal Enuresis Is Not Caused by Dreaming

Nocturnal enuresis, or bed-wetting, was once considered a dream-related disorder; so were sleepwalking and night terrors. However, as a result of recent laboratory studies made possible by the physiological discoveries outlined in Chapter 49, these common disturbances of sleep in the young have all been found to occur independently of normal stage REM dream periods.

Bed-wetting is common in children, especially boys, and young adults. Its incidence has been estimated at 3%–6% for the general population, 15% for "nervous" children, and 30% for institutionalized children. Idiopathic or essential enuresis (whose cause is not known) is correlated with decreased bladder capacity and is now widely believed, despite lack of experimental proof, to be related to a maturational lag in neurological control. Sometimes bed-wetting may be due to urinary tract anomalies, cystitis, diabetes mellitus, diabetes insipidus, or epilepsy.

In a typical enuretic episode, the sleeper awakes to find himself in soaked bedclothes, and can report little else. On the other hand, an observer can usually note a preceding period of agitated sleep, including gross body movements, succeeded by several seconds of tranquility and apparent continuation of sleep, followed in turn by enuresis. Immediately after the incident, it is difficult to waken the sleeper, who is confused, disoriented even to the extent of denying that the bed is wet, and unable to recall any dreams.

Laboratory studies have confirmed that few enuretic episodes (3 of 22 in one study) are related to REM sleep. The initial trigger of an enuretic episode (the early body movements) is most often associated with EEG patterns of stage 4 non-REM sleep, and this is followed by a rapid

emergence from the deeper stages of non-REM sleep. Micturition occurs in stage 4, 3, 2, or 1, depending upon the length of the period of calm intervening between the initial body movements and enuresis. The dreams often reported by patients to parallel enuresis are observed in the laboratory only if the subject is allowed to sleep into the next REM episode, during which the sensations arising from the wet bedclothes may be incorporated into the dream.

Somnambulism Is a Non-REM Phenomenon

In the typical sleepwalking episode, the sleeper sits up quietly, gets out of bed, and walks about rather unsteadily at first, with the eyes open and with a blank facial expression. Soon the somnambulist's behavior becomes more coordinated and complex—avoiding objects, dusting tables, or going to the bathroom, and occasionally mumbling or speaking incoherently. It is difficult to attract the sleepwalker's attention. There may be monosyllabic replies to questions. If left alone, the sleeper usually goes back to bed and upon awakening recalls little of the night's activities or of dreaming. Until recently, somnambulism was almost universally interpreted as "acting out" dream activity.

In the laboratory, sleepwalking occurs almost always in stage 3 or 4 non-REM sleep. In an early study, 25 sleepwalkers were observed for 5 nights each. During this time, 41 incidents occurred, all initiated during the deepest stages of non-REM sleep. Given the intense descending inhibition of spinal motor neurons and consequent paralysis during REM sleep, it would seem only reasonable that somnambulistic episodes are unrelated to REM episodes.

Later studies have confirmed that sleepwalking occurs exclusively during non-REM sleep, most frequently in the first third of the night when stages 3 and 4 predominate. In a remarkable study by A. Jacobson and co-workers, all-night EEG records revealed that high-voltage, slow-wave patterns often *commenced* as the sleeper began the nocturnal ramblings (Figure 50–3).

Enuresis and somnambulism both originate in non-REM sleep and also show similar family histories. One-third of the military recruits who had enuresis also had a personal history of sleepwalking, while another one-fourth said that someone in their family sleepwalked. As with enuresis, somnambulism is more common in children than adults, and its decline with age parallels the normal decrease in the proportion of sleep time spent in stage 4 non-REM sleep.

Night Terrors, Nightmares, and Terrifying Dreams Occur in Different Stages of Sleep

Upsetting dreams may occur during either REM or non-REM sleep. Moreover, they possess, often to an exaggerated degree, the physiological and psychological charac-

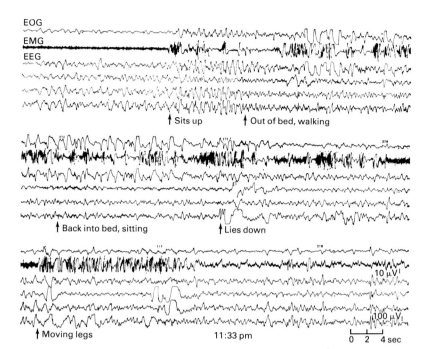

EOG
EMG
EEG

↑ Sits up   ↑ Out of bed, walking

50–3 Electrooculogram (EOG), electromyogram (EMG), and EEG records of a sleepwalking incident observed under laboratory conditions. A high-voltage, slow-wave EEG pattern commences as the sleepwalker sits up in bed, and non-REM sleep patterns are maintained throughout the episode. (Adapted from Jacobson et al., 1965.)

↑ Back into bed, sitting   ↑ Lies down

10 μV

100 μV

↑ Moving legs   11:33 pm   0 2 4 sec

teristics of normal REM and non-REM dreams as outlined in Chapter 49. Bad dreams, during both REM and non-REM sleep, may occur either in children or, less frequently, in adults.

The night terror *(pavor nocturnus)* attack in children is perhaps the best characterized. Usually within 30 min of falling asleep the child abruptly sits up in bed, screams, and appears to be staring wide-eyed at some imaginary object. The child's face is covered with perspiration, and breathing is laborious. In the same manner that sleepwalkers appear to be oblivious to external stimuli, consoling stimuli have no effect on the terrorized child. After the attack, which may last 1 or 2 min, dream recall is rare and usually fragmentary. The next morning there is no recollection of the episode. This fragmented pattern of recall reminds one of non-REM mentation. Thus, it was not surprising that, when Henri Gastaut observed night terror episodes in seven children in his laboratory at Marseilles, all attacks occurred during a sudden arousal from stage 3 or 4 non-REM (delta) sleep. There is recent evidence that night terrors may be suppressed by diazepam, and coincident with this is a measurable decline in the amount of stage 4 (delta-wave) non-REM sleep.

A related non-REM phenomenon is also seen in adults, although less frequently. The core symptoms of these non-REM attacks are respiratory oppression, partial paralysis, and anxiety—usually in that sequence. The anxiety is intense, with sweating, a fixed facial expression, dilated pupils, and difficulty in breathing. Dream activity is rarely well structured; it often consists not of a story, but of a poor recollection of a single oppressive situation, such as having rocks piled on the chest. As in

the pavor nocturnus attack in the child, the subject usually has little memory of the attack the next morning. These patients also show greater than normal daytime anxiety. The name of these non-REM attacks in the adult is *incubus*, which, given the root of this Latin word (from *in* and *cubare*, signifying "to lie upon"), is an appropriate term for a phenomenon characterized by respiratory oppression. However, it also seems likely that a description of the same non-REM phenomenon, characterized by extreme anxiety and oppressed breathing, may have been intended as the original meaning of the word *nightmare*. From the Middle Ages and before, many artists and writers believed that nightmares were caused by a nocturnal demon who pressed upon the sleeper's chest. The German word, *Nachtmar*, and the French word, *cauchemar*, both contain the ancient Teutonic root, *mar*, which means "devil." *Cauchemar* also derives from *caucher*, an ancient French verb meaning "to press," thus literally referring to a "pressing devil."

In contrast to the night terrors and nightmares of delta sleep are the more common frightening dreams that occur during normal REM periods in sleepers of all ages. As would be expected from the study of normal REM events, these terrifying dreams contain complex imagery, have a story line, are vividly recalled, and are not accompanied by depressed respiration, but rather by an exaggerated increase in all the phasic activity, including pontine–geniculate–occipital spikes, that normally characterize REM sleep. Because REM sleep becomes more extensive and more physiologically intense as sleep continues, most terrifying REM dreams occur in the early morning hours. Often these terrifying REM episodes are referred to in the vernacular as nightmares.

Whatever the nomenclature, it is clinically useful to distinguish the high-anxiety dream phenomena that occur during REM sleep from those that occur during non-REM stages of sleep. The reasons are that, like other non-REM disturbances such as enuresis and somnambulism, night terrors should (1) decline with age along with delta sleep, and (2) be alleviated by drugs, such as diazepam, that selectively reduce non-REM delta sleep. In contrast, REM sleep time does not change appreciably after childhood, nor is it suppressed by the same drugs. Hence, the prognosis for childhood non-REM disturbances differs from terrifying REM dreams, and the two should be treated differently.

Sleep Apnea May Result in Hyposomnia or Hypersomnia

Another remarkable disturbance of sleep is characterized by the frequent, periodic cessation of respiration. Both the causes of sleep apnea and the presenting complaints of patients suffering from this disorder are extremely broad. It is therefore unlikely that sleep apnea represents a unitary disorder. In some cases of sleep apnea, the shift from wakefulness to sleep is assumed to be associated with a suppression of activity in the medullary respiratory center. This causes the diaphragm and the intercostal muscles to become immobile. In this phase of apnea, which lasts for 15–30 sec, blood oxygen levels fall and carbon dioxide levels rise, eventually stimulating the respiratory center and causing the respiratory muscles to begin functioning again. Often, however, the lungs do not fill with air because the throat has collapsed, perhaps a reflection of the relaxed state of most body muscles during non-REM sleep. The extreme changes in the concentrations of oxygen and carbon dioxide in the blood that develop after 1 min or more without air rouse the sleeper. Muscle tone returns to the throat, and a few noisy, choking gasps refill the lungs. Arousal may last for only a few seconds until the blood gases return to normal. Then the person returns immediately to sleep and the cycle can be repeated—as many as 500 times during the night.

The different types of sleep apnea can sometimes be distinguished in the sleep laboratory: *Central apneas* can be defined by an absence of respiratory effort. Although the upper airway remains open, the diaphragm stops moving and there is no exchange of air. *Upper airway apneas* are defined by a collapse of the upper airway and no air flow, despite persistent respiratory efforts. Whether the apnea involves central nervous system dysfunction or upper airway obstruction, or a combination of both *(mixed apneas)*, these patients all literally stop breathing during their sleep.

Some sleep apnea patients are apparently oblivious of their persistent nocturnal arousals and may actually complain of too much sleep. These patients were first described by Gastaut in Marseilles in 1965, who called their disorder *hypersomnolent apnea syndrome*. Later, Dement described another group of patients with a similarly disturbed sleep pattern who complained instead of

insomnia. Apparently these patients do not habituate to the frequent nocturnal arousals or do not return to sleep immediately after the apnea. Approximately one-third of patients with sleep apnea complain of insomnia and two-thirds of hypersomnia.

Some investigators have proposed sleep apnea as a model for sudden infant death, or crib death syndrome. On the other hand, the mean age of sleep apnea patients who were studied at Stanford University was 52 years, and the youngest patient was 38. Because relatively few physicians are aware of sleep apnea, the actual incidence of the disorder in the general population is still unknown. In almost all diagnosed cases of sleep apnea, a critical factor has been a report from a sleep partner that the subject snored loudly at night. Few drugs have been found effective in combating sleep apnea, although many are under investigation. In those cases not related to the central nervous system, in which the cause may be some form of upper airway obstruction, a tracheotomy has often successfully restored normal sleep.

Narcolepsy: Irresistible Sleep Attacks Are Accompanied by Several REM-Related Symptoms

The principal symptom of narcolepsy is irresistible sleep attacks lasting 5–30 min during the day, which occasionally occur without warning and at behaviorally inappropriate moments. More often, the narcoleptic feels an overwhelming drowsiness preceding the attack and attempts to fight it off. If the patient naps, he awakes refreshed; 15 min is usually sufficient. One serious danger posed by narcolepsy is accidental death, and automobile accidents are a more frequent complication of narcolepsy than of epilepsy. In one study, 40% of the narcoleptic patients questioned admitted that they had fallen asleep while driving.

In the late 1950s, Robert Yoss and David Daly at the Mayo Clinic described a highly idiosyncratic set of symptoms that seemed to characterize narcoleptics from all walks of life and to include virtually all personality types. They discovered that, in addition to sleep attacks, the narcoleptic patient often exhibits an abrupt loss of muscle tone, a swoonlike reaction termed *cataplexy*, during which the patient may fall to the ground and lie there, conscious, for several minutes. Cataplexy usually occurs when the patient becomes emotionally excited, for instance, during laughter or sexual excitement. Two other less frequent symptoms of narcolepsy are *sleep paralysis*, a brief inhibition of muscle tone during the transition from wakefulness to sleep and vice versa, and *hallucinations* (visual or auditory) at the beginning of sleep. The latter symptoms occur in many normal people, but are exaggerated in narcoleptics.

This quartet of symptoms has been interpreted as reflecting the intrusion of the normally inhibited properties of REM sleep into the waking state (sleep attacks and cataplexy) or into the transitions between wakefulness and sleep (sleep paralysis and hallucinations). In

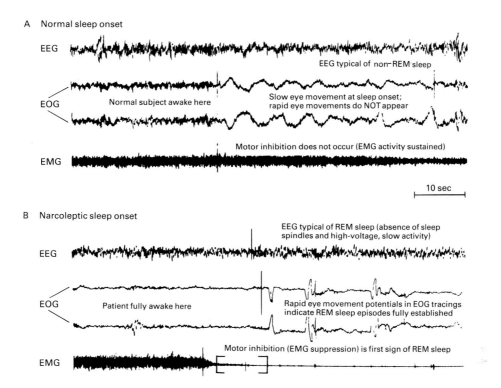

A Normal sleep onset

EEG

EEG typical of non-REM sleep

EOG

Normal subject awake here

Slow eye movement at sleep onset;
rapid eye movements do NOT appear

Motor inhibition does not occur (EMG activity sustained)

EMG

10 sec

B Narcoleptic sleep onset

EEG typical of REM sleep (absence of sleep
spindles and high-voltage, slow activity)

EEG

EOG

Patient fully awake here

Rapid eye movement potentials in EOG tracings
indicate REM sleep episodes fully established

Motor inhibition (EMG suppression) is first sign of REM sleep

EMG

50–4 Narcoleptic patients can enter into REM sleep directly from the waking state. **A.** Sleep onset in the normal person is typified by a gradual change from a waking EEG dominated by alpha activity (10 Hz) to mixed lower frequency patterns coupled with the development of slow, rolling eye movements in the electrooculogram (EOG) and little change in the electromyographic (EMG) recording of muscle tonus. **B.** In the narcoleptic, sleep onset is actually preceded by several seconds of markedly reduced EMG activity (indicated by **brackets** on EMG trace) and then accompanied by conjugate (both traces) rapid eye movements. Sleep-onset REM usually lasts 10–20 min, after which, if the narcoleptic remains asleep, there follows a typical progression through stages 1 to 4 of non-REM sleep. (Adapted from Dement, Guilleminault, and Zarcone, 1975.)

fact, narcoleptic patients can enter directly into REM sleep (Figure 50–4). As a result, *sleep-onset REM* is now considered a fifth defining symptom of narcolepsy.

A sixth and newly discovered sign of narcolepsy is a *decreased voluntary sleep latency.* When tested every 2 hr throughout the day while lying in bed, narcoleptics can usually fall asleep upon request within 2 min, whereas normal subjects take an average of 15 min to get to sleep. Interestingly, the narcoleptic's need for sleep is apparently satiated at a normal rate. Y. Hishikawa and colleagues found that, despite excessive daytime drowsiness, when narcoleptic subjects were asked to sleep as long as possible, they slept no longer than normal.

The cataplexy and sleep paralysis of narcolepsy may have a common neuronal cause. It is possible that both are related to the activation of those brain stem neurons responsible for the massive descending inhibition of spinal motor neurons during stage REM sleep. As we observed in Chapter 49, the loss of muscle tonus during REM sleep does not extend to the eye and middle ear muscles. During the cataplectic attack of the narcoleptic, the patient remains capable of moving his eyes, and can even do so voluntarily in response to questions. During sleep paralysis, patients can also move their eyes. Some

narcoleptics have even learned to terminate the paralysis by vigorous eye movements, followed by fluttering the eyelids and then by moving the facial muscles. They establish a gradual spread of voluntary control using the unparalyzed movements of the eye as an initial base. Sleep paralysis can also be broken immediately by the touch of another.

M. M. Mitler and Dement have found that cataplectic-like behavior can be induced in alert cats by direct microinjections of carbachol, a cholinergic agonist, into the locus ceruleus in the pontine reticular formation. This is the same area whose destruction was found by Jouvet to block motor inhibition during REM sleep (noted in Chapter 49). Like the narcoleptic human, the cataplectic cat could blink its eyes and visually track a moving object, despite the suppression of all other somatic reflexes.

In spite of the ability to fall asleep quickly and to enter the first REM period rapidly, narcoleptics generally show significantly less total REM time than normal and a disturbed sleep architecture. For these reasons, one early hypothesis suggested that the irresistible sleep attacks during the daytime reflected increased pressure to obtain REM sleep. Because stimulant drugs were commonly administered to control the sleep attacks, this proposal was somewhat unsettling. These drugs suppress

REM sleep, and thus it was feared that the treatment might contribute to the illness rather than its cure. However, it now seems that narcolepsy is more complex than a simple state of REM deprivation. Moreover, as outlined in Chapter 49, the consequences of experimental REM deprivation are largely restricted to subsequent sleep periods and intrude very little upon waking behavior.

The symptoms of narcolepsy respond differently to drugs that enhance transmission at central catecholaminergic synapses. The stimulants methylphenidate and δ-amphetamine stimulate the release of newly synthesized transmitter at nerve terminals (and, to a lesser extent, attenuate reuptake) and aid in the control of sleep attacks, but have no effect on the other symptoms of narcolepsy. The tricyclic antidepressant imipramine blocks reuptake of neurotransmitters by presynaptic terminals and prevents cataplexy but has no effect on sleep attacks. Among other drugs that potentiate transmission at monoaminergic synapses, monoamine oxidase inhibitors that prevent the enzymatic destruction of the transmitter substance may improve all four primary narcoleptic symptoms.

There is a strong familial component to narcolepsy, even though onset is usually delayed, often until the second decade. Narcolepsy is not rare. Dement has estimated its incidence in the general population to be approximately 0.07%, which corresponds to about 250,000 Americans. Because many of these cases are not diagnosed, narcoleptics may be subject to unwarranted disapproval for apparent laziness.

Loss of Consciousness: Coma Is Not Deep Sleep

At one time it was common in both the clinical and basic neural sciences to postulate a continuum of consciousness that ranged in graded levels from attention, alertness, relaxation, and drowsiness to sleep, stupor, and coma. It was generally believed that the level of excitation in the ascending reticular activating system determined the level of consciousness. Sensory impulses entering the reticular formation from the different modalities were assumed to merge and lose their specificity within this network of neurons. The reticular formation in turn was thought to act as an energizer and exert a broad facilitatory influence on the rest of the nervous system. A reduction in the amount of impulses from the reticular formation would reduce the overall activity of the brain and consequently result in sleep.

However, with the discovery of the extraordinary amount of neural activity that characterizes sleep, the idea of a neurophysiological continuum from quiescence to excitation had to be abandoned. Moreover, activity of the reticular formation alone does not account for variations in levels of consciousness. As Alf Brodal, one of the major students of the anatomy of the reticular formation, has said, "It would be entirely misleading to consider the reticular formation the 'seat of consciousness.'" Nevertheless, the brain stem reticular core plays a role in many clinical disorders of consciousness.

Transient Losses of Consciousness Can Result from Decreased Cerebral Blood Flow

Fainting, or syncope, most often results from a general reduction in cerebral blood flow, which compromises the ability of the brain to extract oxygen and needed nutrients. This involves a failure of the autoregulatory reflexes of the cerebral vessels (see Appendix IB), which normally maintain a constant blood flow over a wide range of perfusion pressures. Autoregulation may fail if perfusion pressure falls below 60 mm Hg; too precipitous a fall can result from decreased cardiac output or, more frequently, from decreased peripheral resistance, or both. One type of syncope, termed vasovagal, is reflexive in origin and is almost always related to pain, fear, or other emotional stress. In vasovagal syncope, stimulation of the autonomic nervous system usually precedes the drop in blood pressure and the patient is usually aware of "light-headedness" and impending fainting.

Coma Has Many Causes

Sleep and coma differ behaviorally in terms of their arousal threshold, or relative reversibility. They can also be easily distinguished physiologically. Sleep is a highly active neurophysiological state during which cerebral oxygen uptake does not decline from normal waking levels. On the contrary, Seymour Kety found that cerebral oxygen uptake actually increases above normal during REM episodes. In contrast, oxygen uptake falls below the normal resting level in every studied example of coma. Thus, coma may be defined, by exclusion, as a nonsleep loss of consciousness that, unlike syncope, lasts for an extended period. Within the range of this definition, different clinical levels of unconsciousness, including lethargy, loss of sensation, stupor, and coma, have been distinguished clinically in terms of the degree of indifference exhibited by the patient to such common stimuli as talking, shouting, shaking, or noxious prodding. Stupor is a state in which someone is responsive only to shaking, shouting, or noxious stimuli, whereas coma refers to total unresponsiveness.

Two general types of pathological processes may impair consciousness. One consists of a set of conditions that can cause widespread functional depression of the cerebral hemispheres; the other includes more specific conditions that depress or destroy critical brain stem areas. In 1972 Fred Plum and Jerome Posner at Cornell Medical School suggested that diseases causing stupor or coma must either affect the brain widely or encroach upon deep central structures. They classified these diseases into three categories: (1) sub- or infratentorial mass or destructive lesions (such as pontine hemorrhage) that directly damage the central core of the brain stem; (2) supratentorial mass lesions (such as may result from subdural hematomas) that indirectly compress deep diencephalic structures; and (3) metabolic disorders (such as hypoglycemia) that widely depress or interrupt brain functions. In Table 50–1, some of the clinical causes of

Table 50–1. Final Diagnosis in 386 Patients with "Coma of Unknown Etiology"

Diagnosis	Number	Percent of subtype	Percent of total
Supratentorial mass lesions			
Epidural hematoma	2	2.8	
Subdural hematoma	21	30.4	
Intracerebral hematoma	33	47.8	
Cerebral infarct	5	7.3	
Brain tumor	5	7.3	
Brain abscess	3	4.4	
Subtotal	69		17.9
Subtentorial lesions			
Brain stem infarct	37	71.2	
Brain stem tumor	2	3.9	
Brain stem hemorrhage	7	13.5	
Cerebellar hemorrhage	4	7.7	
Cerebral abscess	2	3.9	
Subtotal	52		13.5
Metabolic and diffuse cerebral disorders			
Anoxia or ischemia	51	19.5	
Concussion and postictal states	9	3.5	
Infection (meningitis and encephalitis)	11	4.2	
Subarachnoid hemorrhage	10	3.8	
Exogenous toxins	99	37.9	
Endogenous toxins and deficiencies	81	31.0	
Subtotal	261		67.6
Psychiatric disorders	4		1.0

Source: Adapted from Plum, F., and Posner, J. B. 1980. The Diagnosis of Stupor and Coma, 3rd ed. Philadelphia: Davis.

coma in these three categories are listed along with their relative frequencies of occurrence.

The first questions that usually arise for the physician confronted with a patient in coma are, Where is the lesion and what is the cause? There is another question that is often diagnostically important: In what direction is the process evolving? In coma, the sequence of signs is likely to be as important in revealing the source as the full clinical picture at any given moment. The answers to these questions can often place the disease in one of the above categories and thus reduce the number of inferences required to specify the nature of the disorder. We shall next examine Plum and Posner's major categories.

Infratentorial Lesions. A pathological process that affects the brain stem reticular formation will probably never be restricted to the reticular formation alone. A tumor, vascular disorder, or infection is likely to involve other structures as well, with resulting signs and symptoms described in Chapter 45 that involve cranial nerves, long ascending and descending pathways, and various nuclei. Tumors involving the midbrain and diencephalon may be followed by a loss of consciousness that lasts for

months. The EEG in these patients may show synchronization, suggesting that this type of coma might actually involve normal sleep mechanisms. If these EEG signs are present, the clinical state of stupor might more appropriately be referred to as *hypersomnia.* This often reversible condition may also occur with tumors below the floor of the third ventricle. If the tumor is cystic and is emptied by aspiration, the stupor may promptly disappear. However, in other cases of tumors in the upper midbrain and diencephalon, decerebrate rigidity may be present in addition to loss of consciousness. This pattern may also be seen after occlusion of the basilar artery. Thus, in broad terms, these clinical and EEG patterns are compatible with the view that the upper brain stem and diencephalic regions are concerned with the general activation of the brain, or what is clinically called "crude consciousness."

The role of the lower brain stem in consciousness is less clear. Because the medulla and lower pons regulate respiration and cardiovascular functions, lesions of the lower brain stem are apt to be rapidly fatal. Unconsciousness in these cases is often accompanied by disturbances in breathing, lowered blood pressure, and other brain stem signs (tetraplegia, Babinski signs due to corticospinal tract damage, pinpoint but reactive pupils after disruption of descending sympathetic pathways, and absence of ocular movements). Pontine hemorrhage results in these clinical signs before there are disorders of blood pressure and respiration.

On those rare occasions when patients with extensive lesions of the pons and medulla survive for long periods, the EEG may have a desynchronized pattern, as in the waking state *(alpha coma)*. These clinical findings in humans corroborate the classic experiments in cats performed in 1959 by F. Magni and co-workers. As noted above, they were the first investigators to provide evidence for a region in the caudal brain stem that actively puts the brain to sleep. They tied off cerebral blood vessels so that the arterial supply to the medulla and lower pons was isolated from that of the upper pons, midbrain, and cerebrum (Figure 50–5). Injections of the barbiturate anesthetic thiopental into the rostral brain stem and forebrain (unshaded area of Figure 50–5) anesthetized the cat, as might be expected. However, when only the caudal brain stem (shaded area of Figure 50–5) was anesthetized, the cat awakened as if it had been sleeping. The animal's slow-wave, synchronous EEG was replaced by a desynchronized waking EEG. As described in Chapter 49, the current consensus among sleep investigators is that the structures in the lower pons and medulla responsible for the active induction of non-REM sleep are the midline raphe nuclei or the nucleus of the solitary tract, or both. The solitary nucleus is a pontine structure that receives both taste and visceral information, but it also causes a synchronizing of the cortical EEG when stimulated with low-frequency current.

In short, with regard to the general category of infratentorial lesions, both experimental and clinical observations of limited brain stem dysfunction are consistent with the notion that the subset of reticular neurons that have a tonic activating function upon the cerebrum is not distributed evenly throughout the whole brain stem, but only in the most rostral part.

Supratentorial Lesions. Supratentorial structural lesions (those occurring rostral to the tentorium cerebelli, the dural invagination that separates the posterior cerebrum from the cerebellum) usually cause coma in one of two ways: (1) by destroying a critical amount of cerebral cortex bilaterally, or (2) by subjecting the brain stem and diencephalic structures that lie below the tentorium to compression or traction. If the lesion is unilateral, it may cause transtentorial downward herniation of either the medial temporal lobe *(uncal herniation)* or more medial diencephalic structures *(central herniation)*. As a result of the asymmetry of the lesion, there may be asymmetry of limb movements or tendon reflexes due to involvement of the corticospinal tract. There may also be decerebrate posturing (arms and legs extended) in response to noxious stimuli. This may be due to the compromised function of the rubrospinal and corticospinal systems, which normally exert a net facilitatory effect on flexor muscles, and the consequent release of the vestibulospinal system, which facilitates extensor muscle groups.

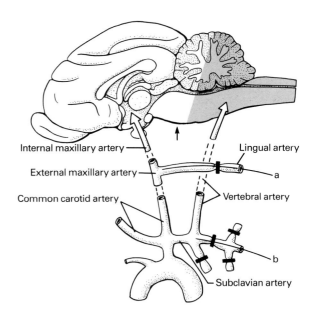

50–5 Procedure for establishing separate perfusion in a cat's brain of either medulla, caudal pons, and posterior cerebellum **(shaded)** or anterior cerebellum, rostral pons, midbrain, and forebrain **(unshaded)**. **Black arrow** indicates level of clamping of the basilar artery that separated the vertebral-basilar arterial circuit **(b)** from the carotid **(a)**. (Adapted from Magni et al., 1959.)

The pupillary response to light is decreased or absent. In uncal herniation, the most sensitive sign is that the ipsilateral pupil is dilated because the third cranial nerve is compressed as it passes through the tentorium, leaving sympathetic influence on the pupil unopposed. In central herniation, one or both pupils tend to be in midposition because the pressure on the midbrain disrupts both parasympathetic and sympathetic pupillary influences. With continuing, long-term compression of the brain stem, eye movements cease, including reflex responses to head rotation and to ice water applied to the tympanic membrane. (The normal response is a forced deviation of the eyes to the opposite side, away from the stimulus.) As brain stem compression moves caudally, a sequence of abnormal respiratory patterns ensues: Cheyne-Stokes breathing characterized by rhythmic waxing and waning of the depth of respiration, with regularly recurring periods of apnea; prolonged periods of hyperventilation; intermittent bouts of irregular or ataxic breathing; and, finally, apnea.

Cerebral infarctions, unless massive and accompanied by considerable brain swelling, do not often cause coma. In fact, the loss of extensive amounts of cerebral tissue (even hemispherectomy) may be sustained without impaired alertness. More important as a cause of coma is brain swelling. Therefore, cerebral hemorrhage is more likely than infarction to cause coma, and it is often accompanied by the typical signs of rostral–caudal transtentorial herniation outlined above. Other supratentorial lesions that commonly cause coma are subdural hematoma, cerebral tumor, or cerebral abscess.

Metabolic Coma. Metabolically caused coma is usually preceded by gradual changes in mentation or cognition. However, in some conditions, such as hypoglycemia, the onset of coma may be abrupt. For obvious reasons, asymmetrical changes in tendon reflexes or other focal signs are less likely in metabolic states than with structural lesions. Common symptoms in metabolic comas are tremor, *asterixis* (rapid loss of postural tone, most easily demonstrated by asking the patient, if sufficiently awake, to extend the wrists), and *myoclonus* (sudden, nonrhythmic jerks of limbs). The respiratory changes in metabolic coma vary with the cause. For instance, opiate drug overdose depresses respiration, while hepatic coma is characterized by hyperventilation. As a rule (which is diagnostically useful), ocular movements are only rarely affected in metabolic coma, unless the coma is quite severe. The pupillary reflex to light is also normally preserved until death, except in comas caused by anoxia or ischemia or by certain toxins, such as atropine.

The causes of metabolic coma are extremely varied and difficult to systematize. They include diffuse brain anoxia or ischemia, hypo- or hyperglycemia, thiamine deficiency, poisons (including ethanol, opiates, barbiturates, heavy metals, and aspirin), acid–base derangements, hyper- or hypocalcemia, pulmonary disease (carbon dioxide narcosis), uremia, liver failure, hypo- or hyperthermia, and meningitis.

The Determination of Cerebral Death Constitutes a Medical, Legal, and Social Decision

Despite improved resuscitative techniques, some comas are not reversible. The peculiar susceptibility of the brain to acute anoxia renders the brain particularly likely to suffer irreparable damage while resuscitative measures may be restoring vitality to less vulnerable organs. The resulting paradox is that of a dead brain in an otherwise living body—a condition beyond deep coma. Legally, physicians determine whether a patient is alive or dead. The development of equipment that artificially maintains respiration and other vital functions and the need of modern transplant surgery for access to viable organs have drawn broad ethical and legal attention to the desirability of agreeing on the medical criteria of cerebral death. In medical practice, the signs of brain death are irreversible coma and lack of spontaneous respiration. The specific criteria used to diagnose brain death differ in different hospitals. One set of criteria was suggested by a task force organized by the National Institute of Neurological and Communicative Disorders and Stroke (Table 50–2). Other sets of criteria were reviewed by Peter Black in 1978.

Because cerebral death usually results from a severe anoxic condition that affects the brain diffusely, the cardinal clinical symptoms (1–4 in Table 50–2) reflect a complete absence of centrally mediated behavioral responses and reflexes, including respiration. However, the criteria were adopted particularly to guard against the false terminal diagnosis of patients made comatose and apneic by reversible drug intoxication or by other lesions that occasionally can mimic cerebral death. One serious and common problem is that persons with self-induced metabolic coma have often taken several drugs, including alcohol, that together may have synergistic effects and may make the identification of drugs in the blood difficult—hence the need for stringent laboratory testing of brain viability.

The most widely used indication of brain death is an isoelectric EEG, or *electrocerebral silence*. This hybrid

Table 50–2. Criteria for Cerebral Death (Brain Death)

Prerequisite: All appropriate diagnostic and therapeutic procedures have been performed

Criteria (to be present for 30 min at least 6 hr after the onset of coma and apnea):
  1. Coma with cerebral unresponsivity (see definition 1)
  2. Apnea (see definition 2)
  3. Dilated pupils
  4. Absent cephalic reflexes (see definition 3)
  5. Electrocerebral silence (see definition 4)

Confirmatory test: Absence of cerebral blood flow

Definitions:
  1. Cerebral unresponsivity—a state in which the patient does not respond purposively to externally applied stimuli, obeys no commands, and does not utter sounds spontaneously or in response to a painful stimulus
  2. Apnea—the absence of spontaneous respiration, manifested by the need for controlled ventilation (that is, the patient makes no effort to override the respirator) for at least 15 min
  3. Cephalic reflexes—pupillary, corneal, oculoauditory, oculovestibular, oculocephalic, ciliospinal, snout, pharyngeal, cough, and swallowing
  4. Electrocerebral silence: an EEG with an absence of electrical potentials of cerebral origin over 2 μV from symmetrically placed electrode pairs over 10 cm apart and with interelectrode resistance between 100 and 10,000 Ω

Source: Adapted from A Collaborative Study of Cerebral Death. Bethesda, Md.: National Institute of Neurological and Communicative Disorders and Stroke, 1977.

term is operationally defined as an EEG record with no biological activity greater than 2 μV between scalp or referential electrode pairs 10 cm or more apart with interelectrode resistance of 100–10,000 Ω (with needle electrodes, 100–100,000 Ω). While the EEG offers the most significant laboratory information concerning cerebral death, an isoelectric EEG does not indicate the location of the lesion. The percentage of patients with brain stem, or infratentorial, lesions showing electrocerebral silence is approximately the same (63%) as those with diffuse cerebral lesions (60%) or focal cortical lesions (62%).

In many European countries, brain death is equated with total cerebral infarction, and the absence of cerebral blood flow is the principal legal sign. Unfortunately, angiography and most other techniques for determining cerebral blood flow are currently too invasive for routine use in patients hovering between life and death. However, in more chronic cases, the demonstration of intracranial circulatory arrest for 30 min should reasonably eliminate the possibility of cerebral viability even if blood flow can then be reestablished. Of 2650 patients surveyed who displayed coma, apnea, and an isoelectric EEG in the absence of drug intoxication and hypothermia, none survived. Thus, empirically, these criteria are conservative. However, judgments about life and death are always made in a social context. In addition to being clinically acceptable, it is also important that the criteria not offend society's notion of what constitutes reasonable assurance of death.

Selected Readings

Black, P. McL. 1978. Brain death (Two parts). N. Engl. J. Med. 299:338–344 and 393–401.

Broughton, R. J. 1968. Sleep disorders: Disorders of arousal? Science 159:1070–1078.

Chase, M., and Weitzman, E. D. 1983. Sleep Disorders: Basic and Clinical Research. New York: SP Medical & Scientific Books.

Dement, W., Guilleminault, C., and Zarcone, V. 1975. The pathologies of sleep: A case series approach. In D. B. Tower (ed.), The Nervous System, Vol. 2: The Clinical Neurosciences. New York: Raven Press, pp. 501–518.

Hauri, P. 1982. The Sleep Disorders, 2nd ed. A Scope Publication. Kalamazoo, Mich.: The Upjohn Company.

Mendelson, W. B., Gillin, J. C., and Wyatt, R. J. 1977. Human Sleep and Its Disorders. New York: Plenum Press.

Plum, F., and Posner, J. B. 1980. The Diagnosis of Stupor and Coma, 3rd ed. Philadelphia: Davis.

Solomon, F., White, C. C., Parron, D. L., and Mendelson, W. B. 1979. Sleeping pills, insomnia and medical practice (summary of report of the Institute of Medicine, National Academy of Sciences). N. Engl. J. Med. 300:803–808.

References

Brodal, A. 1981. Neurological Anatomy in Relation to Clinical Medicine, 3rd ed. New York: Oxford University Press, chap. 6.

A Collaborative Study by NINDS, NIH. 1977. An appraisal of the criteria of cerebral death. A summary statement. J.A.M.A. 237:982–986.

Gastaut, H., and Broughton, R. 1965. A clinical and polygraphic study of episodic phenomena during sleep. In J. Wortis (ed.), Recent Advances in Biological Psychiatry, Vol. 7. New York: Plenum Press, pp. 197–221.

Gastaut, H., Tassinari, C.A., and Duron, B. 1965. Étude polygraphique des manifestations épisodiques (hypniques et respiratoires), diurnes et nocturnes, du syndrome de Pickwick. Rev. Neurol. (Paris) 112:568–579.

Guilleminault, C., Tilkian, A., and Dement, W. C. 1976. The sleep apnea syndromes. Annu. Rev. Med. 27:465–484.

Hishikawa, Y., Wakamatsu, H., Furuya, E., Sugita, Y., Masaoka, S., Kaneda, H., Sato, M., Nan'no, H., and Kaneko, Z. 1976. Sleep satiation in narcoleptic patients. Electroencephalogr. Clin. Neurophysiol. 41:1–18.

Jacobson, A., Kales, A., Lehmann, D., and Zweizig, J. R. 1965. Somnambulism: All-night electroencephalographic studies. Science 148:975–977.

Kales, A., and Kales, J. 1973. Recent advances in the diagnosis and treatment of sleep disorders. In G. Usdin (ed.), Sleep Research and Clinical Practice. New York: Brunner/Mazel, pp. 59–94.

Karacan, I., Thornby, J. I., Anch, M., Holzer, C. E., Warheit, G. J., Schwab, J. J., and Williams, R. L. 1976. Prevalence of sleep disturbance in a primarily urban Florida county. Soc. Sci. Med. 10:239–244.

Kety, S. S. 1960. Sleep and the energy metabolism of the brain. In G. E. W. Wolstenholme and M. O'Connor (eds.), The Nature of Sleep. Boston: Little, Brown, pp. 375–381.

Kupfer, D. J., and Foster, F. G. 1972. Interval between onset of sleep and rapid-eye-movement sleep as an indicator of depression. Lancet 2:684–686.

Magni, F., Moruzzi, G., Rossi, G. F., and Zanchetti, A. 1959. EEG arousal following inactivation of the lower brain stem by selective injection of barbiturate into the vertebral circulation. Arch. Ital. Biol. 97:33–46.

Mendelson, W. B., Cain, M., Cook, J. M., Paul, S. M., and Skolnick, P. 1983. A benzodiazepine receptor antagonist decreases sleep and reverses the hypnotic actions of flurazepam. Science 219:414–416.

Mendelson, W. B., Weingartner, H., Greenblatt, D. J., Garnett, D., and Gillin, J. C. 1982. A clinical study of flurazepam. Sleep 5:350–360.

Mitler, M. M., and Dement, W. C. 1974. Cataplectic-like behavior in cats after micro-injections of carbachol in pontine reticular formation. Brain Res. 68:335–343.

Yoss, R. E., and Daly, D. D. 1957. Criteria for the diagnosis of the narcoleptic syndrome. Proc. Staff Meet. Mayo Clin. 32:320–328.

Localization of Higher Functions and the Disorders of Language, Thought, and Affect

IX

The attempt to localize function in the cerebral cortex dates from the discovery of two types of motor control in specific areas of the frontal lobe: control of expressive speech in the area described by Broca in 1862, and control of voluntary movement in the area studied by Fritsch and Hitzig in 1870. Next came the elucidation of the various primary, secondary, and tertiary sensory cortices—for vision, audition, somatic sensation, and taste—in the occipital, parietal, and temporal lobes. These motor and sensory cortices, however, account for less than one-half of the cerebral cortex in humans. The unattributed areas are called the *association cortex*, a term that grew out of the belief that these parts of the cortex coordinate events arising in the areas specifically dedicated to motor and sensory processes. The association cortex can be divided into three major regions: the prefrontal cortex, which is concerned with higher motor functions, the parietal–temporal–occipital cortex, which is important in higher sensory function, and the limbic cortex, which is important for motivation. All these areas are involved in higher cognitive and affective functioning: in speech, thought, memory, and planning.

Most of the initial evidence relating higher cognitive and affective functions to regions of the association cortex has come from studies of patients with brain damage. In turn, study of patients, and more recently, study of experimental animals with lesions of these areas, have provided new insights into the neuronal mechanisms underlying higher mental functioning. For example, the study of language and its disorders, which began with the work of Broca, is now yielding important information about the logic and limitations of human mental processes.

In this section, we shall review the evidence, based in part on clinical observations, that although specific higher functions are related to specific cortical regions, no higher function is controlled by only a single cortical region. All complex functions are controlled by several different regions working together. Different aspects of consciousness and self-awareness are localized either to the right or to the left hemisphere. This remarkable insight can be deduced from the discovery that the cerebral hemispheres are not simply functional mirror images of each other, but that each has its own specialized capacities.

This background of information on normal cognitive functioning and on disorders of language serves as a basis for considering other disturbances of higher functions such as gesture, thought, and feeling. Diseases involving these functions, particularly the schizophrenias and the depressive disorders, pose great challenges for neurobiology. Can the mechanisms for these disorders be identified and localized to specific areas of the brain?

Irving Kupfermann

Hemispheric Asymmetries and the Cortical Localization of Higher Cognitive and Affective Functions

51

More than a century ago two physicians at the University of Vienna, Franz Joseph Gall and his student Johann Spurzheim, developed a new approach to mental function that they called *cranioscopy,* later renamed *phrenology.* Phrenologists believed that character and personality could be assessed by examining the size and position of specific bumps on the surface of the head. Although extremely popular in the nineteenth century, especially in the United States and Britain, phrenology was later rejected both by the general public and the scientific community. Nevertheless, as we saw in Chapter 1, studies of the aphasias by Pierre Paul Broca, Karl Wernicke, and other clinical neurologists provided strong support for the phrenological perspective that specific higher functions are associated with specific cortical regions. For many years, however, these studies were ignored, and most clinical and experimental neurologists favored the idea that the brain, and particularly the cerebral cortex, acted as a whole.

In the twentieth century this antilocalization view was expounded most forcefully by Karl Lashley, who believed that various parts of the brain are equipotential and that for many functions, virtually any part of the brain could subtitute for any other. Even the proponents of an antilocalization view had to admit, however, that specific sensory and motor functions could be associated with well-defined anatomical loci. Subsequent evidence, which we shall consider in this chapter, indicates that even highly complex brain functions can be attributed to specific brain areas. Localization does not imply, however, that any specific function is exclusively mediated by only one region of the brain. Most functions require the integrated action of neurons located in many regions. *Localization of*

Table 51–1. Major Sensory, Association, and Motor Cortices

Functional designation	Lobe	Location in lobe	Brodmann's area
Primary sensory cortices			
Somatic sensory	Parietal	Postcentral gyrus	1,2,3
Visual	Occipital	Calcarine fissure	17
Auditory	Temporal	Heschl's gyri	41,42
Higher order sensory cortex			
Somatic sensory II	Parietal	Dorsal bank of Sylvian fissure	2 (preinsular portion)
Visual II	Occipital	Occipital gyri	18
Visual III, IIIa, IV, V	Occipital, temporal	Occipital gyri and superior temporal sulcus	18 and area rostral to 18
Visual Inferotemporal Area	Temporal	Anterior and inferior temporal cortex	21,20
Posterior parietal cortex (Somatic sensation, vision)	Parietal	Superior parietal lobule	5 (somatic) 7 (visual)
Auditory	Temporal	Superior temporal gyrus	22
Association cortex			
Parietal–temporal–occipital (Polymodal sensory, language)	Parietal, temporal, and occipital	Junction between lobes	39,40 and portions of 19,21,22,37
Prefrontal (Cognitive behavior and motor planning)	Frontal	Rostral portion of dorsal and lateral surface	Area rostral to 6
Limbic (Emotion and memory)	Temporal, parietal, and frontal	Cingulate and parahippocampal gyri, temporal pole, and orbital surface of frontal lobe	23,24,38,28,11
Higher order motor cortices			
Premotor (including supplementary motor area)	Frontal	Rostral to postcentral gyrus	6
Primary motor cortex			
Motor	Frontal	Precental gyrus	4

function means that certain areas of the brain are more concerned with one kind of function than with others.

Some of the most compelling evidence for localization has come from studies of the *association areas* of the cerebral cortex. These areas include all neocortex other than the regions directly involved in the processing of primary sensory and motor information.[1] The association areas are concerned with the integration of more than one sensory modality and with the planning of movement. The association areas were once considered more extensive than they are now believed to be. As our un-

derstanding of sensory and motor processes has increased, some areas that have been thought to be association cortex have proved instead to be secondary or tertiary sensory or motor areas. Table 51–1 summarizes the major primary and higher order sensory and motor areas and association areas of the cerebral cortex. In this chapter, we shall focus primarily, but not exclusively, on the functions of association cortex.

Because they produce few or no obvious motor or sensory effects when electrically stimulated, the association cortices were at one time called *silent areas.* They were believed to have two main functions: (1) to link the various primary sensory cortices to one another, and (2) to link the sensory cortices to the motor cortices. On the basis of these roles, the association cortices were thought to be the anatomical substrates for the highest brain functions, thought and perception. Modern evidence supports this idea. Not surprisingly, then, the relative extent of the association cortices increases throughout phylogeny, and they reach their greatest size in humans (Figure 51–1).

---

[1]Some classifications divide the association areas into two categories. The first category consists of *sensory association* and *motor association* cortices. These are the higher order (secondary and tertiary) areas devoted to the processing of complex aspects of a *single* sensory modality or motor function. The second category consists of *true association areas,* which are concerned not with one sensory modality but with integrating a variety of sensory, motor, and motivational information. In this textbook we have considered sensory and motor association areas as higher order sensory or motor cortices.

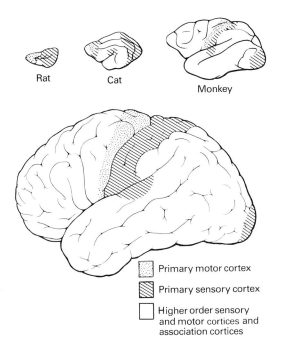

Rat   Cat   Monkey

Primary motor cortex

Primary sensory cortex

Higher order sensory and motor cortices and association cortices

51–1 Drawings (approximately to scale) of the cerebral hemispheres of four mammals. Note the increase both in size and in relative amount of higher order sensory, motor, and association cortices. (Adapted from Thompson, 1975.)

Much of what we know about the function of association areas has come from the study of two types of patients: those with damage to the cortex (due to trauma, cerebrovascular disease, tumors), and those who have undergone brain surgery for a behavioral or neurological disorder. Evidence from the second group of patients has been particularly instructive because each patient has had a relatively well-defined surgical lesion. In some instances insight obtained from clinical studies has been extended by experiments on animals, in which it is possible to make localized lesions and to obtain detailed electrophysiological information.

In this chapter we shall first consider the structure and functions of the association areas. We shall then pay particular attention to the discovery that the human brain, which has many symmetrical features, is actually not perfectly symmetrical. The left and right hemispheres each have their own special capabilities and limitations, and consequently the association areas of the cerebral cortex are not symmetrical either.

The Association Areas Are Involved in Higher Functions

How does information reach an association cortex? As we saw in Chapters 19 and 20, each primary sensory area of cortex is adjacent to and connects with a series of higher order sensory regions. For example, Brodmann's area 17, the primary visual cortex, is adjacent to and interconnects with area 18. Unlike their primary counterparts, the higher order sensory cortices have a much less precise map of the peripheral receptive sheet and are concerned with more complex aspects of sensation. Higher order sensory areas, in turn, project to one or another, or to all three of the major association cortices: the *parietal–temporal–occipital association cortex*, the *prefrontal association cortex*, and the *limbic association cortex* (Figure 51–2).

All three association cortices are involved in several higher functions: complex motor control, sensory perception, cognition, emotional behavior, memory, and language. Nevertheless, a given cortical region appears to specialize in any one or another of these functions. The prefrontal cortex is concerned with higher motor actions, the parietal–temporal–occipital area with higher sensory functions and with language, and the limbic area with memory and with emotional and motivational aspects of

51–2 This schematic drawing of the medial and lateral surface of the human brain shows the regions of the primary sensory and motor cortices, the higher order motor and sensory cortices, and the cortical association areas.

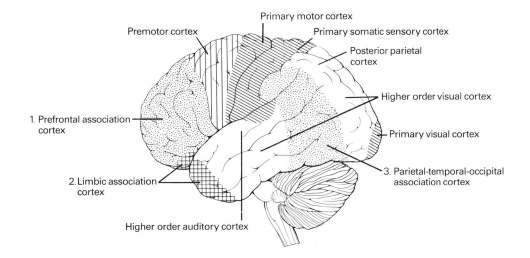

Premotor cortex

Primary motor cortex

Primary somatic sensory cortex

Posterior parietal cortex

Higher order visual cortex

Primary visual cortex

3. Parietal-temporal-occipital association cortex

1. Prefrontal association cortex

2. Limbic association cortex

Higher order auditory cortex

behavior. Let us briefly consider the intracortical connections of these association cortices before turning to the functions of each one.

Intracortical Association Pathways Are Hierarchically Organized

The *parietal–temporal–occipital association cortex* is intercalated between higher order somatic, visual, and auditory areas and receives projections from them. The parietal–temporal–occipital association cortex is therefore thought to link information from several sensory modalities, a step important in the processing of sensory information for perception.

The portion of the *frontal cortex* (Figure 51–2) that is located anterior to the primary motor area has traditionally been divided into two regions: a supplementary or *premotor cortex* (Brodmann's area 6), just anterior to the precentral gyrus, and the *prefrontal cortex*, which is anterior to the premotor cortex and constitutes the association cortex. As noted in Chapter 39, the premotor cortex is important in the initiation of movement. The prefrontal cortex, as we shall see later, is important for the planning of action.

The prefrontal and premotor cortices receive input from various regions of the higher order sensory cortices, as does the parietal–temporal–occipital cortex. Portions

51–3   The intracortical connections of primary motor and sensory cortices, higher order motor and sensory cortices, and association cortices are shown here in a simplified form. The same general pattern is repeated for each of the main primary sensory cortices (for vision, somesthesis, and hearing). For simplicity, a number of intracortical pathways have been omitted (e.g., there are interconnections between prefrontal, parietal–temporal–occipital, and limbic association cortices).

of the higher order sensory cortex that are more closely connected with primary sensory areas project to the premotor cortex (which in turn projects to motor cortex). The areas of the higher order sensory cortex that are less directly connected to primary sensory areas project to the prefrontal cortex (which projects to premotor cortex) (Figure 51–3). These differential patterns of connections permit more precise sensory information to influence the *execution* of movement (by way of successive projections to the premotor and then to the motor cortex) and more abstract sensory information and perception to influence the *planning* of movement (by way of successive projections to the prefrontal cortex, to the premotor cortex, and then to the motor cortex).

The *limbic association cortex* consists of the medial and ventral surfaces of the frontal lobe, the medial surface of the parietal lobe, and portions of the temporal lobe. The limbic association cortex includes the orbitofrontal cortex, the cingulate region, the parahippocampal area, and the anterior tip of the temporal lobe (called the *temporal pole*) (Figure 51–2). It receives a projection from the higher order sensory areas. It sends projections to other cortical regions, including the prefrontal cortex. This provides one pathway by which emotions can affect motor planning.

Even though they are concerned with higher mental functions, all three association areas share organizational principles with the primary sensory and motor cortices. This important discovery emerged from the work of Patricia Goldman and Walle Nauta at the Massachusetts Institute of Technology. They found that the pattern of termination of corticocortical connections between regions of association cortex of the parietal lobe and the frontal lobe in the monkey are organized into distinct, vertically oriented columns. These columns are 200–500 μm wide and extend across all layers of cortex. Thus, columnar organization is not unique to the sensory cortex, but is a general feature of all neocortex; a highly re-

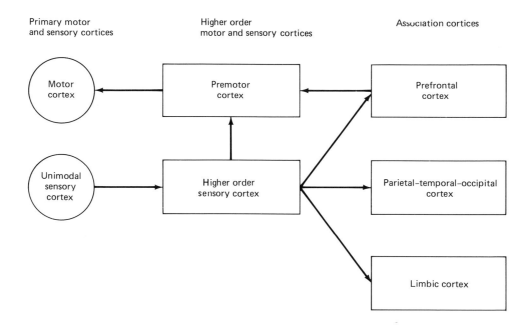

petitive architecture underlies not only simple information processing but also the complex coordination of sensory, motor, and motivational information.

The Association Areas of the Prefrontal Region Are Thought to Be Involved in Cognitive Behavior and Motor Planning

The association functions of the various regions of the frontal cortex are not easily summarized because they are diverse. One important function of the frontal lobes is thought to be related to the capacity of the organism to weigh the consequences of future actions and plan accordingly. The frontal lobes integrate the interoceptive and exteroceptive information that they receive so as to select the appropriate motor response from the many available.

Functional studies on monkeys suggest that the frontal cortex concerned with associative functions can be divided into two main regions: the *prefrontal cortex*, located on the dorsolateral surface of the frontal lobes, and the *orbitofrontal cortex*, located on the medial and ventral surface of the brain. These two regions assume prodigious proportions in lower primates and humans (Figure 51–4). Both regions receive a prominent afferent input from the medial dorsal thalamic nucleus and have a prominent granule cell layer (IV). Both regions therefore are sometimes referred to as the frontal granular cortex, in distinction to the agranular cortex of the motor and premotor areas. The orbitofrontal cortex is part of the limbic association cortex, having direct connections with limbic structures such as the amygdala, and we shall consider it later. In contrast, dorsolateral cortex makes up the prefrontal association cortex. We shall first consider the prefrontal cortex. In the monkey it has three subdivisions (superior prefrontal convexity, inferior prefrontal convexity, and principal sulcus; Figure 51–5), each of which is concerned with a different set of functions.

Lesions of the Principal Sulcus Interfere with Specific Motor Tasks

The principal sulcus is concerned with the strategic planning for higher motor actions, including cognitive tasks. The first evidence leading to our understanding of the cognitive role of the principal sulcus came from a dramatic experiment in the 1930s by Carlyle Jacobsen, working in the laboratory of John Fulton at Yale University. Jacobsen discovered that bilateral removal of the frontal association cortex in primates, an area that includes the principal sulcus, impairs the ability to perform a task involving delayed spatial response. In this experiment, a hungry monkey is shown a piece of food and, while the animal watches, the food is placed randomly under one or the other of two identical opaque containers, one on the left, one on the right. After a delay of 5 sec or longer, the monkey is permitted to select one of the containers. Normal animals quickly learn to select the container covering the food, whereas animals with

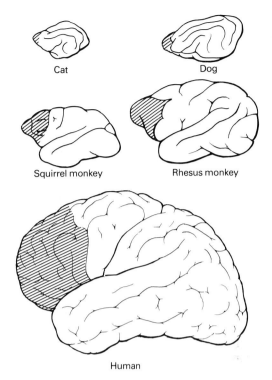

51–4 Proportion of the brain taken up by the frontal association cortex (**hatched area**) in five species (Adapted from Warren and Akert, 1964.)

51–5 The subdivisions of the frontal association cortex of the monkey are shown in two views: **A,** lateral. This view illustrates the dorsoventral surface of the prefrontal lobe, the region of the *prefrontal association cortex.* **B,** ventral and medial. This view illustrates the orbitofrontal cortex, a subdivision of limbic association cortex. (Data from Rosenkilde, 1979.)

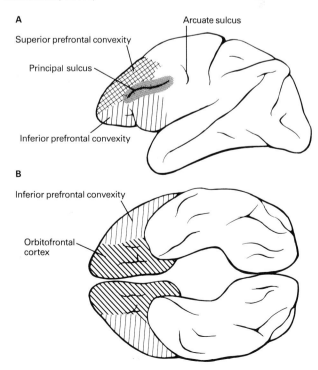

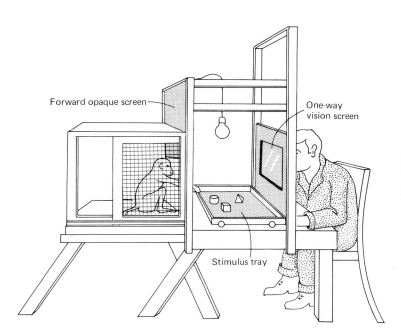

Forward opaque screen

One-way vision screen

Stimulus tray

51–6 The Wisconsin General Testing Apparatus is used to test monkeys in a variety of discrimination and learning problems. (Adapted from Harlow, 1958.)

frontal damage do poorly on this task. The lesioned animals perform well only if there is no delay after the experimenter covers the food. Jacobsen therefore thought that the prefrontal region might be involved in short-term memory. Specifically, he proposed that the frontal association areas are needed for the execution of complex motor tasks in which the essential cues are not available at the time of responding but must be recalled by a short-term memory process.

Subsequent research suggests that this interpretation is correct but that the lesions do not produce a generalized deficit involving all short-term memory; rather, the deficit is specific for certain types of tasks. Furthermore, experiments involving more limited lesions of the frontal association cortex revealed that there is functional heterogeneity of this region. For example, animals with prefrontal lesions also do poorly on a delayed spatial alternation task. In this task, animals must alternate right and left choices between two containers, with a delay interposed between each choice. A relatively small lesion around the principal sulcus is sufficient to produce the deficit in delayed spatial alternation responses. This deficit is highly specific to these tasks and is evident only if the task involves both a delay and a spatial aspect. Animals with a lesion in the principal sulcus have no difficulty with discrimination problems involving no delay or on tasks in which predelay spatial cues are not important. For example, in an apparatus such as that shown in Figure 51–6, the animal can perform well on a visual problem in which it is shown a single visual stimulus and, after a delay, is required to select that cue when it is presented together with another cue.

The idea that the principle sulcus of the prefrontal association cortex is involved in delayed spatial response

tasks is also supported by studies of the activity of single nerve cells in the principal sulcus. Joaquin Fuster at UCLA showed that many neurons in this region increase their firing when a relevant cue is presented during these tasks. They continue to fire throughout the delay period even when the cue is no longer there. In some neurons, the degree of activity is highly dependent on which of several cues is presented to the animal.

John Stamm at the State University of New York at Stony Brook found that electrical stimulation of the prefrontal cortex, which disrupts its normal function, interferes with delayed spatial response tasks, particularly when the stimulation is presented early in the delay period. Finally, Goldman and H. E. Rosvold found that a delayed spatial response task is severely disrupted when the neurotransmitter dopamine is depleted from the principal sulcus by means of localized cortical injection of 6-hydroxydopamine, which selectively destroys neurons that use norepinephrine or dopamine as their transmitter.

These findings are interesting clinically. Delayed spatial response involves a number of conceptual skills: discrimination, short-term memory, and planning and execution of a perceptual–motor task. Since the prefrontal cortex is essential for tasks of this complexity, it is likely to participate in a variety of related cognitive skills. In addition, the prefrontal area of primates and other animals has a particularly prominent dopaminergic innervation and, as discussed above, depletion of dopamine from this area produces effects similar to those of lesions. Thus, it has been suggested that disturbances of this system may contribute to human cognitive disorders such as schizophrenia that are thought to involve alterations in dopaminergic transmission in the brain (see Chapter 53).

Lesions of the Inferior Prefrontal Convexity Interfere with Appropriate Motor Responses

In contrast to lesions of the principal sulcus, lesions of the inferior prefrontal convexity affect all types of delayed responses whether or not they have a spatial element; these lesions appear to interfere with tasks that require the animal to inhibit motor responses at appropriate times. Lesions of the arcuate cortex (a subregion of the premotor cortex), which is just adjacent to the principal sulcus, do not disturb spatial delayed response; however, they diminish the animal's ability to choose among various types of motor responses on the basis of different sensory cues. For example, animals with this lesion have difficulty learning a task in which they must move to the left when an auditory cue comes from above the cage and move to the right when the cue comes from below the cage.

The Association Areas of the Limbic Cortex Mediate Affective Aspects of Emotional Behavior as well as Memory

The limbic association cortex consists of several major subareas located in different lobes: the orbitofrontal cortex, portions of the temporal lobe, and the cingulate gyrus. We shall first consider the orbitofrontal cortex.

The Orbitofrontal Portion of the Limbic Association Cortex Is Concerned with Emotional Behavior

In addition to deficits of delayed responding, Jacobsen and subsequent investigators found that lesions that include the orbitofrontal cortex result in an alteration of the emotional responsiveness of animals. Lesioned chimpanzees no longer exhibited rage and anger when they failed to receive rewards. This alteration in emotional response is not due to damage of the principal sulcus, but to the orbitofrontal cortex, the limbic portion of the frontal cortex. Damage limited to the orbitofrontal cortex decreases the normal aggressiveness and emotional responsiveness of primates. Furthermore, electrical stimulation of the orbitofrontal cortex produces many autonomic responses (increases in arterial blood pressure, dilation of the pupils, salivation, and inhibition of gastrointestinal contractions), suggesting that this area may be involved in a generalized arousal reaction. This interpretation is supported by the observation that orbitofrontal stimulation induces a generalized desynchronization (arousal response) of the cortical electroencephalogram (see Chapter 48) and an increase in plasma cortisol. As discussed in Chapter 46, frontal lesions that include orbitofrontal portions of the limbic association cortex also reduce chronic intractable pain, illustrating still another effect of the limbic cortex on emotional behavior.

Jacobsen reported his observations of the calming effect of frontal cortical lesions (lobotomies) in chimpan-

zees at the Second International Neurology Congress in London in 1935. This report led Egas Moniz, a Portuguese neuropsychiatrist, to suggest that destruction of the frontal–limbic association connections in humans might serve as a treatment for severe mental illness. Moniz collaborated with a neurosurgeon, Almeida Lima, and the first prefrontal lesions were done in Lisbon only a few months after Jacobsen's report.

These early attempts were soon followed by an extensive application of various procedures that involved either ablation of frontal association areas or interruption of the fiber tracts that connect the frontal lobes with subcortical structures or other areas of cortex. These tracts include the *cingulum*, a multifiber bundle in the white matter of the cingulate gyrus that contains aminergic fibers from the brain stem as well as fibers that connect the frontal and parietal lobes with the parahippocampal gyrus and adjacent temporal cortex. A second major tract includes the *thalamocortical projections* from the medial dorsal thalamic nucleus.

The early results of lobotomy appeared favorable. Many patients seemed to show a reduction in anxiety. The results from later, more controlled studies were equivocal. Furthermore, lobotomy was associated with a high incidence of complications, including the development of epilepsy and abnormal personality changes, such as a lack of inhibition on the one hand and a lack of initiative and drive on the other.

However, intellectual capability as measured on conventional tests of intelligence was little affected by these operations even though large lesions were often made. This came as a surprise since it was believed that the huge frontal lobes in humans must in some way be related to higher mental functions, such as abstract thought and reasoning.

Although global intelligence is not greatly affected by frontal lesions (which include prefrontal cortex and premotor cortex), lobotomized patients do show deficits in certain specific tasks. Brenda Milner at McGill University found that patients with frontal lesions experience difficulty in changing strategies when required to do so. For example, they do poorly with the Wisconsin Card Sorting task. This task requires that the individual sort picture cards on the basis of some criterion (such as similar colors or shapes). When the patient solves the problem, the solution is changed, and the patient must select on the basis of a different criterion. The patients with frontal lesions persist with their previously successful solution; they fail to alter their choices, even when informed that their choices are no longer correct. Perseveration and failure to inhibit inappropriate responses are frequently observed in monkeys with frontal lesions, particularly of the inferior prefrontal convexity. Patients with frontal lesions also show difficulty in rapid verbal naming from memory and in performing certain types of pencil-and-paper maze tasks. In addition, studies by Bryan Kolb and his colleagues suggest that these patients may exhibit a generalized decrease in spontaneity of behavior.

After several other well-controlled studies failed to show benefits from psychosurgery, the use of this operation dwindled in the 1950s. In recent years there has been renewed interest in modified forms of psychosurgery based on attempts to make highly localized lesions that might reduce anxiety without producing unfavorable side effects. Several studies suggest that a small lesion limited to the cingulum produces favorable results. Despite the high percentage of patients who show improvement, it is not yet possible to conclude that the improvement is due to surgery rather than to a placebo effect or to spontaneous recovery. In drug studies it is often possible to use the patient as his or her own control by administering the drug and then withdrawing it; but the effects of brain surgery are irreversible. These studies therefore require a matched sample of untreated control patients, and this requirement is rarely fulfilled.

The Temporal Lobe Portion of the Limbic Association Cortex Is Thought to Be Concerned with Memory Functions

In monkeys, lesions of the inferior temporal region, a higher order visual region, result in deficits in the rate of learning of visual tasks. The deficits, which are not due to blindness, are most dramatic when the visual task is complex. For example, inferior temporal lesions interfere with the ability of an animal to improve performance progressively (to develop a learning set) when a long series of related visual problems is presented. In addition to interfering with the *acquisition* of a learned visual task, these lesions interfere with the *retention* or *memory* of visual tasks. Similarly, lesions of the superior temporal cortex of animals result in impaired learning of auditory patterns without producing deafness.

As we saw in Chapter 1, major insights into the functions of the human temporal lobes have come from the work of the neurosurgeon Wilder Penfield. Penfield electrically stimulated various points on the temporal lobe in awake patients before he removed diseased epileptic tissue. As expected, stimulation of the primary auditory areas produced crude auditory sensations. In contrast, stimulation of the superior temporal gyrus produced alterations in the perception of sounds, and auditory illusions and hallucinations. The hallucinations had a rather startling feature. The patients reported that the experience was remarkably real, almost as if they were again actually experiencing a past event. The evocation of complex experiential phenomena after stimulation of the temporal lobes appears to occur only in patients with epilepsy in the temporal lobe; such experiences are relatively specific to the temporal lobe and are not reported when other cortical areas are stimulated.

Many of the patients studied by Penfield and others had a temporal lobe subsequently removed for the treatment of epilepsy. The lesion did not include Wernicke's speech area, but did typically include portions of the hippocampus. The capacities of these patients have been thoroughly studied by Milner. In the few instances in which both the left and the right temporal lobes were removed, patients had a profound and irreversible impairment of the capacity to form certain types of long-term memories (see Chapter 61.)

Milner found that there was also some interference with memory after unilateral removal of the temporal lobe. Compared with the bilateral lesions, the unilateral lesion produced only a mild deficit. Furthermore, the degree of impairment depended on the side of the brain that had the lesion and on the type of material to be memorized. Patients whose left temporal lobe had been removed had difficulty remembering verbal material such as a list of nouns. Patients with a right-sided removal had normal verbal memory but were impaired in their ability to remember patterns of sensory input. When presented with a series of pictures of human faces, some of which were repeated, patients with the right temporal lobe removed had difficulty remembering whether they had previously seen a given face. How much memory was lost depended on the nature of the visual material to be memorized. When given a task involving geometric figures, patients with the right temporal lobe removed did not have this difficulty; given a task involving irregular patterns of line drawings, they did experience difficulty. One possible explanation for these observations is that geometrical patterns can easily be expressed and then stored in a verbal fashion (square, triangle, etc.), but faces and irregular patterns cannot be readily encoded verbally. This general pattern—left-hemisphere lesions impairing the processing of verbal material, and right-hemisphere lesions interfering with the processing of information about sensory patterns—has been repeatedly encountered in studies of brain-damaged patients.

Stimulation (or ablation) of the temporal portion of the limbic association cortex alters emotions. For example, Penfield reported that stimulation of the anterior and medial temporal cortex could produce emotional feelings, particularly fear. The role of the temporal lobes in emotional behavior is also indicated by the finding of a so-called temporal lobe personality in patients with temporal lobe epilepsy. As described in Chapter 1, these patients tend to have an overall deepening of emotional responses. They also have a variety of other personality characteristics that suggest altered emotional responses.

The Association Areas of the Parietal Lobe Are Involved in Higher Sensory Functions and Language

The anterior parietal lobe contains the primary somatic sensory cortex, while the more posterior region contains higher order sensory areas (posterior parietal association area) and an association area of extensive polymodal convergence. Animal studies of the posterior parietal cortex (Brodmann's area 5 and 7) have revealed that lesions in this area produce subtle deficits in the learning of tasks requiring awareness of body image. In addition, there are deficits in certain complex non-body-oriented tasks involving the selection of different objects placed before the animal.

Studies of single cells in the parietal cortex of monkeys by Vernon Mountcastle and his colleagues and by David Robinson, Michael Goldberg, and their colleagues have revealed that certain cells respond to visual stimuli or during visually guided movements. Unlike cells in the visual cortex, the intensity of the response of these cells to a series of identical stimuli is remarkably variable. In particular, the activity of the cell is enhanced when the animal pays attention to the stimulus. These results are consistent with the notion that the parietal cortex is involved in processes associated with attention to the spatial aspects of sensory input and perhaps with the manipulation of objects in space.

Patients with damage to the parietal lobes often show striking deficits, including abnormalities in body image and in perception of spatial relations. In addition, damage to the dominant (usually left) parietal lobe tends to produce *aphasia* (disorder of language, see Chapter 52) and *agnosia* (an inability to perceive objects through normally functioning sensory channels). A particularly dramatic agnosia after damage to the parietal cortex is *astereognosia,* an inability to recognize the form of objects by touch in the absence of any major somatic sensory deficits.

A historically important syndrome associated with damage to the inferior regions of the left parietal cortex is known as *Gerstmann's syndrome.* Patients with Gerstmann's syndrome are characterized by (1) *left-right confusion* (an inability to determine whether a particular part of the body of the examiner is left or right), (2) *finger agnosia* (difficulty in naming fingers when a specific finger is touched, despite the absence of major deficits of finger sensations, (3) *dysgraphia* (a writing disability in the absence of motor or sensory deficits of the upper extremities), and (4) *dyscalculia* (an inability to carry out mathematical calculations). Not all the symptoms are seen in every patient, even in those with large lesions, and consequently this tetrad of symptoms may be of limited diagnostic utility.

Lesions of the nondominant parietal lobe do not cause obvious disturbances of language. Instead, patients with right (nondominant) parietal lobe damage demonstrate a lack of appreciation of the spatial aspects of all sensory input from the left side of the body as well as of external space. Although somatic sensations are relatively intact, the patients sometimes completely ignore half of the body *(neglect syndrome)* and may fail to dress, undress, and wash the affected side. The patients may deny that their arm or leg belongs to them when the limb is passively brought into their field of vision. They may also deny the existence of associated hemiplegia and may attempt to leave the hospital prematurely since they feel that there is nothing wrong with them. Disturbance of the appreciation of external space takes the form of neglect of visual stimuli on that side of the body. These patients sometimes also exhibit a severe disturbance in their ability to copy drawn figures *(constructional apraxia).* In some instances this deficit may be so severe that the patient may draw a figure in which one-half of the body is completely left out.

Patients with a neglect syndrome due to an inferior right parietal lesion can show a deficit in the nonsyntactic processing of language. Kenneth Heilman found that patients with lesions in the inferior right parietal lobe fail to appreciate those aspects of a verbal message that are conveyed by the tone, loudness, and timing of the words (e.g., emotional tone) as opposed to the actual sense of the words. The patients also have difficulty in modulating the sound of their verbal output and convey poorly the nonsyntactic aspects of language. These clinical observations suggest that the right homologue of Wernicke's area may also have a subtle language function dealing with intonation and other nonsyntactic aspects of language.

The Two Hemispheres Are Not Fully Symmetrical and Differ in Their Capabilities

As recently as 1968, it was widely believed that there was no gross asymmetry in the human brain. At that time, Norman Geschwind and Walter Levitsky, at the Harvard Medical School, published the results of a simple experiment. They studied the gross dimensions of 100 human brains, using a camera and a ruler to make measurements of the *planum temporale,* a region on the upper surface of the temporal lobe that includes the classical speech area of Wernicke. The results were clear-cut (Figure 51–7). The left planum was larger in 65% of the brains; the right planum was larger in only 11% of the brains; and in 24% of the brains the left and right sides were approximately equal in size. Later work with a va-

51–7 The planum temporale, shown in a horizontal section in the plane of the Sylvian fissure, is larger in the left hemisphere than in the right in the majority of human brains. (Adapted from Geschwind and Levitsky, 1968.)

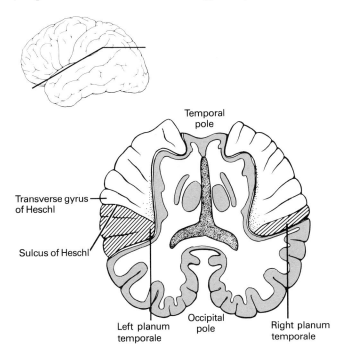

riety of techniques, including computerized tomography, has confirmed these results and established that similar asymmetries are present even in the human fetus. These observations suggest that an inherent anatomical asymmetry may initially favor the left hemisphere for the development of language functions. Once one hemisphere begins to specialize it will excel at that function, which in turn prompts its further development.

In addition to being asymmetrical, the two hemispheres differ in their capabilities—an important discovery in the study of cortical localization. Several techniques have illustrated this hemispheric lateralization in patients without brain damage. One procedure of great clinical importance is the *sodium amytal test*. It was developed to determine the dominant hemisphere for speech functions in order to avoid neurosurgical procedures that might destroy language ability. In this test, the patient is instructed to count aloud. Meanwhile, sodium amytal, a fast-acting barbiturate, is injected into the left or right internal carotid artery. The drug is preferentially carried to the hemisphere on the same side as it is injected and produces a ief period of dysfunction of that hemisphere. When the hemisphere dominant for speech is affected, t patient stops counting and does not respond to the co   nd to continue.

The relationship between hand use and speech lateralization (Table 51–2) was one of the first problems explored with the sodium amytal test. Do left-handed individuals have left-hemisphere speech, as do right-handed people, or do they have right-hemisphere speech? The sodium amytal test has revealed that almost all right-handed people have left-hemisphere speech. Surprisingly, the majority of left-handed people also have left-hemisphere speech; but a significant proportion (15%) have right-hemisphere speech. Furthermore, some left-handed people have control of speech in both the right and left hemispheres. In these people, neither right nor left injections of sodium amytal suppress speech function. Thus, lateralization is weak or absent in some left-handed people.

The sodium amytal test has yielded another unexpected result: unilateral injection of the drug affects not only speech, but also mood. Some studies indicate that the effect on mood is related to the side of injection: left injections tend to produce a brief depression, and right injections, euphoria. The effects have been seen at doses smaller than those needed to block speech. These results

Table 51–2. Linguistic Dominance and Handedness

Handedness	Dominant hemisphere (%)		
	Left	Right	Both
Left or mixed handed	70	15	15
Right handed	96	4	0

Source: Data from Rasmussen and Milner, 1977.

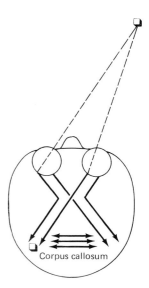

51–8 An image in the right visual field stimulates the left temporal retina and right nasal retina because projections from the nasal retina cross, whereas those from the temporal retina remain uncrossed (shown in a superior view of the brain). The information therefore projects to the left hemisphere, although it can secondarily reach the right hemisphere if the corpus callosum is intact. (Adapted from Sperry, 1968.)

suggest that functions related to mood may also be lateralized to some degree in the human brain. This is consistent with the clinical observation that some patients with damage to the left hemisphere are exceptionally upset about their symptoms. In contrast, patients with damage to the right hemisphere sometimes exhibit a pathological lack of concern for their disability.

Results from several indirect, noninvasive methods correlate well with those from the sodium amytal test. In one test a *tachistoscope* is used. This device presents very brief visual stimuli to the right or left visual hemifield. The stimuli engage either visuospatial processes (e.g., recognizing a face) or verbal processes (e.g., recognizing a word). The nature of the visual pathways is such that the image of a visual stimulus that is restricted to one visual field is projected first to the opposite hemisphere (Figure 51–8). The information is then transmitted, presumably in a slightly degraded form, to the other hemisphere via the corpus callosum. On verbal tasks, right-handed subjects typically perform slightly better when the stimuli are presented to the right visual field, which is contralateral to their verbal hemisphere. In contrast, spatial tasks are performed better when stimuli are presented to the left visual field. Left-handed subjects show greater variability with regard to the visual field superior for the task.

Similar results are obtained with the *dichotic auditory task*, in which lateralization is assessed by simultaneously presenting different auditory stimuli to both ears and determining which ear is better at recognizing the auditory inputs. In right-handed subjects, the left ear tends to be better for nonverbal auditory tasks (e.g., recognition of music), whereas the right ear is better for verbal material. The results of this test suggest that the crossed auditory pathways dominate the functioning of the uncrossed pathways.

Split-Brain Experiments Reveal Important Asymmetries and Show That Consciousness and Self-Awareness Are Not Unitary

Perhaps the most dramatic experimental evidence for the localization of function to one rather than the other hemisphere comes from research on a certain population of epileptic patients—those who have had the corpus callosum and the anterior commissure (the major fiber pathways interconnecting the two hemispheres) cut in an attempt to prevent the spread of epileptic activity from one side of the brain to the other. Studies of these patients show that each hemisphere is capable of functioning independently. Although the right hemisphere is generally mute and cannot communicate verbally about its experience, the mute hemisphere can do many of the things that the verbal hemisphere is capable of doing. Basic processes such as sensory analysis, memory, learning, and calculation can be performed by either hemisphere. The ability of the mute hemisphere is limited, however, when the task involves complex reasoning or analysis.

It seems intuitively obvious that the corpus callosum and other commissures serve to integrate the functions of the two hemispheres. Yet when patients with sectioned hemispheric commissures are observed in a casual manner, it is difficult to tell that there is anything wrong with them. Indeed, early investigators failed to find any deficiencies. By 1940 Warren McCulloch concluded with irony that the only certain role of the corpus callosum was "to aid in the transmission of epileptic seizures from one to the other side of the body" (cited by Sperry in 1964). As recently as 1950 Lashley facetiously reiterated his feeling that the purpose of the corpus callosum "must be mainly mechanical . . . i.e., to keep the hemispheres from sagging."

The functional role of the hemispheric commissures first became apparent in split-brain studies of animals by Ronald Myers and Roger Sperry. In addition to sectioning the corpus callosum, Myers and Sperry limited visual input to one hemisphere by cutting the optic chiasm and thereby destroying the crossed visual fibers. The split-brain animals were trained in complex visual discriminations using one eye; unlike normal animals, when tested with the untrained eye, they behaved as if they were completely naive. In other words, the effects of the training experience were limited to the hemisphere receiving the visual input.

In a classic series of studies, Sperry and Michael Gazzaniga later examined the function of the corpus callosum in humans by carefully studying a group of patients commissurotomized for the treatment of epilepsy. They confirmed the earlier studies on animals and, indeed, under certain experimental conditions demonstrated a severe limitation in the ability of these patients to perform specific tasks that forced one hemisphere to work independently of the other.

One reason these patients do so well in real-life situations is that ordinarily both hemispheres obtain common information that allows integration of function even though direct interhemispheric communication is absent. For example, as the eyes scan the environment, each hemisphere receives a complete representation of the world. Since the optic chiasm is intact in these patients, portions of the same visual images are projected to each hemisphere. However, Sperry and Gazzaniga arranged the experimental situation so that cross-cues were eliminated in patients lacking their corpus callosum. One simple way to accomplish this is to use brief, tachistoscopic visual stimuli that are projected exclusively to either the right or left visual field. Such visual stimuli project only to the opposite hemisphere, for in the absence of callosal fibers the visual information is unable to gain access to the ipsilateral hemisphere (Figure 51–8).

A simple experiment using this technique immediately revealed the deficit. When a subject was presented with an apple in the right visual field and questioned about what he saw, he said—not surprisingly—"apple." When, however, the apple was presented to the left visual field the patient denied having seen anything, or if prompted to give an answer, guessed or confabulated. This is not because the right hemisphere is blind or is unable to remember a simple stimulus. The patient could readily identify the object if he could point to it or, using tactile cues, could manually pick it out from several others presented under a cover (Figure 51–9). In other words, when visual stimuli were limited to the right hemisphere, the patient could not name what he saw but was able to identify the object by nonverbal means. This suggests that although the right hemisphere cannot talk, it indeed can perceive, learn, remember, and issue commands for motor tasks.

Furthermore, the right hemisphere may be capable of primitive understanding of language. For example, many words projected to the right hemisphere can be read and understood. When the letters "D-O-G" were flashed to the left visual field, the patient selected a model of a dog with his left hand. More complicated verbal inputs to the right hemisphere, such as commands, were comprehended relatively poorly. The right hemisphere appears to be almost totally incapable of language output but is able to process simple linguistic inputs.

The right hemisphere is not merely a left hemisphere that lacks verbal capacity, however. In fact, on certain perceptual tasks, the right hemisphere performs better than the left. For example, in a task involving fitting together pieces of colored wooden blocks to make a coherent pattern, patients performed much better with the left hand than with the right. Thus, as indicated earlier, the nonspeech hemisphere is superior on spatial–perceptual problems. This is most evident when the tasks involve manipulation of the environment.

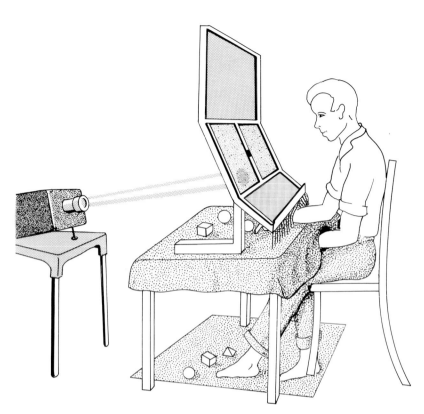

51–9 In this experimental setup, words or images of objects can be briefly flashed on the translucent screens in either the left or right visual field of the commissurotomized subject. The subject can identify the stimuli verbally or nonverbally by palpating and pointing to objects hidden behind the screen. (Adapted from Sperry, 1968.)

There is some indication that in a commissurotomized patient the two hemispheres not only can function independently, but even interfere with each other's function. In block design tasks performed with the nondominant hand (i.e., the hand ipsilateral to the verbal hemisphere), the dominant hand sometimes attempts to interfere, usually impeding the successful solution of the problem. In addition, the dominant hemisphere sometimes initiates verbal comments about the performance of the nondominant hemisphere, frequently exhibiting a false sense of confidence on problems in which it cannot know the solution, since the information was projected exclusively to the nondominant hemisphere.

The above observations have sometimes been interpreted to indicate that patients with split brains function with two independent minds, the left under the control of consciousness, the right perhaps functioning largely unconsciously and automatically. In these patients, either hemisphere is capable of directing behavior. Which hemisphere gains control seems to depend on which hemisphere is best suited for the type of task to be performed. This is seen clearly in experiments with chimeric figures of faces in which, for example, the right half of the face is male and the left half is female (Figure 51–10). Commissurotomized patients, when shown this chimeric figure with a fixation point directly in the middle, verbally report that the face is that of a man; but if asked to point to the face when shown a series of whole faces, they point to a female face. Presumably, either hemisphere is capable of pointing; nevertheless, the

more competent right hemisphere appears to control this task. When the task requires a verbal answer, of which the right hemisphere is incapable, the left hemisphere controls the task.

Each hemisphere has its own strengths as well as weaknesses with regard to a given task. Certain tasks are best performed in an analytic mode, in which the problem is broken down into logical elements. This type of task is well suited to verbal encoding. On the other hand, other tasks may be best performed not by sequential analysis but by some type of simultaneous processing of the whole input. For example, we ordinarily recognize a familiar face not by determining that it has or does not have given features such as a mustache, glasses, and small nose, but rather by some process by which all these elements are integrated into a single perception. The face simply looks familiar or not familiar. If we had to verbalize how we recognize a face, we would find it difficult and time-consuming.

In a greatly oversimplified but didactically useful way, we may think of our brains as consisting of a left hemisphere that excels in intellectual, rational, verbal, and analytical thinking, and a right hemisphere that excels in perceiving and in emotional, nonverbal, and intuitive thinking. The left hemisphere appears to do best at tasks involving declarative memory, while the right hemisphere may be more specialized for tasks involving reflexive memory (see Chapter 61). Each hemisphere is, in principle, capable of independent function, but integration of function is normally maintained by means of ex-

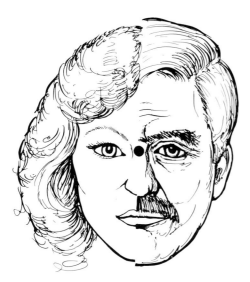

51–10 Chimeric figures such as that illustrated here have been used in experiments with commissurotomized patients to clarify the circumstances under which each hemisphere exerts dominant control. After fixating on the dot in the center of the figure, the patient is asked either to describe verbally what he sees or to point to a face that matches the one he sees. When a verbal response is required, the left hemisphere predominates; since the left hemisphere receives its input from the right visual field, the patient reports seeing the face of a man. In the pointing task, the right hemisphere (which receives input from the left visual field) exerts dominant control, and the patient responds by pointing to the face of a woman.

tensive commissural connections. The experiments with split-brain patients illustrate that consciousness, self-awareness, and other higher processes are not unitary or indivisible; rather, they seem to represent a mosaic of capabilities that are integrated and unified by extensive interconnections between the component parts.

Why Is Function Lateralized?

The question as to why lateralization of function exists in the human brain involves two major issues: First, how does lateralization develop within the life span of the individual? Second, what functional advantages, if any, does lateralization confer? We shall consider each of these questions in turn.

Although it has long been thought that hemispheric dominance is not present in young children, recent analyses of verbal deficits in children who have sustained left- or right-hemisphere damage suggest that left dominance is already present at the earliest onset of language. Nevertheless, in sharp contrast to adults, children who sustain damage to the left hemisphere—even substantial damage—usually show significant recovery of language in later life. Although one hemisphere is specialized for language in children, the other hemisphere has plastic

capabilities and can assume these functions if the hemisphere competent for language is nonfunctional.

In the developing individual, either hemisphere can attain linguistic competence. Why then does the left hemisphere become dominant in the great majority of people? It is likely that, at least in part, dominance develops in the left hemisphere because of an inherent anatomical asymmetry in the human brain, which is even present in the human fetus. As mentioned earlier, this asymmetry may initially favor the left hemisphere for language functions. Specialization of function in turn prompts further development in that area.

One means by which it was hoped to obtain insight into the possible advantages or disadvantages of lateralization of function was by studying the capacities of left-handed individuals, since a relatively high proportion of them appear to lack distinct lateralization. Nevertheless, careful studies of populations of normal individuals have not found any deficits in left-handed people. Curiously, a number of studies have indicated that in various clinical populations with behavioral problems there is a slightly greater incidence of individuals who are left handed or who exhibit incomplete lateralization. An above normal incidence of left-handedness has been reported among patients with epilepsy, cerebral palsy, stuttering, mental retardation, and dyslexia. One possible reason for increased left-handedness in certain clinical populations is that there may be a slightly increased incidence of brain damage in left-handed compared with right-handed individuals. When (and if) early brain damage produces a switch of handedness, it will result in a greater number of right to left switches than left to right, since there is a much greater incidence of right handedness. Of course, the overwhelming majority of left-handed individuals do not have brain damage. Although on theoretical grounds cerebral lateralization should provide for more efficient function, as yet there are no conclusive data establishing this point.

Whatever factors promote lateralization of function, they are not limited to humans. Anatomical asymmetry of the brain has been demonstrated in other animals, including the great apes, monkeys, cats, rats, and birds. This is particularly well documented in birds that learn their song by listening to other birds (see Chapter 60). In studies of canaries, Fernando Nottebohm at Rockefeller University found that a lesion in the avian equivalent of the left cortex severely disrupts song production, whereas a right lesion has less effect (Figure 51–11). After a left lesion, there can be recovery of song; there is no recovery if a right lesion is then made. This suggests that the right hemisphere can mediate singing when the left hemisphere is damaged.

As in humans (see Chapter 58), there are interesting sex differences in this animal model of hemispheric dominance. Centers for vocal control are larger in male birds, which learn to sing by reference to auditory information, than in females, which normally do not sing. Several of the song control areas in the left hemisphere

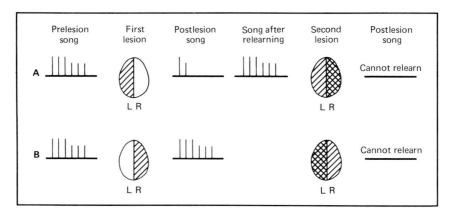

51–11 Effects of a first (**hatched side**) and second (**cross-hatched side**) unilateral brain lesion on song in birds. **A.** When the first lesion was on the left side the song was disturbed, although it could be relearned. **B.** When the first lesion was on the right side the song was not affected. In both cases the song was lost and could not be relearned after the second lesion. The vertical lines represent a simplified sound spectogram of the songs.

contain neurons that bind testosterone. In the canary it has been shown that the presence or absence of circulating testosterone modulates the amount of singing during the life span of the bird.

An Overall View

Analysis of behavioral function indicates that even the most complex functions of the brain can be topographically localized to some extent. This has great clinical importance and explains why certain syndromes—including those concerned with higher functions—are characteristic of disease in specific regions of the brain. It is unlikely, however, that any complex behavior—especially higher functions such as thought, perception, and language—will ever be understood in terms of a single region of the brain apart from considering the relationship of that region to other regions. As Lashley and others recognized, assigning functions to specific regions of the brain presents something of a philosophical problem, since no part of the nervous system functions in the same way alone as it does in concert with other parts. Furthermore, when a part of the brain is removed, the behavior of the animal is more a reflection of the capacities of the remaining brain than of the part of the brain that was removed. Nevertheless, approaching the nervous system by reducing its activities into anatomically discrete units has given us many clues about the contribution of individual parts to the functioning of the whole.

Selected Readings

Fulton, J. F. 1951. Frontal Lobotomy and Affective Behavior: A Neurophysiological Analysis. New York: Norton.

Geschwind, N. 1979. Specializations of the human brain. Sci. Am. 241(3):180–199.

Goldman-Rakic, P. S. 1981. Development and plasticity of primate frontal association cortex. In F. O. Schmitt, F. G. Worden, G. Adelman, and S. G. Dennis (eds.), The Organization of the Cerebral Cortex. Cambridge, Mass.: MIT Press, pp. 69–97.

Hardyck, C., and Petrinovich, L. F. 1977. Left-handedness. Psychol. Bull. 84:385–404.

Kolb, B., and Whishaw, I. Q. 1980. Fundamentals of Human Neuropsychology. San Francisco: Freeman.

Milner, B. 1974. Hemispheric specialization: Scope and limits. In F. O. Schmitt and F. G. Worden (eds.), The Neurosciences: Third Study Program. Cambridge, Mass.: MIT Press, pp. 75–89.

Pandya, D. N., and Seltzer, B. 1982. Association areas of the cerebral cortex. Trends Neurosci. 5:386–390.

The frontal lobes—uncharted provinces of the brain. (Special issue introduced by P. S. Goldman-Rakic.) 1984. Trends Neurosci. 7:403–454.

Valenstein, E. (ed.) 1980. The Psychosurgery Debate; Scientific Legal, and Ethical Perspectives. San Francisco: Freeman.

References

Brozoski, T. J., Brown, R. M., Rosvold, H. E., and Goldman, P. S. 1979. Cognitive deficit caused by regional depletion of dopamine in prefrontal cortex of rhesus monkey. Science 205:929–932.

Fuster, J. M. 1980. The Prefrontal Cortex: Anatomy, Physiology, and Neuropsychology of the Frontal Lobe. New York: Raven Press.

Gazzaniga, M. S., and LeDoux, J. E. 1978. The Integrated Mind. New York: Plenum Press.

Geschwind, N., and Levitsky, W. 1968. Human brain: Left–right asymmetries in temporal speech region. Science 161:186–187.

Goldman, P. S., and Nauta, W. J. H. 1977. Columnar distribution of cortico-cortical fibers in the frontal association, limbic, and motor cortex of the developing rhesus monkey. Brain Res. 122:393–413.

Harlow, H. F. 1958. Behavioral contributions to interdisciplinary research. In H. F. Harlow and C. N. Woolsey (eds.), Biological and Biochemical Bases of Behavior. Madison: University of Wisconsin Press, pp. 3–23.

Jacobsen, C. F. 1935. Functions of frontal association area in primates. Arch. Neurol. Psychiatry 33:558–569.

Lashley, K. S. 1950. In search of the engram. Symp. Soc. Exp. Biol. 4:454–482.

Levy, J., Trevarthen, C., and Sperry, R. W. 1972. Perception of bilateral chimeric figures following hemispheric deconnexion. Brain 95:61–78.

Milner, B. 1968. Visual recognition and recall after right temporal-lobe excision in man. Neuropsychologia 6:191–209.

Moniz, E. 1936. Tentatives Opératoires dans le Traitement de Certaines Psychoses. Paris: Masson.

Mountcastle, V. B., Lynch, J. C., Georgopoulos, A., Sakata, H., and Acuna, C. 1975. Posterior parietal association cortex of the monkey: Command functions for operations within extrapersonal space. J. Neurophysiol. 38:871–908.

Myers, R. E. 1955. Interocular transfer of pattern discrimination in cats following section of crossed optic fibers. J. Comp. Physiol. Psychol. 48:470–473.

Nottebohm, F. 1979. Origins and mechanisms in the establishment of cerebral dominance. In M. S. Gazzaniga (ed.), Handbook of Behavioral Neurobiology, Vol. 2: Neuropsychology. New York: Plenum Press, pp. 295–344.

Penfield, W. 1958. Functional localization in temporal and deep Sylvian areas. Res. Publ. Assoc. Res. Nerv. Ment. Dis. 36:210–226.

Rasmussen, T., and Milner, B. 1977. The role of early left-brain injury in determining lateralization of cerebral speech functions. Ann. N.Y. Acad. Sci. 299:355–369.

Robinson, D. L., Goldberg, M. E., and Stanton, G. B. 1978. Parietal association cortex in the primate: Sensory mechanisms and behavioral modulations. J. Neurophysiol. 41:910–932.

Rosenkilde, C. E. 1979. Functional heterogeneity of the prefrontal cortex in the monkey: A review. Behav. Neural Biol. 25:301–345.

Sperry, R. W. 1964. The great cerebral commissure. Sci. Am. 210(1):42–52.

Sperry, R. W. 1968. Mental unity following surgical disconnection of the cerebral hemispheres. Harvey Lect. 62:293–323.

Stamm, J. S. 1969. Electrical stimulation of monkeys' prefrontal cortex during delayed-response performance. J. Comp. Physiol. Psychol. 67:535–546.

Thompson, R. F. 1975. Introduction to Physiological Psychology. New York: Harper & Row.

Tucker, D. M., Watson, R. T., and Heilman, K. M. 1977. Discrimination and evocation of affectively intoned speech in patients with right parietal disease. Neurology 27:947–950.

Warren, J. M., and Akert, K. (eds.). 1964. The Frontal Granular Cortex and Behavior. New York: McGraw-Hill.

Richard Mayeux and Eric R. Kandel

Natural Language, Disorders of Language, and Other Localizable Disorders of Cognitive Functioning

52

In Chapter 51 we reviewed evidence for the localization of various higher functions in the brain. In this chapter we shall focus on language, one of the most important human cognitive functions. Language is particularly interesting from a neurobiological point of view because its specific and localized organization has given us the keenest insight into the functional architecture of the dominant hemisphere of the brain. The study of language also represents a striking example of how neurobiology might be able to improve our understanding of broadly humanistic issues. Analysis of language requires several disciplines ranging from anthropology and linguistics to developmental and clinical studies in humans. As a result, language offers an especially vivid illustration of the fundamental interconnectedness of the widely divergent areas of science required to study human behavior.

Artificial language, natural language, and indeed all human and animal communication have in common three features: form, content, and use. *Form* refers to the system of signals: the dictionary of sounds and words (or gestures), the combination of sounds (or gestures), and the syntax used to convey messages. *Content* refers to the message of the communication, the ideas that are coded by the language. In human conversation, the content is what a person says and what others understand that person to say. *Use* refers to how people or animals use the message or respond to it in different contexts. Use, therefore, includes nonlinguistic as well as linguistic aspects of communication.

Each feature of language seems to involve a different aspect and perhaps even a different level of neural organization. Thus, language form depends on the neuronal machinery for generating motor behavior—for vocalization and for gesture—as well as on the neural representation of grammatical speech. Content involves a different and higher neural representation, that of images, ideas, concepts, and the neural translation of these ideas into the units of form—into gesture or vocalization. Usage involves still more complex neural representations, those of individual identity and of a perception of social context.

In humans, certain diseases selectively interfere with one or another of these dimensions. Form can be affected by disease of the cerebellum resulting in dysarthria or by lesions of the cerebral cortex resulting in Broca's aphasia. Content is disturbed in Wernicke's aphasia, in conduction aphasia, and in schizophrenia. Use is affected dramatically in the aprosodias, and in the disorders of affect or thought found in some psychiatric illnesses.

In this chapter we shall consider the distinctive features of human language and examine why animal research has increased understanding of human linguistic competence only modestly. However, much has been learned about language from two sources: from the study of language acquisition in children and from neurological disorders of language. We shall therefore review the major findings on the development of language and then examine in some detail the clinical disorders of speech,

reading, writing, and gesture. This family of disorders can now be understood by means of a rather simple neuroanatomical model of language developed originally by Karl Wernicke in the nineteenth century and expanded recently by Norman Geschwind. This model tries to account for various aspects of speech-related disorders and illustrates for each of them the importance of anatomical localization. Abetted by a coherent conceptual scheme, by progress in psycholinguistics, and by the development of powerful imaging techniques, clinical studies of cognitive functions have advanced remarkably in the last fifteen years and have contributed importantly to our understanding of human language and other cognitive processes.

Just before his untimely death in 1984, Geschwind and his colleague Antonio Damasio described this progress as follows:

As late as the mid 1960s, the standard view regarding cerebral dominance for language stated that it had no anatomical correlates, that it did not exist in other species, and that its evolution in humans could not be studied. Such a position . . . implied the neglect or active rejection of the older anatomical studies of dominance . . . . But the discoveries of the past 15 years have proven that each of these standard views was false and have opened up entirely new avenues of study.

It is with these avenues that we shall be concerned here.

All Human Languages Share Four Distinctive Features

All human languages—their form, content, and use—are thought to have distinctive features that separate them from other forms of communication. Human languages are creative, structured, meaningful, and interpersonal. Let us consider briefly each of these features in turn (for a more detailed discussion, see Gleitman and Gleitman, 1981).

The *creative* aspect of language is obvious. We do not learn a language simply by memorizing a large number of stock sentences—rather, we create original sentences with every new thought we speak. As listeners, we readily interpret the sentences spoken by others.

Language is *structured* by a set of rules. We construct sentences grammatically even though we may not apply the rules consciously. We speak agrammatically only infrequently.

Language is *meaningful* (or *representational*). The purpose of structure in language is to permit ideas to be represented and expressed clearly. Words and their arrangement into sentences are a means, and often the only easy means, for communicating ideas. The main purpose of grammar is to allow different meanings to emerge from the various relationships of words in a sentence.

Finally, we use language in an *interpersonal* way; its purpose is to allow one human being, one human brain, to interact with another.

In addition to sharing these four features, human languages throughout the world have other similarities. Vocalizations in all of the world's languages use only a small fraction of the sounds that humans are capable of making. Speech sounds that are used for speech perception are called *phonemes*, perceptual units from which speech sequences are composed. No single language uses all possible phonemes, but each selects from the same pool of speech sounds. Furthermore, all human languages employ a grammatical structure. In all languages, two levels of structure can usually be distinguished: (1) the combination of phonemes to form syllables and words, and (2) the combination of words to form phrases and sentences.

Animal Models of Human Language Have Been Largely Unsatisfactory

Effective approaches to a neural analysis of cognitive and other behavioral functions have often been dependent on animal models. In language, as in other areas, considerable effort has been expended in developing these models. For animal models to be useful in studying human language, there must be points of analogy between animal and human communication. To what extent, then, does the communication of other species share the four features that characterize human language? Animals as simple as crickets and bees have an elementary natural language. Birds that produce song have a more elaborate one (see Chapter 60). These forms of communication are interpersonal (or more broadly, interindividual), but their structure, meaning, and creativity are extremely limited.

What about the closest relatives of human beings, the nonhuman primates? Do they have creative language? Can they be used to study human speech? In the past few decades, opinion on this question has swung back and forth several times. In the 1930s it was generally thought that chimpanzees could learn to speak if they were raised in a home as human children are. With this idea in mind, William and Lorna Kellogg raised a chimpanzee, Gua, with their own child. The chimpanzee adopted many human behaviors, understood a few spoken commands, and mastered a few hand gestures, but never learned to speak. After this and other failures, the pendulum swung to the other side. By the early 1960s, chimpanzees were thought to lack the intellectual capacity for language. Noam Chomsky, a linguist at the Massachusetts Institute of Technology, wrote in 1968: "Anyone concerned with the study of human nature and human capacity must somehow come to grips with the fact that all normal humans acquire spoken language whereas acquisition of even the barest rudiments is quite beyond the capacity of an otherwise intelligent ape."

Shortly thereafter it was discovered that the vocal apparatus of chimpanzees is unable to produce the full range of human sounds. The possibility remained, however, that chimpanzees might show a capacity for language if they did not have to produce speech sounds. In a significant advance, Allen and Beatrice Gardner cir-

cumvented the need for sound production and trained a female chimpanzee named Washoe to use signs borrowed from American Sign Language, the language of the American deaf. Within 4 years, Washoe achieved a substantial vocabulary of 160 words, including signs for objects ("bird," "hand"), attributes ("blue," "green," "different"), and modifiers ("more," "less"). Although these results demonstrate that chimpanzees can learn words, the vocabulary they acquire is much smaller than that of a human infant. A child of four has a vocabulary of more than 3000 words, as compared with Washoe's 160.

The mere ability to use words as symbols is an impressive achievement and raises the next question: Can chimpanzees have structured language? Do they know any rules of grammar? The simplest rules relate to propositional thought and dictate who did what to whom. Can chimpanzees understand and express the relation among the doer, the action, and the one to whom the action is done?

To explore the concept of causation, David Premack trained a chimpanzee, Sarah, to communicate with plastic chips. In these experiments Premack tried to preserve many features that are universal in natural languages. He taught Sarah to interpret commands given by a row of chips and to use the chips to construct her own sentences. Sarah eventually learned negatives, questions, the words for "same" or "different," the expression "is the name of," compound sentences, and "if–then" statements. Most interesting were experiments in which Premack showed Sarah pairs of objects in which the second was a transformed version of the first (an apple and an apple cut into pieces; a dry towel and a wet towel). Sarah was then asked to select one of several other objects that would explain the transformation (for example, a knife and a bowl of water) and insert it between these pairs. She made the appropriate choice about 80% of the time. In other words, Sarah appeared to understand that a knife is necessary to cut the apple into pieces and that water will make the towel wet.

Thus, chimpanzees (and probably gorillas as well) seem to be able to use language in a rudimentary fashion. They can learn a limited number of words and they have some structured propositional thought. It is not certain, however, that they can go beyond that. For example, there is no evidence as yet that chimpanzees can use syntax, the rules that organize words into sentences, or that they can acquire a system of rules that allows them to recognize different arrangements of the same set of words and thereby express different ideas with them. Thus, Washoe can use words such as "Washoe, me, banana," but most students of language think that she cannot distinguish "me give Washoe banana" from "Washoe give me banana." Indeed, most linguists are struck by the imitative and mechanical nature of the language acquired by chimpanzees.

Although the analogy between language in chimpanzees and the structured and creative language of humans seems weak, this work does show that apes (and simpler animals, as we now have good reason to believe) share with humans certain cognitive capabilities such as knowledge of causality. Whether these capabilities play a special role in linguistic competence, however, remains controversial.

Because animal models have a limited role in the study of human language, students of language have relied primarily on anthropological, developmental, and clinical studies.

What Is the Origin of Human Language?

Although it is difficult to pinpoint the time or way in which language evolved, some cerebral structures that are necessary or prerequisite for language appear to have arisen early in human evolution. This important conclusion has come from the work of Marjorie LeMay at the Harvard Medical School, who examined the endocranial casts of human fossils. In most individuals, the left hemisphere is dominant for language and the cortical speech area of the temporal lobe (the planum temporale) is larger in the left than right hemisphere. Since important gyri and sulci often leave an impression upon the skull, LeMay searched the fossil record for the morphological asymmetries associated with speech in modern humans and found them in Neanderthal man (dating back 30,000 to 50,000 years) and in Peking man (dating back 300,000 to 500,000 years). The left hemisphere is also dominant for the recognition of species-specific cries in Japanese macaques, and asymmetries similar to those of humans are present in brains of modern day great apes, such as the chimpanzee. Whether these anatomical and functional asymmetries originally evolved for language, for other forms of communication, or for an entirely different function, is not known.

Although the anatomical structures that are prerequisites for language may have arisen early (perhaps as much as 500,000 years ago), many students of language believe that language *per se* emerged rather *late* in the prehistoric unrecorded period of human existence (about 100,000 years ago) and that perhaps it arose only *once.* According to this view, all human languages are thought to have arisen from a single language first spoken in the eastern part of Africa.

Given the cortical asymmetry of the great apes, we can ask: Did human language evolve from apelike communication? Since human evolution is itself not understood, and since apes, as we have seen, have only rudimentary language capabilities, these questions remain embedded in speculation. Two classes of theories have been advanced: gestural and vocal.

Gestural theories propose that language evolved from a system of gestures that emerged when certain apes assumed an erect posture, freeing the hands for social communication. Vocal communication may then in turn have arisen to free the hands for purposes other than communication. *Vocal theories* contend that humans evolved from apes who had an extensive group of instinctive calls for signifying distress, elation, and courting. Initially, these calls were not voluntarily controlled by the user. According to this theory, a change occurred about 100,000 years ago in the structure of the mouth, jaw, and vocal tract that made it possible to produce different sounds reliably and thereby allowed the ancestors of modern man to exercise control over the form of their calls. They became able to use their calls in different combinations, in *creative* ways. Soon thereafter, these ancestors of modern man dispersed over the earth and the subsequent geographical isolation encouraged the development of different languages. The possibility that language originated in this way from a single source might explain why all human languages have so many features in common.

Alternatively, language may have emerged from neither gesture nor vocalization alone, but from a combination of the two processes. If this were the case, it might be related to the still inexplicable correlation of verbal language and hand dominance (gesture) being jointly lateralized in the left hemisphere.

Is the Capability for Human Language an Innate Cognitive Skill or Is It Learned?

Although the acquisition of language clearly involves learning, a number of arguments have recently been marshalled to indicate that a surprisingly large component of language acquisition is innate. These arguments come from two sources: from studies of the neurobiology of language and from studies of language development in children.

First, as we saw in Chapter 51, speech function is localized; it is predominantly represented in the left hemisphere. Not only do almost all right-handed individuals have a left-hemisphere dominance for speech, but most left-handed people also show a left-hemisphere dominance, although left-handed people often have additional speech functions in the right hemisphere.

Second, the localization of speech in the left hemisphere seems to be related to anatomical differences between the two hemispheres. For example, the planum temporale, the specialized area of the temporal lobe that is committed to speech and includes Wernicke's area, is larger in the left hemisphere in most right-handed people (see Figure 51–7).

Third, this anatomical asymmetry in the planum temporale is present early in development, by the thirty-first week of gestation, suggesting that aspects of cortical specialization for language are innate.

Fourth, infants at birth are sensitive to the acoustic distinctions crucial for the comprehension of all human languages. Indeed, some of this sensitivity later is lost as language is acquired. Although a single language does not utilize all possible phonemes, newborns readily recognize even those phonetic distinctions that are not important in their native language. For example, most adult Japanese cannot perceive the difference between the sounds of "r" and "l." Japanese infants, however, can distinguish these sounds, but they lose this ability as they mature. Peter Eimas of Brown University has suggested that the

Table 52–1. Stages of Development in English That Are Thought to Apply to the Acquisition of All Human Language

Average age		Language ability
6 mon		Beginning of distinct babbling
1 yr	1-word speaker	Language understanding; 1 or more poorly pronounced words
1½ yr		30–50 words used singly, but child cannot link them to make phrases; simple nouns, adjectives, and action verbs. Child does not use functors (the, and, can, be) necessary for syntax.
2 yr	2-word (telegraphic) speaker	50 to several hundred words in the vocabulary, and there is much use of 2-word phrases. These phrases are ordered according to syntax. There are propositional rules.
2½ yr		Many combinations of 3 or more words. Functors begin to appear. There are also many grammatical errors and idiosyncratic expressions. Good understanding of language
3 yr		Vocabulary of about 1000 words; few errors
4 yr		Close to adult speech competence

Source: Based on Lenneberg, E. H. 1967. Biological Foundations of Language. New York: Wiley; and Gleitman, L., and Gleitman, H. 1981. Languages: In H. Gleitman (ed.), Psychology. Norton, Chapter 10.

neural basis of this decline in perceptual ability is similar to that underlying the loss of visual acuity in kittens raised in a restricted visual environment (see Chapter 57).

Finally, there are impressive and universal regularities in the acquisition of language. This presumably reflects the maturation of the human brain (although there are as yet no studies that correlate language acquisition with specific maturation of areas related to language). For example, the acquisition of language by children in all cultures follows a similar series of stages. Children progress from babbling to one-word speech, to two-word speech with syntax, to complex speech (Table 52–1). Some children progress through these stages faster than others, but the average age for each stage is the same for all cultures. Moreover, in all cultures, language development (as manifested by the ability to acquire a new language) is reduced dramatically after puberty. Although there is a progression through a sequence of stages, this sequence is not correlated simply with the amount of language to which a child is exposed. When parents make an extra effort to teach their children to speak, the children usually do not produce their first word, first phrase, or first sentence much ahead of schedule. Even retarded children go through the same stages of language acquisition as do normal children, only more slowly. However, the stage that they have reached at the age of puberty generally proves to be their final stage. If a retarded child has reached only the two-word stage at puberty, additional training will allow the child to learn more words but it is not likely to help the child advance to the stage of using sentences.

Any theory of language has to explain the emergence early in development of cortical areas specialized for language as well as the universal stages in language acquisition, both of which support the idea that humans have an innate predisposition for language. A theory of language must also explain how children learn the rules of language when all they hear are utterances. Children hear language from their parents and from others in the course of casual conversation. No one lectures to them about the rules that govern these utterances. When children do form sentences, we know that they have extracted the correct rules, the underlying logic of the language, from these casual conversations. Moreover, children in different language cultures all end up knowing the same fundamental grammatical rules.

Children, therefore, must infer grammar from the speech that they hear around them. There are so many potential forms of language that if a child had to consider all of them, learning a language would be impossible. Although details of language may be learned, Chomsky argues that children must have some special innate knowledge that allows them to restrict dramatically the number of possible grammars that they have to consider. Chomsky conceives of an infant learning language by testing a genetically determined system of grammatical rules against the evidence the infant receives from its linguistic environment. These grammatical rules or *language universals* reflect an innately determined set of neural mechanisms that limit the possible characteristics of a natural language and of a natural grammar. Chomsky assumes that children learn a natural language readily because they already possess innate knowledge—an innate capability—of these language universals. When exposed to a language with these universals, a child learns it avidly. In contrast, Chomsky argues that a language that violated these universals would be unlearnable.

On the basis of these several findings, linguists and psychologists have suggested that the mechanisms for the universal aspects of language are determined by the structure of the human brain and follow from its development. According to this view, the human brain is prepared for the control of speech by its developmental program. However, the particular language spoken and the dialect and accents in that language are determined by the social environment.

The question now being debated by linguists is whether the constraints that we see in language reflect a specific linguistic capability or whether they simply reflect a general cognitive limitation of learning. Chomsky argues that the constraints are specific to language, but many psychologists disagree. The question thus takes the form: Do linguistic universals of the sort manifest in the complex structure and meaning of language derive from cognitive universals that are more general? There has been as yet no compelling demonstration that the universals of language need be unique. Children can follow abstract rules: they can distinguish between causative and noncausative actions even before they learn language. Indeed, one of the key ideas to come from the study of language in chimpanzees is that certain cognitive universals, such as knowledge of causality, need not be specific to language but might depend on the more general capability to use symbols.

A challenge to the neurobiological approach to cognition and language is to address these problems in humans. A first approach has come from the study of patients. Researchers working with aphasic patients are asking two sorts of questions: One, do disorders of language disrupt only linguistic abilities, or do they also interfere with related cognitive processes? Two, what are the neural structures that underlie the mental grammar of language universals?

Aphasias Are Disorders of Human Language That Also Interfere with Other Cognitive Processing

The aphasias are acquired disturbances of language that result from insult (vascular damage, trauma, or tumor) to specific regions of the brain, almost invariably specific regions of the cerebral cortex. The language disorder caused by cerebral damage is not a uniform, overall reduction in language ability. Rather, lesions in different parts of the cerebral cortex selectively disturb particular aspects of language. Furthermore, these disorders involve more than a breakdown in the production and comprehension of verbal language: aphasia affects other cognitive and intellectual skills to some degree. For example,

as we shall see later, some aphasic patients have difficulty not only comprehending speech but also reading (Wernicke's aphasia). Other aphasic patients have difficulty expressing thoughts in written as well as in spoken language (Broca's aphasia). Such selective language disruptions that occur when particular parts of the cortex are damaged afford unusual insights into how the brain is organized for language.

Aphasia is distinguished from disorders of speech such as *dysarthria* and *dysphonia* that result from weakness or incoordination of the muscles controlling the vocal apparatus. *Dysarthria*, a disturbance in articulation, and *dysphonia*, a disturbance in vocalization, are simply disorders of the mechanical process of speech. These disturbances do not basically affect language comprehension or expression. Patients with cerebellar disorders who are dysarthric, or those with Parkinson's disease who are dysphonic, retain their language capacity despite a severe speech impediment. In contrast, the hallmark of aphasia is a disturbance in language capacity, involving comprehension, production, or both, that is not attributable to a speech impediment.

The Aphasias Can Be Understood on the Basis of the Wernicke–Geschwind Model for Language

There is no universally accepted classification for the various aphasias. We shall describe here a useful classification developed by Norman Geschwind based on Wernicke's model for language and gesture. The reader should refer to the essential anatomical structures involved in language (Figure 52–1) to aid in distinguishing various types of aphasia.

This model for language, which has formed much of the basis for the modern understanding of aphasia (and we shall see below, for other cognitive disorders), can best be illustrated by considering the following task: the naming of a visual object (Figure 52–2). According to the Wernicke–Geschwind model, naming an object is thought to involve transfer of visual information from the retina to the lateral geniculate nucleus, and from there to the primary visual cortex, Brodmann's area 17;

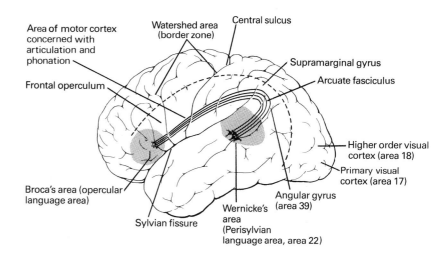

52–1 Primary language areas of the brain.
Broca's area is the motor–speech area adjacent to the motor cortex that controls the movements of articulation, facial expression, and phonation. Wernicke's area lies in the posterior superior temporal lobe and includes the auditory comprehension center. Wernicke's and Broca's areas are joined by a fiber tract called the *arcuate fasciculus.*

the information then travels to higher visual cortex, area 18, and then to a specific region (the *angular gyrus*—Brodmann's area 39) of the parietal–temporal–occipital association cortex. This region is thought to be concerned with the association of different sensory modalities—visual, auditory, and tactile. From here the information is projected to Wernicke's area in the superior posterior temporal lobe (Brodmann's area 22), where the auditory perception of the word is formed and where memory images are stored that represent the word as seen or heard. Once the pattern is formed, it is conveyed, by means of the *arcuate fasciculus*, to Broca's area, where the perception of language is translated into the grammatical structure of a phrase and where the memory for word articulation is stored. This information about the sound pattern of the phrase is then conveyed to the facial area of the motor cortex, which controls articulation, so that the words that name the visual object can be spoken.

The Wernicke–Geschwind model makes a number of interesting predictions. First, it predicts the outcome of a lesion in Wernicke's area. Visual images or words reaching the visual or auditory cortex fail to activate Wernicke's area and thus fail to activate the remainder of the language system. A spoken word may not be processed perceptually and may not be understood; consequently, the task may not be comprehended. Second, the model predicts that a lesion in Broca's area produces a very different disorder. A patient with this lesion has relatively normal comprehension of both written and spoken language, but speech and verbal communication are abnormal because the muscular articulation pattern for

52–2 This schematic view of a horizontal section of the human brain at the level of the corpus callosum shows the probable sequence of neural transmission that occurs when a person names a visual object. (Adapted from Patton, Crill, and Swanson, 1976.)

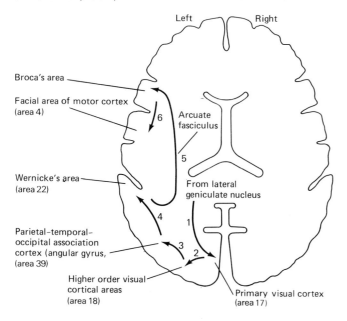

sound and for the grammatical structure of language are never passed on to the motor cortex. Third, the model predicts that a lesion in the arcuate fasciculus disconnects Wernicke's area from Broca's; as a result, verbal communication now is disordered because the visual or auditory pattern is not conveyed to the part of the brain involved with language production.

In the following discussion we shall consider the major clinical syndromes in terms of this simple model. However, patients may not always present in an exact manner because the lesions producing cortical damage are not always highly circumscribed. Aphasia occurs most frequently after strokes: 40% of major vascular disorders in the cerebral hemispheres produce language disorders. Other common etiologies of aphasia include trauma, brain tumors, and degenerative processes, such as Alzheimer's disease. Studies of patients with discrete vascular lesions have played the major role in the elaboration of our understanding of aphasia because these lesions tend to be nonprogressive and the regional anatomy follows known vascular territories.

Six Clinical Syndromes of Aphasia Can Be Distinguished and Related to Different Anatomical Loci

Wernicke's Aphasia

Wernicke's aphasia is characterized by a deficit in comprehension of language. The lesion usually involves the left posterior and superior portions of the temporal lobe (Wernicke's area, Figure 52–1). Whereas comprehension is severely impaired, verbal output is *fluent:* it is normal in rate, rhythm, and melody. However, patients may use the wrong word or combination of words *(paraphasia)*. Language may be excessive; this phenomenon has been called *press of speech* or *logorrhea*. These patients tend to add additional syllables to words and additional words to phrases. Despite the abundance of words, their speech often conveys little meaning, however. For example, when asked where he lived, a patient with Wernicke's aphasia replied, "I came there before here and returned there." The neologistic or paraphasic distortions most frequently involve key lexical items (nouns, verbs, adjectives, adverbs), especially nouns. Patients with Wernicke's aphasia fail to convey the ideas that they have in mind, an impairment called *empty speech*. The patients generally are unaware of this failure, probably because language comprehension is impaired. Repetition is also impaired because comprehension is severely disturbed, and naming is usually paraphasic in nature. In addition, patients with Wernicke's aphasia have severe reading and writing disabilities. Except for these symptoms of aphasia, other neurological signs may be absent, but occasionally a right visual field defect is encountered.

Broca's Aphasia

Broca's aphasia involves damage to the motor association cortex in the frontal lobe and usually includes the posterior portion of the third frontal gyrus that forms part of the frontal operculum (Broca's area, Figure 52–1). Comprehension is usually preserved, but language output is impaired and *nonfluent* (verbal output is decreased). This ranges from almost complete muteness to a slowed, deliberate speech that uses very simple grammatical structures. Patients with Broca's aphasia use only key words. They usually express nouns only in the singular, verbs in the infinitive or participle, and they often eliminate articles, adjectives, and adverbs altogether. For example, a patient with Broca's aphasia asked to say "the large gray cat" may say "gray cat."

Psycholinguistic studies of patients with Broca's aphasia have shown that these omissions are even more dramatic in more complex sentences. Here we can see the second characteristic of this defect: a breakdown in the construction and coordination of constituent phrases. Take the sentence: "The ladies and gentlemen are now all invited into the dining room." A patient with Broca's aphasia may merely be able to say "Ladies, men, room." When asked his occupation, a mailman with Broca's aphasia said "Mail . . . Mail . . . M . . . ." In addition to such "telegraphic" or agrammatical speech, repetition is always impaired in Broca's aphasics, and naming ability may be slightly to moderately impaired. Unlike Wernicke's aphasia, patients with Broca's aphasia are generally aware of these errors.

Although language production is severely compromised in patients with Broca's aphasia, comprehension of spoken language and of written language is usually preserved, because the posterior language regions of Wernicke remain intact. However, patients with Broca's aphasia have difficulty reading aloud, and writing (like speech) is abnormal. Moreover, work by Rita Sloan Berndt and Alfonso Caramazza, at Johns Hopkins University, suggests that Broca's aphasics may also have some difficulty comprehending those aspects of syntax (function words) that they have difficulty producing.

Because Broca's area is located near the motor cortex and the underlying internal capsule, a right hemiparesis and homonymous hemianopsia (loss of vision) is almost always present in this type of aphasia.

Conduction Aphasia

As pointed out in Chapter 1, Wernicke predicted the clinical entity of conduction aphasia when he proposed that an area he had observed in the temporal lobe, concerned with the comprehension of language, projected to Broca's area, presumably related to the expression of language, by means of a pathway that interconnected the two regions. It therefore seemed possible that a lesion could leave both Broca's and Wernicke's areas intact but simply *disconnected* from each other. Subsequent clinical studies verified this prediction. Lesions in the arcuate fasciculus, which interconnects Wernicke's and Broca's areas, lead to conduction aphasia. Damage to the fasciculus occurs with injury of the supramarginal gyrus of the parietal lobe or, less frequently, with injury of the posterior and superior aspect of the left temporal lobe (Figure 52–1).

Although Broca's area is intact, it cannot receive input from Wernicke's area. Like patients with Wernicke's aphasia, patients with conduction aphasia are fluent but have many paraphasic intervals. The degree of fluency may be somewhat less than that seen in Wernicke's aphasia, but comprehension is good. However, damage to the pathways from Wernicke's area (language reception) to Broca's area (language production) greatly impairs the ability to repeat. Other characteristics of conduction aphasia are also consistent with the notion that Broca's and Wernicke's areas have been functionally separated. Naming is severely impaired. Reading aloud is abnormal, but patients can read silently with good comprehension. Writing may also be disturbed; spelling is poor, with omissions, reversals, and even substitutions of letters.

Many patients with conduction aphasia have some degree of apraxia (see below), particularly for limb and facial movements.

Anomic Aphasia

This is a fluent aphasia in which the only disturbance is a difficulty in finding words. This is an unusual form of aphasia that typically follows lesions in the posterior aspect of the left inferior temporal lobe, near the temporal–occipital border. Occasionally, patients with anomic aphasia also have a right superior quadrantanopic visual field defect.

Global Aphasia

Lesions that cause global or total aphasia usually include the entire perisylvian region, thereby compromising both Broca's and Wernicke's areas and the arcuate fasciculus. As a result, patients with global aphasia are unable to speak or comprehend language and cannot read, write, repeat, or name a viewed object. The degree of impairment is variable. A complete right hemiplegia, right hemisensory defect, and usually a right homonymous hemianopsia are present.

Transcortical Aphasias

These aphasias are characterized by two important features: preserved repetition of spoken language and a lesion outside the perisylvian language centers. These aphasias most often result from damage to the brain at the junctions of the vascular territories of the middle, anterior, and posterior cerebral arteries—a region known as the *border zone* or *watershed area* (Figure 52–1).

Transcortical motor aphasia is a nonfluent aphasia. The patient will attempt conversation but can release only a few syllables. In striking contrast, these patients are able to repeat words and phrases well. Comprehension of language is usually normal, as is reading (both silently and aloud), but writing may be impaired. The lesion is usually anterior to Broca's area in the frontal lobe.

Transcortical sensory aphasia is a fluent aphasia with defective comprehension. The patient cannot read or write and has a marked difficulty in word finding, but is able to repeat spoken language easily and fluently. This type of aphasia usually results from a lesion in the parietal–temporal–occipital junction.

A combination of transcortical motor and transcortical sensory aphasias produces *mixed transcortical aphasia* or *isolation of the speech area*. This is an extremely rare disorder. The patient is unable to speak unless spoken to, but then answers easily, although the response is usually a direct echo of the examiner's words, or so-called *echolalia*. The patient is not competent in any other language function.[1]

Aprosodias Are Disorders of the Melodic Intonation of Language and Its Perception

We have so far considered some of the cognitive components of language. However, human language and, more generally, human communication have important affective components as well. These components include the musical intonation of speech *(prosody)*, emotional gesturing, prosodic comprehension, and comprehension of emotional gesturing.

Elliott Ross at the University of Texas in Dallas has recently found that certain affective components of language, including prosody and emotional gesturing used in verbal communication, differentially rely on the specialized processes of the right hemisphere. The term *aprosodia* refers to a disturbance in these affective components of language that are associated with right-hemisphere damage. The functional–anatomical organization of the right hemisphere seems to mirror the organization of propositional language in the left hemisphere. Thus, patients with anterior right-hemisphere lesions are unable to communicate or are "nonfluent" in the affective content of their verbal output, whereas patients with posterior lesions do not appear to recognize or comprehend the affective content of language. These studies, while controversial, suggest an important relationship between affect and language.

Some Disorders of Reading and Writing Can Also Be Accounted for by the Wernicke–Geschwind Model

Reading difficulties fall into two categories: (1) *congenital reading difficulties* (these difficulties in first acquiring the ability to read are called the *dyslexias*), and (2) *acquired reading difficulties* (called *acquired dyslexias* or *alexias*). We shall first focus on the *alexias* because they are particularly instructive for understanding language and illustrate interesting extensions of the Wernicke–Geschwind model of language.

Alexias and Agraphias Are Acquired Disorders of Reading and Writing

These disorders are quite remarkable because they demonstrate that small, circumscribed lesions of the brain in an adult can selectively destroy the capability to read, write, or both, without interfering with speech or other cognitive functions. This remarkable discovery was made by the French neurologist Jules Dejerine, who described word blindness in two classic papers published in rapid succession in 1891 and in 1892. In the first paper Dejerine described a patient with a disorder of both reading and writing (alexia with agraphia). The second patient had a pure word or reading disorder—alexia without agraphia.

Word Blindness Accompanied by Writing Impairment: Alexia with Agraphia. The patient whom Dejerine first encountered could speak and understand spoken language, but could not read (alexia) or write (agraphia). Autopsy of this and subsequent cases revealed that alexia with agraphia is usually associated with lesions of the angular or supramarginal gyri of the parietal–temporal–occipital association cortex. As we saw in Chapter 51, this association cortex is concerned with integrating visual, auditory, and tactile information—a necessary prerequisite for speech comprehension. Once integrated, the information is then conveyed from this association cortex to the speech areas of the temporal lobe and then to those of the frontal lobe. When the association cortex of the angular or the supramarginal gyrus is damaged, patients cannot read or write because they cannot elaborate visual symbols into phonetic or written language. Similarly, the patients cannot recognize words spelled out loud, nor can they spell. These patients also are unable to recognize letter blocks by manual palpation because the angular and supramarginal gyri also mediate the transfer of kinesthetic information to language areas.

Pure Word Blindness: Alexia without Agraphia. Dejerine's second patient could speak perfectly well. An intelligent and highly articulate man, he suddenly observed one day that he could not read a single word! He could comprehend spoken language and could write, but he could neither read nor understand written language, including that which he himself had written. The patient was able, however, to derive meaning from words spelled aloud and was able to spell correctly. Even though he could not comprehend written words, he could copy

---

[1]We have considered here only aphasias due to cortical damage. *Subcortical aphasia* can occur with subcortical lesions that do not involve the cerebral cortex, but the internal capsule or putamen instead. The lesions causing the clinical syndromes are not as localized as those described above. The most common cause of subcortical aphasia is vascular disease.

Three distinct syndromes have been observed with lesions to the left internal capsule or putamen. A patient with an anterior subcortical lesion has slow, dysarthric, and diminished verbal output with a hemiparesis,

yet retains good comprehension of language. A posterior lesion in this area will result in poor comprehension and fluent, even excessive language (logorrhea), as seen in Wernicke's aphasia. Hemiplegia is also present in this disorder. Patients with lesions that involve the entire internal capsule will be globally aphasic and have a dense hemiplegia and sensory loss. The subcortical aphasias can resemble the clinical syndromes mentioned above, but there are also important differences. For example, repetition may be preserved in some patients with anterior or posterior subcortical lesions.

them correctly and could recognize and understand them by manual palpation of the individual letters.

The patient was blind in the right visual field (indicating damage to the left visual cortex) but otherwise had normal visual acuity. Postmortem examination of this and subsequent patients revealed damage to two structures: (1) the left occipital (visual) cortex and (2) the *splenium*, the posterior portion of the corpus callosum, which carries visual information between the two hemispheres by interconnecting area 18 of the occipital cortex of one hemisphere with that of the other.

Damage to the left occipital cortex abolished perception by the left hemisphere by causing loss of vision in the right visual field. As a result, the patient could see only his left visual field using his intact right occipital cortex. Although the visual information could still be processed by the right hemisphere, damage to the splenium prevented its transfer to the angular gyrus (of the parietal–temporal–occipital association cortex) and to language areas of the left hemisphere.

As might be predicted from the location of the lesion, a number of patients have selective deficits in visual perception due to damage in the visual 4 portion of Brodmann's area 18 (see Chapter 30). For example, 50% of patients with pure alexia have either a *color agnosia* (they are capable of matching colors but cannot name or identify them) or an *achromatopsia* (they perceive form but cannot perceive color and therefore see objects only as shades of gray).

Subsequently, John Trescher and Frank Ford extended Dejerine's findings by noticing that surgical disruption of the splenium results in the loss of reading ability in the left but not right visual field. In contrast, section of the *anterior* portion of the corpus callosum (which does not transmit visual information) does not interfere with reading. However, patients with the anterior portion of the corpus callosum transected cannot write with their left hand (controlled by the right hemisphere), because it no longer has access to the left-hemisphere language centers. The patients also cannot name objects held in the left hand because the somesthetic information does not reach the language areas in the left hemisphere.

Phonetic Symbols and Ideographs Are Localized to Different Regions of the Cerebral Cortex. Some of the more interesting disturbances in reading and writing capabilities occur in the Japanese language, which has two distinct systems of writing. One writing system, Kana, is syllabic: words are represented by a series of phonetic symbols (Kana letters). There are 71 letters in the Kana system. The other writing system, Kanji, is in good part ideographic: words are presented by one or more ideographic characters derived from Chinese. There are over 40,000 Kanji characters. Although Kana words are articulated syllable by syllable and are not easily identified at a glance, each Kanji character simultaneously represents both a sound and a meaning.

Because these two writing systems rely on phonemic processing to differing degrees, one might expect that certain focal lesions might affect reading or writing in one system but not the other. This is in fact the case. Both systems rely on language centers in the left hemisphere, but they are processed by different intrahemispheric mechanisms. Lesions of the angular gyrus of the parietal–temporal–occipital association cortex severely disrupt reading of Kana (syllabic) script, but leave comprehension of Kanji (ideographic) script largely intact. Moreover, whereas such lesions can disrupt reading of Kanji to some degree, the disruption entails primarily phonemic processing—the patients may be unable to read the word aloud, but they can accurately explain its semantic meaning. The same word written in Kana script does not elicit an overall global semantic understanding. These observations support the interpretation that the angular gyrus of the left hemisphere serves to link the visual and auditory representation of words. Other dissociations between the processing of Kana and Kanji scripts also occur and have provided further insights into the mechanisms of information processing in the production and comprehension of language.

Dyslexia and Hyperlexia Are Developmental Disorders of Reading

Congenital (or developmental) dyslexia is a disability that emerges in early life and is characterized by a difficulty in learning to read. Dyslexia is a broad category that may encompass a variety of disorders, but all share certain features. For example, dyslexia is more common in left-handers than in right-handers and in boys than in girls. Except for the reading impairment, the cognitive and intellectual capacities of these children are usually normal or even superior. Children with dyslexia seem particularly impaired in phonemic skills—the ability to associate visual symbols with the sounds they represent. However, they can usually understand other signs or symbols of communication, such as traffic signs or words that have a distinctive visual appearance (such as the Coca-Cola trademark). Indeed, Paul Rozin and his colleagues at the University of Pennsylvania have found that American dyslexic children can easily learn to read English when it is represented by characters that depict entire words rather than a sequence of phonetic symbols. The specificity of this disorder and the parallels to alexic disorders caused by strokes have led to the suggestion that dyslexia might result from abnormalities in connections between visual and language areas or in language areas themselves.

Dyslexic children also exhibit a strong tendency to read a word from right to left (confusing words like "was" and "saw") and have particular difficulties with letters whose orientations are important for their identification (for example, p, q, b and d). Similar orientational mistakes occur in writing. These characteristic errors and the disproportionate percentage of left-handers among dyslexics led Samuel Orston to suggest that dyslexia might involve a deficit in the development of dominance by the left hemisphere. Albert Galaburda and Thomas Kemper have recently provided evidence supporting this hypothesis. Galaburda and Kemper found that the normal hemispheric size discrepancy in the planum temporale was much reduced in dyslexic males. In addition, the left planum temporale exhibited striking cytoarchitectonic abnormalities, including an incomplete segregation of cell layers. In contrast, the right hemisphere appeared normal. These observations suggested that in male dyslexic patients, normal migration of neurons to the left cortex had been slowed during development. Similar irregularities have now been noted in female dyslexic patients.

Geschwind made the intriguing (but controversial) proposal that the development of anomalous dominance features and other functional abnormalities may result from either the presence of excessive testosterone or an unusual sensitivity to testosterone during fetal life. Since, as we have seen in Chapter 58, males are exposed to more testosterone in utero than females, they are more likely to be affected, and in fact are more likely to be left-handed, to be dyslexic, and to exhibit other language disorders, such as stuttering and autism. Dyslexics also tend to greater than average spatial skills (a right-hemisphere function), and a disproportionate number of artists, musicians, and mathematicians are left-handed.

A complementary disorder to dyslexia is *hyperlexia*. Whereas the dyslexic child may be normal except for a reading disability, the hyperlexic child is severely deficient in almost all areas but exhibits a striking capacity for oral reading. The child begins to read at an early age, perhaps 3 to 4 years old, without any appreciable training, and will read out loud compulsively. However, hyperlexic children give no evidence of comprehending what they have read. The neural basis for this disorder is not known, although it has been proposed that brain areas responsible for phonemic decoding have become overdeveloped at the expense of other brain regions.

Apraxia Is a Disorder in the Execution of Gesture and Learned Movements

Apraxia, originally defined by the German neurologist Hugo Liepmann at the end of the nineteenth century, is a disorder in the understanding of complex motor commands and the execution of certain *learned* movements. The term *apraxia* is not used for disorders of movement in which only execution of complex skills is impaired, but refers specifically to *deficits in the cognitive (or ideomotor) components of learned movements*. The disorder cannot be explained by weakness, incoordination, sensory loss, poor verbal comprehension, or inattention to the command. Its relationship to aphasia is an important one. Many aphasics are also apraxic, and the anatomical basis for this cognitive impairment can be explained by the Wernicke–Geschwind model as well. The most common form of apraxia is called *ideomotor apraxia*.

A patient with *ideomotor apraxia* is not able to carry out a motor command for movements that normally are done with ease, such as saluting, or pretending to flip a

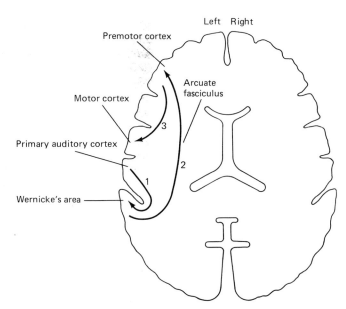

52–3 Schematic view of a horizontal section of the human brain illustrating the probable sequence of neural transmission when a person is asked to raise the right hand.

coin or use a hammer. The movements that the apraxic patient carries out resemble the correct movement but inaccurately.

Ideomotor apraxia can be understood in terms of the anatomical pathways by which movements are normally carried out in response to verbal cues (Figure 52–3). Consider as an example a patient asked to raise the right hand. According to the Wernicke–Geschwind view, the verbal request is processed by the auditory cortex and then projected to Wernicke's area in the left posterior temporal lobe. From there, the information is thought to be conveyed through the left parietal lobe to the left premotor cortex by means of the arcuate fasciculus. From the premotor cortex the information is transmitted to the arm area of the motor cortex, which gives rise to the pyramidal tract, whose fibers activate the nerve cells in the spinal cord controlling the muscles of the arm and hand.

A similar sequence must occur when a patient is asked to raise the left hand. In this case, however, the information now must be transmitted across the corpus callosum from the left premotor cortex to the premotor cortex in the right hemisphere and, from there, to the right supplementary motor cortex (Figure 52–4). A lesion of the corpus callosum therefore will allow the patient to carry out commands relating to the right side of the body (because these commands are processed within the left hemisphere), but not commands relating to the left side of the body. Similar symptoms result from lesions of the left premotor cortex; in addition, these lesions produce right hemiplegia. As also illustrated in Figure 52–4, interhemispheric callosal transmission occurs between the premotor cortices (from the left premotor to the right premotor cortex) and perhaps also between Wernicke's

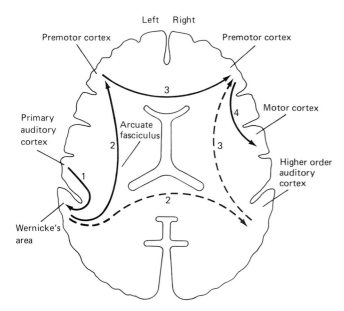

52–4 This schematic view of a horizontal section of the human brain shows the probable intrahemispheric and transcallosal pathways for voluntary movement when a person is asked to raise the left hand. Callosal transmission occurs from the left to the right premotor area. A second callosal pathway is postulated to connect Wernicke's area in the left hemisphere with the homotopic auditory association area in the right hemisphere **(broken line).** This second pathway is then thought to connect with the premotor area of the right hemisphere.

area and the auditory association cortex in the right hemisphere (the existence of the latter pathway is debatable; it is therefore indicated by a broken line in Figure 52–4). A lesion involving the pathways between Wernicke's area, the premotor cortex, Broca's area, or the corpus callosum would then result in ideomotor apraxia. A patient with Wernicke's aphasia, however, is unable to comprehend, and consequently would not be included in the definitions of apraxia suggested by Liepmann.

Three examples of ideomotor apraxia are easily recognized.[2] Much like conduction aphasia and pure word blindness, each of the ideomotor apraxias results from a

---

[2]Other forms of apraxia do exist, but are much less common than ideomotor apraxia. *Ideational apraxia* is an inability to carry out a required sequence of activities on command. It occurs in patients with various disorders of the cerebral cortex, such as Alzheimer's disease, or patients with parietal lobe lesions of either hemisphere. *Constructional apraxia* usually involves difficulty in drawing or copying simple figures or building with blocks or sticks in a three-dimensional fashion. Its anatomical correlate is poorly defined, but it may occur in patients with lesions in either parietal lobe, with diffuse cerebral disorders, or with basal ganglia dysfunction. *Dressing apraxia* involves an inattention to part of one's body and can be either unilateral or general. Unilateral dressing apraxia, in which the patient fails to dress or groom one-half of the body, can occur with disease in either cerebral hemisphere or with unilateral subcortical damage. General dressing apraxia, in which the patient is unable to manipulate clothing appropriately, is seen with right-hemisphere or nondominant parietal lobe disorders and with degenerative disorders, such as Alzheimer's disease.

disconnection syndrome, a lesion that interrupts fiber tracts connecting one cortical region with another. Two of these apraxias are associated with aphasias—conduction aphasia and Broca's aphasia.

Patients with conduction aphasia usually do not have paralysis or sensory loss, and comprehension remains intact. But there is an associated limb and often buccofacial apraxia. The lesion in conduction aphasia involves the arcuate fasciculus of the left parietal lobe and disrupts the processing of the information from Wernicke's area to Broca's area and to the premotor cortex. This disruption occurs because the lesion prevents the command that is heard and understood in Wernicke's area from being transmitted to the premotor cortex via the arcuate fasciculus.

Patients with Broca's aphasia retain the ability to comprehend verbal information but may fail to respond correctly to a command to use the nonparalyzed left arm even though they have understood the command. This apraxic disorder appears to result from the destruction of the callosal fibers at their origin in the cells of the left premotor cortex. Damage in this area prevents impulses that begin in the left premotor cortex from reaching their corresponding area in the right premotor cortex. These patients may also fail to carry out certain commands requiring facial movements, such as "stick out your tongue," "blow," or "cough." This symptom is explained by the destruction of the facial area of the motor cortex of the left hemisphere, which produces a paralysis on the right side of the face; furthermore, impulses from the left supplementary premotor facial area cannot traverse the corpus callosum to the corresponding area in the right hemisphere.

There is also a rare type of ideomotor apraxia that occurs with surgical, and sometimes vascular, destruction of the anterior two-thirds of the corpus callosum. With this lesion, the motor association cortices of both hemispheres remain intact but the lesion prevents transcallosal transmission of impulses. This results in a curious clinical situation in which the patient is unable to carry out commands with the left hand but can perform them perfectly well with the right hand.

An Overall View

Human language represents our highest cognitive function. In both its written and spoken forms, it is one of the major links connecting one person to another as well as to the historical record of civilization. As a result, in the study of language, neural science bridges biology and the humanities. Given this special opportunity, we may well ask, "What can neurobiologists say to psychologists and humanists that can inform them about the nature of the human cognitive process?"

The first and the single most important insight is that language is localizable to one of the two hemispheres. Second, the hemispheric asymmetry that ultimately gave rise to language emerged early in human evolution and already existed some 300,000 years ago. Third, language is not a single capability but a family of capabilities of which two major ones—comprehension and expression—can now be separated out by their distinctive regional localization. Fourth, as first suggested by Wernicke, profound aphasia can result by simply disconnecting these two regions. This demonstration elegantly reveals that precise interconnections are as important for the highest forms of mentation as they are for the simplest reflexes. Moreover, the ability to localize major components of language to different anatomical regions has led to the development of a simple but heuristically powerful explanatory model of language, the Wernicke–Geschwind model, which can readily be extended to account for a family of language-related disorders as well as disorders of gesture. Fifth, the capability for language seems to be present at birth, and aspects of the universal features of language are thought to derive from restraints imposed by the biological structure of the cortical regions concerned with language in the left hemisphere.

Despite these insights, however, the neurobiological understanding of language is very rudimentary. The Wernicke–Geschwind model is a beginning in the localization of cognitive functioning, but it is only a beginning. It has, however, provided an important bridge between the modern analysis of language and its disorders by psycholinguists and the neuroanatomical localization of language function. Moreover, modern imaging techniques such as computerized tomography, evoked potentials, positron emission tomography, and magnetic resonance imaging, in conjunction with careful clinical examinations (such as those described in the postscript below), should substantially enhance our future understanding of the anatomical and physiological bases of cognitive function.

Postscript:
A Clinical Exercise in Distinguishing the Aphasias

Even though there are a number of different aphasias, it is possible to determine the type of aphasic disorder in a simple neurological examination of almost any alert, cooperative patient. The examination of the aphasic patient must include an evaluation of the following six capabilities: spontaneous speech or verbal output, ability to repeat words and phrases, comprehension of spoken language, ability to name objects, reading and writing abilities, and learned movement (Table 52–2). The following sections more fully describe how those traits that we have seen in the preceding sections to be characteristic of some aphasias can be elicited from patients in the course of examining the higher cognitive functioning.

Is Spontaneous Speech Fluent or Nonfluent?

One of the most striking features of aphasia is abnormal spontaneous speech during conversation or in response to questions or picture descriptions. Spontaneous speech is described either as nonfluent or fluent. *Nonfluent language* is characterized by a decreased verbal output (50

words or fewer per minute). Verbal communication is sparse, poorly articulated, abnormal in rhythm and melody *(dysprosodic)*, and consists of short or incomplete sentences and phrases. There may be difficulty in initiating and continuing the flow of speech, manifested by hesitations, pauses, and perseverations. Phrases are reduced in length and may contain only one or two words, usually nouns *(telegraphic speech)*.

Patients with nonfluent aphasia usually are damaged in the frontal lobe anterior to the central sulcus (Rolandic fissure). This condition is referred to as *anterior aphasia*. Examples of anterior aphasia in Table 52–2 are both *Broca's aphasia* and *transcortical motor aphasia*. Broca's aphasia is the most common form of nonfluent aphasia; the lesion that produces this disturbance usually includes Broca's area (the motor–speech area).

Fluent language is normal in output and rate. As a result, fluent aphasia may be difficult to detect because the patient is able to speak at a normal rate. However, fluent aphasics may have difficulty retrieving a content word: "You know what I mean . . . it's a thing you put into the . . . to open the . . . the thing you carry in your pocket." This circumlocution that occurs when a specific word is needed and is actively being sought is a frequent symptom, but not necessarily indicative of fluent aphasia. The patient may substitute general or less specific words, such as "thing," for the name of a specific object. The verbal output of the fluent aphasic patient is frequently characterized by empty speech and long sentences that have few substantive words. Patients with fluent aphasia may also be paraphasic, using the wrong word or wrong sound within a word. For example, a patient may say, "I combed my hair with a toothbrush," or refer to a wallet as a "billhold." The patient may also make up new words or *neologisms*, which are unrecognizable, such as "transmo" for radio.

Patients with fluent aphasia usually have damage posterior to the central sulcus. This condition is referred to as *posterior aphasia*. Examples of posterior aphasias noted in Table 52–2 are *Wernicke's, conduction,* and *transcortical sensory aphasias*.

Can the Patient Repeat Words or Phrases?

The ability to repeat words or phrases is important diagnostically. Patients with damage to the perisylvian area are deficient in word repetition skills. Damage to the perisylvian area affects Wernicke's area, Broca's area, and the arcuate fasciculus, which interconnects them (Figure 52–1). The disruption of repetition with a lesion of the arcuate fasciculus occurs because the auditory pattern does not reach Broca's area, which communicates with the motor cortex. Patients with lesions involving the supramarginal gyrus also are impaired in sentence repetition, as are those with lesions in Wernicke's area. However, patients with lesions peripheral to the opercular language zone maintain their ability to repeat words or phrases.

The examination of an aphasic patient should include sentences for repetition that are phonetically complex as well as sentences that are syntactically complex. Asking

Table 52–2. Clinical Characteristics of Aphasias

Type	Verbal output	Repetition	Comprehension	Naming	Associated signs	Lesion
Broca's	Nonfluent	Impaired	Normal	Marginally impaired	RHP, apraxia of the left limbs and face	Left posterior inferior frontal
Wernicke's	Fluent	Impaired	Impaired	Impaired	± RHH	Left posterior superior temporal
Conduction	Fluent	Impaired	Normal	Impaired (paraphasic)	± RHS, apraxia of all limbs and face	Left parietal
Global	Nonfluent	Impaired	Impaired	Impaired	RHP, RHS, RHH	Left frontal temporal parietal
Anomic	Fluent	Normal (anomic)	Normal	Impaired	None	Left posterior inferior temporal, or temporal–occipital region
Transcortical Motor	Nonfluent	Normal	Normal	Impaired	RHP	Left medial frontal or anterior border zone
Sensory	Fluent	Normal	Impaired	Impaired	± RHH	Left medial parietal or posterior border zone
Mixed (isolation)	Nonfluent	Normal	Impaired	Impaired	RHP, RHS	Left medial frontal parietal or complete border zone

Abbreviations: RHP, right hemiparesis; RHH, right homonymous hemianopsia; RHS, right hemisensory defect.

patients who are otherwise mute to repeat single words is often useful for eliciting verbalization, but repetition of sentences is the critical discriminator. For example, when asked to repeat the word "arithmetic," a patient with a conduction aphasia said, "a-ric-a-won," but when asked to repeat "Today is a nice day," he said "Today is today, today."

How Well Can Language Be Comprehended?

Comprehension can be tested by having a patient follow commands or answer questions. This can be assessed while the patient's history is being taken, or even in conversation. In some patients with severe nonfluent aphasia, the answers to "yes/no" questions should be evaluated.

Disturbances of comprehension are either phonetic, semantic, or both. One area critical for phonemic processing is located directly in Wernicke's area. Consequently, patients with Wernicke's aphasia are unable to hear individual phonemes or combinations of phonemes accurately. Some patients may not be able to perceive the sound of the word or associate it with meaning. This type of deficit may occur when the center for auditory language comprehension is damaged, and it is characteristic of Wernicke's and some transcortical sensory aphasias.

A disturbance of semantic comprehension is charac-

terized by an inability to understand specific words or the specific meanings of words. This is seen in patients with conduction aphasia. However, the association of perceived sound of the word with meaning is dependent on the area of the parietal–temporal–occipital junction. Since Wernicke's aphasia often includes this area in the left hemisphere, defects of both the phonetic and semantic levels of processing may be present.

Is There Difficulty in Naming?

Difficulty in naming or finding the correct word is called *anomia*. It is common to all forms of aphasia. When it is the only demonstrable language deficit, the syndrome is referred to as *anomic aphasia*. There is evidence that patients with anterior aphasia can generate names more easily when seeing or touching an object than in their spontaneous speech, while patients with anomia resulting from temporal or parietal lobe lesions have difficulty naming an object seen or touched. However, the inability to name an object is not necessarily associated with the inability to comprehend the same object by name; the latter deficit would be a disturbance in comprehension.

The type of anomia varies with the anatomical location of the lesion. *Word production anomia* is seen with Broca's aphasia. The patient is unable to produce the correct word even though it may be known. *Word selection anomia* occurs in patients with lesions at the posterior–temporal–occipital junction (anomic aphasia). The patient produces a paraphasic error or even a neologism. One patient referred to a harmonica as "a hand penny orchestra." *Semantic anomia* occurs with lesions in the dominant angular gyrus of the parietal lobe (for example, conduction aphasia) and results in both a productive word-finding problem and a perceptual impairment in word-finding; for example, the patient may not correctly identify the category or type of word to use. Occasionally, *modality-specific (tactile, visual, auditory)* or *category-specific* anomia results from lesions in the parietal–occipital or occipital region. An example of this is *color anomia* (the inability to name colors correctly), caused by a lesion in the left occipital lobe and in the splenium of the corpus callosum.

Are There Associated Disturbances of Reading and Writing?

Patients with aphasia usually exhibit deficits in written language similar to their deficits in spoken language. These similarities support the interpretation that aphasias represent true disturbances in language function and are not simply perceptual or motor disorders. For example, in patients with Wernicke's aphasia, writing is fluent but abnormal, and reading comprehension is poor, although some patients may retain the ability to read text aloud without comprehending its meaning. In patients with Broca's aphasia, both writing and speech are nonfluent. Comprehension of written material, while not entirely normal, is greater than in Wernicke's aphasia, but the ability to read aloud is disrupted.

Are There Other Associated Signs?

Other neurological signs can also help localize the area of disturbance in most aphasic patients. For example, patients with anterior aphasia almost always have a right hemiparesis that is usually worse in the arm and face than in the leg. On the other hand, patients with a posterior aphasia may have no fixed neurological sign. However, some patients with posterior aphasia have a hemisensory disturbance or visual field defect, as do patients with alexia without agraphia syndrome (Table 52–2).

Selected Readings

Benson, D. F. 1979. Aphasia, Alexia, and Agraphia. New York: Churchill Livingstone.

Benson, D. F., and Geschwind, N. 1976. The aphasias and related disturbances. In A. B. Baker and L. H. Baker (eds.), Clinical Neurology, Vol. 1. New York: Harper & Row, Chapter 10.

Chomsky, N. 1968. Language and the mind. Psychol. Today 1(9):48–68.

Critchley, M. 1979. The Divine Banquet of the Brain and Other Essays. New York: Raven Press.

Damasio, A. R. and Geschwind, N. 1984. The neural basis of language. Annu. Rev. Neurosci. 7:127–147.

Gardner, R. A., and Gardner, B. T. 1969. Teaching sign language to a chimpanzee. Science 165:664–672.

Geschwind, N. 1965. Disconnexion syndromes in animals and man. Brain 88:237–294, 585–644.

Geschwind, N. 1974. Problems in the anatomical understanding of the aphasias. In N. Geschwind (ed.), Boston Studies in the Philosophy of Science, Vol. 16: Selected Papers on Language and the Brain. Dordrecht, Holland: Reidel.

Geschwind, N., and Fusillo, M. 1966. Color-naming defects in association with alexia. Arch. Neurol. 15:137–146.

Geschwind, N., Quadfasel, F. A., and Segarra, J. M. 1968. Isolation of the speech area. Neuropsychologia 6:327–340.

Gleitman, L. R., and Gleitman, H. 1981. Language. In H. Gleitman (ed.), Psychology. New York: Norton, Chapter 10.

Heilman, K. M., and Scholes, R. J. 1976. The nature of comprehension errors in Broca's, conduction and Wernicke's aphasics. Cortex 12:258–265.

Kellogg, W. N. 1968. Communication and language in the home-raised chimpanzee. Science 162:423–427.

LeMay, M. 1976. Morphological cerebral asymmetries of modern man, fossil man, and nonhuman primate. Ann. N.Y. Acad. Sci. 280:349–366.

Lenneberg, E. H. 1967. Biological Foundations of Language. New York: Wiley.

Liepmann, H. 1914. Bemerkungen zu v. Monakows Kapitel "Die Lokalisation der Apraxie." Monatsschr. Psychiatr. Neurol. 35:490–516.

Naeser, M. A., Alexander, M. P., Helm-Estabrooks, N., Levine, H. L., Laughlin, S. A., and Geschwind, N. 1982. Aphasia with predominantly subcortical lesion sites. Arch. Neurol. 39:2–14.

Miller, G. A. 1981. Language and Speech. San Francisco: Freeman.

Patton, H. D., Sundsten, J. W., Crill, W. E., and Swanson, P. D. 1976. Introduction to Basic Neurology. Philadelphia: Saunders.

Premack, D. 1976. Intelligence in Ape and Man. Hillsdale, N.J.: Erlbaum.

Ross, E. D. 1981. The aprosodias. Arch. Neurol. 38:561–569.

Schwartz, M. F. 1985. Classification of language disorders from a psycholinguistic viewpoint. In J. Oxbury, R. Whurr, M. Coltheart, and M. Wyke (eds.), Aphasia. London: Butterworth.

Skinner, B. F. 1957. Verbal Behavior. New York: Appleton-Century-Crofts.

References

Benson, D. F. 1978. Neurological correlates of aphasia and apraxia. In W. B. Matthews and G. H. Glaser (eds.), Recent Advances in Clinical Neurology, Number 2. Edinburgh: Churchill Livingstone, pp. 163–175.

Benson, D. F., Sheremata, W. A., Bouchard, R., Segarra, J. M., Price, D., and Geschwind, N. 1973. Conduction aphasia. Arch. Neurol. 28:339–346.

Berndt, R. S., and Caramazza, A. 1980. A redefinition of the syndrome of Broca's aphasia: Implications for a neuropsychological model of language. Appl. Psycholinguistics 1:225–278.

Bloom, L. 1970. Language Development: Form and Function in Emerging Grammars. Cambridge, Mass.: MIT Press.

Bloom, L., and Lahey, M. 1978. Language Development and Language Disorders. New York: Wiley.

Bloomfield, L. 1933. Language. New York: Holt, Rinehart and Winston.

Brown, R. 1973. A First Language: The Early Stages. Cambridge, Mass.: Harvard University Press.

Bruner, J. 1983. Child's Talk: Learning to Use Language. New York: Norton.

Chomsky, Noam. 1972. Language and Mind, 2nd ed. New York: Harcourt Brace Jovanovich.

Damasio, H., and Damasio, A. R. 1980. The anatomical basis of conduction aphasia. Brain 103:337–350.

Dejerine, J. 1891. Sur un cas de cécité verbale avec agraphie, suivi d'autopsie. C. R. Séances Mem. Soc. Biol. 43:197–201.

Dejerine, J. 1892. Contribution a l'étude anatomo-pathologique et clinique des différentes variétés de cécité verbale. C. R. Séances Mem. Soc. Biol. 44:61–90.

Eimas, P. D. 1985. The perception of speech in early infancy. Sci. Am. 252(1):46–52.

Galaburda, A. M., and Kemper, T. L. 1979. Cytoarchitectonic abnormalities in developmental dyslexia: A case study. Ann. Neurol. 6:94–100.

Gardner, H. 1974. The Shattered Mind: The Person After Brain Damage. New York: Knopf.

Geschwind, N. 1967. The varieties of naming errors. Cortex 3:97–112.

Geschwind, N. 1971. Current concepts: Aphasia. N. Engl. J. Med. 284:654–656.

Geschwind, N. 1975. The apraxias: Neural mechanisms of disorders of learned movement. Am. Sci. 63:188–195.

Iwata, M. 1984. Kanji versus Kana: Neuropsychological correlates of the Japanese writing system. Trends Neurosci. 74:290–293.

LeMay, M., and Culebras, A. 1972. Human brain—morphologic differences in the hemispheres demonstrable by carotid arteriography. N. Engl. J. Med. 287:168–170.

LeMay, M., and Geschwind, N. 1978. Asymmetries of the human cerebral hemispheres. In A. Caramazza and E. B. Zurif (eds.), Language Acquisition and Language Breakdown: Parallels and Divergencies. Baltimore: Johns Hopkins University Press, pp. 311–328.

Orton, S. T. 1937. Reading, Writing and Speech Problems in Children. New York: Norton..

Rozin, P., Poritsky, S., and Sotsky, R. 1971. American children with reading problems can easily learn to read English represented by Chinese characters. Science 171:1264–1267.

Saffran, E. M. 1982. Neuropsychological approaches to the study of language. Br. J. Psychol. 73:317–337.

Trescher, J. H., and Ford, F. R. 1937. Colloid cyst of the third ventricle. Arch. Neurol. Psychiatry 37:959–973.

Edward J. Sachar

Disorders of Thought:
The Schizophrenic Syndromes

53

Some of the most exciting developments in modern psychiatry have come from the contributions of neurobiology to our understanding of normal and abnormal mental processes. Insights from neurobiology—such as those we encountered in the study of language and hemispheric dominance—have provided a new dimension to our understanding of the nature of our normal conscious experience and our perceptions of ourselves and of the outside world. For example, work on cortical localization has shown that conscious experience is not unitary: we experience different things and carry out different aspects of conscious mentation with the left and the right hemispheres. As a result of these advances, neurobiology is beginning to be in a position to address disorders of thinking and emotion. In this and the next chapter we shall focus on the two most serious mental illnesses, schizophrenia and the affective disorders—diseases that involve serious disturbances in self-awareness, self-perception, state of feeling (or affect), and social interaction.

In addition to being interesting scientifically, schizophrenia and the affective disorders are of great social importance. They are the major causes of psychiatric hospitalization, and their victims fill about 20% of all hospital beds occupied throughout the country. Before the advent of psychotherapeutic agents, the two diseases alone accounted for *half* of *all* hospital bed occupancy. Advances in biochemical understanding and in psychopharmacological treatment have led to an enormous reduction in hospitalization and in human suffering.

The Diagnosis of Mental Illnesses Must Meet Certain Criteria

As we have seen in our discussions of neurological diseases such as myasthenia gravis, research on any illness requires first that the illness be reliably diagnosed. Diagnosis in psychiatry is generally more difficult than in other branches of medicine because the symptoms of mental illness are expressed in behavior, cognition, and subjective feelings, which are considerably more difficult to quantify than pulse, temperature, and blood pressure. This problem is reflected in current difficulties in achieving consensus in independent evaluations of mental symptoms. Furthermore, there are as yet few psychiatric disorders in which the clinical diagnosis has been correlated with demonstrable pathology. The biological defects underlying many of these disorders do not involve the gross anatomical changes seen in most neurological diseases; rather, they probably involve more subtle structural and molecular changes, perhaps akin to those that cause myasthenia gravis. The search for such biological defects has been hampered by the lack of satisfactory animal models for schizophrenia and affective disorders.

To establish a diagnostic category, three criteria should initially be met: (1) a group of symptoms must be identified that can be reliably assessed; (2) these symptoms must be shown to cluster together in certain patients, forming a syndrome; and (3) the group of symptoms must effectively distinguish these patients from others.

The proposed diagnostic category must then be validated against one or more independent measures. Five measures are commonly used to provide this validation.

1. *Clinical course.* A diagnosis is borne out by showing that patients with a particular syndrome also follow a characteristic clinical course (for example, a progressive unremitting social deterioration, or recurrent cycles of recovery followed by relapse of the same type of symptoms).
2. *Natural history.* Diagnosis is validated if the syndrome occurs at a characteristic age or is associated with a specific precipitant.
3. *Response to specific treatment.* The accuracy of a diagnosis may be established by response to treatment. A syndrome may respond relatively specifically to one class of drugs and not to another. Pharmacological specificity has recently proved to be an extremely important validator.
4. *Genetic pedigree.* Validation can be obtained if it can be shown that blood relatives or twins of the patients have a disproportionately higher incidence of the same disorder than the population at large.
5. *Biochemical or hormonal abnormalities.* The demonstration of biological abnormalities associated with the condition provides powerful validation.

The most severe mental disturbances show a clinical course marked by *psychotic episodes*. These are characterized by a loss of reality testing, with profound misinterpretations of perception *(hallucinations)* or markedly aberrant beliefs *(delusions)*. Psychotic episodes are characteristic of both the schizophrenic diseases and the affective disorders. Schizophrenia, which we shall consider in this chapter, is the most crippling of the psychotic illnesses and primarily strikes teenagers and young adults.

Schizophrenia Can Now Be More Accurately Diagnosed

Recent advances in the classification of mental disease have led to the development of rigorous criteria for the reliable diagnosis of schizophrenia and for distinguishing it from other disorders with psychotic episodes that have similar features. These advances—exemplified in the third and greatly revised edition of the *Diagnostic and Statistical Manual of Mental Disorders (DSM-III)*, published in 1980 by the American Psychiatric Association—form the basis of the standard definition of schizophrenia in the United States.

The improved criteria for diagnosing schizophrenia have emerged only gradually from decades of research that began in the early part of the twentieth century with the careful clinical observations of two great pioneers, Emil Kraepelin in Germany and Eugen Bleuler in Switzerland. After observing hundreds of patients, Kraepelin and Bleuler identified two major clinical syndromes that were associated with psychotic episodes and characteristic long-term outcomes. Kraepelin described an illness that he called *dementia praecox* (precocious deterioration of the intellect) because of its early age of onset, usually in adolescence, and his belief that the disease usually followed a progressive course of mental decline leading to *dementia*, a dramatic deterioration of intellectual performance. Kraepelin was careful to distinguish this illness from *manic depressive psychoses*, which have different symptoms and follow a different course characterized not by progressive deterioration but by remissions and relapses.

Bleuler dropped the term dementia praecox because he found some patients in whom the onset occurred in adulthood and because occasional cases remitted. In a detailed analysis of the symptoms, Bleuler came to the conclusion that the disease is probably not a single entity but a group of closely related diseases that are not characterized by a deterioration of the intellect but by a splitting of the cognitive sides of the personality from the affective or emotional side. Bleuler therefore called the disease *schizophrenia*, a splitting of the mind. (This is not to be confused with multiple or split personalities, a rare disease in which a person alternately assumes two or more identities.) A person suffering from schizophrenia may show inappropriate affect by laughing while recounting a tragic event or may show no emotion (a *flattening of affect*) when telling of a joyous experience.

Much of the work following that of Kraepelin and Bleuler has differentiated schizophrenia more clearly from other psychotic disorders that have similar features by using the validating methods described above. In the past, a variety of other mental illnesses have sometimes been confused with schizophrenia or lumped into a common diagnostic category with it. These include manic depressive illness, brief reactive psychoses, paranoid states, and psychoses associated with drug intoxication. Now, on the basis of the modern criteria, each of these disorders can be distinguished and separated from schizophrenia.

The current criteria of schizophrenia require that a patient be continuously ill for at least 6 months and that one or more of the following groups of symptoms be present:

1. Bizarre delusions (for example, of being persecuted or having one's feelings, thoughts, and actions controlled by an outside force).
2. Auditory hallucinations (for example, hearing voices commenting on one's actions).
3. A disorder of thought, consisting of incoherence, loss of the normal association between ideas, or marked poverty of speech accompanied by a loss of emotional responsiveness (flattening of affect) or less specific delusions and hallucinations.

Schizophrenic patients may also exhibit bizarre behavior, unusual postures, mannerisms, or rigidity.

Schizophrenia is characterized by one or more episodes of psychosis, separated by long intervening periods in which the patient is not overtly psychotic but nonetheless is still isolated socially, has a flat affect, lacks motivation, and behaves eccentrically. These distorted behavior patterns are referred to as *residual symptoms*; because of their persistence, in many ways they are the most crippling part of the illness. The 6-month period of illness required for a definitive diagnosis includes the psychotic phase and a time during which there are either prodromal (warning) or residual nonpsychotic symptoms. *Prodromal signs* include social withdrawal, impairment in role-function, odd behavior and ideas, and neglect of personal hygiene. In diagnosing schizophrenia it is important to exclude an affective disorder or an organic mental syndrome. The prognosis of schizophrenia is generally (but not always) poor; often psychotic relapses are frequent, and social functioning decreases progressively as the years go by.

Rather than viewing the purely psychotic episodes and the residual symptoms as different phases of the *same* disease, some students of schizophrenia have proposed that the disorder be divided into two different overlapping syndromes: positive-symptom schizophrenia, in which the symptoms of the psychotic episodes predominate, and negative-symptom schizophrenia, in which the residual symptoms predominate.

Patients said to have *positive-symptom* schizophrenia (the more common of the two forms) manifest blatant psychotic symptoms, such as delusions, hallucinations, and markedly bizarre or disorganized behavior. These positive symptoms tend to respond well to treatment with antipsychotic medication (discussed below). Positive symptoms are often prominent in patients who had functioned relatively well before they became ill and who then improve after an episode of psychosis. Patients said to have *negative-symptom* schizophrenia have symptoms characterized by an absence of certain normal mental functioning. They show a poverty of speech, flattening of affect, poor social adjustment, and impaired attention. These symptoms tend to respond less well to antipsychotic drugs, and when they are predominant, they are indicative of a poorer outcome. As we shall see below, some investigators have proposed that positive symptoms may be due to a specific neurochemical lesion, perhaps involving dopaminergic transmission within the limbic system, whereas negative symptoms might result from more diffuse, and possibly more profound structural brain lesions akin to those seen in dementia.

The distinction between positive and negative symptoms in schizophrenia, which we shall consider in more detail later, reconciles the earlier ideas of Bleuler by arguing that schizophrenia is indeed a group of disorders, of which some lead to a deterioration of the intellect (negative-symptom schizophrenia) and others do not (positive-symptom schizophrenia). We shall here focus primarily on positive-symptom schizophrenia.

There Is an Important Genetic Component to Schizophrenia

The search for the causes of schizophrenia is at present one of the most exciting in psychiatric research. For many years, clinicians and researchers have suspected that schizophrenia is caused by a genetic abnormality. Nonetheless, many clinicians have also argued that social factors, such as poor parenting, contribute importantly to the disorder.

Some of the earliest direct evidence that genes are important to the development of schizophrenia was provided by Franz Kallmann of the New York State Psychiatric Institute at Columbia University. Approximately 1% of the general population suffers from schizophrenia. Except for Ireland, northern Yugoslavia, and parts of Scandinavia, which have slightly higher rates, this figure is fairly uniform throughout the world even though different definitions of schizophrenia are used by clinicians in different countries. Kallmann found that the incidence of schizophrenia among parents, children, and siblings of patients with the disease is much higher than that seen in the general population. Although work following Kallmann's contribution has indicated that the rates may vary somewhat, there is now agreement that approximately 10%–15% of these relatives themselves have schizophrenia (compared with 1% in the population at large). Thus the evidence is strong that the disease tends to run in families. A genetic basis for the disease cannot simply be inferred from the increased incidence in fami-

Table 53–1. Diagnoses of Schizophrenia or Related Disease in Relatives of Schizophrenic Adoptees and in Relatives of Control Adoptees[a]

Psychiatric diagnoses	Biological relatives		Adoptive relatives	
	Schizophrenic	Control	Schizophrenic	Control
Chronic schizophrenia	2.9[b]	0	1.4	1.1
Latent schizophrenia	3.5	1.7	0	1.1
Schizophrenia, uncertain subtype	7.5[b]	1.7	1.4	3.3
Total	14.0[b]	3.4	2.7	5.5

Source: Adapted from Kety et al., 1975.
[a]Expressed as a percentage of total biological and adoptive relatives.
[b]Statistically significant.

lies, however. As Seymour Kety, one of the major investigators of the genetics of mental illness, has observed, not all conditions that run in families are necessarily genetic—wealth and poverty run in families, and even nutritional deficiencies like pellagra used to run in families.

To distinguish genetic from environmental factors—or nature from nurture—Kallmann and other investigators developed several other research designs. One method was to compare the rates of illness in monozygotic and dizygotic twins. Identical (monozygotic) twins have essentially identical genetic material, whereas fraternal (dizygotic) twins share only half of their genetic material and are equivalent to siblings in the genetic sense. Therefore, identical twins should be more or less identical in their tendency to develop an illness such as schizophrenia if the disease is caused entirely by genetic factors. The tendency for twins to have the same illness rates is called *concordance*. The studies on twins established that the concordance rate for schizophrenia in identical twins is about 50%, but it is only about 10% in fraternal twins—about the same as for siblings. If schizophrenia were caused by the genetic abnormalities alone, then the concordance rate of identical twins would be nearly 100%. The 50% rate indicates that genetic factors are not the only cause, but because schizophrenia is five times more likely in identical than in fraternal twins, genetic factors must be nevertheless important.

Some critics argue that the increased concordance rate in identical twins might be partly explained by the psychological trauma of having a schizophrenic identical twin. To address this issue, and to disentangle further the effects of nature and nurture, Leonard Heston studied patients in the United States and David Rosenthal, Paul Wender, and Kety studied patients in Denmark by using a new method, the adopted offspring technique. Heston, Kety, and their colleagues studied adopted children whose biological parents suffered from schizophrenia and compared the rates of schizophrenia in these children to those of adopted children born of normal parents. Since all of the children were adopted, social factors were well controlled. These children were reared apart from their biological parents in homes where the adoptive parents were free of psychiatric illness, so the environmental effects of being reared by an ill or well parent were eliminated.

These studies have consistently found an increased rate of schizophrenia in the adopted children of schizophrenic parents as compared with adopted children of nonschizophrenic parents. The difference in rate—about 10%–15%—is the same as was observed in the earlier family studies by Kallmann and others. In control samples the rate was the same as in the general population (Table 53–1). These studies also found that even when not overtly schizophrenic, the children of schizophrenic parents tended to be odd; they showed social isolation and poor rapport with people, and had a rambling and tangential speech. The children of schizophrenic parents also tended to be suspicious, to have eccentric beliefs, and to engage in obsessional or magical thinking. This group of symptoms, which has been called the *schizotypal personality disorder*, may represent a nonpsychotic condition that is genetically related to schizophrenia.

The genetic studies have revolutionized our thinking about schizophrenia. Many earlier observations suggested that schizophrenia is a disorder caused primarily by psychosocial and environmental factors, particularly by pathological parenting. For example, it was observed that mothers of schizophrenic patients were often odd individuals with disturbed patterns of thinking and of communicating. The investigators in these earlier studies probably were mistaking the signs of a *hereditary disorder* that affects both parent and child for a *pathogenic* psychosocial interaction between parent and child. In reality, both genes and environment are involved inextricably.

Specific Drugs Are Effective in the Treatment of Schizophrenia

The evidence from genetic research that there is a specific inherited cause of some cases of schizophrenia was soon supplemented by insights into the nature of the dis-

A
Phenothiazine derivatives

Phenothiazine nucleus

	R_1	R_2
		Aliphatic
Chlorpromazine	—Cl	$-CH_2-CH_2-CH_2-N(CH_3)_2$
Trifluopromazine	$-CF_3$	$-CH_2-CH_2-CH_2-N(CH_3)_2$
		Peperidine
Thioridazine	$-SCH_3$	$-CH_2-CH_2-$ (piperidine ring with N—CH$_3$)
Mesoridazine	$-\overset{O}{\underset{\|}{S}}-CH_3$	$-CH_2-CH_2-$ (piperidine ring with N—CH$_3$)
Piperacetazine	$-\overset{O}{\underset{\|}{C}}CH_3$	$-CH_2-CH_2-CH_2-N$ (piperidine ring) $-CH_2-CH_2-OH$
		Piperazine
Prochlorperazine	—Cl	$-CH_2-CH_2-CH_2-N$ (piperazine) $N-CH_3$
Trifluoperazine	$-CF_3$	$-CH_2-CH_2-CH_2-N$ (piperazine) $N-CH_3$
Butaperazine	$-\overset{O}{\underset{\|}{C}}(CH_2)_2CH_3$	$-CH_2-CH_2-CH_2-N$ (piperazine) $N-CH_3$
Perphenazine	—Cl	$-CH_2-CH_2-CH_2-N$ (piperazine) $N-CH_2-CH_2-OH$
Fluphenazine	$-CF_3$	$-CH_2-CH_2-CH_2-N$ (piperazine) $N-CH_2-CH_2-OH$
Acetophenazine	$-\overset{O}{\underset{\|}{C}}CH_3$	$-CH_2-CH_2-CH_2-N$ (piperazine) $N-CH_2-CH_2-OH$
Carphenazine	$-\overset{O}{\underset{\|}{C}}CH_2CH_3$	$-CH_2-CH_2-CH_2-N$ (piperazine) $N-CH_2-CH_2-OH$
Thiopropazate	—Cl	$-CH_2-CH_2-CH_2-N$ (piperazine) $N-CH_2-CH_2-O-\overset{O}{\underset{\|}{C}}-CH_3$

order that were derived from neuropharmacology. Antipsychotic drugs introduced during the 1950s were found to be very effective in treating the symptoms of schizophrenia, and these drugs shed further light on the nature of the underlying pathological process.

Until the 1950s no treatment was specifically effective for schizophrenia. The introduction of reserpine and, particularly, in 1954, of the phenothiazines (beginning with chlorpromazine), followed by butyrophenones (e.g., haloperidol) and then other chemical classes of antipsy-

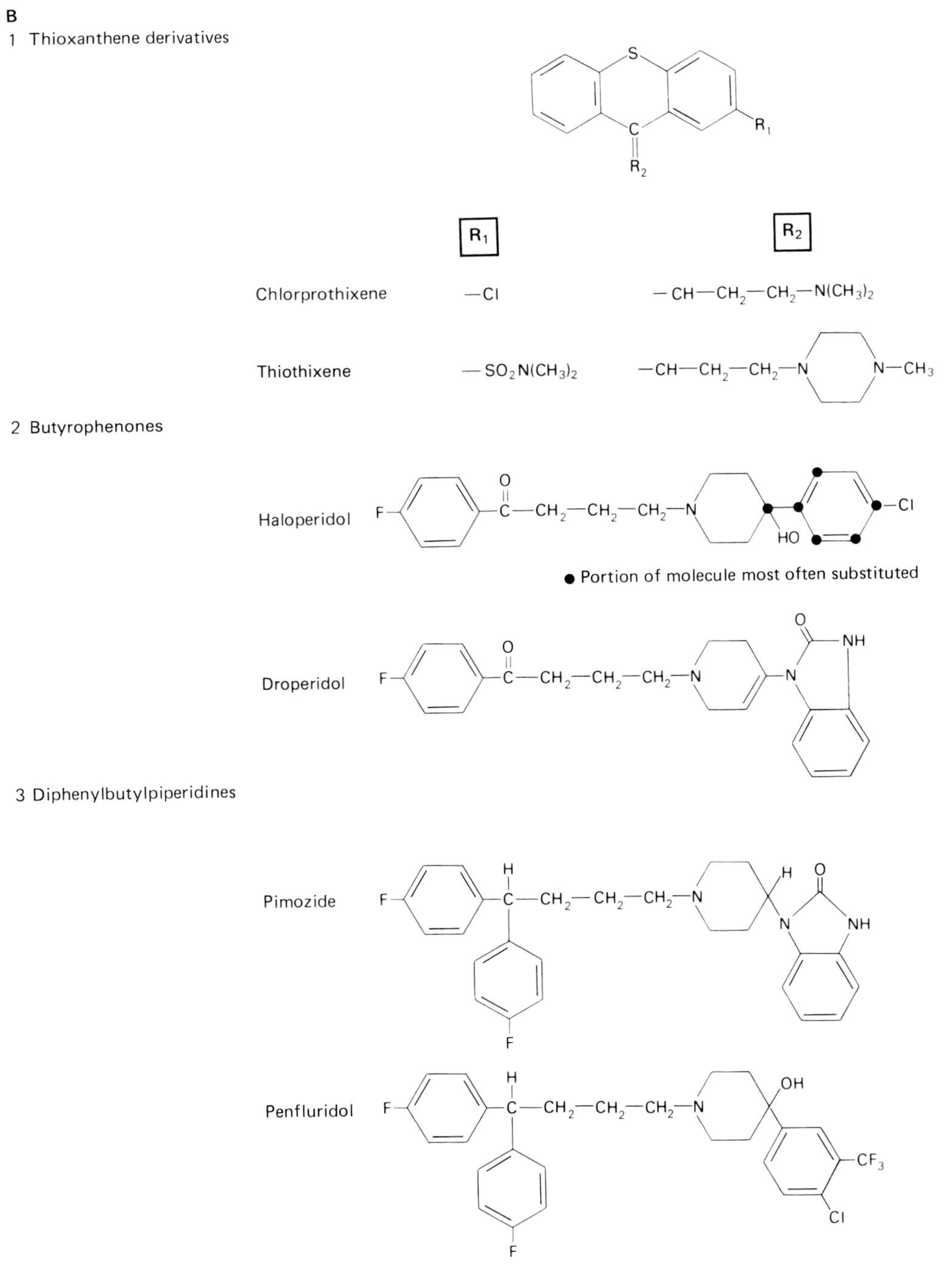

B
1 Thioxanthene derivatives

| R₁ | R₂ |

Chlorprothixene $-Cl$ $-CH-CH_2-CH_2-N(CH_3)_2$

Thiothixene $-SO_2N(CH_3)_2$ $-CH-CH_2-CH_2-NN-CH_3$

2 Butyrophenones

Haloperidol

● Portion of molecule most often substituted

Droperidol

3 Diphenylbutylpiperidines

Pimozide

Penfluridol

53–1 Drugs used to treat schizophrenia. An aromatic (benzene-type) moiety is indicated in some of the structures. **A.** Structural relationships of phenothiazines. **B.** Structural relationships of thioxanthene derivatives, butyrophenones, and diphenylbutylpiperidines. (Adapted from Kety et al., 1975.)

chotic drugs (e.g., thioxanthenes) (Figure 53–1), dramatically improved the treatment of the psychotic phase of schizophrenia. Originally it was believed that these drugs were primarily tranquilizers, calming patients without unduly sedating them. These agents do have a fast effect, calming the acutely agitated, excited, assaultive patient within hours. However, by 1964 it was established that the drugs also have a delayed but powerful therapeutic effect on the positive symptoms of schizophrenia: over several weeks, they improve or abolish the delusions,

Table 53–2. Differential Response of Schizophrenic Symptoms to Phenothiazines

Symptoms of schizophrenia	Response
Primary	
Thought disorder	+ + +
Blunted affect	+ + +
Withdrawal	+ + +
Autistic behavior	+ + +
Accessory	
Hallucinations	+ +
Paranoid ideation	+
Grandiosity	+
Hostility, belligerence	0
Nonschizophrenic	
Anxiety, tension, agitation	0
Guilt, depression	0

Source: Adapted from Klein and Davis, 1969.

hallucinations, and some types of disordered thinking (Table 53–2). Maintaining remitted patients on antipsychotic medication also sharply reduces the rate of relapse.

Antischizophrenic Drugs Affect Dopaminergic Transmission

The effectiveness of the antipsychotic drugs suggests that positive-symptom schizophrenia may result from a biochemical defect in the brain, the nature of which may be inferred from the mode of action of the drugs. The first clue to the cellular action of these drugs came from an analysis of their major side effects. The drugs often produce a syndrome resembling parkinsonism (hence the term *neuroleptic,* meaning an agent that stimulates the nervous system). As in parkinsonism, this drug-induced extrapyramidal syndrome is reversed by anticholinergic agents. Because parkinsonism is thought to be due to a deficiency in dopaminergic transmission (see Chapter 40), this side effect suggested that antischizophrenic drugs interfere with the action of dopaminergic neurons. Following an initial suggestion by the Swedish pharmacologist Arvid Carlsson, a series of investigations established that despite differences in their chemical structure (Figure 53–1), all the effective antischizophrenic agents interfere with dopaminergic transmission and that they do this mostly by blocking dopamine receptors (Figure 53–2). Moreover, almost all drugs that block dopaminergic transmission have therapeutic effects in schizophrenia. Thus, although each of the antischizophrenic drugs acts

53–2 The therapeutic potency of antipsychotic drugs approximates their relative ability to inhibit dopamine release and bind to dopamine receptors. **A.** Drugs are arranged along the horizontal axis in terms of the average daily dose prescribed for schizophrenia; **horizontal bars** indicate the range of clinical doses. Along the vertical axis is a measurement of the inhibition of dopamine release from presynaptic cells, by

equal amounts of each drug. (From Seeman and Lee, 1975.) **B.** The clinical potencies of neuroleptic drugs are compared with potencies of the same drug doses in displacing ^{3}H-haloperidol from dopamine receptor sites in vitro in calf caudate nucleus membranes. Ordinate **IC$_{50}$**, drug concentration required to displace 50% of specific ^{3}H-haloperidol binding. (From Seeman et al., 1976.)

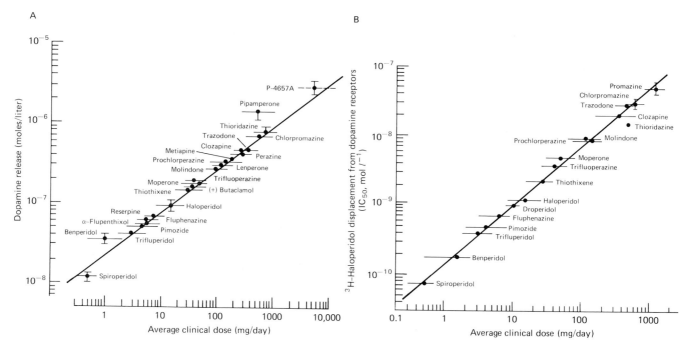

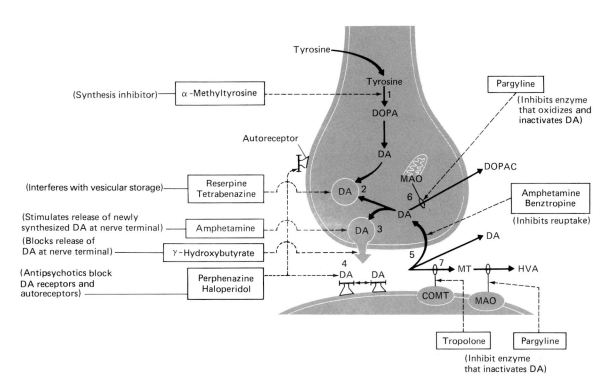

53–3 The key steps in the synthesis and degradation of dopamine (**DA**) and the sites of action of various psychoactive substances are shown in this dopaminergic synapse. (Adapted from Cooper, Bloom, and Roth, 1982.)

1: Enzymatic synthesis. The conversion of tyrosine to DOPA by tyrosine hydroxylase is blocked by the competitive inhibitor α-methyltyrosine and other tyrosine hydroxylase inhibitors.

2: Storage. Reserpine and tetrabenazine interfere with the uptake and storage of dopamine by the storage granules. The depletion of dopamine produced by reserpine is long-lasting and the storage granules appear to be irreversibly damaged. Tetrabenazine also interferes with the uptake and storage mechanism of the granules, but only transiently.

3: Release. γ-Hydroxybutyrate effectively blocks the release of dopamine by blocking impulse flow in dopaminergic neurons. Amphetamine administered in high doses releases dopamine, but most of the releasing ability of amphetamine appears to be related to its ability to effectively block dopamine reuptake.

4: Receptor interaction. The antipsychotic drugs such as perphenazine and haloperidol are dopamine receptor-blockers that are particularly effective on the D2 and the autoreceptors.

5: Reuptake. Dopamine has its action terminated by being taken up into the presynaptic terminal. Amphetamine, as well as the anticholinergic drug benztropine, is a potent inhibitor of this reuptake mechanism.

6: Monoamine oxidase (**MAO**). Dopamine present in a free state within the presynaptic terminal can be degraded by the enzyme MAO, which appears to be located in the outer membrane of the mitochondria. Dihydroxyphenylacetic acid (**DOPAC**) is a product of the action of MAO and aldehyde oxidase on dopamine. Pargyline is an effective inhibitor of MAO. Some MAO is also present outside the dopaminergic neuron.

7: Catechol-O-methyltransferase (**COMT**). Dopamine can be inactivated by the enzyme COMT, which is believed to be localized outside the presynaptic neuron. Tropolone is an inhibitor of COMT.

somewhat differently on the central nervous system, interference with dopaminergic transmission appears to be a common feature of all the antipsychotic agents.

Four key observations implicate blockage of dopaminergic transmission in the action of antischizophrenic drugs: *first,* antischizophrenic agents are ligands for dopamine receptors. When tested in cell-free binding assays with membranes isolated from nervous tissue, they displace dopamine and other neuroleptics. More persuasively, the milligram-for-milligram potency of the antipsychotic drugs in binding to dopamine receptors in filter assays closely approximates the relative therapeutic potency of these agents (Figure 53–2). Originally these drugs were thought to exert their action by blocking all dopamine receptors equally. Recent evidence suggests, however, that there are at least two (and perhaps several) types of dopamine receptor. One type (called *dopamine receptor D1*) *activates* adenylate cyclase (the enzyme that converts ATP to cyclic AMP; see Chapter 14). This receptor is located postsynaptically and has a low affinity for most types of antipsychotic drugs. A second type of receptor (called *dopamine receptor D2*), also located postsynaptically, is linked to a regulatory protein that *inhibits* adenylate cyclase activity. The D2 receptor has a high affinity for all antipsychotic drugs and is thought to be one of these sites where these drugs exert their major actions.

In addition to the D1 and D2 receptors on the postsynaptic target cells of dopaminergic neurons, the dopaminergic neurons themselves have an *inhibitory autoreceptor*. (This receptor type is not yet well characterized but is not linked to an adenylate cyclase.) These autoreceptors are thought to be the second site where the antipsychotic drugs exert their actions. These receptors are located on the cell body and on the presynaptic terminals of the dopaminergic neuron and control both the rate of firing and the release of dopamine by the action potentials that invade the terminal (Figure 53–3).

The *second* observation implicating blockage of dopaminergic transmission stems from the initially paradoxical finding that antischizophrenic drugs lead to increased concentrations of dopamine's breakdown product (homovanillic acid, HVA) in the cerebrospinal fluid and other body fluids. These drugs must therefore increase the firing of dopaminergic neurons, which has recently been shown to be at least partly caused by blocking the inhibitory dopamine autoreceptor or by some other inhibitory feedback effect.

Third, dopaminergic agonists—such as L-dihydroxyphenylalanine (L-DOPA), amphetamine, and apomorphine—cause a characteristic stereotyped behavioral syndrome in animals. In rats this syndrome involves sniffing and gnawing, and in higher animals such as monkeys it involves bizarre repetitive acts very much like those observed in amphetamine addicts. Amphetamine psychosis is the closest drug model to schizophrenia that has been observed in humans. Antischizophrenic drugs appear to act as a selective antidote not only to this stereotyped behavior in animals, but also to amphetamine psychosis in humans, providing further support for the relationship between dopamine and schizophrenia.

Fourth, neuroleptics stimulate the secretion of prolactin by the pituitary, often causing nursing women to discharge excess milk even after the child has been weaned. Dopamine appears to be the major substance inhibiting prolactin secretion, acting at the D2 receptors in the pituitary gland. Thus, measuring levels of prolactin in human beings is a simple means of monitoring effects on the dopamine receptors in the pituitary. These effects also support the idea that antischizophrenic drugs act by blocking dopaminergic transmission.

The antischizophrenic drugs do not act only on dopaminergic transmission. Some agents affect other transmitter systems. For example, chlorpromazine has some blocking action on the receptor for norepinephrine and for serotonin, and all phenothiazines cause a secondary increase in the synthesis of monoamine transmitters. However, these actions do not correlate with clinical potency and may be responsible instead for some of the side effects of the drugs.

A Dopamine Hypothesis of Schizophrenia Has Been Proposed

Two types of evidence have led to the development of the hypothesis that schizophrenia results from an excess of dopaminergic transmission. The first type, described above, is that antischizophrenic drugs act on dopamine receptors. The second is that dopamine agonists (Figure 53–4) and other drugs that enhance the action of dopamine (cocaine, amphetamine, and L-DOPA) can induce psychotic syndromes resembling paranoid schizophrenia.

Several molecular mechanisms might explain the disease: (1) too much dopamine is released by dopaminergic neurons; (2) dopaminergic receptors are hypersensitive to the normal amount of dopamine released; (3) the number of dopaminergic receptors is increased, leading to a functional increase in sensitivity to a normal amount of dopamine; (4) an antagonistic neurotransmitter system is underactive; or (5) there is a malfunction of a feedback pathway (neuronal or hormonal) that controls a component of the dopamine system.

These possibilities are listed to indicate that a variety of cellular mechanisms might alter synaptic transmission and that we need to be cautious about simplifying

53–4 Chemical structures of dopamine agonists.

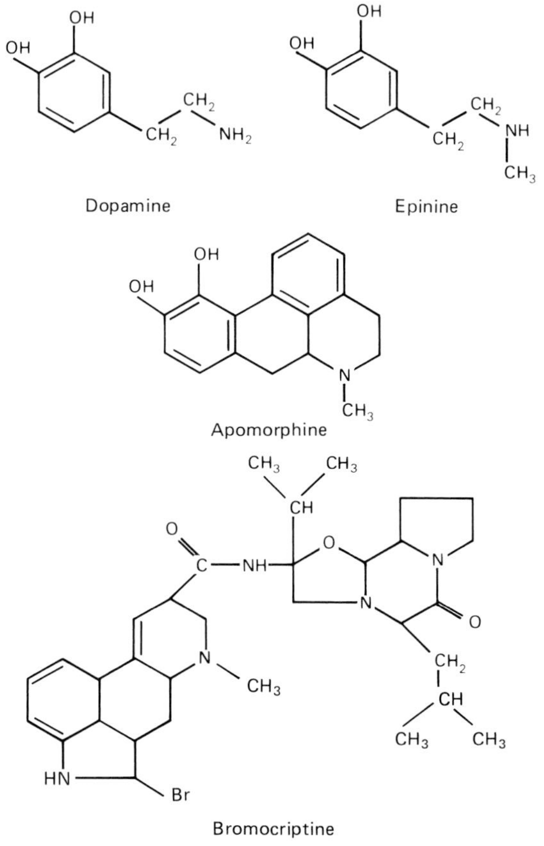

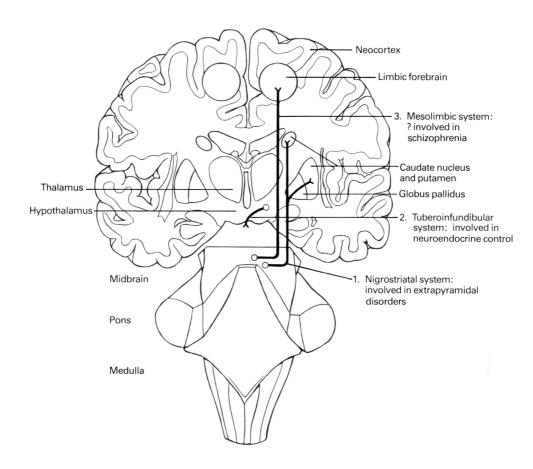

Neocortex

Limbic forebrain

3. Mesolimbic system:
   ? involved in
   schizophrenia

Caudate nucleus
and putamen

Globus pallidus

2. Tuberoinfundibular
   system: involved in
   neuroendocrine control

1. Nigrostriatal system:
   involved in extrapyramidal
   disorders

Thalamus

Hypothalamus

Midbrain

Pons

Medulla

hypotheses. At the moment, there is no compelling evidence that excessive activity of dopaminergic neurons (or any other disturbance of dopaminergic transmission) underlies schizophrenia. Nevertheless, the idea has received some indirect support. Several investigators have demonstrated an increased number of D2 receptors in tissue from the brains of schizophrenics studied at autopsy. This increase has been noted in the caudate nucleus, nucleus accumbens (part of the limbic system), and olfactory tubercle. Moreover, this observation of increased D2 receptors has been extended to the brains of schizophrenic patients who have never been treated with any type of medication, so that the finding cannot be explained as a secondary effect of drug treatment.

The Neuropathology of Schizophrenia Might Be Located in the Mesolimbic Dopaminergic System

The possibility that dopaminergic transmission is disturbed in schizophrenia raises further questions. There are many components to the dopamine system in the brain. Which component is critical for schizophrenia? The suggestion that a disorder in dopaminergic transmission is involved in schizophrenia is analogous to knowing that a disorder of cholinergic transmission is in-

53–5 There are three major central dopaminergic tracts.

volved in myasthenia gravis without knowing that the defect is located at the synapse between motor neurons and voluntary muscle. In schizophrenia (as in depressive disorders, which will be considered in Chapter 54), the challenge is to move from an initial set of pharmacological clues to more precise anatomical localization.

Formaldehyde-induced histofluorescence microscopy (see Chapter 13) has been very helpful in this regard. It has revealed that there are three principal (and several minor) dopaminergic systems in the brain (Figure 53–5): the nigrostriatal, mesolimbic, and tuberoinfundibular.

The *nigrostriatal system* involves dopaminergic cell bodies located in the substantia nigra with axons that project primarily to the putamen and the caudate nucleus. As was pointed out in Chapter 40, partial degeneration of this system contributes importantly to the pathogenesis of Parkinson's disease. This may also be the system involved in the long-term side effects of antipsychotics, known as *tardive dyskinesia,* as well as other, short-term side effects such as hand tremor and rigidity of muscles.

In the *mesolimbic system*, dopaminergic cell bodies are located in the ventral tegmental area of Tsai, medial and superior to the substantia nigra. The axons of these cells project to the limbic system—specifically to the mesial components, the nucleus accumbens, the olfactory tubercle, the nuclei of the stria terminalis, and parts of the amygdala—and to the lateral septal nuclei, the mesial frontal, anterior cingulate, and entorhinal cortex.

In the *tuberoinfundibular system*, dopaminergic cell bodies in the arcuate nucleus of the median eminence project their axons to the pituitary stalk. This system is important for prolactin regulation.

The role of the limbic system in emotions and in memory (see Chapters 46 and 61) and the superficial similarity between schizophrenia and certain types of psychomotor epilepsy have encouraged the speculation that a dysfunction in the mesolimbic system may be involved in the etiology of schizophrenia. Among the projections of the mesolimbic dopaminergic system, the projection to the nucleus accumbens is receiving the most attention. This is because of the suggestion that the nucleus accumbens and its related structures serve as *gates or filters* for information concerned with affect and with certain types of memory projections from the hippocampus to other parts of the brain (hypothalamus and frontal cortex), and that the dopaminergic projection modulates the flow of neural activity through this filter network. The nucleus accumbens is located between the anterior pole of the caudate nucleus, the olfactory tubercle, and the septum. This nucleus (as well as the other targets of the mesolimbic dopaminergic projection) receives massive converging input from the hippocampus and the amygdala, and projects in turn to the septum, hypothalamus, and frontal lobe—areas that might well be involved in schizophrenia.

There Are Important Weaknesses in the Dopamine Hypothesis

There are, however, problems with the dopamine hypothesis of schizophrenia from both a conceptual and a clinical point of view. Conceptually, it is difficult to extrapolate from the mechanisms of action of a therapeutic agent to the causal mechanisms of the disease, since pharmacological manipulation may produce changes that compensate for the disease without directly affecting the disordered mechanism itself. For example, the primary defect in Parkinson's disease is a decrease in dopamine, but the symptoms are alleviated by anticholinergic drugs. This issue can be further illustrated by referring to a simple model (Figure 53–6). Consider the hypothetical situation of four presynaptic neurons converging on a postsynaptic neuron, with each presynaptic neuron releasing a different transmitter (transmitters A, B, and C and dopamine). Transmitter A and dopamine inhibit the postsynaptic cell, whereas transmitters B and C excite it. If schizophrenia resulted from a defect in neuron A or its

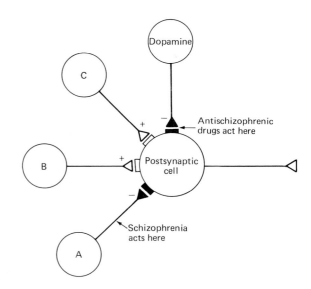

53–6 This scheme shows how an antischizophrenic drug could ameliorate a neural imbalance due to excessive inhibitory action on a particular set of neurons, such as might be caused by schizophrenia, without directly acting on the neurons that are disordered by the disease. Assume that schizophrenia is due to a synaptic imbalance at a particular neural structure as a result of inhibition exceeding excitation due to overactivity of inhibitory neuron A. Blocking the effectiveness of a parallel dopaminergic inhibitory neuron could ameliorate the disease by reducing the net inhibition converging on the postsynaptic cell. (Adapted from R. Zigmond, personal communication.)

transmitter that caused an excess of this inhibitory transmitter to act on the postsynaptic cell, one might improve the symptoms by simply blocking the action of dopamine, the other inhibitory transmitter, because this intervention would reduce net inhibition onto the postsynaptic cell. However, this model could easily prove inadequate. For instance, the dopamine neuron and neuron A might have very different inputs converging on them. If so, inhibiting dopaminergic transmission might not be an effective treatment. Even this simple example illustrates that a correlation between excess dopamine and schizophrenia is not sufficient to allow a conclusion about the underlying cause of the disease. Information on the molecular basis of the disease is thus incomplete.

From a clinical standpoint, the time course of action of antipsychotic drugs also must be explained. These drugs block dopamine receptors rapidly, but the schizophrenic psychosis remits gradually over several weeks. This disparity suggests that blocking dopaminergic transmission may have secondary consequences on other neuronal systems, consequences that evolve over a period of several weeks. Furthermore, neuroleptics are most effective in treating or preventing blatant positive symptoms, such as hallucinations and delusions. They are relatively ineffective for the defect or negative symptoms—low motivation, shallow affect, and social incompetence—that constitute such a serious aspect of schizophrenia. The drugs do not worsen the negative syndrome, but they do not alleviate it; indeed, there is as yet no effective treatment for the negative aspects of the disease, which in many schizophrenics precede the first psychotic episode and later dominate. This observation lends further support to the idea that this category of schizophrenia should be separated from that in which the positive symptoms predominate.

Negative Symptoms of Schizophrenia May Have Other Causes

Although the dopamine hypothesis is perhaps the most influential theory of the cause of schizophrenia, other mechanisms may be involved. Disturbances in other neurotransmitter systems in the brain, including the peptides, have been suggested as being important.

However, except for the dopaminergic disturbance, the only other convincing clues about the nature of the disease have come from anatomical studies of patients with predominantly negative-symptom schizophrenia. Computerized tomography has revealed that some schizophrenic patients suffer from diffuse atrophy of the brain: this atrophy involves the cerebral cortex and the cerebellum, and leads to ventricular enlargement. The discovery of ventricular enlargement has now been thoroughly documented and is often associated with the negative symptoms of schizophrenia (poverty of speech, affective flattening, retardation, and asociality). These patients often have a history of poor social functioning before the onset of schizophrenic symptoms, suggesting that the disease starts early in life. They also have cognitive impairments, and they respond poorly to neuroleptic drugs. Ventricular enlargement, although characteristic of this particular group of patients, is not present in all patients suffering from negative-symptom schizophrenia, nor is it specific to this disease. For example, this abnormality also occurs in patients with dementia of the Alzheimer's type.

Are There Two Distinct but Overlapping Forms of Schizophrenia?

By providing clear evidence that some patients with negative symptoms have atrophy of the brain and enlargement of the ventricles, brain imaging techniques have made a dramatic impact on the study of schizophrenia. On the basis of these studies a new hypothesis has been suggested for classifying major subtypes within the broad category of schizophrenia. According to this view, one type of schizophrenia is characterized by predominately positive symptoms such as delusions and hallucinations. This type is thought to have an underlying pathophysiology involving excessive dopaminergic transmission in the limbic system. The other type, a minority type, is

characterized by predominately negative symptoms, and is thought to be due to diffuse neuronal loss as reflected by brain atrophy shown on computerized tomography scanning.

Other techniques for brain imaging, such as the use of positron emission tomography, magnetic resonance imaging, and studies of cerebral blood flow are now being applied in research on schizophrenia. These techniques should help to clarify the specific anatomical systems involved in both the positive- and negative-symptom forms of schizophrenia.

Selected Readings

Andreasen, N. C., Olsen, S. A., Dennert, J. W., and Smith, M. R. 1982. Ventricular enlargement in schizophrenia: Relationship to positive and negative symptoms. Am. J. Psychiatry 139:297–302.

Creese, I., Sibley, D. R., Hamblin, M. W., and Leff, S. E. 1983. The classification of dopamine receptors: Relationship to radioligand binding. Annu. Rev. Neurosci. 6:43–71.

Crow, T. J. 1980. Molecular pathology of schizophrenia: More than one disease process? Br. Med. J. 280:66–68.

Hart, B. D. 1962. The Psychology of Insanity. Cambridge, England: Cambridge University Press.

Klein, D. F., Gittelman, R., Quitkin, F., and Rifkin, A. 1980. Diagnosis and Drug Treatment of Psychiatric Disorders: Adults and Children, 2nd ed. Baltimore: Williams & Wilkins.

Reveley, A. M., Reveley, M.A., Clifford, C. A., and Murray, R. M. 1982. Cerebral ventricular size in twins discordant for schizophrenia. Lancet 1:540–541.

Snyder, S. H. 1982. Neurotransmitters and CNS disease: Schizophrenia. Lancet 2:970–974.

Weinberger, D. R., Wagner, R. L., and Wyatt, R. J. 1983. Neuropathological studies of schizophrenia: A selective review. Schizophr. Bull. 9:193–212.

References

Bleuler, E. 1911. Dementia Praecox or the Group of Schizophrenias. J. Zinkin (trans.). New York: International Universities Press, 1950.

Carlsson, A. 1974. Antipsychotic drugs and catecholamine synapses. J. Psychiatr. Res. 11:57–64.

Cooper, J. R., Bloom, F. E., and Roth, R. H. 1982. The Biochemical Basis of Neuropharmacology, 4th ed. New York: Oxford University Press.

Creese, I. 1982. Dopamine receptors explained. Trends Neurosci. 5:40–43.

Davis, J. M., and Garver, D. L. 1978. Neuroleptics: Clinical use in psychiatry. In L. L. Iversen, S. D. Iversen, and S. H. Snyder (eds.), Handbook of Psychopharmacology, Vol. 10: Neuroleptics and Schizophrenia. New York: Plenum Press, pp. 129–164.

Heston, L. L. 1970. The genetics of schizophrenic and schizoid disease. Science 167:249–256.

Kallmann, F. J. 1938. The Genetics of Schizophrenia. New York: Augustin.

Kety, S. S., Rosenthal, D., Wender, P. H., Schulsinger, F., and Jacobsen, B. 1975. Mental illness in the biological and adoptive families of adopted individuals who have become schizophrenic: A preliminary report based on psychiatric interviews. In R. R. Fieve, D. Rosenthal, and H. Brill (eds.), Genetic Research in Psychiatry. Baltimore: Johns Hopkins University Press, pp. 147–165.

Klein, D. F., and Davis, J. M. 1969. Diagnosis and Drug Treatment of Psychiatric Disorders. Baltimore: Williams & Wilkins.

Kraepelin, E. 1909. Dementia Praecox and Paraphrenia. From Kraepelin's Text-Book of Psychiatry, 8th ed. R. M. Barclay (trans.). Edinburgh: Livingstone, 1919.

Matthysse, S. W., and Kety, S. S. (eds.). 1975. Catecholamines and Schizophrenia. Oxford: Pergamon Press.

Nauta, W. J. H., Smith, G. P., Faull, R. L. M., and Domesick, V. B. 1978. Efferent connections and nigral afferents of the nucleus accumbens septi in the rat. Neuroscience 3:385–401.

Roberts, P. J., Woodruff, G. N., and Iversen, L. L. (eds.). 1978. Advances in Biochemical Psychopharmacology, Vol. 19: Dopamine. New York: Raven Press.

Seeman, P., and Lee, T. 1975. Antipsychotic drugs: Direct correlation between clinical potency and presynaptic action on dopamine neurons. Science 188:1217–1219.

Seeman, P., Lee, T., Chau-Wong, M. and Wong, K. 1976. Antipsychotic drug doses and neuroleptic/dopamine receptors. Nature 261:717–719.

Edward J. Sachar

Disorders of Feeling: Affective Diseases

54

Mental illnesses involving depression and mania are called *affective disorders* because a prominent aspect of these illnesses is a disturbance of affect—mood or state of feeling. One type of affective disorder, major depression, was described by Hippocrates. He proposed that moods depend upon the balance of four humors—blood, phlegm, yellow bile, and black bile—and attributed depression to an excess of black bile ("melancholia"). Though his explanation of the etiology of depression seems fanciful today, Hippocrates was correct in asserting that the most profound psychological disorders arise from physiological processes.

Efforts to update Hippocrates' original psychobiological formulation were hindered until recently by an inability to diagnose depressive states precisely. As Freud pointed out in 1917 in a paper entitled "Mourning and Melancholia," "Even in descriptive psychiatry the definition of melancholia is uncertain; it takes on various clinical forms (some of them suggesting somatic rather than psychogenic affections) that do not seem definitely to warrant reduction to a unity." In the past two decades, criteria for classifying affective disorders have been developed on the basis of the strategies for validating diagnostic categories outlined in Chapter 53. From the welter of human conditions involving unhappiness, misery, grief, disappointment, and despair have emerged certain depressive syndromes that are readily distinguishable. In this chapter, we shall focus on two of these syndromes: the major depressive disorders of the unipolar (recurrent depressive) and bipolar (manic depressive) types.

The Clinical Features of Major Depressive Disorders Suggest a Defect in the Hypothalamus

Unipolar (Recurrent Depressive) Disorders

The clinical features of unipolar major depression can be briefly summarized. Untreated, the usual episode of depression lasts 4–12 months and is characterized by a pervasive dysphoric (unpleasant) mood and a generalized loss of interests and the ability to experience pleasure. In Hamlet's words: "How weary, stale, flat, and unprofitable seem to me all the uses of this world!" The diagnosis also requires several additional symptoms: disturbed sleep (usually insomnia, with early morning awakening), diminished appetite, loss of energy, decreased sex drive, psychomotor agitation (restlessness) or retardation (slowing down of thoughts and actions), difficulty in concentrating, and guilty, pessimistic, and suicidal thoughts. These symptoms may reach unmanageable proportions. Although not required for diagnosis, other common symptoms are constipation, decreased salivation, and a diurnal variation in severity of symptoms—they are usually worse in the morning. In addition to the inclusion criteria, there are exclusion criteria; for example, there should be no signs of schizophrenia or neurological disease. When the syndrome is defined in this manner, at any given time about 4% of the world's population suffers from depression—8,000,000 people in the United States alone.

Severe depression can be profoundly debilitating. In extreme cases, patients may cease to eat or to maintain basic personal cleanliness. Because they are so passive, severely depressed people are a relatively low suicide risk; the risk increases significantly as they begin to recover.

Several features of depression suggest that an intrinsic regulatory defect underlies this disorder. Many of the characteristic symptoms point to a disturbance of functions that are regulated, at least in part, by the hypothalamus: pervasive disorders of mood, appetite, sexual drive, sleep, and autonomic and motor activity (see Chapters 46 and 47). When these features are prominent, the syndrome is called *endogenous depression* or *melancholia*. The insomnia of endogenous depression is associated with characteristic sleep abnormalities (as recorded by the electroencephalogram) that are not seen in ordinary patients suffering from insomnia, although they are sometimes seen in patients with other forms of depression.

Although the median age is approximately 40 years, the first episode of the illness can occur at almost any age. Indeed, young children can develop depression, and the disorder is not uncommon in adolescence. Women are affected about two to three times more often than men. In at least 60% of episodes in both sexes, no significant psychosocial precipitating factors are evident. Even in those cases in which a psychosocial precipitant is found, once the condition is established, it typically appears to be autonomous; it is relatively unresponsive to psychotherapy or environmental changes. In contrast, as we shall see below, treatment with medication or electroconvulsive therapy is quite effective. Although some people suffer only a single episode, the illness is often recurrent.

Bipolar (Manic Depressive) Disorders

Patients with bipolar disorders suffer both depressive and manic episodes. The illness affects men and women equally, and the average age of onset is a decade younger than that of unipolar depression. The depressions are clinically similar to those seen in unipolar illness. The mania is characterized by an elevated, expansive, or irritable mood lasting at least 1 week, associated with several of the following symptoms: overactivity, overtalkativeness, increased energy and libido, pressure of ideas, grandiosity, distractibility, decreased need for sleep, and reckless involvements. In severe cases the patients are delusional.

As in unipolar depression, the bipolar syndrome suggests an impairment of hypothalamic functions, with disturbances in mood, energy, appetite, sleep, and sexual function. Most episodes have no detectable psychosocial precipitant. The bipolar disorder is also a recurrent illness, and subsequent affective episodes of both types occur about twice as often as in unipolar disease.

There Is a Strong Genetic Predisposition for the Major Depressions

As in schizophrenia, genetic factors are important in both unipolar and bipolar affective disorders. The morbidity rate of depression in first-degree relatives (parents, siblings, and children) of patients with depressive illness is much higher than that seen in the general population. As with schizophrenia, the overall concordance rate for identical twin pairs is approximately 50%; the rate for fraternal twins is approximately 10% (the same as for siblings).

Seymour Kety, Paul H. Wender, and David Rosenthal have extended their studies of schizophrenia in adopted people and studied the adoptive and biological families of adoptees with manic depressive disorders. They again investigated the genetic predisposition by evaluating the biological relatives and the environmental contribution by evaluating the adoptive relatives. These investigators found a higher rate of affective illness in the biological parents of adoptees who grew up to develop manic depressive illness than in their adoptive parents or in the biological and adoptive parents of mentally healthy adoptees. As might be expected, the incidence of suicide among biological relatives of adoptees who suffered from depression was 6–10 times higher than among the relatives of normal adoptees (Figure 54–1).

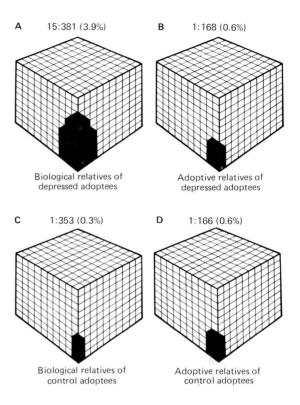

A   15:381 (3.9%)

Biological relatives of
depressed adoptees

B   1:168 (0.6%)

Adoptive relatives of
depressed adoptees

C   1:353 (0.3%)

Biological relatives of
control adoptees

D   1:166 (0.6%)

Adoptive relatives of
control adoptees

54–1 Incidence of suicides among biological and adoptive relatives of depressed patients. There is a higher incidence of suicide among biological relatives of adoptees who suffered from bipolar depression (**A**) than among their adoptive relatives (**B**) and among the biological (**C**) and adoptive (**D**) relatives of mentally healthy adoptees. Each ratio shows the number of relatives who committed suicide with respect to the total number of relatives. (Adapted from Kety, 1979.)

Furthermore, monozygotic twins reared apart have a concordance rate of 40%–60% (similar to the concordance of those reared together). As with schizophrenia, however, the presence of many discordant identical twin pairs indicates that nongenetic contributing factors influence the susceptibility to affective disorders. The precise mode of genetic transmission is still unclear. Transmission does not follow a classic single-gene Mendelian pattern and may be polygenic.

There Are Effective Somatic Treatments for Depression

There are two effective treatments for major unipolar and bipolar depression: electroconvulsive therapy (ECT) and antidepressant drugs. Of the two, electroconvulsive therapy has been used for a longer period of time—over four decades. Although generally antidepressants would be used first in the treatment of major depression, electroconvulsive therapy is very effective. It produces full remission or marked improvement in about 90% of patients with well-defined major depression.

The critical therapeutic factor in electroconvulsive therapy is the induction of a generalized seizure. A motor seizure is not necessary or desirable for therapeutic results, and modern electroconvulsive therapy is always given under anesthesia with complete muscle relaxation. Approximately 4–12 treatments (on the average 6–8), given at 2-day intervals over a 2–4 week period, usually

suffice to produce a complete remission of symptoms. As might be predicted from our knowledge of seizure activity (Chapter 48), electroconvulsive therapy creates many temporary changes in brain function. Although the mechanism of its therapeutic action is still not understood, it may be related to changes in aminergic receptor sensitivity, as we shall see below.

The most widely used antidepressant drugs fall into two major classes: the *monoamine oxidase inhibitors*, such as phenelzine (Figure 54–2), and the *tricyclic compounds*, such as imipramine, so named for their three-ring molecular structure (Figure 54–3). Both the monoamine oxidase inhibitors and the tricyclic antidepressants produce remission or marked improvement in about 70% of patients with major depression. When high doses are given (and blood drug levels are monitored to ensure proper concentrations), the success rate with tricyclic drugs may reach 85%, approaching the effectiveness of electroconvulsive therapy. Bipolar depressives occasionally become manic during treatment with either class of antidepressant. Although a few patients begin to improve immediately, there is usually a lag of 1–3 weeks before the symptoms of depression begin to improve, and 4–6 weeks are generally required for full response.

Lithium salts are effective in terminating manic episodes. Maintenance lithium therapy is of significant prophylactic value in preventing or attenuating recurrent manic and depressive episodes, especially the former. Antischizophrenic drugs (see Chapter 53) are also quite effective in terminating manic episodes. These antischi-

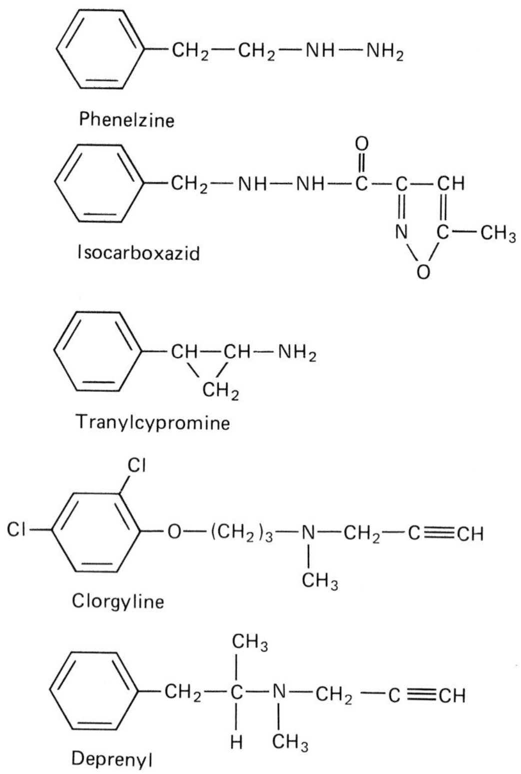

54–2 Clinically useful MAO inhibitors are diverse chemically. It is thought that these drugs act by decreasing the catabolism of biogenic amines in the brain, thereby making more neurotransmitter available for release at central synapses. The antidepressant effects of the drugs take several weeks to develop fully.

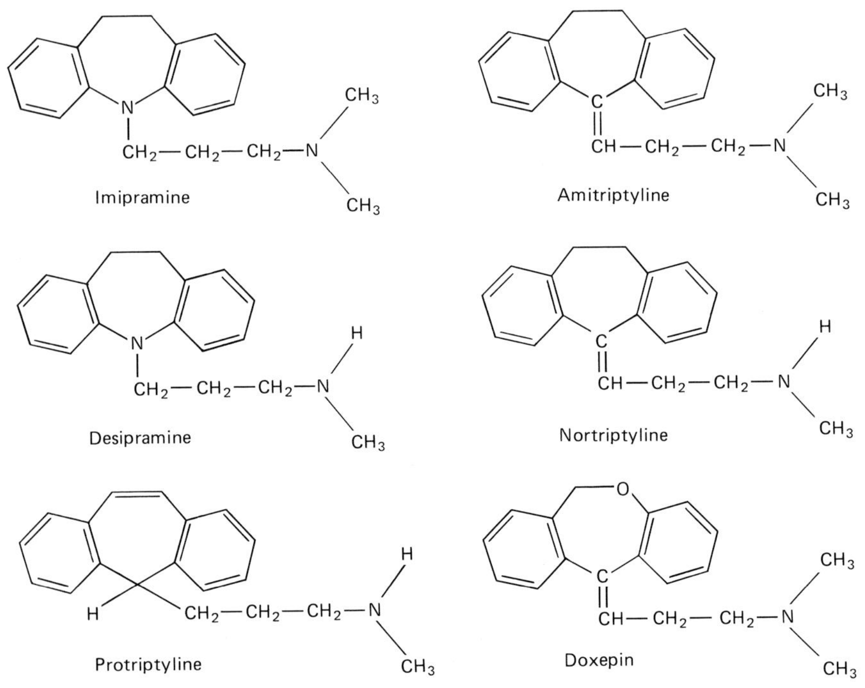

zophrenic agents are used frequently in combination with tricyclic drugs to treat psychotic depression (depression accompanied by delusions and hallucinations).

A Biogenic Amine Hypothesis of Depression Has Been Proposed

The most generally accepted idea about the nature of depression is that it involves a functional deficiency in monoamines, although currently this biogenic amine hypothesis is undergoing critical re-examination and modification. According to this hypothesis, depression is caused by a functional deficiency of brain serotonin or norepinephrine, or both, and the antidepressants work by increasing the availability of either or both amines (Figure 54–4). Mania was initially believed to result from the overactivity of noradrenergic systems, but this simple explanation no longer appears adequate. As discussed in Chapters 13 and 15, norepinephrine is synthesized from tyrosine, and serotonin from tryptophan in appropriate neurons. The transmitters are packaged in storage granules, and when the neuron is stimulated, they are released from the terminals into the synaptic cleft by means of exocytosis. After interacting with postsynaptic receptors, both norepinephrine and serotonin are actively taken up into the presynaptic terminals to be packaged again in vesicles or to be catabolized by the mitochondrial enzyme monoamine oxidase.

The idea that biogenic amines are reduced in depression derives from studies of the effects of various drugs on the serotonergic and noradrenergic systems of the brain. The first support for the biogenic amine

54–3 These tricyclic drugs are modifications of phenothiazine (see 53–1). They have immediate and long-term effects: blockage of the uptake of biogenic amine neurotransmitters is evident soon after administration, as are many of the side effects. Dry mouth is especially common because all of the tricyclics are potent anticholinergic agents. Antidepressant action usually begins 4 days to 3 weeks after starting the medication.

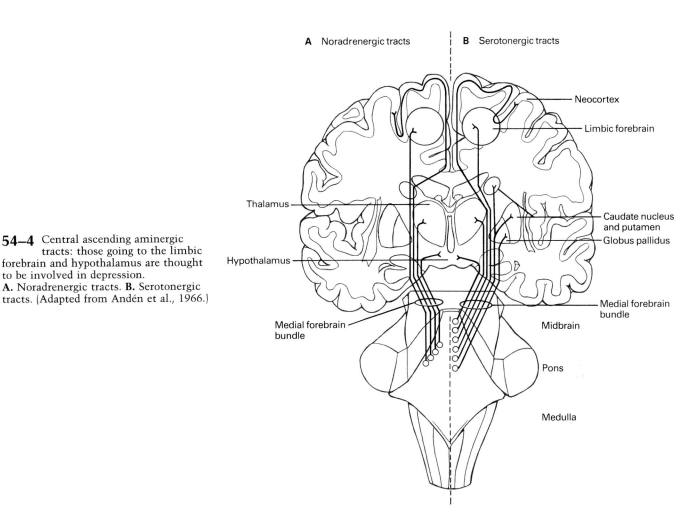

A Noradrenergic tracts | **B** Serotonergic tracts

Neocortex

Limbic forebrain

Thalamus

Caudate nucleus and putamen

Globus pallidus

Hypothalamus

Medial forebrain bundle

Medial forebrain bundle

Midbrain

Pons

Medulla

54–4 Central ascending aminergic tracts: those going to the limbic forebrain and hypothalamus are thought to be involved in depression.
A. Noradrenergic tracts. **B.** Serotonergic tracts. (Adapted from Andén et al., 1966.)

hypothesis came from the observation, in 1950, that reserpine—a Rauwolfia alkaloid then used extensively in the treatment of hypertension—precipitated depressive syndromes in about 15% of treated patients. This finding had a parallel in animal studies, in which reserpine produced a depressionlike syndrome consisting of motor retardation and sedation. Soon after these observations, Bernard Brodie and his colleagues at the National Institutes of Health showed that reserpine inactivates aminergic storage granules and therefore depletes the brain of serotonin and norepinephrine by releasing these neurotransmitters from their intracellular vesicles. The transmitters, released into the cytoplasm, are unprotected and consequently become vulnerable to degradation by monoamine oxidase (Figure 54–5).

Inhibitors of monoamine oxidase such as iproniazid were later found to be effective antidepressants. Iproniazid was initially developed to treat tuberculosis. In the course of clinical trials it was noted that some depressed tuberculosis patients experienced mood elevations when treated with this drug. Iproniazid was next tried in depressed nontubercular patients and found to be effective.

Monoamine oxidase inhibitors increase the content of serotonin and norepinephrine in the brain by decreasing the degradation of these transmitters by monoamine oxidase (Figure 54–5). In animals, monoamine oxidase inhibitors have also been found to prevent the biochemical and behavioral sedative effects of reserpine.

Further support for the view that monoamine oxidase inhibitors exercise their therapeutic action by increasing the functional availability of biogenic amines came with the discovery of a second class of effective antidepressants—the tricyclic compounds. These agents were found to block the active reuptake of released serotonin and norepinephrine by serotonergic and noradrenergic neurons, thereby prolonging the period over which the transmitters persist and act in the synaptic cleft.

Additional evidence has come from the use of still other pharmacological agents that affect aminergic transmission. For example, precursors of serotonin and norepinephrine can ameliorate depression: L-tryptophan can potentiate the therapeutic effect of monoamine oxidase inhibitors, and, recently, 5-hydroxytryptophan, the immediate precursor of serotonin, has also been found to

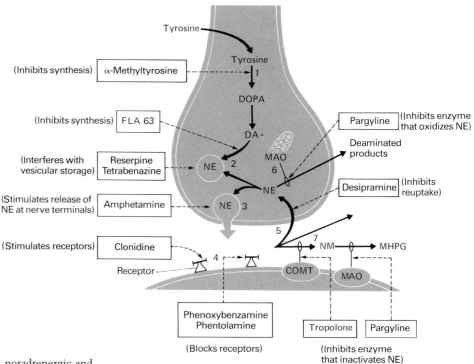

A Noradrenergic synapse

54–5 This schematic model of central noradrenergic and serotonergic neurons indicates the possible sites of drug action.

A. Noradrenergic synapse

Step 1. Enzymatic synthesis:
  a. Tyrosine hydroxylase reaction blocked by the competitive inhibitor α-methyltyrosine.
  b. Dopamine **(DA)** β-hydroxylase reaction blocked by a dithiocarbamate derivative, Fla-63-bis-(1-methyl-4-homopiperazinyl-thiocarbonyl)-disulfide **(FLA-63)**.

Step 2. Storage: Reserpine and tetrabenazine interfere with the uptake–storage mechanism of the amine granules. The depletion of norepinephrine **(NE)** produced by reserpine is long-lasting and the storage granules are irreversibly damaged. Tetrabenazine also interferes with the uptake–storage mechanism of the granules.

Step 3. Release: Amphetamine appears to cause an increase in the net release of norepinephrine, probably primarily by its ability to block the reuptake.

Step 4. Receptor interaction: Clonidine is a very potent receptor-stimulating drug. Phenoxybenzamine and phentolamine are effective α-receptor blocking agents. Recent experiments have indicated that these drugs also have a presynaptic site of action.

Step 5. Reuptake: Norepinephrine has its action terminated by being taken up into the presynaptic terminal. The tricyclic drug desipramine is a potent inhibitor of this uptake mechanism.

A (continued)

Step 6. Monoamine oxidase **(MAO)**: Norepinephrine or dopamine present in a free state within the presynaptic terminal can be degraded by the enzyme MAO, which appears to be located in the outer membrane of mitochondria. Pargyline is an effective inhibitor of MAO.

Step 7. Catechol-O-methyltransferase **(COMT)**: Norepinephrine can be inactivated by the enzyme COMT, which is believed to be localized outside the presynaptic neuron. Tropolone is an inhibitor of COMT. The normetanephrine **(NM)** formed by the action of COMT on norepinephrine can be further metabolized by MAO and aldehyde reductase to 3-methoxy-4-hydroxyphenylglycol **(MHPG)**. The MHPG formed can be further metabolized to MHPG sulfate by the action of a sulfotransferase found in the brain.

B. Serotonergic synapse

Step 1. Enzymatic synthesis: Tryptophan is taken up into the serotonin-containing neuron and converted to 5-hydroxytryptophan **(5-OH-tryptophan)** by the enzyme tryptophan hydroxylase. This enzyme can be effectively inhibited by p-chlorophenylalanine and α-propyldopacetamide. The next synthetic step involves the decarboxylation of 5-OH-tryptophan to form serotonin **(5HT)**.

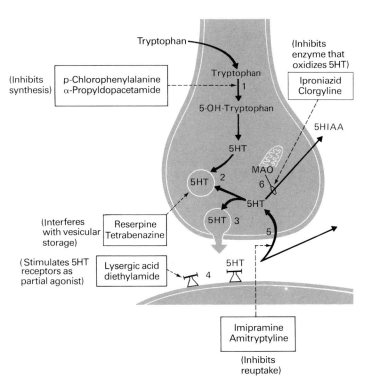

B Serotonergic synapse

B *(continued)*

Step 2. Storage: Reserpine and tetrabenazine interfere with the uptake–storage mechanism of the amine granules, causing a marked depletion of serotonin.

Step 3. Release: At present there is no drug available that selectively blocks the release of serotonin. However, lysergic acid diethylamide, because it has the ability to block or inhibit the firing of serotonergic neurons, causes a reduction in the release of serotonin from the nerve terminals.

Step 4. Receptor interaction: Lysergic acid diethylamide acts as a partial agonist at serotonergic synapses in the central nervous system. A number of compounds have also been suggested to act as receptor-blocking agents at serotonergic synapses, but direct proof of these claims at the present time is lacking.

Step 5. Reuptake: Considerable evidence now exists to suggest that serotonin may have its action terminated by being taken up into the presynaptic terminal. The tricyclic drugs with a tertiary nitrogen such as imipramine and amitryptyline appear to be potent inhibitors of this uptake mechanism.

Step 6. Monoamine oxidase (**MAO**): Serotonin present in a free state within the presynaptic terminal can be degraded by the enzyme MAO, which is located in the outer membrane of mitochondria. Iproniazid and clorgyline are effective inhibitors of MAO. (Adapted from Cooper, Bloom, and Roth, 1982.)

act as an antidepressant. Although L-DOPA is not a particularly effective antidepressant, it can precipitate manic or hypomanic episodes in patients with bipolar depression. Amphetamine, which releases catecholamines from nerve endings and, to a lesser extent, blocks their reuptake, transiently elevates mood in normal people and in some depressed patients. Triiodothyronine (T3), a hormone that is thought to sensitize catecholamine receptors in the brain, potentiates the antidepressant effect of moderate doses of tricyclics. In short, the effects of various agents on monoamine synthesis (L-tryptophan, *p*-chlorophenylalanine), storage (reserpine), release (amphetamine), degradation (monoamine oxidase inhibitors), and reuptake (tricyclics), as well as on receptor sensitivity (triiodothyronine), all implicate monoaminergic dysfunction in the affective disorders.

Other studies have focused on measuring the metabolites of serotonin and norepinephrine in depressed patients and controls. Because these transmitters do not cross the blood–brain barrier, the concentrations of their metabolites are measured in body fluids such as the cerebrospinal fluid and used as an index of transmitter metabolism in the brain. Marie Åsberg of the Karolinska Institute in Sweden found that the concentration of the major metabolite of serotonin, 5-hydroxyindole acetic acid (5-HIAA), is reduced in the spinal fluid of about half of all severely depressed patients studied, particularly in those who were suicidal.

It has been argued that biogenic amines are the transmitters used by the parts of the brain involved in motivation and pleasure. As described in Chapter 47, studies on animals suggest that certain systems in the brain are concerned with positive motivation (or the perception of pleasure) because electrical stimulation in these areas creates a state in which the animals actively seek further electrical stimulation. These pathways are made up primarily of catecholaminergic neurons. The pervasive loss of the feeling of pleasure in depressed patients might be related to disturbances in these systems.

The Original Biogenic Amine Hypothesis Is Undergoing Major Revision

Although these psychopharmacological and biochemical observations provide circumstantial support for the biogenic amine hypothesis, several important issues remain to be clarified. For example, many studies have evaluated the changes in the concentration of biogenic amine transmitter metabolites in peripheral body fluids; their concentrations, however, are difficult to relate to brain levels of these transmitters. A decrease in a neurotransmitter metabolite in the periphery could be produced by decreased synthesis of the transmitter in the brain, decreased transmitter release, or increased degradation of the transmitter; and there could be several causes of each. Furthermore, if the neurochemical disturbance in depression involves only a relatively small brain region (as is likely), it would be extraordinarily difficult to assess the specific alteration of transmitter metabolism in that region by measuring the combined metabolites coming from all areas of the brain. Although some alterations have been noted, subtle alterations of greater functional consequence may have been overlooked.

In addition, the biogenic amine hypothesis fails to account for certain clinical phenomena. For example, the time course for inhibition of monoamine oxidase by some inhibitors is slow, which is consistent with the slow onset of the clinical response. As soon as they are applied, the tricyclic agents, however, block the high-affinity reuptake systems for serotonin and norepinephrine, but the clinical response to these drugs is observed only 2–3 weeks after treatment is started. In addition, the tricyclic drugs vary widely in their relative abilities to block serotonin or norepinephrine reuptake, yet their clinical efficacies in depressed patients are all about the same, particularly if doses are adjusted to achieve the proper blood concentrations.

Some clues to resolving the discrepancy between the time course of the clinical effects of tricyclic drugs and their rapid action on uptake have come from the realization that these agents also affect processes other than uptake. The search for chronic effects of antidepressant drugs on nerve cells has revealed striking changes in the long-term sensitivity of various monoamine receptors. Particularly instructive is that effective treatments of depression—electroconvulsive therapy, as well as antidepressants of almost every class—reduce the sensitivity of β-adrenergic receptors. These treatments produce *down-regulation* of these receptors; they reduce the total number of postsynaptic receptors and thereby they also reduce the activity of norepinephrine-stimulated adenylate cyclase. Similarly, antidepressants also decrease the sensitivity of certain serotonin receptors (5-HT$_2$) by down-regulation. These changes are associated with decreases in synaptic strength.

In addition to the effects on postsynaptic receptors, long-term administration of tricyclic drugs causes a decrease in the number of presynaptic receptors. In contrast to down-regulation of the *post*synaptic receptors, down-regulation of the *pre*synaptic autoreceptors (which nor-

mally inhibit release) would enhance synaptic function. Perhaps the predominant effect of tricyclics is on the presynaptic receptors, and this action underlies the therapeutic response.

It is clear from these considerations that the earlier simple version of the catecholamine hypothesis—little or too much of a particular neurotransmitter—is no longer tenable. No satisfactory revised theory has yet emerged. Nonetheless, brain serotonergic and noradrenergic pathways are strongly implicated in the chemical pathology of affective disorders and in the clinical response to therapeutic agents.

There Are Disordered Neuroendocrine Functions in Depression

The many clinical signs of hypothalamic disturbance in depression suggest that hypothalamic modulation of neuroendocrine activity might also be affected. Indeed, the neurotransmitter systems most strongly implicated in depression—serotonergic and noradrenergic—also play important roles in neuroendocrine regulation. One of the best-established neuroendocrine disturbances in severe depression is a hypersecretion of cortisol from the adrenal cortex, secondary to excessive secretion of ACTH (adrenocorticotropin) by the pituitary. In normal people the secretion of cortisol follows a definite circadian rhythm, in which secretion peaks at 8:00 a.m. and virtually ceases in the evening and early morning hours. In contrast, about one-half of depressed patients secrete excessive amounts of cortisol, primarily during the afternoon and evening (Figure 54–6). This afternoon and evening hypersecretion is sometimes resistant to feedback suppression by the potent synthetic corticosteroid *dexamethasone*, which acts to depress ACTH. This disturbance of cortisol secretion in depression is not dependent on stress, and it is rarely found in other psychiatric disorders. Cortisol secretion returns to normal with clinical recovery.

Norepinephrine inhibits the action of corticotropin-releasing factor and of ACTH. Since depletion of norepi-

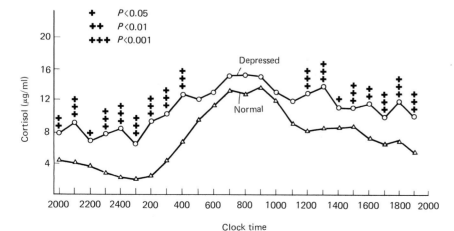

54–6 The mean hourly plasma cortisol concentration over a 24-hr period for seven unipolar depressed patients is compared with the mean for 54 normal subjects. Each data point represents the mean cortisol concentration during the preceding hour. **Plus signs** indicate the significance of differences between depressed and normal values for each hour.

nephrine leads to the hypersecretion of ACTH and cortisol, the hypersecretion of cortisol in depression may be secondary to a functional depletion of norepinephrine in the hypothalamus. In support of this idea, small intravenous doses of amphetamine (a norepinephrine releaser) have been found to lower cortisol levels rapidly to normal in endogenously depressed patients.

Another characteristic endocrine abnormality in depression is a blunted response of growth hormone to hypoglycemia induced by a standard dose of insulin. The growth hormone response can also be blunted by blockers and depletors of norepinephrine and serotonin. Thus, a wide variety of studies has suggested neuroendocrine abnormalities in depression, probably stemming from an underlying dysfunction in the noradrenergic system that regulates this hypothalamic–pituitary function.

Many of these neuroendocrine tests are still considered to be experimental, but the dexamethasone suppression test has been used as a diagnostic assay of depression because at least 40% of rigorously diagnosed depressed patients show abnormalities on this test. The test is not diagnostic, however. Patients suffering from dementia, anorexia nervosa, bulimia, alcohol withdrawal, or weight loss also have a positive dexamethasone suppression test. Dexamethasone suppression is sometimes used jointly with the sleep electroencephalogram for diagnostic purposes. Just as a substantial number of depressed patients fail to show normal suppression when given dexamethasone, so, too, many depressed patients show characteristic abnormalities in their sleep patterns as measured by electroencephalography. These abnormalities consist primarily of shortened REM latency and increased REM density during the first half of the night. In addition, some evidence of sleep discontinuity is found in more than 50% of depressed patients.

An Overall View

Although our understanding of the biochemical mechanisms of depression is only elementary, the clinical features, genetics, pharmacology, hormonal abnormalities, and biochemistry suggest that major depressive illness is a transmitter disorder with a genetic component primarily affecting the hypothalamus and probably involving monoamine pathways in an important way. Although the precise mechanisms that cause the defect and their mode of hereditary transmission still remain obscure, the rapid developments in this field in less than two decades encourage optimism that the molecular basis of major depressive illness will soon be elucidated.

Selected Readings

Carroll, B. J., Feinberg, M., Greden, J. F., et al. 1981. A specific laboratory test for the diagnosis of melancholia. Arch. Gen. Psychiatry 38:15–22.

Davis, J. M., and Mass, J. W. (eds.). 1983. The Affective Disorders. Washington, D.C.: American Psychiatric Press.

Kety, S. S. 1979. Disorders of the human brain. Sci. Am. 241(3):202–214.

Murphy, D. L., Campbell, I., and Costa, J. L. 1978. Current status of the indoleamine hypothesis of the affective disorders. In M. A. Lipton, A. DiMascio, and K. F. Killam (eds.), Psychopharmacology: A Generation of Progress. New York: Raven Press, pp. 1235–1247.

Sachar, E. J., Asnis, G., Halbreich, U., Nathan, R. S., and Halpern, F. 1980. Recent studies in the neuroendocrinology of major depressive disorders. Psychiatr. Clin. North Am. 3:313–326.

Schildkraut, J. J. 1978. Current status of the catecholamine hypothesis of affective disorders. In M. A. Lipton, A. DiMascio, and K. F. Killam (eds.), Psychopharmacology: A Generation of Progress. New York: Raven Press, pp. 1223–1234.

Van Praag, H. M. 1982. Neurotransmitters and CNS disease: Depression. Lancet 2:1259–1264.

Winokur, G. 1978. Mania and depression: Family studies and genetics in relation to treatment. In M. A. Lipton, A. DiMascio, and K. F. Killam (eds.), Psychopharmacology: A Generation of Progress. New York: Raven Press, pp. 1213–1221.

References

Andén, N.-E., Dahlström, A., Fuxe, K., Larsson, K., Olson, L., and Ungerstedt, U. 1966. Ascending monoamine neurons to the telencephalon and diencephalon. Acta. Physiol. Scand. 67:313–326.

Åsberg, M., Träskman, L., and Thorén, P. 1976. 5-HIAA in the cerebrospinal fluid. A biochemical suicide predictor? Arch. Gen. Psychiatry 33:1193–1197.

Cooper, J. R., Bloom, F. E., and Roth, R. H. 1982. The Biochemical Basis of Neuropharmacology, 4th ed. New York: Oxford University Press.

Everett, G. M., and Toman, J. E. P. 1959. Mode of action of Rauwolfia alkaloids and motor activity. In J. H. Masserman (ed.), Biological Psychiatry. New York: Grune & Stratton, pp. 75–81.

Foucault, M. 1961. Madness and Civilization: A History of Insanity in the Age of Reason. R. Howard (trans.). New York: Pantheon Books, 1965.

Freud, S. 1917. Mourning and melancholia. In The Collected Papers, Vol. IV. New York: Basic Books, 1959, pp. 152–170.

Klibansky, R., Panofsky, E., and Saxl, F. 1964. Saturn and Melancholy. London: Nelson.

Pletscher, A., Shore, P. A., and Brodie, B. B. 1956. Serotonin as a mediator of reserpine action in brain. J. Pharmacol. Exp. Ther. 116:84–89.

Development, Critical Periods, and the Emergence of Behavior

X

Our understanding of the adult nervous system and its control of behavior has been considerably enhanced by research into the development of the brain. Behavior is dependent on specific interconnections between nerve cells; developmental studies elucidate how these patterns of connections are established and how they are maintained. The nervous system develops in a series of ordered steps that are precisely timed, with a temporal sequence that is characteristic of each neural structure. As a result, each neuron connects only with certain target cells and not with others. In addition, the connections often are formed only at specific regions of the target cells.

It is now obvious that the total genetic information available to an animal—perhaps 10^5 genes in mammals—is not sufficient to specify the total number of neuronal interconnections that are made—perhaps 10^{15}. The limited amount of genetic information available provides strong confirmation for the idea that the development of the nervous system must also involve *epigenetic* processes that sequentially activate and modulate specific portions of the genetic program within the developing cells.

Epigenetic influences arise either from within the embryo or from the external environment. Events in the internal environment include surface interactions between cells, the diffusion of molecules over long distances or between neighboring cells and the release of hormones into the blood stream. The external environment includes nutritive factors, sensory and social experiences, and learning. Many internal and external factors impinge upon the developing cell. The actions of several of these factors are thought to be critical for enabling a neuron to differentiate appropriately.

Each signal presumably is specific chemically, temporally, and possibly also topographically. To be effective, a signal often has to act on the cell at a particular stage of development.

In the next series of chapters we shall consider the development of the brain in a broad context. In addition to examining the early stages of development, we shall look at how the interactions with the external world, and the social and sensory environment, validate the precision of the connections. We shall see that depriving an animal of a normal social, physical, or hormonal environment during an early, critical period can later have profound consequences for maturation of the brain and therefore of behavior. We shall also consider how internal factors, such as androgenic hormones, continue to determine structural aspects of the brain during early postpartum development. Finally, in the context of development, we shall consider the aging of the brain.

Samuel Schacher

Determination and Differentiation in the Development of the Nervous System

55

How does a single cell, the fertilized egg, give rise to so many types of cells? This is a central question in developmental biology. A distinctive aspect of this question arises for the neurobiologist: How do the various types of neurons develop and, in particular, how do they interconnect with such precision? In other tissues of the body, the identity of cells is specified by the genes that the cell expresses, the specific proteins that it makes, and the interaction of the cell with its neighbors. Beyond the fact that a cell must be located in its appropriate organ and belong to a certain class of cells, the precise position of a cell generally is not particularly important. Often, the cell is a member of a homogeneous population of similar cells, all of which interface with each other in similar ways. A beta cell will secrete insulin no matter where in the pancreas it is located. For neurons, however, position within the organ is critical. The properties of each neuron in the brain are determined not only by the chemical messengers that it releases, but also by its location and interconnections within the brain. The function of a cholinergic neuron in a motor nucleus of the spinal cord is quite different from that of a cholinergic neuron in the retina or in the cortex of the temporal lobe. A cholinergic neuron in each of these positions connects and interacts with different groups of neurons, and these interactions, as we have seen, determine the functioning of a cell.

Thus, the development of the nervous system can be viewed in terms of three key questions: (1) How do nerve cells originate? (2) How do the cells differentiate their appropriate properties in the appropriate position within the nervous system? (3)

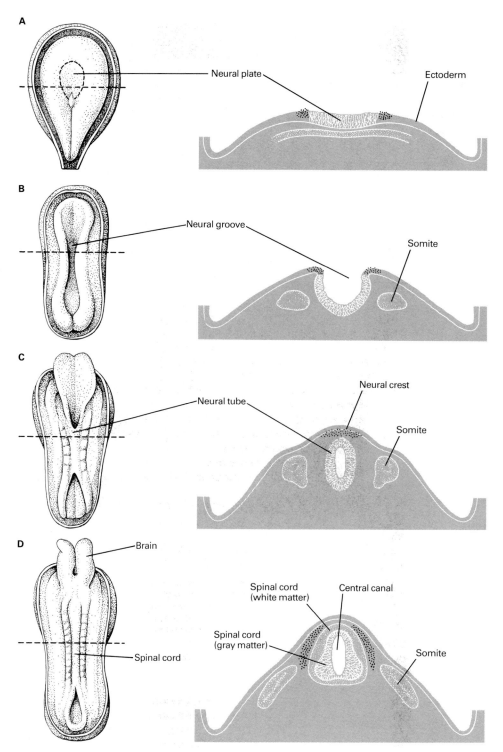

55–1 The nervous system originates from the ectoderm of a human embryo during the third and fourth weeks after conception. **Left,** external view of the developing embryo. **Right,** corresponding cross-sectional view at about the middle of the future spinal cord. **A.** The central nervous system develops from the neural plate, a flat sheet of ectodermal cells on the dorsal surface of the embryo. **B.** The plate folds to form the neural groove. The vertebral column and segmental musculature derive from the somites. **C.** The groove closes into a hollow structure called the neural tube. The structures of the brain develop from the anterior portion of the neural tube, whereas the spinal cord develops from the posterior portion. **D.** The open central canal persists throughout the development of the entire central nervous system. In the spinal cord it becomes very slender, but at the head end it widens to form the ventricles, or cavities, of the brain. (Adapted from Cowan, 1979.)

How do neurons form correct connections with one another to generate appropriate behavior? In this chapter, we shall consider the first two questions. In Chapter 56 we shall consider how appropriate synapses are formed to generate behavior.

Nerve cells originate by means of an initial step in development called *determination*, which ensures that a certain cell population will give rise to the cells of the nervous system (the neurons and the glia). A second step, *differentiation*, ensures that the cells descending from the determined population give rise to specific populations and subpopulations of neurons characteristic of the various regions of the nervous sytstem, and that these neurons proliferate and migrate to the appropriate location and ultimately make highly specific connections with their targets. These two broad steps of development can in turn be subdivided into many sequential cellular processes controlled by spatially and temporally precise signals. The location of the cell and the timing of these signals restrict the options available to cells in achieving their final differentiated state. Because the development of any one cell or brain structure appears to result from a great number of essentially independent sequential and vectorial steps, the process of differentiation becomes irreversible at some point during its course.

Fundamental to modern biology is the view that the structure and function of a cell or an organ—and its activities or behavior—are specified by genes. The sequential cellular processes underlying differentiation are therefore partly controlled by *intrinsic factors*, or mechanisms within the cell that turn its genes on and off. However, with the development of eukaryotic cells, the expression of the genetic blueprint, the *phenotype*, is always shaped to some degree by *extrinsic*, or *epigenetic*, factors arising in the cell's environment. In this chapter we shall examine how, during the stages of determination and differentiation, genetic and epigenetic signals interact in the development of the nervous system.

Determination of Nervous Tissue Occurs Through an Interaction between Mesoderm and a Special Region of Ectoderm

The cells of the nervous system originate from the *ectoderm*, the outer layer of the embryo (Figure 55–1). Within the ectoderm, the cells that will become neurons and glia derive from a specific sheet, called the *neural plate*, which contains about 125,000 cells. This sheet of cells folds into a long, hollow, tubelike structure, called the *neural tube*. From the rostral part of the neural tube, three swellings emerge that are the precursors of the three major regions of the brain (Figure 55–2)—the forebrain (the cerebral cortex and the basal ganglia), the midbrain, and the hindbrain (medulla, pons, and cerebellum). The caudal part of the neural tube gives rise to the spinal cord.

Determination, the transformation of precursor ectodermal cells into cells that ultimately give rise to the

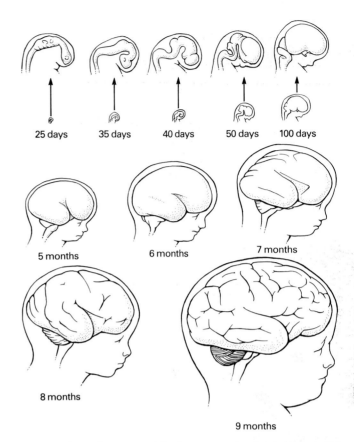

55–2 The embryonic and fetal stages in the development of the human brain are shown viewed from the side. (The first five embryonic stages, 25–100 days, are shown enlarged to an arbitrary common size to clarify their structural details. The drawings of the brain from 5 to 9 months are all scaled to be approximately four-fifths life size.) The three main parts of the brain (the forebrain, midbrain, and hindbrain) originate as prominent swellings at the head end of the early neural tube (see 40-day embryo). In human beings, the cerebral hemispheres eventually overgrow the midbrain, medulla, and pons, and also partly obscure the cerebellum. The characteristic convolutions and invaginations of the brain's surface do not begin to appear until about the middle of gestation. Assuming that the fully developed human brain contains on the order of 100 billion neurons and that virtually no new neurons are added after birth, one can calculate that neurons must be generated in the developing brain at an average rate of more than 250,000/min. (Adapted from Cowan, 1979.)

nervous system (the so-called *neuroectoderm*), is accomplished by the end of the gastrula stage of embryogenesis (Figure 55–3). Once embryonic cells are determined, their ability to differentiate into other tissues is severely restricted. For example, if prospective neuroectoderm is removed from an early gastrula stage embryo and transplanted to a different region in a host embryo, it will differentiate into skin, muscle, or gut depending on its new location in the host embryo. By the end of gastrulation, however, transplanted neuroectoderm can only become neural tissue.

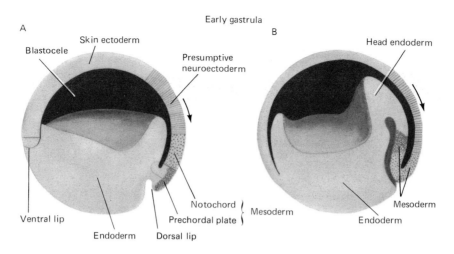

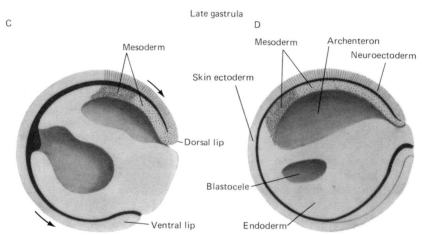

55–3 Gastrulation is the process by which the early embryo acquires its three germ layers. During gastrulation, a portion of the ectoderm invaginates the spherical early gastrula to become the mesoderm, as in this example from an amphibian. Ectoderm cannot differentiate into neural tissue without this underlying mesodermal layer. **A.** In early gastrula, mesoderm cells lie on the surface of the embryo and begin to

migrate toward the dorsal lip. **B.** Mesoderm cells migrate inward and underneath the ectoderm. **C and D.** Mesoderm cells continue to migrate beneath the neuroectoderm so that prechordal plate mesoderm lies underneath rostral neuroectoderm and notochord lies underneath caudal neuroectoderm. (Adapted from Saunders, 1970.)

Underlying Mesoderm Leads to Neural Induction of Neuroectoderm

Determination of the neuroectoderm occurs by a process called *neural induction.* In the early part of this century, Hans Spemann in Germany, working on amphibian embryos, showed that determination of neuroectoderm is induced by the underlying embryonic mesoderm that is formed during gastrulation. Spemann and Hilde Mangold transplanted prospective mesoderm into the embryonic cavity *(blastocele)* of an early gastrula host embryo (Figure 55–4A). Because of the cellular migrations that occur during gastrulation, the transplanted mesoderm came to lie underneath ectoderm that normally would give rise to epidermis of the trunk (Figure 55–4B). As development continued, however, the ectoderm of the trunk epidermis was induced by the underlying mesoderm to develop into nervous tissue (Figure 55–4C).

The presence of underlying mesoderm is essential for the determination of neuroectoderm. In the early 1930s, Johannes Holtfreter, also working in Germany, developed techniques that prevented the normal inward invagination and migration of prospective mesoderm during gastrulation. In the presence of hypertonic salt solutions, the prospective mesoderm fails to move inward and beneath the ectoderm (Figure 55–5) but, rather, moves away from it. The resulting *exogastrulated* embryo develops some normal mesodermal structures (*somites,* precursor cells for the vertebral column and segmental musculature, and the *notochord,* a rod-shaped group of cells that defines the primitive axis of the body), but fails to develop a nervous system (Figure 55–5).

The investigations of Spemann and Holtfreter demonstrated that the interaction between mesoderm and ectoderm is important in determining the neuroectoderm of the nervous system. This now raises the question:

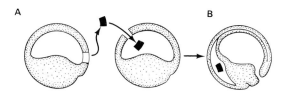

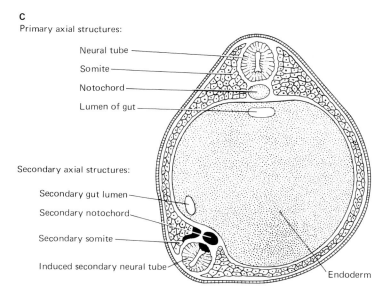

C

Primary axial structures:

Neural tube

Somite

Notochord

Lumen of gut

Secondary axial structures:

Secondary gut lumen

Secondary notochord

Secondary somite

Induced secondary neural tube

Endoderm

55–4 Spemann and Mangold demonstrated the role of mesoderm in neural induction. **A.** They transplanted precursor mesoderm from one gastrula into the embryonic cavity of another early gastrula host. **B.** The transplanted mesoderm came to underlie ectoderm that would normally develop into trunk epidermis. **C.** During development, the transplanted mesoderm induced this ectoderm to develop instead into a secondary set of axial structures, including neural tissue. (Adapted from Saunders, 1970.)

What is the nature of this interaction? The early work of Holtfreter and the later work of Saxen and Toivonen indicated that neuroectoderm is induced by one or more factors released from mesoderm. For example, cultured explants of embryonic ectoderm differentiate into neural tissue if they are cultured together with embryonic mesoderm. Neural induction still occurs if filters with pore sizes ranging from 0.1 to 0.8 μm are placed between the embryonic ectoderm and mesoderm. These filters prevent direct physical contact between the tissue layers and also block the passage of subcellular organelles such as ribosomes or synaptic vesicles, but the filters do not prevent the diffusion of most macromolecules between the tissues. Further experiments using filters with even smaller pores have indicated that the inducers may be peptides; induction is blocked when the pore size is so small that it prevents passage of molecules with molecular weights greater than 1000.

Neural Induction Produces a Regional Specification of the Neuroectoderm That Is Irreversible

A second feature of the interaction between mesoderm and ectoderm during gastrulation is the development of *regional specificity* along the anterior–posterior axis. As a result, the major divisions of the nervous system—forebrain, midbrain, hindbrain, and spinal cord—are specified in the neuroectoderm.

This regional specification of the nervous system along the anterior–posterior axis of the embryo occurs

55–5 If the mesoderm is prevented from invaginating and instead moves away from the ectoderm, the exogastrulated embryo fails to develop a nervous system. (Adapted from Bodemer, 1968.)

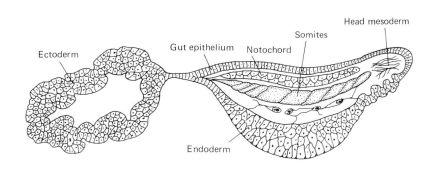

Ectoderm

Gut epithelium

Notochord

Somites

Head mesoderm

Endoderm

early in development, before the neural tube has formed and before most of the nervous system has been generated. At this point, only a few cells have actually begun to differentiate neuronal properties. After neuroectoderm has been specified, however, the imposed regional specification cannot be reversed. Thus, if a specified neuroectoderm is transplanted into a host embryo in an inverted position, so that specified forebrain neuroectoderm is placed in a posterior part of the host embryo, the transplanted nervous tissue does not conform to its new orientation but develops as initially programmed. The specified, transplanted forebrain structure continues to develop as forebrain even though it is now located in a posterior portion of the host embryo.

Thus, the processes of neural induction and regional specification determine the overall regional organization of the entire nervous system. These two processes in turn specify the types of neurons that will later differentiate within a given region of the central nervous system. However, subsequent signals can still modulate the local details critical for later steps in differentiation: the specific properties of neuronal populations and their interconnections.

Differentiation Occurs in Three Phases

After the nervous system has been determined and its axis, and thus its regions, have become specified, the cells of each region begin to differentiate. Differentiation involves three important phases: (1) proliferation and generation of specific classes of neurons; (2) migration of cells to characteristic positions; and (3) maturation of cells and the development of specific interconnections. In this chapter, we shall consider the first two phases. Maturation and the formation of specific connections will be considered in Chapter 56.

Proliferation Occurs in Specific Locations and at Specific Times

Cell Proliferation Occurs in Each Region of the Brain at a Particular Germinal Zone

The neural tube is formed when the lips of the invaginated neural plate fuse in the dorsal midline and the structure separates from the surface of the ectoderm (Figure 55–1C). Fusion of the neural tube first takes place in the prospective cervical region, and later extends rostrally and caudally. Only after the neural tube has closed does cell proliferation start. At first, the neural tube consists of a single layer of epithelial cells. Once proliferation begins, this layer rapidly becomes thicker. Throughout the epithelium of the neural tube, cell proliferation takes place in characteristic areas called *germinal zones.* For most regions of the central nervous system, the germinal zone is located adjacent to the surface of one of the cavities that will become the ventricular system of the brain.

55–6 Actively dividing cells in the germinal zone show characteristic movements of their nuclei that can be described in terms of four stages of the cell cycle: G_1, S, G_2, and M. The nuclei are positioned in the ventricular zone in the G_1 phase of the cell cycle. During DNA synthesis (S phase), the nuclei are positioned in the marginal zone. The nuclei then migrate toward the ventricular surface during the G_2 phase, retract their processes, and undergo mitosis (M phase). The daughter cells can either resume the mitotic cycle and enter the G_1 phase of the cell cycle or stop dividing and migrate away from the ventricular zone. (Adapted from Sauer, 1935.)

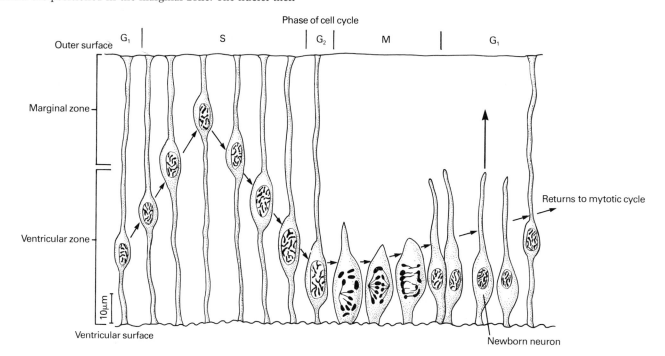

Phase of cell cycle

Outer surface G_1 S G_2 M G_1

Marginal zone

Ventricular zone

Returns to mytotic cycle

10μm

Ventricular surface

Newborn neuron

Within the epithelium of the germinal zone, actively dividing, undifferentiated *stem cells* undergo characteristic oscillatory movements during the course of the cell cycle that leads to cell division (Figure 55–6). During this cycle, the nucleus of an actively dividing stem cell first migrates toward the outer surface of the epithelium (called the *marginal zone*) and then moves back toward the ventricular surface, into the *ventricular zone*. The nucleus undergoes DNA replication only when it moves away from the ventricular lining toward the marginal surface of the epithelium. Once its DNA has replicated, the nucleus moves back to the ventricular zone. The cell then retracts its processes and divides. After cell division, the two daughter cells send out their processes and the nuclei return to the outer surface of the epithelium to replicate their DNA once again. Why does the nucleus undergo these oscillatory movements? One possibility is that movement allows the nucleus to be exposed in an appropriate temporal sequence to different cytoplasmic factors located in different regions of the cell.

After several divisions, a stem cell loses its ability to divide. The postmitotic cell then leaves the germinal zone and migrates to its appropriate position, either as an immature neuron (that never again divides, with the exceptions noted below), or as a glial cell precursor (that can divide). As we shall see in Chapter 56, an intense burst of proliferation results in an overproduction of neurons; in most regions of the nervous system cell death reduces the number of neurons to the final normal population size.

Certain Neurons Proliferate Again after Migration

Although most neurons that migrate are postmitotic and will never again divide, there are three exceptions that are particularly interesting and important. First, in the forebrain, nerve cells leave the ventricular zone and migrate to a special region called the *subventricular zone*, which lies between the ventricular zone and the intermediate zone (Figure 55–7). In the subventricular zone, the neurons proliferate again to give rise to the small neurons and glial cells of the basal ganglia and related deep nuclear structures as well as to some cells of the cerebral cortex. Second, cells that have migrated from the ventricular zone to the subventricular region of the hindbrain undergo still another migration to reach the pial surface of the cerebellum, where they proliferate to form the granule cells and the other interneurons of the cerebellum. Third, neurons that derive from the cells of a distinct germinal structure, the *neural crest*, are generated primarily after the crest cells have migrated to their final destination.

Different Types of Cells Are Generated at Different Times: The Role of Cell Lineage

Every neural structure, especially complex ones such as the cerebral cortex or the spinal cord, has not one but many types of cells. Each cell type (e.g., motor neuron, interneuron, or glia) is generated typically during only one period of development. We do not yet know what

55–7 Progressive thickening of the wall of the developing brain. At the earliest stage (**1**) the wall consists only of a simple (pseudostratified) epithelium, in which the ventricular zone contains the cell bodies and the marginal zone contains only the extended outer cell processes. When some of the cells lose their capacity for synthesizing DNA and withdraw from the mitotic cycle, they form a second layer, the intermediate zone (**2**). In the forebrain, the cells that pass through this zone aggregate to form the cortical plate, the region in which the various layers of the cerebral cortex develop (**3**). The cortical cell layers develop in an inverted fashion, so that cells in deeper layers (i.e., layer VI) develop first. The cells in the superficial layers must migrate past older cells to reach their appropriate position. At the latest stage (**4**), the original ventricular zone remains as the ependymal lining of the cerebral ventricles, and the comparatively cell-free region between this lining and the cortex becomes the subcortical white matter, through which nerve fibers enter and leave the cortex. The subventricular zone is a second proliferative region in which many glial cells and some neurons in the forebrain are generated. (Adapted from Jacobson, 1978.)

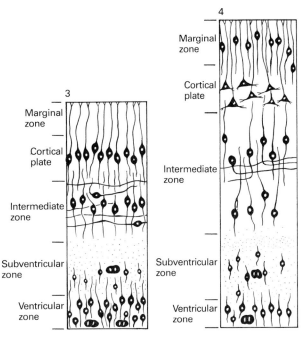

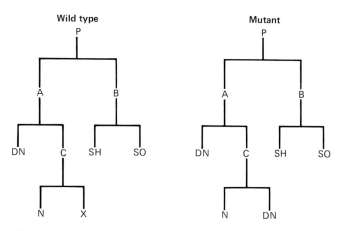

Wild type

Mutant

55-8 Neurotransmitter phenotype is not strictly determined by lineage. Some dopaminergic neurons in *C. elegans* are derived from a cell lineage scheme as shown here. In the wild type, the left daughter cell (**A**) of stem cell **P** gives rise to one daughter cell that differentiates as a dopaminergic neuron (**DN**) and daughter cell **C**. Cell **C** in turn gives rise to a nondopaminergic neuron (**N**) and another cell that soon dies (**X**). In the mutant, the cell that normally dies in the wild type differentiates as a dopaminergic neuron. The right daughter cell of stem cell **P** (**B**) gives rise to a sheath cell (**SH**) and a socket cell (**SO**). (Adapted from Horvitz, 1981.)

determines the time frame for generating the various cell types, but part of the answer may lie in the type of cell lineage to which a neuron belongs. Most of the information that we have about the role of cell lineage in the differentiation of neurons has come from studies on several invertebrate species. The nervous systems of invertebrates are experimentally suitable for cell lineage studies because they contain a much smaller number of neurons than those of vertebrates. Particularly informative studies have been carried out on the nematode, *Caenorhabditis elegans*, by Sidney Brenner, John Sulston, and their colleagues at the MRC unit in Cambridge, England; on the grasshopper by Michael Bate and his colleagues at Cambridge, England, and Corey Goodman at Stanford University; and on the leech by Gunther Stent and colleagues at the University of California at Berkeley. Three major principles have emerged from these studies:

1. A stem cell can give rise to several types of neurons with different functions. For example, in the nematode a single stem cell can give rise to motor neurons as well as sensory neurons, and it can give rise to neurons that use different transmitters (Figure 55–8).
2. The cell types generated from a given stem cell are generally invariant and occupy characteristic positions in the cell lineage. For example, in the grasshopper, two identified serotonergic neurons are always generated from an early cell division of a particular stem cell (labeled NB7-3). As a result, cells with similar functions share a common genealogy.

3. Some neurons are derived uniquely from a given stem cell. As a result, specific progeny neurons will be missing if a particular stem cell is destroyed before it divides. In the grasshopper, ablation of the serotonergic NB7-3 stem cell results in the absence of the two serotonergic cells. Neighboring stem cells cannot regulate their generation of specific neurons to restore the presence of the serotonergic neurons.

These studies indicate that particular neurons are generated at different times. The studies also extend the concept of regional specificity to the level of individual neurons and the stem cells from which these neurons derive. As we shall see later, however, in certain cases the final phenotype of the neuron may be changed by local environmental signals.

Migration Affects Cell Differentiation

Studies of the neural crest and of the cerebellum illustrate how migration affects the differentiation of nerve cells and how neural structures develop.

Cells of the Neural Crest Are Influenced by Their Local Environment

While the neural tube is closing, some cells at the dorsal margins of the neural plate separate from the neural tube to form the neural crest (Figure 55–1C). Cells from the neural crest migrate to populate the entire embryo. The rostral part of the neural crest gives rise both to neurons and to glial cells that form a variety of structures: the neurons that will make up the ganglia or cranial nerves V, VII, VIII, IX, X, the parasympathetic autonomic ganglia of the digestive tract, the ciliary ganglion, Schwann cells, melanocytes, and the meninges of the pia-arachnoid (which covers the diencephalon and telencephalon). The caudal neural crest gives rise to dorsal root ganglia, the sympathetic autonomic ganglia, the chromaffin cells of the adrenal medulla, and the ganglia of the postumbilical intestinal tract.

Because of the diversity of its cell types and their wide distribution in the mature animal, the neural crest is an interesting experimental system for examining the effects of cell migration and local environment on neuronal development. Nicole Le Douarin and her colleagues in Paris have shown that the local environment in which the migrating crest cells ultimately find themselves greatly influences the subsequent development of their specific biochemical properties. To carry out her pioneering experiments, Le Douarin developed a natural marking technique for determining the source of neurons derived from neural crest cells. The technique is based on the histologically detectable differences between the structure of the nuclei in two species of birds: quail and chick. These differences allowed her to transplant "naturally marked" neural crest cells from one region in a donor species to another in the host species and to identify the transplanted cells by their characteristic nuclei.

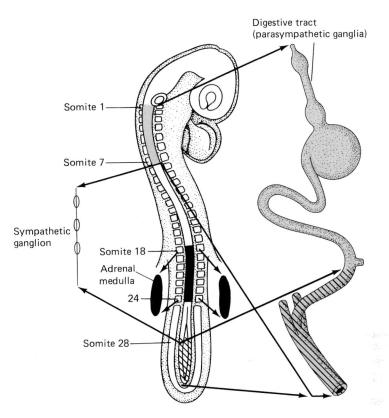

55–9 Different regions of the neural crest give rise to parasympathetic neurons of the digestive tract and adrenergic cells of the adrenal medulla. The parasympathetic neurons of the digestive tract are derived from neural crest cells in the anterior (somite region 1–7) and posterior (below somite 28) portion of the neural tube. The sympathetic ganglia are derived from crest cells in somite region 7–28. The adrenergic cells of the adrenal medulla are derived from crest cells in the somite region 18–24. (Adapted from Le Douarin et al., 1975.)

In the first group of experiments, Le Douarin determined which regions of the neural crest give rise to the sympathetic and parasympathetic nervous systems (Figure 55–9). She transplanted specific quail neural tube regions (with the associated neural crest) to corresponding positions in the host chick embryos. She later examined the mosaic embryos for the location of quail cells and found that the parasympathetic ganglia are derived from crest cells that come from the anterior portion (somite levels 1–7) and the posterior portion (below somite 28) of the neural tube. In contrast, the ganglia of the sympathetic nervous system are derived from neural crest cells at the intermediate level (somite levels 7–28).

Le Douarin then asked the following question: Is the fate of a neural crest cell that is destined to be either a sympathetic neuron (synthesizing norepinephrine) or a parasympathetic neuron (synthesizing acetylcholine) determined before or after migration to the appropriate sites? To answer this question, she transplanted regions of quail neural tube (including the associated neural crest) to heterotypic regions of the chick embryo. For example, she took neural crest cells from somite region 18–24 (the sympathetic precursor region) in the quail and transplanted them to somite region 1–7 (a parasympathetic region) in the chick (Figure 55–10A). The transplanted quail cells migrated along routes typical of crest cells from somite region 1–7. These cells ended up in parasympathetic ganglia and functioned as parasympathetic neurons, releasing acetylcholine as their transmitter.

A similar reversal in transmitter biosynthesis was observed when presumptive parasympathetic crest cells from quail (anterior neural crest) were transplanted to somite region 16–26 (sympathetic and adrenal medulla) in chick embryos (Figure 55–10B). The quail cells migrated to the adrenal medulla and differentiated adrenergic properties. These experiments indicated that the route of migration for the different neuronal elements is determined by their position in the neural crest. Moreover, the final differentiated state of the crest cells is *not* determined before migration; rather, it is strongly influenced by the interaction between the migrating cells and the environment both along the migration route and at the final destination.

Le Douarin's work with embryos has been extended into dissociated cell culture in a series of elegant experiments with immature sympathetic neurons by Edwin Furshpan, David Potter, and Paul Patterson and their colleagues at the Harvard Medical School and by Mary and Richard Bunge at Washington University. Immature sympathetic neurons normally maintain their adrenergic properties in culture and synthesize norepinephrine. However, if the neurons are cultured together with a variety of nonneural cells that are targets for parasympathetic innervation, they develop cholinergic properties: they contain choline acetyltransferase, synthesize acetylcholine, and make effective cholinergic synapses on appropriate targets.

The conversion from one neurotransmitter to the other may include an intermediate step in which the

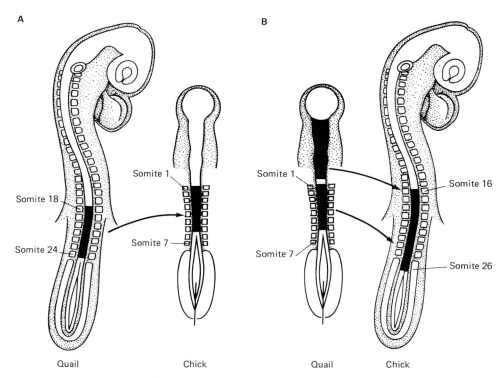

55–10 Heterotypic transplantation of quail neural tube and crest into chick embryos demonstrates the role of the local environment in cell migration and differentiation.
A. Neural cells from somite region 18–24, which normally migrate to the adrenal medulla and synthesize norepinephrine, are transplanted to somite region 1–7, which gives rise to cells that migrate to form the parasympathetic ganglia of the digestive tract and synthesize acetylcholine. The transplanted cells migrate to the digestive tract and develop cholinergic properties. **B.** Crest cells that normally migrate to the digestive tract and synthesize acetylcholine are transplanted into a region in which cells typically migrate to the adrenal medulla (somite region 16–26) and synthesize norepinephrine. The transplanted cells migrate to the adrenal medulla and develop adrenergic properties. (Adapted from Le Douarin et al., 1975.)

cells in culture synthesize and release *both* acetylcholine and norepinephrine. This has been demonstrated by Furshpan and his colleagues, who developed a microculture system consisting of a single immature sympathetic neuron cocultured with cardiac myotubes. Initially, these neurons release only norepinephrine at their target cells. After 2 weeks in culture, some of the neurons show synaptic interactions with the muscle cells that are characteristic of both types of transmitter. Electrical stimulation of these neurons produces both inhibition (cholinergic action) and excitation (adrenergic action), and these effects are blocked selectively by cholinergic and adrenergic blocking drugs. Moreover, the neurons do not have to be in direct contact with the nonneural cells for the cholinergic properties to appear. The nonneural cells secrete a substance into the medium, and this diffusible factor, which is not yet completely characterized, can itself cause sympathetic neurons to develop cholinergic properties. Thus, these experiments indicate that the choice of transmitter that a neural crest cell will synthesize and release is not completely preprogrammed; rather, the environment in which the developing neuron finds itself can affect the expression of its transmitter-

synthesizing capabilities. An extrinsic chemical factor is critical in activating (or repressing) genes that control the synthesis of acetylcholine or norepinephrine.

Cellular Interactions Aid Migration in the Cerebellar Cortex

As we have seen, the cerebellar cortex is a well-characterized network consisting of five classes of precisely interconnected neuronal elements (see Chapter 39). Studies of the development of the cerebellar cortex have illustrated features that appear to be quite general and apply to other cortical structures, including the neocortex of the cerebral hemispheres. First, young (postmitotic) neurons leave their germinal zone and typically migrate past older cells to reach their final position (as occurs, for example, in the thickening of the wall of the brain; Figure 55–7). Second, the migration and final position of the neurons may be influenced by the intimate interaction between the migrating cells and a particular type of glial process, the *radial glial fibers*. These processes are extensions of a type of glia called *Bergmann astrocytes*, which span the entire length of the cerebellar cortex.

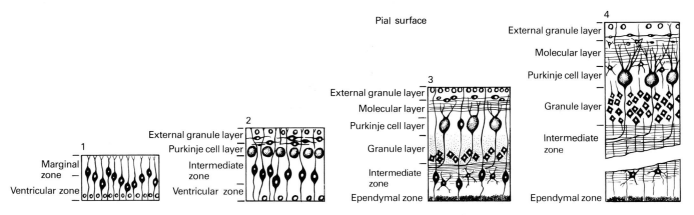

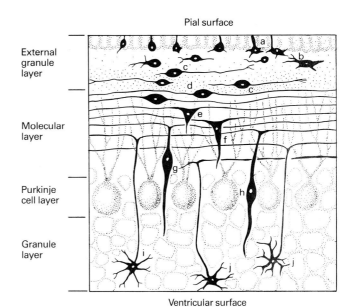

55-11 Cell migration and differentiation during the development of the cerebellar cortex. At the earliest stage (**1**), the developing cerebellum has two zones, the ventricular zone and the marginal zone. The ventricular zone contains the cell bodies of actively dividing neurons, and the marginal zone contains their processes. As cells become postmitotic (**2**), they migrate through the intermediate zone and form the Purkinje cell layer. At this time, cells migrating along the pial surface form a second germinal zone, the external granule layer. As development continues (**3 and 4**), the Purkinje cells develop their dendritic processes, and cerebellar interneurons migrate from the external granule layer and differentiate their processes to form the molecular and granule layers. The germinal zone bordering the ventricle is now called the ependymal zone, which gives rise to ependymal cells lining the ventricle, the glial cells, and the neurons of the deep cerebellar nuclei. (Adapted from Jacobson, 1978.)

During development, the cerebellar cortex is elaborated into several histologically distinct zones (Figure 55–11). Initially, there is a single germinal zone at the surface of the fourth ventricle (the *ventricular zone*), with a *marginal zone* above it. This germinal zone gives rise to the Purkinje cells and the Golgi cells. These large neurons, the first to develop in the cerebellar cortex, migrate from the ventricular zone through the marginal *intermediate zone* to form the Purkinje cell layer. The germinal zone of the fourth ventricle also gives rise to a group of precursor neurons that migrate to the pial surface to form a second germinal zone, called the *external granule layer*. These neuronal precursor cells proliferate extensively and generate the three major interneurons of the cerebellum: the basket cells and stellate cells of the molecular layer, and the granule cells of the granule layer. The birth of these interneurons coincides with the stage when the Purkinje cell layer is nearly completed and the Purkinje cells have begun to spin out their primary dendritic processes. The neurogenesis of the interneurons of the molecular layer—basket and stellate cells—is completed first (at birth in primates), whereas the granule cells continue to be generated afterward (for periods of 6 months to 2 years after birth in primates).

The development of the granule, basket, and stellate cells illustrates the importance of cellular interactions in neuronal differentiation. To reach the final destination in the granule layer, the granule cells must migrate from the external granule layer across the molecular and Purkinje cell layers (Figure 55–12). As the granule cell becomes bipolar, with its processes oriented parallel to the

55-12 After proliferating in the external granule layer, cerebellar granule cells must migrate to the granule layer. As a granule cell becomes postmitotic (**a**) in the external granule layer, it begins to spin out bipolar processes (**b, c, d**) that are parallel to the pial surface and perpendicular to the Purkinje cell dendrites. The cell extends a third process (**e, f**) into the molecular layer, and the cell body moves along this growing process (**g, h**) through the molecular and Purkinje layers to reach its final position (**i, j**) in the granule layer. (Adapted from Jacobson, 1978.)

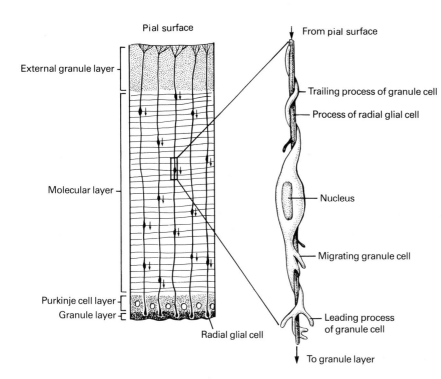

55–13 Granule cells migrate through the molecular and Purkinje cell layers along radially oriented processes of glial cells (Bergmann astrocytes). The cell bodies of the radial glial cells are located near the junction of the Purkinje and granule cell layers. (Adapted from Rakic, 1971.)

pial surface and perpendicular to the Purkinje cell dendrites, the granule cell extends a third process into the molecular layer. The granule cell body then moves along the extended process, leaving the bipolar processes behind to form the parallel fibers. These parallel fibers are the axons of granule cells that make synaptic contacts with the dendritic spines of Purkinje cells. The direction of growth of the cytoplasmic process in the molecular layer and the movement of the cell body are guided through the intervening layers by radial glial fibers formed by the processes of Bergmann astrocytes (Figure 55–13). These glial cells, generated in the ventricular zone, have their cell bodies positioned just beneath the Purkinje cell layer, and they project radially oriented fibers to the pial surface. The migrating granule cells then move along these fibers until they reach the granule layer.

Pasko Rakic, now at Yale University, and Richard Sidmon, at Harvard University, have suggested that the interaction between migrating granule cells and radial glial fibers may be essential for the survival and normal development of the granule cells. This idea is supported by observations made on an autosomal recessive mutation in mice known as *weaver*. Animals with this mutation show muscular weakness, unsteadiness of movement, and severe tremor. The cerebellum of a weaver mouse is extensively depleted of granule cells. This deficiency does not result from decreased proliferation of granule cells in the external granule layer, but from an inability of granule cells, once generated, to migrate to their appropriate position. Electron-microscopic analysis of homozygous and heterozygous weaver mice reveals either

extensive degeneration of radial glial fibers before the granule cells begin to migrate, or glial fibers whose orientation across the cerebellar cortex is widely aberrant. These changes in the radial glial fibers may explain the degeneration of granule cells found at the junction of the external granule layer and the molecular layer as well as in the molecular layer itself. The granule cells are normal in areas in which radial glial fibers are present and properly oriented, and these areas show little granule cell degeneration.

The basket cells and stellate cells of the molecular layer arrive at their final position in a different manner. Interneurons of the molecular layer become postmitotic and remain as round cells at the junction of the molecular layer and the external granule layer. As more parallel fibers are formed by the granule cells, the postmitotic interneurons of the molecular layer begin to extend bipolar processes perpendicular to the parallel fibers. As additional parallel fibers are formed around the interneuron cell bodies and their bipolar processes, the interneurons become fixed in place. The bipolar processes now branch upward or downward to maximize the number of parallel fiber contacts. For example, the earliest interneurons generated, the basket cells (Figure 55–14A), come to be positioned close to the Purkinje cell bodies on a shallow bed of recently formed granule cell parallel fibers. Additional parallel fibers are laid down externally and at right angles to the basket cells and fix the basket cell bodies in position. Now the dendrites of the basket cells lengthen enormously by growing externally toward the pial surface, making contacts with an increasing number of parallel fibers.

55–14 Basket and stellate cells are fixed in position by parallel fibers from granule cells. **A.** The cell body of the basket cell becomes fixed in position close to Purkinje cell bodies by granule cell parallel fibers that are laid down perpendicular to the bipolar processes of the basket cell (**plane ab**). When its position is fixed, its dendrites lengthen toward the pial surface, contacting large numbers of parallel fibers. **B.** Stellate cells become fixed within the molecular layer and grow dendrites in both directions perpendicular to the plane of the parallel fibers (**ab**) to contact older and new parallel fibers. (Adapted from Rakic, 1973.)

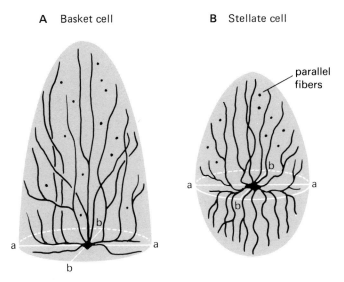

A   Basket cell   B   Stellate cell

parallel fibers

Interneurons that are generated later are fixed in position in the middle of the molecular layer and become stellate cells. These cells can grow dendrites internally toward the Purkinje cell layer to make contacts with older parallel fibers, and externally toward the pial surface to make contacts with new parallel fibers (Figure 55–14B). The manner in which basket and stellate cells develop suggests that they do not originate as separate types of neurons but as one type of cell whose mature position and phenotype are influenced by the time of generation and by local interactions with granule cell parallel fibers.

An Overall View

During the course of development, neurons must express a specific set of genes and differentiate appropriate neuronal properties (transmitter-synthesizing and -processing enzymes, receptor proteins, and ion channel proteins) and ultimately form specific connections with one another and peripheral targets. For the developing neuron to make appropriate connections, it must elaborate axons that project to the correct target tissue and select cells in that target with which to form synapses. The choices that neurons make in selecting their targets may also be influenced by local environmental cues.

The last stage in this process—the formation of specific connections—is not entirely a function of the later stages of development. Neuronal specificity derives not from a single step of recognition but from a program of development that is the result of two large groups of processes. First, there is the overall developmental sequence that includes determination, differentiation, proliferation, cell migration, axonal outgrowth, dendrite elaboration, cell death, and neuronal recognition. Each of these phases is patterned in space and time by the various con-

trolling factors. Second, as we shall see in Chapters 56 and 57, synaptic connections are finally stabilized by the appropriate environmental conditions in postembryonic life. The challenging tasks remain of delineating further the interconnections of the brain and determining how environmental cues act on the genes to achieve this remarkable organization.

Selected Readings

Cowan, W. M. 1979. The development of the brain. Sci. Am. 241(3):112–133.

Goodman, C. S., Bate, M., and Spitzer, N. C. 1981. Embryonic development of identified neurons: Origin and transformation of the H cell. J. Neurosci. 1:94–102.

Goodman, C. S., and Pearson, K. G. 1982. Neuronal development: Cellular approaches in invertebrates. Neurosci. Res. Program Bull. 20:777–942.

Jacobson, M. 1978. Developmental Neurobiology, 2nd ed. New York: Plenum Press.

Le Douarin, N. 1982. The Neural Crest. Cambridge, England: Cambridge University Press.

Patterson, P. H. 1978. Environmental determination of autonomic neurotransmitter functions. Annu. Rev. Neurosci. 1:1–17.

Rakic, P. 1971. Neuron-glia relationship during granule cell migration in developing cerebellar cortex. A Golgi and electron-microscopic study in Macacus rhesus. J. Comp. Neurol. 141:283–312.

References

Bodemer, C. W. 1968. Modern Embryology. New York: Holt, Rinehart and Winston.

Brenner, S. 1974. The genetics of *Caenorhabditis elegans.* Genetics 77:71–94.

Furshpan, E. J., MacLeish, P. R., O'Lague, P. H., and Potter, D. D. 1976. Chemical transmission between rat sympathetic neurons and cardiac myocytes developing in microcultures: Evidence for cholinergic, adrenergic, and dual-function neurons. Proc. Natl. Acad. Sci. U.S.A. 73:4225–4229.

Horvitz, H. R. 1981. Neuronal cell lineages in the nematode *Caenorhabditis elegans*. In D. R. Garrod and J. D. Feldman (eds.), Development in the Nervous System. Cambridge, England: Cambridge University Press, pp. 331–346.

Le Douarin, N. M., Renaud, D., Teillet, M. A., and Le Douarin, G. H. 1975. Cholinergic differentiation of presumptive adrenergic neuroblasts in interspecific chimeras after heterotopic transplantations. Proc. Natl. Acad. Sci. U.S.A. 72:728–732.

Rakic, P. 1973. Kinetics of proliferation and latency between final cell division and onset of differentiation of cerebellar stellate and basket neurons. J. Comp. Neurol. 147:523–546.

Rakic, P., and Sidman, R. L. 1973. Weaver mutant mouse cerebellum: Defective neuronal migration secondary to abnormality of Bergmann glia. Proc. Natl. Acad. Sci. U.S.A. 70:240–244.

Sauer, F. C. 1935. Mitosis in the neural tube. J. Comp. Neurol. 62:377–405.

Saunders, J. W., Jr. 1970. Patterns and Principles of Animal Development. New York: Macmillan.

Spemann, H. 1938. Embryonic Development and Induction. New Haven: Yale University Press.

Toivonen, S., Tarin, D., and Saxen, L. 1976. The transmission of morphogenetic signals from amphibian mesoderm to ectoderm in primary induction. Differentiation 5:49–55.

Weisblat, D. A., Harper, G., Stent, G. S., and Sawyer, R. T., 1980. Embryonic cell lineages in the nervous system of the glossiphoniid leech *Helobdella triserialis*. Dev. Biol. 76:58–78.

Eric R. Kandel

Synapse Formation, Trophic Interactions between Neurons, and the Development of Behavior

56

Behavior depends on the formation of appropriate interconnections among neurons in the brain. In Chapter 55, we saw how neurons first become determined and how they migrate to their final position and begin to differentiate. In this chapter we shall focus on the subsequent stages of neuronal differentiation. Specifically, we shall examine one of the critical questions in developmental neurobiology: How do neurons form appropriate synaptic connections? Stable synaptic connections result from a sequence of events that can be analyzed in terms of five mechanistic questions:

1. How do neurons within a given population acquire information about their final position in the brain, and how do they use cues based on position to select where to send their axons?
2. How do outgrowing axons find their correct and appropriate target cells?
3. How, having found one another, do the processes of two neurons form a functioning connection?
4. Once they have formed a synapse, how do the two interacting pre- and postsynaptic neurons use their functioning synapse to influence each other's subsequent program of differentiation and survival?
5. How precise are the connections made between the cells of the nervous system?

In analyzing the steps in synapse formation we shall also consider the degree to which the functions of the nervous system and the expression of behavior are determined by genes and by developmentally programmed maturation on the one hand and by environmentally induced learning on the other. We shall examine the extent to which neural connections result from invariant processes of regulation, growth, and differentiation, and the extent to which they are formed as a result of experience and learning.

In the late 1920s and early 1930s psychologists believed that most of the connections between neurons in the brain are not inherently determined. These psychologists maintained that the genetic program alone produces a central nervous system that is an unorganized network capable only of random interactions. From this unformed state, behavioral feedback from trial-and-error learning would be required to produce a coherent neural organization. According to this view, a particular class of cells might, in principle, be capable of forming connections with any one of many targets. The exact connections formed by the cells would be directed by learning, that is, by the pattern of stimulation that the organism receives from its external environment. In contrast to this early view, many modern neurobiologists believe that the complexity of the brain demands a specific developmental program that restricts from the outset which targets a particular class of neurons will innervate. These two views have given rise to two theories of development that, by analogy to constitutional law, may be called the loose and the strict constructionist views. According to *loose constructionists*, there is only a limited developmental program, and learning plays a key role in the formation of synaptic connections. According to *strict constructionists*, there is an extensive genetic and developmental program in synapse formation and a more limited role for learning.

Information about Final Position Is Important for Establishing Precise Connections in the Central Nervous System

Let us begin by considering one of the central questions in nervous system development: How precise are the steps by which a nerve cell seeks and finds another nerve cell? The best evidence for the specificity of nerve cell connection comes from experiments on the visual system by Roger Sperry, now at the California Institute of Technology.

Sperry was intrigued with the questions: How is the visual system put together? How do nerve fibers know how to grow to their appropriate place, and how precise are the interconnections that they form? Working with frogs, salamanders, and goldfish because of their remarkable capacity for regeneration, Sperry found that when he cut the optic nerve it would regenerate completely, leading to full restoration of vision. Even though a scar formed in the nerve after it was cut, regenerating fibers found their way through the scar, and, on the other side, made the synaptic contacts necessary for normal vision.

Using the optic nerve of goldfish, Sperry next carried out other experiments on connectional specificity. To understand these experiments, we first must appreciate some of the experimental advantages of the visual system of the goldfish (Figure 56–1). In the goldfish, optic nerve fibers cross completely in the optic chiasm. All of the fibers from the right eye cross to the left, and most connect to the left optic tectum, a structure that is analogous to the mammalian superior colliculus. After leaving the retina, the fibers sort into two divisions: the medial and the lateral optic tracts. Fibers from the dorsal retina run in the lateral tract to the ventral part of the tectum, while fibers from the ventral retina run in the medial tract to the dorsal tectum. Fibers from the anterior retina join one tract or the other to reach the tectum and then leave that tract late as they continue on to the posterior tectum, where they terminate; fibers from the posterior retina leave the tracts early to enter the anterior part of the tectum, where they terminate. Fibers first enter the superficial parallel layer of the tectum, and then exit from this layer by dipping down into an underlying plexiform layer. Fibers arising from the outer periphery of the retina exit from the parallel layer and dip down to the plexiform layer soon after entering the tectum; those from more central points along a given retinal radius delay their entrance into the plexiform layer until they reach the central zones of the tectum.

Thus, the normal pathways of optic nerve fibers are complicated, and regenerating optic nerve axons are confronted with several consecutive points of decision com-

56–1 In the visual system of the goldfish, axons of the ganglion cells in the retina of the right eye cross completely in the optic chiasm to end in the left optic tectum. Axons from ganglion cells in the dorsal retina run in the lateral optic tract to end in the ventral tectum, whereas axons from the ventral retina run in the medial tract and end in the dorsal tectum. Moreover, axons from the anterior retina enter both tracts to terminate in the posterior tectum, while axons from the posterior retina enter both tracts to end in the anterior part of the tectum.

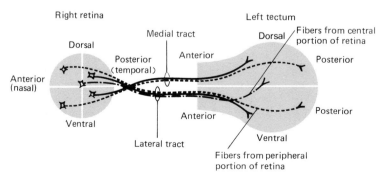

parable to a type of multiple-Y maze. To return to the tectum by its original pathway, a regenerating axon must make several correct decisions in sequential order: (1) It must correctly select either the medial or the lateral tract. (2) It must then make a series of selections along the circumference of the tectum and decide whether to turn radially into the parallel layer of the tectum or continue to push ahead tangentially in the main tract. (3) When it enters the parallel layer of the tectum and advances from the periphery to the center, the fiber must again decide whether to continue to grow centrally within the parallel layer or to dip downward into the plexiform layer. (4) Finally, after entering the plexiform layer, the different types of retinal fibers must select the proper neuron upon which to synapse. This selection must be made with reference not only to tectal topography and directionality in vision, but also to the detection of color and shapes.

Sperry took advantage of this system of multiple decision points in an elegant experiment in which he severed the optic nerve and at the same time removed large portions of retina. Severing the optic nerve led to degeneration of the distal portion of all axons running from cell bodies in the retina to the tectum. In removing an area of retina, Sperry removed the cell bodies of some of those axons and thus ensured that there would be no regeneration from the retinal region. Then he determined what happened to axons regenerating from the remaining part of the retina to assess the extent to which regenerating fibers are able to duplicate the normal pathways from specific areas of the retina to corresponding regions of the tectum.

Sperry first destroyed the dorsal part of the retina and asked: How specific is preference for tract? He found that even though fibers coming from the ventral part of the retina had a choice of tracts, they chose only the appropriate medial tract and entered the dorsal tectum (Figure 56–2A, 1). No fibers entered the lateral tract, and the ventral tectum remained unoccupied. Similarly, when he destroyed the ventral part of the retina and cut the optic nerve, the axons from the dorsal retina chose the lateral tract and went to the ventral tectum (Figure 56–2A, 2).

In still another set of experiments, Sperry tested the preference of regenerating fibers for the point of entrance into the tectum along its circumference. When the anterior (nasal) part of the retina was excised, the severed fibers from the posterior (temporal) retina split into two groups: one group entered the medial tract and the other entered the lateral tract. Axons from both tracts entered and reinnervated the anterior regions of the tectum and did not extend into the posterior region (Figure 56–2B, 1). When the posterior (temporal) half of the retina was removed, the regenerating fibers from both ventral and dorsal quadrants of the anterior (nasal) retina split into two groups: one group entered the medial tract and the other entered the lateral tract. Within both tracts, most of the fibers remained in the tract until they approached the posterior region of the tectum, where they dipped into the tectum to enter the plexiform layer (Figure 56–2B, 2).

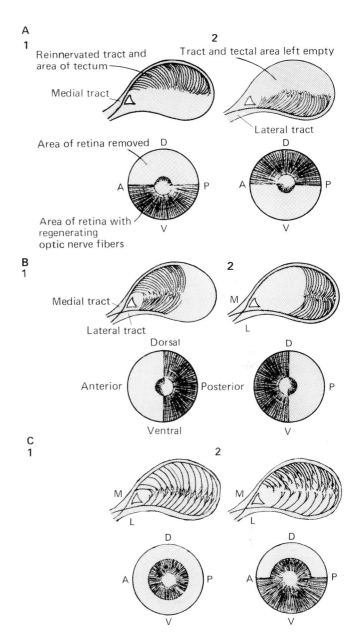

56–2 Three experiments by Sperry illustrate the precision with which outgrowing axons of regenerating retinal ganglion cell fibers connect with appropriate regions of the contralateral tectum in the goldfish. **D**, dorsal; **V**, ventral; **A**, anterior; **P**, posterior; **M**, medial; **L**, lateral.

A. After complete nerve section and ablation of either the dorsal **(1)** or ventral **(2)** hemiretina, regenerating nerve fibers show a preference for the appropriate division of the optic tract (lateral or medial) and site in the tectum (dorsal or ventral).

B. After removal of the anterior (nasal) **(1)** or posterior (temporal) **(2)** hemiretina, the regenerating nerve fibers show a correct preference for the appropriate point of entrance into the tectum along its circumference.

C. After removal of the entire peripheral retina **(1)** or only the dorsal part of the peripheral retina **(2)**, the regenerating nerve fibers show a correct preference for the appropriate point of entrance into the plexiform layer. (Adapted from Attardi and Sperry, 1963.)

Sperry also tested whether regenerating axons, after they enter the parallel layer of the tectum, show any preference for the point of entrance into the underlying plexiform layer. When the peripheral retina was removed, the outgrowing fibers from the central retina entered the tectum through both the medial and lateral tracts, but once having entered the tectum, the fibers from each tract did not descend into the plexiform layer until after they had reached the central zone (Figure 56–2C, 1). The fibers from the central retina bypassed the entire margin of the optic tectum, although the outgrowing nerve fibers have many opportunities to make contacts among the dense populations of neurons, and possibly glia and capillaries, in the optic tectum. Of these many opportunities, the fibers ultimately refused all but the appropriate ones. Incorrect zones in the tectum were consistently bypassed and left unoccupied.

Recent work indicates that the precise specificity demonstrated in Sperry's experiments represents only the final outcome of a prolonged and complex regenerative process, during which adjustments are constantly being made. Fujisawa and his colleagues used injections of horseradish peroxidase to mark regenerating neurons histochemically and showed that the initial searching, finding, and interconnecting are not precisely programmed; rather, the outgrowing axons actually wander over other tectal areas before homing in on the appropriate target. Moreover, although the initial outgrowth may follow the correct path, synapses also form along the way; however, these contacts are broken with time as further correction occurs. Even though the correct choices are ultimately made, the neurons appear to reach the final state through many provisional (and often incorrect) paths. Thus, the specificity encountered in these regeneration experiments is relative, not absolute.

As might be expected from the precise organization of the fiber tracts in the goldfish visual system, a great deal of specificity has also been found to govern the *initial* outgrowth of developing neurons. Particularly strong evidence for such specificity has come from studies by W. Maxwell Cowan and James Kelly on chick embryos and by Lynn Landmesser on the outgrowth of motor neurons to skeletal muscles. Here again, however, specificity is not absolute. For example, during the initial outgrowth of connections between eye and tectum in frogs, the retina continues to grow by gradually adding neurons in concentric annuli. At the same time, the optic tectum grows by adding neurons only at its caudal and medial borders. Despite this mismatch in modes of growth, the retinal ganglion cells form an organized map on the tectum quite early and retain that map throughout development and into maturity. This finding led Michael Gaze and his colleagues in England to propose that the connections that are initially formed in the tectum are not permanent but shift caudally during development until growth is complete. This notion has now received direct support from Martha Constantine-Paton at Princeton University; she found that during the early stages of development, retinal ganglion cells continually change the tectal neurons with which they form contacts.

The work of Gaze and co-workers and of Constantine-Paton suggests that, in addition to the ultimate specificity evident in Sperry's experiments, developmental systems also show a secondary capability to adjust and fine tune their connections in response to later cues. Thus, the evidence from both development and regeneration in the adult can best be understood in terms of two sequential stages: First, there is a *matching stage.* The process of matching is based on selective recognition of the proper target cells by the outgrowing axons of the presynaptic neurons. This is clearly evident in Sperry's work, in which appropriate regions of the retina and tectum are matched and interconnected to produce the overall features of the retinotopic map. The matching stage is followed by a *sorting and adjustment stage,* in which interactions between nearby afferent terminals refine the map and increase its precision.

What mechanisms underlie the early matching and the later fine tuning? At least five kinds of mechanisms are thought to be important:

1. *Chemical coding of pre- and postsynaptic cells.* Both the outgrowing nerve cells and their target cells are chemically marked according to their position.
2. *Pathfinding by reading substrate cues.* Outgrowing axons are guided to their target by following cues along the pathway.
3. *Selective recognition of the target by the outgrowing axon.* Specific patterns of connections are formed by intrinsic chemical recognition mechanisms.
4. *Adjustments in the size of the population by means of cell death and synapse elimination.*
5. *Fine tuning of connections through activity, competition, and other interactive processes.*

The first three mechanisms are thought to be essential for the initial matching of the outgrowing axons to their target. We shall consider them first. We shall then examine the last two mechanisms, which are thought to be important for the later steps of connection formation: sorting and adjustment.

The Initial Mapping of Connections Is Thought to Involve Three Sequential Processes

The Outgrowing Presynaptic Nerve Cells and Their Target Cells Are Chemically Coded to Mark Their Position

From his experiments on retinotectal connections, Sperry concluded that the nerve cells in both the eye and the tectum are coded for position along two axes, and that each cell is marked in relation to its neighbors. He further suggested that, as a result of these topographic labels, retinal ganglion cells acquire the capability to recognize appropriate tectal cells. He postulated that this recognition (he called it *affinity*) is based on molecular markers that derive from the position of the neurons' cell bodies in the retina. The neurons in the optic tectum undergo parallel differentiation and acquire complementary markers according to their position in the tectum.

To determine whether neurons actually have this postulated positional specificity, Sperry displaced a group of neurons from their normal position, allowed them to form connections, and then determined whether the new connections were appropriate to the cells' original position or to their new position. He assumed that neurons become specified according to their relative position in the retina or tectum at a particular time during their development. If the neurons had acquired their specificity before being displaced, they would be expected to form connections appropriate to their original position. Thus, in examining this problem, Sperry specifically addressed the broad question that we posed at the beginning of this chapter: To what degree are connections between neurons determined by built-in developmental programs, and to what degree are they due to patterns of impulses or to experience?

In amphibians, it is possible to cut the optic nerve and rotate the eyeball on its optic axis by 180°. The eye then heals in the new position and the fibers regenerate and reform connections with cells in the optic tectum. Sperry tested the precision of the connections behaviorally. He examined the visual motor responses of frogs whose eyes had been rotated and found that *these normally accurate responses were now consistently misguided by 180°*. For objects lying in the original upper anterior (now posterior) visual field, the animal consistently reached in the direction of its original lower posterior (now anterior) field (Figure 56–3). These maladaptive responses persist and are never corrected, indicating that, despite their current and persistent *behavioral inappropriateness*, the optic nerve fibers regenerate to the tectal nerve cells to which they were *originally connected* (and for which they were originally appropriate). This inability to re-educate the visual system suggests that the general pattern of neural connections in this system is laid down in an invariant manner without regard for the adaptiveness of the functional effect.

Further evidence for positional specificity was provided by Marcus Jacobson, then at Johns Hopkins University. He demonstrated that the retina has two gradients that develop independently. Jacobson rotated the eye cups of early larval amphibian embryos before the optic nerve grew out, long before the connections between eye and brain developed. He found that if the eye is rotated before stage 29 (an early developmental stage) the eye cup forms a normal projection; he concluded that retinal position has not been specified by stage 29. Rotation 10 hr later, at stage 30, leads to a normal dorsal–ventral retinal axis but causes inversion of the anterior–posterior retinal axis. The position of the anterior–posterior axis has therefore become specified by this stage. Rotation at stage 31, 10 hr later still, leads to total inversion, indicating that both axes have now been specified. Thus, although before stage 29 the retinal cells are not specified, after stage 29 the two retinal axes are rapidly specified within 24 hr. Stages 29 and 30 therefore constitute a *critical period* in development after which retinal specification becomes irreversible. *Critical periods are a common feature of the development of the ner-*

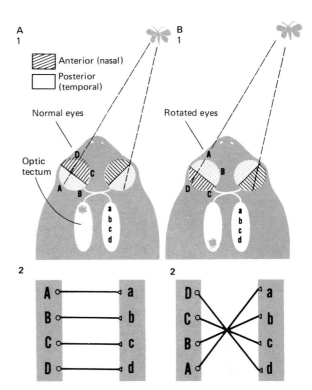

56–3 Rotation of the eye illustrates that visual connections in the frog are not determined by experience. Eyes and optic tecta first viewed from above (**1**) and then in a schematic representation (**2**). **A.** In the normal eyes, the projections of a fly in front of the frog are indicated on retinal points (**A, B, C, D**) and as these four points are projected on the tectum (**a, b, c, d**). **B.** After the eyes are rotated 180°, the neural connections between the retina and the tectum remain the same, so that the animal's visual perceptions are consistently incorrect by 180°. (Adapted from Lund, 1978.)

vous system. As we have seen before and shall see again later, critical periods have been found in the development of other parts of the nervous system and even in the types of behaviors they control (for social and perceptual skills, see Chapter 57; for sexual differentiation, see Chapter 58).

It seems improbable that every single cell in the retina has a unique protein marker that distinguishes it from all other cells because there are not enough genes to code for the large number of proteins that would be required for all the retinal cells (about 100,000 in the frog), much less for all their connections, which are 100 to 1000 times more numerous still. Most likely, the cells are marked by quantitative differences. For example, it is possible to conceive of a cell surface label that would operate as follows: two morphogenetic gradients operating at right angles impose coordinates on the retina. Two gradients in the tectum similarly mark each tectal cell in a complementary way. Each gradient represents the distribution of the same surface molecule, perhaps a glycoprotein. Each marker is produced by neurons at one end of an axis of cells, and it diffuses from one cell to another along the axis by means of the gap junctions that connect one cell to another during development (see Chapter 9). The substance is freely diffusible between the cells, and a certain fixed proportion of the molecules is retained by each cell so that the cells closest to the site of production retain the most molecules and those farthest away take up the least. Once taken up by the cell, the substance alters the properties of the surface membrane of that cell in a characteristic way (Figure 56–4).

Intriguing support for the notion that gradients of surface molecules can exist in the eye comes from G. David Trisler, Michael Schneider, and Marshall Nirenberg at the National Institutes of Health. Using monoclonal antibodies raised against chick retina, they discovered an antigen that is distributed in a gradient along the dorsal–ventral axis of the retina. Although there is as yet no evidence linking this immunological marker to the specificity of connections found in the retinotectal system, its distribution is consistent with the idea that positional information could be encoded in *molecular* terms.

An alternative to a cell surface label that is favored by Gaze and several others is that each cell occupies a specific position in the retina as a result of a *temporal* sequence determined by its birthdate and time of migra-

tion. The axons of the cells then become arranged in the optic nerve according to the position of the cell body in the retina, and the axons, in turn, impose this order on the tectum.

Outgrowing Axons Are Guided to Targets by Cues Distributed along the Pathway

Sperry postulated that once position is specified, the retinal ganglion cells begin to spin out their axons. The outgrowing axons are then guided to appropriate zones in the tectum by a series of chemical and mechanical cues. The detailed mechanisms by which axons go to one region rather than another are poorly understood. It seems likely that axons follow cues, although the nature of these cues differs in different parts of the nervous system. It is well known that axons readily follow a variety of physical cues that are provided by the nonneural substrate. Axons also receive cues from neighboring axons, and it is probable that the outgrowing nerve fibers navigate by continuously responding to surface signals embedded in the substrate of cellular elements that they traverse.

What are these signals? How might they work? As first shown by Santiago Ramón y Cajal, the movement of axons is determined by their *growth cones*, expansions of the tip of the growing axon that generate the

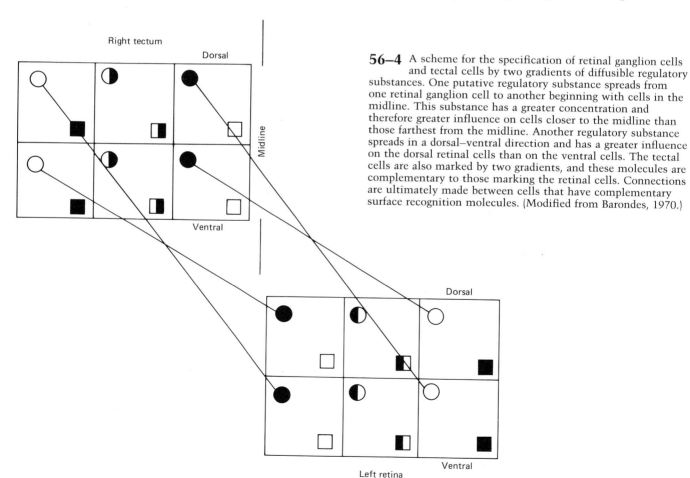

56–4 A scheme for the specification of retinal ganglion cells and tectal cells by two gradients of diffusible regulatory substances. One putative regulatory substance spreads from one retinal ganglion cell to another beginning with cells in the midline. This substance has a greater concentration and therefore greater influence on cells closer to the midline than those farthest from the midline. Another regulatory substance spreads in a dorsal–ventral direction and has a greater influence on the dorsal retinal cells than on the ventral cells. The tectal cells are also marked by two gradients, and these molecules are complementary to those marking the retinal cells. Connections are ultimately made between cells that have complementary surface recognition molecules. (Modified from Barondes, 1970.)

mechanical force that pulls the axon forward. The motility of growth cones is punctuated by cycles of protrusion, adhesion, and contraction, and it is likely that the physical substrate over which a fiber grows out contributes cues that guide the growth cone to its target. Substrates vary in adhesiveness, and that selective adhesion can guide the direction of the outgrowing process. Variations in the texture and shape of the available surfaces on which the processes grow may produce regional differences in the adhesion between the growth cone and the substrate that determine the direction of growth.

Consistent with this idea is the recent work by Gerald Edelman and his colleagues at Rockefeller University, who have been characterizing a population of *nerve cell adhesion molecules*. These are large glycoproteins with molecular weights of 180,000–250,000 that contain large amounts of the ionically charged sugar, sialic acid. Different regions of the brain are thought to contain different forms of the adhesion molecules, distinguished by different sugar residues.

In addition to adhesiveness, the growth cones might also sense more specific recognition molecules. For example, specific receptors on the surface of the outgrowing growth cones might recognize molecules on the surface of the cells forming the substrate. Alternatively, a signal molecule might be secreted by a substrate cell and internalized by the outgrowing cell; the molecule could then act from within the second cell to influence the direction of neurite outgrowth.

All of the pathfinding mechanisms we have so far considered are local; all involve cell–substrate interaction. None quite explains how axons find their way over great distances. Rita Levi-Montalcini, working in Rome, has thrown some light on this vexing problem. She injected into the brain of a young rat a protein called *nerve growth factor* (which we shall consider in more detail later) and found that axons of sympathetic neurons, which normally do not invade the central nervous system, grew into the brain in great abundance, presumably following chemical tracks created by the diffusion of nerve growth factor from the site of injection.

Nerve growth factor can also direct the outgrowth of the processes of sympathetic or dorsal root ganglion neurons in tissue culture. Ross Gundersen and John Barrett at the University of Miami have shown that the growth cones of sensory neurons in tissue culture turn in the direction of a pipette that releases nerve growth factor. The orientation of these processes is determined by the concentration gradient of the growth factor, suggesting that the growth cones can sense and respond to gradients of chemical signals; nerve growth factor and other chemotactic signals might thereby guide outgrowing fibers to their appropriate targets.

Thus, the direction pursued by the growth cones of an outgrowing axon is influenced by a variety of cues that range from (1) simple differences in the texture and stickiness of the substrate, to (2) rather precise molecular cues from recognition molecules imbedded in the surface membrane of the cells over which the growth cone

moves, to (3) diffusible gradients set up by a distant source.

The Outgrowing Axons Selectively Recognize the Target Cells

Sperry suggested that retinal neurons form synaptic connections preferentially with selected tectal neurons that have complementary cytochemical affinities. The incoming axon recognizes specific cues for appropriate synapse formation. Sperry proposed that the synapse is formed not only on an appropriate cell, but at a specific topographic portion of the cell's surface. It is not known how this is accomplished. In the case of the nerve–muscle synapse, glycoproteins (such as fibronectin, laminin, and chondronectin) or proteoglycans in the basement membrane located in the extracellular region (the *extracellular matrix*) of the synapse are thought to provide some of the cues.

If the actual wiring of connections is programmed and specific (except for some fine tuning), the critical aspects of the basic wiring should be present at birth or at least before the animal has a chance to learn about its environment. David Hubel and Torsten Wiesel found that in both the cat and the monkey there is at birth a precise topographical organization of the visual field in the retina, the lateral geniculate nucleus, and area 17 of the visual cortex. In addition, the response properties seen in the adult are largely present in newborn animals. Although, as we shall see below, some fine details of the interactions between neurons (and between neurons and muscle) are regulated by experiential factors, the recognition of one cell by another seems to be quite specific and to require preexisting information on the part of both the pre- and postsynaptic cells. The mechanisms for this recognition are not known, however. One attractive idea is that each outgrowing nerve fiber finds its way by means of a series of clues, by trial and error. Gap junctions or some other means of exchanging information between two cells might develop, to allow the exchange of cues between the pre- and postsynaptic cells. Once a chemical synapse is established, the chemical and electrical properties of both the pre- and postsynaptic elements can be further modulated by cellular interactions that make the connection work optimally.

The Final Stages of Synapse Formation Are Thought to Involve Numerical Matching and Fine Tuning Through Competition and Activity

The final steps in synapse formation and stabilization involve two major interactions between the outgrowing nerve fiber and the target: (1) the matching of the size of the population of presynaptic neurons and their targets by cell death, synapse retraction, and competition for growth substance, and (2) fine tuning of connections by competition and activity. Although each of the steps has now been examined in many systems, they have been studied best in the synapse between motor neurons and muscle because the synapse is so simple and accessible.

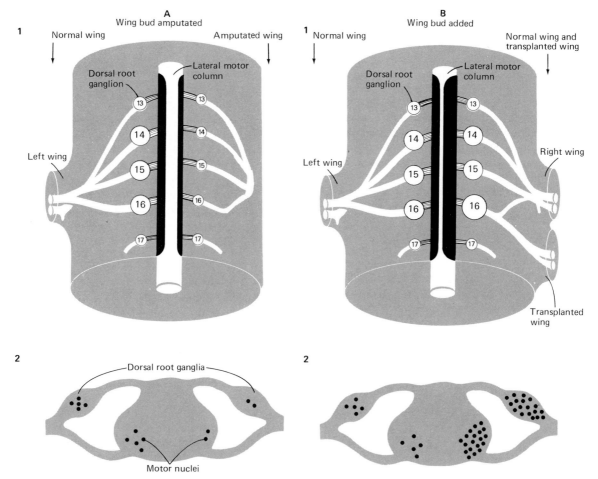

56-5 Cell death of the outgrowing neurons is regulated by the number of available target cells. For example, in the chick embryo illustrated here, the number of target cells available influences the number of surviving sensory and motor neurons. **A.** When a wing bud of a chick embryo is amputated, the population of motor neurons in the ventral horn and afferent neurons in the dorsal root ganglia destined to connect to the wing bud is greatly reduced compared with normal. **B.** When an extra wing bud is added to the same side as a normal one, a greater number of motor and afferent neurons survive. **A1** and **B2.** Longitudinal view of the spinal cord showing the motor neurons of the lateral motor columns and the afferent regions of the dorsal root ganglia. **A2** and **B2.** Cross-sectional view at one level of the spinal cord and dorsal root. (From Hamburger, 1934.)

The Size of the Target Population Influences the Number of Surviving Neurons

The size of the target population of cells is a major factor in modulating the relation between the outgrowing neurons and their targets. The study of the influence of a target muscle on the outgrowing motor neuron began with a classic set of experiments by Ross Harrison (who also developed the technique of tissue culture) and by Viktor Hamburger and Rita Levi-Montalcini (Figure 56-5). By removing a limb bud in chick embryos (or by adding extra limb buds), Hamburger and Levi-Montalcini manipulated the size of the target field of innervation to which the outgrowing nerves were directed. In a typical experiment, a chick embryo is surgically deprived of one bud on the third day of incubation, about 24 hr before the outgrowing axons from the motor neurons reach the limb. As a result, a scar forms. As the axons of the motor neuron grow out, they at first look quite normal. However, when the outgrowing axons encounter the scar rather than the muscle, they fail to find a signal produced by the target. Lacking this signal, the motor neurons shrivel up and die. There is massive degeneration of the motor cells destined to innervate the amputated limb (Figure 56-5A).

During normal development an excess of motor neurons is generated in the period of motor cell proliferation. About one-half of these potential motor neurons die as nerve–muscle synapses are established, perhaps because they do not form functional contacts, so that the population of motor cells is reduced to the number found in the normal adult. Ablation of the limb bud accentuates the normally occurring cell death and causes all the motor neurons that would have innervated the limb to die.

If, instead, a second limb bud is added to one side of the embryo, the size and number of motor neurons greatly increase on that side (Figure 56–5B). The existence of a greater field of innervation leads to the ultimate survival of more cells than usual because fewer cells die.

Thus, targets in the periphery profoundly influence the survival of the motor neurons. One mechanism by which the number of presynaptic neurons can be regulated by the size of the target is the competition of innervating neurons for some signal from the target that will determine survival. Unless neurons grow out and receive a critical signal from the muscle, perhaps by forming successful synapses on the muscle, they die. To survive, a motor neuron must compete with other outgrowing neurons for this restricted nutrient that can be obtained only by making successful contacts with a target muscle cell.

Some Early Synaptic Contacts Are Later Retracted

Not only does the target regulate the number of neurons that survive, but it also controls the number of synapses that each surviving cell makes (Figure 56–6). Synapse control, which is independent of reduction in nerve cell number, occurs afterward. In this process some synapses that were initially formed are eliminated. For example, whereas adult muscle fibers are generally innervated by only one axon, embryonic muscle is innervated by several. After a few weeks, the number of motor axons is reduced through a process of competition based on factors that initially favored one axon over another (for example, an axon that was active and made its contacts early would be likely to survive at the expense of an axon that formed its contacts later). The remaining axon now often increases the number of synaptic contacts on the target (Figure 56–6A). Dale Purves and J. W. Lichtman have shown that a similar developmental regulation of synaptic contacts occurs at neuron–neuron contacts in autonomic ganglia. Certain synapses are eliminated, even though the overall number of contacts increases, because the axons that remain form more synaptic contacts than they had before the inappropriate axons had retracted (Figure 56–6B). An important function of the elimination of certain synapses is to ensure that the connections that are retained are quantitatively as well as qualitatively correct.

Whereas cell death serves to match the population of neurons to the population of target cells, synapse elimination serves to make the pattern of innervation precise. The competitive basis of these developmental readjustments of synaptic connections is thought to be related to the trophic support that the innervating axons receive from their target cells.

Max Cowan and his colleagues have shown that these regressive phenomena are also prominent features of the development of the central nervous system. Here process and synapse elimination is often not restricted to the axon terminal, nor does it function simply to fine-tune a set of initial connections. Rather, process and synapse

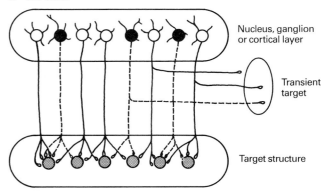

A Cell death

Nucleus, ganglion or cortical layer

Transient target

Target structure

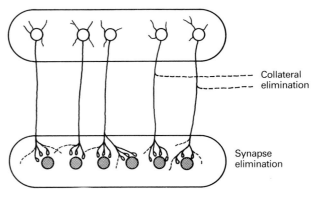

B Process elimination

Collateral elimination

Synapse elimination

56–6 Cell death and the elimination of processes and synapses are important regressive events in development. **A.** Cell death is responsible for matching the size of a population of presynaptic neurons so that it is appropriate to the size of the target population. **B.** Synapse and process elimination regulates the number of contacts that a given axon makes on its target and is responsible for the exclusion of inappropriate collateral processes. After some of the synaptic connections in the neonate are eliminated, the remaining presynaptic fibers increase the number of their contacts on the target cell. (Adapted from Cowan and O'Leary, 1984).

elimination can eliminate axon collateral processes and have important consequences for modifying or even eliminating components of neural pathways (Figure 56–6B).

Nerve Growth Factor Is an Example of a Trophic Signal

What trophic signal might the postsynaptic cell be emitting to encourage the survival of the newly differentiated motor neurons? The best available clue comes from the studies of Levi-Montalcini and her colleagues on developing sympathetic neurons. In 1951 Levi-Montalcini and Hamburger discovered that implantation of a mouse sarcoma into a 3-day chick embryo resulted in a significant innervation of the sarcoma by cells of the sympathetic ganglia. They showed that this increased growth was

A Nerve growth factor prohormone
   (M$_r$ ~ 130,000)

B Monomer of β subunit (nerve growth factor)

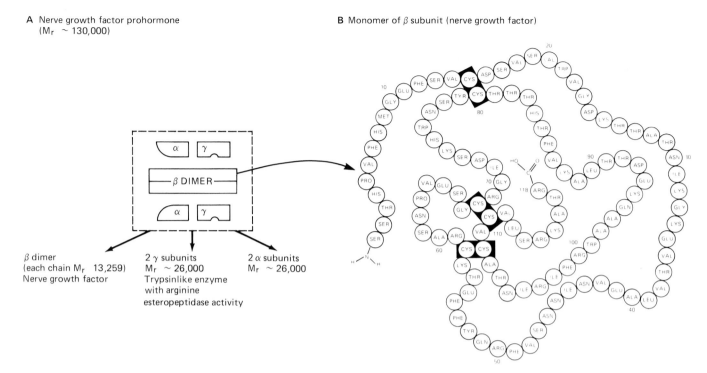

β dimer
(each chain M$_r$ 13,259)
Nerve growth factor

2 γ subunits
M$_r$ ~ 26,000
Trypsinlike enzyme
with arginine
esteropeptidase activity

2 α subunits
M$_r$ ~ 26,000

56–7 The active component of nerve growth factor is the beta subunit of a large prohormone. **A.** The prohormone is cleaved into the five subunits, which represent three types of peptides: 2 alphas, 1 beta, and 2 gammas. (Courtesy of D. Ishii.) **B.** The amino acid sequence of a monomer of the beta subunit, which is the active growth-promoting component of the larger protein precursor. (From Angeletti and Bradshaw, in Patterson and Purves, 1982.)

caused by the diffusible substance that they called *nerve growth factor* (NGF). Although its mode of action is not known, nerve growth factor is critical for the development and maintenance of sympathetic neurons as well as the sensory neurons of the dorsal root ganglia. Administration to newborn animals of antibody raised against nerve growth factor causes sympathetic ganglia to atrophy. (This treatment is therefore called an *immunosympathectomy*.) In contrast, administration of nerve growth factor stimulates the outgrowth of processes from sympathetic neurons, and its presence enhances and often is essential for the survival of embryonic sympathetic neurons. Moreover, Ian Hendry, Leslie Iversen, Levi-Montalcini, Hans Thoenen, Louis Reichardt and their colleagues have found that nerve growth factor is synthesized and released by the target cells innervated by sympathetic neurons. (The submaxillary salivary gland of some vertebrates is a particularly good storage depot.) Nerve growth factor is then taken up by the terminals of sympathetic neurons by pinocytosis and carried by fast retrograde axonal transport to the cell body, where it acts by altering gene expression.

Nerve growth factor is a protein that is synthesized in target cells as part of a larger prohormone. NGF contains three types of subunits—alpha, beta, and gamma. It has a molecular weight of 130,000 and a stoichiometry of two alpha, one beta, and two gamma subunits (α$_2$βγ$_2$) (Figure 56–7). The gamma subunit is a proteolytic en-

zyme that is thought to be involved in the processing of the prohormone; the alpha subunit inhibits this protease. The beta subunit alone is responsible for its biological activity on nerve cells. The beta subunit is a dimer with a molecular weight of about 26,000; each of its monomeric units is a polypeptide chain made up of 118 amino acids (Figure 56–7B). There is some homology in amino acid sequence between the beta subunit and insulin, another hormone that enhances growth. These similarities suggest that both proteins belong to the same family and may have evolved from a common precursor molecule, perhaps a growth-promoting protein (see Chapter 13).

During normal development about one-third of the dorsal root ganglion cells and sympathetic neurons die. Hamburger and Levi-Montalcini have shown that when NGF is present in abundance it rescues sympathetic and dorsal root ganglion cells that would otherwise die, suggesting that these cells die when they lack this growth factor.

Unlike sympathetic neurons and the sensory cells in the dorsal root ganglia, motor neurons do not require this particular nerve growth factor. However, Mark Gurney at the University of Chicago has recently isolated a growth factor that appears important for the outgrowth of processes and the survival of motor neurons. Therefore, most developmental neurobiologists think that NGF is only one of many growth factors that are likely to be discovered in the near future.

We have discussed examples in which the target influences the outgrowing neuron. Also important in development are situations in which the outgrowing neuron influences its target. A good example is the effect of activity in the motor neuron on the properties of skeletal muscle.

Activity Can Influence the Distribution of the Acetylcholine Receptor in the Muscle Membrane

Acetylcholine receptors of vertebrate skeletal muscles normally are confined to the region of the end-plates. Here the density exceeds 20,000 receptor molecules/μm^2. In contrast, a few micrometers away the density of receptors falls to extremely low levels, less than $50/\mu m^2$. Julius Axelsson and Stephen Thesleff in Sweden and Ricardo Miledi in England found that if the nerve is cut and allowed to degenerate, acetylcholine receptors are no longer restricted to the end-plate, but are distributed in the membrane of the extrajunctional regions all over the muscle fiber (Figure 56–8). The density of receptors in the extrajunctional region never quite reaches the density of the denervated end-plate. This diffuse distribution of new receptors does not represent the unmasking of occult receptors; rather, it reflects the synthesis of new receptors and their insertion into the membrane.

Three other observations are related to the appearance of new receptors: (1) If the muscle is reinnervated, the extrajunctional receptors disappear. The receptors again become restricted to the region of the end-plate. (2) Embryonic muscle is diffusely sensitive to acetylcholine. Once it becomes innervated, however, its sensitivity to acetylcholine becomes restricted to the end-plate region. (3) A muscle fiber innervated by one nerve fiber can no longer be innervated by another. Thus, once synapse formation has occurred, restriction of chemosensitivity may be one of the several mechanisms that prevent other nerve axons from forming synapses on the muscle.

What restricts the insertion of acetylcholine receptors following innervation and what leads to the insertion of new receptors in response to denervation? One early notion was that the transmitter substance (acetylcholine) or some other (trophic) substance flows from nerve to muscle and is responsible for restricting the acetylcholine receptors. When the nerve is cut, the substance stops flowing and new receptors are inserted into the extrajunctional membrane. Although this view was generally accepted and, for a while, influential, Terje Lømo and Jean Rosenthal have shown it to be only partly correct. The appearance of receptors in the extrajunctional region after denervation is mostly due to *disuse*, the lack of muscle contraction normally produced by activity in the nerve. Similarly, activity (use) of the muscle accounts in large part for the decrease in the receptor density in the extrajunctional region of innervated muscle.

Activity, however, does not account for all of the restriction. For example, if muscle activity is prevented by applying to the nerve a cuff of tetrodotoxin, which blocks the voltage-sensitive Na^+ channels and thereby nerve

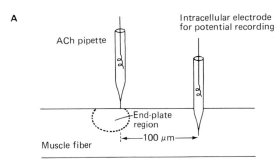

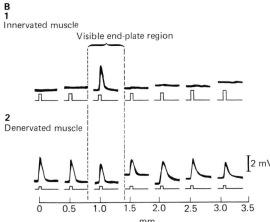

56–8 The distribution of acetylcholine (**ACh**) receptors is increased following denervation. **A.** The distribution of the ACh receptor can be mapped by applying a small amount of acetylcholine iontophoretically through an extracellular electrode (pipette) at various points along the muscle. **B.** Intracellular recordings show depolarizing responses when acetylcholine is applied to a region of the muscle membrane containing receptors. **1:** In innervated muscle, the receptors are largely restricted to the end-plate. **2:** After denervation, receptors are also found in the extrasynaptic membrane of the muscle fiber. (Adapted from Axelsson and Thesleff, 1959.)

impulse activity, the spread of acetylcholine receptors is not as great as when the nerve is cut. (The presence of acetylcholine receptors is assayed by the binding of α-bungarotoxin, a substance that binds specifically with the acetylcholine receptor; see Chapter 14.) Furthermore, simulation of the electrical activity of normal innervation cannot completely restrict the acetylcholine receptors to the end-plate zone of denervated muscle. Part of the restriction of the receptors seems to require the passage of some (as yet unspecified) substance from nerve to muscle.

Gerald Fischbach at Washington University found that, during the development of synapses in cell culture, cholinergic axons rapidly induce clusters of acetylcholine receptors at the site where transmitter is released onto skeletal muscle. This clustering of receptors at high density is also thought to be induced by one or more unidentified substances released by the motor axon. Fischbach, Thomas Podleski at Cornell University, and Phillip Nelson at the National Institutes of Health have isolated a

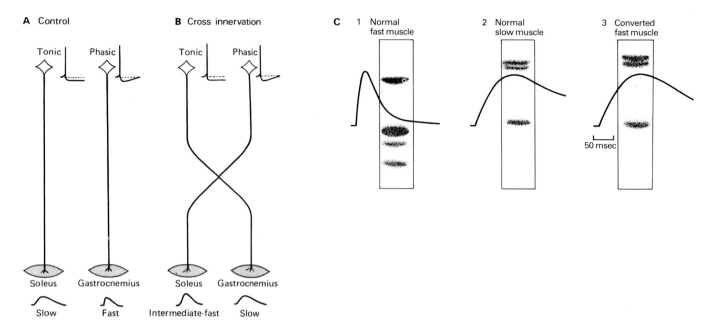

56–9 Cross innervation of motor axons to slow and fast muscle transforms the contractile properties of the muscles. **A.** Control preparations. **B.** A cross-innervated preparation produced by surgically cross-anastomosing the axon of tonic (slow) motor neurons to fast muscle and vice versa. The unique characteristics of the two species of motor neurons do not change after cross innervation; however, fast muscles are completely transformed to slow muscles and slow muscles are changed into an intermediate form. **C.** Changing the pattern of stimulation alters contractile proteins of muscle, as illustrated in SDS gels of the myosins from muscle. **1** and **2** illustrate the gel pattern for myosin from normal fast and slow muscle, respectively. **3** illustrates the gel for fast muscle that has been stimulated for 20 weeks at frequencies characteristic of a slow motor neuron. Both the contractile response and the myosin pattern have now come to resemble those of a slow muscle. (Part **C** adapted from Salmons and Sréter, 1976.)

peptide from brain and spinal cord that is present in cholinergic neurons and that increases the number of receptor clusters by 40-fold.

Activity Can Influence the Speed of Muscle Contraction

As we have seen in the discussion of muscles and their receptors (Chapter 34), adult cats and other mammals have two types of muscles that can be distinguished on the basis of color and by speed of contraction: fast (pale) and slow (red). Fast muscles (also called twitch muscles) depend on glycolytic metabolism, whereas slow muscles, rich in myoglobin, depend on aerobic respiration. Fast muscles are involved in phasic contractions; slow muscles are involved in postural adjustment. The relationship of motor neurons to muscle has been studied by John C. Eccles, who found that motor neurons and muscles have matching properties. Motor neurons that innervate fast muscles have a rapid conduction velocity and a brief hyperpolarizing afterpotential and can therefore fire rapidly at 30–60 impulses/sec. Motor neurons that innervate slow muscles conduct slowly and have a larger afterpotential. These motor neurons fire more slowly, at 10–20 impulses/sec.

Newborn kittens have only slow muscles. Their muscles differentiate into fast or slow over a period of weeks after birth. How does this differentiation occur? Do the motor neurons determine the properties of the muscle, or does the muscle determine the properties of the motor neurons? To examine this question Arthur J. Buller, John C. Eccles, and Rosamond Eccles switched nerves and muscles surgically and found that the neurons, independent of the muscles they innervated, retained their properties. In contrast, the muscles changed their contractile properties when their innervation was changed. A fast muscle was converted to a slow muscle as a result of being innervated by a slow motor neuron, and slow muscles likewise converted to faster muscles (Figure 56–9). This transformation is remarkable for two reasons. First, as this experiment illustrates, the differentiation into fast or slow muscle is not an irreversible process that occurs only once in the developmental history of the organism; the process of differentiation is maintained continuously throughout life. A change in innervation at any time will lead to the redifferentiation of the muscle. Second, the fast and slow muscles differ in their myosin light chains. The initial differentiation and the subsequent redifferentiation involve an alteration in gene expression. Thus, the nervous system can control which light chain gene is expressed by the muscle!

What is responsible for this step in redifferentiation, this change in gene expression? Is there a chemical influence that flows from the nerve to the muscle, perhaps something released in conjunction with the neurotransmitter? Or is the signal simply the pattern or speed of contraction that the neuron imposes on the muscle? Lømo, R. H. Westgaard, and H. A. Dahl found that at least part of the differentiation of muscle is determined by the pattern of activity, i.e., the frequency of contraction. Thus, motor innervation is critical for the differentiation of fast and slow muscles because it determines the rate at which the muscle will contract.

An Overall View

Studies of the development of the brain and of behavior support a modified constructionist view, according to which the major connections of the nervous system are established under genetic and developmental control. Developmental sequences are not rigid, however, and can be influenced by the environment and by experience. They depend crucially on a series of optimally timed cellular interactions. These interactions include three that map the presynaptic population onto the target: (1) molecular marking of the two populations according to position; (2) guiding the growth cone to its target; and (3) ensuring, by means of at least low-grade recognition, that the outgrowing axon reaches the correct region in the target. This initial matching is then followed by a series of shaping adjustments thought to involve competition for limited growth factors. Finally, there is further fine tuning through activity. Moreover, although the initial establishment of the connection occurs in the absence of learning, as we shall see in the next section (Part XI), learning is important for subsequent fine tuning and maintenance as well as for regulating the strength of the connections.

Selected Readings

Attardi, D. G., and Sperry, R. W. 1963. Preferential selection of central pathways by regenerating optic fibers. Exp. Neurol. 7:46–64.

Barde, Y. -A., Edgar, D., and Thoenen, H. 1983. New neurotrophic factors. Annu. Rev. Physiol. 45:601–612.

Cowan, W. M. 1979. The development of the brain. Sci. Am. 241(3):112–133.

Cowan, W. M. 1982. A synoptic view of the development of the vertebrate central nervous system. In J. G. Nicholls (ed.), Repair and Regeneration of the Nervous System. Dahlem Konferenzen. Berlin: Springer, pp. 7–24.

Cowan, W. M., and O'Leary, D. D. M. 1984. Cell death and process elimination: The role of regressive phenomena in the development of the vertebrate nervous system. In K. J. Isselbacher (ed.), Medicine, Science and Society. New York: Wiley, pp. 643–668.

Edds, M. V., Jr. 1967. Neuronal specificity in neurogenesis. In G. C. Quarton, T. Melnechuk, and F. O. Schmitt (eds.), The Neurosciences: A Study Program. New York: Rockefeller University Press, pp. 230–240.

Gundersen, R. W., and Barrett, J. N. 1980. Characterization of the turning response of dorsal root neurites toward nerve growth factor. J. Cell Biol. 87:546–554.

Gurney, M. E. 1984. Suppression of sprouting at the neuromuscular junction by immune sera. Nature 307:546–548.

Jacobson, M. 1978. Developmental Neurobiology, 2nd ed. New York: Plenum Press.

Landmesser, L. T. 1980. The generation of neuromuscular specificity. Annu. Rev. Neurosci. 3:279–302.

Landmesser, L. 1984. The development of specific motor pathways in the chick embryo. Trends Neurosci. 7:336–339.

Letourneau, P. C. 1983. Axonal growth and guidance. Trends Neurosci. 6:451–455.

Levi-Montalcini, R. 1975. NGF: An uncharted route. In F. G. Worden, J. P. Swazey, and G. Adelman (eds.), The Neurosciences: Paths of Discovery. Cambridge, Mass.: MIT Press, pp. 245–265.

Lømo, T., and Westgaard, R. H. 1976. Control of ACh sensitivity in rat muscle fibers. Cold Spring Harbor Symp. Quant. Biol. 40:263–274.

Lund, R. D. 1978. Development and Plasticity of the Brain. New York: Oxford University Press.

Margolis, R. U., and Margolis, R. K. (eds.). 1979. Complex Carbohydrates of Nervous Tissue. New York: Plenum Press.

Patterson, P. H., and Purves, D. (eds.). 1982. Readings in Developmental Neurobiology. Cold Spring Harbor, New York: Cold Spring Harbor Laboratory.

Purves, D., and Lichtman, J. W. 1985. Principles of Neural Development. Sunderland, Mass.: Sinauer Associates.

Reichardt, L. F. 1984. Immunological approaches to the nervous system. Science 225:1294–1299.

Sanes, J. 1983. The role of extracellular matrix in neural development. Annu. Rev. Physiol. 45:581–600.

Stent, G. S. (ed.). 1977. Function and Formation of Neural Systems. Dahlem Konferenzen. Berlin: Springer.

Weeds, A. G., Trentham, D. R., Kean, C. J. C., and Buller, A. J. 1974. Myosin from cross-reinnervated cat muscles. Nature 247:135–139.

References

Axelsson, J., and Thesleff, S. 1959. A study of supersensitivity in denervated mammalian skeletal muscle. J. Physiol. (Lond.) 147:178–193.

Barondes, S. H. 1970. Brain glycomacromolecules and interneuronal recognition. In F. O. Schmitt (ed.), The Neurosciences: Second Study Program. New York: Rockefeller University Press, pp. 747–760.

Buller, A. J., Eccles, J. C., and Eccles, R. M. 1960. Interactions between motoneurones and muscles in respect of the characteristic speeds of their responses. J. Physiol. (Lond.) 150:417–439.

Cajal, S. R. 1929. Étude sur la Neurogenèse de Quelques Vertébrés. Trans. by L. Guth as Studies on Vertebrate Neurogenesis. Springfield, Ill.: Thomas, 1960.

Cowan, W. M., Fawcett, J. W., O'Leary, D. D. M., and Stanfield, B. B. 1984. Regressive events in neurogenesis. Science 225:1258–1265.

Edelman, G. M. 1984. Cell-adhesion molecules: A molecular basis for animal form. Sci. Amer. 250(4):118–129.

Fujisawa, H., Tani, N., Watanabe, K., and Ibata, Y. 1982. Branching of regenerating retinal axons and preferential selection of appropriate branches for specific neuronal connections in the newt. Dev. Biol. 90:43–57.

Gaze, R. M., Keating, M. J., and Chung, S. H. 1974. The evolution of the retinotectal map during development in Xenopus. Proc. R. Soc. Lond. [Biol.] 185:301–330.

Gaze, R. M., Keating, M. J., Ostberg, A., and Chung, S.-H. 1979. The relationship between retinal and tectal growth in larval *Xenopus:* Implications for the development of retino-tectal projection. J. Embryol. Exp. Morphol. 53:103–143.

Hamburger, V. 1934. The effects of wing bud extirpation on the development of the central nervous system in chick embryos. J. Exp. Zool. 68:449–494.

Hamburger, V. 1977. The developmental history of the motor neuron. The F. O. Schmitt Lecture in Neuroscience. Neurosci. Res. Program Bull. [Suppl.] 15:1–37.

Hamburger, V., and Levi-Montalcini, R. 1949. Proliferation, differentiation and degeneration in the spinal ganglia of the chick embryo under normal and experimental conditions. J. Exp. Zool. 111:457–501.

Harrison, R. G. 1935. On the origin and development of the nervous system studied by the methods of experimental embryology. Proc. R. Soc. Lond. [Biol.] 118:155–196.

Hendry, I. A., Stöckel, K., Thoenen, H., and Iversen, L. L. 1974. The retrograde axonal transport of nerve growth factor. Brain Res. 68:103–121.

Horton, J. C., Greenwood, M. M., and Hubel, D. H. 1979. Non-retinotopic arrangement of fibres in cat optic nerve. Nature 282:720–722.

Jacobson, M. 1968. Development of neuronal specificity in retinal ganglion cells of *Xenopus.* Dev. Biol. 17:202–218.

Jessell, T. M., Siegel, R. E., and Fischbach, G. D. 1979. Induction of acetylcholine receptors on cultured skeletal muscle by a factor extracted from brain and spinal cord. Proc. Natl. Acad. Sci. U.S.A. 76:5397–5401.

Kelly, J. P., and Cowan, W. M. 1972. Studies on the development of the chick optic tectum. III. Effects of early eye removal. Brain Res. 42:263–288.

Levi-Montalcini, R. 1952. Effects of mouse tumor transplantation on the nervous system. Ann. N.Y. Acad. Sci. 55:330–343.

Lømo, T., and Rosenthal, J. 1972. Control of ACh sensitivity by muscle activity in the rat. J. Physiol. (Lond.) 221:493–513.

Lømo, T., Westgaard, R. H., and Dahl, H. A. 1974. Contractile properties of muscle: Control by pattern of muscle activity in the rat. Proc. R. Soc. Lond. [Biol.] 187:99–103.

Miledi, R. 1960. The acetylcholine sensitivity of frog muscle fibres after complete or partial denervation. J. Physiol. 151:1–23.

Reh, T. A., and Constantine-Paton, M. 1984. Retinal ganglion cell terminals change their projection sites during larval development of *Rana pipiens.* J. Neurosci. 4:442–457.

Salmons, S., and Sréter, F. A. 1976. Significance of impulse activity in skeletal muscle type. Nature 263:30–34.

Sperry, R. W. 1951. Mechanisms of neural maturation. In S. S. Stevens (ed.), Handbook of Experimental Psychology. New York: Wiley, pp. 236–280.

Thoenen, H., Otten, U., and Schwab, M. 1979. Orthograde and retrograde signals for the regulation of neuronal gene expression: The peripheral sympathetic nervous system as a model. In F. O. Schmitt and F. G. Worden (eds.), The Neurosciences: Fourth Study Program. Cambridge, Mass.: MIT Press, pp. 911–928.

Trisler, G. D., Schneider, M. D. and Nirenberg, M. 1981. A topographic gradient of molecules in retina can be used to identify neuron position. Proc. Natl. Acad. Sci. U.S.A. 78:2145–2149.

Ullrich, A., Gray, A., Berman, C., Coussens, L., and Dull, T. J. 1983. Sequence homology of human and mouse β-NGF subunit genes. Cold Spring Harbor Symp. Quant. Biol. 48:435–442.

Yoon, M. G. 1976. Topographic polarity of the optic tectum studied by reimplantation of the tectal tissue in adult goldfish. Cold Spring Harbor Symp. Quant. Biol. 40:503–519.

Eric R. Kandel

Early Experience, Critical Periods, and Developmental Fine Tuning of Brain Architecture

57

The brain is a precisely wired device that performs a series of logical operations on the sensory input it receives from a variety of receptors. This information is processed into coherent patterns of activity that we call thoughts and feelings. On the basis of these patterns (our perception of the external and internal world), the brain is capable of initiating action.

Although the structure of the brain is, to an important degree, specified by genetic and developmental processes, the pattern of interconnections between neurons also depends upon experience. Indeed, the brain is remarkably plastic: it is readily capable of changing its performance and even its strategies as a result of experience. At certain stages in development, the integrative action of the brain and, at a cellular level, its very structure, are dependent on its interaction with the environment.

The influence of the environment on the brain and, therefore, on behavior varies with age. Abnormal environmental experience or patterns of stimulation usually have more profound effects at early stages of development than at later ones. In this chapter we shall first examine how early experience influences the development of the immature brain. In Chapter 62, we shall consider how later experience, such as learning, influences the adult brain.

There Is a Critical Period in the Development of Normal Social and Perceptual Competence

As we saw in Chapter 56, there are critical periods in the development of the brain. These irreversible points of choice commit nerve cells to differentiate along one path or another. There are similar critical periods in the development of instinctive behavior—for example, in the acquisition of sexual identity (see Chapter 58). Recent experiments, ranging from very complex ones in human infants to relatively simple ones in experimental animals, have demonstrated that there are also critical periods in the development of social and perceptual competence. During these periods the infant must interact with a normal environment if further development is to proceed normally.

A particularly well-studied example of a critical period in the acquisition of a normal behavior is *imprinting*, a form of learning encountered in birds and examined in detail by the Austrian ethologist Konrad Lorenz. Just after birth, birds quickly learn to become attached to a prominent moving object, typically the mother, in their environment. This imprinting is important for the protection of the hatchling. Like one-trial learning, it is acquired rapidly, and once acquired it generally does not disappear. However, imprinting can be acquired only during a critical period (which in some species lasts a few hours) early in postnatal development. Imprinting, therefore, illustrates the close relationship between development and learning.

The clearest way to show that certain social or perceptual stimuli are important for development is to deprive an infant of these stimuli and to examine the consequences on later perceptual or social performance. Although ethics prevents scientists from carrying out deprivation experiments on human infants, deprivation has sometimes been imposed, often unintentionally, by parents or by public institutions. There are a few reliable histories of wild children who survived abandonment in the forest or jungle and who later were returned to civilization. (One particularly striking case was the French child Victor, who was discovered in 1800 and whose story inspired the film *The Wild Child*, directed by François Truffaut.) Anecdotal evidence also abounds about newborn infants who were left unattended during the major part of each day, being fed but not otherwise cared for. As might be expected, severely deprived children are socially misfit and usually are forever irreclaimable. The social behavior of these abandoned children is abnormal, and they often are mute and incapable of learning language.

The first coherent evidence that social interaction with other humans is essential for the normal development of infants came in the 1940s with the classic studies of the psychoanalyst René Spitz, who worked in New York. Spitz compared the development of infants raised in a foundling home for abandoned children with the development of infants raised in a nursing home attached to a women's prison. Both institutions were clean, and adequate food and medical care were provided. The babies in the nursing home were all cared for by their mothers, who, because they were in prison and away from their families, tended to shower affection on their infants in the limited time allotted to them each day. In

contrast, in the foundling home the infants were cared for by nurses, each of whom was responsible for seven babies. As a result, children in the foundling home had much less contact with other human beings than those in the prison's nursing home. The two institutions also differed in another respect. In the nursing home the cribs were open, and the infants could readily watch the activity in the ward; they could see other babies play and observe their mothers and the staff go about their business. In the foundling home the bars of the cribs were covered by sheets that prevented the infants from seeing outside. This dramatically reduced the infants' environment. In short, the babies in the foundling home lived under conditions of relative sensory and social deprivation.

Spitz followed a group of newborn infants at each of the two institutions throughout their early years. At the end of the first 4 months, the infants in the foundling home scored better than those in the nursing home on several developmental tests. This suggested to Spitz that genetic factors did not favor the infants in the nursing home. However, 8 months later, at the end of the first year, the motor and intellectual performance of the children in the foundling home had fallen far below that of those in the nursing home, and many had developed a syndrome that Spitz called *hospitalism* (now often called *anaclitic depression*). These children were withdrawn, showed little curiosity or gaiety, and were prone to infection. (They appeared to have acquired a socially induced form of immunodeficiency syndrome.) During their second and third years, children in the nursing home were similar to children raised in normal families at home: they walked well and talked actively. In contrast, the development of the children in the foundling home was delayed. Only 2 of 26 children in the foundling home were able to walk, only these 2 spoke at all, and even they could say only a few words. Normal children at this age are agile, have a vocabulary of hundreds of words, and speak in sentences.

Although Spitz's pioneering studies were not well controlled (and have often been criticized for their methodology), several aspects of his work have been confirmed in later, more carefully controlled studies, and most students of infant development now agree that Spitz's conclusions are basically correct. Severe social and sensory deprivation in early childhood can have catastrophic consequences for later development. In contrast, isolation later in life (although often unpleasant) is much better tolerated. The studies by Spitz thus stand as a landmark; they define a paradigm that has since been applied repeatedly and profitably.

Isolated Young Monkeys Do Not Develop Normal Social Behavior

Spitz's work was carried one important step further in the 1960s when Harry and Margaret Harlow at the University of Wisconsin developed an experimental model of human social deprivation by rearing monkeys in isolation. They found that newborn monkeys isolated for 6 months to 1 year were physically healthy but behaviorally devastated. These monkeys crouched in a corner of their cages and rocked back and forth like severely disturbed (autistic) children. They did not interact with other monkeys, nor did they fight, play, or show any sexual interest. Whereas a 6-month period of social isolation during the first 1.5 years of life produces a persistent and serious behavioral alteration, a comparable period of isolation later in life is innocuous. Thus, in monkeys, as in humans, there is a critical period for social development.

The Harlows next sought to determine the factors that need to be introduced into the isolation experience to prevent the development of the isolation syndrome. They found that the syndrome could be partially reversed by giving an isolated monkey a surrogate mother—a cloth-covered wooden dummy. This elicited clinging behavior in the isolated monkey but was insufficient for the emergence of fully normal social behavior. Social development would occur normally only if, in addition to a surrogate mother, the isolated animal had contact for a few hours each day with a normal infant monkey who spent the rest of the day in the monkey colony. More recently, Stephen Suomi and Harry Harlow found that the isolation syndrome can sometimes be reversed fully by contact with certain monkeys (who might be considered monkey psychotherapists) with special personality traits, such as unflagging gregariousness. These monkeys persistently engage the isolate in social and aggressive behavior until the isolate begins to respond.

Early Sensory Deprivation Alters Perceptual Development

Early deprivation does not have to be so all-encompassing as social isolation to have behavioral consequences. For example, there is also a critical period in the development of normal perception. Even restricted sensory deprivation may have dire consequences. In 1932 Marius von Senden in Germany reviewed the world literature on cataracts in the newborn. Cataracts are opacities of the lens that interfere with the optics of the eye but not with the nervous system; they can be fully corrected surgically in the infant. Von Senden discovered several children who were born with binocular cataracts that were removed much later in life (from ages 10 to 20). Because of the cataracts, these children were deprived of patterned vision. When their cataracts were later removed, these patients could recognize colors but they had difficulty in recognizing shapes and patterns.

The idea that normal sensory experience is required for normal perceptual development was supported by the work of the American psychologist Austin Riesen, who raised newborn monkeys in the dark for the first 3–6 months. When these monkeys were later introduced to a normal visual world, Riesen found that they could not discriminate even simple shapes. It took weeks or even months of training to teach them to distinguish a circle from a square, whereas normal monkeys learn such discrimination in days. Thus, the development of normal perception—the capacity to distinguish between objects in the visual world—requires exposure to patterned visual stimulation early in development.

There Are Cellular Correlates of Sensory Deprivation in Experimental Animals

How is this perceptual development accomplished? Can we begin to understand how the interaction between the perceptual environment and the brain during the critical period influences the functioning of individual nerve cells?

An important step toward understanding the development of perception was made by Torsten Wiesel and David Hubel of the Harvard Medical School in an imaginative series of studies on newborn kittens and monkeys. Wiesel and Hubel examined the effects of visual deprivation on cellular responses in area 17 of the visual (striate) cortex.

In normal humans, as well as in monkeys and cats, the two eyes function together so that the world appears as one even though it is seen with two eyes that project slightly different images on two retinas. We are able to see an object as one entity because when the eyes are normally aligned, their convergence ensures that the images of the object will be cast on corresponding positions on the two retinas. This process is called *fusion.* Even with optimal convergence, however, fusion is not perfect for objects that lie out of the plane of fixation, at different distances from the eyes. This small amount of *noncorrespondence* (binocular disparity) is exceedingly important for function because it is interpreted by the visual system as a difference in depth. Through the combination of fusion and noncorrespondence, we see the visual world in three dimensions—a property of vision called *stereopsis.*

By recording from single cells at various points in the visual pathway to determine whether they could respond to inputs from both eyes, Hubel and Wiesel discovered where fusion of visual images begins. They found that cells in the retina, the lateral geniculate nucleus, and layer IVc of the cerebral cortex respond only to input from one eye or the other. In the monkey, binocular interaction begins at the level of the cortex—specifically, in the cells *above and below* (but not including) layer IVc (Figure 57–1). Convergence of input from the two eyes is first apparent in cells in these layers. Moreover, a number of investigators—including Horace Barlow, Colin Blakemore, and Jack Pettigrew at the University of California at Berkeley, Peter Bishop in Australia, and Gian Poggio at Johns Hopkins University—have found special groups of cortical cells that specifically sense noncorrespondence; these cells presumably mediate depth perception.

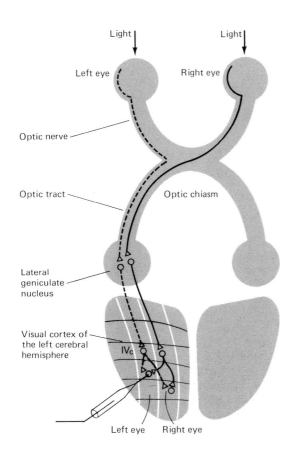

57–1 The input from the two eyes is segregated up to the level of the visual cortex. The retinal ganglion cells of each eye project to separate layers of the lateral geniculate nucleus. The axons of cells in the lateral geniculate nucleus form synaptic connections with neurons in layer IVc of the primary visual (striate) cortex. Cortical neurons in layer IVc are organized in two sets of ocular dominance columns that each receive input from only one eye, but, as Wiesel and Hubel found by making systematic extracellular recordings, the axons of the cells in layer IVc go to adjacent columns as well as the upper and lower layers in the same column. As a result of these connections, the input becomes mixed so that most cells in the upper and lower layers of the cortex receive information from both eyes.

Thus, most cells above and below layer IVc respond to an appropriate stimulus presented to either eye; only a small proportion of cells respond exclusively to the left or the right eye (Figure 57–2A and B). However, if a monkey is raised from birth up to 6 months of age with one eyelid sutured closed, the animal will have permanently lost useful vision in that eye after the occluding sutures are removed. Electrical recordings from the retinal ganglion cells in the deprived eye and from cells in the lateral geniculate nucleus that receive the projections from that eye indicate that these cells have normal receptive fields and respond to visual stimuli projected onto the deprived eye. In contrast, in the visual cortex most cells no longer respond to the deprived eye. The very few cortical cells that can be driven from the deprived eye *are insufficient for visual perception* (Figure 57–2C, 2). Not only has the deprived eye lost its ability to drive most cortical neurons, but this loss is permanent and irreversible. Consistent with other developmental processes that involve a critical period, similar visual deprivation in an adult has no effect on later visual perception and no effect on the visual response of cortical cells to stimulation of one or the other eye. Yet, during the peak of the critical period, as little as one week of deprivation will lead to complete loss of vision and of cortical responsiveness.

Recall from Chapters 28 and 29, and Figure 29–1, that axons from the principal cells in the lateral geniculate nucleus receiving input from each eye terminate in sep-

arate and alternating bands of area 17 of the visual cortex, principally within layer IVc. These endings are the anatomical basis for cortical ocular dominance columns of equal size for each eye (Figure 57–3). The cells in layer IVc then project to cells that lie in higher and lower layers of adjacent columns. These projections from layer IVc equip the cortical layers above and below to process convergent input from the two eyes.

By depriving newborn monkeys of input from one eye, Hubel, Wiesel, and Simon LeVay could examine whether visual deprivation also alters the architecture of the ocular dominance columns in the cerebral cortex. They injected labeled amino acids into one or the other eye and, using autoradiography, observed the transport of the label to the cortex. After closure of one eye, they found that the columns receiving input from the normal eye were greatly widened at the expense of those receiving input from the deprived eye (Figure 57–3B and C).

Here, then, is direct evidence that sensory deprivation early in life can alter the structure of the cerebral cortex! In 1965, when Hubel and Wiesel first discovered the existence of a critical period for binocular interaction, they had only a physiological indication of the effect of sensory deprivation. With the anatomical techniques then available, they were unable to find any morphological change in the visual cortex. Only after the development of autoradiographic labeling techniques involving axonal transport for mapping neuronal connections (see Chapter

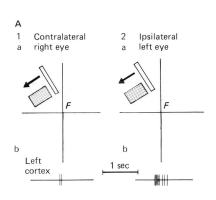

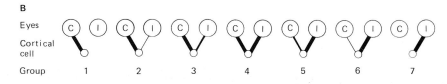

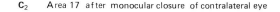

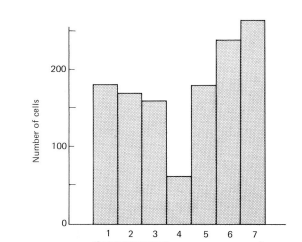

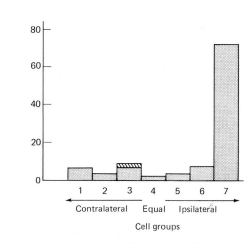

57–2 Binocular interaction and plasticity in area 17 of the monkey's visual cortex.

A. The response of a typical neuron in the visual cortex of the left hemisphere to a diagonal bar of light moving to the left across the cell's receptive field **(shaded rectangle).** The visual fields as seen by the right eye **(1a)** and the left eye **(2a)** are drawn separately for clarity, although the two are superimposed in normal vision. The fields in the two eyes are similar in orientation, position, shape, and size and respond to the same form of stimulus (in this case a moving bar). The action potential recordings below show that the cortical cell responds more effectively when the stimulus is presented to the ipsilateral eye **(2b)** than to the contralateral eye **(1b)**. F indicates the location of the foveal region, the region of greatest visual acuity in the visual field.

B. Ocular dominance groups. On the basis of the responses of the sort illustrated in **A,** Hubel and Wiesel divided the response properties of cortical nuerons into seven ocular

dominance groups. If a cell **(small circles)** in the visual cortex is influenced only by the contralateral eye **(C),** it falls into group 1. If it receives input only from the ipsilateral eye **(I),** it falls into group 7. For the intermediate groups, one eye may influence the cell much more than the other (groups 2 and 6), or the differences may be slight (groups 3 and 5). According to these criteria, the cell in **A** would fall into group 6.

C. Ocular dominance histograms in normal and monocularly deprived monkeys. **1:** This histogram is based on 1256 cells recorded from area 17 in the left hemisphere of normal adult and juvenile monkeys. The cells in layer IV that received only monocular input were excluded. Most cells responded to input from both eyes. **2.** This histogram was obtained from the left hemisphere of a monkey in which the right (contralateral) eye had been closed from age 2 weeks to 18 months but was then reopened. Most of the cells responded only to stimulation of the ipsilateral eye. The **hatched area** represents cells with abnormal responses. (Adapted from Hubel and Wiesel, 1977.)

14), were Hubel and Wiesel able, in 1972, to demonstrate the structural features of the disturbance. Thus, the studies of Hubel, Wiesel, and LeVay illustrate that we are just beginning to develop the techniques to explore the structural organization of the brain and its possible al-

terations by experience and by disease. It will be interesting in the future to see whether social deprivation of the sort studied by Harlow and co-workers leads to a deterioration or distortion of connections in other areas of the brain.

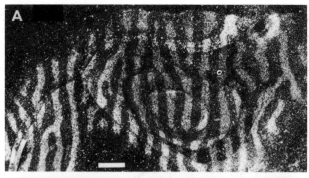

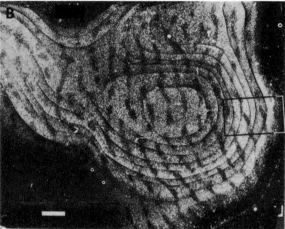

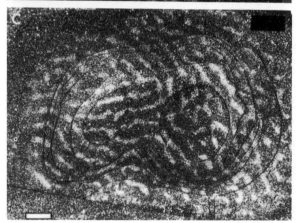

57–3 Visual deprivation of one eye reduces the size of the ocular dominance columns for that eye in the visual cortex of the monkey.

A. Ocular dominance columns in a normal adult. The right eye had been injected 10 days earlier with the radiolabeled amino acid *proline* (that is, incorporated into protein), mixed with the labeled sugar *fucose* (that is, incorporated into glycoprotein). This autoradiograph is of a tangential section through the dome-shaped area 17 of the right hemisphere and was made with the technique of dark-field microscopy, in which the labeled processes are illuminated by white grains and distinguished against the black background. Here the radioactivity can be seen forming white stripes, which correspond to the terminals in layer IV of afferents from the lateral geniculate nucleus that carry input from the injected eye. The alternating dark stripes correspond to geniculate afferents from the uninjected eye. The section goes through layer V, which is seen as the dark oval central area.

B. A comparable section through the visual cortex of an 18-month old monkey whose right eye had been closed at 2 weeks of age. The label was injected into the open eye. The plane of section cuts across layer VI which is seen as the central oval shape. The white stripes of label correspond to the open eye, the narrower dark stripes to the eye that had been closed.

C. A section comparable to that in part **B** from an 18-month old animal whose right eye had been shut at 2 weeks. In this case, however, the label was injected into the eye that had been closed, giving rise to narrow white stripes in the cortex and expanded dark ones. **Scale bars** in all parts, 1 mm. (Adapted from Hubel, Wiesel, and LeVay, 1977).

Loss of Responsiveness of Cortical Neurons to the Closed Eye Results from Altered Competition between Inputs

How are these structural alterations brought about? One factor that could account for the shrinkage of ocular dominance columns receiving input from the closed eye is that the connections from the closed eye are not optimally used. Perhaps use, the generation of action potentials, is critical for the maintenance of connections between the cells of the lateral geniculate nucleus and the neurons in layer IVc of the striate cortex. To test this idea, Hubel and Wiesel closed both eyes in kittens. If *activity* were important, one would expect that closing *both* eyes would weaken the connections of the two eyes equally and prevent cortical cells from being driven by *either* eye. One might then also expect complete loss of all ocular dominance columns. The effects should be similar to those produced by closing one eye except that they should be much more severe and apply equally to both eyes.

In fact, this is not at all what happens! Cortical neurons of cats reared with both eyes closed are still driven by *both* eyes, and the ocular dominance columns are *still* segregated anatomically. Not only does binocular lid closure not exaggerate the effects of monocular closure; it does not even simulate them. The effects of binocular closure are much less severe than those of monocular closure. In contrast to the effects of closing one eye of a kitten during the critical period, a comparable week of *binocular* lid closure has little effect on subsequent vision. Binocular lid closure must last for many months before cellular function and columnar architecture begin to be impaired. These differences illustrate that monocular lid closure does not produce its effects merely by altering use, but presumably by putting the closed eye at a competitive disadvantage with respect to the open eye. The maintenance of the normal anatomical segregation of the ocular dominance columns seems to require a competition between the two eyes, a competition that depends not on the absolute level of activity, but on a *balance of activity* in both sets of lateral geniculate fibers ending on the cortical cells in layer IVc. The effects of monocular lid closure are presumably due to a selective reduction of activity in the geniculate cortical pathway driven by one eye, thereby altering the ability of this pathway to compete equally for representation on common cortical cells.

To explore further the possible role of balanced activity in competition, Wiesel and Hubel interfered with this balance in another way. Rather than causing the cells from one eye to fire more effectively than those of the other, they simply caused the cells from the two eyes to fire out of synchrony. They cut one extraocular muscle, the lateral rectus, and produced an experimental strabismus, or squint—a condition in which the two eyes are not fully aligned. Sectioning this muscle causes the eye to deviate inward. After surgery (performed 3–5 weeks after birth), the eyes move normally except for the misalignment. When the critical cortical neurons of cats or monkeys with strabismus were examined 1 year later, binocular interactions were absent. Cells in the striate cortex responded to either one eye or the other but not to both, and anatomical studies (so far done only in cats) showed that the columns were more sharply defined than normal, indicating an exaggeration of the separation that normally characterizes the terminations of the geniculate neurons from the two eyes. In animals with strabismus both eyes receive the same amount of stimulation and the animal sees normally with each eye, but the two retinas never receive the same image at the same time. As we have seen, most cortical cells are not driven equally by the two eyes but respond more effectively to one eye or the other. The lack of synchrony between the eyes confers an advantage on the eye that had initially been more effective at firing a given binocular cortical cell and allows that eye to gain complete control. Thus, balanced competition between the two eyes is indeed necessary for the maintenance of the normal anatomical segregation of the ocular dominance columns.

Michael Stryker and Sheri Strickland at the University of California at San Francisco have now demonstrated directly the importance of synchronous activity.

They blocked all impulse activity in the optic nerve by injecting tetrodotoxin into each eye of kittens between the ages of 2 and 8 weeks. They then stimulated the optic nerve electrically with implanted electrodes. When the two nerves were stimulated synchronously (as happens when both eyes are open), both eyes were later able to drive cortical neurons. In contrast, when the nerves were driven equally but *asynchronously* (as is the case with squint), most cortical cells were later driven by only one eye or the other but not by both. The formation and maintenance of normal binocular vision seems to require *synchronous and balanced electrical activity* in the pathways from the two eyes.

Balanced Competition Is Important for Segregating Inputs into the Cortical Columns during Normal Development

How does the altered competition that results from monocular visual deprivation produce changes in the width of ocular dominance columns in layer IVc of the visual cortex? Do monocular visual deprivation and the consequent imbalance of activity interfere with the normal development of columns, or does deprivation act on already formed columns by causing connections from the nondeprived eye to sprout and those from the deprived eye to retract? To answer these questions, we need to know the state of the columns at birth. If the columns are fully formed at birth, closing one eye might cause the fibers from the normal eye to invade the columns of the deprived eye by sprouting new terminals. However, if at birth the fibers from each eye overlap extensively in layer IVc and retract only later to form the columns, a competitive process might operate during the first weeks after birth to regulate this sequential retraction. Closing and therefore reducing the activity from one eye may then disrupt the competitive balance and put the terminals of the deprived eye at a selective disadvantage. As a result, the terminals from the deprived eye would retract more than normal.

Studies in the monkey and in the cat by Pasko Rakic, now at Yale University, and by Hubel and Wiesel and their associates, LeVay, Stryker, and Carla Shatz, support the second possibility. In the monkey, the ocular dominance columns are present at birth but only in a rudimentary form; the columns do not fully crystallize until the afferent fibers from the lateral geniculate nucleus become completely segregated 6 weeks after birth. In the cat, segregation of afferent fibers from the lateral geniculate occurs later (Figure 57–4 and Table 57–1).[1]

---

[1]The development of the visual cortex of the monkey is similar to that of the cat, but it differs in the *timing* of the segregation of the afferent fibers from the lateral geniculate nucleus to the cortex with respect to birth and eye opening. As a result, the periods of susceptibility to monocular deprivation are different in the two species. Whereas in the monkey the afferents begin to segregate 6 to 3 weeks *prenatally*, in the cat the segregation does not begin until much later—2 to 3 weeks *postnatally*.

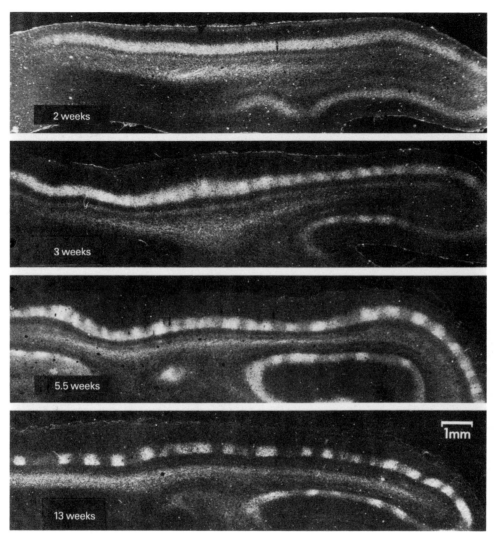

57–4 Ocular dominance columns develop postnatally in the cat. These dark-field autoradiographs (horizontal sections, midline at the top, anterior to the left) illustrate four developmental stages of the visual cortex ipsilateral to an eye that was injected with ^{3}H-proline. The geniculocortical afferents serving the injected eye are labeled by transneuronal transport. At about two weeks (15 days) of postnatal age the afferents are spread uniformly along layer IV, completely intermingled with the (unlabeled) afferents serving the contralateral eye. At 3 weeks and 5.5 weeks the emerging columns are gradually becoming visible but only as modest fluctuations in labeling density. At 13 weeks, the borders of the labeled bands become more sharply defined as the afferents progressively aggregate into clumps—the anatomical basis for the physiologically described ocular dominance columns. (From LeVay, Stryker, and Shatz, 1978.)

Table 57–1. Stages in the Development of Ocular Dominance Columns in the Monkey

Stage	Time period
Beginning of afferent fiber segregation	6–3 weeks prenatal
Beginning of critical period	Birth
Height of sensitivity to monocular deprivation	From birth to 6 weeks postnatal
Nearly complete afferent segregation	3–6 weeks
End of layer IVc susceptibility to monocular deprivation	6–8 weeks
End of susceptibility of upper and lower layers of cortex to monocular deprivation	6 months to 1 year postnatal

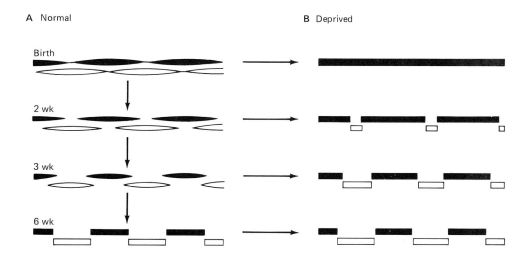

57–5 Scheme proposed by Hubel, Wiesel, and LeVay to explain the effects of eye closure on columns in layer IVc; it is based on the assumption that the segregation of the eyes is not complete until some weeks after birth (as demonstrated by experiments in monkeys). The **filled shapes** represent the terminations of geniculate afferents in layer IVc corresponding to one eye; the **open shapes** represent the terminations from the other eye. In each, the width is intended to represent the presumed density of the terminals. The two sets of columns should be superimposed but are shown one above the another for clarity. The thickness of these bands indicates the relative density of terminals at each point along layer IVc.

A. According to this model, some periodic and regular variation in density of the afferent fibers already is present at birth, reflecting the rudiments of what will later become ocular dominance columns (Figure 57–3A). Because of the normal competition between the eyes, the weaker input at any given point declines and the stronger is strengthened. The normal result is a progressive retraction as the sparse terminals die out

entirely. The way this might work is as follows. During the normal formation of the ocular dominance columns, two mutually opposed processes interact. The first, a *spreading process,* is concerned with establishing for the afferent fibers from *each* eye a complete topographical map within the same cortical space. This spreading mechanism is completed long before birth. The second, a *grouping process,* begins 3–6 weeks before birth. An interactive mechanism among the fibers from each eye tries to group the fibers from one eye and segregate them from fibers from the other eye. By 6 weeks after birth, this grouping process has led to a compromise whereby each area in layer IVc is alternately divided into fiber groups first from one eye then from the other eye.

B. If an eye is deprived (**open shapes**), the consequences depend on when that deprivation occurs. Deprivation at birth leads to complete dominance by the open eye (**filled shapes**) because little segregation has occurred at this point. Deprivation at 2, 3, and 6 weeks has a progressively weaker effect on the ocular dominance columns since they become more segregated with time. (From Hubel, Wiesel, and LeVay, 1977.)

One possible model for normal development (based on observations in the monkey) is illustrated in Figure 57–5A. At birth, the sets of terminals representing the two eyes have arrived in layer IVc but have not yet completely separated out into the distinct bands characteristic of fully segregated columns because initially the projection from each eye tries to form its own topographical map within the full cortical space of layer IVc. In the first few weeks after birth the competitive interaction that takes place between the two eyes causes the ocular dominance columns to crystallize into mature form as the two initially intermingled sets of incoming axons segregate and sort themselves out, presumably by the selective retraction of one or the other set of terminals (similar to the process of synapse retraction that we considered in Chapter 56). This retraction and sorting does not require form vision but seems to depend on balanced and synchronous spontaneous activity in the receptors, retinal ganglion cells, and afferent pathways from the two eyes.

Why do some terminals retract and others do not? Perhaps at birth there is a random or, more likely, a developmentally determined difference in the density of the terminals made by each eye on common target cells in layer IVc of the cortex (as indicated in Figure 57–5A). As a result, there will be a local competitive advantage on common target cells for those sets of connections that initially are the more numerous and effective, and a corresponding disadvantage for the less numerous sets: the latter sets of terminals would therefore be more likely to regress.

Seen from this perspective, the role of balanced competition is to allow two populations of afferent fibers to share effectively a common neural space, in this case, layer IVc. In the absence of balanced competition the afferent fibers from each of the two eyes would attempt to spread and form their own complete topographical map within the single neural space. This is indeed what happens in early stages of development when the incoming fibers overlap extensively. This is also what happens in

A

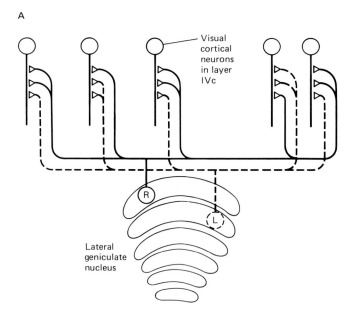

B

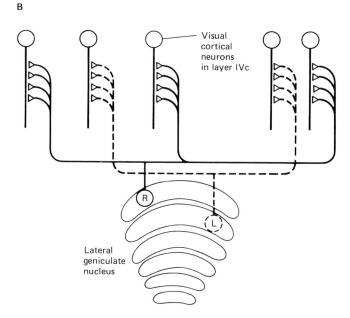

57–6 The process of segregation of ocular dominance columns in the monkey cortex has been demonstrated by labeling of individual geniculate neurons.

A. Early in development, the afferent axons from the cells in the lateral geniculate nucleus innervated by the right (**R**) and left (**L**) eye converge on common cortical neurons in layer IVc of the visual (striate) cortex. Because of genetic or possibly random developmental processes, this convergence is slightly biased so that alternating groups of cells clustered in layer IVc (illustrated here as single cells) tend to receive slightly more input from geniculate cells serving one rather than the other eye—indicated here as two synaptic endings rather than one.

B. As a result of the initial intrinsic bias illustrated in **A**, the geniculate cells that have slightly more powerful connections edge out competing cells from the other eye and gain complete dominance over the cortical cells. The resulting primary input from one or the other eye over adjacent and alternating cell groups gives rise to the characteristic stripes apparent in the autoradiographs. (See also Figures 57–3 and 57–4.) (Based on Gilbert and Wiesel, 1983.)

lower vertebrates (such as frogs and fish) where each eye projects completely to the opposite side of the brain (Chapter 56). Balanced competition is thought to accomplish two things: it *opposes spreading* of fibers and *enhances grouping* of fibers. By opposing the initial tendency for spreading, balanced competition amplifies the initial difference present in the strength of the two inputs, so that the weaker input at any point will decline until the overlap between the two sets of afferents is eliminated, leading to the almost complete segregation of the terminals. By enhancing grouping, balanced competition further causes the fibers from each eye to become clustered and thereby to become even more segregated from the fibers from the other eye.

What are the axons from the neurons in the lateral geniculate nucleus competing for? Clearly, they are competing for control of common cortical cells. But what does this mean in molecular terms? One attractive possibility—in view of the argument we considered in Chapter 56—is that the intermingled afferents are competing for a trophic factor, perhaps a peptide much like nerve growth factor, secreted by the cortical neurons in layer IVc. Perhaps this growth factor is released only by the target cells if the incoming afferents are synchronously active. The afferent fibers with the more extensive contacts might then take up more of the factor and therefore be able to maintain their contacts at the expense of afferent fibers with fewer contacts.

A Normal

Ocular dominance columns

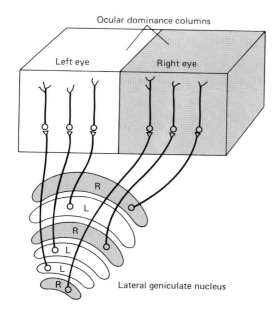

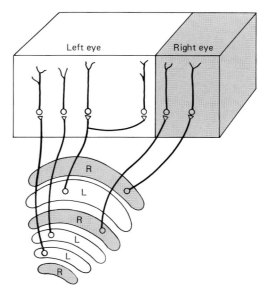

Lateral geniculate nucleus

57–7 This drawing illustrates schematically how closing of one eye might lead to changes in the ocular dominance columns in the visual (striate) cortex.

A. Ocular dominance columns are normally equal in size for each eye.

B. After the right eye has been closed, the columns devoted to the right eye are narrow compared with those of the left eye.

One hypothesis to account for these changes is indicated in the drawing. According to this scheme, closing one eye changes the balance between the open and the closed eye so that the geniculate cells receiving input from the closed eye regress and lose some of their connections with cortical cells, whereas the geniculate cells receiving input from the open eye sprout and connect to cortical cells previously occupied by geniculate neurons from the other eye.

The Development of Ocular Dominance Can Be Followed by Injecting Single Geniculate Axons with a Marker Substance

It is possible to test the model of Figure 57–5 by injecting a marker into the axons of single geniculate neurons in the kitten and to follow anatomically the segregation of the ocular dominance columns during development. This has been done by Charles Gilbert and Wiesel, now at Rockefeller University. They found that in the early postnatal period a single geniculate afferent gives off numerous branches to areas covering several future ocular dominance columns for each eye (Figure 57–6A). As the geniculate neuron matures, there is a selective loss of alternate axon branches, so that ultimately a given axon innervates ocular dominance columns serving one eye and leaves gaps for the columns serving the opposite eye (Figure 57–6B).

In an experimental animal deprived monocularly during the critical period, the axons of the geniculate cells from the closed eye retract and become trimmed to an abnormal extent, while the terminals from the normal eye fail to become trimmed and continue to occupy the territory that they normally would have relinquished. At slightly later stages during the critical period, when the ocular dominance columns are almost fully segregated, a second mechanism seems to come into play. Monocular

closure still causes an expansion and contraction of the columns, but now an additional factor operates that was absent earlier in development: sprouting. Axons appear to sprout into the territory that they had earlier vacated in favor of the now deprived eye (Figure 57–7).

Columns Can Be Induced in Brain Regions Lacking Them by Establishing Appropriate Competition

If ocular dominance columns arise from the competition between two sets of afferent fibers for representation on common cortical neurons in a single neural space, then it should be possible to induce the formation of columns where columns normally are not present simply by establishing competition between two sets of innervating axons. Margaret Law and Martha Constantine-Paton at Princeton University have examined this possibility in developing frogs.

In the frog, most of the retinal ganglion cells send their axons to the opposite side of the brain, where they terminate in the optic tectum and establish a precise map of the visual world. Here there is no competition and, indeed, this map has no columnar organization. To establish a potential source of competition, Law and Constantine-Paton transplanted a third eye

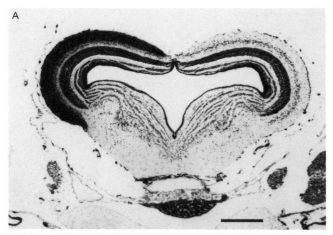

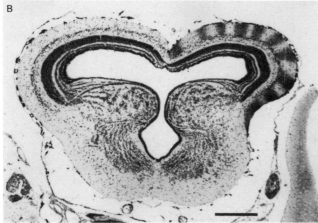

57–8 Ocular dominance columns are induced by transplanting a third eye in frogs. Autoradiographs of a coronal section through the midbrain of two frogs.

A. Normal frog. The left eye was injected with ^{3}H-proline 3 days before the animal was killed. The photograph of entire superficial neuropil of the right optic lobe (**left side** of the picture) is filled with silver grains, indicating the region occupied by synaptic terminals from the labeled (contralateral) eye.

B. Three-eyed frog. The normal right eye was injected with ^{3}H-proline. The left optic lobe of this animal (**right side** of the picture) was innervated by the labeled eye as well as the supernumerary eye. The normally continuous retinotectal synaptic zone of the contralateral eye has consequently been divided into regularly spaced bands of terminal neuropil. Bar indicates 400 μm. (From Constantine-Paton, 1981.)

into a region of the head near one of the normal eyes. The retinal ganglion cells of the transplanted eye sent out axons that terminated in the contralateral optic tectum. This projection was mapped by injecting a radioactive tracer into the transplanted eye. The axons from the transplanted eye formed a columnar system of terminals that alternated in a regular array with terminals from the normal eye (Figure 57–8). Thus, in the optic tectum, as in the cerebral cortex, columnar organization results when two sets of identically specified presynaptic terminals are forced to compete for the same population of postsynaptic cells in a common neural space. Because of this competition, fibers that are thought to make early (and therefore presumably more extensive) contact on a given cell retain their connections, whereas the fibers that make later and less extensive contact retract. The end result is that each set of fibers retracts from some cells and not others, thereby establishing comparable and alternating zones of dominance. As is the case with the mammalian visual system, the formation of these columns in the frogs requires balanced competition and synchronous activity in the two pathways. Columns do not form when activity is blocked by tetrodotoxin.

The Development of Ocular Dominance Columns Is an Important Model for Understanding the Development of Behavior

Research on the development of ocular dominance columns provides an important bridge between the study of the development of the nervous system on the level of single nerve cells and the development of behavior. For example, Jack Pettigrew has found that toward the end of the fourth postnatal month, neurons in the visual cortex of cats mature and become sensitive to ocular disparity. In addition, recent psychophysical studies by Richard Held and his colleagues at the Massachusetts Institute of Technology have shown that stereopsis also emerges in human infants toward the end of the fourth postnatal month, a time when the ocular dominance columns become completely segregated. Thus, the capability for stereoscopic vision seems to begin with the maturation of the ocular dominance columns.

In a larger sense, it is becoming clear that, as with other aspects of behavior, the development of form perception and of the binocular vision necessary for depth perception requires that an individual undergo a number of developmental stages in the course of postnatal life.

Each of these stages leads to one or more developmental decisions, many of which are irreversible. The developmental decisions made during maturation require appropriate sensory input from the environment to validate, shape, and update normal developmental processes. Consequently, the effects of deprivation are most severe during a restricted and well-defined period of time early in postnatal life.

It should be emphasized, however, that critical periods generally do not have *sharp* time boundaries. Even when the critical period has ended for one region of the brain, or even for one layer within a cortical region (such as layer IVc), there is still an opportunity for competition in other layers, so that residual plasticity continues for some time. In the visual cortex of the monkey, for example, layer IVc reaches the end of its period of susceptibility to monocular deprivation at 8 weeks, whereas the upper and lower layers continue to be susceptible for almost the entire first year (Table 57-1). Perhaps each cortical area and each layer within each area has its own timetable for segregation of connections and its own distinctive critical period. This might account for the great complexity in the disturbances of development. Thus, certain untoward environmental experiences, such as visual deprivation, that interfere with the development of a primary sensory region of the brain produce their behavioral consequences early in postnatal development, whereas other experiences, such as social deprivation, exert their actions later.

The existence of several discrete stages in the formation of the ocular dominance columns is likely to represent a general feature of development. Indeed, different cortical areas might have quite different timetables. If this were so it might explain two important features of intellectual and behavioral development: (1) why certain capabilities—such as those for language, music, or mathematics—usually must be developed well before puberty if they are to develop at all; and (2) why traumatic insults at certain stages of postnatal life affect one aspect of perceptual or character development while insults at other periods in development affect other aspects of behavior.

Studies of Development Are Important Clinically

Studies of maternal deprivation provide a striking example of how genes and developmental programs (nature) and experience (nurture) interact inextricably in early life and how environmental deprivation can dramatically alter developmental processes. In addition to providing insights into the mechanisms governing development, these studies and others on simpler developmental processes have obvious clinical relevance. Changes in clinical treatment have resulted, for example, from studies of strabismus and its consequences for the development of visual perception. Children with strabismus initially have good vision in each eye. However, because they cannot fuse the images in the two eyes, these children often tend to favor one eye, fixating and attending with it. As a result, these children often lose useful vision in

the neglected eye. In the past, ophthalmologists waited until such children were 8–9 years old, long after the critical period, to correct the strabismus. Thanks to the work of Hubel and Wiesel, ophthalmologists now surgically correct the strabismus very early, when normal binocular vision can still be restored.

Selected Readings

Harlow, H. F. 1958. The nature of love. Am. Psychol. 13:673–685.

Held, R. 1985. The Development of Binocularity. Trends Neurosci. In press.

Hubel, D. H., and Wiesel, T. N. 1977. Ferrier Lecture: Functional architecture of macaque monkey visual cortex. Proc. R. Soc. Lond. [Biol.] 198:1–59.

Knudsen, E. I. 1984. The role of auditory experience in the development and maintenance of sound localization. Trends Neurosci. 7:326–330.

Leiderman, P. H. 1981. Human mother–infant social bonding: Is there a sensitive phase? In K. Immelmann, G. W. Barlow, L. Petrinovich, and M. Main (eds.), Behavioral Development. Cambridge, England: Cambridge University Press, pp. 454–468.

Rakic, P. 1981. Development of visual centers in the primate brain depends on binocular competition before birth. Science 214:928–931.

Riesen, A. H. 1958. Plasticity of behavior: Psychological aspects. In H. F. Harlow and C. N. Woolsey (eds.), Biological and Biochemical Bases of Behavior. Madison: University of Wisconsin Press, pp. 425–450.

References

Constantine-Paton, M. 1981. Induced ocular-dominance zones in tectal cortex. In F. O. Schmitt, F. G. Worden, G. Adelman, and S. G. Dennis (eds.), The Organization of the Cerebral Cortex. Cambridge, Mass.: MIT Press, pp. 47–67.

Gilbert, C. D., and Wiesel, T. N. 1983. Clustered intrinsic connections in cat visual cortex. J. Neurosci. 3:1116–1133.

Harlow, H. F., Dodsworth, R. O., and Harlow, M. K. 1965. Total social isolation in monkeys. Proc. Natl. Acad. Sci. U.S.A. 54:90–97.

Hubel, D. H., Wiesel, T. N., and LeVay, S. 1977. Plasticity of ocular dominance columns in monkey striate cortex. Philos. Trans. R. Soc. Lond. [Biol. Sci.] 278:377–409.

Lane, H. 1976. The Wild Boy of Aveyron. Cambridge, Mass.: Harvard University Press.

LeVay, S., and Stryker, M. P. 1979. The development of ocular dominance columns in the cat. In J. A. Ferrendelli (ed.), Aspects of Developmental Neurobiology, Society for Neuroscience Symposia. Vol. 4. Bethesda, Md.: Society for Neuroscience, pp. 83–98.

LeVay, S., Stryker, M. P., and Shatz, C. J. 1978. Ocular dominance columns and their development in layer IV of the cat's visual cortex: A quantitative study. J. Comp. Neurol. 179:223–244.

LeVay, S., Wiesel, T. N., and Hubel, D. H. 1980. The development of ocular dominance columns in normal and visually deprived monkeys. J. Comp. Neurol. 191:1–51.

LeVay, S., Wiesel, T. N., and Hubel, D. H. 1981. The postnatal development and plasticity of ocular-dominance columns in the monkey. In F. O. Schmitt, F. G. Worden, G. Adelman, and S. G. Dennis (eds.), The Organization of the Cerebral Cortex. Cambridge, Mass.: MIT Press, pp. 29–45.

Lorenz, K. 1965. Evolution and Modification of Behavior. Chicago: University of Chicago Press.

Poggio, G. F., and Fischer, B. 1977. Binocular interaction and depth sensitivity in striate and prestriate cortex of behaving rhesus monkey. J. Neurophysiol. 40:1392–1405.

Rakic, P. 1976. Prenatal genesis of connections subserving ocular dominance in the rhesus monkey. Nature 261:467–471.

Rakic, P. 1977. Prenatal development of the visual system in rhesus monkey. Philos. Trans. R. Soc. Lond. [Biol. Sci.] 278:245–260.

Spitz, R. A. 1945. Hospitalism: An inquiry into the genesis of psychiatric conditions in early childhood. Psychoanal. Study Child 1:53–74.

Spitz, R. A. 1946. Hospitalism: A follow-up report on investigation described in Volume 1, 1945. Psychoanal. Study Child 2:113–117.

Spitz, R. A., and Wolf, K. M. 1946. Anaclitic depression: An inquiry into the genesis of psychiatric conditions in early childhood, II. Psychoanal. Study Child 2:313–342.

Stryker, M. P., and Strickland, S. L. 1984. Physiological segregation of ocular dominance columns depends on the pattern of afferent electrical activity. Invest. Ophthalmol. Visual Sci. [Suppl.] 25:278 (ARVO abstracts).

Suomi, S. J., and Harlow, H. F. 1975. The role and reason of peer relationships in rhesus monkeys. In M. Lewis and L. A. Rosenblum (eds.), Friendship and Peer Relations. New York: Wiley, pp. 153–185.

von Senden, M. 1932. Space and Sight. (P. Heath, trans.) Glencoe, Ill.: Free Press, 1960.

Wiesel, T. N., and Hubel, D. H. 1963. Single-cell responses in striate cortex of kittens deprived of vision in one eye. J. Neurophysiol. 26:1003–1017.

Dennis D. Kelly

Sexual Differentiation
of the Nervous System

58

Most behavioral and perceptual functions of the nervous system are common to both sexes. The maintenance of higher animal species, however, requires separate and coordinated contributions from the two sexes. Reproductive behavior is also governed by strong ontogenetic restrictions. The demands of conceiving and nurturing a new member of the species are such that the responsibility is withheld from the very young and the very old, and is reserved for an intermediate age when the organism has reached maturity but has not yet lost strength and vigor. The emergence of sexually dimorphic behaviors is based on anatomical, physiological, and behavioral differences that are ultimately directed by the nervous system and produced by neuronal networks that are sexually differentiated and influenced by developmental events. Sex-linked neural differentiation also extends to many nonreproductive behaviors.

Sexual differentiation is another example of the developmental plasticity of the brain: The genetic make-up (nature) of the organism determines the range of potential for the individual, but the environment (nurture) shapes the final outcome. Characteristic of such developmental plasticity is the existence of a *critical time period* during which specific interactions between the growing brain and its environment (internal as well as external) mold future behavioral capacities. Critical periods reflect the sequential nature of the growth process; at each stage of development a choice is made between alternatives. Once a time-dependent critical choice is made, it becomes difficult or impossible to reverse the process.

Reproductive Behaviors Are Sexually Dimorphic

Although vertebrate mating behavior is richly varied, ethologists have described a fundamental pattern of copulatory behaviors that is common to warm-blooded animals and that shows strong sexual dimorphism. (The term *dimorphism* refers to the existence of two distinct forms within a species; *sexual dimorphism* of behavior refers to different forms of behaviors shown by males and females.) According to this pattern, mating involves three states:

1. The orientation and courtship of two partners, generally involving both the identification of an appropriate mate and some signal of readiness.
2. Certain clear-cut, gender-specific postural adjustments by which the female exposes her genitals and the male attains intromission.
3. Mutual genital reflexes that lead to insemination.

We may take the mating pattern of ring doves as a specific example. During courtship, the male dove bows and coos; the partners interlock beaks and strut around cooing and charging. Abruptly, the female assumes a posture that makes her oviduct accessible to the male. She spreads her wings, extends her tail, and flexes her legs. The male dove mounts from the rear, and, as an aid in attaining intromission, clasps the feathers on the back of

his partner's neck with his beak. In this position, the doves copulate by pelvic thrusts.

The mating posture of vertebrate animals shows extraordinary cross-species homologies. For this reason neurobiologists have used mounting and lordosis as the behavioral markers for neural differentiation. Male rats, guinea pigs, rabbits, cats, and monkeys perform with remarkable similarity—mounting the female from the rear, clasping the back of the neck in their mouths, and, after gaining intromission, thrusting with the pelvis. Female behavior is also highly organized, but more species specific. For example, in the mating posture the female rat pauses and crouches tensely, but then interrupts the pauses with darting movements to various areas of the cage. When mounted or touched from the rear, she exhibits a lordotic elevation of the rump.

In the limited behavioral repertoires of lower forms of animals, apparently gender-specific courtship behaviors often serve other purposes. Either sex may exhibit both male and female copulatory patterns in environmental circumstances that have little to do with reproduction. For instance, both sexes use the female sexual posture as a submissive gesture during intraspecific encounters for dominance.

Gonadal Hormones Influence the Sexual Differentiation of the Brain

The mature gonads of males and females produce different steroid sex hormones. Is it possible that testicular hormones produce male behavior and ovarian hormones

58–1 Estrogen induces sexual receptivity in female ovariectomized rats in a dose-dependent manner. After eight daily subcutaneous injections of estradiol benzoate, receptivity was measured by the lordosis quotient (the number of lordotic responses of the subject, divided by the number of mounts, multiplied by 100). (Data from Bermant and Davidson, 1974.)

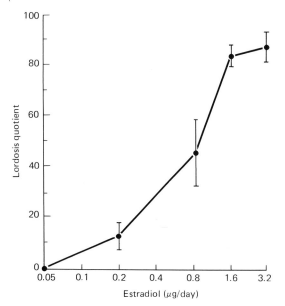

produce female behavior equally well in adult males and females? If so, the sex-related patterns of behavior could be explained by the type of hormones that are present in the body of the adult organism. This reasoning underlies the theory of *hormone specificity*, now known to be an oversimplification. An alternative view, for which there is now good evidence, is the theory of *developmental host specificity*. According to this view, during a specific perinatal critical period, certain target tissues in the brain develop a sensitivity to the hormone appropriate to one sex or the other. Besides inducing selective responsiveness to hormones, events during the same critical period create in the brain a gender-specific, organizational blueprint, which in adulthood will lead to the expression of appropriate sexual behaviors in response to hormonal stimulation.

In the adult, the primary influence of circulating steroid sex hormones is to activate sexual responses. Thus, administration of estrogen increases sexual receptivity in female rats in an orderly, dose-dependent manner (Figure 58–1). However, in the developing organism (particularly the fetus), sex steroids primarily influence the differentiation of specific body tissues in males and females, including parts of the brain. Both male and female genotypes are thought to be compatible with either brain sex phenotype. To a remarkable degree, the brain sex phenotype is determined largely by exposure to specific steriod hormones during a critical period early in life. Clinical evidence suggests that the brain of a developing fetus is essentially undifferentiated and bipotential. The brain of the fetus (and later of the individual) always assumes the female form and psychosocial orientation unless this course is prevented by the action of male hormones.

What is the nature of this clinical evidence? Two informative syndromes arise from spontaneously occurring hormonal deficiencies during early human development. In a congenital anhormonal condition known as *Turner's syndrome*, gonadal tissue does not form. The syndrome characteristically is found in a phenotypic female who, because of the lack of gonads, fails to show the pubertal changes associated with adolescence. Many cases therefore are not discovered until adolescence. If these patients are treated with ovarian hormones during adolescence, they respond as normal females. Moreover, the sexual preference and libido of such individuals seem to parallel closely those of a heterosexual female. The important point, however, is that patients with Turner's syndrome are not genetic females (XX), but neither are they genetic males (XY). Evidence from karyotypes indicates that most of them possess only one chromosome, which in humans is always an X chromosome (having only a Y chromosome is lethal).

The second genetic anomaly involves individuals incapable of responding to androgens. This condition, called the *androgen insensitivity syndrome*, is an X-linked recessive gene defect that is transmitted by heterozygous females to half of their male offspring. Such offspring cannot reproduce, so the syndrome occurs only

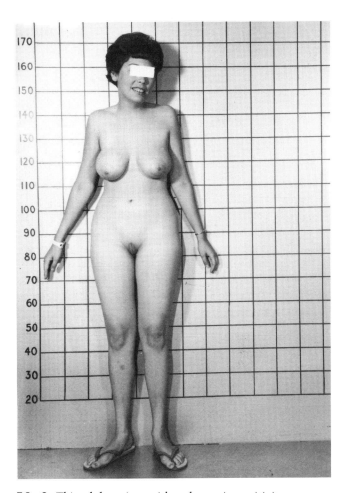

58–2 This adult patient with androgen insensitivity syndrome is a genetic XY male. Female pubertal development occurred, with no exogenous hormonal treatment, under the influence of estrogens normally secreted by the testes. (From Money and Ehrhardt, 1972.)

in genetic males. Because these genetic males cannot respond to the androgens they produce, they are indistinguishable from phenotypic females in their external appearance, as well as in their heterosexual orientation and libidinal interests. The body morphology of an adult genetic male with this syndrome is shown in Figure 58–2. This condition is also known clinically as *testicular feminization*. This is an unfortunate misnomer, for the testes of these individuals appear normal morphologically and are not feminizing in any way; nor do they secrete hormones that resemble the hormones of the ovary. Although the testes of individuals with testicular feminization remain undescended, the temporal pattern of their secretions throughout development is essentially the same as that of normal males.

Recent studies on mutant mice and rats that—like patients with androgen insensitivity syndrome—are selectively insensitive to androgens have demonstrated that the deficiency is characterized by absent (or undetectable) intracellular androgen receptors. Estrogen receptors are unaffected. Thus, despite normal production of androgens by the testes, cells do not respond to any androgens throughout the development of the individual with testicular feminization.

The implication drawn from these clinical states is that the female form and its psychosexual orientation can develop in the absence of hormonal influences from the gonads. Moreover, the pattern of female development is not restricted to a female genotype. Individuals who are genetically male can develop as females under special circumstances. To integrate these clinical phenomena with experimental observations on the sexual differentiation of the organism in utero, we must first consider the hormonal environment in which fetuses of both sexes develop.

Perinatal Hormones Affect the Sexual Differentiation of the Developing Organism

In considering the development of gender identity, it is important to distinguish between homotypical and heterotypical steroid sex hormones. *Homotypical hormones* are hormones of a given sex administered to an individual of the same sex—for example, androgens to a male. *Heterotypical hormones* are those of one sex given to the other sex. These terms may also be applied to gender-specific behaviors: *homotypical behavior patterns* are those appropriate to the reference gender and *heterotypical behavior patterns* are those appropriate to the opposite sex.

Fetal Exposure to Male Hormones Causes Hermaphroditism in Genetic Females

During pregnancy the fetuses of both sexes are normally exposed to the high levels of circulating estrogens in the maternal blood. Since estrogen is homotypical for female fetuses and heterotypical for male fetuses, the following question has arisen: What would happen if this normal relationship were reversed in an experimental animal, bringing female fetuses under heterotypical hormone influences? In early experiments, Charles Phoenix and co-workers found that injecting high doses of testosterone into the mother has two consequences for the female offspring. First, they are born as hermaphrodites: their external genitalia are indistinguishable from those of normal males, but female tissues are also present in the abdomen. Thus, exposure to an unusual amount of male hormone during the fetal period markedly distorts organ development in the female, partially reversing the differentiation of the peripheral sex apparatus. The second and more intriguing effect is that the adult sexual behavior of hermaphroditic females is also altered. When subsequently treated with estrogen and progesterone, such genotypic female guinea pigs show some elements of homotypical sexual behaviors—lordosis, for example—but their capacity for this behavior is greatly reduced as

compared with normal control females. On the other hand, these animals display much more mounting behavior than a normal female. When treated with testosterone as adults, these hermaphroditic females display a degree of heterotypical mounting comparable to that of normal males, and the female pattern of lordosis is suppressed.

Steroid Hormones Influence Perinatal Development Only during Critical Periods

As we have seen, the developing nervous system of either gender is bipotential. A female pattern of anatomical and behavioral organization can emerge in either an anhormonal or maternal-dominated prenatal environment. The emergence of the male pattern, however, requires the influence of androgens. If androgens are needed for the development of normal male fetuses, where in the uterine environment do androgens come from? Most experiments on this question have been carried out in the rat, which has a 21-day gestation period. These studies show that the male testes begin to synthesize androgens as early as the 13th day of fetal development, and androgen secretion continues in newborn rats until the 10th day after birth.

The possibility that the androgens produced by the immature gonads of the developing male rat are responsible for further masculinization can be checked simply by removing the testes. Even though castration on the day of birth deprives the male rat of testicular androgens only for little more than one-half of the period that these hormones are normally present, it has profound effects on the sexual development of genotypic male rats: rats castrated between 1 and 5 days of age develop the behavioral characteristics of genotypic females. If they are injected with estrogen and progesterone as adults, they display lordotic behavior when mounted by normal males. In contrast, males that are castrated later in development, after 10 or more days of age, show little or no tendency to display lordosis under comparable conditions.

There is additional evidence that perinatal male hormones affect subsequent sexual behavior by influencing the developing central nervous system rather than the peripheral sexual apparatus. Both males and females secrete two *gonadotropins* (or gonad-stimulating hormones) from the anterior pituitary: *luteinizing hormone* (LH) and *follicle-stimulating hormone* (FSH). In males these hormones are secreted at a steady level. In females, surges of the hormones underlie the cyclical activities of the reproductive tract.

In 1962 Charles Barraclough and Roger Gorski demonstrated that the female cyclical secretion of gonadotropin by the pituitary does not depend directly on the genetic sex of the animal, but rather on the absence of androgen during the perinatal period. As we saw, this critical period in the rat includes the first week after birth. Under normal circumstances, cyclical secretion is prevented from developing in the male by his own andro-

Table 58–1. Adult Gonadotropin Secretion Patterns in Rats Subjected to Neonatal Endocrine Manipulation

Genetic sex	Treatment	Age when treated	Adult luteinizing hormone secretion pattern
Female	None	—	Cyclical
	Testosterone[a]	4 days	Noncyclical
	Testosterone[a]	16 days	Cyclical
Male	None	—	Noncyclical
	Castration	1 day	Cyclical
	Castration	7 days	Noncyclical

Source: Adapted from Raisman, 1974.

[a]Single injection of 1.25 mg testosterone propionate.

gens. A recent experiment by Geoffrey Raisman illustrates this point (Table 58–1). Treatment of the normal genetic female rat with a single dose of androgen on the fourth day of postnatal life permanently abolishes the ability to ovulate in the adult. Conversely, a male castrated within 1 day of birth can exhibit cyclic ovulation and behavioral estrus if he receives transplanted ovaries as an adult. The same manipulations carried out after the critical period do not affect the normal development and expression of the adult function proper to the genetic sex of the animal.

Timing of the Critical Period Varies in Different Species

As we saw above, the critical period for the androgenization of the rat nervous system is perinatal, extending from a few days before birth to 10 days after birth. However, species vary widely in the developmental critical periods during which their brains are maximally sensitive to gonadal hormones. Some general conclusions can be drawn from a consideration of the critical periods presented in Table 58–2.

In most species the critical period for sexual differentiation corresponds to the period when the gonads of the normal male are active. In rats, the specialized *testicular Leydig cells* generally are differentiated between days 16 and 18 after conception. In human male fetuses the testes are most active between the 12th and the 22nd weeks after conception. During the first 6 weeks of postnatal life, there is also a second period of androgen secretion.

The Brain Can Be Androgenized by Many Natural and Experimental Compounds

The critical developmental period for sexual differentiation corresponds to a period of sensitivity to a broad spectrum of steroids, many of which are not normally present in the body. Experimental masculinization of the brain may result from exposure to such functionally diverse hormones as testosterone, androstenedione, estradiol, and diethylstilbestrol (DES), and even drugs, such as barbiturates, and pesticides, such as dichlorodiphenyltrichloroethane (DDT).

Paradoxically, the principal active hormone that determines the natural male brain pattern in newborn rats is estradiol, one of the female sex hormones. Even though the hormone that reaches the brain is testosterone, much of it is converted there to estradiol by enzymes in the nerve cells that are the targets of sexual

Table 58–2. Critical Periods for Sexual Differentiation of Several Mammals

Species	Gestation period (days)	Critical period (days after conception)
Hamster	16	Postnatal
Mouse	19–20	Prenatal and postnatal
Rat	21–23	18–27
Ferret	42	Postnatal
Dog	58–63	Prenatal and postnatal
Guinea pig	63–70	30–37
Sheep	145–155	30–90
Rhesus monkey	146–180	40–60

Source: Adapted from Goy and McEwen, 1980; MacLusky and Naftolin, 1981.

differentiation. When administered in experiments in vivo, estradiol has been found to be eight times more effective than testosterone in androgenization. This raises a question for which we do not as yet have an answer: Why do high maternal estrogen levels not suffice to androgenize normal female fetuses in utero?

Sexually Differentiated Brains Have Different Physiological Properties and Behavioral Tendencies

Does a brain that mediates male behaviors differ from one that mediates female behaviors? If so, what are the properties of a masculinized brain? First, an androgenized brain exhibits a tonic secretory pattern of luteinizing hormone, whereas the pattern of the female brain is cyclic. One hypothesis for the cellular basis of this sexual endocrine difference involves neurons in the preoptic area of the hypothalamus. In normal females the estrogen secreted by growing ovarian follicles regulates these preoptic cells, which, as we shall see in a later section, contain steroid receptors within their cell bodies. In response to estrogen, these estrogen-sensitive cells, or those to which they are synaptically connected, increase their secretion of luteinizing hormone–releasing hormone (LHRH), which prompts a surge in the production of luteinizing hormone (LH) by the anterior pituitary. Luteinizing hormone–releasing hormone is a decapeptide that regulates the release of both LH and follicle-stimulating hormone (FSH), and thus it is also known as gonadotropin-releasing hormone (GnRH). In females the steroid sensitivity of the preoptic cells is cyclical. In the androgenized brain, these preoptic cells appear to be refractory to hormonal activation, and even their direct electrical stimulation fails to alter luteinizing hormone release by the pituitary.

Second, although in both sexes receptor molecules for steroid sex hormones develop within cells located in similar brain regions, the distribution and steroid-concentrating properties of these cells differ slightly in androgenized and nonandrogenized brains. Steroid-binding cells are found in the hypothalamus (particularly in the preoptic area), amygdala, midbrain, and spinal cord (where their distribution differs most markedly between the sexes). There are also a few steroid-binding cells in the frontal cortex, which, in the rat, disappear as the animal matures. As we shall see later, these cortical sites may be important for the differentiation of nonreproductive but sexually dimorphic behavioral capabilities.

Unlike receptors for neurotransmitter substances (see Chapter 14), steroid receptors are not components of the neuron's external membrane. Experiments using radioactively labeled gonadal steroids have shown that instead the hormones bind to specific intracellular receptor proteins in the cytoplasm of the sexually differentiated target cell (Figures 58–3 and 58–4). The hormone–protein complex then enters the cell's nucleus and interacts with specific genes, thereby altering gene expression in the target cell.

Although receptors for both estrogen and testosterone exist in the brains of both sexes, Richard Whalen and J. Massicci at the University of California found differences in the degree to which nuclei of hypothalamic cells bind and retain estrogen in the two sexes: the nuclei of female rats take up more radiolabeled estrogen and retain it longer than those of the male.

58–3   An autoradiographic method is used to identify the location of steroid target neurons in ovariectomized rats. Two hours after radioactively labeled estradiol is injected (1) the rat's brain is removed (2) and frozen (3). In a darkroom, frozen sections of the brain are placed against a photographic emulsion and stored for several months (4). Electrons from the decaying tritium atoms expose silver atoms in the emulsion (5). The densest accumulation of tritiated estradiol molecules is found in the nuclei of cells whose distribution in the brain is shown in Figure 58–4. (Adapted from McEwen, 1976.)

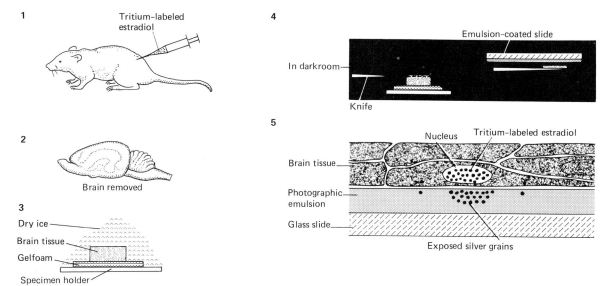

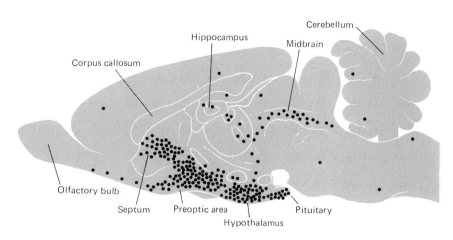

58–4 The regional distribution of estradiol-sensitive neurons in the brain of an albino rat is shown in a sagittal section just adjacent to the midline. Within the hypothalamus the greatest concentration of receptor sites (**dots**) is in the preoptic-suprachiasmatic area and the arcuate-ventromedial area. These are the areas responsible for controlling the release of luteinizing hormone by the pituitary. In more lateral sections (not shown) the amygdala and orbitofrontal cortex also appear as targets. (Adapted from McEwen, 1976.)

Third, the mature animal with an androgenized brain exhibits male mounting behavior when exposed to androgens administered systemically or implanted directly into the anterior hypothalamus. On the other hand, the behavior of adult males that were castrated during the critical period cannot be changed by androgens. However, when castrates receive replacement androgens during the critical period, this later behavioral demasculinization is prevented. A dramatic example of remasculinization in rats is shown in Figure 58–5 (broken line).

A fourth and separate property of mature androgenized brains is that they show little behavioral response to estrogens. In normal males there is an active suppression of the lordotic response, which in adult feminine brains may be elicited by estrogen. The display of adult lordosis following priming with estrogen is not genetic; it is either established or inhibited by the perinatal hormonal environment. This has been demonstrated in male rats in the castration-replacement paradigm shown in Figure 58–5 (solid line): early androgen replacement during the critical period effectively suppressed adult heterotypical behavior in response to estrogen.

Although the critical periods for activating male ejaculatory behavior and suppressing lordotic behavior appear to be roughly comparable in Figure 58–5, Whalen and David Edwards, then at the University of California, have provided strong evidence that the suppression in masculinized brains of heterotypical, female behavior patterns (*defeminization*) is a separate process from the active organization of homotypical male behavior patterns (*masculinization*). They castrated neonatal male rats and administered replacement therapy during the critical period that consisted *only* of injections of *androstenedione*, an androgen produced primarily by the adrenal gland and also by the gonads of both sexes. As adults these animals displayed a blend of male and female behavior. In addition to having different sensitivities to hormones, the two independent processes—masculinization and defeminization—occur at slightly different times in the developmental sequence.

Finally, events during the critical period result in strong sex differences in the nonreproductive behavioral repertoires of prepubertal juveniles. Because the prepubertal period is relatively anhormonal, these gender-specific behavior patterns do not depend on either sensitivity to, or activation by, steroid hormones. Masculinized male rhesus monkeys show more rough-and-tumble play, more aggressive encounters with other males, and less maternal imitative behaviors than females. Androgenized and nonandrogenized individuals also show consistent differences in the proportion of time that they play with members of their same brain sex.

58–5 The adult sexual behavior of neonatally castrated rats depends on the age at which testosterone replacement therapy is given. Therapy was administered to six groups at different ages. When the androgens were replaced within 2 days of birth, the castrated males exhibited appropriate malelike responses (**broken line**) in the presence of testosterone in adulthood. However, as the interval between castration and replacement increased, the remasculinizing effect of early androgen replacement therapy declined. Female sexual behavior was measured in terms of a lordosis quotient: the percentage of mounts by a stud male that elicited lordosis in the castrated test animal (**solid line**). (Adapted from Beach, Noble, and Orndoff, 1969.)

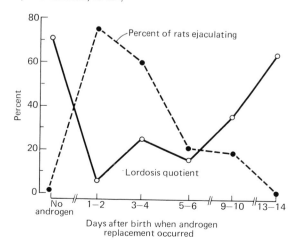

Perinatal Hormones Also Determine the Degree to Which Sex-Linked Behaviors Are Expressed by Normal Males and Females

Events during the critical period for sexual differentiation of the nervous system do not result in complete androgenization or complete feminization. Intermediate degrees are both possible and normal. Moreover, the same set of perinatal events that differentiate the brains and behaviors of males and females might also be responsible for determining the natural, graded range of these behaviors within normal male and female populations.

In humans there is considerable variability in the amounts of testosterone and estrogen to which a developing normal fetus is exposed. Do these perinatal variations affect the degree to which sex-linked behaviors are expressed later in adulthood? Evidence for this possibility has come primarily from studies on rodents, which produce litters containing many pups. Positioning in the uterus is sexually random. Frederick vom Saal has shown that female fetal mice that come to lie between two male fetuses during the course of their uterine development have a higher concentration of testosterone in both their blood and amniotic fluid than do females that develop between one male and one female or between two other females. The three types of females, defined by their intrauterine position as next to 2 males, 1 male, or zero males (2M, 1M, 0M), differ during later life in many characteristics, including activity levels, aggressiveness, and acceptability as mating partners to males. Although females that develop between two males reproduce normally, they display erratic estrus cycles, begin to mate later, and cease to bear young earlier than females that develop between two females. Thus, normal variations in the reproductive life spans of female mice appear to be related directly to position in the uterus and hence to variation in exposure to sex hormones.

Intrauterine position also has an important effect on variations of certain male characteristics. The size and weight of the testes of males that develop between two other males are greater than those of males not surrounded by male siblings. Physiologically, the seminal vesicles of males surrounded by two male siblings are more sensitive to testosterone. Lower doses of testosterone are required to induce aggression in adult neonatally castrated males that developed between two male siblings than in similarly castrated adults that developed between two females.

All of the behavioral variations displayed by 2M, 1M, and 0M offspring fall within the accepted, normal range of masculine or feminine behaviors. Indeed, together these subgroups define the normal range of behavioral expression in the whole population. The ways in which the 2M, 1M, and 0M offspring differ from each other are the same as those by which the two sexes differ from each other. The degree to which a normal male or female displays a sexually differentiated behavior or function may be determined by perinatal hormonal mechanisms similar to those that differentiate the two sexes from one another. Individual differences in any behavior containing sexually dimorphic components might be due, at least in part, to hormonal exposure during the critical period.

Sexual Differentiation Is Reflected in the Structure of Certain Neurons

Is there a morphological basis for the androgen-dependent process in the developing central nervous system that underlies the gender-specific patterns of behavioral organization? Some morphological sex differences exist in the ultrastructure of cellular and synaptic organelles, in synaptic and dendritic organization, and even in the gross volume of defined cell groups. The size of the cell nucleus differs for cells in the preoptic area and ventromedial hypothalamus of males and females, as do the size of neuronal processes and synaptic terminals in the arcuate nucleus and the density of dendritic fields in the preoptic area.

In 1971, Raisman and Pauline Field first studied the ultrastructure of a sexually distinct synaptic organization of afferents to the preoptic area of the hypothalamus. They suggested that the relative apportionment of synapses on dendritic spines versus shafts might represent different patterns of connections in the two sexes, and thereby serve as a mechanism of sexual differentiation. Until that time, most scientists believed that exposure to perinatal steroids primarily altered the responsivity of the central nervous system, not its pattern of connection.

Perhaps the most salient morphological sex difference in mammals was described in rats by Gorski and his associates. Both the size and the number of neurons in a limited portion of the medial preoptic nucleus in the preoptic hypothalamic forebrain region are greater in males than in females. This region is now called the *sexually dimorphic nucleus of the preoptic area* (Figure 58–6). The striking sexual difference in this densely staining area is differentiated during the perinatal period and is not dependent on the continued presence of gonadal hormones in the adult. C. D. Jacobson and Gorski have shown that the size and number of neurons in the sexually dimorphic nucleus first increase in the male rat around the time of birth, and this trend continues throughout the first 10 days of postnatal life. It is not yet known what is controlled by the sexually dimorphic nucleus in the rat. Preliminary evidence suggests a role in the organization and expression of male sexual behaviors.

The human preoptic area has not yet been examined quantitatively, but some clear-cut sexual differences in the anatomy of the human brain have been found already. For example, the adult corpus callosum is sexually dimorphic. Marie-Christine de Lacoste and Ralph Holloway found that its cross-sectional surface area relative to brain weight is larger in females. These sexual differences in the corpus callosum are also present in fetal brains. There, the maximal sexual divergence in mor-

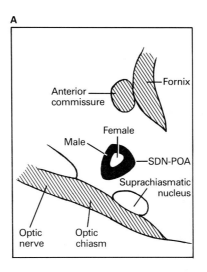
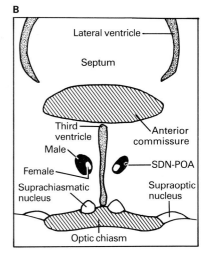

58–6 Localization of the sexually dimorphic nucleus of the preoptic area (**SDN-POA**) of the rat brain. **A.** Sagittal plane. **B.** Coronal plane. Note that the volume of the SDN-POA in the female is completely contained within that of the male. (From Gorski et al., 1978.)

phology appears to develop between 18 and 26 weeks of gestation, a period that roughly corresponds to the peak of androgen production.

We are not yet able to identify the functional or behavioral correlate for any of the morphological sex differences that occur in various species in the superior cervical ganglion, the amygdala, the dorsal hippocampus, and the orbital frontal cortex, but there is one example of a sex difference in the spinal cord that can be correlated directly with a sexually dimorphic behavior. Testicular androgen released during the critical period differentiates a set of behavioral penile reflexes in the male rat. Expression of these spinal behavioral reflexes in the adult is dependent on androgen. Examination of the spinal cord of male rats reveals that androgen-concentrating motor neurons innervate two striated muscles that assist in moving the penis. In female rats, the same muscles are either absent or vestigial, as is the corresponding spinal motor nucleus. However, as described in an elegant series of experiments by Stephen Breedlove and Arthur Arnold, a single properly timed neonatal injection of testosterone is capable of masculinizing the spinal cord of female rats.

Cellular Mechanisms Involved in the Development of Sex Differences in the Brain Can Be Studied in Vitro

The diversity of the structural differences we have just described makes it difficult to formulate a general idea of the cellular mechanism underlying sexual dimorphism. One possibility, suggested by the work of C. Dominique Toran-Allerand at Columbia University, is that morphological sex differences reflect the growth-promoting effects of gonadal steroids on specific populations of neurons.

Toran-Allerand has been able to maintain cultures of hypothalamic slices from newborn mouse brains for long periods in vitro. In her initial experiments, she exposed one-half of each slice to the androgenizing steroids—testosterone or estradiol—while the other half served as a control. When she removed the meninges of the explant, she found a marked increase in the outgrowth of neurites (new axons and dendrites) in a small proportion of cells in the slices that were exposed to an androgenizing agent (Figure 58–7). The morphological response of target cells to androgens also included extensive new branching of existing processes. The stimulation of neuritic growth by androgen is dose dependent. Low concentrations of steroid resulted in sparse outgrowth. Not all neurons are sensitive to steroids. The growth-promoting effects of gonadal steroids were especially pronounced in cells located in the anterior preoptic region and in an area called the infundibular–premammillary region.

The principal implication of these developmental studies in tissue culture is that the different neuronal organization imposed on the brains of males and females by sex steroids may result from alterations in the growth rate of axons and dendrites of select steroid-sensitive cells. During the critical period, steroid sex hormones might bias the rate of axonal differentiation in different regional populations and thereby ultimately affect neural circuitry. Since the amount of postsynaptic space is limited and constant, sexual differentiation of neural connections could occur as a result of changes in the balance of competition for postsynaptic sites between axonal populations of different origins. For example, if the partition of postsynaptic space between dendritic spines and shafts is determined competitively in time, the rate of growth of incoming neurites from different nuclear groups could determine the synaptic organization of the hypothalamus in the two sexes. In the context of competition, the emergence of a female pattern of neural or-

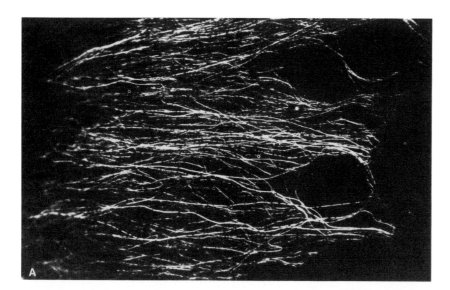

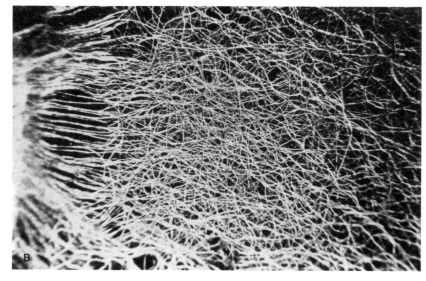

58–7 Photomicrographs of mirror slices of hypothalamic explants from the same newborn mouse demonstrate steroid sensitivity in this region. **A.** The control culture shows silver-impregnated neurites coursing outward in hairlike wisps from the margin of the explant. **B.** The neuritic growth of the homologue exhibits an extraordinarily dense plexus formation and extends well beyond the control. This growth was stimulated by the addition of estradiol (100 ng/ml) to the fluid bathing the culture. (From Toran-Allerand, 1978.)

ganization would not represent a primordial property of nervous tissue or the passive emergence of an intrinsic state; rather, both male and female patterns of neuronal organization may require equally active morphological mechanisms.

A Wide Range of Behaviors Is Influenced by Sex Differences in the Organization of the Brain

We have so far focused mainly on the dimorphic reproductive behaviors of males and females as the primary behavioral markers of brain sex. Several recent, converging lines of evidence suggest, however, that the repertoire of behaviors that are influenced by the perinatal hormonal environment may extend beyond the domain of reproductive behaviors. We shall now consider this research in the context of two questions: (1) What other types of behavior might be influenced by sex differences in the cellular organization of the brain? (2) To what ex-

tent might sexually differentiated neural organization, and its consequent behavioral biases, be influenced by environmental events?

Aggressive Behaviors: Stimuli Differ for the Two Sexes

Gonadal hormones are important in activating adult aggressive behavior and in establishing social dominance. The term *agonistic* is often applied to this repertoire of within-species behaviors that include escape, threat, and both offensive and defensive fighting, but not predation of other species.

In most rodent species, males but not females will attack intruders. This offensive aggression is enhanced by prior social isolation, and its activation in the normal male adult depends on the presence of androgens, in a dose-dependent fashion. In an early and influential study, Edwards found that neonatal castration reduces the adult expression of this type of aggressiveness, even in the presence of high doses of testosterone. As with other behaviors that are differentiated during the critical period in rodents, castration at 1 day of age is more effective than at 6 days or later. Edwards also discovered that androgenized female mice, tested after receiving testosterone as adults, display a masculine, offensive pattern of aggressiveness against male intruders. As a result, it was first thought that aggression is an androgen-dependent behavior that is organized during the critical period as part of the broad process of masculinization.

The problem with this view is that the females of most species are also normally aggressive, although in different situations, such as when protecting their young. The stimuli that elicit aggressive behavior differ in the two sexes, and the earlier experiments on the sexual differentiation of aggressive behavior preferentially studied environmental situations that favored male forms of aggression. Joseph DeBold and Klaus Miczek demonstrated that during lactation normal female mice greatly increase aggressive biting of intruders. Interestingly, the presence of a familiar male in the cage greatly increases maternal aggressiveness toward intruders, as well as the protectiveness of the mother toward her pups. The enhancement of maternal aggression by a male partner depends on the presence of testosterone *in the male*. The company of a castrated male partner does not facilitate the female's aggressiveness unless he is implanted with testosterone. As we might predict, the development of this characteristically female pattern of maternal aggression is dependent on the *absence* of androgens during the critical period. We may conclude, therefore, that exposure of the developing central nervous system to androgen must result in (1) the eventual adult expression of male forms of aggression (masculinization), and (2) the active suppression of female forms of aggressive behavior (defeminization). Like reproductive behaviors, agonistic behaviors appear to be organized during the same critical period along sexually differentiated lines.

Cognitive Behaviors: The Development of the Monkey Cortex Is Sexually Dimorphic

Patricia Goldman-Rakic has shown in rhesus monkeys that a clear-cut sexual dimorphism exists in the developmental processes that underlie certain cognitive functions of the frontal lobes. In both infant and adult male monkeys, but only in adult female monkeys, lesions of the orbital prefrontal cortex result in impaired performance on a wide variety of tests involving spatial discrimination and delayed responses. In contrast, identical lesions in infant females do not induce similar deficits until the animal has reached an age of 15–18 months. Thus the effects of orbital prefrontal lesions are age dependent, and the age at which this part of the cortex becomes involved in spatial learning differs markedly between the sexes. The earlier participation of the masculine frontal cortex in object-reversal learning may also be related to the subsequent superiority shown by male monkeys in these learning tasks as adults. Prenatal exposure of developing female monkey fetuses to androgens eliminates this sex difference in the performance of the adults and also results in a malelike susceptibility in infancy to orbital prefrontal lesions. Thus, the frontal cerebral cortex of the monkey is sexually dimorphic in its rate of development— a fact that may be related to the existence of steroid-sensitive neurons in the frontal cortex of infant rats, which, as McEwen has shown, disappear by puberty.

Human Cerebral Asymmetries Display Sexual Dimorphism

The specialization of cognitive functions in the left and right cerebral hemispheres of the mature human brain has been described in detail in Chapter 51. In brief, the left hemisphere in most right-handed individuals is specialized for language and related serial processing of information, whereas the right hemisphere is specialized for a variety of nonverbal processes, including three-dimensional visualization, mental rotation, face recognition, and understanding the meaning of facial expressions. Important in the present context is the suggestion, supported by several lines of recent evidence, that the brains of the two sexes may differ in their patterns of cognitive asymmetry. As with the development of prefrontal cortical functions in the monkey, there is even evidence that the two sexes differ in the rate of maturation of cognitive functions in the two hemispheres.

In a particularly interesting experiment, Sandra F. Witelson used a behavioral test that involved tactile perception to assess the relative participation of the two hemispheres in spatial processing. Children were given 10 sec to palpate simultaneously, out of view, two different shapes, one with each hand, using only the index and middle fingers. The children then tried to identify the objects that they had felt from pictures. In adults, tactile shape discrimination depends mainly on the right hemisphere, and to make the test as dependent as possible on the right hemisphere, Witelson designed her stimuli to be meaningless shapes, not readily labeled. Boys performed in a manner consistent with right-hemisphere specialization (left hand superiority) as early as the age of 6, regardless of their level of proficiency, which largely overlapped that of girls. Girls showed evidence of bilateral representation (no clear hand superiority) until the age of 13, suggesting that boys develop a greater hemispheric specialization at an earlier age. Therefore, over an extended period of development, a sex difference may exist in the hemispheric allocation of cognitive functions.

Witelson also pointed out that sexual dimorphism in the neural organization underlying cognition may have educational implications. For instance, reading is considered to involve both spatial and linguistic processing. The brains of boys and girls may be differentially organized for these cognitive processes at the time when they are learning to read. Different approaches in teaching reading, such as the look-see and phonetic methods—which stress different cognitive strategies and, by inference, depend on different neural structures—may not be equally effective in girls and boys.

If the right hemisphere in girls is not specialized for a particular cognitive function, then it may retain greater plasticity for a longer period than that of males. Clinical impressions are consistent with this idea. Language functions appear to transfer more readily to the right hemisphere in females than in males after damage to the left hemisphere in childhood. The extended plasticity of the young female brain also suggests that females may have a lower incidence of developmental disorders associated with left-hemisphere dysfunction. Developmental dyslexia, developmental aphasia, and infantile autism are more frequent in males. In all of these syndromes, language deficits are dominant symptoms.

There is recent evidence that cerebral asymmetries differ in the two sexes not only in their rate of maturation, but also in the ultimate degree to which they develop in the adult. J. Inglis and J. S. Lawson demonstrated that in male neurological patients there is a strong association between the nature of cognitive deficits observed and the side of the brain that has been injured: verbal functions are disordered with left-hemisphere lesions, and nonverbal functions with right-hemisphere lesions. In female neurological patients, this association is much weaker, suggesting that the adult female brain is functionally less asymmetrical than the male brain.

These sex differences in the susceptibility of the developing human brain to early damage and in the adult pattern of cerebral asymmetry have not yet been related to perinatal hormonal events, nor have the typically observed sex differences in cognitive abilities (males often score higher in tests of mathematical reasoning and in understanding spatial relationships, females higher in tests of verbal fluency and in the meaning of facial expressions).

Although our understanding of sex differences in human neural organization is still limited, it seems clear that the range of gender-typical behavioral biases that may be related to perinatal events is quite broad and that biologically based sex differences are not limited to reproductive behavior.

Human Sexuality Also Depends upon Learning

It is often tempting to view any intrinsic biological control mechanism, such as the perinatal differentiation of the nervous system, as representing a fixed, relatively permanent constraint upon behavior. In reality, however, there are few fixed action patterns in the human repertoire. Although strongly biased by neural organization, most behaviors remain flexible and open to modification. For example, even though we inherit a finely tuned regulatory system for food consumption and body weight, certain nonpathological life experiences can override the homeostat for body weight and produce obesity in oth-

erwise normal individuals. A person may develop a passionate interest in fine food and wines, may get a job as a restaurant critic, and so on. The brain is also outfitted with intrinsic circuits for modulating aggressive and other emotional behaviors; nevertheless, without apparent neuropathology, individuals can become pacifists or terrorists for ideological reasons. Similarly, there is ample social evidence that the neural organization of reproductive behaviors, while *biased* by hormonal events during a critical perinatal period, certainly does not exert an immutable influence over adult sexual behavior or even over an individual's psychosexual orientation. Within the life of the individual, religious, social, or economic motives can prompt biologically similar people to become celibates, swingers, prostitutes, or rapists.

While the research outlined in this chapter alerts us to the idea that perinatal hormones influence sexuality in adulthood, it would be a mistake to ignore the influence of learning. A single dramatic example may suffice to remind us of the overriding role of life experiences in molding human sexuality. This case history, reported by John Money and Anke Ehrhardt, involves a set of monozygotic male twins who, besides sharing an identical genetic constitution, were presumably exposed to the same hormonal environment in utero. During circumcision at the age of 7 months, the penis of one of the boys was accidentally removed by electrocautery. After discussions with the parents, 4 months later the child was reassigned as a girl, and surgical reconstruction of the genitalia was begun. The subsequent experience of the family with their new daughter was later summarized by the mother:

The mother stated that her daughter by four and a half years of age was much neater than her brother, and in contrast with him, disliked to be dirty: "She likes for me to wipe her face. She doesn't like to be dirty, and yet my son is quite different. I can't wash his face for anything . . . . She seems to be daintier. Maybe it's because I encourage it . . . . One thing that really amazes me is that she is so feminine. I've never seen a little girl so neat and tidy as she can be when she wants to be . . . . She is very proud of herself, when she puts on a new dress, or I set her hair. She just loves to have her hair set . . . . She just loves it."

Even allowing for a mother's natural bias, the behavioral plasticity shown by an individual adjusting to a new sexual role is impressive.

Selected Readings

Bardin, C. W., and Catterall, J. F. 1981. Testosterone: A major determinant of extragenital sexual dimorphism. Science 211:1285–1294.

Goy, R. W., and Goldfoot, D. A. 1975. Neuroendocrinology: Animal models and problems of human sexuality. Arch. Sex. Behav. 4:405–420.

Goy, R. W., and McEwen, B. S. 1980. Sexual Differentiation of the Brain. Cambridge, Mass.: MIT Press.

Hines, M. 1982. Prenatal gonadal hormones and sex differences in human behavior. Psychol. Bull. 92:56–80.

MacLusky, N. J., and Naftolin, F. 1981. Sexual differentiation of the central nervous system. Science 211:1294–1303.

Pfaff, D. W., and McEwen, B. S. 1983. Actions of estrogens and progestins on nerve cells. Science 219:808–814.

Robinson, T. E., Becker, J. B., Camp, D. M., and Mansour, A. 1985. Variation in the pattern of behavioral and brain asymmetries due to sex differences. In S. D. Glick (ed.), Cerebral Lateralization in Non-Human Species. Orlando, Fla.: Academic Press.

Toran-Allerand, C. D. 1984. On the genesis of sexual differentiation of the central nervous system: Morphogenetic consequences of steroidal exposure and possible role of α-fetoprotein. In G. J. De Vries, J. P. C. De Bruin, H. B. M. Uylings, and M. A. Corner (eds.), Sex Differences in the Brain: The Relation Between Structure and Function. Prog. in Brain Res. 61:63–98.

References

Ayoub, D. M., Greenough, W. T., and Juraska, J. M. 1983. Sex differences in dendritic structure in the preoptic area of the juvenile macaque monkey brain. Science 219:197–198.

Baack, J., de Lacoste-Utamsing, C., and Woodward, D. J. 1982. Sexual dimorphism in human fetal corpora callosa. Soc. Neurosci. Abstr. 8:213.

Barraclough, C. A., and Gorski, R. A. 1962. Studies on mating behaviour in the androgen-sterilized female rat in relation to the hypothalamic regulation of sexual behaviour. J. Endocrinol. 25:175–182.

Beach, F. A., Noble, R. G., and Orndoff, R. K. 1969. Effects of perinatal androgen treatment on responses of male rats to gonadal hormones in adulthood. J. Comp. Physiol. Psychol. 68:490–497.

Bermant, G., and Davidson, J. M. 1974. Biological Bases of Sexual Behavior. New York: Harper & Row.

Breedlove, S. M., and Arnold, A. P. 1980. Hormone accumulation in a sexually dimorphic motor nucleus of the rat spinal cord. Science 210:564–566.

Breedlove, S. M., Jacobson, C. D., Gorski, R. A., and Arnold, A. P. 1982. Masculinization of the female rat spinal cord following a single neonatal injection of testosterone propionate but not estradiol benzoate. Brain Res. 237:173–181.

DeBold, J. F., and Miczek, K. A. 1981. Sexual dimorphism in the hormonal control of aggressive behavior of rats. Pharmacol. Biochem. Behav. [Suppl. 1] 14:89–93.

de Lacoste-Utamsing, C., and Holloway, R. L. 1982. Sexual dimorphism in the human corpus callosum. Science 216:1431–1432.

Edwards, D. A. 1968. Mice: Fighting by neonatally androgenized females. Science 161:1027–1028.

Goldman, P. S., Crawford, H. T., Stokes, L. P., Galkin, T. W., and Rosvold, H. E. 1974. Sex-dependent behavioral effects of cerebral cortical lesions in the developing rhesus monkey. Science 186:540–542.

Gorski, R. A., Gordon, J. H., Shryne, J. E., and Southam, A. M. 1978. Evidence for a morphological sex difference within the medial preoptic area of the rat brain. Brain Res. 148:333–346.

Inglis, J., and Lawson, J. S. 1981. Sex differences in the effects of unilateral brain damage on intelligence. Science 212:693–695.

Jacobson, C. D., and Gorski, R. A. 1981. Neurogenesis of the sexually dimorphic nucleus of the preoptic area in the rat. J. Comp. Neurol. 196:519–529.

McEwen, B. S. 1976. Interactions between hormones and nerve tissue. Sci. Am. 235(1):48–58.

Money, J., and Ehrhardt, A. A. 1972. Man & Woman, Boy & Girl. Baltimore: Johns Hopkins University Press.

Phoenix, C. H., Goy, R. W., Gerall, A. A., and Young, W. C. 1959. Organizing action of prenatally administered testosterone propionate on the tissues mediating mating behavior in the female guinea pig. Endocrinology 65:369–382.

Raisman, G. 1974. Evidence for a sex difference in the neuropil of the rat preoptic area and its importance for the study of sexually dimorphic functions. Res. Publ. Assoc. Res. Nerv. Ment. Dis. 52:42–49.

Raisman, G., and Field, P. M. 1971. Sexual dimorphism in the preoptic area of the rat. Science 173:731–733.

Toran-Allerand, C. D. 1978. Gonadal hormones and brain development: Cellular aspects of sexual differentiation. Am. Zool. 18:553–565.

vom Saal, F. S., and Bronson, F. H. 1980. Sexual characteristics of adult female mice are correlated with their blood testosterone levels during prenatal development. Science 208:597–599.

Whalen, R. E., and Edwards, D. A. 1967. Hormonal determinants of the development of masculine and feminine behavior in male and female rats. Anat. Rec. 157:173–180.

Whalen, R. E., and Massicci, J. 1975. Subcellular analysis of the accumulation of estrogen by the brain of male and female rats. Brain Res. 89:255–264.

Witelson, S. F. 1976. Sex and the single hemisphere: Specialization of the right hemisphere for spatial processing. Science 193:425–427.

Lucien Côté

Aging of the Brain and Dementia

59

Age robs us of all things, even the mind

(Virgil, *Eclogues* IX, line 51)

Virgil's observation is as true today as it was when he wrote it over 2000 years ago. The maximum number of years that human beings can live has not increased significantly, but the average human life expectancy has increased markedly, especially since the turn of this century. This increase is largely due to medical advances such as the reduction in infant mortality, the development of vaccines, and the availability of antibiotics, drugs that lower blood pressure, and other forms of medical treatment. In 1900 the average life expectancy was 47 years. Now a man's life expectancy is approximately 71 years and a woman's, 78 (Figure 59–1). Moreover, life expectancy continues to increase. During the decade between 1968 and 1979 it rose at a rate of 1 month per year for all people over 50. In particular, there has been a significant decrease in both heart disease and stroke because of advances in our knowledge of these diseases, the development of new drugs, better control of blood pressure, and increased emphasis on proper diet, salt intake, weight control, exercise, and activity. However, as we shall see, this increase in life expectancy has unmasked a new epidemic: *dementia*, a deterioration of mental function. Dementia accompanies aging in certain susceptible individuals. These individuals constitute a minority, but a substantial and increasing proportion, of the aging population.

Most gerontologists (scientists interested in the biological, psychological, and social problems of aging) agree that lengthening the life span of humans has little merit if the quality of life is not preserved. The ultimate goal of research on aging is not only to lengthen life, but also to maintain and enhance its quality.

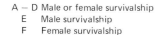

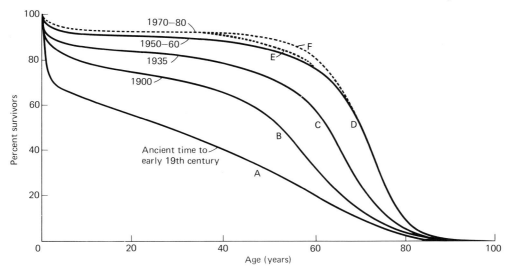

59–1 Human survivorship trends from ancient times to the present. These idealized curves illustrate the rapid approach to the limiting rectangular curve that has occurred during the past 150 years. The major factors responsible for these transitions are listed above the graph. Note that life expectancy for males has changed only slightly since 1950 in the 50 + age group. However, female survivorship has improved significantly during this period, at least in part because of better treatment of reproductive system malignancies. (Adapted from Strehler, 1975.)

In this chapter we shall examine what is known of the molecular mechanisms of aging, focusing in particular on the aging brain and on some illnesses characteristic of age that produce severe memory loss and intellectual deterioration.

Several Hypotheses Have Been Proposed for the Molecular Mechanisms of Aging

Several lines of evidence suggest that aging occurs as the result of changes in informational macromolecules. At least three hypotheses have been advanced that relate aging to changes in DNA and RNA. Zhores Medvedev proposed a redundant message theory, according to which mutations and chromosomal anomalies accumulate with age. As these errors accumulate in functioning genes, reserve (redundant) sequences, containing the same information on DNA molecules, take over until the redundancy is exhausted. Senescence then follows. On the other hand, Bernard Strehler and his colleagues suggested that aging is part of a larger developmental sequence. Just as some genes program phases of embryonic development, others program the aging processes in the organism. Strehler proposed that the changes of old age result from the normal expression of a genetic program that begins at conception and ends in death. A third hypothesis, supported by many researchers on aging, maintains that the genetic apparatus does not contain a program for senescent changes per se, but that errors in duplication of DNA increase with age because of random damage and insults that occur with time (wear and tear, radiation effects, and so on). When a significant number of errors accumulates, abnormal mRNA and protein molecules are formed, and these cannot function normally. The burden of errors results in senescence.

A particularly intriguing variant of these ideas, based upon the work of Leonard Hayflick, is that cells possess a biological clock that dictates their life span. Hayflick has found that normal human fibroblasts grown in culture divide regularly until they cover the entire surface of the culture flask. If the cells are transferred in equal numbers to two flasks containing fresh medium they divide until they again become confluent. Normal cultured human fibroblasts can double only a limited number of times (about 50 times) over a period of 7–9 months. Starting at around the 35th passage, their rate of division begins to slow down; eventually they stop dividing and die. Fibroblasts from older human donors double significantly fewer times than those obtained from human embryos. The number of cell doublings is roughly related to the age of the donor whose cells are used.

The longevity of the species from which fibroblasts are obtained also is a factor in dictating the number of possible passages. Fibroblasts from mouse embryos (whose expected life span is 3 years) divide about 15 times before they die; fibroblasts from humans (with a life span of 70–80 years) divide about 50 times; and those from Galapagos tortoises (with a life span of 175 years) divide about 90 times. Thus, the number of passages is also roughly related to the longevity of the species.

If nuclei from young fibroblasts are interchanged with those of old fibroblasts (a transfer technique made possible by using cytochalasin B and centrifugation), the newly formed hybrid cells divide according to the age of the nuclei and not of the cytoplasm. Thus the biological clock seems to be located in the nucleus of the fibroblast. These and other studies indicate that at least some aspects are intrinsic or genetic.

Dementia Is Prominent in the Clinical Syndromes of Aging

No matter what the fundamental processes that underlie senescence are, the consequences of aging in the human brain can be devastating when they impair normal mental functions. Most people age without substantial loss of intellectual powers, but this is not true for all people. About 11% of people in the United States over 65 years of age show mild to severe mental impairment. Moreover, there is about a 2% per year increase in dementia from age 75 on. As a result, approximately 25% of people 80 years of age have significant dementia. The total number of people involved is staggering. *One million people in the United States are seriously demented.* An estimated 120,000 patients die each year of severe dementia, and thus dementia is the fourth most common cause of death in humans (after cancer, heart disease, and stroke). Given more effective modes of treatment for cancer and heart disease in the future, the average life span of humans is expected to increase significantly and reach about 120 years. This achievement may be of dubious value, since the incidence of dementia rapidly increases with every added year of life.

The word *dementia* denotes a progressive decline in mental function, including acquired intellectual skills. It can be caused by many abnormal processes and therefore lacks diagnostic specificity. Alzheimer's disease is the major cause of dementia, accounting for or contributing to about 70% of all cases of dementia. Bernard Tomlinson and G. Henderson have shown that only about 15% of cases of dementia result from multiple infarcts (many little strokes). Thus, contrary to the popular notion held in the past, "hardening of the arteries of the brain" is not the main cause of dementia (although in some cases hardening of the arteries may add to and aggravate the cause of Alzheimer's disease). The remaining 15% of cases of dementia are caused by factors that can potentially be corrected by treatment. These treatable diseases include infections of the brain and the meninges, nutritional diseases (such as vitamin deficiencies), endocrine and metabolic diseases, intracranial mass lesions, chronically increased intracranial pressure, and normal pressure hydrocephalus.

Presenile and senile dementia of the Alzheimer's type constitute the same disease entity. They are indistinguishable both pathologically and clinically except for the age of onset. The presenile form of Alzheimer's disease has its onset before the age of 60; the senile form begins after. Alzheimer's disease is usually insidious in onset and often becomes obvious to the family after the patient has undergone a period of minor stress. The early manifestations include forgetfulness, untidiness, transient confusion, periods of restlessness and lethargy, and errors in judgment. Recent memory is impaired, although remote memory is often not lost and may even be enhanced. Patients lose interest in current events, and eventually they are restricted to a wheelchair or bed. Although the course of the illness is highly variable, it may be 5–10 years before the patient with Alzheimer's disease reaches the final stage, marked by mental emptiness and loss of control of all body functions. Alzheimer's disease reduces a person's normal remaining life expectancy by about one-half.

Alzheimer's disease is common in patients with Down's syndrome (mongolism), in whom it typically occurs at an early age. However, Alzheimer's disease primarily is a disease of the aging.

Five Characteristic Cellular Changes of Aging Occur with Increased Frequency in Dementia

There are many types of microscopic changes in the brains of aged humans. Five of these are particularly prominent and important because they occur with greater frequency in dementia. These are: the accumulation of lipofuscin granules, granulovacuolar organelles, neuritic plaques, and neurofibrillary tangles, and changes in cell bodies and dendrites.

Lipofuscin granules are pigmented subcellular organelles that autofluoresce green, yellow, or brown (Figure 59–2). These granules accumulate in the cytoplasm of neurons as humans age. They are thought to be large end-stage lysosomes that accumulate recycled membrane and other cellular debris that cannot be further catabolized by the neuron. There is no evidence that the accumulation of these large granules impairs the function of the neurons. The rate of accumulation with age seems to be characteristic for certain cell groups. For example, neurons of the olivary and dentate nuclei of the human brain contain lipofuscin granules in the first decade of life. By age 60 the granules occupy most of the cell body of these neurons. On the other hand, the cells of the globus pallidus contain little lipofuscin until late in life. We still have no idea what accounts for these differences between cell types.

Granulovacuolar organelles accumulate with age in the cytoplasm and dendrites of degenerating nerve cells of the hippocampus and adjacent cortex (Figure 59–3). Each vacuole has an outer membrane with a small dense granule in its center. These organelles are much more numerous in brains of Alzheimer's patients than in age-matched, nondemented people.

Neuritic (senile) plaques are most dense in the hippocampus but they are also found in parts of the neocortex (Figure 59–4). Plaques are seen in brains of nondemented old people but are much more common in

59–2 A large aggregate of lipofuscin **(arrow)** occupies a major portion of the cell body of this spinal cord motor cell. Hematoxylin and eosin stain. (From Duffy, 1976.)

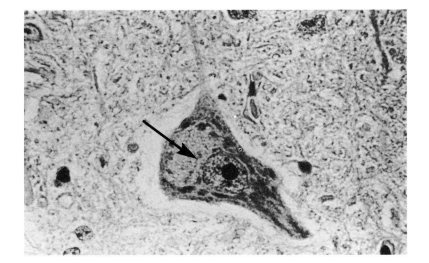

59–3 Granulovacuolar organelles have accumulated in the cytoplasm of this neuron. Each organelle consists of a small vacuole with a central argyrophilic granule **(arrow).** (From Duffy, 1976.)

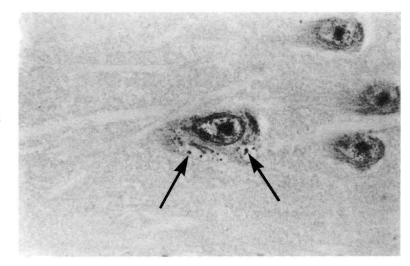

59–4 A senile plaque consists of masses of granular and filamentous argyrophilic material and has an amorphous core containing amyloidlike material. Bielschowsky silver stain. (From Duffy, 1976.)

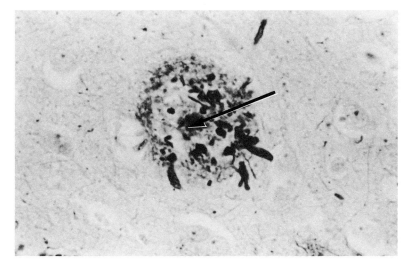

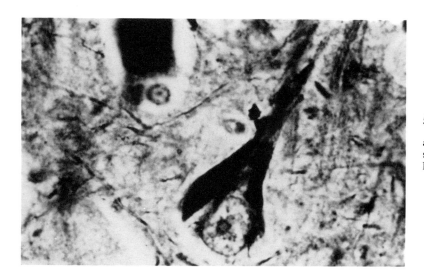

59–5 Neurofibrillary degeneration occurs in nerve cells of the cerebral cortex. Large bundles of abnormal twisted tubules with a marked affinity for silver give the jet-black appearance seen with the Bielschowsky silver stain. (From Duffy, 1976.)

Alzheimer's disease. These extracellular plaques, which are about 5–100 μm in diameter, are best visualized with reduced silver stains. They are composed of a central core of amyloid surrounded by masses of neural processes undergoing various degrees of degenerative change. Glial cells form their outer margins. The precursors of these plaques are small groups of enlarged neurites containing clusters of mitochondria and lysosomes.

Neurofibrillary tangles (Alzheimer's bodies; Figure 59–5) are one of the most common histological features of the neuronal cell bodies in brains of patients with Alzheimer's disease (but they can also be present in post-

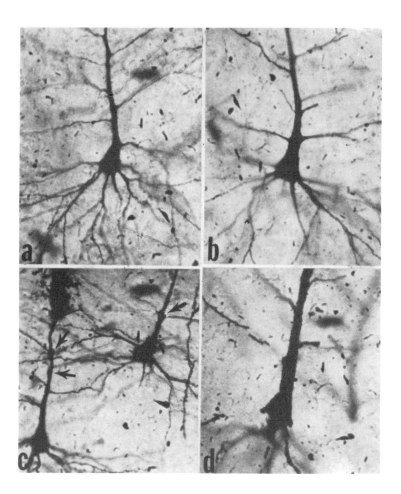

59–6 Very early senescent changes in pyramidal cells of the prefrontal cortex. **A** and **B.** These pyramidal cells from the third and fifth layers in an 83-year-old patient are presumably within normal limits. **C.** These third-layer pyramidal cells from a 96-year-old patient show early swelling of the cell bodies and lumpiness developing in dendrite shafts **(arrows).** **D.** This third-layer pyramidal cell from an 83-year-old man shows swelling, especially of the apical shaft, and a loss of most basilar dendrites. Golgi impregnation. × 220. (From Scheibel and Scheibel, 1975.)

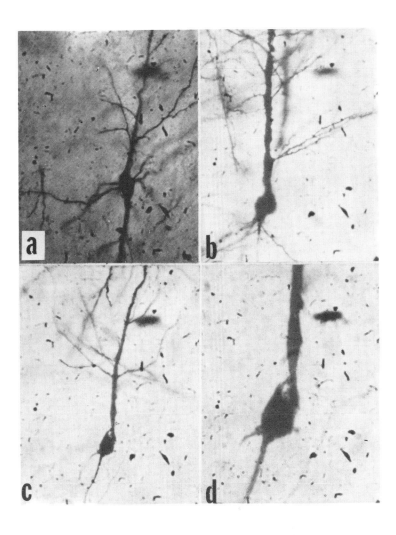

59–7 Progressive senile changes in cortical spindle cells. **A.** This fourth-layer spindle cell from the superior temporal gyrus of an 89-year-old man appears normal. × 220. **B.** This spindle cell shows irregular swelling of the cell body and apical process with partial loss of deep process. × 220. **C** and **D.** A lower fourth-layer spindle cell from the superior temporal gyrus of a 96-year-old man shows irregular swelling of the soma and apical process and partial loss of horizontal branches. Golgi impregnation: part **C** × 220; part **D** × 440. (From Scheibel and Scheibel, 1975.)

encephalitic parkinsonism and in amyotrophic lateral sclerosis). A few neurofibrillary tangles are frequently found in nondemented, aged individuals. It is believed that these organelles derive from the fibrillar proteins that constitute the normal cytoskeleton of neurons (see Chapter 4) but that they have been chemically modified. Neurofibrillary tangles chiefly consist of paired helical fibers, measuring about 25 nm in diameter at their widest, which constrict at about 80-nm intervals to a width of about 10 nm. Each helical fiber is made up of a pair of filaments slightly greater than 10 nm in diameter. Even though somewhat thicker than neurofilaments, these fibers might be a degraded type of intermediary filament. Because neurofibrillary tangles contain small amounts of normal neurofilaments as well as other cytoskeletal proteins, it has been difficult to interpret the cross-reactivity that has been observed when neurofibrillary tangles have been studied with immunocytochemical methods using antibodies raised against various normal cytoskeletal proteins as antigens.

It has been difficult to study Alzheimer's disease in the laboratory because the pathology of this socially important disorder has not yet been produced in experimen-

tal animals. Neurofibrillary tangles are unique to human brain: in no other animal have these lesions been found. Injection of alumina into the brains of laboratory animals induces a lesion that superficially resembles the neurofibrillary tangle. These lesions lack the paired helical fibers characteristic of the human tangles, however, and consist entirely of disordered neurofilaments.

Profound changes in the cell body and dendrites of neurons lead to a loss of dendrites with age, especially in demented individuals (Figures 59–6 and 59–7). Arnold Scheibel and others have observed that initially there is swelling and distortion of the somatic and dendritic silhouette, followed by progressive loss of dendrites (Figure 59–8). These changes may be closely related to the increased choking of the cytoplasmic space with abnormal pathological inclusions. Loss of dendrites would severely diminish synaptic interactions and decrease the capacity for neurons to process information. These changes are thought by some investigators to be better indices of neural aging than all other histological findings described thus far.

The morphological changes seen in Alzheimer's disease are also found to some degree among the nonde-

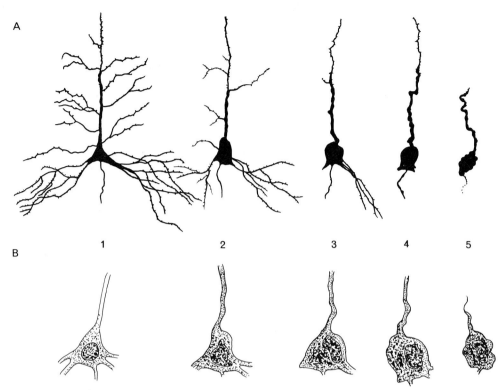

59–8 Progression of senile changes in cortical pyramidal cells. The cell body and apical process swell and become distorted and there is a gradual loss of dendrites. Shown here are schematic representations of how these cells would look with (**A**) Golgi impregnation and (**B**) Bielschowsky stain. (Adapted from Scheibel and Scheibel, 1975.)

mented aged, but in dementia the number of lesions is much greater and they have a different distribution. By age 80 the brain normally has decreased in weight by less than 15%; but in demented patients the extent of decrease usually is much greater. In addition, in dementia the cortical gyri are thin and the sulci prominent. In some patients, however, the functional deficit is even greater than these atrophic changes would indicate, suggesting that much of the tissue without gross lesions is also abnormal.

It is therefore important to ask whether Alzheimer's disease is only an accelerated process of aging or a pathological process quite distinct from normal aging. Similarly, is Parkinson's disease, which occurs in the middle and later years of life, an accelerated aging process in a discrete area of the brain, the basal ganglia? These questions are best approached biochemically.

Characteristic Biochemical Changes Take Place in the Brain with Aging

A major impediment to research on human aging has been the difficulty of obtaining brain tissue for analysis. Animal studies are not satisfactory for this analysis be-

cause there are many species differences in the aging process of the brain. For example, mice show relatively little change in brain weight, water content, and DNA concentration with increasing age. In contrast, humans and other primates show a significant loss in brain weight and increase in DNA with senescence. Primates such as rhesus monkeys are difficult to study because of their long life span and prohibitive cost. Studies of time-dependent biochemical changes associated with aging in humans are therefore best carried out in human brain.

By age 80, total brain protein is reduced by 30%. Concomitantly, there is a progressive increase in total DNA, presumably caused by proliferation of glial cells (gliosis), and only a slight increase in water content. Lipid constituents (neural fats, cerebrosides, and phosphatides) decrease minimally with age.

Acetylcholine, dopamine, norepinephrine, serotonin, γ-aminobutyric acid (GABA), and other neurotransmitters are synthesized and degraded by enzymes and act by binding to receptors (see Chapters 13 and 14). Age-related alterations in the synthesis and degradation of neurotransmitters and their receptors could explain some of the characteristics of senescence: altered sleep pattern, mood, appetite, neuroendocrine functions, motor activity, and memory. With age, there are indeed drastic reductions in the enzymes involved in the synthesis of dopamine and norepinephrine in human brain. Similar but less severe changes occur in the activities of enzymes crucial to acetylcholine synthesis. Some recent studies also have demonstrated reductions with age in the receptors for dopamine, norepinephrine, and acetylcholine in various regions of the human brain.

These general patterns of chemical changes appear to be characteristic for normal aging; however, *diseases* of aging, such as parkinsonism, Huntington's disease, and dementia, are often accompanied by more selective changes, specific to one or a very few transmitter systems. We have already seen that neurotransmitter function is impaired in Parkinson's disease (Chapter 40). There is a profound reduction in the amount of dopamine in a discrete system of the brain (the extrapyramidal motor system). Similarly, in Huntington's disease, another degenerative disease, the levels of glutamic acid decarboxylase activity, GABA, and choline acetyltransferase activity are sharply reduced.

Alzheimer's Disease Involves Selective Loss of Cholinergic Neurons in the Basal Forebrain

Of all the changes in transmitter-related proteins in the brain, one of the most dramatic involves the cholinergic neurons. The first hint of a selective loss of cholinergic neurons in Alzheimer's disease came in the mid-1970s when several investigators showed a 60%–90% loss of choline acetyltransferase activity in the cerebral cortex, hippocampus, and related areas. Choline acetyltransferase catalyzes the synthesis of acetylcholine and is a marker for cholinergic neurons. This important observation was puzzling because cell counts of the neocortex and hippocampus of patients with Alzheimer's disease did not reveal major reductions in numbers of neurons when compared with age-matched controls. The disappearance of large amounts of the transferase without a parallel loss in the number of cell bodies implied that the main source of choline acetyltransferase was in the presynaptic terminals of neurons whose cell bodies were extrinsic to the cortex and hippocampus.

Studies in experimental animals resolve this paradox. These studies show that most of the massive cholinergic projection to the neocortex and hippocampus come from the cholinergic neurons in *nucleus basalis of Meynert* (which is located beneath the globus pallidus in the substantia innominata of the basal forebrain). In humans, the nucleus basalis is larger than in other species and is a major component of the substantia innominata. Lesions in the basal forebrain of rats reduce the choline acetyltransferase activity in the neocortex 60%–70%. The cholinergic neurons located in the nucleus basalis receive afferents from many sources, including the hypothalamus, amygdala, peripeduncular nucleus, midbrain, and other brain stem nuclei, and they project diffusely to the neocortex, entorhinal cortex, amygdala, hippocampus, olfactory bulbs, thalamus, hypothalamus, and brain stem. The nucleus basalis is therefore believed to play a central role in integrating subcortical function and influencing neocortical activity.

Donald Price, Joseph Coyle, and Mahlon DeLong at Johns Hopkins University examined the nucleus basalis in patients with Alzheimer's disease and observed a profound (75%) and selective degeneration of neurons within this nucleus as compared with age-matched controls. This finding is the first to link a biochemically and anatomically distinct population of neurons to dementia. However, there is mounting evidence that other transmitter systems—for example, biogenic amines and neuropeptides such as somatostatin and substance P—are also involved in Alzheimer's disease.

Unfortunately, there is no specific treatment for Alzheimer's disease. Attempts to improve the mental status of the patient by administering a precursor to acetylcholine such as choline or lecithin, a rich source of choline, have been unsuccessful. Although studies in animals indicate that the amounts of acetylcholine in the brain can be increased with the administration of these precursors, it does not seem to help in Alzheimer's disease. This suggests that in Alzheimer's disease cholinergic neurons are no longer able to synthesize acetylcholine. Cholinergic and other transmitter agonists are now being tested.

One Form of Dementia Is of Viral Origin

One form of dementia is thought to be of viral origin. *Jakob-Creutzfeldt disease* is a relatively rare subacute spongiform encephalopathy seen in adults that is characterized clinically by dementia, myoclonic jerks, and often ataxia. The disease is transmissible to chimpanzees and humans and is due to a virus that is thought to have a long incubation or latency period in nerve cells before its activity becomes expressed. These viruses are therefore called *slow viruses.*

An Overall View

Although it is one of the eternal interests of mankind, the process of aging is not yet understood. The scientific information now at hand is limited and consists of clinical and pathological clues, fragmentary ideas about mechanisms, and some uncertain hypotheses. Modern gerontologists believe that the aging process, like other mechanisms in neurobiology, will become clearer when approached with the insights and techniques of cell biology and biochemistry. As the average age of the population increases, dementia of the Alzheimer type is reaching epidemic proportions. A breakthrough in understanding the cause and treatment of Alzheimer's disease is necessary if we are to avert a growing medical crisis.

Selected Readings

Hayflick, L. 1975. Current theories of biological aging. Fed. Proc. 34:9–13.

Katzman, R. (ed.) 1983. Biological Aspects of Alzheimer's Disease. Cold Spring Harbor, New York: Cold Spring Harbor Laboratories, Banbury Reports, Vol. 15.

Roth, M. 1978. Diagnosis of senile and related forms of dementia. In R. Katzman, R. D. Terry, and K. L. Bick (eds.), Aging, Vol. 7: Alzheimer's Disease: Senile Dementia and Related Disorders. New York: Raven Press, pp. 71–85.

Samorajski, T., and Ordy, J. M. 1972. Neurochemistry of aging. In C. M. Gaitz (ed.), Advances in Behavioral Biology, Vol. 3: Aging and the Brain. New York: Plenum Press, pp. 41–61.

Tomlinson, B. E., and Henderson, G. 1976. Some quantitative cerebral findings in normal and demented old people. In R. D. Terry and S. Gershon (eds.), Aging, Vol. 3: Neurobiology of Aging. New York: Raven Press, pp. 183–204.

Whitehouse, P. J., Price, D. L., Struble, R. G., Clark, A. W., Coyle, J. T., and DeLong, M. R. 1982. Alzheimer's disease and senile dementia: Loss of neurons in the basal forebrain. Science 215:1237–1239.

Wiśniewski, H. M., and Terry, R. D. 1973. Morphology of the aging brain, human and animal. Neurobiological Aspects of Maturation and Aging. Prog. Brain Res. 40:167–186.

References

Boyd, W. D., Graham-White, J., Blackwood, G., Glen, I., and McQueen, J. 1977. Clinical effects of choline in Alzheimer senile dementia. Lancet 2:711.

Côté, L. J., and Kremzner, L. T. 1983. Biochemical changes in normal aging in human brain. In R. Mayeux and W. G. Rosen (eds.), Advances in Neurology, Vol. 38: The Dementias. New York: Raven Press, pp. 19–30.

Dastur, D. K., Lane, M. H., Hansen, D. B., Kety, S. S., Butler, R. N., Perlin, S., and Sokoloff, L. 1963. Effects of aging on cerebral circulation and metabolism in man. In J. E. Birren, R. N. Butler, S. W. Greenhouse, L. Sokoloff, and M. R. Yarrow (eds.), Human Aging: A Biological and Behavioral Study. Public Health Service Publ. No. 986. Washington, D.C.: U.S. Government Printing Office, pp. 57–76.

Davies, P., and Maloney, A. J. F. 1976. Selective loss of central cholinergic neurons in Alzheimer's disease. Lancet 2:1403.

Duffy, P. E. (ed.). 1976. Tumors of the Nervous System. Philadelphia: Davis.

Etienne, P., Gauthier, S., Johnson, G., Collier, B., Mendis, T., Dastoor, D., Cole, M., and Muller, H. F. 1978. Clinical effects of choline in Alzheimer's disease. Lancet 1:508–509.

Gajdusek, D. C. 1978. Slow infections with unconventional viruses. Harvey Lect. 72:283–353.

Gibbs, C. J., Jr., Gajdusek, D. C., Asher, D. M., Alpers, M. P., Beck, E., Daniel, P. M., and Matthews, W. B. 1968. Creutzfeldt-Jakob disease (spongiform encephalopathy): Transmission to the chimpanzee. Science 161:388–389.

Hayflick, L. 1980. The cell biology of human aging. Sci. Am. 242(1):58–65.

Marsden, C. D., and Harrison, M. J. G. 1972. Outcome of investigation of patients with presenile dementia. Br. Med. J. 2:249–252.

McGeer, E., and McGeer, P. L. 1976. Neurotransmitter metabolism in the aging brain. In R. D. Terry and S. Gershon (eds.), Aging, Vol. 3: Neurobiology of Aging. New York: Raven Press, pp. 389–403.

Medvedev, Zh. A. 1972. Repetition of molecular-genetic information as a possible factor in evolutionary changes of life span. Exp. Gerontol. 7:227–238.

Perry, E. K., Perry, R. H., Blessed, G., and Tomlinson, B. E. 1977. Necropsy evidence of central cholinergic deficits in senile dementia. Lancet 1:189.

Price, D. L., Whitehouse, P. J., Struble, R. G., Clark, A. W., Coyle, J. T., DeLong, M. R., and Hedreen, J. C. 1982. Basal forebrain cholinergic systems in Alzheimer's disease and related dementias. Neurosci. Comment. 1(2):84–92.

Scheibel, M. E., and Scheibel, A. B. 1975. Structural changes in the aging brain. In H. Brody, D. Harman, and J. M. Ordy (eds.), Aging, Vol. I: Clinical, Morphologic, and Neurochemical Aspects in the Aging Central Nervous System. New York: Raven Press, pp. 11–37.

Signoret, J. L., Whiteley, A., and Lhermitte, F. 1978. Influence of choline on amnesia in early Alzheimer's disease. Lancet 2:837.

Strehler, B., Hirsch, G., Gusseck, D., Johnson, R., and Bick, M. 1971. Codon-restriction theory of aging and development. J. Theor. Biol. 33:429–474.

Strehler, B. L. 1975. Implications of aging research for society. Fed. Proc. 34:5–8.

Walford, R. L. 1974. Immunologic theory of aging: Current status. Fed. Proc. 33:2020–2027.

White, P., Hiley, C. R., Goodhardt, M. J., Carrasco, L. H., Keet, J. P., Williams, I. E. I., and Bowen, D. M. 1977. Neocortical cholinergic neurons in elderly people. Lancet 1:668–671.

Genes, Environmental Experience, and the Mechanisms of Behavior

XI

The study of neural science is concerned with normal human mental activity, the biological basis of individual action and thought. As we saw in Part X, behavior emerges gradually as the brain develops. At first, the development of the brain is largely under the control of genetic and developmental programs. Influences from the environment begin to exert their effect in utero, but they become of prime importance only after birth. Consequently, a knowledge of innate (genetic and developmental) as well as environmental determinants is needed to understand any behavior fully. This knowledge is also essential for developing rational therapeutic strategies for the treatment of mental disorders.

In considering innate factors in the control of behavior, we shall first focus on aspects of behavior that are heritable. Clearly, a behavior per se is not inherited: it is DNA that is inherited. The DNA of genes codes for proteins that are important for the development, maintenance, and regulation of neural circuits that produce behavior. We shall then examine the interaction of genetic and environmental factors in determining behavior.

In considering behavior, we shall see that careful and quantitative analysis of stimuli and of responses is important because responses are the *observable* indices of behavior. Stimuli and responses can be manipulated experimentally and measured objectively. By emphasizing *observable actions*, behaviorists focus research on the questions: What does an organism do and how does it do it? An extreme behaviorist view is that observable indices of behavior are synonymous with mental life. This view narrowly defines psychic life in terms of the scientific techniques available for studying it and denies the existence of consciousness as well as unconscious mentation, feelings, and motivation.

However—as has been emphasized by cognitive psychologists and by psychoanalysts—in addition to actions, humans and other higher animals also possess knowledge of the surrounding world and of past events. Thus, we need also to ask the following question: What does the organism know and how does it come to know it? How is that knowledge represented in the brain? Is the representation of conscious mental activity or knowledge different from that of unconscious activity?

The field of neural science has not yet been particularly helpful in analyzing the richness of internal representation recognized by cognitive psychologists as intervening between stimulus and response, or of the dynamic mental processes experienced by all of us that traditionally have been discussed from the framework of psychoanalysis or cognitive psychology. Much less has neural science been able to address the subjective sense of individuality, will, and purpose that is a common feature of Western culture. Despite our inability to deal with these aspects of behavior experimentally, they are the issues most crucial to us as scientists, as clinicians, and as people. In the past, ascribing a particular aspect of behavior to an unobservable mental process essentially excluded the problem from direct laboratory study because the complexity of the brain posed a barrier to any complementary biological analysis. As the nervous system becomes accessible to a cellular analysis of behavior, however, certain internal representations of environmental experiences can be explored in a controlled experimental manner, as we illustrate in the chapters of this section. This progress encourages us in the belief that elements of cognition relevant to humans can now be explored directly and need no longer be merely inferred.

In modern neural science, the disciplines of neurophysiology, anatomy, cell biology, and psychology meet. Along with astute clinical observation, neural science is providing renewed support for the idea first proposed by the Hippocratic physician over two millennia ago that the appropriate study of the mental processes begins with the study of the brain. Cognitive psychology and psychoanalytic theory have been valuable because they recognize the diversity and complexity of human mental experience—they discern the importance of both genetic and learned factors in determining how the world is represented mentally, and they postulate that behavior is based on that representation. By emphasizing mental structure and internal representation, psychoanalysis served as a source of modern cognitive psychology, a psychology that has stressed the logic of mental operations and of internal representations. Experimental cognitive psychology and clinical psychotherapy now need to be strengthened by insights into the cellular neurobiology of behavior. The task for the years ahead is to produce an empirical neuropsychology that—though still concerned with problems of internal representation, dynamics, and subjective states of mind—is firmly grounded in neural science.

Irving Kupfermann

Genetic Determinants of Behavior

60

Behavior results from the interaction of genetic (or innate) and environmental factors. The relative importance of the two factors varies, but even the most stereotyped behavior can be modified by the environment, and the most plastic behavior, such as language, is influenced by innate factors. Because genetic factors provide the substrate on which the environment acts, we shall consider the innate determinants of behavior first. In the next two chapters, we shall examine the process of learning, by which experience can modify behavior.

We shall begin by reviewing historical and current ideas about the innate determinants of behavior and then consider possible neural mechanisms underlying certain types of innate behaviors in animals. We shall address four questions: What aspects of behavior are inherited? How do genes exert control over behavior? How do genetic processes interact with the environment? And finally, which aspects of human behavior are predominantly innate?

The Concept of Instinct: Are Aspects of Behavior Genetically Determined?

Traditionally, instinctive behavior, behavior that has not been learned, has been regarded as the component of behavior directly related to genetic endowment. A consideration of instinct is therefore a good starting point for examining the genetic determinants of behavior. The concept of instinct has a long and controversial history. Antecedents to the notion of instinct can be traced to the beginning of history. The ancient Greek philosophers and, later, Christian theologians sought to exalt humans and to set them apart from lower animals by arguing that much human behavior can be guided by reason, whereas the behavior of animals is entirely the result of *natural instincts,* a term that came to be applied to complex, unlearned behaviors.

These early explanations of human and animal behavior were not based on systematic experimental observations. Modern scientific usage of the term *instinct* dates to the latter part of the nineteenth century and the influential writings of Charles Darwin. Darwin's work on the evolution of species indicated that there are no sharp discontinuities between the evolution of humans and simpler animals. Darwin therefore suggested that the behavior of animals is guided not only by instinct but also by primitive forms of the same reasoning processes that guide human behavior. More important, Darwin argued that since humans evolved from simpler animals, human behavior also must be guided by instincts. These notions were soon amplified by psychologists who saw in the concept of instinct a way to explain much of human behavior on the basis of a few underlying principles. For example, Sigmund Freud suggested that all normal and abnormal human behavior is powerfully shaped by two fundamental instincts, or inner, genetically determined sets of strivings: a life (or sexual) instinct, and a death (or aggressive) instinct. Freud maintained that these instincts provide an innate mental force that energizes all behavior. In 1908 William McDougall published an influential book entitled *An Introduction to Social Psychology,* in which he postulated that humans have up to a dozen instincts: flight, repulsion, curiosity, pugnacity, self-abasement, self-assertion, parenting, reproduction, desire for food, gregariousness, acquisition, and construction.

These systematic theories about human instincts were soon challenged by John Watson and other members of the school of behaviorism. Behaviorists rejected the idea that the best way to understand behavior is by studying the mind or the inner forces that determine behavior. They argued that only the observable aspects of behavior can be studied, not its inner mechanisms. The behaviorists pointed out that the notion of instinct as used by Freud, McDougall, and other psychologists referred to *unlearned inner strivings and propensities that guide behavior.* Viewed in this way, instincts are unobservable mechanisms, that is, intervening variables that are invoked to explain behavior.

Behaviorists argued against the utility of unobservable mentalistic concepts such as instincts or inner strivings. They insisted that a true science of behavior must deal only with observable responses and not with inferred phenomena such as thoughts, propensities, ideas, images, or inner strivings. The behaviorists further maintained that psychologists who attempted to explain behavior by relying on the concept of instincts were merely renaming phenomena and explaining nothing. Thus, human aggressiveness was supposedly explained by an aggressive instinct, generosity was due to an instinct of altruism, and so forth.

Most behaviorists also had difficulty with the notion of instinctive behavior as *completely* unlearned acts. Although some behaviorists admitted that stereotyped unlearned motor patterns might exist in lower animals, they pointed out that it can never be proved that a given behavior is completely free of learning. Even if one carefully observes an organism and controls its environment, there may be unsuspected sources of environmental stimuli that allow the animal to learn. The more radical behaviorists felt that all behavior could be explained on the basis of simple reflexes that could be modified by experience. Under the pervasive influence of behavioristic philosophy, most experimental psychologists in the United States abandoned the consideration of innate determinants of behavior and focused almost exclusively on the study of learning. In many instances, processes that were formerly called *instincts* were renamed *drives* (for example, hunger, sex, thirst, and curiosity) and were studied without commitment or reference to whether they originated from innate factors or learning.

Ethologists Define Instincts as Inborn Motor Patterns

During the period from 1920 to 1950, when psychologists in the United States had rejected the theory of instinctive behavior, European zoologists such as Konrad Lorenz and Nikolaas Tinbergen began a series of studies that laid the groundwork for what today is known as *ethology*—the comparative study of behavior, with particular emphasis on its mechanisms, ontogenesis, and evolution. This approach emphasizes the study of behavior under natural conditions.

Ethologists advanced the study of instincts in two ways. First, whereas previous scientists had speculated about the role of instinct in behavior, the ethologists were the first to observe and experiment systematically on inborn behavior. Second, they limited their biological studies of instinct to inborn stereotyped *sequences of observable motor movement that are unlearned.* These studies, carried out in a wide variety of species, led to a partial reconciliation of the older mentalistic concepts of instinct and the antiinstinct philosophy of the behaviorist movement.

While acknowledging some of the criticisms directed at the concept of instinct as unlearned behavior, ethologists pointed out that it is difficult to explain some behaviors of lower animals on the basis of learning alone. For example, a female bird that has been isolated from other birds since hatching is still able to build a perfect nest as an adult and can clean and care for its young. Such behavior could not have been learned while the animal was maturing. Ethologists emphasized, however, that instinctive behavior is not completely unaffected by the environment, as all behavior is the result of the interaction between the genetic endowment of the animal and the internal and external environments. Nevertheless, just as physical structures can be inherited, so certain behaviors appear to be inherited, and a consideration of genetic factors in behavior is useful for clarifying the concept of instinct. According to the ideas of the ethologists, asking whether a behavior is instinctive is equivalent to asking whether the behavior is inherited. Seen from this standpoint, the problem of instinct reduces to the question: Is it possible to inherit behavior?

Can Behavior Be Inherited?

Psychologists have traditionally considered behavior to be the result of the operation of the mind. At one time the mind was thought to be spiritual, and it was difficult to envisage how it could be inherited. As we have seen in earlier chapters, most neural scientists now believe that the mind represents a set of processes or functions. According to this view, the mind is not an entity of any kind, but rather a set of functions carried out by the brain. Mind is what the brain does, just as walking is one of the things that legs do. If mind and behavior are functions of the brain, it becomes easy to see how behavior can be affected by genetic factors, as is the function of every other organ of the body.

Nevertheless, there has been great resistance to the notion that behavior, particularly human behavior, can be inherited. Part of the reason for this resistance has been a mistaken notion of what inheritance of behavior really means. Take, for example, the question: Is mental illness inherited? So posed, the question implies that a complex behavioral disorder is controlled entirely by a set of genes that are inherited. This is almost never the case. The expression of inherited factors nearly always depends on an interaction of genetic and environmental factors. Thus, you can inherit genes that program you to grow tall, but if you are not raised with the appropriate diet you will be short. Although learning may or may not be important for the expression of a genetic factor, one or more environmental factors (for example, appropriate nutrition, light, etc.) will be important. *Innate or inborn behaviors are responses that are not highly dependent on specific learning experiences in which information is extracted from the environment.* However, there is no sharp distinction between learned and innate behaviors. There is instead a continuous gradation, from stereotyped responses that are almost independent of the animal's history, to responses that are highly sensitive to environmental factors. What the ethologists call *instinctive behaviors are a special class of innate behaviors that consist of relatively complex sequences of responses.* Instinctive behaviors are now often termed *species-specific behaviors* because they characterize a given species, much as do morphological or physiological features. In the following sections we shall consider several examples of the influence of environment on the expression of genetic information related to behavior.

Sign Stimulus and Fixed Action Pattern Are Two Key Concepts in the Analysis of Species-Specific Behavior

In the course of investigating examples of rigid behavioral patterns that seem to require minimal experience for their expression, Lorenz, Tinbergen, and other ethol-

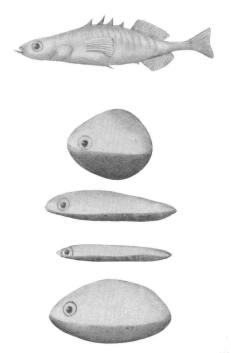

60–1 These models of the stickleback fish were used to identify the sign stimulus of mating and attack responses in this species. The **top model** is an accurate imitation of the male but lacks a red belly; the **next four models,** which have a red underside, are more frequently attacked by other males than the top model. (Adapted from Tinbergen, 1951.)

ogists developed a theoretical orientation based, in part, on two useful concepts: sign stimulus and fixed action pattern. Complex inborn behavioral patterns in lower animals typically are activated by specific stimulus conditions; the effective stimulus is called a *sign stimulus* or *releaser.* Behavioral analysis has shown that animals, given a complex stimulus condition, often respond to certain very specific features of a situation rather than to the condition as a whole.

The role of sign stimuli is illustrated by a now classic series of studies by Tinbergen on the sexual behavior of the stickleback fish. During the mating season the male stickleback develops a bright red abdomen. The red abdomen provokes fighting responses from other males but elicits approach responses from females. The nature of the stimulus was characterized by the use of wax models. A model resembling a stickleback in every detail except the red belly did not elicit a response (Figure 60–1). On the other hand, a model that had a red underside, but otherwise did not resemble a stickleback, effectively released fighting behavior in males and mating behavior in females. Although the patch of red was a necessary condition for the stimulus to be effective, it was not sufficient. The red patch also had to occupy a specific location. When the same model was turned upside down, it no longer elicited fighting responses. A similar analysis has revealed that the swollen abdomen of the female serves as a sign stimulus for the male and triggers mating behavior. Because the sign stimuli eliciting mating or attack responses are effective even in animals that have been raised in total isolation, they are considered to be innately determined.

Species-specific behavioral sequences typically begin with a phase of *appetitive behavior*, which consists of highly variable responses that aid the animal in finding appropriate environmental stimuli or a goal object (for example, mate, food, water, or nesting material). Appetitive behavior is followed by a phase of *consummatory behavior*, which consists of a series of relatively stereotyped movements, termed *fixed action patterns*. Each fixed action pattern is a behavioral sequence that is triggered by an environmental cue (the sign stimulus).

A fixed action pattern resembles a reflex in that it is a behavioral response elicited by a specific stimulus and its expression does not require previous learning. It differs from a simple reflex in that it is more complex and is preceded by a phase of appetitive behavior. In addition, for fixed action patterns the nervous system produces a complex transformation of the input. Whereas the strength and duration of reflex responses often closely reflect the features of the evoking stimulus, the duration, latency, and intensity of fixed action patterns generally are not precisely related to the stimulus parameters (Figure 60–2). Also, unlike reflex responses, a fixed action pattern sometimes can occur in the absence of any eliciting stimuli. This kind of behavior is referred to as *vacuum activity*. Finally, apparently inappropriate fixed action patterns can occur when an animal is in a situation that elicits conflicting responses. For example, faced with a choice to fight or flee, a cat might momentarily groom itself instead. Such responses are referred to as *displacement activities*.

Fixed Action Patterns Are Generated by Central Programs

What is the neural basis of complex fixed action patterns? Does the central nervous system impose the properties of the entire pattern and does the stimulus act primarily to release its expression? Or are fixed action patterns merely complex series of reflexes, with the guiding stimuli provided by the animal's proprioceptive input? The idea that each reflex in a series of responses produces proprioceptive or other sensory input that elicits the next reflex response was championed by Charles Sherrington.

To approach this issue experimentally, it is necessary to eliminate all sources of peripheral sensory input that could provide the cues needed for the series of reflexes. This experiment has been done in several invertebrates in which the nervous system is removed from the animal. The isolated nervous system thus receives no sensory feedback, but it remains alive, and its neurons are easily studied by intracellular recording electrodes. As we shall see below, the nervous systems of certain invertebrates contain *command neurons*, which elicit complex behavioral sequences when stimulated. Experiments of this type have been done on flying, walking, swimming, and feeding responses in insects, crustaceans, and molluscs. In all of these animals, the isolated nervous system can generate the same sequence of motor output shown by the intact specimen. Sensory input typically modifies the strength or frequency of the central program, but the essential pattern does not require timing cues from sensory feedback.

Evidence that central motor programs exist for fixed action patterns has also been obtained in vertebrates. The data indicating a central program for locomotion in the cat were outlined in Chapter 37. Many other responses,

60–2 The intensity and duration of a stimulus affects reflexes but not fixed action patterns. Three hypothetical responses to three types of stimuli are shown: **a,** a weak and brief stimulus; **b,** a strong and brief stimulus, and **c,** a still stronger and prolonged stimulus. **A.** A simple reflex, for example, pupillary constriction elicited by a light. **B.** A fixed

action pattern, such as courtship behaviors in fish or birds, in response to an appropriate sign stimulus. Note that the simple reflex response reflects the nature of the stimulus, whereas the fixed action pattern is triggered by the stimulus but the nature of the response is not closely linked to the nature of the stimulus.

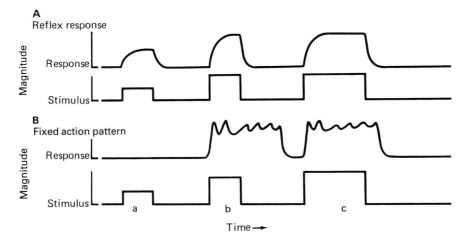

some quite complex, appear to involve built-in motor programs in vertebrates. These include swallowing, biting, grooming, orgasm, coughing, yawning, vomiting, and the startle reflex. Swallowing is a well-studied example. This response is triggered by stimulation of the pharynx. Once triggered, the behavior involves a complex sequential activation of at least 10 different muscle groups (Figure 60–3). Robert Doty and James Bosma examined the reflex control of swallowing in the dog by looking at the pattern of muscle contraction (elicited by the electrical stimulation of pharyngeal nerves) before and after anesthetizing the pharynx or inactivating the various muscles either surgically or by application of a local anesthetic. Nothing that was done to alter or eliminate sources of peripheral feedback produced a significant change in the motor sequence of swallowing. However, different levels of arousal or different degrees of pharyngeal stimulation could alter the strength and duration of the motor output. Thus, in swallowing, as in locomotion, the details of the pattern can be modified by external sensory feedback even though the basic pattern is internally generated.

Certain complex behaviors of vertebrates, as well as invertebrates, consist of combinations of different fixed action patterns in sequence. For example, John Fentress found that grooming behavior in mice involves four actions directed toward the face, belly, back, and tail. Grooming of the face is associated with six stereotyped action patterns, including licking, single or parallel strokes with the forepaws, and shuddering of the body. The various patterns do not occur in random sequences, but in a predictable order, although the order is not absolutely fixed.

What are the neural mechanisms responsible for triggering fixed action patterns? In 1938 C. A. G. Wiersma at the California Institute of Technology reported the important discovery that in crayfish, a complete, complex motor output can be triggered by stimulating specific command neurons. The firing of a single command neuron can elicit a complex defensive response involving dozens of different muscles. Command neurons have divergent synaptic outputs that excite or inhibit a population of follower neurons. These follower cells in turn are interconnected to generate specific patterns of motor output.

In mammals there is no evidence for unique neurons that can function as command neurons do in invertebrates. Nevertheless, it is tempting to suggest that a group of specific cells in mammals may constitute a command system that functions like a single command neuron of invertebrates and triggers preprogrammed motor acts. Recent evidence indicates that, even in invertebrates, many complex motor acts are not triggered by single command neurons; rather, parts of the complete act are triggered by individual cells. Just as the generation of a perception depends on several feature detectors operating in parallel, the generation of a complex motor act may involve the operation of several command neurons or command systems, each of which is responsible for some limited aspect of the movement.

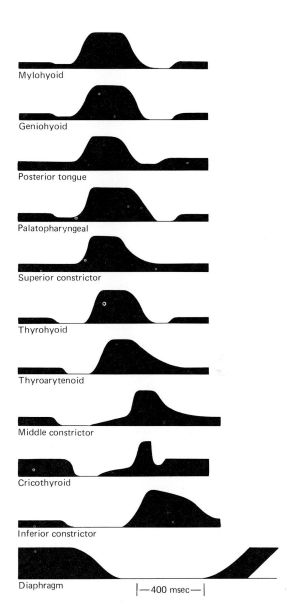

60–3 This schematic summary of electromyographic activity during swallowing in the dog demonstrates the complex sequential activation of various muscles in this fixed action pattern. The height of the line for each muscle indicates the intensity of the action observed, ranging from complete inactivity to the maximum occurring in deglutition. (Adapted from Doty and Bosma, 1956.)

Certain command systems appear to be driven by neural mechanisms that are tuned to specific features of sensory input, for example, the red abdomen of the stickleback fish. Ethologists refer to this type of mechanism as an *innate releasing mechanism*. The nature of innate releasing mechanisms is largely unknown. We do know, however, that individual neurons of the sensory systems of vertebrates can respond to highly specific features of sensory input (see Chapter 29), and it is reasonable to assume that neurons of this type are important elements of innate releasing mechanisms. A simplified model of

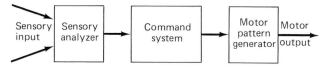

60–4 Simplified model of the neural organization that may underlie fixed action patterns.

the possible neural basis of fixed action patterns is shown in Figure 60–4. Feature detection neurons, as part of a sensory system or an innate releasing mechanism, are excited by specific sensory input and provide excitation to command neurons or command systems. The command system, in turn, triggers a central motor program that generates a stereotyped behavioral sequence.

The Role of Genes in the Expression of Behavior Can Now Be Studied Directly

Given that certain aspects of behavior are innate, how do genes code for behavior? The current revolution in molecular genetics has made it possible not only to delineate more precisely the central issues discussed in this chapter, but also to look at simple instances in which the relationship between genes and behavior is unambiguous.

Clearly, genes do not code for behavior in a direct one-to-one way; a single gene cannot code for a single behavior. Behavior is generated by neural circuits involving many nerve cells. Genes code for specific proteins, and many different proteins—both structural and enzymatic—are required for the development of a neural circuit.

The fact that many genes are required does not mean, however, that individual genes are not critical for the expression of a behavior. The importance of genes for behavior can best be demonstrated in simple animals, such as the fruit fly *Drosophila*, in which mutations of single genes can be easily studied. Such studies show that mutations of single genes can produce abnormalities of learned behavior (see Chapter 62) as well as instinctive behaviors such as courtship or locomotion. A particularly interesting and well-studied behavioral mutant of *Drosophila*, called *shaker*, makes spontaneous, non-functional movements. The abnormal movements are due to prolonged action potentials in nerve and muscle cells. These abnormal action potentials result from a single gene mutation that deprives *shaker* of a particular K^+ channel (the early K^+ channel discussed in Chapter 8). In *Drosophila* this K^+ channel contributes importantly to the rapid repolarization of the action potential.

Genes are essential not only for producing the appropriate neural circuitry of a behavior, but also for *regulating the expression of the behavior* in the adult because genes code for the structural proteins necessary to maintain the neuronal circuitry as well as for enzymes—

including the transmitter-synthesizing enzymes that are essential for normal synaptic transmission. Moreover, genes directly code for peptide hormones and modulators that trigger or inhibit the expression of behavior. For example, a complete behavioral sequence—a fixed action pattern—can be triggered by a peptide hormone acting on the appropriate command elements in the neural circuitry.

An illustration of how genes can switch on a behavioral sequence comes from the study of egg laying in the invertebrate *Aplysia*. Egg laying is a fixed action pattern with appetitive and consummatory phases. The appetitive phase includes cessation of walking, inhibition of feeding, and head waving. This is followed by an all-or-none consummatory phase consisting of deposition of the egg string. The consummatory phase and several aspects of the appetitive repertory are triggered by a basic peptide hormone, called *egg-laying hormone*, that is released by a cluster of identified neurons, the *bag cells*. The egg-laying hormone acts directly on the smooth muscle of follicles in the ovotestes to initiate egg laying by a mechanism analogous to the action of oxytocin on the uterine musculature of mammals. In addition, the hormone excites and inhibits identified neurons throughout the nervous system of the animal.

Although the egg-laying hormone itself consists of only 36 amino acids, its gene encodes a precursor polyprotein consisting of 271 amino acid residues. Thus, the synthesis of egg-laying hormone is similar to that of several well-studied neuropeptides in vertebrates, such as the proopiomelanocortin family of peptides that were considered in Chapter 13. Since the egg-laying hormone is synthesized as part of a larger precursor molecule, before it can be released it must be cleaved from the larger molecule at pairs of basic amino acid residues that flank its own sequence. Indeed, the precursor contains eight pairs of basic residues that serve as cleavage sites flanking other neuroactive peptides.

What are the functions of the peptides? Three peptides have now been isolated from the precursor, and each appears to be coordinately released with the egg-laying peptide. At least two of these peptides function as neurotransmitters that alter the activity of specific neurons: the idea is attractive that each of these peptides is responsible for regulating a different behavioral component of egg laying.

These studies allow us to explore in a behavioral context the more general question that we examined in Chapter 13: Why are polyproteins used as precursors for peptide hormones and transmitters? One reason is that polyproteins provide a mechanism for coordinated expression and release. The coordinated release of diverse peptides in various combinations may be important in orchestrating different aspects of a behavior. By means of their several constituent peptides, polyproteins can ensure that the various neuronal circuits responsible for the different facets of a stereotyped behavior are activated in a coherent manner.

Thus, in certain experimentally advantageous behaviors it is now possible to relate specific genes to particular proteins in specific neural circuits and even to the controlling elements that act on those neural circuits to regulate the expression of a behavior.

Higher Mammals and Humans Seem to Have Certain Innate Behavioral Patterns

Most research on innate behavior has been done on non-mammalian species, but considerable evidence indicates that mammals, including primates, also exhibit innate behaviors. A particularly elegant example is the work done with monkeys by Gene Sackett at the University of Wisconsin. Sackett tried to determine whether the behavioral responses to a specific visual stimulus are innate. He raised individual monkeys in complete isolation from their mothers and other monkeys. When these animals were given an opportunity to look at various types of photographs, they greatly preferred images of other infant monkeys over nonmonkey images. Until they were 10 weeks old, they preferred pictures of monkeys over other pictures even if the monkey in the picture showed threatening gestures. As they matured, however, their preference for monkeys with threatening gestures diminished abruptly. They began to be disturbed by photographs of threatening monkeys but not by other types of images. Sackett's experiments clearly demonstrate that primates have innate releasing mechanisms.

What is the role of innate factors in determining human behavior? Because there are inherent and ethical limitations on the study of humans, no definitive conclusions are yet possible. It is generally thought that *the primary determinants of such complex human activities as warfare, marriage, and religion presumably are largely the result of learning and culture*, but the degree to which these activities may be influenced by innate factors is unknown. Although learning plays an enormous role in human behavior, and humans have no clear-cut complex series of inborn behaviors such as those seen in lower animals, the comparative data we shall consider here and the studies on the hormonal determinants of gender identity considered in Chapter 58 indicate that *there also are innate determinants of human behavior*. Four types of data support this conclusion: (1) the evidence for genetic factors influencing human behavior, (2) the universality of certain human behavioral patterns, (3) the existence of motor patterns that resemble fixed action patterns, and (4) the existence of relatively complex motor patterns in the absence of any obvious specific learning experiences.

Certain Human Behavioral Traits Have a Hereditary Component

Unfortunately, discussions about the role of genetic factors in human behavior can readily provoke polemics because this issue has profound social, ethical, and political implications. It is beyond the scope or purpose of this textbook to review these aspects of the problem in detail. Nevertheless, the point we try to illustrate here is that all behavior, including human behavior, is mediated by components whose formation and organization are controlled by genes, and therefore must to some extent be under genetic control.

There is substantial evidence for hereditary factors in human behaviors, particularly in severe mental illnesses such as schizophrenia. For many years neurobiologists were uneasy with the idea that schizophrenia, with its extreme disorder of thought and perception, is entirely due to the influence of a faulty environment. Studies of identical twins and of adopted individuals have now demonstrated conclusively that there is an important genetic component to this behavioral disorder (see Chapter 53). Although the evidence from studies of twins links heredity and schizophrenia, the same evidence proves that nongenetic factors are also important.

Intelligence is another area of human behavior in which there is evidence for genetic factors. Although it is not clear exactly what is measured by intelligence tests, there is wide agreement (but not complete unanimity) that scores on intelligence tests are partly a function of inherited factors. Several forms of severe mental retardation are linked to genetic factors. For example, Down's syndrome, or mongolism, is known to be caused by the presence of an extra autosome, chromosome 21. Phenylketonuria, a metabolic disorder that also leads to mental retardation, is due to an autosomal recessive gene that codes for a type of phenylalanine hydroxylase with reduced enzymatic activity; this reduced activity results in abnormally high levels of phenylalanine in the body fluids.

Many Human Behaviors Are Universal

All humans display many similar behaviors regardless of differences in their environmental or cultural backgrounds. These behaviors include the deep tendon reflexes, the eyeblink response, and startle reflexes. In addition, we have common basic drives and needs, such as hunger, thirst, and sex. Equally important and widespread are human needs not related to simple tissue deficits. For example, to varying degrees, people of all cultures need social contact and variety of sensory experience.

One of the best examples of a complex set of human behaviors that is universal is emotional expression, first studied systematically by Darwin. Facial expressions of anger, fear, disgust, and joy are generally recognized even between people from cultures that have had no contact. Thus, the recognition of certain emotional expressions probably has a strong innate component. Furthermore, the facial motor patterns themselves tend to be similar in diverse cultures.

Humans also exhibit behavioral patterns that appear to be analogous to the vacuum or displacement activities

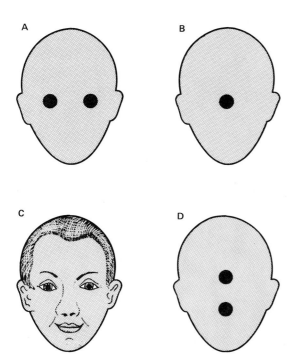

60—5 Patterns such as these are used to study the sign stimuli that elicit smiling in young babies. In babies of about 6 weeks of age, patterns **A** and **D** are more effective than **B** and **C**. Thus, the critical features appear to be multiple spots of high contrast. As the babies mature, the dot patterns become progressively less effective in eliciting a smile, while the face image (**C**) becomes more effective. (Adapted from Ahrens, 1954.)

of animals. For example, during conflict situations or periods of stress, people, like animals, often exhibit grooming behavior such as stroking their hair or scratching.

Stereotyped Sequences of Movements Resemble Fixed Action Patterns

Many emotional expressions, such as the startle response and smiling, involve a stereotyped sequence of movements. Smiling in human infants appears to be controlled by a specific sign stimulus. The eliciting stimulus has been studied by the use of models, similar to the colored wax models that have been used to study mating behavior in fish. Although young infants smile in response to a smiling human face, studies with inanimate models indicate that the response is not to the face as a whole, but rather to certain specific features (Figure 60–5). Contrasting elements (eyes, in the case of a real face) appear to be particularly important. As the child matures, however, other elements of the face assume increasing significance. Even in adults, eyes appear to function in some ways as a sign stimulus. A striking example is the brow flash response, studied by Irenaus Eibl-Eibesfeldt in several cultures. This stereotyped response,

which many of us are unaware that we use, consists of a rapid raising and dropping of the eyebrows. In widely different cultures, it occurs as part of a greeting response between individuals who know each other.

Certain Complex Patterns Require Little or No Learning

Although there are numerous examples of widespread behavioral patterns in humans that are unlikely to be entirely learned, in many instances the precise role of learning is difficult to assess. The role of learning can be studied in animals by raising them in restricted environments. In humans these types of experiments are not possible, but we can gain insights from "natural" experiments. For example, babies who are blind at birth have a limited opportunity to learn facial expressions, yet their facial responses can appear normal. Blind babies who smile in response to a sound may even turn their eyes toward the source of the sound. Other examples of abilities and disabilities in humans with limited environmental experiences are discussed in Chapter 57.

The Brain Sets Limits on the Structure of Language

The ability to speak sets humans apart from other animals. Languages differ greatly from culture to culture, and one might therefore conclude that language is not affected by innate determinants; but this is clearly not so. The nature of language is limited and shaped by the nature of our sensory–motor apparatus. For example, languages do not utilize frequencies of sound that we cannot hear or produce. More important, as we saw in Chapter 52, Noam Chomsky at the Massachusetts Institute of Technology and many other linguists have accounted for the fact that widely different languages share common principles of grammar by proposing that the structure of languages is determined by conceptual constraints imposed by the structure of the brain.

It is difficult to experiment on humans to clarify the interaction of environmental factors and biological constraints in the development of language. However, several models of animal communication now exist, although some question remains as to whether animal communication is a true form of language. Nonhuman primates can be taught a form of limited communication using sign language. Birds have a natural song, which is clearly not language in the human sense, but which nevertheless is a highly complex auditory output that serves a primitive communicative function. Studies of bird song by Masakazu Konishi, by P. Marler and W. J. Hamilton, III, and by W. H. Thorpe provide a fascinating and instructive example of the interaction of innate factors with the environment. Early investigators posed the question: Does a bird learn its song from other birds or is the song inborn? The question has no simple answer:

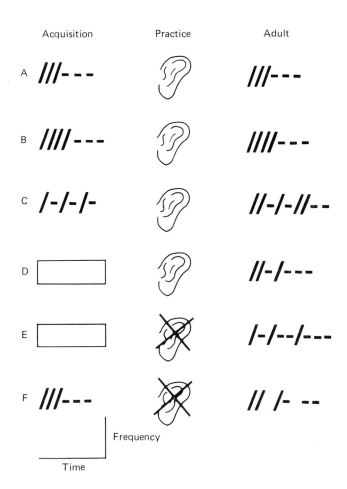

Acquisition	Practice	Adult

A

B

C

D

E

F

Frequency

Time

60—6 Acquisition of bird song in birds such as the chaffinch. Each group of traces represents a schematized sound spectrogram of the nature of the song the bird was exposed to (**Acquisition** period) or the nature of the song the bird sang as an **Adult.** The abscissa of each trace indicates time, the ordinate frequency. (For example, the song illustrated in **A** consists of three brief notes of ascending frequency followed by three notes of constant frequency.) Songs are acquired during initial exposure in the first few months of life (acquisition period). During the **Practice** period parts of the acquired song are sung, but the full song does not appear until the bird is an adult. The figure shows six types of experiments in which birds were exposed to different song patterns or no song (**rectangle**) during the acquisition phase. The role of auditory feedback during the practice phase was studied by deafening the birds in some experiments (**crossed out ear**).

A and **B.** The normal adult sings a song that is similar to the one heard during the early acquisition phase. **C.** However, there are constraints on exactly what can be learned. When the young bird is exposed to an "unusual" song (i.e., very different from what is commonly heard in the wild), the adult song does not bear a close resemblance to that originally heard. **D.** Birds that do not hear any song during the acquisition phase nevertheless develop a song that is somewhat similar to the normal pattern (shown in **A** and **B**). **E.** If, however, the birds cannot hear themselves during the practice period, the song is highly abnormal. **F.** If birds hear a normal pattern during acquisition but cannot hear themselves during practice, their song is close to normal. Experiments **D** and **E** suggest that, even if not exposed to an appropriate song during acquisition, the birds can, in effect, teach themselves the appropriate song if they have feedback telling them how they sound. Thus the birds have a built-in template that "tells" them how the song should sound. As illustrated by experiments **A, B, C,** and **F**, the built-in template can be modified, within limits, by experience.

there are great differences between birds. In chickens, normal sound production occurs even when animals are raised in isolation and never hear another bird. On the other hand, in songbirds, such as the chaffinch or white-crowned sparrow, the song is distorted if the animal is raised in isolation.

In 1965, Konishi made the remarkable discovery that if certain songbirds were deafened at birth, their adult song was even more distorted than if they were raised in isolation (Figure 60–6). This suggests that to perfect their song these birds must hear themselves sing. They must therefore have a built-in auditory template against which the song they produce is compared. This template is present even if the bird never hears another bird, because even the song of deafened birds is not random, but resembles, although imperfectly, the normal song. When given a chance to hear a song, the bird produces a more normal song. Variations in the song that a young bird hears result in similar variations in its own adult song but only within certain narrow limits. Most songbirds do not learn to imitate songs that deviate too far from their normal song commonly encountered in the wild.

These observations show that *biological constraints* set limits on the effects that the environment can have.

In recent years there has been a growing appreciation that biological constraints operate not only in the learning of bird song but in all learning, including complex human learning.

Selected Readings

Boakes, R. 1984. From Darwin to Behaviourism. Cambridge: Cambridge University Press.

Camhi, J. M. 1984. Neuroethology. Nerve Cells and the Natural Behavior of Animals. Sunderland, Mass.: Sinauer Associates.

Delcomyn, F. 1980. Neural basis of rhythmic behavior in animals. Science 210:492–498.

Eibl-Eibesfeldt, I. 1970. Ethology: The Biology of Behavior. E. Klinghammer (trans.). New York: Holt, Rinehart and Winston.

Fieve, R. R., Rosenthal, D., and Brill, H. (eds.). 1975. Genetic Research in Psychiatry. Baltimore, Md.: Johns Hopkins University Press.

Gould, J. L. 1982. Ethology: The Mechanisms and Evolution of Behavior. New York: Norton.

Hirsch, J. (ed.). 1967. Behavior-Genetic Analysis. New York: McGraw-Hill.

Kupfermann, I., and Weiss, K. R. 1978. The command neuron concept. Behav. Brain Sci. 1:3–39.

Lewontin, R. 1982. Human Diversity. New York: Scientific American Books.

Manning, A. 1972. An Introduction to Animal Behavior, 2nd ed. Reading, Mass.: Addison-Wesley.

Salkoff, L., and Wyman, R. 1983. Ion channels in *Drosophila* muscle. Trends Neurosci. 6:128–133.

Scheller, R. H., Jackson, J. F., McAllister, L. B., Schwartz, J. H., Kandel, E. R., and Axel, R. 1982. A family of genes that codes for ELH, a neuropeptide eliciting a stereotyped pattern of behavior in Aplysia. Cell 28:707–719.

References

Ahrens, R. 1954. Beitrag zur Entwicklung des Physiognomie- und Mimikerkennens. Z. Exp. Angew. Psychol. 2:412–454, 599–633.

Chomsky, N. 1957. Syntactic Structures. The Hague: Mouton.

Darwin, C. 1872. The Expression of the Emotions in Man and Animals. London: Murray.

Doty, R. W., and Bosma, J. F. 1956. An electromyographic analysis of reflex deglutition. J. Neurophysiol. 19:44–60.

Fentress, J. C. 1972. Development and patterning of movement sequences in inbred mice. In J. A. Kiger, Jr. (ed.), The Biology of Behavior. Corvallis: Oregon State University Press, pp. 83–131.

Freud, S. 1940. An Outline of Psychoanalysis. J. Strachey (trans.). New York: Norton, 1949.

Kety, S. S., Rosenthal, D., Wender, P. H., and Schulsinger, F. 1968. The types and prevalence of mental illness in the biological and adoptive families of adopted schizophrenics. In D. Rosenthal and S. S. Kety (eds.), The Transmission of Schizophrenia. Oxford: Pergamon Press, pp. 345–362.

Konishi, M. 1965. The role of auditory feedback in the control of vocalization in the white-crowned sparrow. Z. Tierpsychol. 22:770–783.

Lorenz, K. Z. 1950. The comparative method in studying innate behaviour patterns. Symp. Soc. Exp. Biol. 4:221–268.

Marler, P., and Hamilton, W. J., III. 1966. Mechanisms of Animal Behavior. New York: Wiley.

McDougall, W. 1908. An Introduction to Social Psychology. London: Methuen, 1960. New York: Barnes & Noble, 1960.

Sackett, G. P. 1966. Monkeys reared in isolation with pictures as visual input: Evidence for an innate releasing mechanism. Science 154:1468–1473.

Sherrington, C. 1947. The Integrative Action of the Nervous System, 2nd ed. New Haven: Yale University Press.

Thorpe, W. H. 1956. Learning and Instinct in Animals. Cambridge, Mass.: Harvard University Press.

Tinbergen, N. 1951. The Study of Instinct. Oxford: Clarendon Press.

Watson, J. B. 1930. Behaviorism, rev. ed. New York: Norton.

Wiersma, C. A. G. 1938. Function of the giant fibers of the central nervous system of the crayfish. Proc. Soc. Exp. Biol. Med. 38:661–662.

Irving Kupfermann

Learning

61

In Chapter 60 we considered how inborn and environmental factors interact to produce behavior. The environmental factor most important in altering behavior in humans is learning. *Learning* is the acquisition of knowledge about the world. *Memory* is the retention or storage of that knowledge. The study of learning has taught us about the logical capabilities of the brain and is therefore an objective and powerful approach to evaluating mental processing. In the study of learning we can ask several related questions: What types of environmental relationships are learned most easily? What conditions optimize learning? How many different forms of learning are there? What are the stages of memory formation?

Learning is a process that can occur in the absence of overt behavior but its occurrence can only be inferred by seeing changes in behavior. The overt behavioral changes, and the other changes that cannot be detected simply by the organism's overt behavior, all reflect alterations in the brain produced by learning. For this reason, although learning has been very fruitfully studied by purely behavioral techniques, many of the fundamental questions about learning will require direct examination of the brain.

The study of learning is central to the understanding of both normal and abnormal behavior. Learning is thought to contribute to the genesis of certain mental and somatic diseases, and the principles governing learning that have emerged from laboratory studies are used in the treatment of patients with these diseases. Moreover, behavioral techniques based on learning are now used widely in neurobiological and clinical research to assess the effects of brain lesions and drugs.

Psychologists study learning by exposing organisms to information about the world, usually specific types of controlled sensory experiences. By this means, two major procedures (or paradigms) have been discovered, which give rise to two major classes of learning: nonassociative learning and associative learning. In *nonassociative learning* the organism is exposed once or repeatedly to a single type of stimulus. This procedure provides an opportunity for the organism to learn about the properties of that stimulus. In *associative learning* the organism learns about the relationship of one stimulus to another (classical conditioning) or about the relationship of a stimulus to the organism's behavior (operant conditioning).

Certain Elementary Forms of Learning Are Nonassociative

The most common forms of learning are nonassociative and include habituation and sensitization. *Habituation*, first systematically studied by the Russian biologist Ivan Pavlov, is a decrease in a behavioral reflex response to a repeated, nonnoxious stimulus. An example of habituation is the failure of a person to show a startle response to a loud noise that has been regularly presented. In *sensitization* (or *pseudoconditioning*) there is an increased reflex response to a wide variety of stimuli for a period of time after an intense or noxious stimulus has been delivered. A sensitized animal responds more vigorously to a mild tactile stimulus after it has received a painful pinch. Moreover, a sensitizing stimulus can override the effects of habituation. For example, after a startle response to a noise has become habituated, it can be restored by delivering a strong pinch. This process is called *dishabituation*. Sensitization and dishabituation occur whether or not the intense stimulus is presented soon after the weaker stimulus; no close association between the two stimuli is needed.

Not all examples of nonassociative learning are simple. There are many types of more complex learning in which there is no obvious associational element, although hidden forms of association may be present. These types of learning include *sensory learning*, in which a continuous record of sensory experience is formed, and *imitation learning*, which includes aspects of the acquisition of language.

Classical Conditioning Involves Associating a Conditioned and an Unconditioned Stimulus

There are many types of associative learning. One useful way to classify them is on the basis of the experimental procedures used to establish the learning. Two experimental paradigms have been extensively studied and used clinically: classical and operant conditioning. Associative learning also often occurs in forms that do not readily fit into an operant–classical schema.

Classical conditioning was introduced into behavioral science by Ivan Pavlov at the turn of the century, when he recognized that learning frequently consists of the ac-

quisition of responsiveness to a stimulus that originally was ineffective. Aristotle had earlier suggested the theory that learning involves the association of ideas, a proposal developed further by John Locke and the British empiricist philosophers, the forerunners of modern psychologists. Pavlov's brilliant insight was to combine the philosophers' concept that *learning involves the association of ideas* with Charles Sherrington's concept of the *reflex act*. With this framework Pavlov was able to deal with unobserved mental phenomena—ideas—and to study them objectively by examining behavioral acts, which are external and observable phenomena. Pavlov's theories marked a permanent shift in the study of learning from introspective inferences about unobservable ideas to the objective analysis of stimulus and response. According to Pavlov, what animals and humans learn is not the association of ideas but the association of stimuli.

The essence of classical conditioning is the pairing of two stimuli, an unconditioned stimulus, or US, and a conditioned stimulus, or CS. The *conditioned stimulus*, such as a light or tone, is chosen because it produces either no overt responses or weak responses unrelated to the response that eventually will be learned. On the other hand, the *unconditioned stimulus*, such as food or a shock to the leg, is chosen because it always produces an overt response, the *unconditioned response*, such as salivation or leg withdrawal. Indeed, the reason the response is called unconditioned is because it is innate; it is produced by the eliciting (unconditioned) stimulus without learning. When the conditioned stimulus is repeatedly followed by the unconditioned stimulus in a precise temporal sequence, the conditioned stimulus begins to elicit responses, called *conditioned responses*, that resemble the unconditioned responses. The conditioned stimulus ultimately becomes an anticipatory signal for the occurrence of the unconditioned stimulus, and the animal responds to the conditioned stimulus as if it were preparing for the unconditioned stimulus.

Thus, classical conditioning is a means by which animals learn to predict relationships between events in the environment. For example, if a light is followed repeatedly by the presentation of meat, after several learning trials the animal will respond to the light in the same way as it responds to meat: the light itself will produce salivation. The conditioned response is not precisely identical to the unconditioned response, but the two responses are so similar that it is useful to think of conditioning as a process by which the animal learns to react to the conditioned stimulus as a substitute for the unconditioned stimulus. Classical conditioning is further subdivided into appetitive conditioning and defensive conditioning: if the unconditioned stimulus is rewarding (food, water), the conditioning is considered *appetitive*; if the stimulus is noxious (shock), it is considered *defensive*.

As previously mentioned, Pavlov regarded classical conditioning not only as a way to study learning but also as a way to approach the mind—the inner workings of the brain. He was keenly aware that if he could train animals to respond selectively to stimuli, he could discover which aspects of a stimulus an animal is capable of recognizing and processing. For example, psychologists have explored whether an animal can recognize and distinguish colors by determining whether lights of different colors can serve as discriminative stimuli for classical conditioning. During *discriminative training*, one conditioned stimulus (CS⁺) is presented in association with reinforcement on some trials. On other trials, another conditioned stimulus (CS⁻) is presented but is never followed by reinforcement. If the CS⁺ and CS⁻ are similar in certain respects, the animal will initially exhibit generalization; that is, it will show conditioned responses to both the reinforced and nonreinforced stimuli. If the animal can discriminate between the stimuli, then after continued training it will show conditioned responses primarily or exclusively to the CS⁺ and not to the CS⁻. By appropriately manipulating the hue and intensity of visual stimuli, psychologists can determine whether the animal is responding to color rather than to differences in brightness. By this means they can determine the perceptual capacities of any animal capable of being conditioned.

An important principle of conditioning is that an established conditioned response decreases in intensity or probability of occurrence if the conditioned stimulus is repeatedly presented without the unconditioned stimulus. This process is known as *extinction*. Thus, a light that has been paired with an unconditioned stimulus of food will gradually cease to evoke salivation if the light is repeatedly shown in the absence of food. Extinction is just as important an adaptive mechanism as conditioning, because a continued response to cues that are no longer significant is not in the animal's best interest. The available evidence indicates that extinction does not simply involve the fading of previous learning; rather, during the extinction process the animal learns something new—the conditioned stimulus no longer predicts that the unconditioned stimulus will occur; instead, it comes to predict that the unconditioned stimulus will *not* occur.

Conditioning Involves the Learning of Predictive Relationships

Until quite recently, many animal psychologists thought that classical conditioning depends only on temporal contiguity. According to this view, each time a conditioned stimulus is followed by a reinforcing or unconditioned stimulus, an internal stimulus–response or stimulus–stimulus bond is strengthened, until eventually the bond becomes strong enough to produce conditioning. The only relevant variable determining the strength of conditioning was thought to be the number of contiguous CS–US events. This theory is inadequate for two reasons: first, it does not make sense from an adaptive point of view. If animals learned to derive predictive information simply from the occurrence of two events in

close temporal contiguity, they might develop erroneous notions about the true causal relationship between signals in the environment. Second, a substantial body of empirical evidence indicates that learning cannot be adequately explained by such simple contiguity.

A striking example of the inadequacy of simple contiguity to produce conditioning is the so-called blocking phenomenon, discovered by Leon Kamin at Princeton University. Kamin discovered blocking by carrying out a three-part experiment. First, he conditioned a stimulus, a light, by pairing it repeatedly with an aversive unconditioned stimulus, a strong electric shock. He then assessed conditioning by determining the ability of the light to suppress ongoing behavior (a reflection of its ability to evoke a strong conditioned fear response in the animal similar to that initially evoked by the electrical shock). In the second part of the blocking experiment, Kamin presented the conditioned stimulus simultaneously with a new stimulus, a tone, and the light-tone compound stimulus was then repeatedly paired with the shock. When now, in the third part of the experiment, Kamin presented the tone alone, he found that little or no conditioning had occurred to the tone. Despite repeated pairings of the light-tone compound stimulus with shock, the tone, when presented alone, failed to suppress behavior and did not evoke a fear response. These findings are consistent with Robert Rescorla and Alan Wagner's theory of classical conditioning, according to which the amount of conditioning on a trial is dependent on the degree to which the unconditioned stimulus is unexpected. If the unconditioned stimulus is completely unexpected because it has not been previously paired with a conditioned stimulus, maximal learning can occur. But when the unconditioned stimulus is fully expected because it is already well predicted by the conditioned stimulus, learning reaches an asymptote and no further learning can occur. Thus, the tone component of the light-tone stimulus is an ineffective conditioning stimulus because the other element of the compound conditioned stimulus (the light) already successfully and fully predicts the occurrence of the unconditioned stimulus. This notion has been formalized in simple mathematical terms by Rescorla and Wagner, and predicts a surprising number of the properties of classical conditioning.

Another line of experiments also demonstrates the inadequacy of simple contiguity in producing conditioning and has revealed that classical conditioning develops best when, in addition to *contiguity*, there is also a *contingency*—a truly predictive relationship—between the conditioned stimulus and the unconditioned stimulus. If an animal is presented with a long sequence of conditioned and unconditioned stimuli each occurring randomly and completely independently, some contiguous CS–US sequences will occur just by chance. Nevertheless, a conditioned response to the CS does not develop. Clearly, the animal is not just counting the number of CS–US pairings, but rather is determining the *overall correlation* or *predictive relationship* between the CS and US. In fact, if a stimulus is presented repeatedly so that it specifically does *not* occur in association with a US, that stimulus comes to predict the absence of the US. When that stimulus is later paired with a US, conditioning occurs only very slowly, presumably because the animal must first unlearn the previous predictive property of the stimulus. In some instances stimuli that have been associated with the absence of the US actually acquire *inhibitory* properties, and their presence can suppress the occurrence of behavioral responses. Thus, in addition to being paired in time, the CS and reinforcer (the US) need to be positively correlated; the CS must indicate an increased probability that the US will occur.

These considerations suggest why animals and humans acquire classical conditioning so readily. It appears likely that animals exhibit classical conditioning, and perhaps all forms of associative learning, because *the brain has evolved to enable animals to distinguish events that reliably and predictably occur together from those that are unrelated.* In other words, the brain has evolved as a detector of causal relationships in the environment.

All animals that exhibit associative conditioning, from snails to humans, seem to learn by detecting environmental contingencies rather than detecting the simple contiguity of a CS and US. Why is the recognition of contingent relationships similar in humans and in simpler animals? One good reason lies in the conservation that is characteristic of evolution and in the consequences of evolutionary pressure on adaptation. All animals, regardless of habitat and heritage, face common problems of adaptation and survival, problems for which learning and flexible decision-making are useful. When different species face common environmental pressures, they often manifest similar patterns of adaptation. These patterns are likely to involve homologous mechanisms because a successful biological solution to an environmental challenge, once evolved in a common primitive ancestor, continues to be inherited as long as it remains useful.

What environmental conditions might have shaped or maintained a common learning mechanism in a wide variety of species? To function effectively, animals need to recognize certain key relationships between external events. They must be able to recognize and distinguish prey from predators; they must search out food that is nutritious and avoid food that is poisonous. There are two ways in which an animal arrives at such knowledge. As discussed in Chapter 60, the correct information can be preprogrammed into the animal's nervous system. The ability to choose correctly among alternatives can also be acquired through learning. Genetic and developmental programming may suffice for all of the behavior of very simple organisms, such as parasites, but more complex animals must be capable of extensive learning to cope efficiently with varied or novel situations. Complex animals need to recognize order in the world. An effective way to do this is to be able to detect causal or predictive relationships between stimulus events, or between behavior and subsequent stimuli.

Operant Conditioning Involves Associating an Organism's Own Behavior with a Subsequent Reinforcing Environmental Event

A second major paradigm of associative learning, introduced by Edward Thorndike of Columbia University, is *operant conditioning* (sometimes called *instrumental conditioning* or *trial-and-error learning*). In a typical laboratory example of operant conditioning, an investigator begins by placing a hungry rat in a test chamber that has a lever protruding from one wall. Because of previous learning as well as innate response tendencies and random activity, the rat will occasionally press the lever. If the rat promptly receives food when it presses the lever, its subsequent rate of lever pressing will increase above the spontaneous rate. The animal can be described as having learned that a certain response (lever pressing) among the many it has made (for example, grooming, rearing, and walking) is rewarded with food. With this information, whenever the rat is hungry and finds itself in the same chamber, it is likely to make the appropriate response.

If we think of classical conditioning as the formation of a predictive relationship between two stimuli (the conditioned stimulus and the unconditioned stimulus), operant conditioning can be considered to consist of the formation of a predictive relationship between a response and a stimulus. Unlike classical conditioning, which is restricted to specific reflex responses that are evoked by specific identifiable stimuli, operant conditioning involves behaviors (called *operants*) that apparently occur spontaneously or with no recognizable eliciting stimuli. Thus, operant behaviors are said to be emitted rather than elicited, and when the behaviors produce favorable changes in the environment (that is, when they either are rewarded or lead to the removal of noxious stimuli), the animal tends to repeat them. This process is known as *reinforcement*; it encompasses the more general observation that behaviors that are rewarded tend to be repeated at the expense of behaviors that are not, while behaviors followed by aversive, though not necessarily painful, consequences *(punishment)* are generally not repeated. Experimental psychologists agree that this simple idea, called the *law of effect*, probably reflects an important principle that governs much voluntary behavior.

Superficially, operant and classical conditioning appear to be dissimilar, involving completely different stimulus and response relationships. However, the laws that govern operant conditioning and those that govern classical conditioning are quite similar, suggesting that the two forms of learning are manifestations of a common underlying neural mechanism. For example, in both forms of conditioning, timing is critical: typically, the reinforcer must closely follow the operant response. If the reinforcer in operant conditioning is delayed, only weak conditioning occurs. Similarly, in classical conditioning, the learning is generally poor when there is a long delay between the conditioned and the unconditioned stimulus. Finally, predictive relationships are equally important in both types of learning. In classical conditioning the animal learns that a certain stimulus predicts a subsequent event. In operant conditioning the animal learns to predict the consequences of its own behavior.

Food-Aversion Conditioning Illustrates How Biological Constraints Help Determine the Efficacy of Reinforcers

The two forms of associative learning discovered by Pavlov and Thorndike—classical conditioning and operant conditioning—are so general and so prominent that for many years it was thought that classical conditioning could occur simply by arbitrarily associating any two stimuli or, in the case of operant conditioning, any response and any reinforcer. Recent studies have indicated, however, that there are important biological (evolutionary) constraints on learning. As we have seen, animals generally learn to associate stimuli that are relevant to their survival; they will not learn to associate events that are biologically meaningless. These findings illustrate nicely a principle we have encountered in the study of the development of behavior. The brain is not a *tabula rasa,* but has inherent predispositions toward the detection and manipulation of certain environmental contingencies. For example, not all reinforcers are equally effective with all stimuli. This principle is dramatically illustrated in studies of *food aversion* (also called *bait shyness,* as it seems to be the means by which animal pests such as rats and mice learn to avoid poisoned bait foods). If a distinctive taste stimulus, such as vanilla, is followed by nausea produced by a poison, an animal will quickly develop a strong aversion to the taste of vanilla. Unlike most other forms of conditioning, food aversion develops even when the unconditioned stimulus (poison-induced nausea) occurs with a delay of up to hours after the conditioned stimulus (specific taste). This makes biological sense, since the ill effects of naturally occurring toxins usually follow ingestion only after some delay.

The food-aversion paradigm has been applied in the treatment of chronic alcoholism. The patient is first given alcoholic beverages to smell and taste, and then a powerful emetic such as apomorphine. The pairing of alcohol and nausea rapidly results in aversion to alcohol. Food-aversion learning has several other important implications in medicine. First, it may be a means by which people unintentionally learn to regulate their diets to avoid the unpleasant consequences of inappropriate or nonnutritious food. Second, the malaise associated with certain forms of cancer may induce aversion conditioning to foods in the ordinary diet of the patient. This, in part, might account for depressed appetites in cancer patients. Furthermore, the nausea that follows chemotherapy for cancer can produce aversion to foods that were tasted shortly before the treatment.

For most species, including humans, food-aversion conditioning is restricted to *taste stimuli* associated with subsequent *illness.* Food aversion develops poorly, or not at all, if the salient taste is followed by a painful stimulus. Conversely, if a visual or auditory stimulus, instead of a taste stimulus, is paired with nausea, an animal does not develop an aversion to that stimulus. Thus, the choice of an appropriate reinforcer depends on the nature of the response to be learned. Evolutionary pressures have predisposed the brains of different species of animals to learn an association between certain stimuli, or between a certain stimulus and a response, much more readily than between others. Within a given species, genetic and experiential factors also can modify the effectiveness of a reinforcer. The results obtained with a particular class of reinforcer vary enormously from species to species and from individual to individual within a species, particularly in humans.

Conditioning Is Used as a Therapeutic Technique

Various psychotherapeutic procedures involve reeducation of the patient in the context of a trusting relationship with the therapist. Aspects of therapeutic change are likely to involve components of classical and operant conditioning, but the specific contribution that each of these procedures makes to therapy has been delineated in only a few relatively simple instances.

Classical Conditioning Has Been Applied in Systematic Desensitization

The process of extinction, characteristic of classical conditioning, may underlie the therapeutic changes resulting from a clinical technique known as *systematic desensitization* (although other interpretations of this method have been offered). Systematic desensitization was introduced into psychiatry by Joseph Wolpe, a South African physician who used it to decrease neurotic anxiety or phobias evoked by certain definable environmental situations, such as heights, crowds, or public speaking. The patient is first taught a technique of muscular relaxation. Then, over a period of days, the patient is told to imagine a series of progressively more severe anxiety-provoking situations while using relaxation to inhibit any anxiety that might be elicited. At the end of the series, the strongest potentially anxiety-provoking situations can be brought to mind without anxiety. This desensitization, induced in the therapeutic situation, often generalizes to real-life situations that the patient encounters.

Operant Conditioning Has Been Used to Treat Severe Behavioral Problems

Principles of operant conditioning also have been applied to the management of psychiatric disorders. One important therapeutic application is in the management of severely disturbed institutionalized patients with behavioral problems, such as shouting obscenities, messiness, or poor hygienic habits. The goal of conditioning these patients is to increase the frequency of positive, constructive behaviors. These behaviors are first defined precisely, and an effective reinforcement is found (compliments, privileges, money, or food). Nurses and orderlies are then trained to provide reinforcements when the patients behave in the desired way.

Biofeedback is another form of operant conditioning that has proved useful clinically. Biofeedback is used to enhance (or suppress) responses of which the patient is unaware. The behavior of interest, such as very slight muscle contractions in a stroke patient, is recorded by an electronic device that provides the patient with immediate reinforcement in the form of an auditory or visual cue signaling that the response has occurred.

Learning and Memory Can Be Classified as Reflexive or Declarative on the Basis of How Information Is Stored and Recalled

The classification of associative learning into either operant or classical conditioning is based on the experimental procedures used to establish the conditioning. This distinction is therefore useful to clinicians or experimentalists who wish to apply a well-defined, reproducible methodology to their work. Alternative classification schemes of learning are based not on what the experimenter does, but rather on the type of knowledge acquired by the subject. These classifications cut across the operant–classical distinction and take into account that a single procedure may produce different forms of learning depending on how the experimental subject codes and recalls the information that is learned. Endel Tulving, at the University of Toronto, was one of the first to appreciate that the memory for many different types of learning can be divided into two categories. Different authors have used various terms to reflect this dichotomy or closely related dichotomies. For our purposes, we shall refer to the two categories as *reflexive* and *declarative* memory. Later in this chapter, we shall consider evidence indicating that these two types of memory can be differentially affected by brain damage and that they may involve different neuronal systems of the brain.

Reflexive memory has an automatic or reflexive quality, and its formation or readout is not dependent on awareness, consciousness, or cognitive processes such as comparison and evaluation. Reflexive memory accumulates slowly through repetition over many trials. This type of memory is expressed primarily by improved performance on certain tasks and is poorly expressed by declarative sentences. Examples of reflexive memory include perceptual and motor skills and the learning of procedures and rules, such as those of grammar. Reflexive memory, however, is not limited to learning of procedures and skills. Certain verbal learning tasks, if repeated often enough, assume the characteristics of reflexive learning. These tasks can then be performed automatically without the participation of other cognitive devices.

Declarative memory depends on conscious reflection for its acquisition and recall, and it relies on cognitive processes such as evaluation, comparison, and inference. Declarative memory encodes information about specific autobiographical events as well as the temporal and personal associations for those events. It often is established in a single trial or experience, and it can be concisely expressed in verbal declarative statements, such as "I saw a yellow canary yesterday." Declarative memory involves the processing of bits and pieces of information that the brain can then use to reconstruct past events or episodes. As we noted above, in certain instances declarative memory may be transformed into the reflexive type by constant repetition. For example, learning to drive a car at first involves conscious cognitive processes, but eventually driving becomes automatic and nonconscious.

How do elementary forms of learning such as classical conditioning fit into this reflexive and declarative scheme? Although classical conditioning often results in reflexive memory, even this ostensibly simple form of conditioning may, under some circumstances, lead to declarative memory and involve mediation by cognitive processes. Consider the following experiment. A subject lays his hand, palm down, on an electrical grill; a light (conditioned stimulus) is turned on and he is immediately shocked on a finger. His finger withdraws (unconditioned response), and, after several light–shock conditioning trials, he withdraws his finger when the light alone is presented. The subject has been conditioned; but what exactly has been conditioned? It appears as though the light is triggering a specific pattern of muscle activity that results in withdrawal. However, what if the subject now places his hand on the grill upside down, and the light is presented? If a specific pattern of muscle activity has been conditioned, the light should produce a response that moves the finger *into* the grill. On the other hand, if the subject has acquired the information that the light means grill shock, he may make a different response appropriate to that information. In fact, when this experiment is done, the subject moves his finger *away* from the grill; that is, he makes an adaptive response, even though it involves motor movements antagonistic to the original ones. Therefore, the subject did not originally learn a fixed response to a fixed stimulus, but, rather, acquired information that the brain could use to solve specific problems.

In another study of the nature of declarative memory, researchers analyzed remembered versions of previously learned stories. The versions that the subjects recalled were shorter and more coherent, and they contained reconstructions not present in the original. The subjects were unaware of where they were substituting, and they often felt most certain about the reconstructed part. The subjects were not confabulating; they were merely recalling in a way that interpreted the original material so it made sense.

Observations such as these lead us to believe that the accumulation of knowledge about past events is an *active* process involving cognitive events. Initially, what goes into the memory store is a representation of information that has been changed as a result of processing by our perceptual apparatus. Optical illusions illustrate that we do not perceive the world precisely as it is but, rather, as a modified version that is altered on the basis of past experience as well as on principles and limits of perceptual analysis. Moreover, once the information is stored, what is recalled from the declarative memory store is not a faithful reproduction of the internal store. Recall of declarative memory involves a process in which past experiences are used in the present as clues to help the brain reconstruct a significant past event. During this reconstruction, the brain uses a variety of cognitive processes—comparison, inferences, shrewd guesses, and suppositions—to generate a consistent and coherent picture.

The Neural Basis of Memory Can Be Summarized in Four Principles

Although the literature on the neurobiology of memory is extensive, much of what is known can be summarized in just four principles: (1) memory has stages and is continually changing; (2) long-term memory may be represented by physical changes in the brain; (3) the traces for memories are localized in multiple regions throughout the nervous system; and (4) reflexive and declarative memories may involve different neuronal circuits. Here we shall consider information obtained by gross techniques, such as brain lesions, electrical stimulation, and drugs. Studies of the cellular mechanisms of learning will be considered in Chapter 62.

Memory Has Stages

It is an old clinical observation that a person who has been knocked unconscious can have selective memory loss for events that occurred shortly before the blow *(retrograde amnesia)* and shortly after regaining consciousness *(anterograde amnesia)*. This phenomenon has been documented thoroughly in animal studies using such traumatic agents as electroconvulsive shock, physical trauma to the brain, and drugs that depress neuronal activity or inhibit protein synthesis in the brain. Clinical studies also indicate that brain trauma can produce amnesia that is particularly prominent for recent events, typically within a few days of the trauma. Thus, recently acquired memories are readily disrupted, whereas older memories remain quite undisturbed. Once something has been learned, the extent of potential retrograde amnesia—the span of time during which memory is labile—varies from several seconds to several years, depending on the nature and strength of the learning and on the species of animal.

Studies of memory disruption have contributed to a commonly used model of the memory storage system (Figure 61–1). Input to the brain is processed into a short-term memory store. This information is later transformed by some process into a more permanent long-term store. To complete the model, a system has been

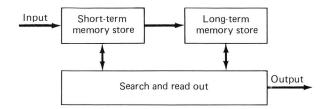

61–1 Model of memory storage system.

added that functions to search the memory store and to read out the information as demanded by specific tasks. In this model, interference with the retention of previous experience can occur either by partial destruction of the contents of a memory store or by disruption of the search and read-out mechanism. In traumatic amnesia, at least part of the interference must be due to a disturbance of the search and read-out mechanism. This conclusion stems from the observation that, after trauma, some memory for once-forgotten events gradually returns. If the stored memory had been completely destroyed, it obviously could not have been recovered.

Observations of patients undergoing a series of electroconvulsive shocks for the treatment of depression have confirmed and extended the findings of experiments made on animals. Larry Squire and his associates at the University of California Veterans Hospital studied patients who had been given shock therapy. They used a memory test that could reliably quantify the degree of memory for relatively recent events (1–2 years old), old events (3–9 years old), and very old events (9–16 years old). Patients were asked to identify various television programs that were broadcast during a single year between 1957 and 1972. The patients were initially tested and then tested again (with a different set of television programs) after the electroconvulsive shock therapy. The results of this experiment are shown in Figure 61–2. Both before and after shock therapy, correct memory for the programs steadily decreased with time after the memory was first formed. This is a reflection of the all-too-familiar process of forgetting. After the shock therapy, however, the patients showed a significant but transitory memory loss for programs that had gone off the air 1 or 2 years previously, but their memory for the older programs was the same as it was before the shock therapy.

One interpretation of these observations is that the read-out of recent memories is easily disrupted until the memories have been converted into a long-term memory form. Once converted, they are relatively stable, but with time, even without external trauma, there is a gradual loss of the stored information or a diminished capacity to retrieve it. Thus the memory process, at least as assessed by susceptibility to disruption, is *always undergoing continual change with time.*

Several experiments on the effects of drugs on learning support the idea that the memory process is time dependent and is subject to modification when the memory is first formed. James McGaugh and associates at the

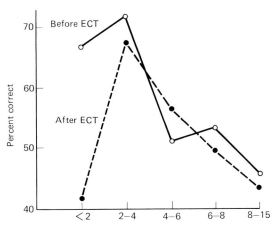

61–2 Recent memories are more susceptible to disruption by electroconvulsive shock therapy (**ECT**) than older memories. Patients were tested on their ability to recognize correctly the name of television programs that were on the air during 1 year between 1957 and 1972. Testing was done before and after the patients received ECT for treatment of depression. After the ECT, the patients showed a significant (but transitory) loss of memory for recent programs (1–2 years old) but not for old programs. (Adapted from Squire, Slater, and Chace, 1975.)

University of California at Irvine have shown in animals that subconvulsant doses of excitant drugs such as strychnine can improve the retention of learning even when the drug is administered after the training trials. If the drug is given to the animal *soon* after training, retention tested the next day is facilitated. If, however, the drug is given several hours after training, it has no effect.

Long-term Memory May Be Represented by Plastic Changes in the Brain

How is information stored? One type of very brief short-term memory for visual events, called *iconic memory*, is probably due to brief retinal afterimages that follow exposure to visual stimuli. If a person is briefly allowed to view a matrix of many letters and numbers, he can accurately recall specific elements of the matrix; but, unlike most forms of learning, accuracy of recall diminishes extremely rapidly, typically in less than 1 sec. The time before accuracy diminishes can be extended by increasing the brightness of the visual stimulus, and the time course for the decline of accuracy parallels the decay of the visual afterimages. Photochemical processes in the retina can account for visual afterimages. Thus, one very simple form of short-term memory appears to be encoded by a transient physical change in the sensory receptor.

Slightly longer lasting short-term memory that persists for minutes to hours could be mediated by a variety of short-term neural plastic events that we considered in Chapter 11, such as posttetanic potentiation and presynaptic inhibition.

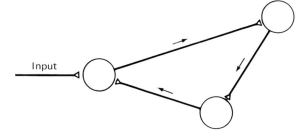

61–3 A reverberating circuit might be used to encode short-term memory. Brief excitatory input can produce long-lasting neural activity through the circulation of spikes among neurons that excite one another.

Another possible mechanism for encoding short-term memory is the storage of information in the form of ongoing neural activity that is maintained by excitatory feedback connections between neurons (Figure 61–3). This type of activity could reverberate within a closed loop of neurons and might be sustained for some period of time. The idea of reverberatory circuits is interesting because it does not involve any enduring physical changes in nerve cells; the memory for the event is maintained simply by ongoing neuronal activity. There are few experiments to support this notion, and it seems unlikely that this will prove to be a common mechanism for memory.

But how is long-term memory stored? How are changes maintained for years? Two possibilities exist. First, but not likely, is the possibility that reverberating circuits like those postulated to underlie short-term memory may persist and represent long-term memory as well. The second possibility is that long-term memory is related to some *plastic* rather than *dynamic* change— that is, to a permanent functional or structural change in the brain. A simple experiment can distinguish between these alternatives. If all neuronal activity is temporarily stopped, memories represented by the dynamic mechanism of reverberating circuits should be permanently abolished. Neuronal activity can be silenced by the use of deep anesthesia, by anoxia, or by cooling the brain. When this is done, short-term or recent memories are disrupted, but older memories are not. Thus, it is safe to conclude that at least older memories are not mediated by reverberatory activity but, more likely, involve physical changes in the brain. Because of the enduring nature of memory, it seems reasonable to postulate that in some way the changes must be reflected in long-term alterations of the connections between neurons. We shall consider this question again in Chapter 62.

Memory Traces Are Often Localized in Different Places Throughout the Nervous System

Whatever their nature, it seems clear that the memory traces for many different types of learning are not localized to any one brain structure. Pavlov, the father of physiological studies of learning, believed that all learning processes are limited to the neocortex. The psychologist Karl Lashley, at Harvard University, spent most of his scientific career making lesions in the cortex to define precisely where the representation of learning (called the *engram*) was located. He never succeeded. Lashley and others found that although cortical lesions can seriously disrupt learning, animals can relearn certain tasks even when they are completely decorticated. Classical conditioning of certain simple reflexes can be mediated by the spinal cord even after it has been isolated surgically from the brain, as was first shown by P. S. Shurrager and Elmer Culler in 1940. Thus, many and perhaps all regions of the nervous system appear to contain neurons with the properties of plasticity needed for memory storage.

Even for a simple learning task, several parallel channels of information are used. There is ample opportunity, therefore, for information to be stored in different regions of the brain. For example, David Cohen at the State University of New York at Stony Brook, in studies of conditioned heart rate response in pigeons, found that any one of three visual pathways can sustain the learned response.

Parallel processing may explain in part why a given limited lesion does not eliminate specific learning, but a more important factor may reside in the very nature of the learning process. As we have seen from behavioral studies, learning involves neither the simple formation of stimulus–response bonds nor a faithful reproduction of sensory experience. Although the physical changes representing learning are likely to be localized to specific neurons, the complex nature of learning ensures that these neurons are widely distributed in the nervous system. Therefore, even after extensive lesions, some trace can remain. Furthermore, the brain has the capacity to take even the limited information remaining, work it over, and reconstruct a good reproduction of the original.

Reflexive and Declarative Memories May Involve Different Neuronal Circuits

Although many memory traces are typically widely distributed, some learning tasks are profoundly affected by circumscribed lesions of the brain. The most striking evidence indicating that specific brain structures can exert specific effects on learning comes from studies of the cerebellum and of the temporal lobes. These studies suggest the intriguing hypothesis that the brain may possess two classes of neural circuits, one of which is concerned with reflexive memory, the other with declarative memory.

Reflexive Memory. Lesions to several regions of the brain have been found to affect simple classically conditioned responses, and these regions probably represent loci for reflexive types of learning. For example, lesions of the amygdala interfere with conditioned heart rate responses, apparently by interrupting pathways close to the motor end of the reflex arc. Another example of a specific lesion affecting a classically conditioned response comes

from the research of Richard Thompson, David McCormick, and their associates at Stanford University. They have been studying the eyeblink (or nictitating membrane) protective reflex in rabbits. By pairing an auditory stimulus with a puff of air to the eye, a conditioned eyeblink reflex can be established to the auditory stimulus. The conditioned response is totally abolished by a lesion to the medial dentate and lateral interpositus nuclei of the cerebellum. After this region is lesioned, the previously effective conditioned auditory stimulus is no longer capable of producing an eyeblink, although the unconditioned eyeblink response that follows the unconditioned stimulus (air puff) remains intact. These results have been confirmed and extended by Mitchell Glickstein in London and John Moore and his colleagues at the University of Massachusetts. Furthermore, the dentate-interpositus nuclei also show learning-dependent increases in neuronal activity that closely parallel the development of the conditioned behavioral response. The results of these experiments, taken as a whole, indicate that the cerebellum plays an essential role in mediating conditioned eyeblink and perhaps other simple forms of classical conditioning.

Declarative Memory. In humans, lesions of the temporal lobe and closely associated structures of the limbic system or of the diencephalon dramatically affect learning. These lesions have weak effects on specific prior memories; they primarily interfere with the retention of new ones. Thus, these structures are not themselves registers or banks for memory storage, but are somehow involved in the process by which memories are placed into storage or are retrieved and read out from storage.

A significant clue that the temporal lobes are important for memory came from the observations by the neurosurgeon Wilder Penfield at the Montreal Neurological Institute. In the course of temporal lobe surgery for the control of epilepsy, Penfield electrically stimulated the exposed temporal lobes in fully conscious patients. The patients reported vividly experiencing past events. For example, stimulation of one point on the temporal lobe caused a patient to hear a specific melody that she believed she had heard in the past. Repeated stimulation of the same point evoked successive experiences of hearing the same melody.

Additional evidence of a role for the temporal lobes in memory has come from the study of a few epileptic patients who underwent bilateral removal of the hippocampus and associated structures in the temporal lobes. Brenda Milner found that these patients exhibit a profound and irreversible deficit of recent memory. They lose the capacity to form new long-term memories, but previously acquired long-term memories remain relatively intact; for example, they remember their names and how to talk. Short-term memory is also unaffected; but the transition from short-term to long-term memory is virtually absent for most types of learning. For example, if the patient was told to remember the number 7, he could repeat the number immediately. If, however, the patient was distracted, even briefly, he had no recollection of the number. The extent of the deficit is indicated by the observation that one patient failed to recognize individuals whom he had known closely for years. In addition to anterograde amnesia, these patients often show some retrograde amnesia; that is, they have a loss of memories that were stored and available for recall before surgery. Often, memories lost retrogradely because of lesions or trauma gradually return, but anterograde amnesia is permanent.

An amnesic syndrome superficially similar to that seen in patients who have undergone bilateral removal of temporal lobe structures occurs in patients suffering from *Korsakoff's psychosis*. This disease, which results from chronic alcoholism and its nutritional deficiency, is characterized by confusion and severe memory deficits. Patients with Korsakoff's psychosis exhibit pathological changes in diencephalic structures that are part of the limbic system. Typically, they have damage to the mammillary bodies of the hypothalamus as well as to the medial dorsal nucleus of the thalamus. Careful study of the precise nature of the deficit in patients with Korsakoff's psychosis supports the idea that the memory deficit is due, at least in part, to defective encoding at the time of original learning rather than exclusively to a defect in the retrieval mechanism. Patients with Korsakoff's psychosis learn slowly, but once the material is learned, they appear to forget at a normal rate.

Elizabeth Warrington and Lawrence Weiskrantz in England have found that when patients with Korsakoff's psychosis are given a list of words to remember, they do poorly on a simple recall task, but their performance is greatly improved when retention is tested by the use of prompts or partial cues. For example, their performance is normal if, following the original learning, they are tested for retention by a completion task rather than being asked simply to recall the words. In the completion task the patients are given a list of letter sequences, each of which has the first few letters of a word in the original list. Then, on the basis of their memory for the words in the original list, the patients must complete the words.

Peter Graf, George Mandler, and Patricia Haden, at the University of California, found that this disjunction between performance on simple recall and completion tests can be demonstrated in normal subjects with no memory defects if the subjects are required to learn a list of words in a task that minimizes the opportunity to understand the meaning of the word. In this experiment, a list of 20 words was presented with the instruction to detect certain vowels in the words. The subjects were not asked to memorize the words or to understand their meaning. After the vowel detection task, they were unable to recall the words in the list. However, like the patients with Korsakoff's psychosis, the subjects were able to recall many of the words if they were given the initial letters of the words and were asked to complete them. Subjects in a second group were presented with a list of words and were instructed to determine if they liked each word, a task that requires an understanding of its se-

mantic content. These subjects subsequently remembered the words just as well on simple recall as on a completion task. These findings support the suggestion that patients with Korsakoff's psychosis fail to encode the semantic component of material properly on initial learning.

Reflexive Versus Declarative Memory in Amnesic Patients. A remarkable finding in studies of amnesic patients, either with temporal lobe or diencephalic damage, is that they can learn certain tasks perfectly well. Although these patients cannot master tasks involving declarative memory, they perform well on tasks involving reflexive memory. A given learning task often involves aspects of both types of learning, and in these instances amnesic patients remember some aspects of the problem, but not others. Thus, if the patient is given a highly complex mechanical puzzle to solve, the patient may learn it as quickly as a normal person but on questioning will not remember seeing the puzzle or having worked on it previously. In other words, amnesic patients can learn a complex skill and yet be unable to recall the specific events that allowed them to learn the rules and procedures that make up the skill. Furthermore, even in instances in which they remember some experience of the past, the experience lacks the feeling of familiarity that accompanies recall in normal individuals.

Warrington and Weiskrantz suggested that the fundamental deficit of amnesic patients is due to some type of disconnection between memory storage systems and a cognitive mediational system in the brain that aids in the retrieval and storage of memory. It is possible that in amnesic patients the cognitive system functions normally, but it lacks access to the declarative learning system. Therefore, amnesic patients often show totally unimpaired intelligence and yet are virtually incapable of new declarative learning. This idea helps explain why amnesic patients, when they perform a particular task, are often not aware that they actually had learned it a few days or weeks earlier.

A major challenge confronting the neurobiology of learning is to determine how reported alterations in the brain are causally related to behavioral changes. A second task is to determine the mechanisms underlying the relevant plastic changes. To this end, a number of simplified vertebrate and invertebrate animal preparations are being investigated, and some of the information deriving from these studies is reviewed in Chapter 62.

Selected Readings

Dickinson, A. 1980. Contemporary Animal Learning Theory. Cambridge, England: Cambridge University Press.

Domjan, M., and Burkhard, B. 1982. The Principles of Learning and Behavior. Monterey, Calif.: Brooks/Cole.

Hilgard, E. R., and Bower, G. H. 1975. Theories of Learning, 4th ed. Englewood Cliffs, N. J.: Prentice-Hall.

Kandel, E. R. 1983. From metapsychology to molecular biology: Explorations into the nature of anxiety. Am. J. Psychiatry 140:1277–1293.

Kanfer, F. H., and Phillips, J. S. 1970. Learning Foundations of Behavior Therapy. New York: Wiley.

Klatzky, R. L. 1980. Human Memory. Structures and Processes. 2nd ed. San Francisco: W. H. Freeman.

Lashley, K. S. 1950. In search of the engram. Symp. Soc. Exp. Biol. 4:454–482.

Mackintosh, N. J. 1983. Conditioning and Associative Learning. Oxford: Clarendon Press.

Rescorla, R. A. 1978. Some implications of a cognitive perspective on Pavlovian conditioning. In S. H. Hulse, H. Fowler, and W. K. Honig (eds.), Cognitive Processes in Animal Behavior. Hillsdale, N. J.: Erlbaum, pp. 15–50.

Squire, L. R., Cohen, N. J., and Nadel, L. 1984. The medial temporal region and memory consolidation: A new hypothesis. In H. Weingartner and E. S. Parker (eds.), Memory Consolidation: Psychobiology of Cognition. Hillsdale, N.J.: Erlbaum, pp. 185–210.

Thompson, R. F., Berger, T. W., and Madden, J., IV. 1983. Cellular processes of learning and memory in the mammalian CNS. Annu. Rev. Neurosci. 6:447–491.

Woody, C. D. (ed.). 1982. Conditioning: Representation of Involved Neural Functions. New York: Plenum Press.

Yates, A. J. 1970. Behavior Therapy. New York: Wiley.

References

Cohen, D. H. 1982. Central processing time for a conditioned response in a vertebrate model system. In C. D. Woody (ed.), Conditioning: Representation of Involved Neural Functions. New York: Plenum Press, pp. 517–534.

Glickstein, M., Hardiman, M. J., and Yeo, C. H. 1983. The effects of cerebellar lesions on the conditioned nictitating membrane response of the rabbit. J. Physiol. (Lond.) 341:30P–31P.

Graf, P., Mandler, G., and Haden, P. E. 1982. Simulating amnesic symptoms in normal subjects. Science 218:1243–1244.

McGaugh, J. L., and Herz, M. J. 1972. Memory Consolidation. San Francisco: Albion.

Milner, B. 1966. Amnesia following operation on the temporal lobes. In C. W. M. Whitty and O. L. Zangwill (eds.), Amnesia. London: Butterworths, pp. 109–133.

Moore, J. W., Desmond, J. E., and Berthier, N. E. 1982. The metencephalic basis of the conditioned nictitating membrane response. In C. D. Woody (ed.), Conditioning: Representation of Involved Neural Functions. New York: Plenum Press, pp. 459–482.

Pavlov, I. P. 1927. Conditioned Reflexes: An Investigation of the Physiological Activity of the Cerebral Cortex. G. V. Anrep (trans.). London: Oxford University Press.

Penfield, W. 1958. Functional localization in temporal and deep Sylvian areas. Res. Publ. Assoc. Res. Nerv. Ment. Dis. 36:210–226.

Rescorla, R. A., and Wagner, A. R. 1972. A theory of Pavlovian conditioning: Variations in the effectiveness of reinforcement and nonreinforcement. In A. H. Black and W. F. Prokasy (eds.), Classical Conditioning II: Current Research and Theory. New York: Appleton-Century-Crofts, pp. 64–99.

Shurrager, P. S., and Culler, E. 1940. Conditioning in the spinal dog. J. Exp. Psychol. 26:133–159.

Squire, L. R., Slater, P. C., and Chace, P. M. 1975. Retrograde amnesia: Temporal gradient in very long term memory following electroconvulsive therapy. Science 187:77–79.

Thompson, R. F., McCormick, D. A., Lavond, D. G., Clark, G. A., Kettner, R. E., and Mauk, M. D. 1983. The engram found? Initial localization of the memory trace for a basic form of associative learning. Prog. Psychobiol. Physiol. Psychol. 10:167–196.

Thorndike, E. L. 1911. Animal Intelligence: Experimental Studies. New York: Macmillan.

Tulving, E. 1984. Précis of elements of episodic memory. Behav. Brain Sci. 7:223–268.

Warrington, E. K., and Weiskrantz, L. 1982. Amnesia: A disconnection syndrome? Neuropsychologia 20:233–248.

Wolpe, J. 1958. Psychotherapy by Reciprocal Inhibition. Stanford, Calif.: Stanford University Press.

Eric R. Kandel

Cellular Mechanisms of Learning
and
the Biological Basis of Individuality

62

Throughout this book we have emphasized that behavior is determined by the functioning of the brain and that mental illness reflects the brain's malfunction. All functions of the brain, in turn, represent an interaction between genetic and developmental processes on the one hand and environmental factors such as learning on the other. Here, we shall again examine the role of learning and memory in the generation of behavior, but now focusing on the mechanisms whereby learning alters the structure and function of nerve cells and their interconnections.

Some of the most characteristic aspects of behavior result from the ability to learn from experience. We are what we are largely because of what we have learned and remember about our world. Learning also has broad cultural ramifications and extends beyond the individual to the transmission of culture from generation to generation. Learning is a major vehicle for behavioral adaptation and for social progress. Moreover, since the performance of most behaviors involves some aspect of learning and memory, experience contributes at least partly to many psychological disorders. Thus, insofar as psychotherapeutic intervention is successful in treating neurotic mental illnesses, it presumably works because treatment creates an educational experience that allows people to change.

As we have seen in Chapters 60 and 61, some of the most challenging problems in neural science lie at the interface between the study of mental processes and biology. In recent years cognitive psychology and neurobiology have matured independently and, in the process, have moved closer together. As a result, we are now beginning to benefit from the increase in explanatory power that often occurs when two disparate disciplines begin to converge on a common ground. The rewards of this merger are evident particularly in the study of memory and learning. Animal studies are yielding insights into mental processes from the behavioral to the molecular levels and are providing the foundation for a science of mentation that promises ultimately to revolutionize our understanding of behavior and its abnormalities.

Much progress in the cellular study of learning and memory has recently been made by examining elementary forms of learning: habituation, sensitization, and classical conditioning. These elementary behavioral modifications have been analyzed both in simple vertebrate preparations, such as the isolated spinal cord or brain slice, and in the nervous systems of invertebrates.

Habituation Involves a Depression of Synaptic Transmission

As we saw in Chapter 61, *habituation* is a decrease in the strength of a behavioral response that occurs when an initially novel eliciting stimulus is repeatedly presented. When an animal encounters a new stimulus it first responds with a series of orienting reflexes. With repetition of the stimulus, if it is neither rewarding nor noxious, the animal reduces and ultimately suppresses its responses. Habituation is probably the most ubiquitous of all forms of learning. Through habituation, animals and humans learn to ignore stimuli that have lost novelty or meaning, thus freeing themselves to attend to stimuli that are important. Habituation is thought to be the first learning process to emerge in human infants and is used to study the development of intellectual processes such as attention, perception, and memory in the newborn. The psychologist Michael Lewis, working at Columbia University, found that the ability of 1-year-old infants to habituate to the repeated presentation of a visual stimulus correlates well with various measures of intelligence obtained at 4 years of age.

The first approach to studying habituation in an animal model was made by Charles Sherrington in 1906. While studying the behavior underlying posture and locomotion, he observed that certain reflex forms of behavior—such as the flexion withdrawal of a limb to stimulation of the skin—habituated with repeated stimulation and that recovery occurred only after many seconds of rest. Sherrington suggested that the habituation of the withdrawal reflex is due to a functional decrease in the effectiveness of the set of synapses through which the motor neurons for the behavior have been repeatedly activated.

This problem was later investigated again by W. Alden Spencer and Richard Thompson at the University of Oregon. They found close behavioral parallels between habituation of the spinal reflexes in the cat and habituation of more complex behavioral responses in humans. The cellular studies by Spencer and Thompson in the isolated spinal cord provided the first evidence that habituation involves changes in synaptic effectiveness. By recording intracellularly from motor neurons, they found that habituation results in a decrease in the synaptic activity onto the motor neurons of the reflex. However, as we saw in Chapter 35, the interneuronal organization of the spinal cord is quite complex, making it difficult to study the detailed cellular mechanisms of habituation in the flexion reflex. As a result, the further investigation of habituation has required still simpler systems in which the behavioral response can be accounted for by a series of known monosynaptic connections.

The most complete analysis of habituation has been carried out by Vincent Castellucci, Irving Kupfermann, and Eric Kandel at Columbia University. They studied an invertebrate, the marine snail *Aplysia californica*, which has a simple nervous system containing only 10^5 cells.

62–1 In the neural circuit of the gill-withdrawal reflex in the marine snail *Aplysia,* a key site of plasticity that underlies habituation is the synapse between the terminals of the sensory neurons and the central target cells—the interneurons and the motor neurons. In this circuit there are about 24 mechanoreceptor sensory neurons that innervate the siphon skin, only one of which is illustrated here for simplicity. These sensory cells project onto a cluster of six motor neurons that innervate the gill. In addition, the sensory neurons also excite a group of interneurons, which in turn synapse on the motor neurons.

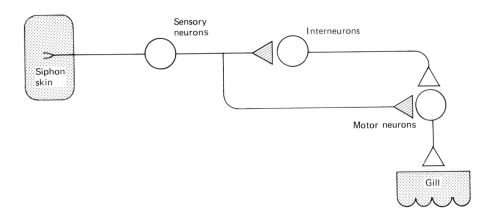

Aplysia has a reflex for withdrawing its respiratory organ, the *gill*, and its *siphon* (a small fleshy spout above the gill used to expel seawater and waste). This reflex is similar to the leg-flexion reflex mediated by the spinal cord that was studied by Spencer and Thompson. The gill and siphon withdraw if a mild tactile stimulus is delivered to the siphon. With repeated stimulation, this reflex withdrawal habituates. As we shall see later, this response can also be sensitized and classically conditioned.

Whereas the neural circuit, or wiring diagram, of the flexion reflex in the cat is complex, that for gill withdrawal is simple. The reflex has an important monosynaptic component consisting of a group of motor neurons that mediate the behavior and a group of sensory neurons that synapse on the motor neurons (Figure 62–1). There are also several excitatory and inhibitory interneurons upon which the sensory neurons converge and that in turn synapse on the motor neurons. In response to a novel stimulus, the sensory neurons generate large excitatory postsynaptic potentials in the interneurons and motor cells. These excitatory postsynaptic potentials summate both temporally and spatially and cause the motor cells to discharge strongly, leading to a brisk withdrawal of the gill. As the stimulus is repeatedly presented, the synaptic potentials produced by the sensory neurons in the interneurons and in the motor cells become progressively smaller; fewer action potentials are therefore generated in the motor cells, and the behavior is reduced. Finally, the postsynaptic potentials generated by the sensory neurons become very small and fail to elicit action potentials in the motor neurons, at which point no behavior is produced. The memory for habituation is stored as a persistent reduction in the effectiveness of the synaptic connections between the sensory and motor neurons. This reduction leads to a diminished behavioral response that lasts for several hours.

Analyzing the mechanisms underlying habituation, Castellucci, Marc Klein and Kandel found that the decrease in synaptic transmission results, in part, from a prolonged shutting off (inactivation) of the Ca^{++} channel in the presynaptic terminal, leading to a decrease in Ca^{++} influx and a diminished output of chemical transmitter. After the reflex is habituated, a tactile stimulus to the skin still activates the sensory neurons, and an action potential still propagates into the terminals of the neurons. However, because the Ca^{++} channels are partly inactivated, less Ca^{++} flows into the terminals with each action potential. Since, as we saw in Chapter 11, transmitter release depends on the influx of Ca^{++} into the terminals with each action potential, less transmitter is released (Figure 62–4B). The Ca^{++} is thought to function in transmitter release by allowing the vesicles that contain the transmitter to be mobilized into release sites at active zones and to bind to the surface membrane there—a necessary step for exocytosis. Thus, in this simple case, short-term memory for a learning task is due not to reverberating activity in a closed chain of neurons (Chapter 61), but to a functional, or plastic, change in the strength of a previously existing set of connections. This

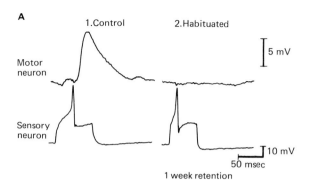

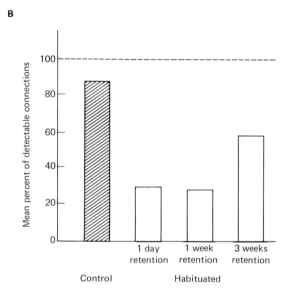

62–2 Long-term habituation is reflected physiologically by a dramatic depression of synaptic effectiveness between the sensory and motor neurons in *Aplysia*. **A.** Comparison of a synaptic connection between a sensory neuron and the motor neuron L7 in a control (untrained) *Aplysia* (**1**) and in an *Aplysia* that had been subjected to long-term habituation training (**2**). Control animals show an effective synaptic potential, whereas the synaptic connection in habituated animals is undetectable even 1 week after training.
B. Histogram illustrating a decrease, as compared to control, of mean percentage of detectable connections in habituated animals at several points in time after long-term habituation training: 1 day, approximately 1 week, and approximately 3 weeks. (Adapted from Castellucci, Carew, and Kandel, 1978.)

seems to be a general mechanism of habituation since a similar process accounts for short-term habituation of escape responses in crayfish and cockroaches.

What are the limits of this plasticity? How much can the effectiveness of a given synapse change and how long can the change last? Memory can be either short term, lasting for minutes or hours, or long term, lasting for days, weeks, or years. Can changes in synaptic effectiveness also give rise to long-term memory? Whereas a single training session of 10 stimuli in *Aplysia* leads to short-term habituation that can last for hours, 4 or more repeated training sessions produce long-term habituation that lasts up to 3 weeks. Castellucci, Thomas Carew, and Kandel have compared the connections between the sensory neurons and the motor neurons in control animals with those in animals examined at various times after they acquired long-term habituation. In the control animals, 90% of the sensory neurons made electrophysiologically detectable connections onto the motor neurons (Figure 62–2). In contrast, both 1 day and 1 week after long-term habituation, the detectable connections with the motor cells were reduced to 30%; the rest of the connections had been inactivated to such a degree that they could not be demonstrated with electrophysiological techniques.

Thus, short- and long-term changes in synaptic efficacy can underlie certain instances of short- and long-term memory. Moreover, this plastic capability is quite specific to a particular set of synapses. Most synaptic connections in the nervous system of *Aplysia* are not at all affected by a pattern of stimulation that leads to the learning of habituation. However, at a crucial synapse such as that identified in the withdrawal reflex—a synapse that has evolved to mediate the consequences of experience and learning—a relatively small amount of stimulation can produce long-term changes in synaptic strength.

Sensitization Involves an Enhancement of Synaptic Transmission

Sensitization is a more complex form of learning than habituation: it is the enhancement of an animal's reflex responses as a result of the presentation of a strong or noxious stimulus. In contrast to habituation, sensitiza-

tion causes an animal to pay attention to a variety of stimuli, even previously innocuous ones, because they are potentially accompanied by painful or dangerous consequences. Sensitization, like habituation, can last from minutes to days and weeks, depending on the pattern of stimulation.

At the cellular level, sensitization in *Aplysia* also involves an alteration of synaptic transmission at the synapses made by the sensory neurons on the motor neurons and interneurons. The same synaptic locus can therefore be regulated in opposite ways by opposing forms of learning: its activity can be depressed by habituation and enhanced by sensitization. In sensitization, however, another mechanism comes into play. This mechanism is *presynaptic facilitation*, which is mediated by an axoaxonic synapse, a synapse on a synapse (Figure 62–3). The sensitizing stimuli activate a group of facilitating interneurons, which synapse on or near the terminals of the sensory cells. These facilitating neurons enhance transmitter release from sensory neuron terminals by causing an increase in the amount of cyclic adenosine 3′, 5′-monophosphate (cyclic AMP) in the sensory neurons. Because experimental application of serotonin mimics the actions of the facilitating interneurons and the natural sensitizing stimuli, and because the terminal regions of the sensory neurons receive serotonergic innervation, some of the facilitators are thought to be serotonergic.

To understand how an elevation in the concentration of cyclic AMP enhances transmitter release from sensory neuron terminals, it may be helpful to review the steps involved in neurotransmission. As an action potential propagates toward the synaptic terminals of the sensory neurons, it begins to depolarize the terminals and open up

62–3 Presynaptic facilitation is a feature of the mechanism of sensitization of the gill-withdrawal reflex in *Aplysia*. Stimuli to the tail activate neurons that excite facilitating interneurons. The facilitating cells (some of which are thought to utilize serotonin as their transmitter, as indicated by the dense-core vesicles in their terminal) in turn end on the synaptic terminals of the sensory neurons from the siphon skin, where they enhance transmitter release by means of presynaptic facilitation.

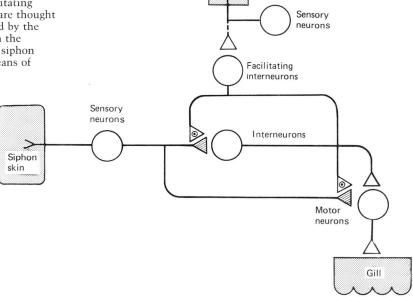

A Control   B Habituation   C Sensitization

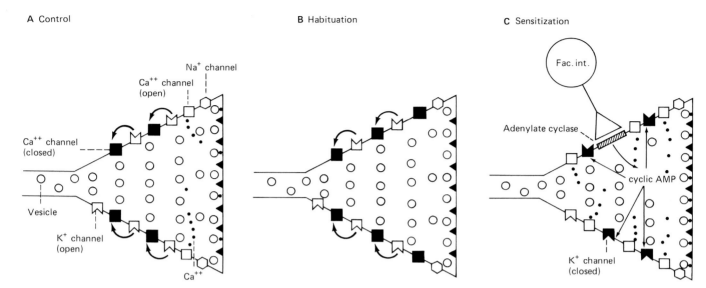

62–4 These schematic models of presynaptic terminals show the mechanisms of short-term habituation and sensitization. **A.** In the control state an action potential in the sensory neuron opens up a number of Ca^{++} channels in parallel with the Na^+ channels of the membrane. As a result, some Ca^{++} flows into the terminals and allows a certain number of transmitter-containing synaptic vesicles to bind to release sites and be released. The opening of the K^+ channel repolarizes the terminal and prevents other Ca^{++} channels from opening (indicated by **arrows**). **B.** Repeated action potentials in the terminals, leading to habituation, decrease the number of open Ca^{++} channels in the sensory terminal and, at the limit, may shut them down altogether. The resulting depression in Ca^{++} influx functionally inactivates the synapse

by decreasing mobilization to active zone release sites and by preventing synaptic vesicles from binding the external membrane, a necessary step for release by exocytosis. **C.** Sensitization is produced by interneurons, some of which are thought to be serotonergic. Serotonin and other facilitating transmitters act on an adenylate cyclase in the terminals, which converts ATP to cyclic AMP. Cyclic AMP, in turn, acts to decrease the repolarizing K^+ current and leads to a broadening of the action potential. The increase in the duration of the action potential prolongs the time during which Ca^{++} channels can open, leading to a greater influx of Ca^{++}, and therefore to increased transmitter release. (Adapted from Klein and Kandel, 1978.)

the Na^+ channels, thereby producing more depolarization and generating an action potential in the terminal. The depolarizing component of the action potential in the terminal then opens up voltage-gated Ca^{++} channels and allows a certain amount of Ca^{++} to come into the cell. The depolarizing component of the action potential also opens up several classes of K^+ channels; the resulting efflux of K^+ repolarizes the action potential and closes the Ca^{++} channels. Thus, the activation of the Na^+ and K^+ channels not only generates the action potential and determines its duration, but also opens the Ca^{++} channels and determines how long they remain open. Serotonin and other facilitating transmitters released by the facilitating interneuron stimulate sensory neuron terminals to increase their level of cyclic AMP, which works to prolong the action potential in these terminals by decreasing a component of the K^+ current that normally shuts it off. When the action potential is prolonged, the Ca^{++} channels stay open longer, and more Ca^{++} is able to enter the terminals and participate in transmitter release (Figure 62–4). In addition, serotonin and cyclic AMP lead to a change in the way that Ca^{++} is handled within the cell so as to aid in the mobilization of transmitter vesicles and thereby amplify its effect.

Sensitization Can Now Be Understood in Molecular Terms

On the basis of pharmacological and biochemical studies, Klein, Castellucci, Robert Hawkins, Steven Siegelbaum, Lise Bernier, James Schwartz, and Kandel have pieced together the likely sequence of biochemical steps that occur as a result of sensitization (Figure 62–5). According to this model, serotonin, which is thought to be released by some of the facilitating neurons in the gill and siphon withdrawal reflex, activates a serotonin receptor in the membrane of the presynaptic terminal of the sensory neuron. The serotonin receptor engages a coupling protein (G-protein), which in turn activates an adenylate cyclase. Stimulation of the adenylate cyclase increases the concentration of cyclic AMP within the terminal. Cyclic AMP then activates a protein kinase—an enzyme thought to be the common site of action for cyclic AMP in eukaryotic cells. Protein kinases add phosphate groups to proteins, thereby changing their charge and consequently their shape. This process, called *phosphorylation*, can lead to either an increase or a decrease in the activity of a protein (see Chapter 14). In the case of sensitization the activated protein kinase has been shown to

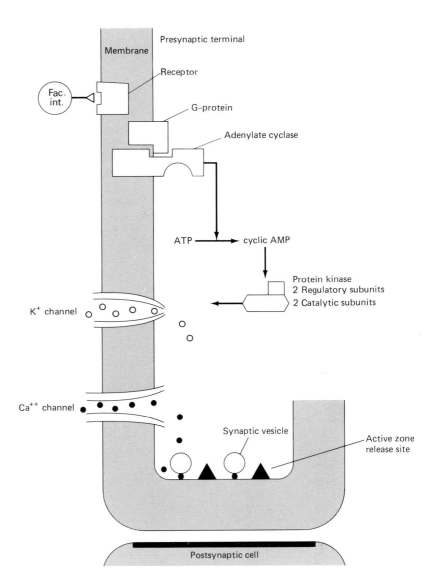

62–5 Postulated biochemical steps of presynaptic facilitation underlying sensitization. The action of serotonin and other facilitating transmitters leads to a closure of a special class of K^+ channels, and a consequent increase in Ca^{++} influx. The facilitating transmitters activate a receptor that engages a coupling protein, called the G-protein, that increases the activity of the enzyme adenylate cyclase. The adenylate cyclase converts ATP to cyclic AMP, and thus increases the level of cyclic AMP in the terminal of the sensory neuron. The cyclic AMP activates an enzyme called the cyclic AMP-dependent protein kinase by attaching to its regulatory subunit, which releases its active catalytic subunit. The catalytic subunit then phosphorylates either the K^+ channel directly or a regulatory protein associated with it, thereby changing the conformation of the channel and decreasing the K^+ current. This prolongs the action potential, increases the influx of Ca^{++}, and thus augments transmitter release. The enzyme phosphatase in turn acts to remove the phosphate groups of the K^+ channel modulated by the kinase so that when the concentration of cAMP returns to control level the K^+ channel opens up again.

phosphorylate a novel K^+ channel protein (the serotonin-sensitive K^+ channel) or a protein that is associated with it. This serotonin-modulated K^+ channel has been found to participate selectively in sensitization. Phosphorylation of this channel or associated proteins reduces a component of the K^+ current that normally repolarizes the action potential. Reduction of this current prolongs the action potential and thereby allows Ca^{++} channels to be activated for longer periods of time.

Sensitization Can Reverse the Synaptic Depression of Habituation

Sensitization is an effective form of learning; it so enhances behavioral responsiveness that it can reverse the synaptic and behavioral depression that occurs not only in short-term but even in long-term habituation (Figure 62–6). Thus, synaptic pathways, determined by innate genetic and developmental processes, can be functionally interrupted and then functionally restored (or dishabituated) by simple learning experiences! The training procedures that produce this learning are relatively modest, comparable to the social experience of one person speaking to another. By extension from what we know of the mechanisms of simple forms of learning, we may assume that when two people speak, not only do they make eye contact and voice contact, but through behavior the actions of the neurons in the brain of each person have a direct and long-lasting effect on the functioning of the neurons in the brain of the other.

A

1.Habituated   2.Habituated + sensitized

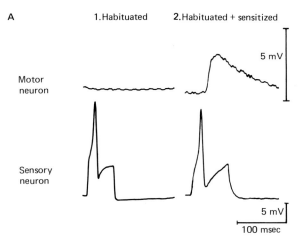

Motor
neuron

Sensory
neuron

5 mV

5 mV

100 msec

B

1.Behavior   2.Synaptic
connections

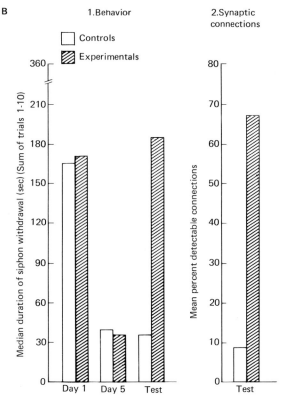

□ Controls

▨ Experimentals

Median duration of siphon withdrawal (sec) (Sum of trials 1-10)

Mean percent detectable connections

Day 1   Day 5   Test

Test

62–6 A sensitizing stimulus to a long-term habituated animal can restore synaptic transmission that had been inactivated by habituation and thereby restore behavioral responsiveness. **A.** A typical inactivated connection from a habituated *Aplysia* (**1**) is compared with a typical excitatory postsynaptic potential from an animal that had previously been habituated but then received a sensitizing stimulus (**2**).
B. Histograms compare the degree of behavioral responsiveness in a control group of long-term habituated animals with that in an identically trained experimental group that received a single sensitizing stimulus after 5 days of habituation training (**1**). Both groups of animals exhibited significant habituation on day 5, compared to day 1. The experimental animals showed significant sensitization after a single sensitizing stimulus; the long-term habituation of the control animals remained unchanged. The physiological correlates of these behavioral data are demonstrated by a summary of 20 experiments in which the number of detectable synaptic connections was determined in control (long-term habituated) animals and in long-term habituated animals that were sensitized (**2**). (Adapted from Carew, Castellucci, and Kandel, 1979.)

Long-term Habituation and Sensitization Produce Morphological Changes

Habituation and sensitization are learning processes that can turn the synapses of specific neurons off and on. In long-term learning, is this functional change accompanied by a morphological change? To answer this question, Craig Bailey and Mary Chen at the College of Physicians and Surgeons of Columbia University have carried out a morphological analysis on the sensory neurons of the gill-withdrawal reflex in *Aplysia*. They injected the sensory neurons with the electron-dense marker horseradish peroxidase and visualized their syn-

aptic terminals with the electron microscope. This technique enabled these investigators to compare synapses that have undergone long-term learning with control synapses. In particular, they analyzed changes both in the number and distribution of synaptic vesicles (the likely storage sites of transmitter quanta) and in the size and extent of active zones (the sites from which transmitter is actually released; see Chapter 12). Active zones contain arrays of submembranous dense particles where the vesicles are positioned and their contents released. The active zones are located in varicose expansions of the axonal processes. However, not all varicosities contain active zones. In sensory neurons from untrained animals, only

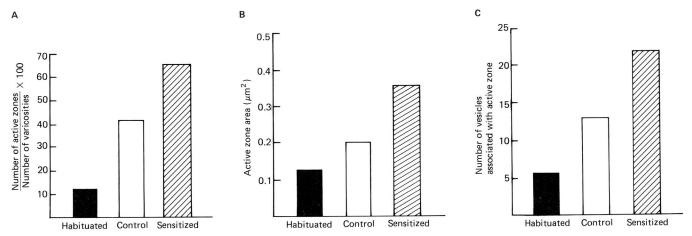

62–7 Long-term habituation and sensitization lead to structural changes in the presynaptic terminals of sensory neurons. These histograms compare the properties of active zones in control animals with those in long-term habituated or sensitized animals. **A.** Number of active zones per varicosity. **B.** Area of active zones. **C.** Number of vesicles associated with active zones. With habituation, the number and size of the active zones and their transmitting capability are smaller than in controls, whereas with sensitization, they are all increased. (Adapted from Bailey and Chen, 1983.)

40% of terminals have active zones; the rest do not. Long-term habituation reduces the presence of active zones to only 10% of the terminals. Moreover, even the few remaining active zones are smaller than in control varicosities. In contrast, sensitization increases the incidence of active zones to 65% of terminals, and the average size of each zone is larger than in control animals (Figure 62–7).

Cell-Biological Studies of Habituation and Sensitization Have Provided Some Basic Insights into the Mechanisms of Learning and Memory

Several points emerge from a consideration of these simple examples of learning and memory. One is that both short- and long-term memory can be localized to particular sites. In these instances, at least, memory is not dependent on widely distributed processes. These memories are also not dependent on reverberating activity in closed neuronal loops. Second, learning need not involve gross anatomical rearrangement in the nervous system. No nerve cells or even synaptic pathways are created or destroyed; rather, learning of habituation and sensitization results from changes in the effectiveness of previously existing chemical synaptic connections. Finally, learning need not depend on special "memory" neurons—or by extrapolation, memory centers in the brain—whose only function is to store information. Learning can result from changes in neurons that also act as integral components of a normal reflex pathway. It is therefore likely that different types of experiences may be stored in a large number of different cells that are involved in a variety of other functions. Learning itself is not necessarily an independent process; rather, it can be a modification of other, already existing processes.

The demonstration of the molecular and structural changes during even these simple forms of learning has required a variety of techniques developed only recently, as well as a variety of simple preparations that are suitable for a cell-biological approach. No wonder, then, that we are only beginning to understand the biological basis of other mental processes and that the analysis of mental disorders such as schizophrenia and depression has so far been beyond our reach. It will be interesting in the future to see whether mental illnesses that result from learning lead to a distortion of the connections in specific areas of the brain.

Classical Conditioning Involves Activity-Dependent Enhancement of Presynaptic Facilitation

As we saw in Chapter 61, classical conditioning is a slightly more complex form of learning than sensitization because the subject is not concerned with learning about the properties of one stimulus (the sensitizing stimulus) but must learn a temporal association between two stimuli. In classical conditioning an initially weak or ineffective conditioned stimulus becomes highly effective in producing a behavioral response after it has been paired in time with a strong unconditioned stimulus. The timing is critical to the outcome. For classical conditioning to work, the conditioned stimulus *must precede* the unconditioned stimulus and it must usually do so by a critical interval of about 0.5 to 1.0 sec. This form of learning is therefore *noncommutative*. It does not work if the conditioned stimulus follows the unconditioned stimulus. Classical conditioning is fascinating because, as we saw earlier, it represents the learning of a fundamental causal relationship. When an animal has been conditioned, it has learned that the conditioned stimulus predicts the

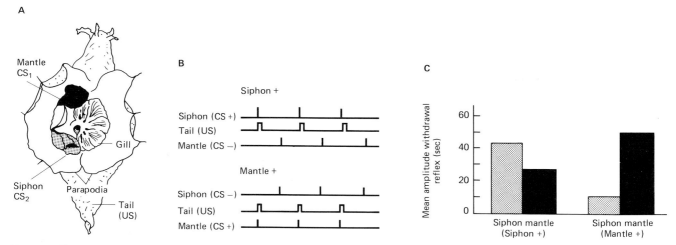

62–8 Differential classical conditioning of gill-withdrawal and siphon-withdrawal reflexes in *Aplysia* illustrates that the paired pathway is enhanced compared to the unpaired pathway. **A.** Dorsal view of *Aplysia* shows the two conditioned stimulus **(CS)** pathways (siphon and mantle shelf) and the unconditioned stimulus **(US)** pathway used for differential conditioning. **B.** The protocol used for differential conditioning involved two groups of animals. The **Siphon⁺** group received a stimulus to the siphon **(CS⁺)** paired with tail shock, and an unpaired stimulus to the mantle **(CS⁻)**. In the **Mantle⁺** group, the stimulus to the mantle was paired **(CS⁺)** and that to the siphon was unpaired **(CS⁻)**. **C.** After differential conditioning, animals receiving **Siphon⁺** training show significantly greater responses to the siphon CS than to the mantle CS; the reverse is true for animals receiving **Mantle⁺** training. (Adapted from Carew, Hawkins, and Kandel, 1983.)

unconditioned stimulus. Thus, through classical conditioning, an organism is able to discriminate *cause and effect relationships* in the environment. In contrast, nonassociative learning such as sensitization does not require temporal pairing of stimuli and does not teach the animal to expect any relationship between stimuli. Often a reflex can be modified by sensitization as well as by classical conditioning. In such cases, the response enhancement produced by classical conditioning is greater or lasts longer than the enhancement produced by sensitization. Moreover, whereas sensitization indiscriminately affects a broad range of defensive responses, classical conditioning enhances only a restricted range of responses appropriate to the pairing of the conditioned stimulus and the unconditioned stimulus.

Carew, Hawkins, Terrell Walters, and Kandel have found that the gill and siphon withdrawal reflex of *Aplysia* can be enhanced by classical conditioning as well as by sensitization. Moreover, the withdrawal reflex is capable of being differentially conditioned. The withdrawal can be elicited by stimulating not only the siphon but also a nearby structure called the mantle shelf. Each of these areas is innervated by its own population of sensory neurons, and each pathway can be activated independently to serve as a conditioned stimulus (Figure 62–8A). These pathways can be differentially conditioned by pairing the unconditioned stimulus (a strong shock to the tail) with stimuli to either the siphon or the mantle shelf and stimulating the other pathway in a way that is unpaired with the tail shock (Figure 62–8B). After such training, the response to stimulation of the paired site is significantly greater than the response to stimulation of the unpaired site (Figure 62–8C).

Unlike nonassociative learning, associative learning requires temporal specificity—a specific timing of stimuli. What then are the cellular mechanisms whereby this temporal pairing of stimuli leads to learning that is both more robust than nonassociative forms and more restricted in its distribution (being limited to the paired pathways)? Hawkins, Carew, Thomas Abrams, and Kandel found that temporal specificity results from a convergence of the conditioned and unconditioned stimuli at the level of individual sensory neurons in the conditioned stimulus pathway. Greater presynaptic facilitation of the sensory neurons—greater depression of the serotonin-sensitive K^+ channel leading to greater influx of Ca^{++} and more transmitter release—occurs in response to the unconditioned stimulus when the sensory neurons have just been active because of exposure to the conditioned stimulus (Figure 62–9). Thus, the facilitation of the connection from a sensory neuron to a follower neuron is amplified if—and only if—the sensory neuron is active just before the arrival of the input from the facilitating neurons that are activated by the unconditioned stimulus. Activity in the sensory neurons that follows the unconditioned stimulus has no effect. Moreover, for facilitation to be amplified, activity in the sensory neurons must precede the unconditioned stimulus by a brief critical period. We have seen in our discussion of neuronal modulation during development and critical periods (Chapters 56 and 57) that activity is often an important step in the fine-tuning of synaptic connections. Here we can see quite clearly that appropriately timed activity is also important for learning in the mature organism.

These experiments indicate that the mechanism of classical conditioning of the withdrawal reflex is actually

A

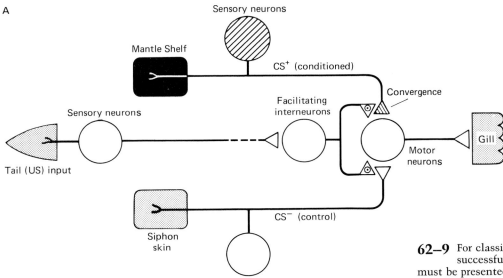

Sensory neurons

Mantle Shelf

CS⁺ (conditioned)

Convergence

Sensory neurons

Facilitating
interneurons

Tail (US) input

Motor
neurons

Gill

Siphon
skin

CS⁻ (control)

Sensory neurons

B

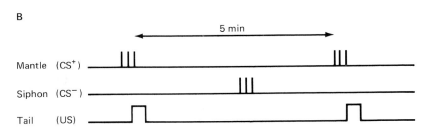

5 min

Mantle (CS⁺)

Siphon (CS⁻)

Tail   (US)

C

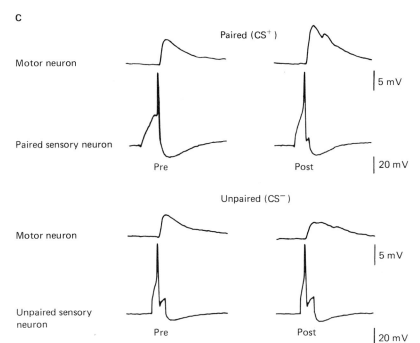

Paired (CS⁺)

Motor neuron

Paired sensory neuron

5 mV

Pre   Post

20 mV

Unpaired (CS⁻)

Motor neuron

Unpaired sensory
neuron

5 mV

Pre   Post

20 mV

50 msec

62–9 For classical conditioning to be successful, the unconditioned (**US**) must be presented shortly after the conditioned stimulus (**CS**). This temporal specificity underlies the associative component of the learning. Temporal specificity has been found to be due to intracellular convergence of the US and CS pathways at a synapse critically involved in mediating the learned response.

A. Wiring diagram of the two pathways involved in differential classical conditioning of the gill-withdrawal reflex. The US, a shock to the tail, excites facilitating interneurons that in turn synapse on the presynaptic terminals of sensory neurons from the two CS pathways, the mantle shelf and siphon. This is the mechanism of sensitization and it affects both pathways equally. Pairing of mantle CS and US causes the mantle CS pathway to be active. Recent activity in the sensory neurons (due to the CS) primes them to respond in a boosted or amplified manner to stimulation by the facilitating interneurons from the US pathway. This is the mechanism of classical conditioning. This mechanism at once amplifies the response of the paired (mantle) pathway and restricts it to that pathway. **B.** Experimental protocol used to compare the response of animals receiving paired presentations of the mantle CS and tail US (**CS⁺**) with that of animals receiving the siphon CS and tail US in a temporally unpaired sequence (**CS⁻**). **C.** Examples of the excitatory postsynaptic potentials produced in a common, identified motor neuron by action potentials from paired and unpaired sensory neurons. Electrical recordings were made before training (**Pre**) and 1 hr after training (**Post**), when facilitation of the excitatory postsynaptic potential from the paired sensory neuron is considerably greater than that from the unpaired neuron.

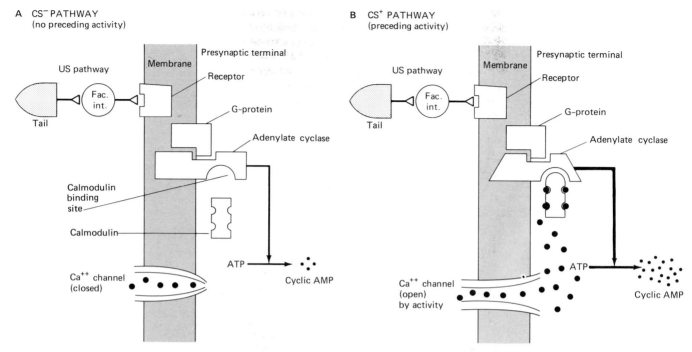

62–10 Model for classical conditioning based on the hypothesis that preceding activity leads to an influx of Ca^{++} in the sensory neurons of the conditioned stimulus (**CS**) pathway, and that Ca^{++} exerts its action by enhancing the activity of that Ca^{++}-dependent adenylate cyclase. **A.** In the unpaired pathway (**CS$^-$**) the sensory neuron does *not* have preceding activity, and its Ca^{++} channels are closed. **B.** In the paired pathway (**CS$^+$**), the preceding activity of the sensory neuron has caused its Ca^{++} channels to open. Increased intracellular Ca^{++} binds to calmodulin, which in turn binds to

the adenylate cyclase, leading to a conformational change in this enzyme; this change promotes the synthesis of a greater amount of cyclic AMP in response to the facilitating transmitter than would occur in the absence of Ca^{++} binding. The greater increase in the level of cyclic AMP in the paired pathway activates more cyclic-AMP-dependent protein kinase, closes more K$^+$ channels, broadens subsequent action potentials, and leads to a substantially greater increase in transmitter release. (From Kandel et al., 1983; Abrams et al., 1983.)

an elaboration of presynaptic facilitation, the mechanism of sensitization of the reflex. The sensory neurons undergo a greater amount of facilitation in response to the facilitating neurons or to experimentally applied serotonin if they were active just before the serotonin or the facilitating neurons act on them. This novel property of presynaptic facilitation is called *activity dependence*.

How is this activity-dependent enhancement of presynaptic facilitation achieved? Abrams and his colleagues found that one of the consequences of activity is to allow Ca^{++} to move into the neuron with each action potential and thereby amplify the synthesis of cyclic AMP by serotonin (Figure 62–10): specifically, the Ca^{++} influx is thought to act through calmodulin to amplify the activation of the adenylate cyclase by the facilitating transmitter. Indeed, most cells of the body have an adenylate cyclase that is independent of Ca^{++}. But many brain cells have a second type of adenylate cyclase that is sensitive to Ca^{++}–calmodulin, and this Ca^{++}–calmodulin-dependent adenylate cyclase generates more cyclic AMP when Ca^{++}–calmodulin is bound to it than when it is not. In *Aplysia* (and as we shall see below in *Drosophila* as well) this second form of adenylate cyclase might be important for classical conditioning.

The cellular mechanisms of classical conditioning seem to be an amplified form of those involved in sensitization, suggesting that there may be a basic molecular alphabet or grammar to elementary forms of learning whereby more complex forms of learning partake of the molecular machinery of simpler forms. According to this view, a variety of distinct forms of behavioral modifications could be achieved by the combinations and permutations of a surprisingly small set of molecular building blocks.

Activity-dependent enhancement may be a general mechanism. Walters and John Byrne at the University of Texas found a similar enhancement for conditioning of the tail-withdrawal reflex in *Aplysia*. Independent studies of classical conditioning in the mollusc *Hermissenda* by Daniel Alkon, in the locust by Graham Hoyle and Marjorie Woollacott, and in cortex of the cat by Charles Woody suggest that modulation of a K$^+$ channel may also be critical for learning in a variety of other animals.

Similar results are now emerging from the application of a different approach. The fruit fly, *Drosophila*, has been used extensively by Seymour Benzer and his colleagues to explore how genes control behavior. Benzer, William Harris, Duncan Byers, Yadin Dudai, and William Quinn have found that the fruit fly can be classically conditioned. Using genetic selection procedures, Quinn, Dudai, and Byers then isolated single-gene mutants that could not learn. Four of these mutants have now been studied in detail and have two interesting features. First, in addition to being unable to learn classical conditioning, some of these mutants cannot learn sensitization. Second, all of the mutants have a defect in the cyclic AMP cascade. One lacks one type of cyclic AMP phosphodiesterase, the enzyme that degrades cyclic AMP. As a result, the fly has abnormally high levels of cyclic AMP that are thought to be out of the range of normal modulation. Other learning mutants have defects

in the serotonin receptor, the biogenic amine transmitters, or the Ca^{++}–calmodulin-dependent adenylate cyclase. Thus, both cell-biological approaches in *Aplysia* and genetic approaches in *Drosophila* indicate that the cyclic AMP cascade is important in elementary forms of learning and memory storage.

The Somatotopic Map in the Brain Is Modifiable by Experience

In Chapter 57 we saw that the structure of columns concerned with ocular dominance in area 17 of the cerebral cortex can be greatly modified by experience during an

62–11 There are multiple representations of the body surface in the primary somatic sensory cortex (Chapter 25). This is illustrated here for the somatic sensory cortex of the owl monkey. There is a separate representation of the hand area in both areas 3b and 1. **A.** The location of these two hand areas is shown in this dorsolateral view of the monkey brain. **B.** The hand of an owl monkey is innervated by the ulnar and median nerves. These nerves serve different territories on the ventral surface of the hand (**part 1**) and are represented in adjacent areas of cortex in each of the two maps—that of area 3b and that of area 1 (**part 2**). The

topographic organization of the cortical map of the ventral surface of the hand is remarkably orderly, as is shown in **part 3** for each of the two areas of the cortex.

Cortex devoted to the representation of the ventral surface of the digits is indicated in **white**; that devoted to the dorsal surface is indicated in **dark shading**. In these cortical maps, the five digits (**D_1 to D_5**) and the four palmar pads (**P_1 to P_4**) are arranged in an orderly sequence and their representations have been numbered in order. The insular (**I**) pads, the hypothenar (**H**) pads, and the thenar (**T**) pads are also indicated. (Adapted from Merzenich and Kaas, 1982.)

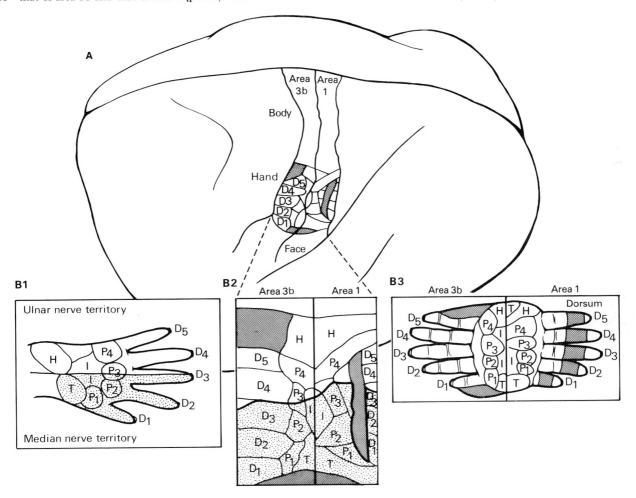

early critical period. If one eye is closed during the peak of the critical period, even for only one week, the columns devoted to that eye shrink and those devoted to the open eye expand. This ability to modify ocular dominance columns is restricted to a relatively short period just after birth, but it raises an intriguing question: To what degree can altered sensory experience in later life produce changes in the architecture of the brain—in the size of cortical columns, or even in the precise details of the various sensory and motor maps? The work we have just reviewed in simple animals indicates that learning produces structural and functional changes in specific nerve cells. In mammals, and especially in humans, in whom each component of function is represented by hundreds of thousands of nerve cells, learning is likely to lead to alterations in many nerve cells and is therefore likely to be reflected in changes in the basic pattern of interconnections characteristic of the various sensory and motor systems. This is indeed what appears to be happening. The most detailed evidence has come from studies on the somatic sensory system.

As we saw in Chapter 25, the primary somatic sensory cortex consists of four Brodmann's areas (1, 2, 3a, and 3b) in the postcentral gyrus. Each of these areas represents a separate map of the body surface (Figure 62–11). Michael Merzenich and J. H. Kaas at the University of California in San Francisco recently found that the cortical maps can change in a systematic and use-dependent manner. They first encountered this phenomenon by exploring the recovery of function after nerve injury in monkeys.

They severed the median nerve in the hand, which innervates the cutaneous receptors on much of the ventral surface of the hand, the palm and the glabrous portions of digits 1, 2, and 3 (Figure 62–11). After cutting the nerve, one would expect those cortical areas committed to denervated parts of the hand to be unresponsive and silent. However, when the cortex was remapped even immediately after denervation, only a portion of the territory devoted to the median nerve was unresponsive. Merzenich and Kaas found that the adjacent cortex had expanded its influence into the denervated cortex: a significant part of the cortical area of the median nerve could now be activated by stimulating the neighboring parts of the hand outside the territory of the median nerve. For example, the region formerly activated by the ventral (palmar) surface of the thumb (digit 1) was now activated by the dorsal (hairy) surface of that finger. Thus, a fragmentary representation of the adjacent region of the dorsum of the thumb immediately expanded and replaced the representation of the ventral surface (Figure 62–12). Moreover, single nerve cells responding to stimuli on the hand in areas outside the territory of the median nerve had restricted, specific, and well-organized receptive fields. These single-cell recordings revealed that the dorsal surface of finger 2 that previously had a small representation in the median nerve territory of the cortex had a much larger territory several weeks after the median nerve had been cut. Similarly, areas on insular pads that previously had a modest representation expanded substantially in the weeks after sectioning of the nerve (Figure 62–13).

62–12 The regions of areas 3b and 1 of the owl monkey cortex that are devoted to the hand can be modified by section of the median nerve. **A.** The normal cortical representations of the hand with the ulnar and median nerves intact are similar to those illustrated in Figure 62–11, part B2. Again, **darkly shaded** areas are representations of the dorsal surface. The ventral surface of the hand is illustrated in **white**. **B.** The areas of cortex deprived of innervation following section of the median nerve are indicated by **stippling**. **C.** Several

months after median nerve section, the two cortical maps have fully reorganized and all cortical territory formerly belonging to the median nerve has been occupied by other innervation. Now, much of the deprived cortex is activated by stimulation of the dorsal digits and the dorsum of the hand. In addition, the cortical representation of the palmar pads has increased. These new inputs are not randomly arranged but are again highly ordered in a new but equally precise topographical map. (From Merzenich and Kaas, 1982.)

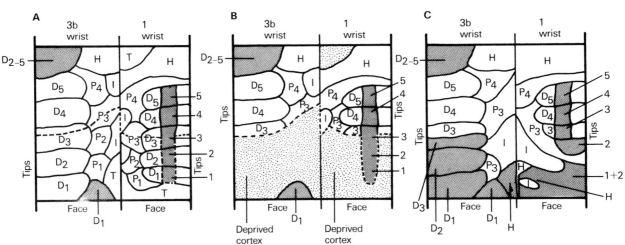

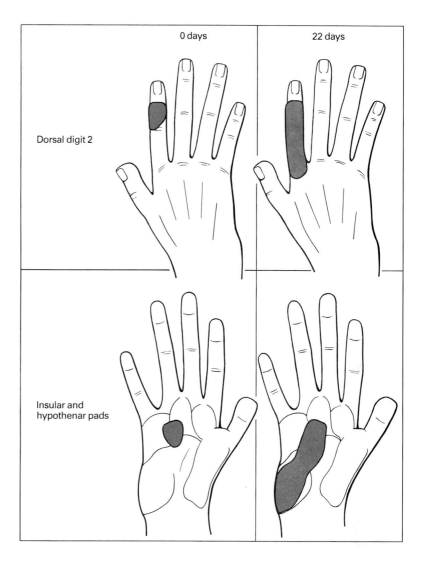

62–13 After the median nerve of a monkey is sectioned and prevented from regenerating, the area of skin represented in the cortical field that previously belonged to the median nerve expands over time. The **shaded** regions represent the total area taken up by receptive fields recorded in area 3b for the dorsum of digit 2 and in areas 1 and 3b for the insular and hypothenar pads immediately **(left)** and 22 days **(right)** after nerve section. (Adapted from Merzenich et al., 1983.)

These findings indicate that the organization apparent in the maps of the somatic and perhaps all sensory systems reflects only part of the total pattern of anatomical connections—the maps reveal only the *dominant* pattern of organization in a particular region of the brain. Other aspects of the pattern of interconnections are revealed or unmasked only when the dominant pathways are inactivated.

The map that is found immediately after cutting the median nerve changes further over the next few days. If the median nerve is not allowed to regenerate, the remaining silent parts of the cortex are taken over and occupied by adjacent normally innervated digits and by parts of the hand innervated by the ulna and radial nerves. Within 3 weeks after nerve section almost all the former cortical territory of the median nerve is reoccupied (Figures 62–12C and 62–13).

Changes in the Somatotopic Map Produced by Learning May Contribute to the Biological Expression of Individuality

The studies of Merzenich and Kaas demonstrate that cortical somatic sensory maps are not static, but dynamic. The maps can expand into functionally vacated sectors to represent the bordering skin regions in finer grain. These changes suggest that even in adult monkeys there is a use-dependent competition for cortical territory. Once a particular input becomes inactive, its representational territory can be captured by inputs from adjacent, normally innervated skin.

The reorganization is manifested in the cortex, but it is likely that the primary change is at a lower level in the brain. As first illustrated by Patrick Wall and David Egger at University College London, reorganization oc-

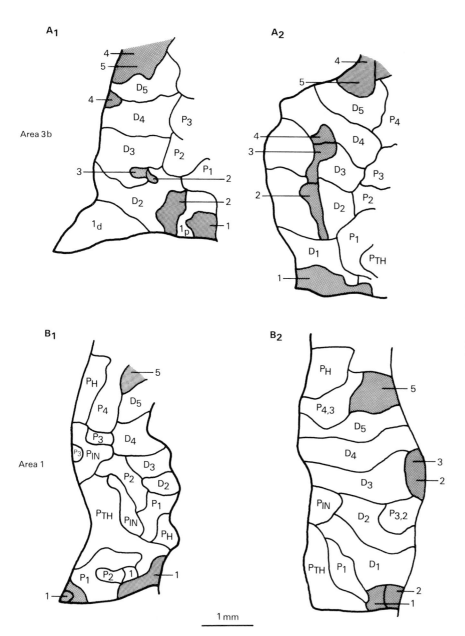

62–14 The cortical maps of the hand surfaces in areas 3b and 1 obtained from two normal owl (**A**) and squirrel (**B**) monkeys illustrate the striking variations that occur naturally from one individual to another. Again, the ventral surface of the hand is indicated in **white.** The dorsal surface is **shaded.** (From Merzenich, 1985.)

curs at least in part at the level of the dorsal column nuclei, which contain the first synapses of the somatic sensory system. Organizational changes are therefore probably a general property of the system and occur throughout the somatic afferent pathway. The fact that anatomical changes occur so early in sensory processing suggests that the substrates of higher mental processing are also labile and capable of influence by experience.

The cortical maps of an adult, and indeed the whole adult sensory system, are probably subject to constant modification on the basis of use or activity of the peripheral sensory pathways. Since all of us are brought up in somewhat different environments and use our bodies and senses differently, it is clear that the architecture of our brains will be shaped in unique ways. This architecture,

in turn, will interact importantly with our unique genetic constitution to shape the biological basis and therefore the psychological expression of our individuality.

Two further studies by Merzenich have provided evidence consistent with this view. First, he studied normal animals and found that the topographical maps vary considerably from one animal to another (Figure 62–14). This study, of course, does not separate the effects of different experiences from the consequences of different heredity. Merzenich and his colleagues therefore investigated the factors that underlie this variability in a second series of experiments. They encouraged monkeys to use their middle fingers at the expense of other fingers in the hand by having the monkey press a rotary disc for food with only these fingers. After several thousand bar presses, the area in the cortex devoted to the middle fingers was greatly expanded. These findings suggest that such practice acts on preexisting patterns of connections and strengthens their effectiveness.

Studies of Neuronal Changes with Learning Provide Insights into Psychiatric Disorders

The demonstration that learning is accompanied by changes in the effectiveness of connections has led us to a new way of viewing the relationship between social and biological processes in the generation of behavior. There is a tendency in medicine and psychiatry to think that biological determinants of behavior act on a different level of the mind than do social and functional determinants. For example, it is still customary to classify psychiatric illnesses into two major categories: organic and functional. *Organic* mental illnesses include the dementias and the toxic psychoses; *functional* mental illnesses include the various depressive syndromes, the schizophrenias, and the neurotic illnesses. This distinction dates to the nineteenth century, when neuropathologists examined the brains of patients coming to autopsy and found gross and readily demonstrable disturbance in the architecture of the brain in some psychiatric diseases but not in others. Diseases that produced anatomical evidence of brain lesions were called organic; those lacking these features were called functional.

The experiments reviewed in this chapter show that this distinction is unwarranted. Everyday events—sensory stimulation, deprivation, and learning—have profound biological consequences, causing an effective disruption of synaptic connections under some circumstances, and a reactivation of connections under others. It therefore is incorrect to imply that certain diseases (organic diseases) affect mentation by producing biological changes in the brain, whereas other diseases (functional diseases) do not. All mental processes are biological and any alteration in those processes is organic.

Rather than making the distinction along biological and nonbiological lines, it is more appropriate to ask the following questions in each type of mental illness: To what degree is this biological process determined by genetic and developmental factors, to what degree is it determined by a toxic or an infectious agent, and to what degree is it environmentally or socially determined? Even in the most socially determined mental disturbances, the end result is biological, since it is the activity of the brain that is being modified. Insofar as social intervention, such as psychotherapy or counseling, works, it must work by acting on the brain, and quite likely on the connections between nerve cells. Moreover, the absence of demonstrable structural changes does not rule out the possiblity that important changes are nevertheless occurring, although they may be undetectable with available techniques. The work of David Hubel and Torsten Wiesel that we reviewed in Chapter 57 and that by Bailey and Chen illustrates nicely that the demonstration of the biological nature of mental functioning will

require more subtle anatomical methodology than the light-microscopic histology of nineteenth-century pathologists. To clarify these issues it will be necessary to develop a neuropathology of mental illness that is based on function as well as on structure. Various new imaging techniques (reviewed in Chapter 22), such as positron emission tomography and magnetic resonance imaging, may allow the noninvasive exploration of the human brain on a cell-biological level—the level of resolution that is required to understand the mechanisms of mentation and of mental disorders.

An Overall View

Cellular studies reviewed here and in Chapters 56 and 57 on synapse development lead one to think of three overlapping ontogenetic stages of synaptic modification. The first stage, that of synapse formation, occurs primarily in the developing animal and is under genetic and developmental control. The second stage, that of validation and fine tuning of newly developed synapses, occurs during critical early periods of development and requires an appropriate pattern of environmental stimulation. The third stage, the regulation of the transient and long-term effectiveness of synapses, occurs throughout later life and is determined by day-to-day experience. One of the implications of this view is that the potentialities for all behaviors of which humans are capable are built into the brain by genetic and developmental mechanisms. Environmental factors and learning bring out these latent capabilities by altering the effectiveness of preexisting pathways, thereby leading to the expression of new patterns of behavior.

It follows from this argument that everything that occurs in the brain—from the most private thoughts to commands for motor acts—represents organic, or biological, processes. We do not yet have the tools to examine complex ideas and feelings on the cellular level, but the pace of neurobiological research is quickening; in the not too distant future we may begin to have a cellular neuropsychology of human mentation and, with it, a new and therapeutically more efficacious approach to mental illness.

The merger of neurobiology and neuropsychology that we have emphasized throughout the chapters of this textbook is filled with promise. We have seen how modern psychology, which has shown that the brain stores an internal representation of experiential events, converges with neurobiology, which has shown that this representation can be understood in terms of individual nerve cells and their interconnections. From this convergence we have gained a new perspective on perception, learning, and memory. We have also seen that the concept of mentation loses none of its power or its beauty when the experimental approach is moved from the domain of psychology into the range of molecular biology. On the contrary, the combined developments in psychology and in neurobiology promise to renew interest in aspects of mentation that until now have been out of experimental reach. Although the earlier behaviorist psychology was content to explore observable aspects of behavior, advances in modern cognitive psychology indicate that investigations that fail to consider internal representations of mental events are inadequate to account for behavior. This recognition of the importance of internal representations, a conclusion intrinsic to psychoanalytic thought, might have been discouraging as recently as 10 years ago, when internal mental processes were essentially inaccessible to experimental analysis. However, subsequent developments in cell and molecular biology have made it feasible to explore elementary aspects of internal mental processes. Thus, contrary to some expectations, biological analysis is unlikely to diminish the interest in mentation or to make mentation trivial by reduction; rather, cell and molecular biology have merely expanded our vision, allowing us to perceive previously unanticipated interrelationships between biological and psychological phenomena.

The boundary between behavior and biology is arbitrary and changing. It has been imposed not by the natural contours of the disciplines, but by lack of knowledge. As our knowledge expands, the biological and behavioral disciplines will merge at certain points, and it is at these points of merger that our understanding of mentation will rest on particularly secure ground. For as we have tried to illustrate in this book, the merger of biology and cognitive psychology is more than a merger of methods and concepts. Ultimately, the joining of these two disciplines represents the emerging conviction that a coherent and biologically unified description of mentation is possible.

Selected Readings

Kandel, E. R. 1984. Steps toward a molecular grammar for learning: Explorations into the nature of memory. In K. J. Isselbacher (ed.), Medicine, Science and Society. Symposia Celebrating the Harvard Medical School Bicentennial. New York: Wiley, pp. 555–604.

Kandel, E. R., and Schwartz, J. H. 1982. Molecular biology of learning: Modulation of transmitter release. Science 218:433–443.

Merzenich, M. M., and Kaas, J. H. 1982. Reorganization of mammalian somatosensory cortex following peripheral nerve injury. Trends Neurosci. 5:434–436.

Merzenich, M. M., Kaas, J. H., Wall, J., Nelson, R. J., Sur, M., and Felleman, D. 1983. Topographic reorganization of somatosensory cortical areas 3B and 1 in adult monkeys following restricted deafferentation. Neuroscience 8:33–55.

Merzenich, M. M., Nelson, R. J., Stryker, M. P., Cyander, M. S., Schoppmann, A., and Zook, J. M. 1984. Somatosensory cortical map changes following digit amputation in adult monkeys. J. Comp. Neurol. 224:591–605.

References

Abrams, T. W., and Kandel, E. R. 1985. Roles of calcium and adenylate cyclase in activity-dependent facilitation, a cellular mechanism for classical conditioning in Aplysia. Neurosci. Abstr.

Abrams, T. W., Carew, T. J., Hawkins, R. D., and Kandel, E. R. 1983. Aspects of the cellular mechanism of temporal specificity in conditioning in Aplysia: Preliminary evidence for Ca^{2+} influx as a signal of activity. Soc. Neurosci. Abstr. 9:168.

Alkon, D. L. 1983. Learning in a marine snail. Sci. Am. 249(1):70–84.

Bailey, C. H., and Chen, M. 1983. Morphological basis of longterm habituation and sensitization in Aplysia. Science 220:91–93.

Benzer, S. 1973. Genetic dissection of behavior. Sci. Am. 229(6):24–37.

Brons, J. F., and Woody, C. D. 1980. Long-term changes in excitability of cortical neurons after Pavlovian conditioning and extinction. J. Neurophysiol. 44:605–615.

Carew, T., Castellucci, V. F., and Kandel, E. R. 1979. Sensitization in Aplysia: Restoration of transmission in synapses inactivated by long-term habituation. Science 205:417–419.

Carew, T. J., Hawkins, R. D., and Kandel, E. R. 1983. Differential classical conditioning of a defensive withdrawal reflex in Aplysia californica. Science 219:397–400.

Carew, T. J., Walters, E. T., and Kandel, E. R. 1981. Classical conditioning in a simple withdrawal reflex in Aplysia californica. J. Neurosci. 1:1426–1437.

Castellucci, V. F., Carew, T. J., and Kandel, E. R. 1978. Cellular analysis of long-term habituation of the gill-withdrawal reflex of Aplysia californica. Science 202:1306–1308.

Castellucci, V. F., and Kandel, E. R. 1974. A quantal analysis of the synaptic depression underlying habituation of the gillwithdrawal reflex in Aplysia. Proc. Natl. Acad. Sci. U.S.A. 71:5004–5008.

Castellucci, V. F., and Kandel, E. R. 1976. Presynaptic facilitation as a mechanism for behavioral sensitization in Aplysia. Science 194:1176–1178.

Castellucci, V. F., Kandel, E. R., Schwartz, J. H., Wilson, F. D., Nairn, A. C., and Greengard, P. 1980. Intracellular injection of the catalytic subunit of cyclic AMP-dependent protein kinase simulates facilitation of transmitter release underlying behavioral sensitization in Aplysia. Proc. Natl. Acad. Sci. U.S.A. 77:7492–7496.

Dudai, Y. 1985. Genes, enzymes, and learning in Drosophila. Trends Neurosci. 8:18–21.

Dudai, Y., Jan, Y.-N., Byers, D., Quinn, W. G., and Benzer, S. 1976. dunce, a mutant of Drosophila deficient in learning. Proc. Natl. Acad. Sci. U.S.A. 73:1684–1688.

Hawkins, R. D., Abrams, T. W., Carew, T. J., and Kandel, E. R. 1983. A cellular mechanism of classical conditioning in Aplysia: Activity-dependent amplification of presynaptic facilitation. Science 219:400–405.

Hoyle, G. 1979. Mechanisms of simple motor learning. Trends Neurosci. 2:153–155.

Kaas, J. H., Nelson, R. J., Sur, M., Lin, C.-S., and Merzenich, M. M. 1979. Multiple representations of the body within the primary somatosensory cortex of primates. Science 204:521–523.

Kandel, E. R., Abrams, T., Bernier, L., Carew, T. J., Hawkins, R. D., and Schwartz, J. H. 1983. Classical conditioning and sensitization show aspects of the same molecular cascade in Aplysia. Cold Spring Harbor Symp. Quant. Biol. 48:821–830.

Klein, M., and Kandel, E. R. 1978. Presynaptic modulation of voltage-dependent Ca^{2+} current: Mechanism for behavioral sensitization in Aplysia californica. Proc. Natl. Acad. Sci. U.S.A. 75:3512–3516.

Lewis, M. 1971. Individual differences in the measurement of early cognitive growth. In J. Hellmuth (ed.), Exceptional Infant, Vol. 2: Studies in Abnormalities. New York: Brunner/Mazel, pp. 172–210.

Livingstone, M. S., Sziber, P. P., and Quinn, W. G. 1984. Loss of calcium/calmodulin responsiveness in adenylate cyclase of *rutabaga*, a Drosophila learning mutant. Cell 37:205–215.

Merzenich, M. M. 1985. Functional "maps" of skin sensations. In C. C. Brown (ed.), The Many Facets of Touch. The summary publication of Johnson & Johnson Pediatric Roundtable #10—Touch. Skillman, N. J.: Johnson & Johnson Baby Products Company, pp. 15–22.

Merzenich, M. M. 1985. Sources of intraspecies and interspecies cortical map variability in mammals: conclusion and hypotheses. In M. J. Cohen and N. C. Spitzer (eds.), Comparative Neurobiology: Modes of Communication in the Nervous System. New York: Wiley (in press).

Merzenich, M. M., Kaas, J. H., Wall, J. T., Sur, M., Nelson, R. J., and Felleman, D. J. 1983. Progression of change following median nerve section in the cortical representation of the hand in areas 3b and 1 in adult owl and squirrel monkeys. Neuroscience 10:639–665.

Quinn, W. G. 1984. Work in invertebrates on the mechanisms underlying learning. In P. Marler and H. Terrace (eds.), Biology of Learning. Dahlem Konferenzen. Berlin: Springer, pp. 197–246.

Sherrington, C. S. 1906. The Integrative Action of the Nervous System. New Haven: Yale University Press. (Reprinted 1947.)

Sherrington, C. S. 1947. The Integrative Action of the Nervous System, 2nd ed. New Haven: Yale University Press.

Shuster, M. J., Camardo, J. S., Siegelbaum, S. A., and Kandel, E. R. 1985. Cyclic AMP-dependent protein kinase closes the serotonin-sensitive K^+ channels of *Aplysia* sensory neurones in cell-free membrane patches. Nature 313:392–395.

Siegelbaum, S. A., Camardo, J. S., and Kandel, E. R. 1982. Serotonin and cyclic AMP close single K^+ channels in *Aplysia* sensory neurones. Nature 299:413–417.

Spencer, W. A., Thompson, R. F., and Neilson, D. R., Jr. 1966. Response decrement of the flexion reflex in the acute spinal cat and transient restoration by strong stimuli. J. Neurophysiol. 29:221–239.

Wall, P. D., and Egger, M. D. 1971. Formation of new connexions in adult rat brains after partial deafferentation. Nature 232:542–545.

Walters, E. T., and Byrne, J. H. 1983. Associative conditioning of single sensory neurons suggests a cellular mechanism for learning. Science 219:405–408.

Woody, C. D., Swartz, B. E., and Gruen, E. 1978. Effects of acetylcholine and cyclic GMP on input resistance of cortical neurons in awake cats. Brain Res. 158:373–395.

Woollacott, M. H., and Hoyle, G. 1976. Membrane resistance changes associated with single, identified neuron learning. Soc. Neurosci. Abstr. 2:339.

Appendix I
Brain Fluids and Their Disorders

Lewis P. Rowland

Blood–Brain Barrier, Cerebrospinal Fluid, Brain Edema, and Hydrocephalus

IA

It is always surprising to realize that the brain—the remarkable organ that makes us what we are—is 80% water, and 20% of that water is extracellular. In addition to the brain (1400 g), the cranial cavity contains blood (75 ml) and cerebrospinal fluid (75 ml). Consideration of brain fluids and the cerebrospinal fluid (CSF) is essential for understanding both the normal functions of the brain and the clinically important alterations in brain functions that arise from derangements in these fluid systems.

Cerebrospinal Fluid Is Secreted by the Choroid Plexus

Most of the CSF is found within the four ventricles, where it is secreted mainly by the *choroid plexus*, which consists of capillary networks surrounded by cuboidal or columnar epithelium (Figure I–1A). The extrachoroidal CSF is secreted by the brain capillaries. CSF flows from the lateral ventricles through the interventricular foramina (of Monro) into the third ventricle. From here it flows into the fourth ventricle through the cerebral aqueduct (of Sylvius) and then through the foramina of Magendie and Luschka into the *subarachnoid space*. The subarachnoid space lies between the arachnoid and the pia mater, which together with the dura mater form the three meninges that cover the brain (Figure I–1B). Within the subarachnoid space, fluid flows down the spinal canal and also upward over the convexity of the brain (Figure I–1A). The CSF flowing over the brain extends into the sulci and the depths of the cerebral cortex in extensions of the subarachnoid space along blood vessels called the *Virchow-Robin spaces*. Small solutes diffuse freely between the extracellular fluid and the CSF in these perivascular spaces and across the ependymal

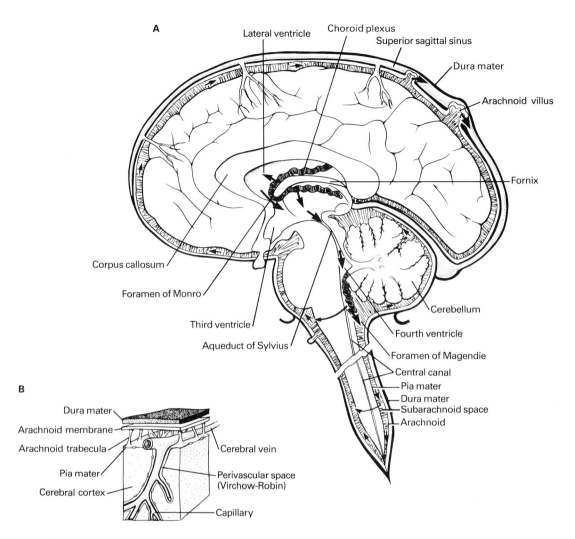

I–1 Distribution of CSF. **A.** Sites of formation, circulation, and absorption of CSF: All spaces containing CSF communicate with each other. There are choroidal and extrachoroidal sources of the fluid within the ventricular system. The CSF circulates to the subarachnoid space and is absorbed into the venous system via the arachnoid villi. The presence of arachnoid villi adjacent to the spinal roots supplements the absorption into the intracranial venous sinuses. **B.** The subarachnoid space is bounded internally by the pia mater and extends along the blood vessels that penetrate the surface of the brain. (Adapted from Kuffler and Nicholls, 1976; and Fishman, 1980.)

lining of the ventricular system, facilitating the movement of metabolites from deep within the hemispheres to cortical subarachnoid spaces and the ventricular system.

The CSF is absorbed through the *pacchionian granulations,* or *arachnoid villi.* These structures are typically found in clusters and appear as grossly visible herniations of the arachnoid membrane through the dura and into the lumen of the superior sagittal sinus and other venous structures (Figure I–1A). The villi themselves are visible only microscopically and their actual structure is still not fully understood. It is not clear whether the essential structure is a membrane that separates CSF and venous blood (a closed system), or a series of tubules within the villus that communicate directly with venous blood (an open system). A third possibility is that vacuoles form within cells of the villus membrane to transport fluid from one side of the cell to the other, a form of "vesicular transport" that combines the characteristics of both a closed and an open system (Figure I–2). In any case, the granulations appear to function as valves that allow one-way flow of CSF from the subarachnoid spaces into venous blood. This one-way flow of CSF is sometimes called *bulk flow* because all constituents of CSF leave with the fluid. Some solutes are also absorbed by the choroid plexus and brain capillaries, clearing metabolites from the brain. The rate of formation of CSF is about 0.35 ml/min or about 500 ml/day.

I–2 It is postulated that giant vacuoles transport CSF within the arachnoid villus. This mechanism could account for the one-way "bulk flow" of CSF from the subarachnoid space to the venous system. The arachnoid cells have tight intercellular junctions. Some vesicles are large enough to encompass red blood cells. (Adapted from Fishman, 1980.)

Specific Permeability Barriers Exist between Blood and Cerebrospinal Fluid and between Blood and Brain

The composition of CSF resembles an ultrafiltrate of blood plasma, but the small differences are significant because they affect brain excitability (Table I–1). The concentrations of potassium, bicarbonate, calcium, and glucose are lower and the pH is lower in CSF than in blood plasma. On the other hand, the CSF contains more magnesium and chloride than plasma. These differences are due to regulation of the constituents of CSF by active transport. The formation of CSF in the choroid plexus seems to involve both capillary filtration and active epithelial secretion. Normally, blood plasma and CSF are in osmotic equilibrium.

Table I–1. Comparison of Serum and Cerebrospinal Fluid

Component	CSF[a]	Serum[a]
Water content (%)	99	93
Protein (mg/dl)	35	7000
Glucose (mg/dl)	60	90
Osmolarity (mOsm/liter)	295	295
Na^+ (meq/liter)	138	138
K^+ (meq/liter)	2.8	4.5
Ca^{++} (meq/liter)	2.1	4.8
Mg^{++} (meq/liter)	2.3	1.7
Cl^- (meq/liter)	119	102
pH	7.33	7.41

Source: Adapted from Fishman, 1980.

[a]Average or representative values.

CSF and extracellular fluids of the brain are in equilibrium, and the ultimate composition of these fluids is a function of the *blood–CSF barrier* or *blood–brain barrier* (these terms are considered equivalent because the extracellular space of the brain is in equilibrium with CSF). The concept of a blood–brain barrier was developed by Paul Ehrlich, who found that the intravenous injection of dyes (such as trypan blue) stained tissues in most organs, but not in the brain. The brain and CSF are selectively excluded by the barrier and are thus normally protected against surging fluctuations in the content of many constituents of the blood.

It is important to recognize that there is not a single, comprehensive barrier; rather, many different systems exist for excluding substances from the brain and, conversely, for transporting substances from blood to CSF or brain and vice versa (Figures I–3 and I–4). For any solute, the efficacy of the exclusion or the transport is determined by *morphological and functional characteristics of brain capillaries* and by the *biochemical and biophysical characteristics of the solute.*

It is not certain why the behavior of brain capillaries differs so much from that of vessels in other organs, but at least three obvious morphological features distinguish brain capillaries (Figure I–5). (1) There are *tight junctions* between capillary endothelial cells in the brain, unlike systemic capillaries. (2) Brain capillaries are surrounded by, and encased in, the glial foot processes of astrocytes. (3) Mitochondria are more numerous in endothelial cells of brain capillaries. These and other factors give the brain capillary endothelium a special quality that prevents many types of molecules from permeating it, making exchange depend instead on different specialized transport mechanisms. Thus, the brain capillary endothelium is

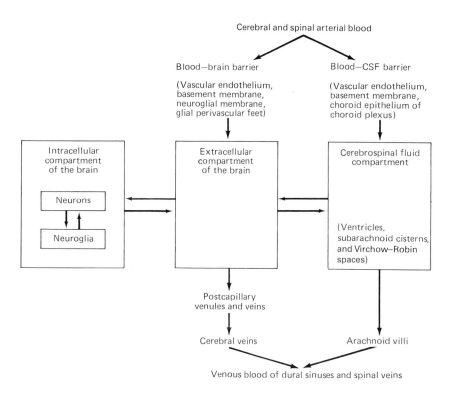

I-3 The structural and functional relationships involved in the blood–brain and blood–CSF barriers. Tissue elements that may participate in forming the barriers are indicated in **parentheses.** Substances entering the neurons and glial cells (i.e., intracellular compartment) must pass through the cell membrane. **Arrows:** direction of fluid flow under normal conditions. (Adapted from Carpenter, 1978.)

functionally more like a secretory membrane than like the capillary endothelium in other organs.

The characteristics of the solute also affect permeability. The size of the molecule is crucial. Small molecules in the blood, such as sucrose (molecular weight 360), enter the brain at a much more rapid rate than large molecules, such as inulin (molecular weight 5000), and both enter more rapidly than any protein. This probably accounts for the fact that the normal level of albumin in CSF is only 0.5% of that in plasma. Many larger proteins do not enter at all; and, under normal conditions, substances that are bound to serum proteins (including bilirubin and many drugs) also do not enter CSF or extracellular fluids of the brain.

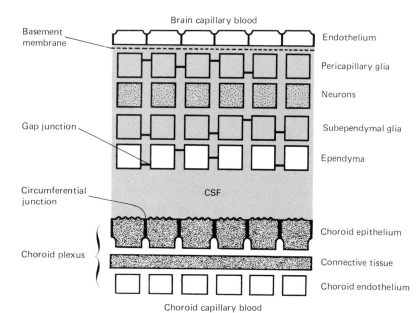

I-4 Cells involved in the exchange of materials among blood, CSF, and intercellular spaces. Molecules are free to diffuse through the endothelial cell layer lining capillaries in the choroid plexus. They are, however, restrained by circumferential junctions between the choroid epithelial cells that secrete CSF. There is also a circumferential seal occluding their passage between the endothelial cells lining brain capillaries (see Figure I–5). These barriers prevent free diffusion of molecules out of the blood. (Adapted from Kuffler and Nicholls, 1976.)

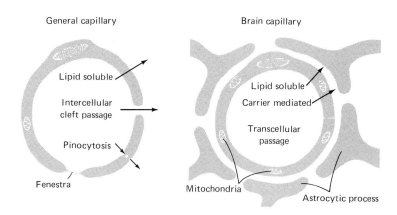

I–5 The ultrastructural features of the capillary endothelial cells of the brain differ from those of general (systemic) capillaries. Note the relative absence of pinocytotic vesicles, the greatly increased number of mitochondria, and the presence of tight junctions in brain capillaries, whereas general capillaries have clefts, fenestrae, and prominent pinocytotic vesicles. (Adapted from Fishman, 1980.)

Lipid solubility also enhances the transport of substances. For example, lipid-soluble substances, such as carbon dioxide, oxygen, and many drugs, enter the brain rapidly. Ionized polar compounds, such as bicarbonate, enter the brain slowly unless there is a specific transport system for them.

The third essential component of the blood–brain barrier comprises the carrier-mediated transport systems for sugars, other metabolites, and some amino acids. The specificity of these transport systems has many practical consequences. For instance, dopamine does not enter the brain from blood plasma, but its precursor, L-dihydroxyphenylalanine (L-DOPA), does enter and has been used effectively to treat parkinsonism (see Chapter 40). Many of these transport systems are bidirectional, mediating the transport of some substances out of the brain and the CSF and into the blood plasma, as well as controlling entry.

The influence of these barrier systems can be understood by considering the actions of penicillin, an important antibiotic used to treat some forms of meningitis. In normal individuals, penicillin is virtually excluded from CSF for at least three reasons: (1) It is an organic acid of low solubility in lipids. (2) In plasma, penicillin is bound to albumin. (3) In the choroid plexus, there is a transport system that moves penicillin out of CSF and into blood. Each of these characteristics limits the amount of penicillin in the CSF under normal circumstances. In meningitis, however, the barrier is less effective and the antibiotic is able to enter in amounts sufficient to be therapeutic.

There are barriers in the capillaries at all levels of the brain and spinal cord, and also in the choroid plexus. As Robert Fishman has pointed out, the permeability barriers provide a *system to preserve homeostasis in the nervous system, facilitating the entry of necessary metabolites, but blocking entry or facilitating removal of unnecessary metabolites or toxic substances.* It is important to recognize the distinction between *net change* in the content of any constituent of CSF and *exchange* between plasma and CSF, which also occurs at all levels. For instance, if radioactive Na^+ or K^+ is present in the plasma, the isotope may appear in the CSF or brain without a change in the total concentration of the ion in either plasma or CSF; radioactive and stable ions would have been exchanged without a net change. Water molecules are also exchanged. Furthermore, both water and solutes of CSF are removed by bulk flow through the pacchionian granulations.

The Blood–Brain Barrier Breaks Down in Some Diseases

In many diseases the blood–brain barrier does not function effectively and substances that are normally excluded may enter the brain—as already illustrated by the example of penicillin. Failure of the barrier has practical implications. For instance, albumin labeled with radioactive iodine has been used to detect brain tumors and other focal brain lesions. Because the barrier within the lesion breaks down, albumin can enter the lesion but does not reach normal parts of the brain. The accumulating radioactivity in the restricted area of the lesion can then be localized by external detectors. Radioactive tracers have now been largely supplanted by computerized tomography, but breakdown of the blood–brain barrier allows iodinated compounds to pass from the blood into the lesions, and can therefore be used to enhance the computerized image.

Stanley Rapoport at the National Institutes of Health found that brief periods of hyperosmolarity can temporarily increase the permeability of the blood–brain barrier, apparently by opening (unzipping) the tight junctions of the capillary endothelial cells. Some investigators are therefore treating brain tumors or infections by administering intracarotid injections of hypertonic solutions of urea, followed by injections of the appropriate antibiotics, chemotherapeutic agents, or specific antibodies. By this means it is sometimes possible to achieve beneficial effects with agents that would otherwise be excluded from the brain. On the other hand, as we shall see below in relation to cerebral edema, pathological alteration of the barrier may have adverse consequences.

Cerebrospinal Fluid Has Multiple Functions

The composition of CSF is in equilibrium with brain extracellular fluid and is therefore important in maintaining a constant external environment for neurons and glia. The CSF also provides a mechanical cushion to protect the brain from impact with the bony calvarium when the head moves. By its buoyant action, the CSF allows the brain to float, thereby reducing its weight from 1400 g in air to less than 50 g in situ. The CSF may also serve as a lymphatic system for the brain and as a conduit for some polypeptide hormones and other substances. The pH of CSF affects both pulmonary ventilation and cerebral blood flow—another example of the homeostatic role of CSF.

The Composition of Cerebrospinal Fluid May Be Altered in Disease

Normally the CSF does not contain *red or white blood cells.* White blood cell counts greater than 5/μl are pathological. In acute bacterial meningitis, the count may reach 5000/μl. Cells may be increased moderately in viral infections or in response to cerebral infarction, brain tumor, or other cerebral tissue damage. Tumor cells in CSF can be collected on filters and identified by their characteristic morphology.

Protein content may be increased by almost any pathological process of the brain or spinal cord, presumably because of changes in vascular permeability to protein. Protein content greater than 500 mg/dl is usually a manifestation of a block in the spinal subarachnoid space by a tumor or other compressive lesion. The gamma globulin content is disproportionately increased to more than 13% of total protein in multiple sclerosis and a few other diseases. Because this may occur without a corresponding increase in blood gamma globulin content, the increase in the CSF is attributed to the production of the immunoglobulins within the brain. In multiple sclerosis, the abnormal immunoglobulins can also be identified as "oligoclonal bands" by electrophoresis.

The concentration of *glucose* is decreased in acute bacterial infections and only exceptionally in viral infections. In chronic diseases, a CSF glucose content less than 40 mg/dl implies a tumor in the meninges, fungal or tuberculous infection, or sarcoidosis. The basis for the reduced CSF glucose content is not clear: it may be due to impaired transport into CSF; to excessive utilization by organisms, blood cells, tumor cells, or the brain itself; or to combinations of these mechanisms.

Cultures of CSF are used to identify the *causal organism* in infections. Other constituents, such as homovanillic acid or cyclic adenosine 3',5'-monophosphate, are being evaluated, but abnormalities have not yet been shown to be diagnostic of specific disorders.

The *gross appearance* of CSF is clinically important. The fluid is normally clear and colorless. It may appear cloudy when it contains many leukocytes. It also can appear grossly bloody or different shades of yellow (xanthochromia) when blood pigments are left behind after a hemorrhage or when CSF protein content is greater than 150 mg/dl, indicating that bilirubin (bound to albumin) has been brought from the plasma to the CSF.

Increased Intracranial Pressure May Harm the Brain

CSF pressure is ordinarily measured by *lumbar puncture*, a procedure in which a needle is inserted through the skin, between the fourth and fifth lumbar vertebrae, and into the lumbar subarachnoid space, with the patient lying sideways (lateral decubitus position). Because the spinal cord extends only to the first lumbar vertebra, there is no risk of injuring the cord. When the CSF flows freely through the needle, the hub of the needle is attached to a manometer and the fluid is allowed to rise. The normal pressure is 65–195 mm CSF (or water), or 5–15 mm Hg.

In measuring the lumbar CSF pressure as a guide to intracranial pressure, it is assumed that pressures are equal throughout the neuraxis. Normally, this is a reasonable assumption. In many pathological states (such as brain tumor or obstruction of CSF pathways), however, this assumption may not be true. For this reason, and also because the lumbar needle cannot be left in place for prolonged periods, catheters are sometimes inserted into the lateral ventricles to measure pressure there. Equally effective are pressure-sensitive transducers that can be inserted under the skull for continuous monitoring of intracranial pressure.

In considering the factors that regulate intracranial pressure, the cranium and spinal canal may be regarded as a closed system. According to the *Monro-Kellie doctrine*, an increase in the volume of any one of the contents of the calvarium—brain tissue, blood, CSF, or brain fluids—must be accompanied by a decrease of another component or there will be a marked increase in intracranial pressure because the bony calvarium rigidly fixes the total cranial volume. If there is a sudden increase in intracranial blood volume—for example, during a voluntary Valsalva maneuver or a sneeze—CSF may surge into the cervical subarachnoid space momentarily, because the dura there has elastic qualities. Increased CSF volume may partially compress cerebral blood vessels. Chronic changes may be compensated for by increased absorption or decreased formation of CSF. When these compensatory mechanisms fail, CSF levels and intracranial pressures rise. Several types of abnormalities lead to this condition and the consequences vary.

Brain Edema Is a State of Increased Brain Volume Due to Increased Water Content

Brain edema may be local (surrounding contusion, infarct, or tumor) or generalized. Local brain edema may cause herniation of brain tissue (cingulate gyrus beneath falx, temporal lobe uncus across tentorium, cerebellar tonsils through foramen magnum, or cerebral cortex outward through calvarial defects after surgery or injury).

Vasogenic Edema Is a State of Increased Extracellular Fluid Volume

Vasogenic edema is the most common form of brain edema. It is attributed to increased permeability of brain capillary endothelial cells, which increases the volume of the extracellular fluid. White matter is affected more than gray matter. Vasogenic edema is revealed in positive isotope brain scans associated with brain tumor, abscess, infarct, or hemorrhage. This distortion of the blood–brain barrier is also responsible for the enhancement or increased density of lesions seen by computerized tomography after intravenous injection of media that contain iodine. Generalized forms of vasogenic edema occur in head injury, lead encephalopathy, and meningitis. Functional manifestations include focal neurological abnormalities, electroencephalographic slowing, intracranial hypertension, and impaired consciousness.

Glucocorticoids are effective in treating vasogenic edema caused by brain tumor or abscess but are of doubtful value in cerebral infarct or pseudotumor (see below). Hypertonic solutions of urea, mannitol, or glycerol may be used to treat vasogenic edema, but these solutions may affect normal brain rather than the focal lesion and, after an initial fall in CSF pressure, a rebound to even higher levels may occur because the solute is not excluded by the defective barrier in the edematous tissue. However, hypertonic solutions are often used in acute situations, as in preparing patients for definitive surgery, or in the diffuse brain edema of head injury or infection. In these conditions, alternative treatments include external drainage of CSF from the ventricles or the administration of barbiturates in doses large enough to depress cerebral metabolism and cerebral blood flow, thereby reducing intracranial volume; both of these treatments are attended by risks and are reserved for extreme conditions.

Cytotoxic Edema Is the Swelling of Cellular Elements

Cytotoxic edema is the intracellular swelling of neurons, glia, and endothelial cells, with a concomitant reduction of brain extracellular space. Cytotoxic edema occurs in hypoxia after cardiac arrest or asphyxia because failure of the ATP-dependent Na–K pump allows Na^+, and therefore water, to accumulate within cells. Another cause of cytotoxic edema is water intoxication, which follows the acute systemic hypo-osmolarity that is caused by the influx of water and is associated with acute Na^+ depletion, or inappropriate secretion of antidiuretic hormone. Under these circumstances water moves from extracellular to intracellular sites. Cytotoxic edema may also accompany other forms of edema in meningitis, encephalitis, and Reye's syndrome.

Interstitial Edema Is Attributed to Increased Water and Sodium in Periventricular White Matter

In interstitial edema, best exemplified by obstructive hydrocephalus, water and Na^+ content increase in periventricular white matter. The most effective treatment of interstitial edema is surgical shunting of CSF to relieve the obstruction. Acetazolamide may reduce CSF formation but does not do so completely; it is of limited value in interstitial edema and of no value in vasogenic edema or cytotoxic edema.

Pseudotumor cerebri or benign intracranial hypertension is thought by some researchers to be a form of interstitial edema, but this has not been proved. In this condition, increased CSF pressure is usually attended by headaches and papilledema. Mental function, however, is not depressed, as often happens in generalized cerebral edema. Moreover, hydrocephalus does not occur in this condition (implying that CSF absorption is not impaired). Thus, the cause of the increased intracranial pressure is uncertain. The condition may persist for months or years, but often seems to be self-limited.

Hydrocephalus Is an Increase in the Volume of the Cerebral Ventricles

Hydrocephalus results from one of three possible causes: oversecretion of CSF, impaired absorption of CSF, or obstruction of CSF pathways.

Oversecretion of CSF is rare but is thought to occur in some functioning tumors of the choroid plexus (papillomas) because removal of the tumor may relieve the hydrocephalus. However, subarachnoid hemorrhage and high CSF protein content also characterize these tumors and could impair the absorption of CSF.

Impaired absorption of CSF could conceivably result from any condition that raises the venous pressure, such as thrombosis and occlusion of cerebral venous sinuses, severe congestive heart failure, or removal of the jugular vein during radical neck dissections for tumors. However, well-documented cases of this type are rare. Impaired absorption is suspected as the cause of the more common communicating hydrocephalus, in which there is no obstruction of CSF flow from the lateral ventricles through the foramina of Luschka and Magendie and all four ventricles are enlarged. In this condition, CSF pressure may be high or normal. In infants, CSF pressure may not rise because the cranial sutures have not yet fused and the cranium can expand. In adults, communicating hydrocephalus may occur in some patients who survive subarachnoid hemorrhage or meningitis. This type of hydrocephalus is attributed to impaired absorption of CSF because of mechanical obstruction or otherwise impaired function of the subarachnoid granulations caused by protein and detritus. A similar mechanism is thought to explain the high CSF pressure in some patients with CSF protein content greater than 500 mg/dl due to acute peripheral neuropathy (Guillain-Barré syndrome) or spinal cord tumor.

Impaired absorption is also held responsible for the syndrome of *normal-pressure hydrocephalus.* This syndrome is of interest because it causes dementia. Dementia is a major, almost epidemic public health problem. The dementia of this disorder is unusual in that it can be relieved by shunting of CSF; however, it is difficult to identify patients who will respond. In addition to dementia, the clinical syndrome comprises unsteady gait and urinary incontinence. In a computerized tomography scan the ventricles are uniformly enlarged and there is no evidence of cortical atrophy or enlargement of the subarachnoid spaces over the convexity of the brain. In normal individuals, if ^{125}I-labeled albumin is injected into the lumbar subarachnoid space the isotope can be traced by a gamma camera up to the arachnoid granulations, but it does not enter the ventricles. In patients with normal-pressure hydrocephalus the label does not follow the normal course to the convexities, may reflux into the ventricles, and takes longer to appear in the blood. In another test, there is an excessive rise of CSF pressure when sterile saline is infused into the lumbar subarachnoid space at a rate of 0.3 ml/min. Unfortunately, no one of these criteria alone reliably predicts a successful response to shunting, and even all of them together may fail to predict the outcome. Why CSF pressure does not rise in this syndrome is also unknown.

Obstruction of CSF pathways may result from tumors, congenital malformations, or scarring. A particularly vulnerable site for all three mechanisms is the narrow cerebral aqueduct of Sylvius. *Aqueductal stenosis* may result from congenital malformations or scarring due to intrauterine infection or hemorrhage. Later in life, the aqueduct may be occluded by tumor. In another condition, obstruction of the outlets of the fourth ventricle by congenital atresia of the foramina of Luschka and Magendie may lead to enlargement of all four ventricles *(Dandy-Walker syndrome).* In early life, the cranial vault enlarges with the ventricles, but after the sutures fuse, cranial volume is fixed.

The ideal treatment of hydrocephalus would be to remove the causative factor. However, this can be done for only the few cases caused by tumors. In other cases, CSF can be diverted past the block or to a new site for absorption. Numerous ingenious surgical procedures have been attempted, but the most popular are ventriculoatrial, ventriculoperitoneal, and lumbar–peritoneal shunts. Complications include infection (meningitis or septicemia), obstruction of either end of the shunt, or subdural hematoma. Drug therapy directed toward decreasing CSF production or enhancing CSF absorption has not been successful in treating hydrocephalus, and ethical questions are raised in the treatment of infants with hydrocephalus and severe cortical atrophy.

Selected Readings

Børgesen, S. E., and Gjerris, F. 1982. The predictive value of conductance to outflow of CSF in normal pressure hydrocephalus. Brain 105:65–86.

Bradbury, M. 1979. The Concept of a Blood–Brain Barrier. New York: Wiley.

Cervós-Navarro, J., and Ferszt, R. (eds.). 1980. Advances in Neurology, Vol. 28: Brain Edema: Pathology, Diagnosis, and Therapy. New York: Raven Press.

Cutler, R. W. P., and Spertell, R. B. 1982. Cerebrospinal fluid: A selective review. Ann. Neurol. 11:1–10.

Fishman R. A., 1975. Brain edema. N. Engl. J. Med. 293:706–711.

Fishman R. A. 1980. Cerebrospinal Fluid in Diseases of the Nervous System. Philadelphia: Saunders.

Flitter, M. A. 1981. Techniques of intracranial pressure monitoring. Clin. Neurosurg. 28:547–563.

Katzman, R., and Pappius, H. M. 1973. Brain Electrolytes and Fluid Metabolism. Baltimore: Williams & Wilkins.

Milhorat, T. H. 1972. Hydrocephalus and the Cerebrospinal Fluid. Baltimore: Williams & Wilkins.

Miller, J. D. 1979. Barbiturates and raised intracranial pressure. Ann. Neurol. 6:189–193.

Rapoport, S. I. 1976. Blood–Brain Barrier in Physiology and Medicine. New York: Raven Press.

Stein, S. C., and Langfitt, T. W. 1974. Normal-pressure hydrocephalus: Predicting the results of cerebrospinal fluid shunting. J. Neurosurg. 41:463–470.

References

Carpenter, M. B. 1978. Core Text of Neuroanatomy, 2nd ed. Baltimore: Williams & Wilkins.

Kuffler, S. W., Nicholls, J. G., and Martin, A. R. 1984. From Neuron to Brain: A Cellular Approach to the Function of the Nervous System, 2nd ed. Sunderland, Mass.: Sinauer.

Shu Chien

Cerebral Blood Flow and Metabolism

IB

Proper functioning of the central nervous system depends on an adequate cerebral blood flow that delivers oxygen, glucose, and other nutrient materials and removes carbon dioxide and other metabolic products. Cerebral circulation is supplied by the internal carotid arteries and the vertebral arteries. The total blood flow to the brain is about 750–1000 ml/min; of this amount about 300 ml flows through each internal carotid and about 100–200 ml flows through the vertebral basilar system. The venous outflow is drained by the internal jugular veins and the vertebral veins. The arterial supply can be studied by angiography, which involves the intra-arterial injection of a radiopaque contrast medium and radiographic examinations. In recent years, digital subtraction angiography has been developed for visualization of cerebral blood supply following intravenous injection of contrast medium. In this discussion of cerebral blood flow we shall consider how it is measured, how it is regulated, and how it varies in health and disease.

The human brain constitutes only 2% of the total weight of the body, but it receives about 15% of the cardiac output, and its oxygen consumption is approximately 20% of that for the total body (Table I–2). These values indicate the high metabolic rate and oxygen requirement of the brain. These needs are met by a correspondingly high rate of blood flow per unit brain weight. The values given in Table I–2 are mean values for the whole brain. As we shall see later, the rates of blood flow and metabolism are greater for gray matter, where the cell bodies of the neurons are located, than for white matter. Since brain tissues contain no more than their fair share of blood volume by weight, the high blood flow reflects a rapid transit time.

Table I–2. Normal Values for Mean Cerebral Blood Flow and Oxygen Consumption

Parameter	Total body	Brain		
		Per 100 g	Total brain	Percent total body
Weight (kg)	70		1.5	2%
Blood flow (ml/min)	5000	50	750	15%
Oxygen consumption (cc/min)	250	3.3	50	20%
Blood volume (ml)	5000	4	60	1.2%

Mean Cerebral Blood Flow and Regional Cerebral Blood Flow Are Measured by Different Techniques

Several methods have been devised to measure cerebral blood flow with relatively noninvasive techniques. These methods have made possible our understanding of the mechanism of regulation of cerebral blood flow in human beings.

Mean Cerebral Blood Flow Is Measured by Arteriovenous Equilibration with Freely Diffusible Inert Gas

The first measurements of cerebral blood flow in humans were done by Kety and Schmidt, who applied the Fick principle using the inert gas, N_2O. In this method the subject is asked to breathe a gas mixture containing 15 percent N_2O, and blood samples are taken at frequent intervals from a systemic artery and from the internal jugular vein. The N_2O diffuses readily across pulmonary alveolar and capillary membranes and enters the systemic circulation. During the early phase of N_2O inhalation, the arterial N_2O concentration (C_a) is higher than the venous N_2O concentration (C_v) emerging from the brain because N_2O readily crosses the capillary and cell membranes and is dispersed in the tissue (Figure I–6, t_1 and t_2). After approximately 10 min of inhalation (Figure I–6, t_{eq}), equilibration of N_2O is achieved between the arterial blood and venous blood, and the blood N_2O concentration ($C_{eq} = C_a = C_v$ at this time, in cubic centimeters N_2O per milliliter blood) is also in equilibrium with that in tissue (C_t, in cubic centimeters N_2O per gram tissue). The two concentrations are related by the tissue–blood partition coefficient (λ, in milliliters per gram):

$$C_t = \lambda C_{eq}.$$

The λ for N_2O partition between brain and blood is approximately 1 ml/gram.

The quantity of N_2O dispersed in the brain at equilibrium is equal to the cumulative difference between the rates of arterial influx of N_2O ($\dot{V}C_a$) and venous efflux of N_2O ($\dot{V}C_v$) during the period of equilibration (from t_0 to t_{eq}). $\dot{V}$ is the rate of blood flow (in milliliters per minute) and it is assumed to be constant during the period of study. Therefore:

$$\frac{\dot{V}}{M} = \frac{\lambda C_{eq}}{\displaystyle\sum_{t_0 \to t_{eq}} (C_a - C_v)}.$$

where M is the brain weight. The cerebral blood flow per unit brain weight ($\dot{V}/M$) can thus be determined by sequential sampling of arterial and internal jugular venous blood and by analysis of their N_2O concentrations throughout the equilibration process during N_2O inhalation. In place of N_2O, other inert gases that are freely diffusible across capillary and cell membranes can also be used for the same determination.

The Kety-Schmidt method provided most of the initial information on the regulation of cerebral blood flow and the metabolism. However, it has several disadvantages: (1) it gives only the mean cerebral blood flow per unit brain weight, without distinguishing between different types of brain tissues (gray matter or white matter) or

I–6 Mean cerebral blood flow is measured by equilibration with N_2O.

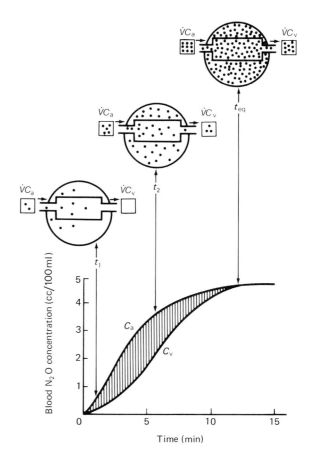

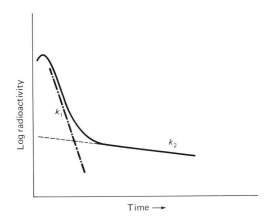

I–7 Semilogarithmic plot of ^{133}Xe radioactivity in the head. The rates of washout k_1 and k_2 represent those from gray matter and from white matter, respectively.

different regions of the brain; (2) the method is invasive, and the painful sensation and discomfort may alter the mean cerebral blood flow; and (3) the procedure requires relatively long periods of time and the analysis of many samples. The N_2O inhalation and arteriovenous sampling method has now been replaced by techniques that allow the determination of regional cerebral blood flow.

Regional Cerebral Blood Flow Is Measured by the Equilibrium Diffusion Technique

Techniques for measuring regional cerebral blood flow usually involve the inhalation or the intravenous or intra-carotid injection of a radioactive diffusible indicator (e.g., ^{133}Xe gas) and the monitoring of intracranial radioactivity by means of extracranial detectors. Because of the noninvasive nature of the inhalation technique, it is the method of choice.

The rate of washout *(k)* of the diffusible indicator from a tissue depends on the rate of blood flow per unit tissue mass *($\dot{V}/M$)* and the tissue–blood partition coefficient *(λ)*:

$$k = (\dot{V}/M)/\lambda$$

Following an intra-carotid bolus injection of the diffusible indicator, the semilogarithmic curve plotting radioactivity against time shows a two-exponential decay (Figure I–7). The later, slower rate of decay (k_2) is attributable to the washout from white matter (w). By extrapolating this slow component back to zero time and subtracting the extrapolated values from the results recorded in the early phase, we obtain the more rapid rate of washout (k_1) from gray matter (g). Thus,

$$(\dot{V}/M)_g = k_1\lambda_g$$

$$(\dot{V}/M)_w = k_2\lambda_w$$

where λ_g ($\simeq$ 0.8 ml/g) and λ_w ($\simeq$ 1.5 ml/g) are the tissue–blood partition coefficients for gray matter and white matter, respectively. Flow per unit mass of gray matter, $(\dot{V}/M)_g$, is approximately four times that of white matter, $(\dot{V}/M)_w$. With the use of the noninvasive inhalation input, these two components cannot be easily resolved by such graphical means. The initial slope, which represents primarily the gray matter blood flow, is usually used as an index of analysis.

By using a detector consisting of multiple monitoring probes, we can obtain the washout curves in different regions of the brain (Figure I–8), and regional cerebral blood flows can be determined with the aid of data storage and computation devices. Regional cerebral blood flow can also be studied by using dynamic computerized X-ray tomography (CT), in which the regional washout of nonradioactive xenon is computed from changes in CT density, following the saturation of brain tissues during a prior period of xenon inhalation.

The determination of regional cerebral blood flow is more valuable than mean cerebral blood flow because many of the physiological changes and clinical abnormalities are confined to a specific region and may not be manifested in the average flow measurements made on the whole brain.

Cerebral Blood Flow Is Affected by Changes in Arterial Pressure and Cerebral Flow Resistance

The brain is an organ with no significant capacity for anaerobic metabolism; its proper functioning depends on an adequate circulatory transport. The regulation of cerebral blood flow $(\dot{V}_b)$ is geared to maintain cerebral metabolism

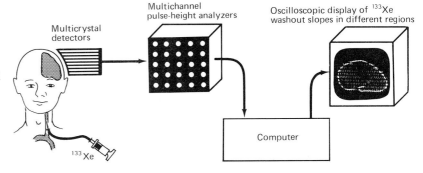

I–8 Instrumentation for determination of regional cerebral blood flow.

and local homeostasis. $\dot{V}_b$ is a function of the pressure gradient and the cerebral vascular resistance (R_b):

$$\dot{V}_b = (P_a - P_{ijv})/R_b$$

where P_a is the arterial pressure and P_{ijv} is the internal jugular venous pressure. The pressure gradient is determined primarily by the arterial pressure, which is regulated within narrow limits under normal conditions by circulatory reflexes and other control mechanisms. Resistance to cerebral flow is a function of the blood viscosity and the size of cerebral vessels. The factors regulating arterial pressure and cerebral flow resistance are briefly described below.

Arterial Pressure Is Regulated by Circulatory Reflexes

Baroreceptor Reflex. Arterial pressure is regulated by many circulatory reflexes, the most important of which are the baroreceptor reflexes. Baroreceptors are located in the aortic arch and carotid sinuses, and the frequency of firing of these receptors varies directly with the arterial pressure as well as with the rate of rise of the arterial pressure. An increase in baroreceptor impulses causes reflex inhibition of sympathetic adrenergic efferents to the cardiovascular system and a reflex stimulation of the cardiac vagus nerve, leading to a decrease in arterial pressure. The baroreceptors are tonically active when arterial pressure is normal. Therefore, a decrease in arterial pressure causes a reduction of baroreceptor impulses and a rise in arterial pressure. It is important to realize that the carotid sinus baroreceptors are located just at the point of inflow to the cerebral circulation. They therefore monitor the perfusion pressure to the brain.

Cerebral Ischemic Response. The baroreceptors cease to discharge when the arterial pressure falls below 50–60 mm Hg. Under these severely hypotensive conditions, vasomotor neurons in the brain are stimulated by the resulting ischemia and cause sympathetic excitation of the cardiovascular system as a last resort to maintain the arterial pressure.

Cerebral Flow Resistance Is Subject to Several Types of Regulation

Factors involved in the control of the resistance are the viscosity of the blood and the size and number of resistance vessels. Because of the approximately fourth-power influence of vessel radius on resistance, it is generally regarded as the predominant regulatory factor in resistance control. The size of the resistance vessels is under the influence of neural control and autoregulation.

Blood Viscosity. A major factor in controlling blood viscosity is the concentration of red blood cells. Anemia causes a decrease in blood viscosity and an increase in cerebral blood flow, with the result that oxygen delivery is maintained at approximately normal levels despite the lowering of oxygen carrying capacity of the blood.

Neural Regulation. There is evidence that the sympathetic adrenergic system can cause cerebral vasoconstriction, but this action is weak under normal conditions compared to that seen in many other parts of the circulation. In hypertensive states, adrenergically induced vasoconstriction of cerebral arteries and arterioles may play an important role in the control of blood flow and the regulation of capillary pressure within normal limits.

Autoregulation (Independent of Vasomotor Neurons). Local metabolic factors, such as an increase in P_{CO_2}, a decrease in pH, or a decrease in P_{O_2}, cause vasodilation ($\downarrow R_b$) and an increase in cerebral blood flow (Figure I–9A). Changes in these metabolic factors in the opposite direction lead to vasoconstriction and a decrease in cerebral blood flow. The influence of P_{CO_2} on cerebral vascular resistance is one of the most important factors controlling cerebral blood flow, and this effect is probably mediated by alterations in perivascular pH. Animal experiments have shown that local concentrations of adenosine and K^+, both of which cause vasodilation, may also play a significant role as metabolic mediators for the autoregulation of cerebral blood flow.

In addition, smooth muscle in small cerebral arteries

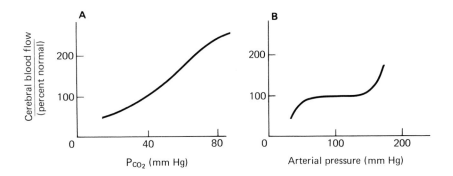

I–9 Autoregulation can alter cerebral blood flow or keep it relatively steady in response to changes in other parameters, with the result of adjusting cerebral blood flow to metabolic demand. **A.** Increased P_{CO_2} causes vasodilation and thus an increase in cerebral blood flow. **B.** Variations in arterial pressure between 60 and 140 mm Hg do not cause a significant change of cerebral flow because of autoregulation.

and arterioles can change its active tension in response to changes in transmural pressure. Thus, an increase in arterial pressure causes vasoconstriction ($\uparrow R_b$), and a decrease in arterial pressure causes vasodilation ($\downarrow R_b$). Therefore, the cerebral blood flow ($\dot{V}_b \cong P_a/R_b$) remains essentially constant for a range of mean arterial pressures from approximately 60 to 140 mm Hg (Figure I–9B).

The brain tissue is enclosed in the rigid cranium together with blood vessels and the cerebrospinal fluid. Variations in either the cerebral blood volume or cerebrospinal fluid volume can, therefore, exert pressure effects on the other components (for discussion of the Monro-Kellie doctrine, see Appendix IA). An increase in cerebrospinal fluid pressure compresses cerebral vessels and increases R_b. The autoregulatory response of arteriolar smooth muscle to this transmural pressure change is to undergo active vasodilation, thus reducing the increase in R_b somewhat.

Cerebral Blood Flow and Metabolism Change under Various Conditions

Mean Cerebral Blood Flow and Metabolism Are Affected by Certain Pathological Conditions

Mean cerebral blood flow and metabolism are not markedly affected by daily activities, such as changes in posture, muscular exercise, mental activity, or sleep. Most general anesthetics cause a reduction in cerebral metabolic rate and a concomitant decrease in cerebral blood flow. Large doses of epinephrine stimulate cerebral metabolism and increase cerebral blood flow. Mean cerebral blood flow decreases with aging, with a negative linear correlation between age (20–70 years) and mean cerebral blood flow in "healthy" subjects. Whether mean cerebral metabolic rate undergoes a parallel decline with age is controversial. Hypertension *per se* does not change cerebral circulation or metabolism unless there are arteriosclerotic changes. Anemia (by decreasing the blood viscosity) and hypoventilation (by causing vasodilation) increase cerebral blood flow, but they have no significant effect on cerebral metabolism. Cerebral metabolism and blood flow both increase in convulsion and are suppressed in coma and barbiturate poisoning. Normal and pathological changes are summarized in Table I–3.

Regional Cerebral Blood Flow and Metabolism Vary with Physiological Activities and Disease

As mentioned, measurements of mean cerebral blood flow and metabolism of the whole brain, which are not affected by daily activities, often do not reflect regional changes. In various types of physical and mental activities, regional cerebral blood flow does increase in appropriate areas of the brain specifically concerned with the activity. For example, blood flow in the occipital lobe increases during visual stimulation and blood flow in the corresponding motor areas increases during limb movements. The areas of brain tissue with increases in re-

Table I–3. Changes in Mean Cerebral Blood Flow and Metabolism Under Various Physiological and Pathological Conditions

Condition	Blood flow[a]	Metabolism[a]
Daily activity		
Posture (effect of standing)	slight $\downarrow$	—
Muscular exercise	—	—
Mental activity	—	—
Sleep	—	—
Drugs		
General anesthetics	$\downarrow$	$\downarrow$
Epinephrine (large dose)	$\uparrow$	$\uparrow$
Old age	$\downarrow$	$\downarrow$ (?)
Diseases		
Sclerosis of cerebral vessels	$\downarrow$	$\downarrow$
Hypertension (noncerebral change)	—	—
Anemia	$\uparrow$	—
Hypoventilation	$\uparrow$	—
Convulsion	$\uparrow$	$\uparrow$
Coma	$\downarrow$	$\downarrow$
Barbiturates	$\downarrow$	$\downarrow$

[a]*Symbols:* $\downarrow$ decrease; $\uparrow$ increase; — no change.

gional cerebral blood flow during a speech test are shown in Figure I–10.

Determinations of regional cerebral blood flow provide information on the local derangement of blood flow in disease states and elucidate the intracerebral redistribution of blood flow in various conditions. An example of this is the response of regional cerebral blood flow to CO_2 inhalation in patients after a cerebral stroke. Inhalation of CO_2 can cause significant increases of the reduced cerebral blood flow in most of the regions studied, but often the region with the lowest resting flow suffers

I–10 Regional cerebral blood flow increases in the shaded areas during a speech test. The activated regions include the mouth–tongue–larynx area of the somatosensory and motor cortex, the supplementary motor area, and the auditory cortex.

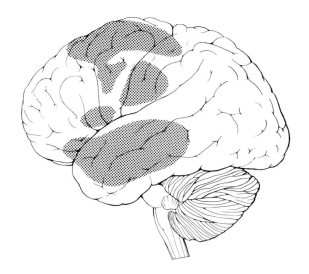

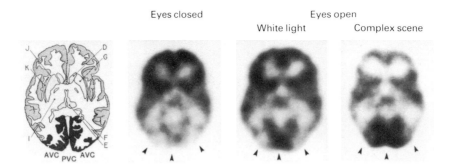

I–11 Positron emission tomographs taken at brain level at 4.4 cm above the orbitalmeatal plane. The sketch at the left was made from actual brain slices to illustrate some of the cerebral structures at the cross-sectional levels of the tomographic study. **D**, Head of the caudate nucleus; **E**, thalamus; **F**, posterior horn of the lateral ventricle; **G**, putamen and globus pallidus; **I**, internal capsule; **J**, external capsule;

PVC, primary visual cortex; **AVC**, associative visual cortex. Positron emission tomographs obtained during an eyes-closed control period and following visual stimulation with white light and complex scene. Increasing gray scale is proportional to the glucose metabolic rate, with black being the highest. (Adapted from Phelps et al., 1983.)

a further decrease in flow upon inhalation of CO_2. This reflects a loss of the vasodilation response to CO_2 in the most severely affected region. When vasodilation is induced by CO_2 in other regions, the blood flow through the undilated region decreases because blood flow is shunted to the dilated areas. This phenomenon is referred to as intracerebral steal.

The technique of *positron emission tomography* (Chapter 22) can be used to determine regional cerebral blood flow and metabolism of the human brain. Substances containing short-lived positron-emitting radionuclides (e.g., ^{15}O, ^{13}N, ^{11}C, ^{18}F, and ^{77}Kr) are used for this purpose. Positrons (positively charged electrons) interact with electrons to yield annihilation radiation and two photons traveling in opposite directions. With the use of radiation coincidence detectors of the two photons, and with the aid of computerized processing, the brain image of the distribution of the nuclide can be obtained as a function of time.

Positron emission tomography (PET) can be used to measure regional cerebral blood flow following the administration of a diffusible tracer (e.g., inhalation of ^{77}Kr). The regional cerebral blood flow measurements obtained in this manner agree well with those determined with the use of ^{133}Xe.

Regional cerebral metabolism can be quantified by PET using either radiolabeled metabolic substrates (e.g., ^{11}C-glucose) or radiolabeled, metabolically inert analogues of these substrates, e.g., ^{18}F-labeled 2-deoxy-2-fluoro-D-glucose (FDG). Since glucose is the energy source for neurons, cells take up more glucose when they are active than when they are at rest. The FDG is taken up by active cells as if it were glucose; it is phosphorylated, but FDG-6-PO_4 is not a substrate for subsequent metabolism and hence accumulates in the cell. The amount of radioactivity accumulated measures the extent of neuronal activity. This method allows one to localize anatomically regions of functional activity in the brain of living humans in a safe, noninvasive way.

In the gray matter of the cerebral cortex of normal human subjects, the metabolic rate for glucose ranges from approximately 7 mg/100 g/min in the parietal cortex to 10 mg/100 g/min in the visual cortex; the subcortical white matter has a rate of approximately 4 mg/100 g/min.

Sensory activation and performance of motor tasks result in an increase in local glucose metabolism in regions of the brain concerned with such activities. For example, Figure I–11 illustrates the increases in glucose metabolic rate in the visual cortex following visual stimulation.

Positron emission tomography has been used to evaluate regional cerebral metabolism in a variety of pathologic states. In patients with epileptic seizures, PET shows areas of altered glucose metabolic rates that can be correlated with regions of abnormal electroencephalographic activities. The size and distribution of the metabolic defect are typically larger than those of the pathologic lesion determined at autopsy, indicating that PET can detect regions of functional derangement wider than the areas of gross structural alterations.

With the use of PET and $^{15}O_2$, one can measure the regional cerebral oxygen extraction fraction (OEF), which is a function of the arterial O_2 content (AO_2), the regional cerebral metabolic rate for oxygen ($CMRO_2$), and regional CBF:

$$OEF \times AO_2 = CMRO_2/CBF$$

Thus, OEF reflects the relation of oxygen consumption to blood flow. An example of such studies is shown in Figure I–12. Regional CBF and OEF were determined by PET and ^{15}O continuous inhalation (as $^{15}O_2$ and $C^{15}O_2$) in a patient with a left internal carotid occlusion and focal transient ischemic attacks. Preoperative studies showed a marked decrease in CBF (estimated from $C^{15}O_2$) in the region corresponding to the patient's clinical

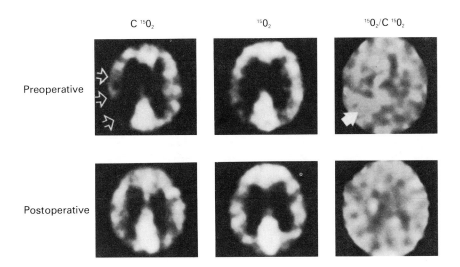

C $^{15}O_2$ $^{15}O_2$ $^{15}O_2/C^{15}O_2$

Preoperative

Postoperative

symptoms (arrows). The increase in oxygen extraction (estimated from $^{15}O_2/C^{15}O_2$) served to compensate for the hypoperfusion, thus minimizing the decrease in $CMRO_2$ and maintaining the functional viability of the ischemic tissue. After bypass surgery, which reestablished the perfusion of the ischemic brain tissues, the postoperative parameters returned to normal and the transient ischemic attacks disappeared.

By simultaneous measurements of cerebral blood flow and metabolism, flow–metabolism mismatch has been found in patients with cerebrovascular disease. For example, in many patients during the first month after a stroke, cerebral blood flow in the infarct region may increase while oxygen consumption decreases; this "luxury perfusion" is associated with a decrease in oxygen extraction. In other patients, cerebral blood flow in the ischemic area decreases either in proportion to or more than the cerebral oxygen consumption. This "misery perfusion" is associated with a normal or increased oxygen extraction. These results indicate that, in acute infarction, one cannot predict the metabolic status, which is the important parameter determining functional viability, from cerebral blood flow measurements alone. Concomitant determinations of blood flow, oxygen consumption, and glucose metabolic rate would allow the evaluation of flow/metabolism matching and also the coupling between oxygen and glucose metabolism.

The recent development of technology in magnetic resonance imaging (MRI) has provided us with a method not only for the imaging of human anatomy, but also for the assessment of biochemical status and physiological functions, and all of these are accomplished in a noninvasive manner without the use of ionizing radiation. The MRI method is based on the spin of the particles (protons and neutrons) in the atomic nuclei about their axes. When placed in a uniform static magnetic field, a portion of the spinning nuclei will be aligned. The application of a smaller external electromagnetic field at an appropriate resonance frequency will cause the spinning

I–12 Cerebral blood flow (CBF), metabolic rate for oxygen ($CMRO_2$) and arteriovenous oxygen extraction ($^{15}O_2/C^{15}O_2$) in a patient with a left internal carotid occlusion studied before and after extracranial–intercranial bypass. Decreasing gray scale is proportional to the parameters measured, with white being the highest. (Adapted from Baron et al., 1981.)

I–13 **A:** ^{31}P spectrum from the brain of a 17-day-old infant suffering from hypotonia, probably due to congenital muscular dystrophy rather than cerebral pathology. **B:** ^{31}P spectrum from the brain of a 6-day-old infant who suffered severe birth asphyxia. (Adapted from Cady et al., 1983.)

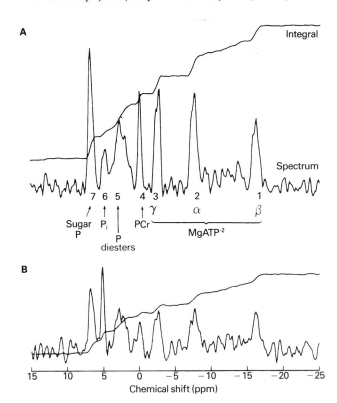

nuclei to precess around the vertical axis, i.e., they rotate around this axis like spinning tops or gyroscopes after having been tipped. This resonance frequency is determined by the gyromagnetic frequency specific for each nucleus species and the strength of the magnetic field. Therefore, by choosing the appropriate frequencies, one can tune in to specific nuclei (e.g., ^1H or ^{31}P) and observe their reactions. Medical images of brain and other tissues have been obtained by using the resonance frequency for ^1H. ^{31}P MRI has been used to study phosphorus metabolism in vivo, especially in muscle. The phosphorus spectrum shows clear peaks for sugar phosphates, inorganic phosphates (P_i), phosphocreatine (PCr), and the different phosphate groups of ATP. An example of such spectra for human infant brains is shown in Figure I–13. The infant with a motor disorder probably muscular in nature (i.e., the brain is presumably normal) has a PCr/P_i ratio of 1.66 (Figure I–13A), whereas this ratio is only 0.45 in the infant with severe birth asphyxia (Figure I–13B). This decrease in PCr/P_i ratio, which was also found in other infants with severe birth asphyxia, reflects the breakdown of phosphocreatine; the ratio increased as the clinical condition improved. The position of the inorganic phosphate peak (Figure I–13) can be used to determine the intracellular pH of brain tissue. The estimated pH in human infant brain is 7.19 ± 0.14 (S.D.), and there is no indication of significant changes in the infants with birth asphyxia. Thus, ^{31}P MRI offers an important noninvasive method for studying energy metabolism and intracellular pH. Such measurements can be made as a function of time, but the present technology does not allow the imaging of ^{31}P spectra on a regional basis comparable to the degree of size discrimination attained in CBF measurement.

Selected Readings

Dawson, M. J., and Wilkie, D. R. 1984. Muscle and brain metabolism studied by ^{31}P nuclear magnetic resonance. In P. F. Baker (ed.), Recent Advances in Physiology. Edinburgh: Churchill Livingstone, pp. 247–276, No. 10.

Fieschi, C., Lenzie, G. L., and Loeb, C. W. (eds.). 1984. Effects of Aging on Regulation of Cerebral Blood Flow and Metabolism. Monographs in Neural Science 11:51–57. Basel: Karger.

Heistad, D. D., and Kontos, H . A. 1983. Cerebral circulation. In J. T. Shepherd and F. M. Abboud (eds.), Handbook of Physiology, Section 2: The Cardiovascular System, Vol. III, Peripheral Circulation and Organ Blood Flow. Bethesda, Md.: American Physiological Society, pp. 137–182.

Ingvar, D. H., and Schwartz, M. S. 1974. Blood flow patterns induced in the dominant hemisphere by speech and reading. Brain 97:273–288.

Reivich, M. 1982. The use of cerebral blood flow and metabolic studies in cerebral localization. In R. A. Thompson and J. R. Green (eds.), New Perspectives in Cerebral Localization. New York: Raven Press, pp. 115–144.

References

Alavi, A., Reivich, M., Jones, S. C., Greenberg, J. H., and Wolf, A. P. 1982. Functional imaging of the brain with positron emission tomography. In L. M. Freeman and H. S. Weissman (eds.), Nuclear Medicine Annual. New York: Raven Press, pp. 319–372.

Baron, J. C., Bousser, M. G., Rey, A., Guillard, A., Comar, D., and Castaigne, P. 1981. Reversal of focal "misery-perfusion syndrome" by extra-intracranial arterial bypass in hemodynamic cerebral ischemia. Stroke 12:454–459.

Cady, E. B., Costello, A. M. de L., Dawson, M. J., Delpy, D. T., Hope, P. L., Reynolds, E. O. R., Tofts, P. S., and Wilkie, D. R. 1983. Non-invasive investigation of cerebral metabolism in newborn infants by phosphorus nuclear magnetic resonance spectroscopy. Lancet 1:1059–1062.

Phelps, M. E., Schelbert, H. R., and Mazziotta, J. C. 1983. Positron computed tomography for studies of myocardial and cerebral function. Ann. Intern. Med. 98:339–359.

Reivich, M., Kuhl, D., Wolf, A., Greenberg, J., Phelps, M., Ido, T., Casella, V., Fowler, J., Hoffman, E., Alavi, A., Som, P., and Sokoloff, L. 1979. The (^{18}F)fluorodeoxyglucose method for the measurement of local cerebral glucose utilization in man. Circ. Res. 44:127–137.

John C. M. Brust

Stroke:
Diagnostic, Anatomical,
and Physiological Considerations

IC

Blood flow to the brain is highly protected, yet the brain remains highly susceptible to disturbances of the blood supply, as reflected in the high incidence of symptomatic cerebral vascular disease. Diseases of the blood vessels are among the most frequent serious neurological disorders, ranking third as a cause of death in the adult population in the United States and probably first as a cause of chronic functional incapacity. Approximately 2,000,000 people living in the United States today are impaired by the neurological consequences of cerebrovascular disease. Many of them are between 25 and 64 years of age.

The term *stroke*, or *cerebrovascular accident*, refers to the neurological symptoms and signs, usually focal and acute, that result from diseases involving blood vessels. Strokes are either *occlusive* (due to closure of a blood vessel) or *hemorrhagic* (due to bleeding from a vessel). Insufficiency of blood supply is termed *ischemia*; if it is temporary, symptoms and signs may clear with little or no pathological evidence of tissue damage. *Ischemia* is not synonymous with *anoxia*, for a reduced blood supply deprives tissue not only of oxygen, but of glucose as well, and, moreover, prevents the removal of potentially toxic metabolites such as lactic acid. When ischemia is sufficiently severe and prolonged, neurons and other cellular elements die; this condition is called *infarction*.

Hemorrhage may occur at the brain surface *(extraparenchymal)*—for example, from rupture of congenital aneurysms at the circle of Willis, causing *subarachnoid hemorrhage.* Alternatively, hemorrhage may be *intraparenchymal*—for example, from rupture of vessels damaged by long-standing hypertension—and may cause a blood clot or *hematoma* within the cerebral hemispheres, in the brain stem, or in the cerebellum. Hemorrhage may be accompanied by ischemia or infarction. The mass effect of an intracerebral hematoma may compromise the blood supply of adjacent brain tissue; or subarachnoid hemorrhage may, by unclear mechanisms, cause reactive vasospasm of cerebral surface vessels, leading to further ischemic brain damage. Infarcted tissue may also become secondarily hemorrhagic.

Although most occlusive strokes are due to atherosclerosis and thrombosis and most hemorrhagic strokes are associated with hypertension or aneurysms, strokes of either type may occur at any age from a legion of causes that include cardiac disease, trauma, infection, neoplasm, blood dyscrasia, vascular malformation, immunological disorder, and exogenous toxins. Diagnostic strategies and treatment should vary accordingly. We shali examine, however, the anatomical and physiological principles relevant to any occlusive or hemorrhagic stroke.

The Blood Supply of the Brain Can Be Divided into Arterial Territories

Figure I–14 is a schematic illustration of the brain's blood vessels. Each cerebral hemisphere is supplied by an *internal carotid artery*, which arises from a common carotid artery beneath the angle of the jaw, enters the cranium through the carotid foramen, traverses the cavernous sinus (giving off the *ophthalmic* artery), penetrates the dura, and divides into the anterior and middle cerebral arteries. The large surface branches of the *anterior cerebral artery* supply the cortex and white matter of the inferior frontal lobe, the medial surface of the frontal and parietal lobes, and the anterior corpus callosum. Smaller penetrating branches supply the deeper cerebrum and

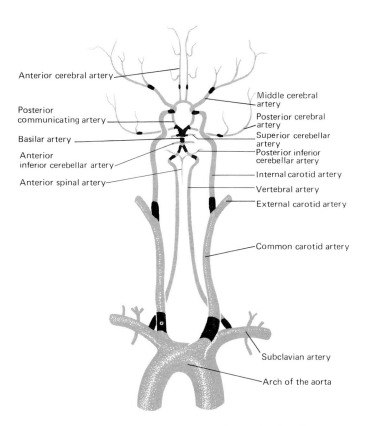

I–14 The blood vessels of the brain. The circle of Willis is made up of the proximal posterior cerebral arteries, the posterior communicating arteries, the internal carotid arteries just before their bifurcations, the proximal anterior cerebral arteries, and the anterior communicating artery. **Dark areas:** common sites of atherosclerosis and occlusion. (Adapted from Barnett, 1982.)

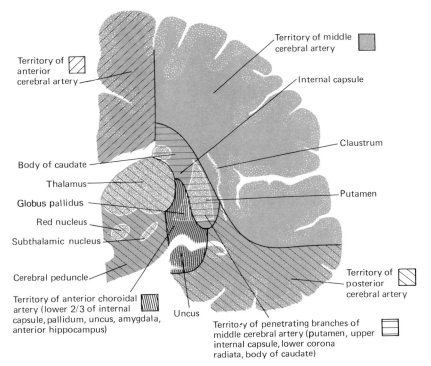

I–15 Cerebral arterial areas. (Adapted from Mohr, Fisher, and Adams, 1980.)

diencephalon, including limbic structures, the head of the caudate, and the anterior limb of the internal capsule. The large surface branches of the *middle cerebral artery* supply most of the cortex and white matter of the hemisphere's convexity, including the frontal, parietal, temporal, and occipital lobes, and the insula. Smaller penetrating branches supply the deep white matter and diencephalic structures such as the posterior limb of the internal capsule, the putamen, the outer globus pallidus, and the body of the caudate. After the internal carotid artery emerges from the cavernous sinus, it also gives off the *anterior choroidal artery*, which supplies the anterior hippocampus and, at a caudal level, the posterior limb of the internal capsule.

Each vertebral artery arises from a subclavian artery, enters the cranium through the foramen magnum, and gives off an *anterior spinal artery* and a *posterior inferior cerebellar artery*. The vertebral arteries join at the junction of the pons and the medulla to form the *basilar artery*, which at the level of the pons gives off the *anterior inferior cerebellar artery* and the *internal auditory artery* and at the midbrain the *superior cerebellar artery*. The basilar artery then divides into the two *posterior cerebral arteries*. The large surface branches of the posterior cerebral arteries supply the inferior temporal and medial occipital lobes and the posterior corpus callosum; the smaller penetrating branches of these arteries supply diencephalic structures, including the thalamus and the subthalamic nuclei, as well as parts of the midbrain.

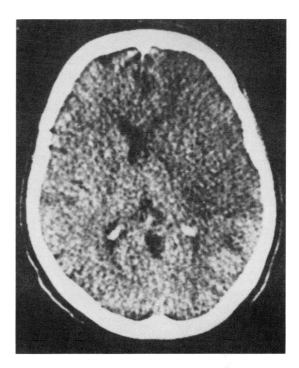

I–17 CT scan showing infarction (**dark area**) in the territory of the middle cerebral artery. (Courtesy of Dr. S. R. Ganti and Dr. Sadek K. Hilal.)

I–16 CT scan showing infarction (**dark area**) in the territory of the anterior cerebral artery. (There is also an infarction, on the same side, in the territory of a major branch of the middle cerebral artery.) (Courtesy of Dr. S. R. Ganti and Dr. Sadek K. Hilal.)

I–18 CT scan showing infarction (**dark area**) in the territory of the posterior cerebral artery. (Courtesy of Dr. S. R. Ganti and Dr. Sadek K. Hilal.)

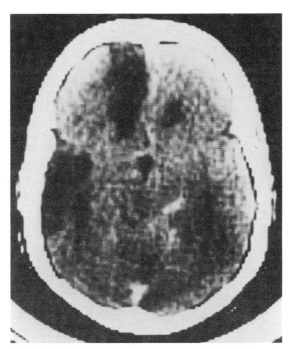

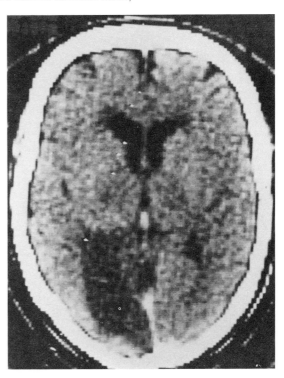

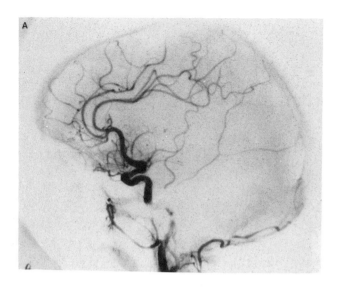

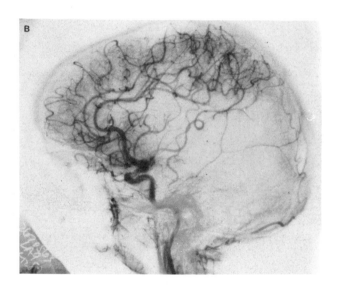

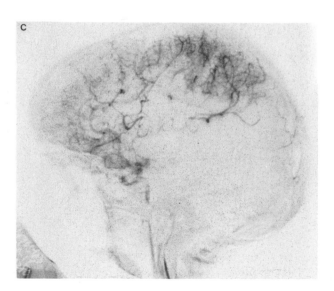

I–19 These angiograms demonstrate the importance of anastomoses in that they allow retrograde filling after occlusion of the middle cerebral artery. **A.** Occlusion of the middle cerebral artery results in no filling in the middle cerebral distribution. **B.** Retrograde filling of middle cerebral artery has begun via distal anastomotic branches of the anterior cerebral artery. **C.** Retrograde filling of middle cerebral artery continues at a time when little contrast material is seen in the anterior cerebral artery. (Courtesy of Dr. Margaret Whelan and Dr. Sadek K. Hilal.)

These arterial territories are shown schematically in Figure I–15. Figures I–16, I–17, and I–18 are computerized tomography (CT) scans demonstrating infarctions in the territories of the anterior, middle, and posterior cerebral arteries, respectively.

Interconnections between blood vessels (anastomoses) protect the brain when part of its vascular supply is compromised. At the *circle of Willis* the two anterior cerebral arteries are connected by the anterior communicating artery, and the posterior cerebral arteries are connected to the internal carotid arteries by the posterior communicating arteries. The protective importance of the circle of Willis is illustrated by the fact that a congenitally incomplete circle, common in the general population, is significantly more common among patients who have had strokes. Other important anastomoses include connections between the ophthalmic artery and branches of the external carotid artery through the orbit, and connections at the brain surface between branches of the middle, anterior, and posterior cerebral arteries. The angiograms in Figure I–19 show occlusion of the middle cerebral artery with retrograde filling through anastomoses.

Clinical Vascular Syndromes May Follow Vessel Occlusion, Hypoperfusion, or Hemorrhage

Infarction Can Occur in the Middle Cerebral Artery Territory

Infarction in the territory of the middle cerebral artery (cortex and white matter) causes the most frequently encountered stroke syndrome, with contralateral weakness, sensory loss, and visual field cut, and, depending on the hemisphere involved, either language disturbance or impaired spatial perception. Weakness and sensory loss affect the face and arm more than the leg because of the somatotopy of the motor and sensory cortex (pre- and postcentral gyri): the face and arm lie on the convexity, whereas the leg resides on the medial surface of the hemisphere. Motor and sensory loss are greatest in the hand, for the more proximal limbs and the trunk tend to have greater representation in both hemispheres. Paraspinal muscles, for example, are hardly ever weak in unilateral cerebral lesions. Similarly, the facial muscles of the forehead and the muscles of the pharynx and jaw are represented bihemispherically and therefore are usually spared. Tongue weakness is variable. If weakness is severe (plegia), muscle tone is usually decreased initially and gradually increases over days or weeks to spasticity with hyperactive tendon reflexes. A Babinski sign, reflecting upper motor neuron disturbance, is usually present from the outset. When weakness is mild, or during recovery, there may be clumsiness or slowness of movement out of proportion to loss of strength; such motor disability may resemble parkinsonian bradykinesia or even cerebellar ataxia.

Acutely, there is often paresis of contralateral conjugate gaze as a result of damage to the convexity of the cortex anterior to the motor cortex (the frontal eye field). The reason this gaze palsy persists for only 1 or 2 days, even when other signs remain severe, is not clear.

Sensory loss tends to involve discriminative and proprioceptive modalities more than affective modalities. Pain and temperature sensation may be impaired or seem altered but are usually not lost. Joint position sense, however, may be severely disturbed, causing limb ataxia, and there may be loss of two-point discrimination, astereognosis (inability to recognize a held object by tactual sensation), or failure to appreciate a touch stimulus if another is simultaneously delivered to the normal side of the body (extinction).

Visual field impairment (homonymous hemianopsia) is the result of damage to the optic radiations, the deep fiber tracts connecting the thalamic lateral geniculate nucleus to the visual (calcarine) cortex. If the parietal radiation is primarily involved, the field cut may be an inferior quadrantanopsia, whereas in temporal lobe lesions quadrantanopsia may be superior.

As we have seen in Chapter 52, in more than 95% of right-handed persons and in the majority of left-handed individuals, the left hemisphere is dominant for language function. Destruction of left opercular (perisylvian) cortex in such patients causes aphasia, which may take a variety of forms depending on the degree and distribution of the damage. Frontal opercular lesions tend to produce particular difficulty with speech output and writing with relative preservation of language comprehension (Broca's aphasia), whereas infarction of the posterior superior temporal gyrus tends to cause severe difficulty in comprehending spoken speech and reading (Wernicke's aphasia). When opercular damage is widespread, there is severe language disturbance of mixed type (global aphasia).

Left-hemisphere convexity damage, especially parietal, may also cause motor apraxia, a disturbance of learned motor acts not explained by weakness or incoordination, with the ability to perform the act when the setting is altered. For example, a patient unable to imitate lighting a match might be able to perform the act normally if given an actual match to strike.

Right-hemisphere convexity infarction, especially parietal, tends to cause disturbances of spatial perception. There may be difficulty in copying simple pictures or diagrams (constructional apraxia), in interpreting maps or finding one's way about (topographagnosia), or in putting on one's clothes properly (dressing apraxia). Awareness of space and the patient's own body contralateral to the lesion may be particularly affected *(hemi-inattention* or *hemineglect).* Patients may fail to recognize their hemiplegia (anosognosia), left arm (asomatognosia), or any external object to the left of their own midline. Such phenomena may occur independently of visual field defects and in patients otherwise mentally quite intact.

Particular types of language or spatial dysfunction tend to follow occlusion, not of the proximal stem of the middle cerebral artery, but of one of its several main pial branches. In such circumstances other signs (e.g., weakness or visual field cut) may not be present. Similarly, occlusion of the Rolandic branch of the middle cerebral artery may cause motor and sensory loss affecting the face and arm without disturbance of vision, language, or spatial perception.

Infarction Can Occur in the Anterior Cerebral Artery Territory

Infarction in the territory of the anterior cerebral artery causes weakness and sensory loss qualitatively similar to that of convexity lesions but affects mainly the distal contralateral leg. There may be urinary incontinence, but it is uncertain whether this is due to a lesion of the paracentral lobule (medial hemispheric motor and sensory cortices) or of a more anterior region concerned with the inhibition of bladder emptying. Damage to the supplementary motor cortex may cause speech disturbance, considered aphasic by some and a type of motor inertia by others. Involvement of the anterior corpus callosum may cause apraxia of the left arm (sympathetic apraxia), which is attributed to disconnection of the left (language-dominant) hemisphere from the right motor cortex.

Bilateral anterior cerebral artery territory infarction (occurring, for example, when both arteries arise anomalously from a single trunk) may cause a severe behavioral disturbance, with profound apathy, motor inertia, and muteness, attributed variably to destruction of the inferior frontal lobes (orbitofrontal cortex), deeper limbic structures, supplementary motor cortices, or cingulate gyri.

Infarction Can Occur in the Posterior Cerebral Artery Territory

Infarction in the territory of the posterior cerebral artery causes contralateral homonymous hemianopsia by destroying the calcarine cortex. Macular (central) vision tends to be spared because the occipital pole, where macular vision is represented, receives blood supply from the middle cerebral artery. If the lesion is on the left and the posterior corpus callosum is affected, there may be alexia (without aphasia or agraphia), attributed to disconnection of the seeing right occipital cortex from the language-dominant left hemisphere. If infarction is bilateral (e.g., following thrombosis at the point where both posterior cerebral arteries arise from the basilar artery), there may be cortical blindness with failure of the patient to recognize that he cannot see (Anton's syndrome), or, as a result of bilateral damage to the inferomedial temporal lobes, memory disturbance.

If posterior cerebral artery occlusion is proximal, the lesion may include, or especially affect, the following structures: the thalamus, causing contralateral hemisensory loss and sometimes spontaneous pain and dysesthesia (thalamic pain syndrome); the subthalamic nucleus, causing contralateral severe proximal chorea

(hemiballism); or even the midbrain, with ipsilateral oculomotor palsy and contralateral hemiparesis or ataxia from involvement of the corticospinal tract or the crossed superior cerebellar peduncle (dentatothalamic tract).

The Anterior Choroidal and Penetrating Arteries Can Become Occluded

Anterior choroidal artery occlusion should, in theory, cause infarction of the posterior limb of the internal capsule, with contralateral hemiparesis, hypesthesia, and hemianopsia; however, such a lesion, often suspected clinically, remains to be demonstrated pathologically.

As mentioned above, the deeper cerebral white matter and diencephalon are supplied by small penetrating arteries—variably called the *lenticulostriates,* the *thalamogeniculates,* or the *thalamoperforates*—which arise from the circle of Willis or the proximal portions of the middle, anterior, and posterior cerebral arteries. These end-arteries lack anastomotic interconnections, and occlusion of individual vessels—usually in association with hypertensive damage to the vessel wall—causes small (less than 1 cm in diameter) infarcts ("lacunes"), which, if critically located, are followed by characteristic syndromes. For example, lacunes in the pyramidal tract area of the internal capsule cause "pure hemiparesis," with arm and leg weakness of equal severity, but little or no sensory loss, visual field disturbance, aphasia, or spatial disruption. Lacunes in the ventral posterior nucleus of the thalamus produce "pure hemisensory loss," with discriminative and affective modalities both involved and little motor, visual, language, or spatial disturbance. Most lacunes occur in redundant areas, e.g., nonpyramidal corona radiata, and so are asymptomatic. If bilateral and numerous, however, they may cause a characteristic syndrome *(état lacunaire)* of progressive dementia, shuffling gait, and pseudobulbar palsy (spastic dysarthria and dysphagia, with lingual and pharyngeal paralysis and hyperactive palate and gag reflexes, plus lability of emotional response, with abrupt crying or laughing out of proportion to mood).

The Carotid and Basilar Arteries Can Become Occluded

Atherothrombotic vessel occlusion often occurs in the internal carotid artery rather than the intracranial vessels. Particularly in a patient with an incomplete circle of Willis, infarction may then include the territories of both the middle and anterior cerebral arteries, with arm and leg weakness and sensory loss equally severe. Another cause of leg weakness and sensory loss in association with a convexity syndrome is occlusion of the middle cerebral artery at its proximal stem; capsular (and other diencephalic) structures supplied by the middle cerebral artery's lenticulostriate branches are then affected in addition to the cortex of the cerebral convexity.

The medial and lateral syndromes of brain stem infarction, which tend to bear annoying eponyms, have been discussed in Chapter 45. To recapitulate briefly, lateral syndromes—for example, following lateral medullary infarction, with vertigo, nystagmus, ipsilateral limb ataxia, loss of pain and temperature sensation on the ipsilateral face and contralateral arm and leg, and ipsilateral ptosis, miosis, and facial anhidrosis (Horner's syndrome)—result from the occlusion of large branches of the vertebral or basilar arteries supplying the lateral brain stem and cerebellum. Medial syndromes—for example, following medial pontine infarction, with ipsilateral abducens, gaze, or facial palsy and contralateral hemiparesis—result from occlusion of small paramedian penetrating vertebral or basilar artery branches.

In fact, most brain stem infarcts follow occlusion of the vertebral or basilar arteries, and the resulting symptoms and signs are less stereotyped than classical descriptions imply. Involvement of the posterior fossa structures in an infarct is suggested by (1) bilateral long tract (motor or sensory) signs, (2) crossed (e.g., left face and right limb) motor or sensory signs, (3) cerebellar signs, (4) stupor or coma (from involvement of the ascending reticular activating system), (5) disconjugate eye movements or nystagmus, including the syndrome of internuclear ophthalmoplegia (medial longitudinal fasciculus syndrome), and (6) involvement of cranial nerves not usually affected by single hemispheric infarcts (e.g., unilateral deafness or pharyngeal weakness).

Diffuse Hypoperfusion Can Cause Ischemia or Infarction

Brain ischemia or infarction may accompany diffuse hypoperfusion (shock), and in such circumstances the most vulnerable regions are often the border zones (watershed areas) between large arterial territories and the end-zones of deep penetrating vessels. Following recovery from, for example, carbon monoxide poisoning or cardiac arrest, a patient may have paralysis and sensory loss in both arms (from bilateral infarction of the cortex at the junction of the middle and anterior cerebral arterial supply, affecting the arm area of the motor and sensory cortex), or disturbed vision or memory (from infarction of occipital or temporal lobes at the junction of middle and posterior cerebral arterial supply). There may also be ataxia (from cerebellar border zone infarction) or abnormal movements such as chorea or myoclonus (presumably from involvement of basal ganglia). Such signs may exist alone or in combination and may be accompanied by a variety of aphasic or other cognitive disturbances.

The Rupture of Microaneurysms Causes Intraparenchymal Hemorrhage

The two most common causes of hemorrhagic stroke—hypertensive intra-axial hemorrhage and rupture of berry aneurysm—tend to occur at particular sites and to cause recognizable syndromes. Hypertensive intercerebral hemorrhage is the result of damage to the same small penetrating vessels which, when occluded, cause lacunes; in this instance, however, the damaged vessels develop weakened walls (Charcot-Bouchard microaneurysms) that eventually rupture. The most common sites are the putamen, thalamus, pons, internal capsule and corona radiata, and cerebellum. Large diencephalic hemorrhages tend to cause stupor and hemiplegia and have a high mortality rate.

With lesions to the putamen, the eyes are usually deviated ipsilaterally (due to disruption of capsular pathways descending from the frontal gaze center), whereas with thalamic hemorrhage the eyes tend to be deviated downward and the pupils may not react to light (due to involvement of midbrain pretectal structures essential for upward gaze and pupillary light reactivity—Parinaud's syndrome). Small hemorrhages may not impair alertness; with thalamic hemorrhage, sensory loss may then be found to exceed weakness. Moreover, CT has shown that small thalamic hemorrhages may cause aphasia when on the left and hemi-inattention when on the right. Figures I–20 and I–21 are CT scans showing a large putaminal and a small thalamic hemorrhage, respectively.

Pontine hemorrhage, unless quite small, usually causes coma (by disrupting the reticular activating sys-

I–20 CT scan showing hemorrhage in the putamen (hematoma is **light area**). (Courtesy of Dr. S. R. Ganti and Dr. Sadek K. Hilal.)

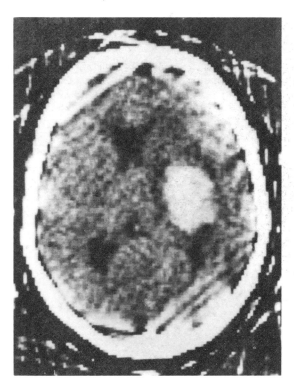

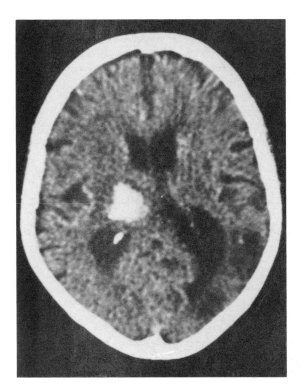

I–21 CT scan showing thalamic hemorrhage (hematoma is **light area**). (There is also infarction of the parietal–occipital area of the opposite hemisphere.) (Courtesy of Dr. S. R. Ganti and Dr. Sadek K. Hilal.)

tem) and quadriparesis (by transecting the corticospinal tract). Eye movements, spontaneous or reflex (e.g., to ice water in either external auditory canal), are absent, and pupils are pinpoint in size, perhaps in part from transection of descending sympathetic pathways and in part from destruction of reticular inhibitory mechanisms on the Edinger-Westphal nucleus of the midbrain. Pupillary light reactivity, however, is usually preserved, for the pathway subserving this reflex, from retina to midbrain, is intact. Respirations may be irregular, presumably from reticular formation involvement. Such a clinical state is nearly always fatal.

Cerebellar hemorrhage, which tends to occur in the region of the dentate nucleus, typically causes a sudden inability to stand or walk (atasia–abasia), with ipsilateral limb ataxia. There may be ipsilateral abducens or gaze palsy, or facial weakness, presumably from pontine compression. Long tract motor and sensory signs, however, are usually absent. As swelling increases, further brain stem damage may cause coma, ophthalmoplegia, miosis, and irregular respiration, with fatal outcome.

The Rupture of Berry Aneurysms Causes Subarachnoid Hemorrhage

Berry aneurysms (not to be confused with hypertensive Charcot-Bouchard aneurysms) are most often found at the junction of the anterior communicating artery with an anterior cerebral artery, at the junction of a posterior communicating artery with an internal carotid artery, and at the first bifurcation of a middle cerebral artery in the Sylvian fissure. Each, upon rupture, tends to cause not only sudden severe headache, but a characteristic syndrome. By producing a hematoma directly over the oculomotor nerve as it traverses the base of the brain, a ruptured posterior communicating artery aneurysm often causes ipsilateral pupillary dilitation with loss of light reactivity. A middle cerebral artery aneurysm may, by either hematoma or secondary infarction, cause a clinical picture resembling that of middle cerebral artery occlusion. After rupture of an anterior communicating artery aneurysm, there may be no focal signs, but only a decreased alertness or some behavioral changes. Posterior fossa aneurysms most often occur at the rostral bifurcation of the basilar artery or at the origin of the posterior inferior cerebellar artery. They cause a wide variety of cranial nerve and brain stem signs. Rupture of an aneurysm at any site may cause abrupt coma; the reason is uncertain but may be related to sudden increased intracranial pressure and functional disruption of vital pontomedullary structures.

Stroke Alters the Vascular Physiology of the Brain

As noted in Appendix IB, brain vessels respond in a unique fashion to changes in arterial pressure or blood gases. Brain arterioles constrict when the blood pressure is raised and dilate when it is lowered (autoregulation). Both of these adjustments tend to maintain optimal cerebral blood flow. The result is that normal individuals maintain a constant cerebral blood flow between mean arterial pressures of approximately 60–160 mm Hg. Above or below these pressures, cerebral blood flow rises or falls linearly.

When arterial P_{CO_2} is raised, brain arterioles dilate, and cerebral blood flow increases; with hypocarbia there is vasoconstriction, and cerebral blood flow decreases. The response is exquisitely sensitive: inhalation of 5% CO_2 increases cerebral blood flow by 50%, and 7% CO_2 doubles it. Changing arterial P_{O_2} causes an opposite and less pronounced response: breathing 100% O_2 lowers cerebral blood flow by about 13%; 10% O_2 raises it by 35%.

The mechanism of these responses is uncertain and controversial, but they serve protective functions, preserving blood flow in the presence of hypotension and increasing the delivery of oxygen and the removal of acid metabolites in the presence of hypoxia, ischemia, or tissue damage. After a stroke, however, cerebral blood flow and the responses to blood pressure or arterial gases are altered.

The term *luxury perfusion* refers to the frequent appearance, after brain infarction, of hyperemia relative to demand. Red venous blood may be seen draining infarcts, and regional cerebral blood flow may or may not be absolutely increased. In addition, there may be vasomotor paralysis, with loss of autoregulation and then blunted responses to changes in P_{O_2} or P_{CO_2}. This kind of physiological abnormality occurs both within and around ischemic lesions. In such patients, carbon dioxide (or other cerebral vasodilators) may produce a paradoxical response, increasing cerebral blood flow in brain regions distant from the infarct without affecting the vessels around the lesion. Blood may therefore be shunted from ischemic to normal brain (intracerebral steal). On the other hand, cerebral vasoconstrictors, by decreasing cerebral blood flow in normal brain without affecting the vessels of ischemic brain, may shunt blood into the area of ischemia or infarction (inverse intracerebral steal or Robin Hood syndrome).

There is controversy about the frequency of these phenomena. Hyperperfusion is not invariable in infarcted brain, and it may coexist with adjacent hypoperfusion. Similarly, intracerebral steal, while probably most common with very large infarcts, is quite unpredictable (particularly in duration) in any single patient. It is also not clear whether increasing cerebral blood flow to infarcted or ischemic areas improves matters by increasing oxygen delivery and the removal of tissue-damaging metabolites or makes matters worse by increasing edema, mass effect, and anastomotic compromise.

Selected Readings

Barnett, H. J. M. 1982. Cerebrovascular diseases. In J. B. Wyngaarden and L. H. Smith, Jr. (eds.), Textbook of Medicine, 16th ed. Philadelphia: Saunders, pp. 2050–2073.

Brust, J. C. M. 1984. Cerebral infarction. In L. P. Rowland (ed.), Merritt's Textbook of Neurology, 7th ed. Philadelphia: Lea & Febiger, pp. 162–168.

Mohr, J. P., Fisher, C. M., and Adams, R. D. 1980. Cerebrovascular diseases. In K. J. Isselbacher, R. D. Adams, E. Braunwald, R. G. Petersdorf, and J. D. Wilson (eds.), Harrison's Principles of Internal Medicine, 9th ed. New York: McGraw-Hill, pp. 1911–1942.

Appendix II
Neuroophthalmology

Peter Gouras

Physiological Optics, Accommodation, and Stereopsis

IIA

The eye resembles a camera with automatic brightness and focus control. It is equipped with rapid, automatic development and renewable film of two different varieties: one, the rod system, is a highly sensitive but coarse-grained achromatic film; the other, the cone system, is a less sensitive but more finely grained color film. The information in this film is analyzed by the visual system—a sophisticated image-processing computer located mainly in the cerebral cortex.

The Lens Focuses an Inverted Image on the Photoreceptors

The basic principles of image formation in the eye depend upon the rules of geometrical optics, first described by Johannes Kepler in the seventeenth century (Figure II–1). As light passes through the eye, an inverted image of the external luminous environment is focused on the retinal photoreceptors that line the back of the eye like photographic film. Unlike most cameras, however, this light-sensitive film is arranged along a spherical rather than a flat surface. The focusing of this image depends upon the transparency of all the intervening structures— the cornea, aqueous humor, crystalline lens, vitreous humor, and neural retina—through which light must pass to reach the photoreceptors.

The optical effects of the neural retina are greatly minimized in its central region—the part of the retina that is used when we look directly at an object. Within this area is a small depression, the central *fovea*, and along the floor of the fovea (the *foveola*) the diameter of the retina is reduced to its thinnest dimension. Light that is not absorbed by the receptor's outer segment travels on to the pigment epithelium and choroid layer. If light from

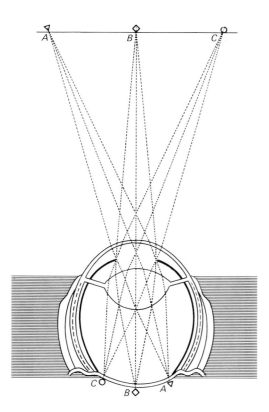

II–1 Formation of the retinal image, according to Descartes. The correct theory had been originated by Kepler. (Adapted from Descartes, 1637.)

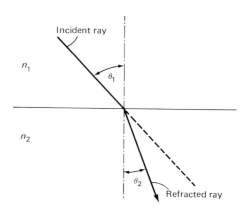

II–2 Snell's law and the index of refraction: the behavior of a light ray as it passes from a medium of lower refractive index (n_1) into one of higher refractive index (n_2). The refractive index of each medium is determined by the ratio n = velocity of light in vacuum/velocity of light in medium. Shorter wavelengths have a higher index of refraction than longer wavelengths in solids and liquids. Upon entering the denser medium, the light ray is bent (refracted) toward the perpendicular. The angle that the light ray forms to a line perpendicular to the surface is θ. For a given wavelength of light and pair of media, the ratio of the sine of the angle of incidence (θ_1) to the sine of the angle of refraction (θ_2) is a constant. This relationship, $n_1 \sin \theta_1 = n_2 \sin \theta_2$, is Snell's law. (Adapted from Ogle, 1961.)

this layer were scattered back onto the retina, image degradation could occur. This is prevented to a large degree by the presence of light-absorbing pigment granules (melanin) that are present both in the processes of pigment epithelial cells that interleaf between the light-sensitive structures of the photoreceptors and in melanocytes found in the choroid.

Light Is Refracted in the Eye

Snell's Law Predicts the Refraction of Light

A guiding principle in image formation by optical systems is the law stated by Snell van Rojen of Leiden in the beginning of the seventeenth century *(Snell's law)*. The essential features of this law are illustrated in Figure II–2. A light ray entering a denser medium (one of higher refractive index[1]) is bent toward a line perpendicular to that surface, such as occurs when light goes from air into glass. If there is no difference in refractive index between the two surfaces, or if the ray itself is perpendicular to the surface, no refraction or bending of the light path occurs. This property of light provides a means of focusing and magnifying visual objects. Any curved object that is

transparent to light and of a different refractive index than air will bend incident light rays. Such objects are called *lenses*, and the cornea and lens of the eye are relevant examples.

In general there are two classes of lenses (Figure II–3): *converging (convex)* and *diverging (concave)*. Convex lenses bring light rays together and concave lenses spread light rays farther apart. That point at which all of the parallel light rays meet after interacting with the lens is called the principal focus or *focal point*. The distance from the center of the lens to the principal focus is called the *focal length* of the lens. The bending or refractive power of a lens is expressed by diopter units. A *diopter* is the reciprocal (in meters) of the focal length of the lens. For example, a 1-diopter lens focuses parallel light at 1 m, and a 2-diopter lens does so at 0.5 m. Converging lenses focus parallel rays on the opposite side of the lens; diverging lenses produce a *virtual focus* (a point from which divergent light rays appear to come but in fact do not) of parallel rays on the same side on which they arrive. Similarly, diverging lenses form virtual images while convex lenses form real images. Distant light rays traveling through a convex lens pass through those points occupied by the image and can be viewed if a screen is placed along this plane. These images are referred to as *real images* and are inverted. The diverging light rays that leave a concave lens, however, do not pass through the points occupied by the image. This *virtual image* is upright and cannot be formed on a screen but can be viewed by looking through the lens.

---

[1]The *refractive index* is the ratio of the velocity of light in a vacuum to its velocity in the medium considered.

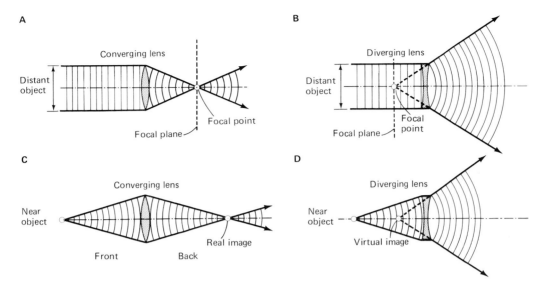

II–3 Focusing of light by converging and diverging lenses.
The refraction of parallel light rays emanating from a distant object is shown for a converging (**A**) and a diverging (**B**) lens; and the refraction of divergent rays arising from a nearby object is shown for a converging (**C**) and a diverging (**D**) lens. The focusing of light by converging lenses (**A** and **C**) produces a real image at a focal point in back of the lens. Light rays

interacting with diverging lenses (**B** and **D**), however, spread apart and never form a real focus. By projecting the paths of these divergent rays (**D**), one finds that they meet at a point in front of the lens known as the virtual focus, which is taken as the focal point of the lens. A virtual image is formed along this plane. (Adapted from Ogle, 1961.)

Thin Lens Formulas Are Derived from Snell's Law

A simplified explanation of image formation by lenses can be obtained by assuming that all lenses are infinitely thin without significant curvature. By applying Snell's law to thin lenses, simple formulas can be derived that provide good approximations to what occurs in real (thick) lenses. Figure II–4A shows how three rays (from an infinite number) emanating from a light source are refracted by a thin convex lens. Ray 1 is parallel to the optical axis of the lens and is refracted through the focal point (F_1) of the lens. Ray 2 is undeviated and travels in a straight line to intersect ray 1 at the image (S') of the light source (S). Ray 3 passes through the other focal point (F_2) of the lens and exits parallel to the optical axis to intersect rays 1 and 2 in the image (S'). According to Snell's law, all the rays from source S within the solid angle that projects through this lens will meet in the image S'. Two of these rays (Figure II–4B) can be used to derive several useful relationships of thin lens optics between the object and image distance and the focal length, where

$$\frac{1}{\text{Object distance}} + \frac{1}{\text{Image distance}} = \frac{1}{\text{Focal length}}.$$

This formula allows one to determine the distance of images of lenses of any focal length. The linear magnification of such lenses can also be obtained:

$$\frac{\text{Image size}}{\text{Object size}} = \frac{\text{Distance of image from the lens}}{\text{Distance of object from the lens}}.$$

II–4 Principle of thin lens formulas. **A.** Refraction of light by a thin convex lens. F_1 and F_2, focal points of lens; S, light source; S', image. **B.** By assuming that the convex lens in **A** is infinitely thin and applying Snell's law to light rays 1 and 2, the image distance can be determined given object distance and focal length. (Although lens power is due to its thickness, as well as refraction by both front and back surfaces, in an infinitely thin lens all refraction can be taken to occur at a single surface.) (Adapted from Ogle, 1961.)

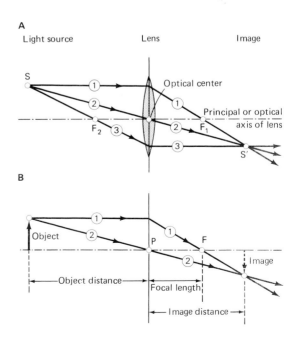

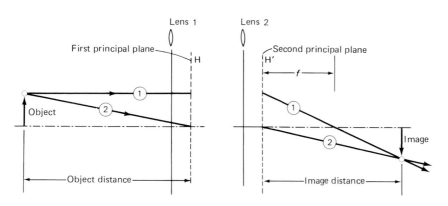

II–5 Application of thin lens formulas to a multiple-lens system. Numerous refracting surfaces of a complex optical system can be reduced to two principal planes, one associated with the object side of the system (**H**), and the other associated with the image side (**H′**). **f:** focal point of the system. (Adapted from Ogle, 1961.)

The following conventions of sign apply to these thin lens equations:

1. Real object and image distances are positive; virtual object and image distances are negative.
2. The focal length of a converging lens is positive; that of a diverging lens is negative.

Most optical systems, such as the eye, are composed of numerous refracting surfaces with different indices of refraction. Any such complex optical system can be reduced to two principal planes: one that pertains to the object side and the other to the image side. Figure II–5 illustrates this for a converging lens system (two lenses). To use the thin lens equation, one measures the object distance to the first principal plane (H) and the image distance to the second principal plane (H′). The principal planes are two of the six cardinal points that define any complex optical system (see below).

Real lenses have significant thickness and curvature that also affect their refractive properties (their ability to bend light). If one restricts the problem to rays that are not too far from the optical axis of a lens, a simplified expression for the image position across such an optical surface is

$$\frac{n_2}{\text{Image distance}} + \frac{n_1}{\text{Object distance}} = \frac{n_2 - n_1}{\text{Radius of curvature of lens}}$$

where n_1 and n_2 are the refractive indices of the media. This expression provides a means of tracing the image position and size across such a refracting surface having significant curvature (R), such as the cornea. One can then redo the calculation for the second surface of the lens and continue the process for multiple optical elements such as those in the eye. The factor $(n_2 - n_1)/R$ is called the *dioptric power of the surface*. If the radius of curvature is a small number (high curvature) and/or the refractive change is large, the dioptric power of the surface is great.

Another consideration that applies to the eye, but not to most optical systems, is the fact that the image is formed within a medium different from that in which the object is usually seen (air). In this case the focal length on the image side of the lens system is different from the focal length on the object side. This arrangement requires the use of another factor, the *nodal points of the optical system*; at the nodal point the angle subtended by the object equals the angle subtended by the image (Figure II–6). The two focal points (anterior and posterior), the two principal points (or planes), and the two nodal points are collectively referred to as the *cardinal points of reference* of any optical system. The dimensions of the critical reference points for the average human eye are shown in Figure II–7; they can be used to analyze the path of light through the eye and to determine quantitative aspects of image formation on the retina. A useful application of the nodal points is in the determination of the size of an object on the retina:

$$\frac{\text{Image size}}{\text{Object size}} = \frac{\text{Distance of image to N′ (17 mm)}}{\substack{\text{Distance of object to N} \\ \text{(distance from cornea + 7.1 mm)}}}$$

If, for example, one wanted to estimate the size of the image on the retina formed by a building 50 m high at a

II–6 Cardinal points of optical reference. The path of light in a complex optical system—i.e., one containing multiple elements with different refracting surfaces—can be accurately traced by simplifying the system to six cardinal reference points and applying the thin lens equations. The six points are the anterior (**F$_a$**) and posterior (**F$_p$**) focal points, the two principal planes (**H, H′**) or points (**P, P′**), and the two nodal points (**N, N′**). n_1 and n_2 are the lower and higher refractive indices, respectively. *a* represents the angle the light rays form with a perpendicular to the optical surface. (Adapted from Ogle, 1961.)

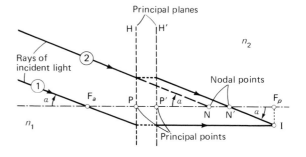

II–7 Dimensions of the six cardinal reference points of the average human eye. Dimensions are given in milliliters. These data can be used to define the properties of light as it travels through the eye and allow the determination of such features as retinal image size. Symbols as in Figure II–6. (Adapted from Ogle, 1961.)

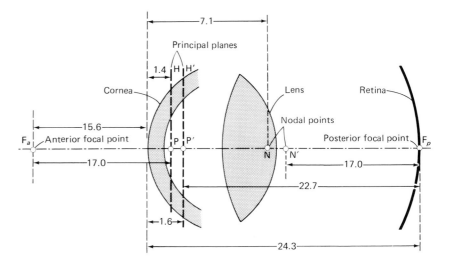

distance of 3 km, then

$$\frac{\text{Retinal image}}{5 \times 10^4 \text{ mm}} = \frac{17 \text{ mm}}{3 \times 10^6 + 7.1 \text{ mm}}.$$

From this calculation the retinal image of the building at this distance is 0.28 mm, a dimension that is slightly less than the diameter of the fovea.

Image Formation in Monocular Vision Has Physical Limitations

Important optical constants of the cornea and lens are presented in Table II–1. The total dioptric power of the eye is not the simple sum of the individual values but also depends upon the distance between each refracting surface. The major change in refractive index occurs at the anterior surface of the cornea, which, combined with the radius of curvature of the cornea, is responsible for most of the dioptric power of the eye. The refractive power of the lens depends mainly on the radius of curvature of both of its surfaces. The refractive index of the lens, increasing from 1.37 at its margin to 1.42 at its

core, makes any simple treatment of this element difficult, but it has the advantage of minimizing spherical and chromatic aberration.

The radius of curvature of the anterior surface of the lens is 10 mm, but, by contraction of the ciliary muscles, it can be reduced to 6 mm, thus providing the lens with the ability to change its dioptric power. The ability to vary the shape of the lens ensures that the focal length remains constant; this is called *accommodation*. *Accommodation provides the major means of modifying the refractive power of the eye, which allows focusing on near objects.* The curvature of the posterior surface of the lens changes relatively little (6–5.5 mm) during accommodation.

Alterations in Refractive Power Affect Image Formation

Normally, with minimum lens curvature, the eye is sharply focused on objects at the horizon (the *far point*) and remains in sharp focus if these objects approach to about 9 m (*emmetropia*; Figure II–8A). Changes in the axial position of images of objects that move to this 9-m point from the horizon are relatively insignificant along the plane of the outer segments of photoreceptors because the retinal image is so small. When objects move closer than this 9 m, however, they are focused beyond the plane of the outer segments, somewhere in the retinal pigment epithelial layer or beyond, and some modification of lens curvature is required to bring them back into focus on the outer segments. Infants can modify their lens curvature to bring objects just beyond their nose into focus, but with age we progressively lose this ability. At about 45 years of age it is no longer possible to focus on objects closer than about an arm's length away without artificial lenses, a condition known as *presbyopia*.

The far points of some eyes are closer than the horizon (*myopia* or *nearsightedness*); parallel rays are focused in front of the retina. Such eyes tend to have longer axial lengths than normal (Figure II–8B), and a patient with

Table II–1. Optical Constants of Normal Eye

	Radius of curvature (mm)	Refractive index Anterior	Refractive index Posterior	Power (diopters)
Cornea				
Anterior	7.8	1	1.376	+48.8
Posterior	6.8	1.376	1.376	−5.9
Lens margin				
Anterior	10.0	1.336	1.386	+7.4
Posterior	−6.0	1.386	1.386	+12.3
Eye + lens				+58.9

Source: Adapted from Westheimer, G., 1980. The eye. In V. Mountcastle (ed.), Medical Physiology, 14th ed., Vol. 1. St. Louis: Mosby, pp. 440–457.

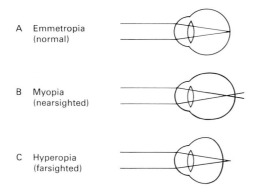

A Emmetropia
   (normal)

B Myopia
   (nearsighted)

C Hyperopia
   (farsighted)

II–8 Refractive errors. **A.** In the normal eye, with the ciliary
muscles relaxed, an image of a distant object is focused
on the retina. As the object distance is reduced, the ciliary
muscles make the lens more convex, thereby keeping the
image on the retina. Refractive errors can occur in the eye,
resulting in abnormal refraction and image focusing in front of
or behind the retina. **B.** In the myopic eye, light rays from a
distant object are focused in front of the retina because the
axial length of the eyeball is too great for its lens. Because the
ciliary muscles cannot reduce the radius of curvature of the
relaxed lens, a diverging lens must be used to reduce this
refraction and correct nearsightedness. **C.** When the length of
the eye is shorter than normal, images of distant objects are
focused at a point beyond the retina (hyperopia). This condition
can be corrected by normal accommodation changes, by
making the lens more convex, or by wearing converging lenses.

this condition needs diverging lenses to see distant objects sharply. The far points of other eyes are farther than
infinity (*hyperopia* or *farsightedness;* Figure II–8C). People with hyperopic eyes may be able to see distant objects
by changing the curvature of the lens (accommodating).
Such eyes tend to have shorter axial lengths than normal
and require converging lenses so that the patient can see
distant objects without accommodating.

Some eyes do not have the same corneal curvature
along different axes *(astigmatism)* and require an axial
correction. Contact lenses can vary corneal refraction by
altering the air–epithelial interface of the cornea directly,
whereas spectacle lenses can only counteract and not
eliminate corneal errors.

The Image Can Be Degraded by Spherical and Chromatic Aberrations

Refracting systems such as the eye have inherent physical limitations that can produce degradation or blurring
of the image. The two major causes of blur in the normal
eye are spherical and chromatic aberration.

Spherical aberration occurs when light rays are refracted more strongly by the periphery than by the center
of a lens (Figure II–9). Nature has made attempts to reduce this problem. The cornea is flatter at its margin
than at its center, and the lens has a higher refractive
index at its center than at its margins. Both of these factors tend to reduce spherical aberration. The directional
selectivity of cones, called the *Stiles-Crawford effect,*
makes the cone (more than the rods) more sensitive to
central or axial rays than to rays passing through the
margins of the lens (Figure II–10). This also minimizes
the effects of lens aberrations on cones. Cones are more
sensitive to blur because they play a much greater role
than rods in fine visual discrimination.

Chromatic aberration is a result of the fact that short
wavelengths are refracted more strongly than long ones
(Figure II–11). This produces differences in both the size
and axial position of chromatically different retinal images formed in white light. Camera lenses are routinely
corrected for this form of aberration by combining lens
elements of different types of glass (crown and flint
glass). The eye has resorted to a different approach to this
important optical problem.

The eye greatly restricts the spectral window within
which it resolves fine visual detail. Insects use ultraviolet light, snakes and perhaps mosquitoes have infrared
detectors, and Superman has X-ray vision, but the human
fovea uses only a small portion of the electromagnetic
spectrum (approximately 500–700 nm), centered near
spectral yellow, for resolving fine detail. This, as we have
seen in Chapter 30, results from the synthesis of three
light-sensitive proteins in cones that are most sensitive
to these wavelengths (red- and green-sensitive cones of
trichromatic color vision). Blue-sensitive cones, as well
as rods (which are most sensitive to shorter wavelengths), are kept out of the central fovea and consequently have little to do with fine visual resolution. In
addition, an inert pigment, macular yellow, which
strongly absorbs blue and violet light (and hence looks
yellow), is deposited in the fovea, and this pigment considerably blocks short wavelengths from affecting foveal
cones. It is mainly at the short-wavelength region of the
spectrum that chromatic aberration is most destructive
to image formation, and it is this spectral region that the
fovea most avoids.

Color vision, which identifies objects by wavelength,
in contrast to mere energy differences across contours
(luminance), becomes more significant as objects become
larger. In color vision all three cone mechanisms act together, with the blue cones assuming a much greater role
than they have in discriminating fine detail.

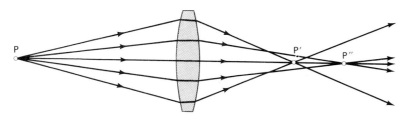

II–9 Spherical aberration. Light rays entering near
the periphery of a spherical lens are refracted
more strongly than those passing through its center.
This results in the focusing of peripheral rays at a
point (**P'**) closer to the lens than central rays (**P''**).

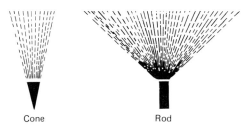

II–10 Directional selectivity of cones. **Dotted lines:** angles that light rays can have and still strongly affect the photoreceptors. The receptive angle of rods is much larger than that of cones; thus cones are less sensitive to rays traversing the periphery of the lens.

Blurs Can Also Be Caused by Diffraction

Peripheral rays, which produce spherical and chromatic aberration blur, can be blocked by pupillary constriction, which consequently increases the depth of field,—the axial range within which an object is still in focus. Excessive pupillary constriction has diminishing returns, however, because of another cause of blur, diffraction (Figure II–12). Diffraction results from the wave nature of light and the interference these waves exert on one another.

Diffraction ultimately determines the limit of spatial resolution, or the minimum resolvable detail of any optical system. The larger the entrance aperture of an optical system, the greater is its resolving power, because of the reduction in diffraction blur. This relationship is reflected in the *numerical aperture*, which is equal to the product of the sine of the half-angle of the cone of rays admitted by the system and the refractive index of the media. The larger the pupillary aperture, however, the greater is the blur caused by spherical and chromatic aberrations. This is the Scylla and Charybdis of the eye. For best resolving power, a pupillary aperture of 2 mm is desirable because it optimally trades off the blur of lens aberrations with that of diffraction. At this pupil size and at the near point (25 cm) the numerical aperture of the

II–11 Chromatic aberration. Light of short wavelength (violet in this diagram) is refracted more strongly than light of longer wavelength (red). The light rays of shorter wavelength are brought to focus at a point closer to the lens than the rays of longer wavelengths. The violet image (**P'Q'**) is therefore smaller than the image formed by red light (**P"Q"**), an effect known as *chromatic change of magnification.*

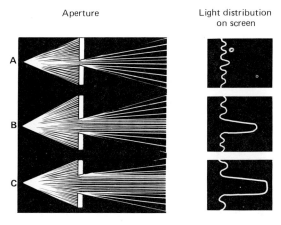

Aperture   Light distribution on screen

II–12 Diffraction. **A.** The aperture is so small that light rays interfere with each other and destroy any image of the source on a screen. **B** and **C.** When the aperture is increased, the effects of diffraction are reduced.

eye is 0.004 and the linear separation of two just resolvable point objects is about 0.1 mm. These resolvable points are not sharply defined geometric spots of light on the retina; each point is a spread of light with a central peak surrounded by a gradually diminishing fall-off. This spreading is due to diffraction, aberration, and scatter in the transmission media. The distance between the centers on the retina for two such resolvable points is about 0.01 mm (10 μm), which is just about the distance between foveal cones. We can actually resolve objects even closer than this if the objects are, for example, broken lines *(vernier acuity).* This is true in part because of the relatively random distribution of cones in the fovea and the convergence of this information onto orientation detectors within the cerebral cortex (Chapter 29).

Ocular Reflexes Adapt the Eye to Changing Conditions

The Pupillary Light Reflex Is an Automatic Brightness Control Mechanism

The pupillary light reflex is a control mechanism similar to those in many cameras. The range of brightness control is limited; it can change retinal illumination by a factor of about 16 (pupillary diameters range from 8 to 2 mm), which is relatively small compared to the enormous operating range of human vision. Going from dim

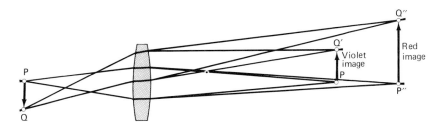

moonlight to bright sunlight alters retinal illumination by a factor of approximately 10^{12}. The importance of the pupillary reflex stems from its rapidity as compared to the slow but much more profound mechanisms of retinal adaptation. Retinal cells and the photoreceptors, in particular, are capable of altering their sensitivity if light levels are too high; this sensitivity loss is traded off for a considerable increase in their speed of response. The neural pathways that mediate the pupillary light reflex are described in Chapter 28.

Accommodation Allows the Eye to Focus up Close

Accommodation is another ocular reflex that employs the pupillary system, in addition to the lens and ocular muscles, to allow the eye to focus on objects closer than the far point. When objects move closer than the far point, they not only go out of focus but also shift position relative to the fovea of each eye. To restore focus and retain stereoscopic vision, three separate processes occur: (1) the curvature of the lens is increased, (2) the pupil constricts toward 2 mm, and (3) the eyes converge.

Lens curvature is altered in a two-stage process—one active, the other passive. In the active process, contraction of the ciliary muscle relaxes tension on the zonular fibers of the lens; in the passive process, the release of tension on the zonular fibers allows the elastic properties of the lens to increase its curvature. The elastic properties of the lens decrease with age; this process starts shortly after birth and progresses throughout life. Its effects are only noticed, however, when it no longer becomes possible to focus on objects held at arm's length.

The signal that induces the accommodation reflex appears to arise mainly from blur in the retinal image. This detection of blur—in contrast to light itself, as in the pu-

II–13 Consensual light response. Monocular illumination results in constriction of the pupil of both the illuminated eye (**1,** direct light response) and the contralateral eye (**2,** consensual light response).

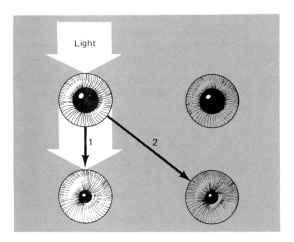

pillary light reflex—requires a much more sophisticated decision. It is for this reason that accommodation involves the visual cortex in its reflex arc. The afferent loop of the accommodation reflex involves optic fibers whose receptive fields are in the fovea. These fibers synapse in the lateral geniculate nucleus, which in turn relays to the visual (striate) cortex. From this point it is not clear how the afferent signals reach the oculomotor nucleus after the decision (mostly unconscious) about blur has been made by the visual cortex. The efferent loop of this reflex is completed by neurons of the oculomotor complex and the message is carried by fibers of the third nerve to the ciliary process, the iris, and the medial recti muscles.

Both the light and the accommodative reflexes can be elicited in both eyes by monocular stimulation, i.e., they are consensual reflexes (Figure II–13). These reflexes are important for diagnostic purposes. The differences in the pathways of the pupillary light and the accommodative reflexes are occasionally highlighted by disease. One of the most notorious of these is the *Argyll Robertson pupil* of the syphilitic patient, in which the pupillary light reflex but not the accommodative reflex is destroyed. In contrast, age destroys the accommodative reflex but not the light reflex.

Binocular Vision Is Important for Depth Perception

All of the preceding discussion has pertained to monocular vision. Although the perception of spatial depth is possible with purely monocular cues, such as motion parallax, perspective, texture gradients, and size, binocular vision creates a totally new visual dimension—*stereopsis*. Stereopsis allows us to perceive a three-dimensional object in spatial depth, an aspect of perception that would be impossible with monocular vision. The eyes view the world from two different vantage points (Figure II–14). The same point on an object but off the point of fixation will not be the same distance from the fovea on each retina. This difference is referred to as a retinal disparity (see Figure II–14). If the object changes its position in depth and consequently the eyes make a vergence movement in order to keep both foveas aligned (see Chapter 43), the retinal disparity values change. The brain must process signals coming from different retinal areas in the two eyes to compute depth and must recalculate this information on the basis of a new set of retinal disparities if the object shifts in depth.

For a given fixation point, there is a locus of points, called the *horopter*, along which images fall on corresponding points of the two retinas. *The Vieth-Müller circle* is an attempt to define the horopter geometrically as a circle that passes through the fixation point and the optical center of each eye (Figure II–15A). This circle deviates from the true horopter because the optical node of the eye does not fall at the geometrical center of the eye, and the center of rotation of the eye does not coincide with this node. Figure II–15B shows the relative posi-

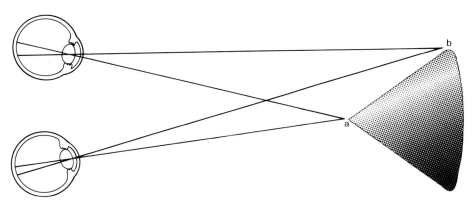

II–14 Binocular disparities are the basis for stereopsis. They arise because the eyes converge slightly, so that their axes of vision meet at a point in the external world (**a**). The point is "fixated." A neighboring point in the world (**b**) will then project to a point on the retina some distance from the center of vision. The distance will not be the same for each eye. (From Poggio, 1984.)

tions of the Vieth-Müller circle and the actual horopter, the areas for stereopsis and for binocular single vision, and the regions where double vision (diplopia) begins. Note that it is possible to have some stereopsis in the presence of diplopia.

The actual locus of positions that induce stereopsis for a given fixation depth in space involves a three-dimensional zone around the horopter, named *Panum's fusional area* after its proposer (1858). It is called a fusional area because objects in this region, lying off the horopter, are seen as single structures in depth. Objects lying outside the fusional area are seen doubly. To see this effect, fix your eyes on the tip of a pencil about 8 inches in front of you. Place your index finger behind the pencil and slowly move the finger away from you. Initially your finger will appear as a single structure, lying further in depth than the pencil. When your arm is fully extended, you should see your finger doubly. It is now outside Panum's fusional area.

For points along the horopter, the area of temporal retina stimulated by light in one eye corresponds to a nasal area in the other eye. This arrangement led Isaac Newton to suggest that there might be a partial decussation of optic nerve fibers from each eye in order to anatomically associate corresponding areas of visual space in the brain. Two centuries later this idea was confirmed by the neuroanatomical demonstration of such a decussation in the human optic chiasm. The neurophysiological work of

David Hubel and Torsten Wiesel has now shown that these corresponding retinal areas are registered by single cells in the visual cortex (Chapter 57).

The decussation of optic nerve fibers along the vertical meridian through the fovea creates an unusual problem for the recombination of corresponding retinal areas around the area of fixation, precisely where stereopsis is best. The unfilled regions are areas of visual space where the corresponding areas of each retina end up in opposite cerebral hemispheres (Figure II–16A). To explain this curious problem in stereopsis, either there is some overlap in the cells subserving the vertical meridian of each eye, or the critical information is relayed from one hemisphere to another via the corpus callosum (Figure II–16B).

When fixation shifts to a different depth in space all the corresponding retinal points must be kept in register with their corresponding unified object detectors (Figure II–15) in the visual cortex by means of an appropriate vergence movement of the eyes. This serves to keep objects fused and thereby prevent diplopia. Different aspects of parallax in a scene cause shifts in the activation of different neighboring parallax detectors (Figure II–15), providing a different perspective of objects in depth. If one considers a particular object that either recedes or advances, its optical magnification on the retina must be considered simultaneously. This movement in depth causes a shift in both the unified object detectors and parallax detectors with different receptive field positions

II–15 The Vieth-Müller horopter circle. **A.** The images of points **P** and **Q** fall on geometrically corresponding points in the two retinas. **B.** The relative positions of the Vieth-Müller circle and the empirical horopter, the overlapping areas for stereopsis and for binocular single vision, and the regions where diplopia begins. (Adapted from Bishop, 1973.)

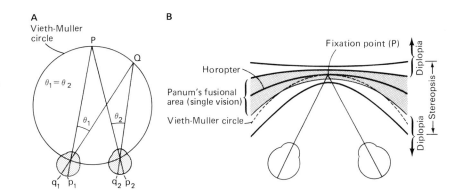

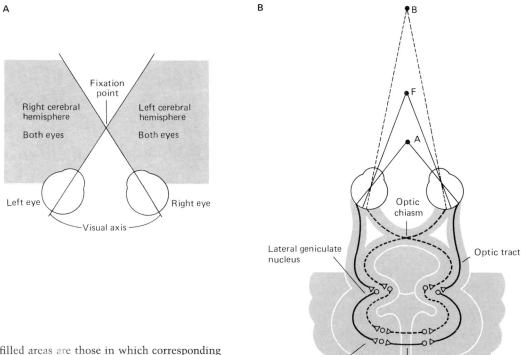

II–16 **A.** Unfilled areas are those in which corresponding retinal areas reach opposite hemispheres of the brain. **B.** Callosal route to bring these corresponding signals together. (Adapted from Bishop, 1973.)

as the contour of the object either shrinks or enlarges on both the retinas of each eye and their corresponding representations in the visual cortex. Physiologically, this resembles a wave of activity moving either inward or outward across different ocular dominance columns (see Figure 29–11) in the visual cortex. This wave must be precisely followed by the vergence oculomotor system in order to maintain a unified image receding or advancing in space. Space and distance must be abstractions of the same activity.

An interesting question about the processing of visual information by the cerebral cortex for stereopsis is whether we neurally process the shape of an object before we put it in proper perspective in depth. Ingenious experiments by Bela Julesz at the Bell Laboratories with computer-generated random dot stereograms, which contain depth clues due to parallax but are devoid of monocular information about the shape of these three-dimensional objects, indicate that the process of stereopsis precedes the stage at which shape is recognized. Thus, stereopsis, like color vision, facilitates object detection in addition to adding a new and aesthetic dimension to visual perception.

How the brain calculates corresponding retinal regions that match for a particular stereo-scene is not yet understood but the experiments of Julesz have provided an important clue. A hypothesis has been developed by David Marr and Tomaso Poggio at the Artificial Intelligence Laboratory at Massachusetts Institute of Technol-

ogy that requires the brain to make several sophisticated assumptions about the visual world it expects to see. This puts constraints on the computations it must perform. One constraint is that a point on a physical surface has only one three-dimensional location at any time; a second is that the variation in depth over a surface is usually smooth and continuous. With these constraints and using neural units with an antagonistic center–surround receptive field organization (Chapter 27), an algorithm has been developed in which local calculations computed asynchronously and in parallel by large numbers of units can now detect objects in Julesz's stereograms. Solving such a problem is a major step toward understanding the way in which the visual brain works.

Selected Readings

Bishop, P. O. 1973. Neurophysiology of binocular single vision and stereopsis. In R. Jung (ed.), Handbook of Sensory Physiology, Vol. 7, Part 3A: Central Processing of Visual Information. Berlin: Springer, pp. 255–305.

Gouras, P. 1972. Light and dark adaptation. In M. G. F. Fuortes (ed.), Handbook of Sensory Physiology, Vol. 7, Part 2: Physiology of Photoreceptor Organs. Berlin: Springer, pp. 609–634.

Julesz, B. 1971. Foundations of Cyclopean Perception. Chicago: University of Chicago Press.

Mach, E. 1913. The Principles of Physical Optics (1926, English translation). Reprint. New York: Dover Publications, 1953.

Moses, R. A. 1975. Accommodation. In R. A. Moses (ed.), Adler's Physiology of the Eye, 6th ed. St. Louis: Mosby, pp. 298–319.

Moses, R. A. 1975. The iris and the pupil. In R. A. Moses (ed.), Adler's Physiology of the Eye, 6th ed. St. Louis: Mosby, pp. 320–352.

Newton, I. 1730. Opticks: or, A Treatise of the Reflections, Refractions, Inflections and Colours of Light, 4th rev. ed. London: William Innys. Reprint. New York: Dover Publications, 1952.

Nishihara, H. K., and Poggio, T. 1982. Hidden cues in random-line stereograms. Nature 300:347–349.

Ogle, K. N. 1961. Optics: An Introduction for Ophthalmologists. Springfield, Ill.: Thomas.

Panum, P. L. 1858. Physiologische Untersuchungen über das Sehen mit zwei Augen. Kiel: Schwerssche Buchhandlung. Cited by Boring, E. G. (1942).

Poggio, T. 1984. Vision by man and machine. Sci. Am. 250(4):106–116.

Westheimer, G. 1972. Visual acuity and spatial modulation thresholds. In D. Jameson and L. M. Hurvich (eds.), Handbook of Sensory Physiology, Vol. 7, Part 4: Visual Psychophysics. Berlin: Springer, pp. 170–187.

Whittaker, E. T. 1951. A History of the Theories of Aether and Electricity, Vol. I The Classical Theories. London: T. Nelson and Sons, rev. & enl. ed.

References

Descartes, R. 1637. La Dioptrique. Leyden: Ian Maire.

Gulick, W. L., and Lawson, R. B. 1976. Human Stereopsis: A Psychophysical Approach. New York: Oxford University Press.

Kepler, J. 1604. Astronomiae Pars Optica. Chap. 5.

Westheimer, G. 1980. The eye. In V. B. Mountcastle (ed.), Medical Physiology, 14th ed., Vol. 1. St. Louis: Mosby, pp. 481–503.

Appendix III
The Flow of Ionic
and Capacitive Current
in Nerve Cells

John Koester

Review of Electrical Circuits

IIIA

Definition of Electrical Parameters

Potential Difference (V or E)
Current (I)
Conductance (g)
Capacitance (C)

Rules for Circuit Analysis

Conductance
Current
Capacitance
Potential Difference

Current Flow in Circuits with Capacitance

Capacitive Circuit
Circuit with Resistor and Capacitor in Series
Circuit with Resistor and Capacitor in Parallel

This section is a review of the basic principles of electrical circuit theory. Familiarity with this material is important for understanding the equivalent circuit model of the neuron that is developed in Chapters 5–9. The section is divided into three parts:

1. The definition of basic electrical parameters.
2. A set of rules for elementary circuit analysis.
3. A description of current flow in circuits with capacitance.

Definition of Electrical Parameters

Potential Difference (V or E)

Electrical charges exert an electrostatic force on other charges: like charges repel, opposite charges attract. As the distance between two charges increases, the force that is exerted decreases. *Work* is done when two charges that initially are separated are brought together: *negative work* is done if their polarities are opposite, and *positive work* if they are the same. The greater the values of the charges and the greater their initial separation, the greater the work that is done (work $= \int_r^o f(r)\, dr$, where f is electrostatic force and r is the initial distance between the two charges). *Potential difference* is a measure of this work. The potential difference between two points is the work that must be done to move a unit of positive charge (1 coulomb) from one point to the other point, i.e., it is the potential energy of the charge. One volt (V) is the energy required to move 1 coulomb a distance of 1 meter against a force of 1 newton.

Current (I)

A potential difference exists within a system whenever positive and negative charges are separated. Such regions of charge separation may be generated by a chemical reaction (as in a battery) or by diffusion between two electrolyte solutions with different ion concentrations across a permeability-selective barrier, such as a cell membrane. If a region of charge separation exists within a conducting medium, then charges move between the areas of potential difference: positive charges are attracted to the region with a more negative potential, and negative charges go to the regions of positive potential. The resulting movement of charges is *current flow*, which is defined as the net movement of positive charge per unit time. In metallic conductors current is carried by electrons, which move in the opposite direction of current flow. In nerve and muscle cells, current is carried by positive and negative ions in solution. One ampere (A) of current represents the movement of 1 coulomb (of charge) per second.

Conductance (g)

Any object through which electrical charges can flow is called an electrical conductor. The unit of electrical conductance is the siemen (S). According to Ohm's law, the current that flows through a conductor is directly proportional to the potential difference imposed across it.[1]

$$I = V \times g$$
Current (A) = Potential difference (V)
$$\times \text{ Conductance (S)}.$$

As charge carriers move through a conductor, some of their potential energy is lost; it is converted into thermal energy due to the frictional interactions of the charge carriers with the conducting medium.

Each type of material has an intrinsic property called conductivity (σ), which is determined by its molecular structure. Metallic conductors have very high conductivities, which means that they conduct electricity extremely well; aqueous solutions with high ionized salt concentrations have somewhat lower values of σ; and oils and fats (lipids) have very low conductivities—they are poor conductors of electricity and are therefore good insulators. The conductance of an object is proportional to σ times its cross-sectional area, divided by its length:

$$g = (\sigma) \times \frac{\text{Area}}{\text{Length}}$$

---

[1]Note the analogy of this formula for current flow to the other formulas for describing flow; e.g., bulk flow of a liquid due to a hydrostatic pressure; flow of a solute in response to a concentration gradient; flow of heat in response to a temperature gradient, etc. In each case flow is proportional to the product of a driving force times a conductance factor.

The length dimension is defined as the direction along which one measures conductance (between *a* and *b*):

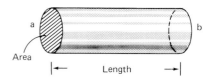

For example, the conductance measured across a piece of cell membrane is less if its length (thickness) is increased, e.g., by myelination. The conductance of a large area of membrane is greater than that of a small area of membrane.

Electrical resistance (R) is the reciprocal of conductance, and is a measure of the resistance provided by an object to current flow. Resistance is measured in ohms (Ω):

$$1 \text{ ohm} = (1 \text{ siemen})^{-1}.$$

Capacitance (C)

A capacitor consists of two conducting plates separated by an insulating layer. The fundamental property of a capacitor is its ability to store charges of opposite sign: positive charge on one plate, negative on the other.

A capacitor made up of two parallel plates with its two conducting surfaces separated by an insulator (an air gap) is shown in Figure III–1A, part 1. There is a net excess of positive charges on plate *x*, and an equal number of excess negative charges on plate *y*, resulting in a potential difference between the two plates. One can measure this potential difference by determining how much work is required to move a positive "test" charge from the surface of *y* to that of *x*. Initially, when the test charge is at *y*, it is attracted by the negative charges on *y*, and repelled less strongly by the more distant positive charges on *x*. The result of these electrostatic interactions is a force *f* that opposes the movement of the test charge from *y* to *x*. As one moves the test charge to the left, across the gap, the attraction by the negative charges on *y* diminishes, but the repulsion by the positive charges on *x* increases, with the result that the net electrostatic force exerted on the test charge is constant everywhere between *x* and *y* (Figure III–1A, part 2). Work (W) is force times the distance (D) over which the force is exerted:

$$W = f \times D.$$

Therefore, it is simple to calculate the work done in moving the test charge from one side of the capacitor to the other. It is the shaded area under the curve in Figure III–1A, part 2. This work is equal to the difference in electrical potential energy, or potential difference, between *x* and *y*.

Capacitance is measured in units called farads (F). The greater the density of charges on the capacitor plates, the greater the force acting on the test charge, and the greater

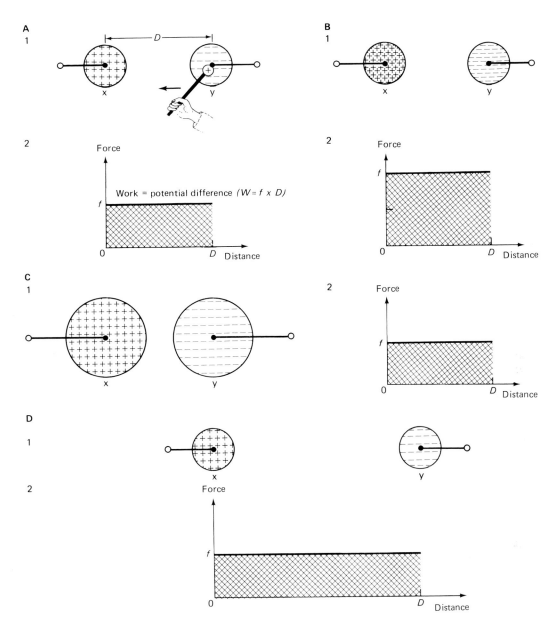

III–1 The factors that affect the potential difference between two plates of a capacitor. **A.** As a test charge is moved between two charged plates (**1**), it must overcome a force (**2**). The work done against this force is the potential difference between the two plates. **B.** Increasing the charge density (**1**) increases the potential difference (**2**). **C.** Increasing the area of the plates (**1**) increases the number of charges required to produce a given potential difference (**2**). **D.** Increasing the distance between the two plates (**1**) increases the potential difference between them (**2**).

is the resulting potential difference across the capacitor (Figure III–1B). Thus, for a given capacitor, there is a linear relationship between the amount of charge (*Q*) stored on its plates and the potential difference across it:

$$Q \text{ (coulombs)} = C \text{ (farads)} \times V \text{ (volts)} \quad \text{(III–1)}$$

where the capacitance, *C*, is a constant.

The capacitance of a parallel-plate capacitor is determined by two features of its geometry: the area (*A*) of the two plates, and the distance (*D*) between them. Increasing the area of the plates increases capacitance, because a greater amount of charge must be deposited on each side to produce the same charge density, which is what determines the force *f* acting on the test charge (Figure III–1A and C). Increasing the distance *D* between the plates does not change the force acting on the test charge, but it does increase the work that must be done to move it from one side of the capacitor to the other

(Figures III–1A and D). Therefore, for a given charge separation between the two plates, the potential difference between them is proportional to the distance. Put another way, the greater the distance is, the smaller is the amount of charge that must be deposited on the plates to produce a given potential difference, and therefore the smaller is the capacitance (Equation III–1). These geometrical determinants of capacitance can be summarized by the equation:

$$C \propto \frac{A}{D}.$$

As shown in Equation III–1, the separation of positive and negative charges on the two plates of a capacitor results in a potential difference between them. The converse of this statement is also true: the potential difference across a capacitor is determined by the excess of positive and negative charges on its plates. In order for the potential across a capacitor to change, the amount of electrical charges stored on the two conducting plates must change first.

Rules for Circuit Analysis

A few basic relationships that are used for circuit analysis are listed below. Familiarity with these rules and conventions will help in understanding the electric circuit examples that follow, and in doing the problems in Appendix IIIB.

Conductance

This is the symbol for a conductor:

A variable conductor is represented this way:

A pathway with infinite conductance (zero resistance) is called a short circuit, and is represented by a straight line:

Conductors in parallel add:

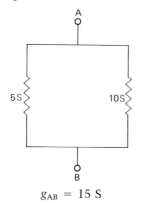

$$g_{AB} = 15 \text{ S}$$

Conductors in series add reciprocally:

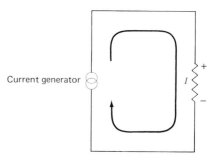

$$\frac{1}{g_{AB}} = \frac{1}{5} + \frac{1}{10} = \frac{3}{10}$$
$$g_{AB} = 3.3 \text{ S}.$$

Resistors in series add, while resistors in parallel add reciprocally.

Current

An *arrow* denotes the direction of current flow (net movement of positive charge).

Ohm's law is

$$I = Vg = \frac{V}{R}.$$

When current flows through a conductor, the end that the current enters is positive with respect to the end that it leaves:

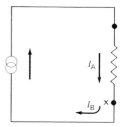

The algebraic sum of all currents entering or leaving a junction is zero (we arbitrarily define current approaching a junction as positive, and current leaving a junction as negative). In this circuit

for junction x,

$$I_A = +5 \text{ A}$$
$$I_B = -5 \text{ A}$$
$$I_A + I_B = 0.$$

In this circuit

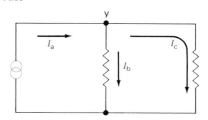

for junction y,

$$I_a = +3 \text{ A}$$
$$I_b = -2 \text{ A}$$
$$I_c = -1 \text{ A}$$
$$I_a + I_b + I_c = 0.$$

Current follows the path of greatest conductance (least resistance). For conductance pathways in parallel, the current through each path is proportional to its conductance value divided by the total conductance of the parallel combination:

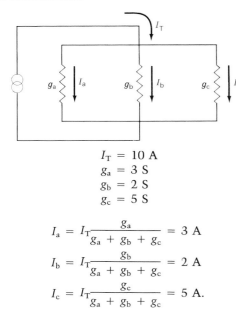

$$I_T = 10 \text{ A}$$
$$g_a = 3 \text{ S}$$
$$g_b = 2 \text{ S}$$
$$g_c = 5 \text{ S}$$

$$I_a = I_T \frac{g_a}{g_a + g_b + g_c} = 3 \text{ A}$$

$$I_b = I_T \frac{g_b}{g_a + g_b + g_c} = 2 \text{ A}$$

$$I_c = I_T \frac{g_c}{g_a + g_b + g_c} = 5 \text{ A}.$$

Capacitance

This is the symbol for a capacitor:

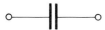

The potential difference across a capacitor is proportional to the charge stored on its plates:

$$V_C = \frac{Q}{C}.$$

Potential Difference

This is the symbol for a battery, or electromotive force. It is often abbreviated by the symbol E.

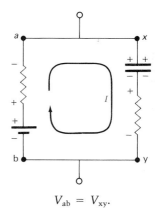

The positive pole is always represented by the longer bar.

Batteries in series add algebraically, but attention must be paid to their polarities. If their polarities are the same, their absolute values add:

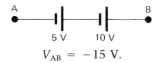

$$V_{AB} = -15 \text{ V}.$$

If their polarities are opposite, they subtract:

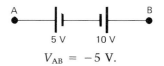

$$V_{AB} = -5 \text{ V}.$$

[The convention used here for potential difference is that $V_{AB} = (V_A - V_B)$.]

A battery drives a current around the circuit from its positive to its negative terminal:

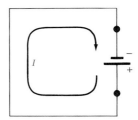

For purposes of calculating the total resistance of a circuit, one may assume that the internal resistance of a battery is zero.

The potential differences across parallel branches of a circuit are equal:

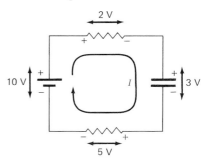

$$V_{ab} = V_{xy}.$$

As one goes around a closed loop in a circuit, the algebraic sum of all the potential differences is zero:

$$2\,V + 3\,V + 5\,V - 10\,V = 0.$$

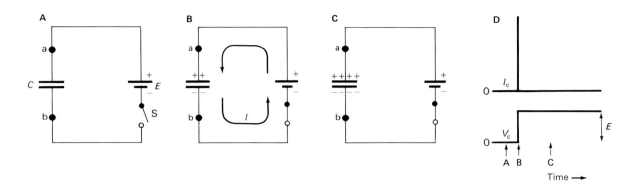

III–2 Time course of charging a capacitor. **A.** Circuit before switch (**S**) is closed. **B.** Immediately after the switch is closed. **C.** After the capacitor has become fully charged. **D.** Time course of changes in I_C and V_C in response to closing of switch.

Current Flow in Circuits with Capacitance

Circuits that have capacitive elements are much more complex than those that have only batteries and conductors. This complexity arises because in capacitive circuits current flow varies with time. The time depen-

dence of the changes in current and voltage in capacitive circuits is illustrated qualitatively in the following three examples.

Capacitive Circuit

Capacitive current does not actually flow across the insulating gap in a capacitor; rather, it results in a build-up of positive and negative charges on the capacitor plates. However, we can measure a current flowing into and out of the terminals of a capacitor. Consider the circuit shown in Figure III–2A. When switch S is closed (Figure

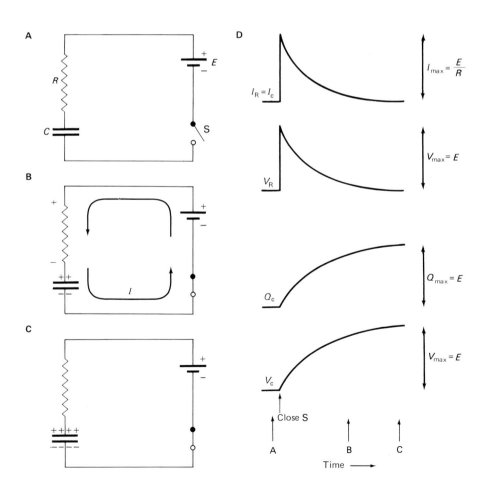

III–3 Time course of charging a capacitor in series with a resistor, from a constant voltage source (**E**). **A.** Circuit before the switch (**S**) is closed. **B.** Shortly after the switch is closed. **C.** After capacitor has settled at its new potential. **D.** Time course of current flow, of the increase in charge deposited on the capacitor, and of the increased potential differences across the resistor and the capacitor.

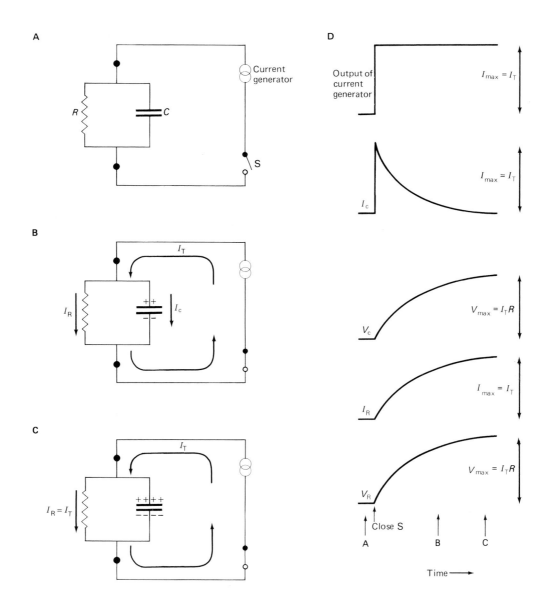

III–4   Time course of charging a capacitor in parallel with a resistor, from a constant current source. **A.** Circuit before switch (**S**) is closed. **B.** Shortly after the switch is closed. **C.** After charge deposited on the capacitor has reached its final value. **D.** Time course of changes in I_C, V_C, I_R, and V_R in response to closing of the switch.

III–2B), a net positive charge is moved by the battery E onto plate a, and an equal amount of net positive charge is withdrawn from plate b. The result is current flowing counterclockwise in the circuit. Since the charges that carry this current flow into or out of the terminals of a capacitor, building up an excess of plus and minus charges on its plates, it is called a *capacitive current* (I_c). Because there is no resistance in this circuit, the battery E can generate a very large amplitude of current, which will charge the capacitance to a value $Q = E \times C$ in an infinitesimally short period of time (Figure III–2D).

Circuit with Resistor and Capacitor in Series

Now consider what happens if one adds a resistor in series with the capacitor in the circuit shown in Figure III–3A. The maximum current that can be generated when

switch S is closed (Figure III–3B) is now limited by Ohm's law ($I = V/R$). Therefore, the capacitor charges more slowly. When the potential across the capacitor has finally reached the value $V_c = Q/C = E$ (Figure III–3C), there is no longer a difference in potential as one goes around the loop; i.e., the battery voltage (E) is equal and opposite to the voltage across the capacitor, V_c. The two thus cancel out, and there is no source of potential difference left to drive a current around the loop. Immediately after the switch is closed the potential difference is greatest, so current flow is at a maximum. As the capacitor begins to charge, however, the net potential difference $(V_c + E)$ available to drive a current becomes smaller, so that current flow is reduced. The result is that an exponential change in voltage and in current flow occurs across the resistor and the capacitor. Note that in this circuit resistive current must equal capacitive current at all times (see Rules for Circuit Analysis, above).

Circuit with Resistor and Capacitor in Parallel

Consider now what happens if we place a parallel resistor and capacitor combination in series with a constant current generator that generates a current I_T (Figure III–4).

When switch S is closed (Figure III–4B), current starts to flow around the loop. Initially, in the first instant of time after the current flow begins, all of the current flows into the capacitor, $(I_T = I_c)$. However, as charge builds up on the plates of the capacitor, a potential difference V_c is generated across it. Since the resistor and capacitor are in parallel, the potential across them must be equal; thus part of the total current begins to flow through the resistor, such that $I_R R = V_R = V_c$. As less and less current flows into the capacitor, its rate of charging becomes slower; this accounts for the exponential shape of the curve of voltage versus time. Eventually, a plateau is reached at which the voltage no longer changes. When this occurs, all of the current flows through the resistor, and $V_c = V_R = I_T R$.

Problem Set for Chapters 5–9

IIIB

1. The diagram below shows the simplified equivalent circuit for a neuron:

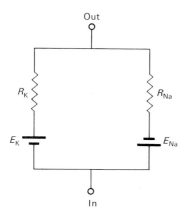

Out

In

$$E_K = -75 \text{ mV}$$
$$E_{Na} = +55 \text{ mV}$$

$$R_K = 0.2 \times 10^6 \ \Omega$$
$$R_{Na} = 5 \times 10^6 \ \Omega$$

a. What is the net electromotive force that drives current around the loop? Draw in an arrow showing the direction of current flow.
b. What is the total resistance around the loop?
c. What is the value of current flowing around the loop?
d. What is the potential difference across R_K? Across R_{Na}? Show on the diagram the polarities of these potential differences.
e. Calculate the potential across the left-hand (K^+) branch. Do the same for the Na^+ branch. What is the membrane potential of the cell?
f. For the circuit shown above, $g_K = 5 \times 10^{-6}$ S and $g_{Na} = 0.2 \times 10^{-6}$ S. Calculate V_m using these values and Equation 6–3, Chapter 6.

2. Assume that for the cell depicted above,

$$g_K = 50 \times 10^{-6} \text{ S}$$
$$g_{Na} = 2 \times 10^{-6} \text{ S}.$$

Calculate V_m.

3. For the cell shown above, assume that

$$g_K = 0.2 \times 10^{-6} \text{ S}$$
$$g_{Na} = 5 \times 10^{-6} \text{ S}$$

(just the opposite of the initial conditions). Calculate V_m.

4. What are the ratios of g_K/g_{Na} for Problems 1, 2, and 3? What does this, along with the values of V_m you just calculated, tell you about the role of the conductances for different ions in determining V_m?

5. Assume that the neuron depicted in Problem 1 has a Na–K pump that works as shown in this diagram:

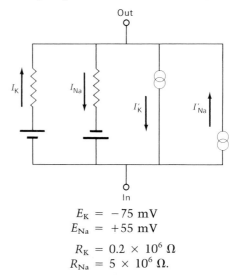

Out

In

$$E_K = -75 \text{ mV}$$
$$E_{Na} = +55 \text{ mV}$$

$$R_K = 0.2 \times 10^6 \ \Omega$$
$$R_{Na} = 5 \times 10^6 \ \Omega.$$

The pump is represented by a pair of constant current generators that generate outward I'_{Na} and inward I'_K. These active currents are opposite to the passive I_{Na} and I_K through the conductance channels. For purposes of calculation these pumps may be assumed to offer infinite resistance to currents generated elsewhere in the circuit. Assume that the pump is *not* electrogenic, and that the cell is in a steady state, i.e., V_m and $[Na^+]_i$ and $[K^+]_i$ are constant. What are the values of I_{Na} and I_K (see Problem 1c)? What are the values of I'_{Na} and I'_K?

6. For the cell depicted in Problem 5, assume that the pump is electrogenic, such that three Na^+ ions are pumped out for each two K^+ ions pumped in. Assume also that the cell is in a steady state (V_m and $[K^+]_i$ and $[Na^+]_i$ are constant).
   a. Given that $I'_{Na} = +25.32 \times 10^{-9}$ A, calculate I_{Na}.
   b. Using this value of I_{Na}, calculate V_m. Compare this with the value calculated in Problem 1e.
   c. Calculate I_K.

7. A neuron has a total membrane capacitance of 10^{-10} F.
   a. How many coulombs of charge are separated across the membrane when the cell has a resting potential of -50 mV?
   b. What is the charge separation across the membrane at the peak of an action potential when $V_m = +50$ mV?
   c. What is the *net* influx of positive charge into the cell during the rising phase of the action potential?
   d. Assume that the cell has a volume of 9.2×10^{-11} liter and the total intracellular concentration of ionic charges is 200 meq. What is the percentage change of the total number of intracellular charges when V_m goes from -50 mV to $+50$ mV at the peak of the spike? (There are 1.04×10^{-5} moles of univalent charge per coulomb.)

8. You are investigating the properties of inputs to the cell shown below:

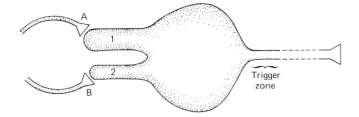

Synapses A and B produce the same depolarization in their respective postsynaptic membranes and are equidistant from the trigger zone. If dendrite 1 has a greater diameter than dendrite 2, which synaptic input will be larger when recorded at the trigger zone?

9. a. What would be the effect on the length constant of an axon of stripping off its myelin sheath?
   b. Why?

10. You are examining the neural circuit shown below:

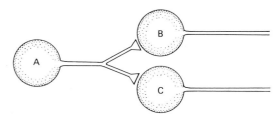

Neuron A excites follower cells B and C. The time constant of cell B is 50 msec and that of cell C is 200 msec.
   a. Neuron A fires in the pattern shown below:

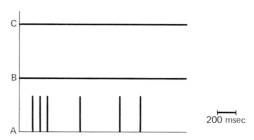

   Sketch the approximate waveforms of the synaptic responses in cells B and C (assume that they do not fire action potentials).
   b. How do the passive properties of neurons B and C affect their ability to integrate signals from presynaptic neurons?

11. An increase in the diameter of an axon will result in an increased conduction velocity because:
   a. membrane capacitance per unit length of axon is increased.
   b. the total number of Na^+ channels is increased.
   c. axoplasmic resistance per unit length of axon is decreased.
   d. membrane resistance per unit length of axon is increased.

12. Neurons A and B have identical geometries, but the membrane resistance of A is 10 times greater than that of B:
   a. A will have a longer time constant than B.
   b. B will have a shorter length constant than A.
   c. A 10-mV synaptic potential generated at the tip of a dendrite will spread toward the trigger zone more effectively in A than in B.
   d. all of the above.

13. Increasing the membrane capacitance (capacitance per unit area of membrane) of a neuron will result in:
   a. an increase in the length constant.
   b. an increase in conduction velocity.

c. an increase in the duration of the synaptic potentials generated in the cell.

d. all of the above.

14. Two excitatory postsynaptic potentials generated 3 msec apart at the tip of a dendrite sum together to produce a subthreshold depolarization of 10 mV at the trigger zone. The chance of these postsynaptic potentials triggering a spike would be greater if:

a. they were generated closer to the cell body.

b. the membrane capacitance (capacitance per unit area) were lower.

15. Consider a dendrite of a neuron with a certain axoplasmic resistance between the dendrite and the neuron's trigger zone. Assume there are synaptic channels open in the dendrite:

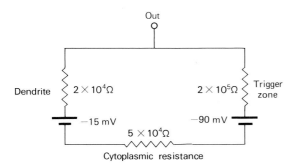

a. What is the current flowing through the cytoplasmic resistance?

b. What is the membrane potential at the trigger zone?

c. What is the membrane potential of the dendrite?

d. Why is the depolarization across the trigger zone less than the depolarization across the synaptic membrane?

16. A nerve cell is represented by the equivalent circuit diagram below. This diagram is simplified in that the Cl^- channels are not represented and the cable properties of the cell are ignored. The active and passive K^+ channels are lumped together in one branch, and the active and passive Na^+ channels are lumped together in a second branch.

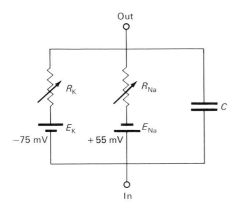

a. Given

$$g_K = 5 \times 10^{-6} \text{ S}$$
$$g_{Na} = 0.2 \times 10^{-6} \text{ S}$$
$$V_m = -70 \text{ mV}$$

for the cell at rest, what is the equation for the potential difference across the Na^+ branch of the circuit (the resting potential)?
Use this equation to calculate I_{Na}.
Using the analogous equation for K^+, calculate I_K.
What is the value of I_c (the capacitive current)?

b. During the rising phase of an action potential in this cell (at P_1), the membrane parameters reach these values:

$$V_m = +20 \text{ mV}$$
$$g_K = 5.13 \times 10^{-6} \text{ S}$$
$$g_{Na} = 200 \times 10^{-6} \text{ S}$$

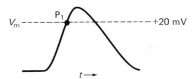

What are the values of I_K, I_{Na}, and I_c?

c. At the peak of the action potential, the membrane parameters are

$$V_m = +50 \text{ mV}$$
$$g_K = 5.263 \times 10^{-6} \text{ S}$$
$$g_{Na} = 131.6 \times 10^{-6} \text{ S}$$

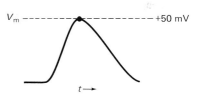

What are the values of I_K, I_{Na}, and I_c?

d. During the falling phase of the spike (P_2), the membrane parameters are

$$V_m = +20 \text{ mV}$$
$$g_{Na} = 33.3 \times 10^{-6} \text{ S}$$
$$g_K = 33.3 \times 10^{-6} \text{ S}$$

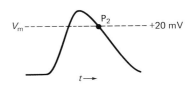

What are the values of I_K, I_{Na}, and I_c?

17. The circuit diagram below shows the synaptic (g_s, E_s) and nonsynaptic, or leakage (g_m, E_m), channels of a neuron. A spike in a presynaptic neuron releases transmitter that causes a brief opening of the synaptic conductance channels (equivalent to closing switch S). The figure on the bottom shows the time course of the change in V_m and of g_s.

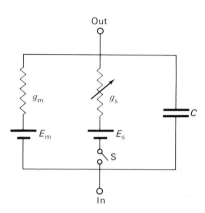

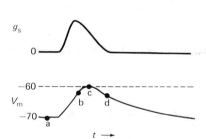

$$g_m = 0.2 \times 10^{-6} \text{ S}$$
$$E_m = -70 \text{ mV}$$
$$E_s = -15 \text{ mV}.$$

a. What is I_c at time a?
b. At time b,

$$g_s = 0.2 \times 10^{-6} \text{ S}$$
$$V_m = -63 \text{ mV}$$

What are the values of I_{gs}, I_{gm}, and I_c?
c. At the peak of the excitatory postsynaptic potential (time c),

$$g_s = 0.044 \times 10^6 \text{ S}$$
$$V_m = -60 \text{ mV}.$$

What are the values of I_{gs}, I_{gm}, and I_c?
d. At time d, during the falling phase, all of the synaptic channels have closed (switch S is open):

$$g_s = 0 \text{ S}$$
$$V_m = -63 \text{ mV}.$$

What are the values of I_{gm}, I_{gs}, and I_c?

18. The circuit diagram below represents a neuron connected to a current generator by an intracellular and an extracellular electrode. Only the passive elements of the membrane (leakage channels and membrane capacitance) are represented.

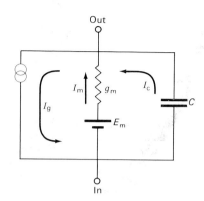

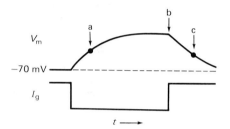

$$E_m = -70 \text{ mV}$$
$$g_m = 0.2 \times 10^{-6} \text{ S}.$$

a. At time a,

$$I_g = 2.8 \times 10^{-9} \text{ A}$$
$$V_m = -63 \text{ mV}.$$

What are the values of I_m and I_c?
b. At time b,

$$I_g = -2.8 \times 10^{-9} \text{ A}$$
$$I_c = 0.$$

What are the values of I_m and V_m?
c. At time c,

$$I_g = 0$$
$$V_m = -66 \text{ mV}.$$

What are the values of I_m and I_c?

19. The K^+ conductance that is turned on in neurons in response to a long depolarizing pulse
   a. is maintained for the duration of the pulse.
   b. precedes the Na^+ conductance.
   c. provides positive feedback that produces additional depolarization.
   d. none of the above.

20. The refractory period is caused by
    a. a residual increase in K$^+$ conductance.
    b. inactivation of Na$^+$ conductance channels.
    c. Na$^+$ pump reversal.
    d. both (a) and (b).

21. Threshold is the value of membrane potential at which
    a. Na$^+$ conductance first turns on.
    b. net ionic current becomes inward.
    c. the action potential becomes an all-or-none, regenerative process.
    d. both (b) and (c).

22. When a voltage-clamped axon is stepped in a depolarizing direction from resting potential (-60 mV) to $+10$ mV for 1 sec,
    a. g_{Na} increases more rapidly than g_K.
    b. the increase in g_{Na} wanes before the end of the pulse.
    c. the net electrochemical driving force for inward I_{Na} will be reduced.
    d. all of the above.

23. Why does one need a voltage clamp to study active membrane conductances?

24. Given that g_{Na} is graded as a function of depolarization, why does an action potential have a sharp threshold?

25. a. Define the reversal potential of a postsynaptic potential.
    b. Must the reversal potential of a postsynaptic potential equal the equilibrium potential of one of the ionic constituents of a neuron?
    c. The reversal potential of an increased conductance excitatory postsynaptic potential is always at a more depolarized level than the threshold for initiating an action potential. True or false?
    d. The reversal potential of a decreased conductance excitatory postsynaptic potential is always at a more depolarized level than the threshold for initiating an action potential. True or false?

26. What are two ways to increase the synaptic current generated by a postsynaptic potential?

27. What single type of ion could produce each of the following synaptic responses:

	Excitatory	Inhibitory
g increases		
g decreases		

28. What would be the effect of a large increase in intracellular Na$^+$ concentration on:
    a. the amplitude of the action potential?
    b. the amplitude of an excitatory postsynaptic potential due to increased g to both Na$^+$ and K$^+$?
    c. the amplitude of an inhibitory postsynaptic potential due to decreased g_{Na}?

29. Do the Na$^+$ currents of the action potential and the excitatory postsynaptic potential use the same channels through the nerve membranes?

Answers to Problem Set

1. a. The Na$^+$ and K$^+$ batteries have the *same* polarity as one goes *around* the loop, so their values add algebraically. Current flows from the positive pole to the negative pole of this battery pair, i.e., clockwise.

    b. $R_{Na} + R_K = 5.2 \times 10^6$ Ω.

    c. $\dfrac{130 \times 10^{-3} \text{ V}}{5.2 \times 10^6 \ \Omega} = 25 \times 10^{-9}$ A, or 25 nA.

    d. $V_{R_K} = (25 \times 10^{-9} \text{ A})(0.2 \times 10^6 \ \Omega) = +5$ mV (inside positive).
    $V_{R_{Na}} = (25 \times 10^{-9} \text{ A})(5 \times 10^6 \ \Omega) = -125$ mV (inside negative).

    e. V_K branch $= V_{Na}$ branch $= V_m = -70$ mV.

    f. $V_m = [(5 \times 10^{-6}$ S$)(-75 \times 10^{-3}$ V$) + (2 \times 10^{-6}$ S$)(+55 \times 10^{-3}$ V$)]/[(5 + 0.2) \times 10^{-6}$ S$]$
    $= -70$ mV.

2. $V_m = -70$ mV.

3. $V_m = +50$ mV.

4. For Problems 1 and 2, $g_K/g_{Na} = 25/1$ and $V_m = -70$ mV.
   For Problem 3, $g_K/g_{Na} = 1/25$ and $V_m = +50$ mV. Thus it is not the *absolute value* of the Na$^+$ and K$^+$ conductances that is important in determining V_m, but rather their values *relative* to each other. For a circuit that has only two branches, V_m will always be closer to the value of the battery of the ion channel type with the greater conductance.

5. From Problem 1c,
$$I_{Na} = -25 \text{ nA}$$
$$I_K = +25 \text{ nA.}$$

Since the cell is in a steady state, I_{Na} and I_K are exactly balanced by I'_{Na} and I'_K; thus,
$$I'_{Na} = +25 \text{ nA}$$
$$I'_K = -25 \text{ nA.}$$

6. a. Since the cell is in a steady state,

$$I_{Na} = -I'_{Na}.$$

Therefore,

$$I_{Na} = -25.32 \text{ nA}.$$

b. $V_m = E_{Na} + R_{Na}I_{Na} = -71.6 \text{ mV}.$
c. Because of the pump's electrogenicity,

$$I'_K = -2/3 \, I'_{Na}.$$

Therefore,

$$I'_K = -16.88 \text{ nA}.$$

Since the cell is in a steady state,

$$I_K = -I'_K = 16.88 \text{ nA}.$$

Note that

$$\frac{I_{Na}}{I_K} = \frac{I'_{Na}}{I'_K} = \frac{3}{2}.$$

7. a. $Q = VC = (10^{-10} \text{ F}) (50 \times 10^{-3} \text{ V}) = 5 \times 10^{-12}$ coulomb.
b. $Q = VC = 5 \times 10^{-12}$ coulomb.
c. 5×10^{-12} coulomb are required to bring V_m from -50 to 0 mV, and another 5×10^{-12} are needed to bring it from 0 up to $+50$ mV. Therefore,

$$Q = 5 \times 10^{-12} + 5 \times 10^{-12} = 10^{-11} \text{ coulomb}.$$

d. The total number of moles of charge that enters is
$(10^{-11} \text{ coulomb}) (1.04 \times 10^{-5} \text{ mole/coulomb}) = 1.04 \times 10^{-16}$ mole.
The original amount of charge in the cell was $(200 \times 10^{-3} \text{ mole/liter}) (9.2 \times 10^{-11} \text{ liter}) = 1.84 \times 10^{-11}$ mole.
Therefore, the percent change in total intracellular charge during the rising phase of the action potential is

$$\frac{1.04 \times 10^{-16}}{1.84 \times 10^{-11}} \times 100 = 0.0006\%.$$

8. Input A. Dendrite 1 has a longer length constant than dendrite 2 because of its larger diameter. The r_m decreases in direct proportion to an increase in dendrite diameter, but r_a decreases in proportion to the diameter squared. Therefore, $\lambda = \sqrt{r_m/r_a}$ is proportional to the square root of the diameter.

9. a. λ would decrease.
b. Because its effective r_m will decrease, and $\lambda = \sqrt{r_m/r_a}$.

10. a.

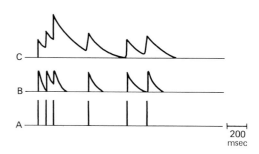

b. Cell C will be more effective than cell B in summing repetitive input.

11. c.

12. d.

13. c.

14. a.

15. a. Find the direction of the current flow:

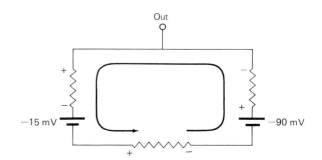

The two batteries oppose each other and the larger (-90 mV) dominates.
Current flow in the loop is

$$I = \frac{V}{R} = \frac{(90 \times 10^{-3} \text{ V}) - (15 \times 10^{-3} \text{ V})}{(2 \times 10^4 + 5 \times 10^4 + 2 \times 10^5 \text{ }\Omega)}$$
$$= \frac{75 \times 10^{-3} \text{ V}}{27 \times 10^4 \text{ }\Omega}$$
$$= 2.78 \times 10^{-7} \text{ A}.$$

b. The membrane potential across the trigger zone is given by

$$V_{in-out} = E_{trig} + (R_{trig} \times I)$$
$$= -[90 \text{ mV} + (2 \times 10^5 \text{ }\Omega) \times (2.78 \times 10^{-7} \text{ A})]$$
$$= -90 \text{ mV} + 55.6 \text{ mV}$$
$$= -34.4 \text{ mV}.$$

c. The membrane potential across the dendrite is given by

$$V_{\text{in—out}} = E_{\text{den}} + (R_{\text{den}} \times I)$$
$$= -15 \text{ mV}$$
$$= + (2 \times 10^4 \ \Omega) \ (-2.78 \times 10^{-7} \text{ A})$$
$$= -15 \text{ mV} - 5.6 \text{ mV}$$
$$= -20.6 \text{ mV}.$$

d. The trigger zone is less depolarized than the dendrite because of the voltage drop across the cytoplasmic resistor:

$$V_{\text{cyt}} = R_{\text{cyt}} \times I$$
$$= (5 \times 10^4 \ \Omega) \ (2.78 \times 10^{-7} \text{ A})$$
$$= 13.9 \times 10^{-3} \text{ V} = 13.9 \text{ mV}$$

This drop is the difference between the two values of V_{m} (dendrite and trigger zone):

$$V_{\text{den}} = V_{\text{cyt}} + V_{\text{trig}}$$
$$-20.6 \text{ mV} = +13.9 \text{ mV} - 34.5 \text{ mV}.$$

16. a.
$$V_{\text{m}} = E_{\text{Na}} + I_{\text{Na}}/g_{\text{Na}}$$
$$I_{\text{Na}} = (g_{\text{Na}}) \times (V_{\text{m}} - E_{\text{Na}}) = -25 \times 10^{-9} \text{ A}$$
$$V_{\text{m}} = E_{\text{K}} + I_{\text{K}}/g_{\text{K}}$$
$$I_{\text{K}} = (g_{\text{K}}) \times (V_{\text{m}} - E_{\text{K}}) = +25 \times 10^{-9} \text{ A}.$$

The current flowing into junction a must equal the current flowing out.

$$I_{\text{K}} + I_{\text{Na}} + I_{\text{c}} = 0.$$

Therefore,

$$I_{\text{c}} = 0.$$

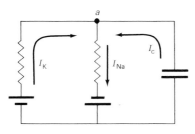

b.
$$I_{\text{K}} = (g_{\text{K}}) \times (V_{\text{m}} - E_{\text{K}})$$
$$= 487 \times 10^{-9} \text{ A}$$
$$I_{\text{Na}} = (g_{\text{Na}}) \times (V_{\text{m}} - E_{\text{Na}})$$
$$= 7000 \times 10^{-9} \text{ A}$$
$$I_{\text{Na}} + I_{\text{K}} + I_{\text{c}} = 0$$
$$I_{\text{c}} = 6513 \times 10^{-9} \text{ A}.$$

c.
$$I_{\text{K}} = 658 \times 10^{-9} \text{ A}$$
$$I_{\text{Na}} = -658 \times 10^{-9} \text{ A}$$
$$I_{\text{c}} = 0.$$

d.
$$I_{\text{Na}} = -1165 \times 10^{-9} \text{ A}$$
$$I_{\text{K}} = 3163 \times 10^{-9} \text{ A}$$
$$I_{\text{c}} = -1998 \times 10^{-9} \text{ A}.$$

Note that when V_{m} is not increasing or decreasing, $I_{\text{c}} = 0$. When V_{m} is changing in a depolarizing direction, I_{c} is outward. When V_{m} is repo-

larizing (or hyperpolarizing), I_{c} is inward. The faster V_{m} is changing, the greater is the absolute value of I_{c}.

17. a. Since V_{m} is not changing at time a, no capacitive current can be flowing.

b.
$$I_{\text{gm}} = +1.4 \times 10^{-9} \text{ A}$$
$$I_{\text{gs}} = -9.6 \times 10^{-9} \text{ A}$$
$$I_{\text{c}} = +8.2 \times 10^{-9} \text{ A}.$$

c.
$$I_{\text{gs}} = -2 \times 10^{-9} \text{ A}$$
$$I_{\text{gm}} = +2 \times 10^{-9} \text{ A}$$
$$I_{\text{c}} = 0.$$

d.
$$I_{\text{gs}} = 0$$
$$I_{\text{gm}} = +1.4 \times 10^{-9} \text{ A}$$
$$I_{\text{c}} = -1.4 \times 10^{-9} \text{ A}.$$

18. a.
$$I_{\text{m}} = +1.4 \times 10^{-9} \text{ A}$$
$$I_{\text{c}} = +1.4 \times 10^{-9} \text{ A}.$$

b.
$$I_{\text{m}} = +2.8 \times 10^{-9} \text{ A}$$
$$V_{\text{m}} = -56 \text{ mV}.$$

c.
$$I_{\text{m}} = +0.8 \times 10^{-9} \text{ A}$$
$$I_{\text{c}} = -0.8 \times 10^{-9} \text{ A}.$$

Note the resemblance between Problems 16b, 17b, and 18a. In all cases, depolarization is occurring because there is a net excess of positive charge flowing into the cell. This net inward ionic current is balanced by an outward capacitive current, which deposits positive charges on the inside of the membrane capacitance. The sources of inward ionic current vary in each of these three cases: it may come through voltage-sensitive ion channels, through synaptic channels, or through an intracellular electrode.

19. a.

20. d.

21. d.

22. d.

23. 1. To separate capacitive and ionic components of membrane current.
    2. To break the regenerative coupling between membrane potential and current.

24. For subthreshold depolarizations, the increase in inward current carried by Na^+ is more than balanced by an increase in outward current by leakage ions (K^+ and Cl^-). For depolarization above threshold, the increase in Na^+ current is greater than the increase in K^+ and Cl^- current, leading to a net inward current and regenerative response.

25. **a.** The membrane potential at which the change in membrane current induced by the change in membrane conductance is zero; that is,

$$I_{EPSP} = g_{EPSP} (V_m - E_{EPSP})$$

For $V_m = E_{EPSP}$,

$$I_{EPSP} = 0.$$

b. No.

c. True.

d. False.

26. **1.** Increase the driving force of the postsynaptic potential by altering the membrane potential (V_m) or by altering the reversal potential (E_{EPSP}).

2. Increase the conductance change produced by the neurotransmitter (g_{EPSP}) because

$$I_{EPSP} = g_{EPSP} (V_m - E_{EPSP}).$$

27.

	Excitatory	Inhibitory
g increases	Na^+	K^+ or Cl^-
g decreases	K^+ or Cl^-	Na^+

28.

a. Decrease amplitude.

b. Decrease amplitude.

c. Decrease amplitude.
In all these cases E_{Na} is reduced.

29. No.

Bibliography

A

Abrams, T. W., and Kandel, E. R. 1985. Roles of calcium and adenylate cyclase in activity-dependent facilitation, a cellular mechanism for classical conditioning in *Aplysia*. J. Neurosci. Abstr. (in press).

Abrams, T.W., Carew, T. J., Hawkins, R. D., and Kandel, E. R. 1983. Aspects of the cellular mechanism of temporal specificity in conditioning in *Aplysia*: Preliminary evidence for Ca^{2+} influx as a signal of activity. Soc. Neurosci. Abstr. 9:168.

Adams, P. 1982. Voltage-dependent conductances of vertebrate neurones. Trends Neurosci. 5:116–119.

Adams, R. D., and Victor, M. 1977. Principles of Neurology. New York: McGraw-Hill.

Adams, R. D., and Victor, M. 1981. Principles of Neurology, 2nd ed. New York: McGraw-Hill, pp. 60–68.

Adrian, E. D. 1928. The Basis of Sensation: The Action of the Sense Organ. London: Christophers.

Adrian, E. D. 1932. The Mechanism of Nervous Action: Electrical Studies of the Neurone. Philadelphia: University of Pennsylvania Press.

Adrian, E. D. 1943. Afferent areas in the cerebellum connected with the limbs. Brain 66:289–315.

Adrian, E. D., and Zotterman, Y. 1926. The impulses produced by sensory nerve-endings. Part 2. The response of a single end-organ. J. Physiol. (Lond.) 61:151–171.

Adrian, R. H., and Bryant, S. H. 1974. On the repetitive discharge in myotonic muscle fibres. J. Physiol. (Lond.) 240:505–515.

Ahrens, R. 1954. Beitrag zur Entwicklung des Physiognomie- und Mimikerkennens. Z. Exp. Angew. Psychol. 2:412–454, 599–633.

Aitkin, L. M., Irvine, D. R. F., and Webster, W. R. 1984. Central neural mechanisms of hearing. In I. Darian-Smith (ed.), Handbook of Physiology, Section 1: The Nervous System, Vol. III, Sensory Processes. Bethesda, Md.: American Physiological Society, pp. 675–737.

Akil, H., Mayer, D. J., and Liebeskind, J. C. 1976. Antagonism of stimulation-produced analgesia by naloxone, a narcotic antagonist. Science 191:961–962.

Akil, H., Watson, S. J., Young, E., Lewis M. E., Khachaturian, H., and Walker, J. M. 1984. Endogenous opioids: Biology and function. Annu. Rev. Neurosci. 7:223–255.

Alavi, A., Reivich, M., Jones, S. C., Greenberg, J. H., and Wolf, A. P. 1982. Functional imaging of the brain with positron emission tomography. In L. M. Freeman (ed.), Nuclear Medicine Annual. New York: Raven Press, pp. 319–372.

Alberts, B., Bray, D., Lewis, J., Raff, M., Roberts, K., and Watson, J. D. 1983. Molecular Biology of the Cell. New York: Garland.

Albuquerque, E. X., Rash, J. E., Mayer, R. F., and Satterfield, J. R. 1976. An electrophysiological and morphological study of the neuromuscular junction in patients with myasthenia gravis. Exp. Neurol. 51:536–563.

Albus, J. S. 1971. A theory of cerebellar function. Math. Biosci. 10:25–61.

Alkon, D. L. 1983. Learning in a marine snail. Sci. Am. 249(1):70–84.

Allen, G. I., and Tsukahara, N. 1974. Cerebrocerebellar communication systems. Physiol. Rev. 54:957–1006.

Amoore, J. E., Johnston, J. W., Jr., and Rubin, M. 1964. The stereochemical theory of odor. Sci. Am. 210(2):42–49.

Anand, B. K., and Brobeck, J. R. 1951. Localization of a "feeding center" in the hypothalamus of the rat. Proc. Soc. Exp. Biol. Med. 77:323–324.

Andén, N.-E., Dahlström, A., Fuxe, K., Larsson, K., Olson, L., and Ungerstedt, U. 1966. Ascending monoamine neurons to the telencephalon and diencephalon. Acta Physiol. Scand. 67:313–326.

Anderson, D. J., and Blobel, G. 1981. *In vitro* synthesis, glycosylation, and membrane insertion of the four subunits of *Torpedo* acetylcholine receptor. Proc. Natl. Acad. Sci. U.S.A. 78:5598–5602.

Andreasen, N. C., Olsen, S. A., Dennert, J. W., and Smith, M. R. 1982. Ventricular enlargement in schizophrenia: Relationship to positive and negative symptoms. Am. J. Psychiatry 139:297–302.

Andres, K. H. 1966. Der Feinbau der Regio olfactoria von Makrosmatikern. Z. Zellforsch. 69:140–154.

Andrews, D. W., Langan, T. A., and Weiner, N. 1983. Evidence for the involvement of a cyclic AMP-independent protein kinase in the activation of soluble tyrosine hydroxylase from rat striatum. Proc. Natl. Acad. Sci. U.S.A. 80:2097–2101.

Appenzeller, O. 1982. The Autonomic Nervous System: An Introduction to Basic and Clinical Concepts, 3rd rev. ed. New York: Elsevier Biomedical Press.

Armstrong, C. M. 1981. Sodium channels and gating currents. Physiol. Rev. 61:644–683.

Arshavsky, Yu. I., Berkinblit, M. B., Fukson, O. I., Gelfand, I. M., and Orlovsky, G. N. 1972. Recordings of neurones of the dorsal spinocerebellar tract during evoked locomotion. Brain Res. 43:272–275.

Arshavsky, Yu. I., Berkinblit, M. B., Fukson, O. I., Gelfand, I. M., and Orlovsky, G. N. 1972. Origin of modulation in neurones of the ventral spinocerebellar tract during locomotion. Brain Res. 43:276–279.

Arshavsky, Yu. I., Berkinblit, M. B., Gelfand, I. M., Orlovsky, G. N., and Fukson, O. I. 1972. Activity of the neurones of the ventral spinocerebellar tract during locomotion. Biophysics 17:926–935.

Artemidorus Daldianus. ca. 140–180 A.D. The Interpretation of

Dreams (Oneirocritica). R. J. White (trans.). Park Ridge, N. J.: Noyes Press, 1975.

Asanuma, H. 1973. Cerebral cortical control of movement. Physiologist 16:143–166.

Asanuma, H. 1981. The pyramidal tract. In V. B. Brooks (ed.), Handbook of Physiology, Section 1: The Nervous System, Vol. II, Motor Control. Bethesda, Md.: American Physiological Society, pp. 703–733.

Asanuma, H., and Sakata, H. 1967. Functional organization of a cortical efferent system examined with focal depth stimulation in cats. J. Neurophysiol. 30:35–54.

Asatryan, D. G., and Feldman, A. G. 1965. Biophysics of complex systems and mathematical models. Functional tuning of the nervous system with control of movement or maintenance of a steady posture.—I. Mechanographic analysis of the work of the joint on execution of a postural task. Biophysics 10:925–935.

Åsberg, M., Träskman, L., and Thoren, P. 1976. 5-HIAA in the cerebrospinal fluid. A biochemical suicide predictor? Arch. Gen. Psychiatry 33:1193–1197.

Ascherl, G. F., Ganti, S. R., and Hilal, S. K. 1980. Neuroradiology for the clinician. In R. N. Rosenberg (ed.), The Science and Practice of Clinical Medicine, Vol. 5: Neurology. New York: Grune & Stratton, pp. 634–718.

Aschoff, J. 1969. Desynchronization and resynchronization of human circadian rhythms. Aerosp. Med. 40:844–849.

Ash, P. R., and Keltner, J. L. 1979. Neuro-ophthalmic signs in pontine lesions. Medicine (Baltimore) 58:304–320.

Attardi, D. G., and Sperry, R. W. 1963. Preferential selection of central pathways by regenerating optic fibers. Exp. Neurol. 7:46–64.

Axelsson, J., and Thesleff, S. 1959. A study of supersensitivity in denervated mammalian skeletal muscle. J. Physiol. (Lond.) 147:178–193.

Ayala, G. F., Dichter, M., Gumnit, R. J., Matsumoto, H., and Spencer, W. A. 1973. Genesis of epileptic interictal spikes. New knowledge of cortical feedback systems suggests a neurophysiological explanation of brief paróxysms. Brain Res. 52:1–17.

Ayoub, D. M., Greenough, W. T., and Juraska, J. M. 1983. Sex differences in dendritic structure in the preoptic area of the juvenile macaque monkey brain. Science 219:197–198.

B

Baack, J., de Lacoste-Utamsing, C., and Woodward, D. J. 1982. Sexual dimorphism in human fetal corpora callosa. Soc. Neurosci. Abstr. 8:213.

Babinski, J. 1896. Sur le réflexe cutané plantaire dans certaines affections organiques du système nerveux central. C. R. Soc. Biol. (Paris) 48:207–208.

Bailey, C. H., and Chen, M. 1983. Morphological basis of long-term habituation and sensitization in Aplysia. Science 220:91–93.

Baitinger, C., Cheney, R., Clements, D., Glicksman, M., Hirokawa, N., Levine, J., Meiri, K., Simon, C., Skene, P., and Willard, M. 1983. Axonally transported proteins in axon development, maintenance, and regeneration. Cold Spring Harbor Symp. Quant. Biol. 48:791–802.

Baker, P. F., Hodgkin, A. L., and Ridgway, E. B. 1971. Depolarization and calcium entry in squid giant axons. J. Physiol. (Lond.) 218:709–755.

Baldissera, F., Hultborn, H., and Illert, M. 1981. Integration in spinal neuronal systems. In V. B. Brooks (ed.), Handbook of Physiology, Section 1: The Nervous System, Vol. II, Motor Control. Bethesda, Md.: American Physiological Society, pp. 509–595.

Baloh, R. W., Furman, J. M., and Yee, R. D. 1985. Dorsal midbrain syndrome: Clinical and oculographic findings. Neurology 35:54–60.

Barchi, R. L. 1982. A mechanistic approach to the myotonic syndromes. Muscle & Nerve 5:S60–S63.

Bard, P. 1928. A diencephalic mechanism for the expression of rage with special reference to the sympathetic nervous system. Am. J. Physiol. 84:490–515.

Bard, P. 1938. Studies on the cortical representation of somatic sensibility. Harvey Lect. 33:143–169.

Bard, P., and Mountcastle, V. B. 1948. Some forebrain mechanisms involved in expression of rage with special reference to suppression of angry behavior. Res. Publ. Assoc. Res. Nerv. Ment. Dis. 27:362–404.

Barde, Y.-A., Edgar, D., and Thoenen, H. 1983. New neurotrophic factors. Annu. Rev. Physiol. 45:601–612.

Barden, H. 1981. The biology and chemistry of neuromelanin. In R. S. Sohal (ed.), Age Pigments. Amsterdam: Elsevier/North-Holland Biomedical Press, pp. 155–180.

Bardin, C. W. and Catterall, J. F. 1981. Testosterone: A major determinant of extragenital sexual dimorphism. Science 211:1285–1294.

Barlow, H. B., Hill, R. M., and Levick, W. R. 1964. Retinal ganglion cells responding selectively to direction and speed of image motion in the rabbit. J. Physiol. (Lond.) 173:377–407.

Barnett, H. J. M. 1982. Cerebrovascular diseases. In J. B. Wyngaarden and L. H. Smith, Jr. (eds.), Textbook of Medicine, 16th ed. Philadelphia: Saunders, pp. 2050–2073.

Baron, J. C., Bousser, M. G., Rey, A., Guillard, A., Comar, D., and Castaigne, P. 1981. Reversal of focal "misery-perfusion syndrome" by extraintracranial arterial bypass in hemodynamic cerebral ischemia. Stroke 12:454–459.

Barondes, S. H. 1970. Brain glycomacromolecules and interneuronal recognition. In F. O. Schmitt (ed.), The Neurosciences: Second Study Program. New York: Rockefeller University Press, pp. 747–760.

Barr, M. L., and Kiernan, J. A. 1983. The Human Nervous System: An Anatomical Viewpoint, 4th ed. Philadelphia: Harper & Row.

Barraclough, C. A., and Gorski, R. A. 1962. Studies on mating behaviour in the androgen-sterilized female rat in relation to the hypothalamic regulation of sexual behaviour. J. Endocrinol. 25:175–182.

Barrett, J. N. 1975. Motoneuron dendrites: Role in synaptic integration. Fed. Proc. 34:1398–1407.

Basbaum, A. I., and Fields, H. L. 1984. Endogenous pain control systems: Brainstem spinal pathways and endorphin circuitry. Annu. Rev. Neurosci. 7:309–338.

Batini, C., Moruzzi, G., Palestini, M., Rossi, G. F., and Zanchetti, A. 1958. Persistent patterns of wakefulness in the pretrigeminal midpontine preparation. Science 128:30–32.

Bauer, G., Gerstenbrand, F., and Rumpl, E. 1979. Varieties of the locked-in syndrome. J. Neurol. 221:77–91.

Baylor, D. A., Fuortes, M. G. F., and O'Bryan, P. M. 1971. Receptive fields of cones in the retina of the turtle. J. Physiol. (Lond.) 214:265–294.

Beach, F. A., Noble, R. G., and Orndoff, R. K. 1969. Effects of perinatal androgen treatment on responses of male rats to gonadal hormones in adulthood. J. Comp. Physiol. Psychol. 68:490–497.

Bear, D. M. 1979. The temporal lobes: An approach to the study of organic behavioral changes. In M. S. Gazzaniga (ed.), Handbook of Behavioral Neurobiology, Vol. 2. New York: Plenum Press, pp. 75–95.

Beidler, L. M. (ed.). 1971. Handbook of Sensory Physiology, Vol. IV: Chemical Senses. Berlin: Springer.

Beidler, L. M. 1980. The chemical senses: Gustation and olfaction. In V. B. Mountcastle (ed.), Medical Physiology, 14th ed., Vol. 1. St. Louis: Mosby, pp. 586–602.

Bennett, M. V. L. 1977. Electrical transmission: A functional analysis and comparison to chemical transmission. In E. R. Kandel (ed.), Handbook of Physiology, Vol. 1: The Nervous System, Part 1. Bethesda, Md.: American Physiological Society, pp. 357–416.

Bennett, M. V. L., and Goodenough, D. A. 1978. Gap junctions, electrotonic coupling, and intercellular communication. Neurosci. Res. Program Bull. 16:371–486.

Bennett, M. V. L., Sandri, C., and Akert, K. 1978. Neuronal gap junctions and morphologically mixed synapses in the spinal cord of a teleost, Sternarchus albifrons (gymnotoidei). Brain Res. 143:43–60.

Benson, D. F. 1978. Neurological correlates of aphasia and apraxia. In W. B. Matthews and G. H. Glaser (eds.), Recent Advances in Clinical Neurology, Number 2. Edinburgh: Churchill Livingstone, pp. 163–175.

Benson, D. F. 1979. Aphasia, Alexia, and Agraphia. New York: Churchill Livingstone.

Benson, D. F., and Geschwind, N. 1976. The aphasias and related disturbances. In A. B. Baker and L. H. Baker (eds.), Clinical Neurology, Vol. 1. New York: Harper & Row, chap. 10.

Benson, D. F. Sheremata, W. A., Bouchard, R., Segarra, J. M., Price, D., and Geschwind, N. 1973. Conduction aphasia. Arch. Neurol. 28:339–346.

Benzer, S. 1973. Genetic dissection of behavior. Sci. Am. 229(6):24–37.

Bergland, R. M., and Page, R. B. 1979. Pituitary–brain vascular relations: A new paradigm. Science 204:18–24.

Berl, S., Puszkin, S., and Nicklas, W. J. 1973. Actomyosin-like protein in brain. Science 179:441–446.

Berman, P. W., and Patrick, J. 1980. Experimental myasthenia gravis: A murine system. J. Exp. Med. 151:204–223.

Berman, P. W., Patrick, J., Heinemann, S., Klier, F. G., and Steinbach, J. H. 1981. Factors affecting susceptibility of different strains of mice to experimental myasthenia gravis. Ann. N. Y. Acad. Sci. 377:237–257.

Bermant, G., and Davidson, J. M. 1974. Biological Bases of Sexual Behavior. New York: Harper & Row.

Bernard, C. 1878–1879. Leçons sur les phénomènes de la vie communs aux animaux et aux végétaux, 2 Vols. Paris: Baillière.

Berndt, R. S., and Caramazza, A. 1980. A redefinition of the syndrome of Broca's aphasia: Implications for a neuropsychological model of language. Appl. Psycholing. 1:225–278.

Berne, R. M., and Levy, M. N. (eds.). 1983. Physiology. St. Louis: Mosby.

Bernstein, J. 1902. Investigations on the thermodynamics of bioelectric currents. Translated from Pflügers Arch. 92:521–562. In G. R. Kepner (ed.), Cell Membrane Permeability and Transport. Stroudsburg, Pa.: Dowden, Hutchinson & Ross, 1979, pp. 184–210.

Bernstein, N. 1967. The Co-ordination and Regulation of Movements. Oxford: Pergamon Press.

Bertler, Å., and Rosengren, E. 1959. Occurrence and distribution of dopamine in brain and other tissues. Experientia 15:10–11.

Betz, V. 1874. Anatomischer Nachweis zweier Gehirncentra. Centrabl. Med. Wiss. 12:578–580, 595–599.

Bever, C. T., Jr., Dretchen, K. L., Blake, G. J., Chang, H. W., Penn, A. S., and Asofsky, R. 1984. Augmented anti-acetylcholine receptor response following long-term penicillamine administration. Ann. Neurol. 16:9–13.

Biernbaum, M. S., and Bowndes, M. D. 1985. Light-induced changes in GTP and ATP in frog rod photoreceptors. Comparison with recovery of dark current and light sensitivity during dark adaptation. J. Gen. Physiol. 85:107–121.

Bilaniuk, L. T., Zimmerman, R. A., Littman, P., Gallo, E., Rorke, L. B., Bruce, D. A., and Schut, L. 1980. Computed tomography of brain stem gliomas in children. Radiology 134:89–95.

Birkmayer, W., and Hornykiewicz, O. (eds.). 1976. Advances in Parkinsonism: Biochemistry, Physiology, Treatment. Fifth International Symposium on Parkinson's Disease, Vienna. Basel: Roche.

Bishop, P. O. 1973. Neurophysiology of binocular single vision and stereopsis. In R. Jung (ed.), Handbook of Sensory Physiology, Vol. 7, Part 3A: Central Processing of Visual Information. Berlin: Springer, pp. 255–305.

Bizzi, E., and Abend, W. 1983. Posture control and trajectory formation in single- and multi-joint arm movements. In J. E. Desmedt (ed.), Motor Control Mechanisms in Health and Disease. New York: Raven Press, pp. 31–45.

Björklund, A., Dunnett, S. B., Stenevi, U., Lewis, M. E., and Iversen, S. D. 1980. Reinnervation of the denervated striatum by substantia nigra transplants: Functional consequences as revealed by pharmacological and sensorimotor testing. Brain Res. 199:307–333.

Björklund, A., and Stenevi, U. 1979. Regeneration of monoaminergic and cholinergic neurons in the mammalian central nervous system. Physiol. Rev. 59:62–100.

Black, P. McL. 1978. Brain death (Two parts). N. Engl. J. Med. 299:338–344 and 393–401.

Blalock, A., Mason, M. F., Morgan, H. J., and Riven, S. S. 1939. Myasthenia gravis and tumors of the thymic region. Report of a case in which the tumor was removed. Ann. Surg. 110:544–561.

Bleuler, E. 1911. Dementia Praecox or the Group of Schizophrenias. J. Zinkin (trans.). New York: International Universities Press, 1950.

Bligh, J. 1973. Temperature Regulation in Mammals and Other Vertebrates. Amsterdam: North-Holland Pub. Co.

Bloom, L. 1970. Language Development: Form and Function in Emerging Grammars. Cambridge, Mass.: MIT Press.

Bloom, L., and Lahey, M. 1978. Language Development and Language Disorders. New York: Wiley.

Bloomfield, L. 1933. Language. New York: Holt, Rinehart and Winston.

Blusztajn, J. K., and Wurtman, R. J. 1983. Choline and cholinergic neurons. Science 221:614–620.

Boakes, R. 1984. From Darwin to Behaviourism. Cambridge, England: Cambridge University Press.

Bodemer, C. W. 1968. Modern Embryology. New York: Holt, Rinehart and Winston.

Boivie, J. J. G., and Perl, E. R. 1975. Neural substrates of somatic sensation. In C. C. Hunt (ed.), MTP International Review of Science. Physiology, Series 1: Neurophysiology, Vol. 3. London: University Park Press, pp. 303–411.

Booth, D. A., Toates, F. M., and Platt, S. V. 1976. Control system for hunger and its implications in animals and man. In D. Novin, W. Wyrwicka, and G. A. Bray (eds.), Hunger: Basic Mechanisms and Clinical Implications. New York: Raven Press, pp. 127–143.

Borbély, A., and Valatx, J.-L. (eds.): 1984. Sleep Mechanisms. Exp. Brain Res. Suppl. 8. Berlin: Springer.

Børgesen, S. E., and Gjerris, F. 1982. The predictive value of conductance to outflow of CSF in normal pressure hydrocephalus. Brain 105:65–86.

Boring, E. G. 1942. Sensation and Perception in the History of Experimental Psychology. New York: Appleton-Century.

Botstein, D., White, R. L., Skolnick, M., and Davis, R. W. 1980. Construction of a genetic linkage map in man using restriction fragment length polymorphisms. Am. J. Hum. Genet. 32:314–331.

Boulant, J. A. 1981. Hypothalamic mechanisms in thermoregulation. Fed. Proc. 40:2843–2850.

Bowker, R. M., Westlund, K. N., Sullivan, M. C., Wilber, J. F., and Coulter, J. D. 1983. Descending serotonergic, peptidergic and cholinergic pathways from the raphe nuclei: A multiple transmitter complex. Brain Res. 288:33–48.

Bowsher, D. 1976. Role of the reticular formation in responses to noxious stimulation. Pain 2:361–378.

Boycott, B. B., and Wässle, H. 1974. The morphological types of ganglion cells of the domestic cat's retina. J. Physiol. (Lond.) 240:397–419.

Boyd, I. A. 1976. The response of fast and slow nuclear bag fibres and nuclear chain fibres in isolated cat muscle spindles to fusimotor stimulation, and the effect of intrafusal contraction on the sensory endings. Q. J. Exp. Physiol. 61:203–253.

Boyd, I. A., and Davey, M. R. 1968. Compositions of Peripheral Nerves. Edinburgh: E & S. Livingstone Ltd.

Boyd, I. A., and Martin, A. R. 1956. The end-plate potential in mammalian muscle. J. Physiol. (Lond.) 132:74–91.

Boyd, W. D., Graham-White, J., Blackwood, G., Glen, I., and McQueen, J. 1977. Clinical effects of choline in Alzheimer senile dementia. Lancet 2:711.

Boynton, R. M. 1979. Human Color Vision. New York: Holt, Rinehart and Winston.

Bradbury, E. M., Radda, G. K., and Allen, P. S. 1983. Nuclear magnetic resonance techniques in medicine. Ann. Intern. Med. 98:514–529.

Bradbury, M. 1979. The Concept of a Blood–Brain Barrier. New York: Wiley.

Breedlove, S. M., and Arnold, A. P. 1980. Hormone accumulation in a sexually dimorphic motor nucleus of the rat spinal cord. Science 210:564–566.

Breedlove, S. M., Jacobson, C. D., Gorski, R. A., and Arnold, A. P. 1982. Masculinization of the female rat spinal cord following a single neonatal injection of testosterone propionate but not estradiol benzoate. Brain Res. 237:173–181.

Bremer, F. 1936. Nouvelles recherches sur le mécanisme du sommeil. C. R. Séances Soc. Biol. Fil. (Paris) 122:460–464.

Brenner, S. 1974. The genetics of *Caenorhabditis elegans*. Genetics 77:71–94.

Brinkman, C. 1984. Supplementary motor area of the monkey's cerebral cortex: Short- and long-term deficits after unilateral ablation and the effects of subsequent callosal section. J. Neurosci. 4:918–929.

Britt, R. H., Herrick, M. K., and Hamilton, R. D. 1977. Traumatic locked-in syndrome. Ann. Neurol. 1:590–592.

Broca, P. 1865. Sur le siége de la faculté du langage articulé. Bull. Soc. Anthropol. 6:377–393.

Brodal, A. 1981. Neurological Anatomy in Relation to Clinical Medicine, 3rd ed. New York: Oxford University Press.

Brodmann, K. 1909. Vergleichende Lokalisationslehre der Grosshirnrinde in ihren Prinzipien dargestellt auf Grund des Zellenbaues. Leipzig: Barth.

Brons, J. F., and Woody, C. D. 1980. Long-term changes in excitability of cortical neurons after Pavlovian conditioning and extinction. J. Neurophysiol. 44:605–615.

Brooke, M. H. 1977. A Clinician's View of Neuromuscular Diseases. Baltimore: Williams & Wilkins.

Brooks, C. McC., Ishikawa, T., Koizumi, K., and Lu, H.-H. 1966. Activity of neurones in the paraventricular nucleus of the hypothalamus and its control. J. Physiol. (Lond.) 182:217–231.

Brooks, V. B. (ed.). 1981. Handbook of Physiology, Section 1: The Nervous System, Vol. II, Motor Control. Bethesda, Md.: American Physiological Society.

Brooks, V. B., and Thach, W. T. 1981. Cerebellar control of posture and movement. In V. B. Brooks (ed.), Handbook of Physiology, Section 1: The Nervous System, Vol. II, Motor Control. Bethesda, Md.: American Physiological Society, pp. 877–946.

Broughton, R. J. 1968. Sleep disorders: Disorders of arousal? Science 159:1070–1078.

Brown, A. G., and Fyffe, R. E. W. 1981. Direct observations on the contacts made between Ia afferent fibres and α-motoneurones in the cat's lumbosacral spinal cord. J. Physiol. (Lond.) 313:121–140.

Brown, R., 1973. A First Language: The Early Stages. Cambridge, Mass.: Harvard University Press.

Brown, R., and Herrnstein, R. J. 1975. Psychology. Boston: Little, Brown.

Brown, T. G. 1911. The intrinsic factors in the act of progression in the mammal. Proc. R. Soc. Lond. [Biol.] 84:308–319.

Brownell, G. L., Budinger, T. F., Lauterbur, P. C., and McGeer, P. L. 1982. Positron tomography and nuclear magnetic resonance imaging. Science 215:619–626.

Brownstein, M. J., Russell, J. T., and Gainer, H. 1980. Synthesis, transport, and release of posterior pituitary hormones. Science 207:373–378.

Brozoski, T. J., Brown, R. M., Rosvold, H. E., and Goldman, P. S. 1979. Cognitive deficit caused by regional depletion of dopamine in prefrontal cortex of rhesus monkey. Science 205:929–932.

Brugge, J. F., and Merzenich, M. M. 1973. Responses of neurons in the auditory cortex of the macaque monkey to monaural and binaural stimulation. J. Neurophysiol. 36:1138–1158.

Bruner, J. 1983. Child's Talk: Learning to Use Language. New York: Norton.

Brust, J. C. M. 1984. Cerebral infarction. In L. P. Rowland (ed.), Merritt's Textbook of Neurology, 7th ed. Philadelphia: Lea & Febiger, pp. 162–168.

Buchtal, F. 1942. The mechanical properties of the single striated muscle fibre at rest and during contraction and their structural interpretation. Dan. Biol. Med. 17:1.

Buckley, K. M., Schweitzer, E. S., Miljanich, G. P., Clift-O'Grady, L., Kushner, P. D., Reichardt, L. F., and Kelly, R. B. 1983. A synaptic vesicle antigen is restricted to the junctional region of the presynaptic plasma membrane. Proc. Natl. Acad. Sci. U.S.A. 80:7342–7346.

Buller, A. J., Eccles, J. C., and Eccles, R. M. 1960. Interactions between motoneurons and muscles in respect of the characteristic speeds of their responses. J. Physiol. (Lond.) 150:417–439.

Bunge, R. P. 1968. Glial cells and the central myelin sheath. Physiol. Rev. 48:197–251.

Burgess, P. R., and Perl, E. R. 1973. Cutaneous mechanoreceptors and nociceptors. In A. Iggo (ed.), Handbook of Sensory Physiology, Vol. 2: Somatosensory System. New York: Springer, pp. 29–78.

Burgess, P. R., Wei, J. Y., Clark, F. J., and Simon, J. 1982. Signaling of kinesthetic information by peripheral sensory receptors. Annu. Rev. Neurosci. 5:171–187.

Burke, R. E., and Rudomin, P. 1977. Spinal neurons and synapses. In E. R. Kandel (ed.), Handbook of Physiology, Vol. 1: The Nervous System, Part 2. Bethesda, Md.: American Physiological Society, pp. 877–944.

Burke, R. E., Rudomin, P., and Zajac, F. E., III. 1976. The effect of activation history on tension production by individual muscle units. Brain Res. 109:515–529.

Burke, R. E., Dum, R. P., Fleshman, J. W., Glenn, L. L., Lev-Tov, A., O'Donovan, M. J., and Pinter, M. J. 1982. An HRP study of the relation between cell size and motor unit type in cat ankle extensor motoneurons. J. Comp. Neurol. 209:17–28.

Burke, R. E., Levine, D. N., Saloman, M., and Tsairis, P. 1974. Motor units in cat soleus muscle: Physiological, histochemical and morphological characteristics. J. Physiol. (Lond.) 238:503–514.

Burnstock, G. 1976. Purinergic receptors. J. Theor. Biol. 62:491–503.

Burnstock, G., Hökfelt, T., Gershon, M. D., Iversen, L. L., Kosterlitz, H. W., and Szurszewski, J. H. 1979. Non-adrenergic, non-cholinergic autonomic neurotransmission mechanisms. Neurosci. Res. Program Bull. 17:377–519.

Burton, H., and Benjamin, R. M. 1971. Central projections of the gustatory system. In L. M. Beidler (ed.), Handbook of Sensory Physiology, Vol. IV: Chemical Senses, Part 2, Taste. Berlin: Springer, pp. 148–164.

Bydder, G. M., Steiner, R. E., Thomas, D. J., Marshall, J., Gilderdale, D. J., and Young, I. R. 1983. Nuclear magnetic resonance imaging of the posterior fossa: 50 cases. Clin. Radiol. 34:173–188.

C

Cady, E. B., Costello, A. M. de L., Dawson, M. J., Delpy, D. T., Hope, P.L., Reynolds, E. O. R., Tofts, P. S., and Wilkie, D. R. 1983. Noninvasive investigation of cerebral metabolism in newborn infants by phosphorus nuclear magnetic resonance spectroscopy. Lancet 1:1059–1062.

Cajal, S. R. 1892. A new concept of the histology of the central nervous system. D. A. Rottenberg (trans.). (See also historical essay by S. L. Palay, preceding Cajal's paper.) In D. A. Rottenberg and F. H. Hochberg (eds.), Neurological Classics in Modern Translation. New York: Hafner, 1977, pp. 7–29.

Cajal, S. R. 1894. La fine structure des centres nerveux. Proc. R. Soc. Lond. 55:444–468.

Cajal, S. R. 1906. The structure and connexions of neurons. In Nobel Lectures: Physiology or Medicine, 1901–1921. Amsterdam: Elsevier, 1967, pp. 220–253.

Cajal, S. R. 1908. Neuron Theory or Reticular Theory? Objective Evidence of the Anatomical Unity of Nerve Cells. M. U. Purkiss and C. A. Fox (trans.). Madrid: Consejo Superior de Investigaciones Científicas Instituto Ramon y Cajal, 1954.

Cajal, S. R. 1909. Histologie du Système Nerveux de l'Homme & des Vertébrés, Vol. 1. L. Azoulay (trans.). Madrid: Instituto Ramon y Cajal, 1952.

Cajal, S. R. 1911. Histologie du Système Nerveux de l'Homme & des Vertébrés, Vol. 2. L. Azoulay (trans.). Madrid: Instituto Ramon y Cajal, 1955.

Cajal, S. R. 1929. Etudes sur la Neurogenèse de Quelques Vertébrés. Trans. by L. Guth as Studies on Vertebrate Neurogenesis. Springfield, Ill.: Thomas, 1960.

Cajal, S. R. 1933. Histology, 10th ed. Baltimore: Wood.

Cajal, S. R. 1937. Recollections of My Life. E. Horne Craigie (trans.). Edited in 2 vols. as Memoirs of the American Philosophical Society, Philadelphia.

Camhi, J. M. 1984. Neuroethology. Nerve Cells and the Natural Behavior of Animals. Sunderland, Mass.: Sinauer.

Cannon, W. B., and Britton, S. W. 1925. Studies on the conditions of activity in endocrine glands. XV. Pseudoaffective medulliadrenal secretion. Am. J. Physiol. 72:283–294.

Caplan, L. R. 1980. "Top of the basilar" syndrome. Neurology 30:72–79.

Carew, T., Castellucci, V. F., and Kandel, E. R. 1979. Sensitization in Aplysia: Restoration of transmission in synapses inactivated by long-term habituation. Science 205:417–419.

Carew, T. J., Hawkins, R. D., and Kandel, E. R. 1983. Differential classical conditioning of a defensive withdrawal reflex in Aplysia californica. Science 219:397–400.

Carew, T. J., Walters, E. T., and Kandel, E. R. 1981. Classical conditioning in a simple withdrawal reflex in Aplysia californica. J. Neurosci. 1:1426–1437.

Carlsson, A. 1959. The occurrence, distribution and physiological role of catecholamines in the nervous system. Pharmacol. Rev. 11:490–493.

Carlsson, A. 1974. Antipsychotic drugs and catecholamine synapses. J. Psychiatr. Res. 11:57–64.

Carpenter, M. B. 1976. Human Neuroanatomy, 7th ed. Baltimore: Williams & Wilkins.

Carpenter, M. B. 1978. Core Text of Neuroanatomy, 2nd ed. Baltimore: Williams & Wilkins.

Carpenter, M. B., and Sutin, J. 1983. Human Neuroanatomy, 8th ed. Baltimore: Williams & Wilkins.

Carroll, B. J., Feinberg, M., Greden, J. F., et al. 1981. A specific laboratory test for the diagnosis of melancholia. Arch. Gen. Psychiatry 38:15–22.

Cassinari, V., and Pagni, C. A. 1969. Central Pain, A Neurosurgical Survey. Cambridge, Mass.: Harvard University Press.

Castellucci, V. F., Carew, T. J., and Kandel, E. R. 1978. Cellular analysis of long-term habituation of the gill-withdrawal reflex of Aplysia californica. Science 202:1306–1308.

Castellucci, V. F., and Kandel, E. R. 1974. A quantal analysis of the synaptic depression underlying habituation of the gill-withdrawal reflex in Aplysia. Proc. Natl. Acad. Sci. U.S.A. 71:5004–5008.

Castellucci, V. F., and Kandel, E. R. 1976. Presynaptic facilitation as a mechanism for behavioral sensitization in Aplysia. Science 194:1176–1178.

Castellucci, V. F., Kandel, E. R., Schwartz, J. H., Wilson, F. D., Nairn, A. C., and Greengard, P. 1980. Intracellular injection of the catalytic subunit of cyclic AMP-dependent protein kinase simulates facilitation of transmitter release underlying behavioral sensitization in Aplysia. Proc. Natl. Acad. Sci. U.S.A. 77:7492–7496.

Catterall, W. A. 1984. The molecular basis of neuronal excitability. Science 223:653–661.

Ceccarelli, B., Hurlbut, W. P., and Mauro, A. 1973. Turnover of transmitter and synaptic vesicles at the frog neuromuscular junction. J. Cell. Biol. 57:499–524.

Cervós-Navarro, J., and Ferszt, R. (eds.). 1980. Advances in Neurology, Vol. 28: Brain Edema: Pathology, Diagnosis, and Therapy. New York: Raven Press.

Chambers, W. W., Liu, C. N., and McCouch, G. P. 1973. Anatomical and physiological correlates of plasticity in the central nervous system. Brain Behav. Evol. 8:5–26.

Changeux, J.-P. 1981. The acetylcholine receptor: An "allosteric" membrane protein. Harvey Lect. 75:85–254.

Changeux, J.-P., Kasai, M., and Lee, C.-Y. 1970. Use of a snake venom toxin to characterize the cholinergic receptor protein. Proc. Natl. Acad. Sci. U.S.A. 67:1241–1247.

Chan-Palay, V. 1979. Combined immunocytochemistry and autoradiography after in vivo injections of monoclonal antibody to substance P and ³H-serotonin: Coexistence of two putative transmitters in single raphe cells and fiber plexuses. Anat. Embryol. 156:241–254.

Chan-Palay, V. 1982. Immunocytochemical and autoradiographic methods to demonstrate the coexistence of neuroactive substances: Cerebellar Purkinje cells have glutamic acid decarboxylase and motilin immunoreactivity, and raphe neurons have serotonin and substance P immunoreactivity. In V. Chan-Palay and S. L. Palay (eds.), Neurology and Neurobiology, Vol. 1: Cytochemical Methods in Neuroanatomy. New York: Liss, pp. 93–118.

Chan-Palay, V., and Palay, S. L. (eds.). 1984. Coexistence of Neuroactive Substances in Neurons. New York: Wiley.

Chase, M., and Weitzman, E. D. 1983. Sleep Disorders: Basic and Clinical Research. New York: SP Medical & Scientific Books.

Cheney, P. D., and Fetz, E. E. 1980. Functional classes of primate corticomotoneuronal cells and their relation to active force. J. Neurophysiol. 44:773–791.

Chiappa, K. H., and Ropper, A. H. 1982. Evoked potentials in clinical medicine. N. Engl. J. Med. 306:1205–1211.

Chomsky, N. 1957. Syntactic Structures. The Hague: Mouton.

Chomsky, N. 1968. Language and the mind. Psychol. Today 1(9):48–68.

Chomsky, N. 1972. Language and Mind, 2nd ed. New York: Harcourt Brace Jovanovich.

Christensen, B. N., and Perl, E. R. 1970. Spinal neurons specifically excited by noxious or thermal stimuli: Marginal zone of the dorsal horn. J. Neurophysiol. 33:293–307.

Clark, R. G. 1975. Manter and Gatz's Essentials of Clinical Neuroanatomy and Neurophysiology, 5th ed. Philadelphia: Davis.

Claudio, T., Ballivet, M., Patrick, J., and Heinemann, S. 1983. Nucleotide and deduced amino acid sequences of Torpedo californica acetylcholine receptor γ-subunit. Proc. Natl. Acad. Sci. U.S.A. 80:1111–1115.

Cleland, B. G., Dubin, M. W., and Levick, W. R. 1971. Sustained and transient neurones in the cat's retina and lateral geniculate nucleus. J. Physiol. (Lond.) 217:473–496.

Coggeshall, R. E., Applebaum, M. L., Fazen, M., Stubbs, T. B., III, and Sykes, M. T. 1975. Unmyelinated axons in human ventral roots, a possible explanation for the failure of dorsal rhizotomy to relieve pain. Brain 98:157–166.

Cohen, B. (ed.) 1981. Vestibular and oculomotor physiology. Ann. N.Y. Acad. Sci. 374:1–892.

Cohen, D. H. 1982. Central processing time for a conditioned response in a vertebrate model system. In C. D. Woody (ed.), Conditioning: Representation of Involved Neural Functions. New York: Plenum Press, pp. 517–534.

Cohen, P. 1982. The role of protein phosphorylation in neural and hormonal control of cellular activity. Nature 296:613–620.

Cole, K. S., and Curtis, H. J. 1939. Electric impedance of the squid giant axon during activity. J. Gen. Physiol. 22:649–670.

A Collaborative Study by NINDS, NIH. 1977. An appraisal of the criteria of cerebral death. A summary statement. J.A.M.A. 237:982–986.

Collins, R. D. 1962. Illustrated Manual of Neurologic Diagnosis. Philadelphia: Lippincott.

Colquhoun, D. 1981. How fast do drugs work? Trends Pharmacol. Sci. 2:212–217.

Conrad, B., Matsunami, K., Meyer-Lohmann, J., Weisendanger, M., and Brooks, V. B. 1974. Cortical load compensation during voluntary elbow movements. Brain Res. 71:507–514.

Conradi, S. 1969. Ultrastructure and distribution of neuronal and glial elements on the motoneuron surface in the lumbosacral spinal cord of the adult cat. Acta Physiol. Scand. [Suppl.] 332:5–48.

Constantine-Paton, M. 1981. Induced ocular-dominance zones in tectal cortex. In F. O. Schmitt, F. G. Worden, G. Adelman, and S. G. Dennis (eds.), The Organization of the Cerebral Cortex. Cambridge, Mass.: MIT Press, pp. 47–67.

Contreras, R. J. 1977. Changes in gustatory nerve discharges with sodium deficiency: A single unit analysis. Brain Res. 121:373–378.

Coombs, J. S., Eccles, J. C., and Fatt, P. 1955. The specific ionic conductances and the ionic movements across the motoneuronal membrane that produce the inhibitory post-synaptic potential. J. Physiol. (Lond.) 130:326–373.

Cooper, J. R., Bloom, F. E., and Roth, R. H. 1982. The Biochemical Basis of Neuropharmacology, 4th ed. New York: Oxford University Press.

Corbit, J. D. 1973. Voluntary control of hypothalamic temperature. J. Comp. Physiol. Psychol. 83:394–411.

Corey, D. P., and Hudspeth, A. J. 1979. Ionic basis of the receptor potential in a vertebrate hair cell. Nature 281:675–677.

Cormack, A. M. 1973. Reconstruction of densities from their projections, with applications in radiological physics. Phys. Med. Biol. 18:195–207.

Costanzo, R. M., and Gardner, E. P. 1980. A quantitative analysis of responses of direction-sensitive neurons in somatosensory cortex of awake monkeys. J. Neurophysiol. 43:1319–1341.

Côté, L. J., and Kremzner, L. T. 1983. Biochemical changes in normal aging in human brain. In R. Mayeux and W. G. Rosen (eds.), Advances in Neurology, Vol. 38: The Dementias. New York: Raven Press, pp. 19–30.

Cotzias, G. C., Van Woert, M. H., and Schiffer, L. M. 1967. Aromatic amino acids and modification of parkinsonism. N. Engl. J. Med. 276:374–379.

Couteaux, R. 1974. Remarks on the organization of axon terminals in relation to secretory processes at synapses. Adv. Cytopharmacol. 2:369–379.

Couteaux, R., Akert, K., Heuser, J. E., and Reese, T. S. 1977. Ultrastructural evidence for vesicle exocytosis. Neurosci. Res. Program Bull. 15:603–607.

Couteaux, R., and Pécot-Dechavassine, M. 1970. Vésicules synaptiques et poches au niveau des "zones actives" de la jonction neuromusculaire. C. R. Hebd. Séances Acad. Sci. Sér. D. Sci. Nat. 271:2346–2349.

Cowan, W. M. 1979. The development of the brain. Sci. Am. 241(3):112–133.

Cowan, W. M. 1982. A synoptic view of the development of the vertebrate nervous system. In J. G. Nicholls (ed.), Repair and Regeneration of the Nervous System. Dahlem Konferenzen. Berlin: Springer, pp. 7–24.

Cowan, W. M., and O'Leary, D. D. M. 1984. Cell death and process elimination: The role of regressive phenomena in the development of the vertebrate nervous system. In K. J. Isselbacher (ed.), Medicine, Science and Society. Symposia celebrating the Harvard Medical School Bicentennial. New York: Wiley, pp. 643–668.

Cowan, W. M., Fawcett, J. W., O'Leary, D. D. M., and Stanfield, B. B. 1984. Regressive events in neurogenesis. Science 225:1258–1265.

Cowey, A. 1981. Why are there so many visual areas? In F. O. Schmitt, F. G. Worden, G. Adelman, and S. G. Dennis (eds.), The Organization of the Cerebral Cortex. Cambridge, Mass.: MIT Press, pp. 395–413.

Crawford, A. C., and Fettiplace, R. 1981. An electrical tuning mechanism in turtle cochlear hair cells. J. Physiol. (Lond.) 312:377–412.

Creese, I. 1983. Dopamine receptors explained. Trends Neurosci. 5:40–43.

Creese, I., Sibley, D. R., Hamblin, M. W., and Leff, S. E. 1983. The classification of dopamine receptors: Relationship to radioligand binding. Annu. Rev. Neurosci. 6:43–71.

Crick, F., and Mitchison, G. 1983. The function of dream sleep. Nature 304:111–114.

Critchley, M. 1979. The Divine Banquet of the Brain and Other Essays. New York: Raven Press.

Cross, B. A., and Green, J. D. 1959. Activity of single neurones in the hypothalamus: Effect of osmotic and other stimuli. J. Physiol. (Lond.) 148:554–569.

Crow, T. J. 1980. Molecular pathology of schizophrenia: More than one disease process? Br. Med. J. 280:66–68.

Crowe, A., and Matthews, P. B. C. 1964. The effects of stimulation of static and dynamic fusimotor fibres on the response to stretching of the primary endings of muscle spindles. J. Physiol. (Lond.) 174:109–131.

Crutcher, M. D., and DeLong, M. R. 1984. Single cell studies of the primate putamen. I. Functional organization. Exp. Brain Res. 53:233–243.

Culp, W. J., and Ochoa, J. (eds.) 1982. Abnormal Nerves and Muscles as Impulse Generators. New York: Oxford University Press.

Curtis, B. A., Jacobson, S., and Marcus, E. M. 1972. An Introduction to the Neurosciences. Philadelphia: Saunders.

Curzon, G. 1977. The biochemistry of the basal ganglia and Parkinson's disease. Postgrad. Med. J. 53:719–725.

Cutler, R. W. P., and Spertell, R. B. 1982. Cerebrospinal fluid: A selective review. Ann. Neurol. 11:1–10.

D

Dählstrom, A., and Fuxe, K. 1964. Evidence for the existence of monoamine-containing neurons in the central nervous system. Acta Physiol. Scand. Suppl. 232:1–55.

Dale, H. 1935. Pharmacology and nerve-endings. Proc. R. Soc. Med. (Lond.) 28:319–332.

Dale, H. H., Feldberg, W., and Vogt, M. 1936. Release of acetylcholine at voluntary motor nerve endings. J. Physiol. (Lond.) 86:353–380.

Dallos, P. 1984. Peripheral mechanisms of hearing. In I. Darian-Smith (ed.), Handbook of Physiology, Section 1: The Nervous System, Vol. III, Sensory Processes. Bethesda, Md.: American Physiological Society, pp. 595–637.

Damasio, A. R., and Geschwind, N. 1984. The neural basis of language. Annu. Rev. Neurosci. 7:127–147.

Damasio, H., and Damasio, A. R. 1980. The anatomical basis of conduction aphasia. Brain 103:337–350.

Daniels, D. L., Williams, A. L., and Haughton, V. M. 1982. Computed tomography of the medulla. Radiology 145:63–69.

Darian-Smith, I. 1982. Touch in primates. Annu. Rev. Psychol. 33:155–194.

Dartnall, H. J. A., Bowmaker, J. K., and Mollon, J. D. 1983. Microspectrophotometry of human photoreceptors. In J. D. Mollon and L. T. Sharpe, (eds.), Colour Vision: Physiology and Psychophysics. New York: Academic Press, p. 69–80.

Darwin, C. 1860. On the Origin of Species by Means of Natural Selection. New York: Appleton.

Darwin, C. 1872. The Expression of the Emotions in Man and Animals. London: Murray.

Dastur, D. K., Lane, M. H., Hansen, D. B., Kety, S. S., Butler, R. N., Perlin, S., and Sokoloff, L. 1963. Effects of aging on cerebral circulation and metabolism in man. In J. E. Birren, R. N. Butler, S. W. Greenhouse, L. Sokoloff, and M. R. Yarrow (eds.), Human Aging: A Biological and Behavioral Study. Public Health Service Publ. No. 986. Washington, D.C.: U.S. Government Printing Office, pp. 57–76.

David, S., and Aguayo, A. J. 1981. Axonal elongation into peripheral nervous system "bridges" after central nervous system injury in adult rats. Science 214:931–933.

Davies, P., and Maloney, A. J. F. 1976. Selective loss of central cholinergic neurons in Alzheimer's disease. Lancet 2:1403.

Davis, B. D. 1985. Perspectives in Biology. Chicago: The University of Chicago Press.

Davis, J. M., and Garver, D. L. 1978. Neuroleptics: Clinical use in psychiatry. In L. L. Iversen, S. D. Iversen, and S. H. Snyder (eds.), Handbook of Psychopharmacology, Vol. 10: Neuroleptics and Schizophrenia. New York: Plenum Press, pp. 129–164.

Davis, J. M., and Mass, J. W. (eds.). 1983. The Affective Disorders. Washington, D.C.: American Psychiatric Press.

Daw, N. W. 1968. Colour-coded ganglion cells in goldfish retina: Extension of their receptive fields by means of new stimuli. J. Physiol. (Lond.) 197:567–592.

Daw, N. W. 1984. The psychology and physiology of colour vision. Trends Neurosci. 7:330–335.

Daw, N. W., Ariel, M., and Caldwell, J. H. 1982. Function of neurotransmitters in the retina. Retina 2:322–331.

Dawson, M. J., and Wilkie, D. R. 1984. Muscle and brain metabolism studied by ^{31}P nuclear magnetic resonance. In P. F. Baker (ed.), Recent Advances in Physiology, No. 10. Edinburgh: Churchill Livingstone, pp. 247–276.

DeArmond, S. J., Fusco, M. M., and Dewey, M. M. 1976. Structure of the Human Brain: A Photographic Atlas, 2nd ed. New York: Oxford University Press.

DeBold, J. F., and Miczek, K. A. 1981. Sexual dimorphism in the hormonal control of aggressive behavior of rats. Pharmacol. Biochem. Behav. 14(Suppl. 1):89–93.

Dejerine, J. 1891. Sur un cas de cécité verbale avec agraphie, suivi d'autopsie. C. R. Séances Mem. Soc. Biol. 43:197–201.

Dejerine, J. 1892. Contribution à l'étude anatomo-pathologique et clinique des différentes variétés de cécité verbale. C. R. Séances Mem. Soc. Biol. 44:61–90.

DeJong, R. N. 1979. The Neurologic Examination, 4th ed. New York: Harper & Row.

de Lacoste-Utamsing, C., and Holloway, R. L. 1982. Sexual dimorphism in the human corpus callosum. Science 216:1431–1432.

Del Castillo, J., and Katz, B. 1954. The effect of magnesium on the activity of motor nerve endings. J. Physiol. (Lond.) 124:553–559.

Del Castillo, J., and Katz, B. 1957. La base "quantale" de la transmission neuro-musculaire. In Microphysiologie comparée des éléments excitables. Colloq. Int. Cent. Natl. Rech. Sci. 67:245–258.

Delcomyn, F. 1980. Neural basis of rhythmic behavior in animals. Science 210:492–498.

DeLong, M. R. 1974. Motor functions of the basal ganglia: Single-unit activity during movement. In F. O. Schmitt and F. G. Worden (eds.), The Neurosciences: Third Study Program. Cambridge, Mass.: MIT Press, pp. 319–325.

DeLong, M. R., and Georgopoulos, A. P. 1981. Motor functions of the basal ganglia. In V. B. Brooks (ed.), Handbook of Physiology, Section 1: The Nervous System, Vol. II, Motor Control. Bethesda, Md.: American Physiological Society, pp. 1017–1061.

Dement, W., and Kleitman, N. 1957. Cyclic variations in EEG during sleep and their relation to eye movements, body motility, and dreaming. Electroencephalogr. Clin. Neurophysiol. 9:673–690.

Dement, W., Guilleminault, C., and Zarcone, V. 1975. The pathologies of sleep: A case series approach. In D. B. Tower (ed.), The Nervous System, Vol. 2: The Clinical Neurosciences. New York: Raven Press, pp. 501–518.

Dement, W. C. 1965. An essay on dreams: The role of physiology in understanding their nature. In New Directions in Psychology II. New York: Holt, Rinehart & Winston, pp. 135–257.

Descartes, R. 1637. La Dioptrique. Leyden: Ian Maire.

Deutsch, J. A., and Howarth, C. I. 1963. Some tests of a theory of intracranial self-stimulation. Psychol. Rev. 70:444–460.

De Valois, R. L. 1960. Color vision mechanisms in the monkey. J. Gen. Physiol. [Suppl. 2] 43:115–128.

De Wied, D., and Gispen, W. H. 1977. Behavioral effects of peptides. In H. Gainer (ed.), Peptides in Neurobiology. New York: Plenum Press, pp. 397–448.

Dickinson, A. 1980. Contemporary Animal Learning Theory. Cambridge, England: Cambridge University Press.

Di Girolamo, M., and Rudman, D. 1968. Variations in glucose metabolism and sensitivity to insulin of the rat's adipose tissue, in relation to age and body weight. Endocrinology 82:1133–1141.

Divac, I., LaVail, J. H., Rakic, P., and Winston, K. R. 1977. Heterogenous afferents to the inferior parietal lobule of the rhesus monkey revealed by the retrograde transport method. Brain Res. 123:197–207.

Dodd, J., Jahr, C. E., Hamilton, P. N., Heath, M. J. S., Matthew, W. D., and Jessell, T. M. 1983. Cytochemical and physiological properties of sensory and dorsal horn neurons that transmit cutaneous sensation. Cold Spring Harbor Symp. Quant. Biol. 48:685–695.

Dogiel, A. S. 1908. Der Bau der Spinalganglien des Menschen und der Säugetiere. Jena: Fischer.

Domjan, M., and Burkhard, B. 1982. The Principles of Learning and Behavior. Monterey, Calif.: Brooks/Cole.

Dokas, L. A. 1983. Analysis of brain and pituitary RNA metabolism: A review of recent methodologies. Brain Res. Rev. 5:177–218.

Doty, R. W., and Bosma, J. F. 1956. An electromyographic analysis of reflex deglutition. J. Neurophysiol. 19:44–60.

Douglas, W. W. 1968. Stimulus-secretion coupling: The concept and clues from chromaffin and other cells. Br. J. Pharmacol. 34:451–474.

Dowling, J. E. 1979. Information processing by local circuits: The vertebrate retina as a model system. In F. O. Schmitt and F. G. Worden (eds.), The Neurosciences: Fourth Study Program. Cambridge, Mass.: MIT Press, pp. 163–181.

Drachman, D. B. 1981. The biology of myasthenia gravis. Annu. Rev. Neurosci. 4:195–225.

Drachman, D. B. 1983. Myasthenia gravis: Immunobiology of a receptor disorder. Trends Neurosci. 6:446–451.

Droz, B. 1963. Dynamic condition of proteins in the visual cells of rats and mice as shown by radioautography with labeled amino acids. Anat. Rec. 145:157–167.

Drucker-Colin, R., Shkurovich, M., and Sterman, N. B. (eds.). 1979. The Functions of Sleep. New York: Academic Press.

Dubner, R., and Bennett, G. J. 1983. Spinal and trigeminal mechanisms of nociception. Annu. Rev. Neurosci. 6:381–418.

DuBois-Reymond, E. 1848–1849. Untersuchungen über thierische Elektricität, Vols. 1, 2. Berlin: Reimer.

Dudai, Y. 1985. Genes, enzymes, and learning in Drosophila. Trends Neurosci. 8:18–21.

Dudai, Y., Jan, Y.-N., Byers, D., Quinn, W. G., and Benzer, S. 1976. dunce, a mutant of Drosophila deficient in learning. Proc. Natl. Acad. Sci. U.S.A. 73:1684–1688.

Duffy, P. E. (ed.). 1976. Tumors of the Nervous System. Philadelphia: Davis.

Du Vigneaud, V. 1956. Hormones of the posterior pituitary gland: Oxytocin and vasopressin. Harvey Lect. 50:1–26.

Dwyer, T. M., Adams, D. J., and Hille, B. 1980. The permeability of the endplate channel to organic cations in frog muscle. J. Gen. Physiol. 75:469–492.

Dyck, P. J. 1982. Diseases of the peripheral nervous system. In J. B. Wyngaarden and L. H. Smith, Jr. (eds.), Cecil Textbook of Medicine, 16th ed. Philadelphia: Saunders, pp. 2153–2165.

Dyck, P. J., Thomas, P. K., Lambert, E. H., and Bunge, R. (eds.). 1984. Peripheral Neuropathy, 2nd ed. Philadelphia: Saunders.

E

Eaton, L. M., and Lambert, E. H. 1957. Electromyography and electric stimulation of nerves in diseases of motor unit. Observations on myasthenic syndrome associated with malignant tumors. J.A.M.A. 163:1117–1124.

Eccles, J. C. 1957. The Physiology of Nerve Cells. Baltimore: The Johns Hopkins Press.

Eccles, J. C. 1964. The Physiology of Synapses. Berlin: Springer.

Eccles, J. 1976. From electrical to chemical transmission in the central nervous system. The closing address of the Sir Henry Dale Centennial Symposium. Notes Rec. R. Soc. Lond. 30:219–230.

Eccles, J. C., Fatt, P., and Koketsu, K. 1954. Cholinergic and inhibitory synapses in a pathway from motor-axon collaterals to motoneurones. J. Physiol. (Lond.) 126:524–562.

Eccles, J. C., Ito, M., and Szentágothai, J. 1967. The Cerebellum as a Neuronal Machine. New York: Springer.

Eccles, R. M., and Lundberg, A. 1959. Synaptic actions in motoneurones by afferents which may evoke the flexion reflex. Arch. Ital. Biol. 97:199–221.

Edds, M. V., Jr. 1967. Neuronal specificity in neurogenesis. In G. C. Quarton, T. Melnechuk, and F. O. Schmitt (eds.), The Neurosciences: A Study Program. New York: Rockefeller University Press, pp. 230–240.

Edelman, G. M. 1984. Cell-adhesion molecules: A molecular basis for animal form. Sci. Am. 250(4):118–119.

Edwards, D. A. 1968. Mice: Fighting by neonatally androgenized females. Science 161:1027–1028.

Ehrlich, P. 1900. On immunity with special reference to cell life. Croonian Lecture. Proc. R. Soc. Lond. 66:424–448.

Ehrlich, P. 1909. On Partial Functions of the Cell. Nobel Lecture. Les prix Nobel en 1908. Stockholm.

Ehrlich, P. 1913. Chemotherapeutics: Scientific principles, methods, and results. Lancet 2:445–451.

Eibl-Eibesfeldt, I. 1970. Ethology: The Biology of Behavior. E. Klinghammer (trans.) New York: Holt, Rinehart and Winston.

Eimas, P. D. 1985. The perception of speech in early infancy. Sci. Am. 252(1):46–52.

Eliasson, S. G., Prensky, A. L., and Hardin, W. B., Jr. (eds.). 1978. Neurological Pathophysiology, 2nd ed. New York: Oxford University Press.

El-Mestikawy, S., Glowinski, J., and Hamon, M. 1983. Tyrosine hydroxylase activation in depolarized dopaminergic terminals—involvement of Ca^{2+}-dependent phosphorylation. Nature 302:830–832.

Elmqvist, D., Hofmann, W. W., Kugelberg, J., and Quastel, D. M. J. 1964. An electrophysiological investigation of neuromuscular transmission in myasthenia gravis. J. Physiol. (Lond.) 174:417–434.

Engel, A. G. 1980. Morphologic and immunopathologic findings in myasthenia gravis and in congenital myasthenic syndromes. J. Neurol. Neurosurg. Psychiatry 43:577–589.

Engen, T. 1982. The Perception of Odors. New York: Academic Press.

Enroth-Cugell, C., and Robson, J. G. 1966. The contrast sensitivity of retinal ganglion cells of the cat. J. Physiol. (Lond.) 186:517–552.

Erb, W. 1883. Handbook of Electro-therapeutics. L. Putzel (trans.). New York: Wood.

Erickson, R. P. 1968. Stimulus coding in topographic and nontopographic afferent modalities: On the significance of the activity of individual sensory neurons. Psychol. Rev. 75:447–465.

Erlanger, B. F., Wassermann, N. H., Cleveland, W. L., Penn, A. S., Hill, B. L., and Sarangarajan, R. 1984. Anti-idiotypic route to antibodies to the acetylcholine receptor and experimental myasthenia gravis. In J. C. Venter, C. M. Fraser, and J. Lindstrom (eds.), Receptor Biochemistry and Methodology, Vol. 4: Monoclonal and Anti-idiotypic Antibodies: Probes for Receptor Structure and Function. New York: Liss, pp. 163–176.

Ernster, L., and Schatz, G. 1981. Mitochondria: A historical review. J. Cell Biol. 91:227s–255s.

Erulkar, S. D., and Rahamimoff, R. 1978. The role of calcium ions in tetanic and post-tetanic increase of miniature end-plate potential frequency. J. Physiol. (Lond.) 278:501–511.

Etienne, P., Gauthier, S., Johnson, G., Collier, B., Mendis, T., Dastoor, D., Cole, M., and Muller, H. F. 1978. Clinical effects of choline in Alzheimer's disease. Lancet 2:508–509.

Evarts, E. V. 1966. Pyramidal tract activity associated with a conditioned hand movement in the monkey. J. Neurophysiol. 29:1011–1027.

Evarts, E V. 1968. Relation of pyramidal tract activity to force exerted during voluntary movement. J. Neurophysiol. 31:14–27.

Evarts, E. V. 1976. Neurophysiological mechanisms in Parkinson's disease. In W. Birkmayer and O. Hornykiewicz (eds.), Advances in Parkinsonism: Biochemistry, Physiology, Treatment. Fifth International Symposium on Parkinson's Disease, Vienna. Basel: Roche, pp. 37–54.

Evarts, E. V. 1981. Role of motor cortex in voluntary movements in primates. In V. B. Brooks (ed.), Handbook of Physiology, Section 1: The Nervous System, Vol. II, Motor Control. Bethesda, Md.: American Physiological Society, pp. 1083–1120.

Evarts, E. V., and Tanji, J. 1976. Reflex and intended responses in motor cortex pyramidal tract neurons of monkey. J. Neurophysiol. 39:1069–1080.

Everett, G. M., and Toman, J. E. P. 1959. Mode of action of Rauwolfia alkaloids and motor activity. In J. H. Masserman (ed.), Biological Psychiatry. New York: Grune & Stratton, pp. 75–81.

F

Falck, B. 1962. Observations on the possibilities of the cellular localization of monoamines by a fluorescence method. Acta Physiol. Scand. [Suppl. 197] 56:6–25.

Falck, B., Hillarp, N. Å., Thieme, G., and Torp, A. 1962. Fluorescence of catechol amines and related compounds condensed with formaldehyde. J. Histochem. Cytochem. 10:348–354.

Fambrough, D. M., and Bayne, E. K. 1983. Multiple forms of $(Na^+ + K^+)$-ATPase in the chicken: Selective detection of the major nerve, skeletal muscle, and kidney form by a monoclonal antibody. J. Biol. Chem. 258:3926–3935.

Fambrough, D. M., Drachman, D. B., and Satyamurti, S. 1973. Neuromuscular junction in myasthenia gravis: Decreased acetylcholine receptors. Science 182:293–295.

Fatt, P., and Katz, B. 1951. An analysis of the end-plate potential recorded with an intra-cellular electrode. J. Physiol. (Lond.) 115:320–370.

Fatt, P., and Katz, B. 1952. Spontaneous subthreshold activity at motor nerve endings. J. Physiol. (Lond.) 117:109–128.

Fawcett, D. W. 1981. The Cell, 2nd ed. Philadelphia: Saunders.

Fechner, G. H. 1860. In D. H. Howes and E. G. Boring (eds.), Elements of Psychophysics, Vol. 1. H. E. Adler (trans.). New York: Holt, Rinehart and Winston, 1966.

Feinberg, I. 1969. Effects of age on human sleep patterns. In A. Kales (ed.), Sleep: Physiology & Pathology. Philadelphia: Lippincott, pp. 39–52.

Feldman, A. G., and Orlovsky, G. N. 1972. The influence of different descending systems on the tonic stretch reflex in the cat. Exp. Neurol. 37:481–494.

Fentress, J. C. 1972. Development and patterning of movement sequences in inbred mice. In J. A. Kiger, Jr. (ed.), The Biology of Behavior. Corvallis: Oregon State University Press, pp. 83–131.

Fernandez, J. M., Neher, E., and Gomperts, B. D. 1984. Capacitance measurements reveal stepwise fusion events in degranulating mast cells. Nature 312:453–455.

Ferrier, D. 1875. Experiments on the brain of monkeys—No. 1. Proc R. Soc. Lond. 23:409–430.

Ferrier, D. 1890. The Croonian Lectures on Cerebral Localisation. London: Smith, Elder.

Ferster, D., and Lindstrom, S. 1983. An intracellular analysis of geniculo-cortical connectivity in Area 17 of the cat. J. Physiol. (Lond.) 342:181–215.

Fertuck, H. C., and Salpeter, M. M. 1974. Localization of acetylcholine receptor by [125]-labeled α-bungarotoxin binding at mouse motor endplates. Proc. Natl. Acad. Sci. U.S.A. 71:1376–1378.

Fesenko, E., Kolesnikov, S. S., and Lyubarsky, A. L. 1985. Induction by cyclic GMP of cationic conductance in plasma membrane of retinal rod outer segment. Nature 313:310–313.

Fetz, E. E., Cheney, P. D., and German, D. C. 1976. Corticomotoneuronal connections of precentral cells detected by postspike averages of EMG activity in behaving monkeys. Brain Res. 114:505–510.

Fields, H. L., and Basbaum, A. I. 1978. Brainstem control of spinal pain-transmission neurons. Annu. Rev. Physiol. 40:217–248.

Fieschi, C., Lenzie, G. L., and Loeb, C. W. (eds.). 1984. Effects of Aging on Regulation of Cerebral Blood Flow and Metabolism. Monogr. Neural Sci. 11:51–57. Basel: Karger.

Fieve, R. R., Rosenthal, D., and Brill, H. (eds.). 1975. Genetic Research in Psychiatry. Baltimore: Johns Hopkins University Press.

Finkel, A. S., and Redman, S. J. 1983. The synaptic current evoked in cat spinal motoneurones by impulses in single group Ia axons. J. Physiol. (Lond.) 342:615–632.

Finkelstein, A., and Mauro, A. 1977. Physical principles and formalisms of electrical excitability. In E. R. Kandel (ed.), Handbook of Physiology, Section 1: The Nervous System, Vol. I, Cellular Biology of Neurons. Bethesda, Md.: American Physiological Society, pp. 161–213.

Fishman, R. A. 1975. Brain edema. N. Engl. J. Med. 293:706–711.

Fishman, R. A. 1980. Cerebrospinal Fluid in Diseases of the Nervous System. Philadelphia: Saunders.

Flannigan, B. D., Bradley, W. G., Jr., Mazziota, J. C., Rauschning, W., Bentson, J. R., Lufkin, R. B., and Hieshima, G. B. 1985. Magnetic resonance imaging of the brain stem: Normal structure and basic functional anatomy. Radiology 154:375–383.

Flitter, M. A. 1981. Techniques of intracranial pressure monitoring. Clin. Neurosurg. 28:547–563.

Flock, Å. 1964. Structure of the macula utriculi with special reference to directional interplay of sensory responses as revealed by morphological polarization. J. Cell Biol. 22:413–431.

Flock, Å. 1965. Transducing mechanisms in the lateral line canal organ receptors. Cold Spring Harbor Symp. Quant. Biol. 30:133–145.

Flourens, P. 1824. Recherces expérimentales sur les propriétés et les fonctions du systéme nerveux, dans les animaux vertébrés. Paris: Chez Crevot.

Forgac, M., and Chin, G. 1985. Structure and mechanism of the (Na^+, K^+) and (Ca^{2+})-ATPases. In P. Harrison (ed.), Topics in Molecular and Structural Biology: Metalloproteins, Vol. 2. New York: Macmillan, pp. 123–148.

Forssberg, H., Grillner, S., and Rossignol, S. 1975. Phase dependent reflex reversal during walking in chronic spinal cats. Brain Res. 85:103–107.

Foucault, M. 1961. Madness and Civilization: A History of Insanity in the Age of Reason. R. Howard (trans.). New York: Pantheon Books, 1965.

Foulkes, D. 1966. The Psychology of Sleep. New York: Scribner's.

Frank, M. 1973. An analysis of hamster afferent taste nerve response functions. J. Gen. Physiol. 61:588–618.

Freud, S. 1891. Zur Auffassung der Aphasien: Eine kritische Studie. E. Stengel (trans.), On Aphasia: A Critical Study. London: Imago, 1953.

Freud, S. 1900–1901. The Interpretation of Dreams, Vols. IV and V. J. Strachey (trans.). London: Hogarth Press and The Institute of Psycho-Analysis, 1953.

Freud, S. 1917. Mourning and Melancholia. In The Collected Papers, Volume IV. New York: Basic Books, 1959, pp. 152–170.

Freud, S. 1933. New Introductory Lectures on Psycho-Analysis, W. J. H. Sprott (trans.). London: Hogarth Press and The Institute of Psycho-Analysis, 1949.

Freud, S. 1940. An Outline of Psychoanalysis. J. Strachey (trans). New York: Norton, 1949.

Freund, H.-J. 1983. Motor unit and muscle activity in voluntary motor control. Physiol. Rev. 63:387–436.

Friedman, M. I., and Stricker, E. M. 1976. The physiological psychology of hunger: A physiological perspective. Psychol. Rev. 83:409–431.

Frisch, D. 1967. Ultrastructure of mouse olfactory mucosa. Am. J. Anat. 121:87–119.

Fritsch, G., and Hitzig, E. 1870. Ueber die elektrische Erregbarkeit des Grosshirns. Arch. Anat. Physiol. Wiss. Med., pp. 300–332. G. von Bonin (trans.). In: Some Papers on the Cerebral Cortex. Springfield, Ill.: Thomas, 1960, pp. 73–96.

Fuchs, A. F. 1967. Saccadic and smooth pursuit eye movements in the monkey. J. Physiol. (Lond.) 191:609–631.

Fuchs, A. F., and Kaneko, C. R. S. 1981. A brain stem generator for saccadic eye movements. Trends Neurosci. 4:283–286.

Fuchs, A. F., and Luschei E. S. 1970. Firing patterns of abducens neurons of alert monkeys in relationship to horizontal eye movement. J. Neurophysiol. 33:382–392.

Fujisawa, H., Tani, N., Watanabe, K., and Ibata, Y. 1982. Branching of regenerating retinal axons and preferential selection of appropriate branches for specific neuronal connection in the newt. Dev. Biol. 90:43–57.

Fulton, J. F. 1951. Frontal Lobotomy and Affective Behavior: A Neurophysiological Analysis. New York: Norton.

Fulton, J. F., and Keller, A. D. 1932. The Sign of Babinski. A Study of the Evolution of Cortical Dominance in Primates. Springfield, Ill.: Thomas.

Fuster, J. M. 1980. The Prefrontal Cortex: Anatomy, Physiology, and Neuropsychology of the Frontal Lobe. New York: Raven Press.

Furshpan, E. J., MacLeish, P. R., O'Lague, P. H., and Potter, D. D. 1976. Chemical transmission between rat sympathetic neurons and cardiac myocytes developing in microcultures: Evidence for cholinergic, adrenergic, and dual-function neurons. Proc. Natl. Acad. Sci. U.S.A. 73:4225–4229.

Furshpan, E. J., and Potter, D. D. 1957. Mechanism of nerve-impulse transmission at a crayfish synapse. Nature 180:342–343.

Furshpan, E. J., and Potter, D. D. 1959. Transmission at the giant motor synapses of the crayfish. J. Physiol. (Lond.) 145:289–325.

G

Gajdusek, D. C. 1978. Slow infections with unconventional viruses. Harvey Lect. 72:283–353.

Galaburda, A. M., and Kemper, T. L., 1979. Cytoarchitectonic abnormalities in developmental dyslexia: A case study. Ann. Neurol. 6:94–100.

Gall, F. J., and Spurzheim, G. 1810. Anatomie et physiologie du système nerveux en général, et du cerveau en particulier, avec des observations sur la possibilité de reconnoître plusieurs dispositions intellectuelles et morales de l'homme et des animaux, par la configuration de leurs têtes. Paris: Schoell.

Galvani, L. 1791. Commentary on the Effect of Electricity on Muscular Motion. R. M. Green (trans.). Cambridge, Mass.: Licht, 1953.

Garcia, J., Hankins, W. G., and Rusiniak, K.W. 1974. Behavioral regulation of the milieu interne in man and rat. Science 185:824–831.

Gardner, H. 1974. The Shattered Mind: The Person After Brain Damage. New York: Knopf.

Gardner, R. A., and Gardner, B. T. 1969. Teaching sign language to a chimpanzee. Science 165:644–672.

Gasser, S. M., Ohashi, A., Daum, G., Böhni, P. C., Gibson, J., Reid, G. A., Yonetani, T., and Schatz, G. 1982. Imported mitochondrial proteins cytochrome b_2 and cytochrome c_1 are processed in two steps. Proc. Natl. Acad. Sci. U.S.A. 79:267–271.

Gastaut, H., and Broughton, R. 1965. A clinical and polygraphic study of episodic phenomena during sleep. In J. Wortis (ed.), Recent Advances in Biological Psychiatry, Vol. 7. New York: Plenum Press, pp. 197–221.

Gastaut, H., Tassinari, C. A., and Duron, B. 1965. Étude polygraphique des manifestations épisodiques (hypniques et respiratoires), diurnes et nocturnes du syndrome de Pickwick. Rev. Neurol. (Paris) 112:568–579.

Gatz, A. J. 1966. Manter's Essentials of Clinical Neuroanatomy and Neurophysiology, 3rd ed. Philadelphia: Davis.

Gay, V. L. 1972. The hypothalamus: Physiology and clinical use of releasing factors. Fertil. Steril. 23:50–63.

Gaze, R. M., Keating, M. J., and Chung, S. H. 1974. The evolution of the retinotectal map during development in Xenopus. Proc. R. Soc. Lond. [Biol.] 185:301–330.

Gaze, R. M., Keating, M. J., Ostberg, A., and Chung, S.-H. 1979. The relationship between retinal and tectal growth in larval Xenopus: Implications for the development of retino-tectal projections. J. Embryol. Exp. Morphol. 53:103–143.

Gazzaniga, M. S., and LeDoux, J. E. 1978. The Integrated Mind. New York: Plenum Press.

Geffen, L. B., and Jarrott, B. 1977. Cellular aspects of catecholaminergic neurons. In E. R. Kandel (ed.), Handbook of Physiology, Vol. 1: The Nervous System, Part 1. Bethesda, Md.: American Physiological Society, pp. 521–571.

Geffen, L. B., and Livett, B. G. 1971. Synaptic vesicles in sympathetic neurons. Physiol. Rev. 51:98–157.

Gellhorn, E. (ed.). 1968. Biological Foundations of Emotion: Research and Commentary. Glenview, Ill.: Scott, Foresman.

George, J. S., and Hagins, W. A. 1983. Control of Ca^{2+} in rod outer segment disks by light and cyclic GMP. Nature 303:344–348.

Gershon, M. D. 1977. Biochemistry and physiology of serotonergic transmission. In E. R. Kandel (ed.), Handbook of Physiology, Vol. 1: The Nervous System, Part 1. Bethesda, Md.: American Physiological Society, pp. 573–623.

Gershon, M. D. 1981. The enteric nervous system. Annu. Rev. Neurosci. 4:227–272.

Geschwind, N. 1965. Disconnexion syndromes in animals and man. Brain 88:237–294, 585–644.

Geschwind, N. 1967. The varieties of naming errors. Cortex 3:97–112.

Geschwind, N. 1969. Problems in the anatomical understanding of the aphasias. In N. Geschwind (ed.), Boston Studies in the Philosophy of Science, Vol. 16: Selected Papers on Language and the Brain. Dordrecht, Holland: Reidel, 1974.

Geschwind, N. 1971. Current concepts: Aphasia. N. Engl. J. Med. 284:654–656.

Geschwind, N. 1974. Selected Papers on Language and the Brain. Dordrecht, Holland: Reidel.

Geschwind, N. 1975. The apraxias: Neural mechanisms of disorders of learned movement. Sci. Am. 63:188–195.

Geschwind, N. 1979. Specializations of the human brain. Sci. Am. 241(3):180–199.

Geschwind, N., and Fusillo, M. 1966. Color-naming defects in association with alexia. Arch. Neurol. 15:137–146.

Geschwind, N., and Levitsky, W. 1968. Human brain: Left–right asymmetries in temporal speech region. Science 161:186–187.

Geschwind, N., Quadfasel, F. A., and Segarra, J. M. 1968. Isolation of the speech area. Neuropsychologia 6:327–340.

Getchell, T. V. 1977. Analysis of intracellular recordings from salamander olfactory epithelium. Brain Res. 123:275–286.

Getchell, T. V., and Shepherd, G. M. 1978. Responses of olfactory receptor cells to step pulses of odour at different concentrations in the salamander. J. Physiol. (Lond.) 282:521–540.

Ghez, C., and Vicario, D. 1978. Discharge of red nucleus neurons during voluntary muscle contraction: Activity patterns and correlations with isometric force. J. Physiol. (Paris) 74:283–285.

Gibbs, C. J., Jr., Gajdusek, D. C., Asher, D. M., Alpers, M. P., Beck, E., Daniel, P. M., and Matthews, W. B. 1968. Creutzfeldt–Jakob disease (spongiform encephalopathy): Transmission to the chimpanzee. Science 161:388–389.

Gilbert, C. D., and Wiesel, T. N., 1979. Morphology and intracortical projections of functionally characterised neurones in cat visual cortex. Nature 280:120–125.

Gilbert, C. D., and Wiesel, T. N. 1983. Clustered intrinsic connections in cat visual cortex. J. Neurosci. 3:1116–1133.

Gilman, A. G., Goodman, L. S., and Gilman, A. (eds.). 1980. The Pharmacological Basis of Therapeutics, 6th ed. New York: Macmillan.

Gilman, S. 1969. The mechanism of cerebellar hypotonia. An experimental study in the monkey. Brain 92:621–638.

Gilman, S., and Winans, S. S. 1982. Manter & Gatz's Essentials of Clinical Neuroanatomy and Neurophysiology, 6th ed. Philadelphia: Davis.

Glaser, G. H. 1979. Convulsive disorders (epilepsy). In H. H. Merritt, A Textbook of Neurology, 6th ed. Philadelphia: Lea & Febiger, pp. 843–883.

Glaser, J. R. 1978. Neuro-ophthalmology. Hagerstown, Md.: Harper & Row.

Gleitman, L. R., and Gleitman, H. 1981. Language. In H. Gleitman (ed.), Psychology. New York: Norton, chap. 10.

Glenney, J. R., Jr., and Glenney, P. 1983. Fodrin is the general spectrin-like protein found in most cells whereas spectrin and the TW protein have a restricted distribution. Cell 34:503–512.

Glickstein, M., Hardiman, M. J., and Yeo, C. H. 1983. The effects of cerebellar lesions on the conditioned nictitating membrane response of the rabbit. J. Physiol. (Lond.) 341:30P–31P.

Gobel, S., and Binck, J. M. 1977. Degenerative changes in primary trigeminal axons and in neurons in nucleus caudalis following tooth pulp extirpations in the cat. Brain Res. 132:347–354.

Goldberg, J. M., and Brown, P. B. 1969. Response of binaural neurons of dog superior olivary complex to dichotic tonal stimuli: Some physiological mechanisms of sound localization. J. Neurophysiol. 31:613–636.

Goldman, D. E. 1943. Potential, impedance, and rectification in membranes. J. Gen Physiol. 27:37–60.

Goldman, P. S., Crawford, H. T., Stokes, L. P., Galkin, T. W., and Rosvold, H. E. 1974. Sex-dependent behavioral effects of cerebral cortical lesions in the developing rhesus monkey. Science 186:540–542.

Goldman, P. S., and Nauta, W. J. H. 1977. An intricately patterned prefronto-caudate projection in the rhesus monkey. J. Comp. Neurol. 171:369–385.

Goldman, P. S., and Nauta, W. J. H. 1977. Columnar distribution of cortico-cortical fibers in the frontal association, limbic, and motor cortex of the developing rhesus monkey. Brain Res. 122:393–413.

Goldman-Rakic, P. S. 1981. Development and plasticity of primate frontal association cortex. In F. O. Schmitt, F. G. Worden, G. Adelman, and S. G. Dennis (eds.), The Organization of the Cerebral Cortex. Cambridge, Mass.: MIT Press, pp. 69-97.

Goldman-Rakic, P. S. 1984. Introduction. The frontal lobes: Uncharted provinces of the brain. Trends Neurosci. 7:425–429.

Goldstein, A., Tachibana, S., Lowney, L. I., Hunkapiller, M., and Hood, L. 1979. Dynorphin-(1-13), an extraordinarily potent opioid peptide. Proc. Natl. Acad. Sci. U.S.A. 76:6666–6670.

Goldstein, K. 1948. Language and Language Disturbances. New York: Grune & Stratton.

Goldstein, M. H., Jr. 1980. The auditory periphery. In V. B. Mountcastle (ed.), Medical Physiology, 14th ed., Vol. 1. St. Louis: Mosby, pp. 428–456.

Golgi, C. 1906. The neuron doctrine—Theory and facts. In Nobel Lectures: Physiology or Medicine, 1901–1921. Amsterdam: Elsevier, 1967, pp. 189–217.

Goodman, C. S., Bate, M., and Spitzer, N. C. 1981. Embryonic development of identified neurons: Origin and transformation of the H cell. J. Neurosci. 1:94–102.

Goodman, C. S., and Pearson, K. G. 1982. Neuronal development: Cellular approaches in invertebrates. Neurosci. Res. Program Bull. 20:777–942.

Goodwin, G. M., McCloskey, D. I., and Matthews, P. B. C. 1972. The contribution of muscle afferents to kinaesthesia shown by vibration induced illusions of movement and by the effects of paralysing joint afferents. Brain 95:705–748.

Gorski, R. A., Gordon, J. H., Shryne, J. E., and Southam, A. M. 1978. Evidence for a morphological sex difference within the medial preoptic area of the rat brain. Brain Res. 148:333–346.

Gould, J. L. 1982. Ethology: The Mechanisms and Evolution of Behavior. New York: Norton.

Gouras, P. 1969. Antidromic responses of orthodromically identified ganglion cells in monkey retina. J. Physiol. (Lond.) 204:407–419.

Gouras, P. 1972. Light and dark adaptation. In M. G. F. Fuortes (ed.), Handbook of Sensory Physiology, Vol. 7, Part 2: Physiology of Photoreceptor Organs. Berlin: Springer, pp. 609–634.

Gouras P. 1984. Color vision. In N. N. Osborne and G. J. Chader (eds.), Progress in Retinal Research, Vol. 3. Oxford: Pergamon Press, pp. 227–261.

Gouras, P., and Kruger, J. 1979. Responses of cells in foveal visual cortex of the monkey to pure color contrast. J. Neurophysiol. 42:850–860.

Gouras, P., and Zrenner, E. 1981. Color vision: A review from a neurophysiological perspective. In D. Ottoson (ed.), Progress in Sensory Physiology 1. Berlin: Springer, pp. 139–179.

Goy, R. W. and Goldfoot, D. A. 1975. Neuroendocrinology: Animal models and problems of human sexuality. Arch. Sex. Behav. 4:405–420.

Goy, R. W. and McEwen, B. S. 1980. Sexual Differentiation of the Brain. Cambridge, Mass.: MIT Press.

Grabiel, A. M. 1984. Neurochemically specified subsystems in the basal ganglia. In D. Evered and M. O'Connor (eds.), Functions of the Basal Ganglia. Ciba Foundation Symposium 107. London: Pitman, pp. 114–149.

Graf, P., Mandler, G., and Haden, P. E. 1982. Simulating amnesic symptoms in normal subjects. Science 218:1243–1244.

Grafstein B., and Forman, D. S. 1980. Intracellular transport in neurons. Physiol. Rev. 60:1167–1283.

Grafstein, B., and Laureno, R. 1973. Transport of radioactivity from eye to visual cortex in mouse. Exp. Neurol. 39:44–57.

Granit, R. 1955. Receptors and Sensory Perception. New Haven: Yale University Press.

Graubard, K., and Calvin, W. H. 1979. Presynaptic dendrites: Implications of spikeless synaptic transmission and dendritic geometry. In F. O. Schmitt and F. G. Worden (eds.), The Neurosciences: Fourth Study Program. Cambridge, Mass.: MIT Press, pp. 317–331.

Gray, E. G. 1959. Axo-somatic and axo-dendritic synapses of the cerebral cortex: An electron microscope study. J. Anat. 93:420–433.

Gray, E. G. 1963. Electron microscopy of presynaptic organelles of the spinal cord. J. Anat. 97:101–106.

Green, D. M., and Wier, C. C. 1984. Auditory perception. In I. Darian-Smith (ed.), Handbook of Physiology, Section 1: The Nervous System, Vol. III, Sensory Processes. Bethesda, Md.: American Physiological Society, pp. 557–594.

Grillner, S. 1973. Locomotion in the spinal cat. In R. B. Stein, K. G. Pearson, R. S. Smith, and J. B. Redford (eds.), Control of Posture and Locomotion. New York: Plenum Press, pp. 515–535.

Grillner, S. 1981. Control of locomotion in bipeds, tetrapods, and fish. In V. B. Brooks (ed.), Handbook of Physiology, Section 1: The Nervous System, Vol. II, Motor Control. Bethesda, Md.: American Physiological Society, pp. 1179–1236.

Grillner, S. 1985. Neurobiological bases of rhythmic motor acts in vertebrates. Science 228:143–149.

Grillner, S., and Shik, M. L. 1973. On the descending control of the lumbosacral spinal cord from the "mesencephalic locomotor region." Acta Physiol. Scand. 87:320–333.

Grillner, S., and Zangger, P. 1975. How detailed is the central pattern generation for locomotion? Brain Res. 88:367–371.

Grob, D. (ed). 1981. Myasthenia Gravis: Pathophysiology and Management. Ann. N.Y. Acad. Sci. 377:1–902.

Gross, C. G. 1973. Visual functions of inferotemporal cortex. In R. Jung (ed.), Handbook of Sensory Physiology, Vol. 7, Part 3B. Berlin: Springer, pp. 451–482.

Groves, P., and Schlesinger, K. 1979. An Introduction to Biological Psychology. Dubuque, Iowa: W. C. Brown.

Guillemin, R. 1978. Control of adenohypophyseal functions by peptides of the central nervous system. Harvey Lect. 71:71–131.

Guilleminault, C., Tilkian, A., and Dement, W. C. 1976. The sleep apnea syndromes. Annu. Rev. Med. 27:465–484.

Gulick, W. L., and Lawson, R. B. 1976. Human Stereopsis: A Psychophysical Approach. New York: Oxford University Press.

Gunderson, R. W., and Barret, J. N. 1980. Characterization of the turning response of dorsal root neurites toward nerve growth factor. J. Cell Biol. 87:546–554.

Gurfinkel', V. S., Surguladze, T. D., Mirskii, M. L., and Tarko, A. M. 1970. Work of human motor units during rhythmic movements. Biophysics 15:1131–1137.

Gurney, M. E. 1984. Suppression of sprouting at the neuromuscular junction by immune sera. Nature 307:546–548.

Gusella, J. F., Wexler, N. S., Conneally, P. M., Naylor, S. L., Anderson, M. A., Tanzi, R. E., Watkins, P. C., Ottina, K., Wallace, M. R., Sakaguchi, A. Y., Young, A. B., Shoulson, I., Bonilla, E., and Martin, J. B. 1983. A polymorphic DNA marker genetically linked to Huntington's disease. Nature 306:234–238.

H

Hall, C. S., and Van de Castle, R. L. 1966. The Content Analysis of Dreams. New York: Appleton–Century–Crofts.

Hamburger, V. 1934. The effects of wing bud extirpation on the development of the central nervous system in chick embryos. J. Exp. Zool. 68:449–494.

Hamburger, V. 1977. The developmental history of the motor neuron. The F. O. Schmitt Lecture in Neuroscience. Neurosci. Res. Program Bull. [Suppl.] 15:1–37.

Hamburger, V., and Levi-Montalcini, R. 1949. Proliferation, differentiation and degeneration in the spinal ganglia of the chick embryo under normal and experimental conditions. J. Exp. Zool. 11:457–501.

Hamill, O. P., Bormann, J., and Sakmann, B. 1983. Activation of multiple-conductance state chloride channels in spinal neurones by glycine and GABA. Nature 305:805–808.

Harden, T. K. 1983. Agonist-induced desensitization of the β-adrenergic receptor-linked adenylate cyclase. Pharmacol. Rev. 35:5–32.

Hardy, M. 1934. Observations on the innervation of the macula sacculi in man. Anat. Rec. 59:403–418.

Hardyck, C., and Petrinovich, L. F. 1977. Left-handedness. Psychol. Bull. 84:385–404.

Harlow, H. F. 1958. Behavioral contributions to interdisciplinary research. In H. F. Harlow and C. N. Woolsey (eds.), Biological and Biochemical Bases of Behavior. Madison: University of Wisconsin Press, pp. 3–23.

Harlow, H. F. 1958. The nature of love. Am. Psychol. 13:673–685.

Harlow, H. F., Dodsworth, R. O., and Harlow, M. K. 1965. Total social isolation in monkeys. Proc. Natl. Acad. Sci. U.S.A. 54:90–97.

Harner, S. G., and Laws, E. R., Jr. 1981. Diagnosis of acoustic neurinoma. Neurosurgery 9:373–379.

Harper, P. S. 1984. Localization of the gene for Huntington's chorea. Trends Neurosci. 7:1–2.

Harris, D. A., and Henneman, E. 1980. Feedback signals from muscle and their efferent control. In V. B. Mountcastle (ed.), Medical Physiology, 14th ed., Vol. 1. St. Louis: Mosby, pp. 703–717.

Harris, G. W. 1955. Neural Control of the Pituitary Gland. Monograph No. 3 of The Physiology Society. London: Arnold.

Harrison, R. G. 1935. On the origin and development of the nervous system studied by the methods of experimental embryology. Proc. R. Soc. Lond. [Biol.] 118:155–196.

Hart, B. D. 1962. The Psychology of Insanity. Cambridge, England: Cambridge University Press.

Hartline, H. K. 1949. Inhibition of activity of visual receptors by illuminating nearby retinal areas in the Limulus eye. Fed. Proc. 8:69.

Harvey, A. M., Lilienthal, J. L., Jr., and Talbot, S. A. 1941. Observations on the nature of myasthenia gravis: The phenomena of facilitation and depression of neuromuscular transmission. Bull. Johns Hopkins Hosp. 69:547–565.

Harvey, A. M., and Masland, R. L. 1941. The electromyogram in myasthenia gravis. Bull. Johns Hopkins Hosp. 69:1–13.

Hassler, R. 1970. Dichotomy of facial pain conduction in the diencephalon. In R. Hassler and A. E. Walker (eds.), Trigeminal Neuralgia. Pathogenesis and Pathophysiology. Stuttgart: G. Thieme, pp. 123–138.

Hauri, P. 1982. The Sleep Disorders, 2nd ed. A Scope Publication. Kalamazoo, Mich.: The Upjohn Company.

Hawkins, R. D., Abrams, T. W., Carew, T. J., and Kandel, E. R. 1983. A cellular mechanism of classical conditioning in Aplysia: Activity-dependent amplification of presynaptic facilitation. Science 219:400–405.

Hayflick, L. 1975. Current theories of biological aging. Fed. Proc. 34:9–13.

Hayflick, L. 1980. The cell biology of human aging. Sci. Am. 242(1):58–65.

Head, H. 1920. Studies in Neurology, Vol. 2, Part IV, The Brain. London: Oxford University Press, pp. 533–800.

Head, H. 1921. Release of function in the nervous system. Proc. R. Soc. Lond. [Biol.] 92:184–209.

Head, H. 1926. Aphasia and Kindred Disorders of Speech, 2 vols. Cambridge, England: Cambridge University Press. Reprint, New York: Hafner, 1963.

Hecaen, H., and Albert, M. L. 1978. Human Neuropsychology. New York: Wiley.

Hecht, S. 1937. Rods, cones, and the chemical basis of vision. Physiol. Rev. 17:239–290.

Heilman, K. M., and Scholes, R. J. 1976. The nature of comprehension errors in Broca's, conduction and Wernicke's aphasics. Cortex 12:258–265.

Heilman, K. M., Scholes, R., and Watson, R. T. 1975. Auditory affective agnosia. Disturbed comprehension of affective speech. J. Neurol. Neurosurg. Psychiatry 38:69–72.

Heimer, L. 1983. The Human Brain and Spinal Cord: Functional Neuroanatomy and Dissection Guide. New York: Springer.

Held, R. 1985. The development of binocularity. Trends Neurosci. (in press).

Heistad, D. D., and Kontos, H. A. 1983. Cerebral circulaton. In J. T. Shepherd and F. M. Abboud (eds.), Handbook of Physiology, Section 2: The Cardiovascular System, Vol. III, Peripheral Circulation and Organ Blood Flow. Bethesda, Md.: American Physiological Society, pp. 137–182.

Helmholtz, H. von. 1850. On the rate of transmission of the nerve impulse. Monatsber. Preuss. Akad. Wiss. Berl., pp. 14–15. Trans. in W. Dennis (ed.), Readings in the History of Psychology. New York: Appleton–Century–Crofts, 1948, pp. 197–198.

Helmholtz, H. L. F. 1877. On the Sensations of Tone (2nd Eng. ed.). New York: Dover, 1954.

Helmholtz, H. von 1911. The Sensations of Vision. In J. P. C. Southall (ed. and trans.), Helmholtz's Treatise on Physiological Optics, Vol. 2. Wash. D.C.: Optical Society of America, 1924. Translated from the 3rd German edition.

Hendry, I. A., Stockel, K., Thoenen, H., and Iversen, L. L. 1974. The retrograde axonal transport of nerve growth factor. Brain Res. 68:103–121.

Henneman, E. 1980. Motor functions of the brain stem and basal ganglia. In V. B. Mountcastle (ed.), Medical Physiology, 14th ed., Vol. 1. St. Louis: Mosby, pp. 787–812.

Henneman, E. 1980. Organization of the spinal cord and its reflexes. In V. B. Mountcastle (ed.), Medical Physiology, 14th ed., Vol. 1. St. Louis: Mosby, pp. 762–786.

Henneman, E. 1980. Skeletal muscle: The servant of the nervous system. In V. B. Mountcastle (ed.), Medical Physiology, 14th ed., Vol. 1. St. Louis: Mosby, pp. 674–702.

Henneman, E., Somjen, G., and Carpenter, D. O. 1965. Functional significance of cell size in spinal motoneurons. J. Neurophysiol. 28:560–580.

Henning, H. 1922. Psychologische Studien au Geschmackssinn. Handbh. Biol. Arbeitsmeth. 6A:627–740.

Herbert, E., Oates, E., Martens, G., Comb, M., Rosen, H., and Uhler, M. 1983. Generation of diversity and evolution of opioid peptides. Cold Spring Harbor Symp. Quant. Biol. 48:375–384.

Hering, E. 1879. Der Raumsinn und die Bewegungen des Auges. In L. Hermann (ed.), Handbuch der Physiologie, Band III, Theil I. Leipzig: F. C. W. Vogel, pp. 343–601.

Hering, E. 1964. Outlines of a Theory of the Light Sense. L. M. Hurvich and D. Jameson (trans.). Cambridge, Mass.: Harvard University Press.

Hertzberg, E. L., Lawrence, T. S., Gilula, N. B. 1981. Gap junctional communication. Annu. Rev. Physiol. 43:479–491.

Hesketh, R. 1983. Inositol trisphosphate: Link or liability? Nature 306:16–17.

Hess, W. R. 1954. Diencephalon: Autonomic and Extrapyramidal Functions. New York: Grune & Stratton.

Heston, L. L. 1970. The genetics of schizophrenic and schizoid disease. Science 167:249–256.

Hetherington, A. W., and Ranson, S. W. 1942. The spontaneous activity and food intake of rats with hypothalamic lesions. Am. J. Physiol. 136:609–617.

Heuser, J. E., and Reese, T. S. 1977. Structure of the synapse. In E. R. Kandel (ed.), Handbook of Physiology, Vol. 1: The Nervous System, Part 1. Bethesda, Md.: American Physiological Society, pp. 261–294.

Heuser, J. E., and Reese, T. S. 1981. Structural changes after transmitter release at the frog neuromuscular juncture. J. Cell Biol. 88:564–580.

Heuser, J. E., Reese, T. S., Dennis, M. J., Jan, Y., Jan, L., and Evans, L. 1979. Synaptic vesicle exocytosis captured by quick freezing and correlated with quantal transmitter release. J. Cell Biol. 81:275–300.

Hikosaka, O., Tanaka, M., Sakamoto, M., and Iwamura, Y. 1985. Deficits in manipulative behavior induced by local injections of muscimol in the first somatosensory cortex of the conscious monkey. Brain Res. 325:375–380.

Hilgard, E. R., and Bower, G. H. 1975. Theories of Learning, 4th ed. Englewood Cliffs, N. J.: Prentice-Hall.

Hille, B. 1977. Ionic basis of resting and action potentials. In E. R. Kandel (ed.), Handbook of Physiology, Section 1: The Nervous System, Vol. I, Cellular Biology of Neurons. Bethesda, Md.: American Physiological Society, pp. 99–136.

Hille, B. 1984. Ionic Channels of Excitable Membranes. Sunderland, Mass.: Sinauer.

Hines, M. 1982. Prenatal gonadal hormones and sex differences in human behavior. Psychol. Bull. 92:56–80.

Hirsch, J. (ed.). 1967. Behavior-Genetic Analysis. New York: McGraw–Hill.

Hishikawa, Y., Wakamatsu, H., Furuya, E., Sugita, Y., Masaoka, S., Kaneda, M., Sato, M., Nan'no, H., and Kaneko, Z. 1976. Sleep satiation in narcoleptic patients. Electroencephalogr. Clin. Neurophysiol. 41:1–18.

Ho, K.-L., and Meyer, K. R. 1981. The medical medullary syndrome. Arch. Neurol. 38:385–387.

Hobson, J. A. 1983. Neurophysiology of dreaming. In M. Monnier and M. Meulders (eds.), Functions of the Nervous System, Vol. 4: Psycho-Neurobiology. Amsterdam: Elsevier, pp. 249–274.

Hobson, J. A., McCarley, R. W., and Wyzinski, P. W. 1975. Sleep cycle oscillation: Reciprocal discharge by two brainstem neuronal groups. Science 189:55–58.

Hodgkin, A. L. 1964. The Conduction of the Nervous Impulse. Springfield, Ill.: Thomas, chap. 4.

Hodgkin, A. L. 1976. Chance and design in electrophysiology: An informal account of certain experiments on nerve carried out between 1934 and 1952. J. Physiol. (Lond.) 263:1–21.

Hodgkin, A. L., and Huxley, A. F. 1952. A quantitative description of membrane current and its application to conduction and excitation in nerve. J. Physiol. (Lond.) 117:500–544.

Hodgkin, A. L., and Katz, B. 1949. The effect of sodium ions on the electrical activity of the giant axon of the squid. J. Physiol. (Lond.) 108:37–77.

Hoffman, D. S., and Luschei, E. S. 1980. Responses of monkey precentral cortical cells during a controlled jaw bite task. J. Neurophysiol. 44:333–348.

Hoffman, P. N., and Lasek, R. J. 1975. The slow component of axonal transport: Identification of major structural polypeptides of the axon and their generality among mammalian neurons. J. Cell Biol. 66:351–366.

Hökfelt, T., and Björklund, A. 1985. Handbook of Chemical Neuroanatomy, Vol. 3: Classical Transmission and the Transmitter Receptors in the CNS, Part 2. Amsterdam: Elsevier Biomedical.

Hökfelt, T., Johansson, O., Ljungdahl, Å., Lundberg, J. M., and Schultzberg, M. 1980. Peptidergic neurones. Nature 284:515–521.

Hökfelt, T., Kellerth, J. O., Nilsson, G., and Pernow, B. 1975. Substance P: Localization in the central nervous system and in some primary sensory neurons. Science 190:889–890.

Hökfelt, T., Lundberg, J. M., Schultzberg, M., Johansson, O., Ljungdahl, Å., and Rehfeld, J. 1980. Coexistence of peptides and putative transmitters in neurons. In E. Costa and M. Trabucchi (eds.), Neural Peptides and Neuronal Communication. New York: Raven Press, pp. 1–23.

Holmes, G. 1939. The cerebellum of man. Brain 62:1–30.

Holtzman, E. 1977. The origin and fate of secretory packages, especially synaptic vesicles. Neuroscience 2:327–355.

Holtzman, E., and Mercurio, A. M. 1980. Membrane circulation in neurons and photoreceptors: Some unresolved issues. Int. Rev. Cytol. 67:1–67.

Holtzman, E., and Novikoff, A. B. 1984. Cells and Organelles, 3rd ed. Philadelphia: Saunders College Publishing.

Homma, S. (ed.). 1976. Understanding the stretch reflex. Prog. Brain Res. 44:1–507.

Hornykiewicz, O. 1966. Metabolism of brain dopamine in human parkinsonism: Neurochemical and clinical aspects. In E. Costa, L. J. Côté, and M. D. Yahr (eds.), Biochemistry and Pharmacology of the Basal Ganglia. New York: Raven Press, pp. 171–185.

Horton, J. C., Greenwood, M. M., and Hubel, D. H. 1979. Non-retinotopic arrangement of fibres in cat optic nerve. Nature 282:720–722.

Horvitz, H. R. 1982. Neuronal cell lineage in the nematode Caenorhabditis elegans. In D. R. Garrod and J. Feldman (eds.), Development of the Nervous System. Cambridge, England: Cambridge University Press, pp. 331–346.

Houk, J., and Henneman, E. 1967. Responses of Golgi tendon organs to active contractions of the soleus muscle of the cat. J. Neurophysiol. 30:466–481.

Houk, J. C. 1979. Motor control processes: New data concerning motoservo mechanisms and a tentative model for stimulus-response processing. In R. E. Talbott and D. R. Humphrey (eds.), Posture and Movement. New York: Raven Press, pp. 231–241.

Houk, J. C., and Rymer, W. Z. 1981. Neural control of muscle length and tension. In V. B. Brooks (ed.), Handbook of Physiology, Section 1: The Nervous System, Vol. II, Motor Control. Bethesda, Md.: American Physiological Society, pp. 257–323.

Hounsfield, G. N. 1973. Computerized transverse axial scanning (tomography): Part 1. Description of system. Br. J. Radiol. 46:1016–1022.

House, E. L., Pansky, B., and Siegel, A. 1979. A Systematic Approach to Neuroscience, 3rd ed. New York: McGraw–Hill.

Houseman, D., and Gusella, J. 1982. Molecular genetic approaches to neural degenerative disorders. In F. O. Schmitt, S. J. Bird, and F. E. Bloom (eds.), Molecular Genetic Neuroscience. New York: Raven Press.

Hoyle, G. 1979. Mechanisms of simple motor learning. Trends Neurosci. 2:153–155.

Hubbard, J. I., Llinás, R., and Quastel, D. M. J. 1969. Electrophysiological Analysis of Synaptic Transmission. Baltimore: Williams & Wilkins.

Hubel, D. H., and Livingstone, M. S. 1981. Regions of poor orientation tuning coincide with patches of cytochrome oxidase staining in monkey striate cortex. Soc. Neurosci. Abstr. 7:357.

Hubel, D. H., and Wiesel, T. N. 1959. Receptive fields of single neurones in the cat's striate cortex. J. Physiol. (Lond.) 148:574–591.

Hubel, D. H., and Wiesel, T. N. 1962. Receptive fields, binocular interaction and functional architecture in the cat's visual cortex. J. Physiol. (Lond.) 160:106–154.

Hubel, D. H., and Wiesel, T. N. 1965. Binocular interaction in striate cortex of kittens reared with artificial squint. J. Neurophysiol. 28:1041–1059.

Hubel, D. H., and Wiesel, T. N. 1972. Laminar and columnar distribution of geniculo-cortical fibers in the macaque monkey. J. Comp. Neurol. 146:421–450.

Hubel, D. H., and Wiesel, T. N. 1977. Ferrier Lecture: Functional architecture of macaque monkey visual cortex. Proc. R. Soc. Lond. [Biol.] 198:1–59.

Hubel, D. H., and Wiesel, T. N. 1979. Brain mechanisms of vision. Sci. Am. 241(3):150–162.

Hubel, D. H., Wiesel, T. N., and LeVay, S. 1977. Plasticity of ocular dominance columns in monkey striate cortex. Philos. Trans. R. Soc. Lond. [Biol. Sci.] 278:377–409.

Hudspeth, A. J. 1983. Transduction and tuning by vertebrate hair cells. Trends Neurosci. 6:366–369.

Hudspeth, A. J., and Corey, D. P. 1977. Sensitivity, polarity, and conductance change in the response of vertebrate hair cells to controlled mechanical stimuli. Proc. Natl. Acad. Sci. U.S.A. 74:2407–2411.

Hughes, J., Smith, T. W., Kosterlitz, H. W., Fothergill, L. A. Morgan, B. A., and Morris, H. R. 1975. Identification of two related pentapeptides from the brain with potent opiate agonist activity. Nature 258:577–579.

Humphrey, D. R. 1979. On the cortical control of visually directed reaching: Contributions by nonprecentral motor areas. In R. E. Talbott and D. R. Humphrey (eds.), Posture and Movement. New York: Raven Press, pp. 51–112.

Hunt, C. C. 1954. Relation of function to diameter in afferent fibers of muscle nerves. J. Gen. Physiol. 38:117–131.

Hunt, C. C., and Kuffler, S. W. 1951. Stretch receptor discharges during muscle contraction. J. Physiol. (Lond.) 113:298–315.

Hunt, C. C., and Perl, E. R. 1960. Spinal reflex mechanisms concerned with skeletal muscle. Physiol. Rev. 40:538–579.

Hurley, J. B., Simon, M. I., Teplow, D. B., Robishaw, J. D., and Gilman, A. G. 1984. Homologies between signal transducing G proteins and ras gene products. Science 226:860–862.

Hursh, J. B. 1939. Conduction velocity and diameter of nerve fibers. Am. J. Physiol. 127:131–139.

Hurvich, L. M. 1972. Color vision deficiencies. In D. Jameson and L. M. Hurvich (eds.), Handbook of Sensory Physiology, Vol. 7, Part 4. Visual Psychophysics. Berlin: Springer, pp. 582–624.

Hurvich, L. M. 1981. Color Vision. Sunderland, Mass.: Sinauer.

Hyvarinen, J., and Poranen, A. 1978. Movement-sensitive and direction and orientation-selective cutaneous receptive fields in the hand area of the post-central gyrus in monkeys. J. Physiol. (Lond.) 283:523–537.

I

Iggo, A., and Andres, K. H. 1982. Morphology of cutaneous receptors. Annu. Rev. Neurosci. 5:1–31.

Imig, T. J., and Adrian, H. O. 1977. Binaural columns in the primary field (A1) of cat auditory cortex. Brain Res. 138:241–257.

Imig, T. J., and Brugge, J. F. 1978. Sources and terminations of callosal axons related to binaural and frequency maps in primary auditory cortex of the cat. J. Comp. Neur. 182:637–660.

Inglis, J., and Lawson, J. S. 1981. Sex differences in the effects of unilateral brain damage on intelligence. Science 212:693–695.

Ingram, V. 1963. The Hemoglobins in Genetics and Evolution. New York: Columbia University Press.

Ingvar, D. H., and Schwartz, M. S. 1974. Blood flow patterns induced in the dominant hemisphere by speech and reading. Brain 97:273–288.

Ischia, S., Luzzani, A., Ischia, A., and Maffezzoli, G. 1984. Bilateral percutaneous cervical cordotomy: Immediate and long-term results in 36 patients with neoplastic disease. J. Neurol. Neurosurg. Psychiatry 47:141–147.

Ito, M. 1984. The Cerebellum and Neural Control. New York: Raven Press.

Iurato, S. 1967. Submicroscopic Structure of the Inner Ear. Oxford: Pergamon Press.

Iwata, M. 1984. Kanji versus Kana: Neuropsychological correlates of the Japanese writing system. Trends Neurosci. 7:290–293.

J

Jack, J. 1979. An introduction to linear cable theory. In F. O. Schmitt and F. G. Worden (eds.), The Neurosciences: Fourth Study Program. Cambridge, Mass.: MIT Press, pp. 423–437.

Jack, J. J. B., Noble, D., and Tsien, R. W. 1975. Electric Current Flow in Excitable Cells. Oxford: Clarendon Press, chaps. 1–5, 7, pp. 276–277.

Jackson, J. H. 1884. The Croonian Lectures on Evolution and Dissolution of the Nervous System. Br. Med. J. 1:591–593, 660–663, 703–707.

Jackson, J. H. 1931–1932. In J. Taylor (ed.), Selected Writings of John Hughlings Jackson, 2 vol. London: Hodder and Stoughton.

Jacobson, A., Kales, A., Lehmann, D., and Zweizig, J. R. 1965. Somnambulism: All-night electroencephalographic studies. Science 148:975–977.

Jacobson, C. D., and Gorski, R. A. 1981. Neurogenesis of the sexually dimorphic nucleus of the preoptic area in the rat. J. Comp. Neurol. 196:519–529.

Jacobsen, C. F. 1935. Functions of frontal association area in primates. Arch. Neurol. Psychiatry 33:558–569.

Jacobson, M. 1968. Development of neuronal specificity in retinal ganglion cells of Xenopus. Dev. Biol. 17:202–218.

Jacobson, M. 1978. Developmental Neurobiology, 2nd ed. New York: Plenum Press.

Jahr, C. E., and Jessell, T. M. 1985. Synaptic transmission between dorsal root ganglion and dorsal horn neurons in culture: Antagonism of monosynaptic and glutamate excitation by kynurenate. J. Neurosci. (in press).

Jan, Y. N., Jan, L. Y., and Kuffler, S. W. 1979. A peptide as a possible transmitter in sympathetic ganglia of the frog. Proc. Natl. Acad. Sci. U.S.A. 76:1501–1505.

Jane, J. A., Yashon, D., DeMeyer, W., and Bucy, P. C. 1967. The contribution of the precentral gyrus to the pyramidal tract of man. J. Neurosurg. 26:244–248.

Jankowska, E., Padel, Y., and Tanaka, R. 1976. Disynaptic inhibition of spinal motoneurones form the motor cortex in the monkey. J. Physiol. (Lond.) 258:467–487.

Jansen, J., and Brodal, A. (eds.). 1954. Aspects of Cerebellar Anatomy. Oslo: Grundt Tanum.

Jessell, T. M., and Iversen, L. L. 1977. Opiate analgesics inhibit substance P release from rat trigeminal nucleus. Nature 268:549–551.

Jessell, T. M., Siegel, R. E., and Fischbach, G. D. 1979. Induction of acetylcholine receptors on cultured skeletal muscle by a factor extracted from brain and spinal cord. Proc. Natl. Acad. Sci. U.S.A. 76:5397–5401.

Jewett, D. L., and Rayner, M. D. 1984. Basic Concepts of Neuronal Function. Boston: Little, Brown.

Joh, T. H., Baetge, E. E., Ross, M. E., and Reis, D. J. 1983. Evidence for the existence of homologous gene coding regions for the catecholamine biosynthetic enzymes. Cold Spring Harbor Symp. Quant. Biol. 48:327–335.

Johansson, R. S., and Vallbo, Å. B. 1983. Tactile sensory coding in the glabrous skin of the human hand. Trends Neurosci. 6:27–32.

Johnson, R. G., Carty, S., and Scarpa, A. 1982. A model of biogenic amine accumulation into chromaffin granules and ghosts based on coupling to the electrochemical proton gradient. Fed. Proc. 41:2746–2754.

Johnson, R. G., and Scarpa, A. 1979. Protonmotive force and catecholamine transport in isolated chromaffin granules. J. Biol. Chem. 254:3750–3760.

Johnson, T. N., and Rosvold, H. E. 1971. Topographic projections on the globus pallidus and the substantia nigra of selectively placed lesions in the precommissural caudate nucleus and putamen in the monkey. Exp. Neurol. 33:584–596.

Jones, E. G., and Cowan, W. M. 1977. Nervous tissue. In L. Weiss and R. O. Greep (eds.), Histology, 4th ed. New York: McGraw–Hill.

Jones, E. G., and Cowan, W. M. 1983. The nervous tissue. In L. Weiss, (ed.), Histology: Cell and Tissue Biology, 5th ed. New York: Elsevier Biomedical, pp. 282–370.

Jones, E. G., Friedman, D. P., and Hendry, S. H. C. 1982. Thalamic basis of place- and modality-specific columns in monkey somatosensory cortex: A correlative anatomical and physiological study. J. Neurophysiol. 48:545–568.

Jones, E. G., and Powell, T. P. S. 1973. Anatomical organization of the somatosensory cortex. In A. Iggo (ed.), Handbook of Sensory Physiology, Vol. 2: Somatosensory System. New York: Springer, pp. 579–620.

Jones, E. G., and Wise, S. P. 1977. Size, laminar and columnar distribution of efferent cells in the sensory-motor cortex of monkeys. J. Comp. Neurol. 175:391–437.

Jonsson, G. 1980. Chemical neurotoxins as denervation tools in neurobiology. Annu. Rev. Neurosci. 3:169–187.

Jouvet, M. 1983. Neurobiology of dream. In M. Monnier and M. Meulders (eds.), Functions of the Nervous System, Vol. 4: Psycho-Neurobiology. Amsterdam: Elsevier, pp. 227–248.

Julesz, B. 1971. Foundations of Cyclopean Perception. Chicago: University of Chicago Press.

K

Kaas, J. H. Merzenich, M. M., and Killackey, H. P. 1983. The reorganization of somatosensory cortex following peripheral nerve damage in adult and developing mammals. Annu. Rev. Neurosci. 6:325–356.

Kaas, J. H., Nelson, R. J., Sur. M., Lin, C.-S., and Merzenich, M. M. 1979. Multiple representations of the body within the primary somatosensory cortex of primates. Science 204:521–523.

Kaas, J. H., Nelson, R. J., Sur, M., and Merzenich, M. M. 1981. Organization of somatosensory cortex in primates. In F. O. Schmitt, F. G. Worden, G. Adelman, and S. G. Dennis (eds.), The Organization of the Cerebral Cortex. Cambridge, Mass.: MIT Press, pp. 237–261.

Kakidani, H., Furutani, Y., Takahashi, H., Noda, M., Morimoto, Y., Hirose, T., Asai, M., Inayama, S., Nakanishi, S., and Numa, S. 1982. Cloning and sequence analysis of cDNA for porcine β-neoendorphin/dynorphin precursor. Nature 298:245–249.

Kales, A., and Kales, J. 1973. Recent advances in the diagnosis and treatment of sleep disorders. In G. Usdin (ed.), Sleep Research and Clinical Practice. New York: Brunner/Mazel, pp. 59–94.

Kallmann, F. J. 1938. The Genetics of Schizophrenia. New York: Augustin.

Kalovidouris, A., Mancuso, A. A., and Dillon, W. 1984. A CT-clinical approach to patients with symptoms related to the V, VII, IX–XII cranial nerves and cervical sympathetics. Radiology 151:671–676.

Kamo, I., Furukawa, S., Tada, A., Mano, Y., Iwasaki, Y., Furuse, T., Ito, N., Hayashi, K., and Satoyoshi, E. 1982. Monoclonal antibody to acetylcholine receptor: Cell line established from thymus of patient with myasthenia gravis. Science 215:995–997.

Kandel, E. R. 1964. Electrical properties of hypothalamic neuroendocrine cells. J. Gen. Physiol. 47:691–717.

Kandel, E. R. 1976. Cellular Basis of Behavior: An Introduction to Behavioral Neurobiology. San Francisco: Freeman, chap. 1.

Kandel, E. R. 1981. Calcium and the control of synaptic strength by learning. Nature 293:697–700.

Kandel, E. R. 1983. From metapsychology to molecular biology: Explorations into the nature of anxiety. Am. J. Psychiatry 140:1277–1293.

Kandel, E. R. 1984. Steps toward a molecular grammar for learning: Explorations into the nature of memory. In K. J. Isselbacher (ed.), Medicine, Science and Society. Symposia Celebrating the Harvard Medical School Bicentennial. New York: Wiley, pp. 555–604.

Kandel, E. R., Abrams, T., Bernier, L., Carew, T. J., Hawkins, R. D., and Schwartz, J. H. 1983. Classical conditioning and sensitization share aspects of the same molecular cascade in Aplysia. Cold Spring Harbor Symp. Quant. Biol. 48:821–830.

Kandel, E. R., and Schwartz, J. H. 1982. Molecular biology of learning: Modulation of transmitter release. Science 218:433–443.

Kaneko, A. 1970. Physiological and morphological identification of horizontal, bipolar and amacrine cells in goldfish retina. J. Physiol. (Lond.) 207:623–633.

Kanfer, F. H., and Phillips, J. S. 1970. Learning Foundations of Behavior Therapy. New York: Wiley.

Karacan, I., Thornby, J. I., Anch, M., Holzer, C. E., Warheit, G. J., Schwab, J. J., and Williams, R. L. 1976. Prevalence of sleep disturbance in a primarily urban Florida county. Soc. Sci. Med. 10:239–244.

Karlin, A. 1983. The anatomy of a receptor. Neurosci. Comment. 1:111–123.

Karlin, A., Holtzman, E., Yodh, N., Lobel, P., Wall, J., and Hainfeld, J. 1983. The arrangement of the subunits of the acetylcholine receptor of Torpedo californica. J. Biol. Chem. 258:6678–6681.

Katz, B. 1966. Nerve, Muscle, and Synapse. New York: McGraw–Hill.

Katz, B. 1969. The Release of Neural Transmitter Substances. Springfield, Ill.: Thomas.

Katz, B., and Miledi, R. 1967a. The study of synaptic transmission in the absence of nerve impulses. J. Physiol. (Lond.) 192:407–436.

Katz, B., and Miledi, R. 1967b. The timing of calcium action during neuromuscular transmission. J. Physiol. (Lond.) 189:535–544.

Katz, B., and Miledi, R. 1970. Membrane noise produced by acetylcholine. Nature 226:962–963.

Katzman, R. (ed.). 1983. Biological Aspects of Alzheimer's Disease. Cold Spring Harbor, New York: Cold Spring Harbor Laboratories, Banbury Reports, Vol. 15.

Katzman, R., and Pappius, H. M. 1973. Brain Electrolytes and Fluid Metabolism. Baltimore: Williams & Wilkins.

Keesey, R. E., Boyle, P. C., Kemnitz, J. W., and Mitchel, J. S. 1976. The role of the lateral hypothalamus in determining the body weight set point. In D. Novin, W. Wyrwicka, and G. A. Bray (eds.), Hunger: Basic Mechanisms and Clinical Implications. New York: Raven Press, pp. 243–255.

Keibel, F., and Mall, F. P. (eds.). 1910–1912. Manual of Human Embryology. 2 vol. Philadelphia: Lippincott.

Kellogg, W. N. 1968. Communication and language in the home-raised chimpanzee. Science 162:423–427.

Kelly, J. P., and Cowan, W. M. 1972. Studies on the development of the chick optic tectum. III. Effects of early eye removal. Brain Res. 42:263–288.

Kelly, J. P., and Van Essen, D. C. 1974. Cell structure and function in the visual cortex of the cat. J. Physiol. (Lond.) 238:515–547.

Kelly, R. B., Deutsch, J. W., Carlson, S. S., and Wagner, J. A. 1979. Biochemistry of neurotransmitter release. Annu. Rev. Neurosci. 2:399–446.

Kennedy, M. B. 1983. Experimental approaches to understanding the role of protein phosphorylation in the regulation of neuronal function. Annu. Rev. Neurosci. 6:493–525.

Kepler, J. 1604. Astronomiae Pars Optica, chap. 5: De modo Visionis. Frankfurt: C. Marnium & Haeredes I. Aubrii, pp. 158–221.

Kety, S. S. 1960. Sleep and the energy metabolism of the brain. In G. E. W. Wolstenholme and M. O'Connor (eds.), The Nature of Sleep. Boston: Little, Brown, pp. 375–381.

Kety, S. S. 1979. Disorders of the human brain. Sci. Am. 241(3):202–214.

Kety, S. S., Rosenthal, D., Wender, P. H., and Schulsinger, F. 1968. The types and prevalence of mental illness in the biological and adoptive families of adopted schizophrenics. In D. Rosenthal and S. S. Kety (eds.), The Transmission of Schizophrenia. Oxford: Pergamon Press, pp. 345–362.

Kety, S. S., Rosenthal, D., Wender, P. H., Schulsinger, F., and Jacobsen, B. 1975. Mental illness in the biological and adoptive families of adopted individuals who have become schizophrenic: A preliminary report based on psychiatric interviews. In R. R. Fieve, D. Rosenthal, and H. Brill (eds.), Genetic Research in Psychiatry. Baltimore: Johns Hopkins University Press, pp. 147–165.

Khanna, S. M., and Leonard, D. G. B. 1982. Basilar membrane tuning in the cat cochlea. Science 215:305–306.

Khodorov, B. I. 1974. The Problem of Excitability. New York: Plenum Press.

Kiang, N. Y.-S. 1965. Discharge Patterns of Single Fibers in the Cat's Auditory Nerve. Cambridge, Mass.: MIT Press.

Kiang, N. Y. S. 1984. Peripheral neural processing of auditory information. In I. Darian-Smith (ed.), Handbook of Physiology, Section 1: The Nervous System, Vol. III, Sensory Processes. Bethesda, Md.: American Physiological Society, pp. 639–674.

Kilpatrick, D. L., Jones, B. N., Lewis, R. V., Stern A. S., Kojima, K., Shively, J. E., and Udenfriend, S. 1982. An 18,200-dalton adrenal protein that contains four [Met]-enkephalin sequences. Proc. Natl. Acad. Sci. U.S.A. 79:3057–3061.

Kimura, K., and Beidler, L. M. 1961. Microelectrode study of taste receptors of rat and hamster. J. Cell. Comp. Physiol. 58:131–139.

Kissileff, H. R., and Van Itallie, T. B. 1982. Physiology of the control of food intake. Annu. Rev. Nutr. 2:371–418.

Klatzky, R. L. 1980. Human Memory. Structures and Processes. 2nd ed. San Francisco: Freeman.

Klein, D. F., and Davis, J. M. 1969. Diagnosis and Drug Treatment of Psychiatric Disorders. Baltimore: Williams & Wilkins.

Klein, D. F. Gittelman, R., Quitkin, F., and Rifkin, A. 1980. Diagnosis and Drug Treatment of Psychiatric Disorders: Adults and Children, 2nd ed. Baltimore: Williams & Wilkins.

Klein, M., and Kandel, E. R. 1978. Presynaptic modulation of voltage-dependent Ca^{2+} current: Mechanism for behavioral sensitization in Aplysia californica. Proc. Natl. Acad. Sci. U.S.A. 75:3512–3516.

Klein, M., Shapiro, E., and Kandel, E. R. 1980. Synaptic plasticity and the modulation of the Ca^{2+} current. J. Exp. Biol. 89:117–157.

Klibansky, R., Panofsky, E., and Saxl, F. 1964. Saturn and Melancholy. London: Nelson.

Klüver, H., and Bucy, P.C. 1937. "Psychic blindness" and other symptoms following bilateral temporal lobectomy in Rhesus monkeys. Am. J. Physiol. 119:352–353.

Klüver, H., and Bucy, P. C. 1939. Preliminary analysis of functions of the temporal lobes in monkeys. Arch. Neurol. Psychiatry 42:979–1000.

Knibestol, M., and Vallbo, Å. B. 1976. Stimulus-response functions of primary afferents and psychophysical intensity estimation on mechanical skin stimulation in the human hand. In Y. Zotterman (ed.), Sensory Functions of the Skin in Primates with Special Reference to Man. Oxford: Pergamon, pp. 201–213.

Knudsen, E. I. 1984. The role of auditory experience in the development and maintenance of sound localization. Trends Neurosci. 7:326–330.

Ko, C.-P. 1984. Regeneration of the active zone at the frog neuromuscular junction. J. Cell Biol. 98:1685–1695.

Koester, J., and Byrne, J. H. (eds.). 1980. Molluscan Nerve Cells: From Biophysics to Behavior. Cold Spring Harbor, N. Y.: Cold Spring Harbor Laboratory.

Kohlerman, N. J., Gibson, A. R., and Houk, J. C. 1982. Velocity signals related to hand movements recorded from red nucleus neurons in monkeys. Science 217:857–860.

Kolb, B., and Whishaw, I. Q. 1980. Fundamentals of Human Neuropsychology. San Francisco: Freeman.

Kolb, H., Mariani, A., and Gallego, A. 1980. A second type of horizontal cell in the monkey retina. J. Comp. Neurol. 189:31–44.

Konishi, M. 1965. The role of auditory feedback in the control of vocalization in the white-crowned sparrow. Z. Tierpsychol. 22:770–783.

Kraepelin, E. 1909. Dementia Praecox and Paraphrenia. From Kraepelin's Textbook of Psychiatry, 8th ed., R. M. Barclay (trans.). Edinburgh: Livingstone, 1919.

Kravitz, E. A. 1967. Acetylcholine, γ-aminobutyric acid, and glutamic acid: Physiological and chemical studies related to their roles as neurotransmitter agents. In G. C. Quarton, T. Melnechuk, and F. O. Schmitt (eds.), The Neurosciences: A Study Program. New York: Rockefeller University Press, pp. 433–444.

Kretz, R., Shapiro, E., Connor, J., and Kandel, E. R. 1984. Posttetanic potentiation, presynaptic inhibition, and the modulation of the free Ca^{++} level in the presynaptic terminals. Exp. Brain Res. [Suppl.] 9:240–256.

Krieger, D. T. 1983. Brain peptides: What, where, and why? Science 222:975–985.

Krieger, D. T., Brownstein, M. J., and Martin, J. D. (eds.). 1983. Brain Peptides. New York: Wiley.

Kries, J. von. 1911. Appendix I. Normal and anomalous colour systems. In J. P. C. Southall (ed. and trans.), Helmholtz's Treatise on Physiological Optics, Vol. 2, pp. 395–425. Washington, D.C.: Optical Society Of America, 1924. Translated from the 3rd German edition.

Kubota, K., and Hamada, I. 1978. Visual tracking and neuron activity in the post-arcuate area in monkeys. J. Physiol. (Paris) 74:297–312.

Kuffler, S. W. 1952. Neurons in the retina: Organization, inhibition and excitation problems. Cold Spring Harbor Symp. Quant. Biol. 17:281–292.

Kuffler, S. W. 1953. Discharge patterns and functional organization of mammalian retina. J. Neurophysiol. 16:37–68.

Kuffler, S. W. 1967. Neuroglial cells: Physiological properties and a potassium mediated effect of neuronal activity on the glial membrane potential. Proc. R. Soc. Lond. [Biol.] 168:1–21.

Kuffler, S. W., and Nicholls, J. G. 1976. From Neuron to Brain: A Cellular Approach to the Function of the Nervous System, 2nd ed. Sunderland, Mass.: Sinauer.

Kuffler, S. W., Nicholls, J. G., and Martin, A. R. 1984. From Neuron to Brain: A Cellular Approach to the Function of the Nervous System, 2nd ed. Sunderland, Mass.: Sinauer.

Kuhar, M. J., and Murrin, L. C. 1978. Sodium-dependent, high affinity choline uptake. J. Neurochem. 30:15–21.

Kupfer, D. J., and Foster, F. G. 1972. Interval between onset of sleep and rapid-eye-movement sleep as an indicator of depression. Lancet 2:684–686.

Kupfermann, I., and Weiss, K. R. 1978. The command neuron concept. Behav. Brain Sci. 1:3–39.

Kuypers, H. G. J. M. 1973. The anatomical organization of the descending pathways and their contributions to motor control especially in primates. In J. E. Desmedt (ed.), New Developments in Electromyography and Clinical Neurophysiology, Vol. 3. Basel: Karger, pp. 38–68.

Kuypers, H. G. J. M. 1981. Anatomy of the descending pathways. In V. B. Brooks (ed.), Handbook of Physiology, Section 1: The Nervous System, Vol. II, Motor Control. Bethesda, Md.: American Physiological Society, pp. 597–666.

L

Land, E. H. 1977. The retinex theory of color vision. Sci. Am. 237(6):108–128.

Landau, W. M., and Clare, M. H. 1959. The plantar reflex in man, with special reference to some conditions where the extensor response is unexpectedly absent. Brain 82:321–355.

Landmesser, L. 1984. The development of specific motor pathways in chick embryo. Trends Neurosci. 7:336–339.

Landmesser, L. T. 1980. The generation of neuromuscular specificity. Annu. Rev. Neurosci. 3:279–302.

Lane, H. 1976. The Wild Boy of Aveyron. Cambridge, Mass.: Harvard University Press.

Lang, B., Newsom-Davis, J., Wray, D., Vincent, A., and Murray, N. 1981. Autoimmune aetiology for myasthenic (Eaton–Lambert) syndrome. Lancet 2:224–226.

Langley, J. N. 1906. On nerve endings and on special excitable substances in cells. Proc. R. Soc. Lond. [Biol.] 78:170–194.

Laporte, Y., and Lloyd, D. P. C. 1952. Nature and significance of the reflex connections established by large afferent fibers of muscular origin. Am. J. Physiol. 169:609–621.

Lashley, K. S. 1929. Brain Mechanisms and Intelligence: A Quantitative Study of Injuries to the Brain. Chicago: University of Chicago Press.

Lashley, K. S. 1950. In search of the engram. Symp. Soc. Exp. Biol. 4:454–482.

Lauterbur, P. C. 1973. Image formation by induced local interactions. Examples employing nuclear magnetic resonance. Nature 242:190–191.

Le Douarin, N. 1982. The Neural Crest. Cambridge, England: Cambridge University Press.

Le Douarin, N. M., Renaud, D., Teillet, M. A., and Le Douarin, G. H. 1975. Cholinergic differentiation of presumptive adrenergic neuroblasts in interspecific chimeras after heterotopic transplantations. Proc. Natl. Acad. Sci. U.S.A. 72:728–732.

Lee, C. Y. 1972. Chemistry and pharmacology of polypeptide toxins in snake venoms. Annu. Rev. Pharmacol. 12:265–286.

Lee, C. Y., and Chang, C. C. 1966. Modes of actions of purified toxins from *elapid* venoms on neuromuscular transmission. Mem. Inst. Butantan. Simp. Internac. 33:555–572.

Lee, T., Seeman, P., Rajput, A., Farley, I. J., and Hornykiewicz, O. 1978. Receptor basis for dopaminergic supersensitivity in Parkinson's disease. Nature 273:59–61.

Lefkowitz, R. J., Stadel, J. M., and Caron, M. G. 1983. Adenylate cyclase-coupled beta-adrenergic receptors: Structure and mechanisms of activation and desensitization. Annu. Rev. Biochem. 52:159–186.

Le Gros Clark, W. E., and Penman, G. G. 1934. The projection of the retina in the lateral geniculate body. Proc. R. Soc. Lond. [Biol.] 114:291–313.

Leiderman, P. H. 1981. Human mother-infant social bonding: Is there a sensitive phase? In K. Immelmann, G. W. Barlow, L. Petrinovich, and M. Main (eds.), Behavioral Development. Cambridge, England: Cambridge University Press, pp. 454–468.

Leigh, R. J., and Zee, D. S. 1983. The Neurology of Eye Movements. Contemporary Neurology Series. Philadelphia: Davis.

LeMay, M. 1976. Morphological cerebral asymmetries of modern man, fossil man, and nonhuman primate. Ann. N.Y. Acad. Sci. 280:349–366.

LeMay, M., and Culebras, A. 1972. Human brain—morphologic differences in the hemispheres demonstrable by carotid arteriography. N. Engl. J. Med. 287:168–170.

LeMay, M., and Geschwind, N. 1978. Asymmetries of the human cerebral hemispheres. In A. Caramazza and E. B. Zurif (eds.), Language Acquisition and Language Breakdown: Parallels and Divergencies. Baltimore: Johns Hopkins University Press, pp. 311–328.

Leng, G., Mason, W. T., and Dyer, R. G. 1982. The supraoptic nucleus as an osmoreceptor. Neuroendocrinol. 34:75–82.

Lenneberg, E. H. 1967. Biological Foundations of Language. New York: Wiley.

Lesky, E. 1976. The Vienna Medical School of the 19th Century. Baltimore: Johns Hopkins University Press.

Letourneau, P. C. 1983. Axonal growth and guidance. Trends Neurosci. 6:451–455.

LeVay, S., and Stryker, M. P. 1979. The development of ocular dominance columns in the cat. In J. A. Ferrendelli (eds.), Aspects of Developmental Neurobiology, Society for Neuroscience Symposia, Vol. 4. Bethesda, Md.: Society for Neuroscience, pp. 83–98.

LeVay, S., Stryker, M. P., and Shatz, C. J. 1978. Ocular dominance columns and their development in layer IV of the cat's visual cortex: A quantitative study. J. Comp. Neurol. 179:223–244.

LeVay, S., Wiesel, T. N., and Hubel, D. H. 1980. The development of ocular dominance columns in normal and visually deprived monkeys. J. Comp. Neurol. 191:1–51.

LeVay, S., Wiesel, T. N., and Hubel, D. H. 1981. The postnatal development and plasticity of ocular-dominance columns in the monkey. In F. O. Schmitt, F. G. Worden, G. Adelman, and S. G.

Dennis (eds.), The Organization of the Cerebral Cortex. Cambridge, Mass.: MIT Press, pp. 29–45.

Levick, W. R., and Thibos, L. N. 1983. Receptive fields of cat ganglion cells: Classification and construction. In N. N. Osborne and G. J. Chader (eds.), Progress in Retinal Research, Vol. 2. Oxford: Pergamon Press, pp. 267–319.

Levi-Montalcini, R. 1952. Effects of mouse tumor transplantation on the nervous system. Ann. N.Y. Acad. Sci. 55:330–343.

Levi-Montalcini, R. 1975. NGF: An uncharted route. In F. G. Worden, J. P. Swazey, and G. Adelman (eds.), The Neurosciences: Paths of Discovery. Cambridge, Mass.: MIT Press, pp. 245–265.

Levin, B. E., and Margolis, G. 1977. Acute failure of automatic respirations secondary to a unilateral brainstem infarct. Ann. Neurol. 1:583–586.

Levy, J., Trevarthen, C., and Sperry, R. W. 1972. Perception of bilateral chimeric figures following hemispheric deconnexion. Brain 95:61–78.

Lewin, R. 1985. Unexpected progress in photoreception. Science 227:500–503.

Lewis, M. 1971. Individual differences in the measurement of early cognitive growth. In J. Hellmuth (ed.), Exceptional Infant, Vol. 2: Studies in Abnormalities. New York: Brunner/Mazel, pp. 172–210.

Lewis, R. S., and Hudspeth, A. J. 1983. Frequency tuning and ionic conductances in hair cells of the bullfrog's sacculus. In R. Klinke and R. Hartmann (eds.), Hearing—Physiological Bases and Psychophysics. Berlin: Springer, pp. 17–24.

Lewontin, R. 1982. Human Diversity. New York: Scientific American Books.

Leyton, A. S. F., and Sherrington, C. S. 1917. Observations on the excitable cortex of the chimpanzee, orang-utan, and gorilla. Q. J. Exp. Physiol. 11:135–222.

Liddell, E. G. T., and Sherrington, C. 1924. Reflexes in response to stretch (myotatic reflexes). Proc. R. Soc. Lond. [Biol.] 96:212–242.

Liddell, E. G. T., and Sherrington, C. S. 1925. Recruitment and some other features of reflex inhibition. Proc. R. Soc. Lond. [Biol.] 97:488–518.

Liddell, E. G. T., and Sherrington, C. 1925. Further observations on myotatic reflexes. Proc. R. Soc. Lond. [Biol.] 97:267–283.

Lieberman, A. R. 1971. The axon reaction: A review of the principal features of perikaryal responses to axon injury. Int. Rev. Neurobiol. 14:49–124.

Liepmann, H. 1914. Bemerkungen zu v. Monakows Kapitel "Die Lokalisation der Apraxie." Monatsschr. Psychiatr. Neurol. 35:490–516.

Light, A. R., and Perl, E. R. 1979. Reexamination of the dorsal root projection to the spinal dorsal horn including observations on the differential termination of coarse and fine fibers. J. Comp. Neurol. 196:117–131.

Liley, A. W. 1956. The quantal components of the mammalian endplate potential. J. Physiol. (Lond.) 133:571–587.

Lincoln, D. W., and Wakerley, J. B. 1974. Electrophysiological evidence for the activation of supraoptic neurones during the release of oxytocin. J. Physiol. (Lond.) 242:533–554.

Lindsley, D. B., Schreiner, L. H., and Magoun, H. W. 1949. An electromyographic study of spasticity. J. Neurophysiol. 12:197–205.

Lindstrom, J. 1979. Autoimmune response to acetylcholine receptors in myasthenia gravis and its animal model. Adv. Immunol. 27:1–50.

Lindstrom, J. 1983. Using monoclonal antibodies to study acetylcholine receptors and myasthenia gravis. Neurosci. Comment. 1:139–156.

Lindstrom, J. 1986. Function and molecular structure of acetylcholine receptor. In A. Engel and B. Q. Banker (eds.), Clinical Myology. New York: McGraw–Hill, chap. 27, in press.

Lindstrom, J. M., and Lambert, E. H. 1978. Content of acetylcholine receptor and antibodies bound to receptor in myasthenia gravis, experimental autoimmune myasthenia gravis, and Eaton-Lambert syndrome. Neurology 28:130–138.

Lisak, R. P., and Barchi, R. L. 1982. Myasthenia Gravis. Philadelphia: Saunders.

Livingstone, M. S., and Hubel, D. H. 1984. Anatomy and physiology of a color system in the primate visual cortex. J. Neuroscience 4:309–356.

Livingstone, M. S., Sziber, P. P., and Quinn, W. G. 1984. Loss of calcium/calmodulin resonsiveness in adenylate cyclase of *rutabaga*, a Drosophila learning mutant. Cell 37:205–215.

Llinás, R. R. 1982. Calcium in synaptic transmission. Sci. Am. 247(4):56–65.

Llinás, R. R. 1984. Comparative electrobiology of mammalian central neurons. In R. Dingledine (ed.), Brain Slices. New York: Plenum Press.

Llinás, R. R., and Heuser, J. E. 1977. Depolarization-release coupling systems in neurons. Neurosci. Res. Program Bull. 15:555–687.

Llinás, R., and Nicholson, C. 1971. Electrophysiological properties of dendrites and somata in alligator Purkinje cells. J. Neurophysiol. 34:532–551.

Llinás, R., Steinberg, I. Z., and Walton, K. 1981. Relationship between presynaptic calcium current and postsynaptic potential in squid giant synapse. Biophys J. 33:323–351.

Lloyd, D. P. C. 1941. The spinal mechanism of the pyramidal system in cats. J. Neurophysiol. 4:525–546.

Lloyd, D. P. C. 1943. Conduction and synaptic transmission of the reflex response to stretch in spinal cats. J. Neurophysiol. 6:317–326.

Lloyd, D. P. C., and Chang, H.-T. 1948. Afferent fibers in muscle nerves. J. Neurophysiol. 11:199–207.

Loewenstein, W. R., and Mendelson, M. 1965. Components of receptor adaptation in a Pacinian corpuscle. J. Physiol. (Lond.) 177:377–397.

Loewi, O. 1960. An autobiographic sketch. Perspect. Biol. Med. 4:3–25.

Loh, Y. P., Brownstein, M. J., and Gainer, H. 1984. Proteolysis in neuropeptide processing and other neural functions. Annu. Rev. Neurosci. 7:189–220.

Lømo, T., and Rosenthal, J. 1972. Control of ACh sensitivity by muscle activity in the rat. J. Physiol. (Lond.) 221:493–513.

Lømo, T., and Westgaard, R. H. 1976. Control of ACh sensitivity in rat muscle fibers. Cold Spring Harbor Symp. Quant. Biol. 40:263–274.

Lømo, T., Westgaard, R. H., and Dahl, H. A. 1974. Contractile properties of muscle: Control by pattern of muscle activity in the rat. Proc. R. Soc. Lond. [Biol.] 187:99–103.

Lorente de No, R. 1933. Anatomy of the eighth nerve. III. General plan of structure of the primary cochlear nuclei. Laryngoscope 43:327–350.

Lorenz, K. Z. 1950. The comparative method in studying innate behaviour patterns. Symp. Soc. Exp. Biol. 4:221–268.

Lorenz, K. 1965. Evolution and Modification of Behavior. Chicago: University of Chicago Press.

Lukes, S. A., Crooks, L. E., Aminoff, M. J., Kaufman, L., Panitch, H. S., Mills, C., and Norman, D. 1983. Nuclear magnetic resonance imaging in multiple sclerosis. Ann. Neurol. 13:592–601.

Lund, R. D. 1978. Development and Plasticity of the Brain. New York: Oxford University Press.

Lundberg, A. 1975. Control of spinal mechanisms from the brain. In D. B. Tower (ed.), The Nervous System, Vol. 1: The Basic Neurosciences. New York: Raven Press, pp. 253–265.

Lundberg, A. 1979. Integration in a propriospinal motor centre controlling the forelimb in the cat. In H. Asanuma and V. J. Wilson (eds.), Integration in the Nervous System. Tokyo: Igaku–Shoin, pp. 47–64.

Lynch, J. C., Mountcastle, V. B., Talbot, W. H., and Yin, T. C. T. 1977. Parietal lobe mechanisms for directed visual attention. J. Neurophysiol. 40:362–389.

M

Mach, E. 1913. The Principles of Physical Optics (1926, Eng. trans.). Reprint, New York: Dover Publications, 1953.

Mach, E. 1866. Über den physiologischen Effect räumlich vertheilter Lichtreize, II. Sitzber. Akad. Wiss. Wien (Math. - Nat. Cl.), Abt. 2, 54:131–144.

Mackintosh, N. J. 1983. Conditioning and Associative Learning. Oxford: Clarendon Press.

MacLean, P. D. 1955. The limbic system ("visceral brain") and emotional behavior. Arch. Neurol. Psychiatry 73:130–134.

MacLusky, N. J., and Naftolin, F. 1981. Sexual differentiation of the central nervous system. Science 211:1294–1303.

Magni, F., Moruzzi, G., Rossi, G. F., and Zanchetti, A. 1959. EEG arousal following inactivation of the lower brain stem by selective injection of barbiturate into the vertebral circulation. Arch. Ital. Biol. 97:33–46.

Magoun, H. W. 1963. Reticulo-spinal influences and postural regulation. In H. W. Magoun (ed.), The Waking Brain, 2nd ed. Springfield, Ill. Thomas, pp. 23–38.

Magoun, H. W., and Rhines, R. 1946. An inhibitory mechanism in the bulbar reticular formation. J. Neurophysiol. 9:165–171.

Makowski, L., Caspar, D. L. D., Phillips, W. C., and Goodenough, D. A. 1977. Gap junction structures. II. Analysis of the X-ray diffraction data. J. Cell Biol. 74:629–645.

Makowski, L., Caspar, D. L. D., Phillips, W. C., Baker, T. S., and Goodenough, D. A. 1984. Gap junction structures. VI. Variation and conservation in connexion conformation and packing. Biophys. J. 45:208–218.

Manning, A. 1972. An Introduction to Animal Behavior, 2nd ed. Reading, Mass.: Addison-Wesley.

Margolis, R. U., and Margolis, R. K. (eds.). 1979. Complex Carbohydrates of Nervous Tissue. New York: Plenum Press.

Mariani, A. P. 1984. Bipolar cells in monkey retina selective for the cones likely to be blue-sensitive. Nature 308:184–186.

Mark, V. H., Ervin, F. R., and Yakovlev, P. I. 1963. Stereotactic thalamotomy. III. The verification of anatomical lesion sites in the human thalamus. Arch. Neurol. 8:528–538.

Marks, J. 1977. Physiology of abnormal movements. Postgrad. Med. J. 53:713–718.

Marks, W. B., Dobelle, W. H., and MacNichol, E. F., Jr. 1964. Visual pigments of single primate cones. Science 143:1181–1183.

Marler, P., and Hamilton, W. J., III. 1966. Mechanisms of Animal Behavior. New York: Wiley.

Marr, D. 1969. A theory of cerebellar cortex. J. Physiol. (Lond.) 202:437–470.

Marr, D. 1982. Vision. San Francisco: Freeman.

Marsden, C. D., and Harrison, M. J. G. 1972. Outcome of investigation of patients with presenile dementia. Br. Med. J. 2:249–252.

Marshall, W. H., and Talbot, S. A. 1942. Recent evidence for neural mechanisms in vision leading to a general theory of sensory acuity. In H. Klüver (ed.), Visual Mechanisms. Lancaster, Pa.: Cattell, pp. 117–164.

Marshall, W. H., Woolsey, C. N., and Bard, P. 1941. Observations on cortical somatic sensory mechanisms of cat and monkey. J. Neurophysiol. 4:1–24.

Martin, A. R. 1977. Junctional transmission. II: Presynaptic mechanisms. In E. R. Kandel (ed.), Handbook of Physiology, Vol. 1: The Nervous System, Part 1. Bethesda, Md.: American Physiological Society, pp. 329–355.

Martin, J. B. 1984. Huntington's Disease: New approaches to an old problem. Neurology 34:1059–1072.

Martin, W. R., Eades, C. G., Thompson, J. A., Huppler, R. E., and Gilbert, P. E. 1976. The effects of morphine- and nalorphine-like drugs in the nondependent and morphine-dependent chronic spinal dog. J. Pharmacol. Exp. Ther. 197:517–532.

Martinez Martinez, P. F. A. 1982. Neuroanatomy: Development and Structure of the Central Nervous System. Philadelphia: Saunders.

Mathews, D. F. 1972. Response patterns of single neurons in the tortoise olfactory epithelium and olfactory bulb. J. Gen. Physiol. 60:166–180.

Matthews, B. H. C. 1933. Nerve endings in mammalian muscle. J. Physiol. (Lond.) 78:1–53.

Matthews, P. B. C. 1964. Muscle spindles and their motor control. Physiol. Rev. 44:219–288.

Matthews, P. B. C. 1972. Mammalian Muscle Receptors and Their Central Actions. Baltimore: Williams & Wilkins.

Matthews, P. B. C. 1981. Muscle spindles: Their messages and their fusimotor supply. In V. B. Brooks (ed.), Handbook of Physiology, Section 1: The Nervous System, Vol. II, Motor Control. Bethesda, Md.: American Physiological Society, pp. 189–228.

Matthysse, S. W., and Kety, S. S. (eds.). 1975. Catecholamines and Schizophrenia. Oxford: Pergamon Press.

Mauk, M. D., Olson, G. A., Kastin, A. J., and Olson, R. D. 1980. Behavioral effects of LH–RH. Neurosci. Biobehav. Rev. 4:1–8.

Mawad, M. E., Silver, A. J., Hilal, S. K., and Ganti, S. R. 1983. Computed tomography of the brain stem with intrathecal metrizamide. Part I: The normal brain stem. Am. J. Neuroradiol. 4:1–11.

Maxam, A. M., and Gilbert, W. 1980. Sequencing end-labeled DNA with base-specific chemical cleavages. Meth. Enzymol. 65:499–560.

Mayer, D. J., and Liebeskind, J. C. 1974. Pain reduction by focal electrical stimulation of the brain: An anatomical and behavioral analysis. Brain Res. 68:73–93.

Mayeux, R., Stern, Y., Côté, L., and Williams, J. B. W. 1984. Altered serotonin metabolism in depressed patients with Parkinson's disease. Neurology 34:642–646.

Mays, L. E., and Sparks, D. L. 1980. Saccades are spatially, not retinocentrically coded. Science 208:1163–1165.

McBurney, D. H. 1984. Taste and olfaction: Sensory discrimination. In I. Darian-Smith (ed.), Handbook of Physiology, Section 1: The Nervous System, Vol. III, Sensory Processes. Bethesda, Md.: American Physiological Society, pp. 1067–1086.

McCloskey, D. I. 1978. Kinesthetic sensibility. Physiol. Rev. 58:763–820.

McCormick, D. A., and Thompson, R. F. 1984. Cerebellum: Essential involvement in the classically conditioned eyelid response. Science 223:296–299.

McDougall, W. 1908. An Introduction to Social Psychology. London: Methuen, 1960. New York: Barnes & Noble, 1960.

McEwen, B. S. 1976. Interactions between hormones and nerve tissue. Sci. Am. 235(1):48–58.

McGaugh, J. L., and Herz, M. J. 1972. Memory Consolidation. San Francisco: Albion.

McGeer, E., and McGeer, P. L. 1976. Neurotransmitter metabolism in the aging brain. In R. D. Terry and S. Gershon (eds.), Aging, Vol. 3: Neurobiology of Aging. New York: Raven Press, pp. 389–403.

McGeer, P. L., Eccles, J. C., and McGeer, E. G. 1978. Molecular Neurobiology of the Mammalian Brain. New York: Plenum Press.

McMahan, U. J., and Kuffler, S. W. 1971. Visual identification of synaptic boutons on living ganglion cells and of varicosities in postganglionic axons in the heart of the frog. Proc. R. Soc. Lond. [Biol.] 177:485–508.

Medvedev, Zh. A. 1972. Repetition of molecular–genetic information as a possible factor in evolutionary changes of life span. Exp. Gerontol. 7:227–238.

Melzack, R., and Wall, P. D. 1965. Pain mechanisms: A new theory. Science 150:971–979.

Mendell, L. M., and Henneman, E. 1971. Terminals of single Ia fibers: Location, density, and distribution within a pool of 300 homonymous motoneurons. J. Neurophysiol. 34:171–187.

Mendell, L. M., Munson, J. B., and Scott, J. G. 1976. Alterations of synapses on axotomized motoneurones. J. Physiol. (Lond.) 255:67–79.

Mendelson, W. B., Cain, M., Cook, J. M., Paul, S. M., and Skolnick, P. 1983. A benzodiazepine receptor antagonist decreases sleep and reverses the hypnotic actions of flurazepam. Science 219:414–416.

Mendelson, W. B., Gillin, J. C., and Wyatt, R. J. 1977. Human Sleep and Its Disorders. New York: Plenum Press.

Mendelson, W. B., Weingartner, H., Greenblatt, D. J., Garnett, D., and Gillin, J. C. 1982. A clinical study of flurazepam. Sleep 5:350–360.

Merritt, H. H. 1979. A Textbook of Neurology, 6th ed. Philadelphia: Lea & Febiger.

Merton, P. A. 1953. Speculations on the servo-control of movement. In G. E. W. Wolstenholme (ed.), The Spinal Cord. London: Churchill Livingstone, pp. 247–255.

Merton, P. A. 1972. How we control the contraction of our muscles. Sci. Am. 226(5):30–37.

Merzenich, M. M. 1985. Functional "maps" of skin sensations. In C. C. Brown (ed.), The Many Facets of Touch. The summary publication of Johnson & Johnson Pediatric Rountable #10—Touch. Skillman, N.J.: Johnson & Johnson Baby Products Company, pp. 15–22.

Merzenich, M. M. 1985. Sources of intraspecies and interspecies cortical map variability in mammals: Conclusions and hypotheses. In M. J. Cohen and N. C. Spitzer (eds.), Comparative Neurobiology: Modes of Communication in the Nervous System. New York: Wiley (in press).

Merzenich, M. M., and Kaas, J. H. 1982. Reorganization of mammalian somatosensory cortex following peripheral nerve injury. Trends Neurosci. 5:434–436.

Merzenich, M. M., Kaas, J. H., Wall, J., Nelson, R. J., Sur, M., and Felleman, D. 1983. Topographic reorganization of somatosensory cortical areas 3B and 1 in adult monkeys following restricted deafferentation. Neuroscience 8:33–55.

Merzenich, M. M., Kaas, J. H., Wall, J. T., Sur, M., Nelson, R. J., and Felleman, D. J. 1983. Progression of change following median nerve section in the cortical representation of the hand in areas 3b and 1 in adult owl and squirrel monkeys. Neuroscience 10:639–665.

Merzenich, M. M., Nelson, R. J., Stryker, M. P., Cyander, M. S., Schoppmann, A., and Zook, J. M. 1984. Somatosensory cortical map changes following digit amputation in adult monkeys. J. Comp. Neurol. 224:591–605.

Merzenich, M. M., and Reid, M. D. 1974. Representation of the cochlea within the inferior colliculus of the cat. Brain Res. 77:397–415.

Meyer-Lohmann, J., Hore, J., and Brooks, V. B. 1977. Cerebellar participation in generation of prompt arm movements. J. Neurophysiol. 40:1038–1050.

Meyerson, B. J. 1979. Hypothalamic hormones and behaviour. Med. Biol. (Helsinki) 57:69–83.

Michael, C. R. 1978a. Color vision mechanisms in monkey striate cortex: Dual-opponent cells with concentric receptive fields. J. Neurophysiol. 41:572–588.

Michael, C. R. 1978b. Color vision mechanisms in monkey striate cortex: Simple cells with dual opponent-color receptive fields. J. Neurophysiol. 41:1233–1249.

Miledi, R. 1960. The acetylcholine sensitivity of frog muscle fibres after complete or partial denervation. J. Physiol. (Lond.) 151:1–23.

Miledi, R., Molinoff, P., and Potter, L. T. 1971. Isolation of the cholinergic receptor protein of Torpedo electric tissue. Nature 229:554–557.

Miles, F. A. 1969. Excitable Cells. London: Heinemann.

Milhorat, T. H. 1972. Hydrocephalus and the Cerebrospinal Fluid. Baltimore: Williams & Wilkins.

Miller, G. A. 1981. Language and Speech. San Francisco: Freeman.

Miller, J. D. 1979. Barbiturates and raised intracranial pressure. Ann. Neurol. 6:189–193.

Miller, J. M., and Towe, A. L. 1979. Audition: Structural and acoustical properties. In T. Ruch, and H. D. Patton (eds.), Physiology and Biophysics, Vol. 1. The Brain and Neural Function, 20th ed. Philadelphia: Saunders, pp. 339–375.

Miller, T. M., and Heuser, J. E. 1984. Endocytosis of synaptic vesicle membrane at the frog neuromuscular junction. J. Cell Biol. 98:685–698.

Milner, B. 1966. Amnesia following operation on the temporal lobes. In C. W. M. Whitty and O. L. Zangwill (eds.), Amnesia. London: Butterworths, pp. 109–133.

Milner, B. 1968. Visual recognition and recall after right temporal-lobe excision in man. Neuropsychologia 6:191–209.

Milner, B. 1974. Hemispheric specialization: Scope and limits. In F. O. Schmitt and F. G. Worden (eds.), The Neurosciences: Third Study Program. Cambridge, Mass.: MIT Press, pp. 75–89.

Mitchell, P. 1961. Coupling of phosphorylation to electron and hydrogen transfer by a chemi-osmotic type of mechanism. Nature 191:144–148.

Mitler, M. M., and Dement, W. C. 1974. Cataplectic-like behavior in cats after micro-injections of carbachol in pontine reticular formation. Brain Res. 68:335–343.

Mohr, J. P., Fisher, C. M., and Adams, R. D. 1980. Cerebrovascular diseases. In K. J. Isselbacher, R. D. Adams, E. Braunwald, R. G. Petersdorf, and J. D. Wilson (eds.), Harrison's Principles of Internal Medicine, 9th ed. New York: McGraw–Hill, pp. 1911–1942.

Moll, L., and Kuypers, H. G. J. M. 1977. Premotor cortical ablations in monkeys: Contralateral changes in visually guided reaching behavior. Science 198:317–319.

Molliver, M. E., Grzanna, R., Lidov, H. G. W., Morrison, J. H., and Olschowka, J. A. 1982. Monoamine systems in the cerebral cortex. In V. Chan-Palay and S. L. Palay (eds.), Neurology and Neurobiology, Vol. 1: Cytochemical Methods in Neuroanatomy. New York: Liss, pp. 255–277.

Money, J., and Ehrhardt, A. A. 1972. Man & Woman, Boy & Girl. Baltimore: Johns Hopkins University Press.

Moniz, E. 1936. Tentatives Operatoires dans le Traitement de Certaines Psychoses. Paris: Masson.

Moore, J. W., Desmond, J. E., and Berthier, N. E. 1982. The metencephalic basis of the conditioned nictitating membrane response. In C. D. Woody (ed.), Conditioning: Representation of Involved Neural Functions. New York: Plenum Press, pp. 459–482.

Moore, R. Y., and Eichler, V. B. 1972. Loss of a circadian adrenal corticosterone rhythm following suprachiasmatic lesions in the rat. Brain Res. 42:201–206.

Moore, R. Y., and Lenn, N. J. 1972. A retinohypothalamic projection in the rat. J. Comp. Neurol. 146:1–14.

Moore-Ede, M. C. 1983. The circadian timing system in mammals: Two pacemakers preside over many secondary oscillators. Fed. Proc. 42:2802–2808.

Morest, D. K. 1964. The laminar structure of the inferior colliculus of the cat. Anat. Rec. 148:314.

Mori, H., Komiya, Y., and Kurokawa, M. 1979. Slowly migrating axonal polypeptides: Inequalities in their rate and amount of transport between two branches of bifurcating axons. J. Cell Biol. 82:174–184.

Moruzzi, G., and Magoun H. W. 1949. Brain stem reticular formation and activation of the EEG. Electroencephalogr. Clin. Neurophysiol. 1:455–473.

Moses, R. A. 1975. Accommodation. In R. A. Moses (ed.), Adler's Physiology of the Eye, 6th ed. St. Louis: Mosby, pp. 298–319.

Moses, R. A. 1975. The iris and the pupil. In R. A. Moses (ed.), Adler's Physiology of the Eye, 6th ed. St. Louis: Mosby, pp. 320–352.

Moss, R. L., and McCann, S. M. 1973. Induction of mating behavior in rats by luteinizing hormone-releasing factor. Science 181:177–179.

Mosso, J. A., and Kruger, L. 1973. Receptor categories represented in spinal trigeminal nucleus caudalis. J. Neurophysiol. 36:472–488.

Mott, F. W., and Sherrington, C. S. 1895. Experiments upon the influence of sensory nerves upon movement and nutrition of the limbs. Preliminary communication. Proc. R. Soc. Lond. 57:481–488.

Moulton, D. G. 1976. Spatial patterning of response to odors in the peripheral olfactory system. Physiol. Rev. 56:578–593.

Mountcastle, V. B. 1957. Modality and topographic properties of single neurons of cat's somatic sensory cortex. J. Neurophysiol. 20:408–434.

Mountcastle, V. B. 1975. The view from within: Pathways to the study of perception. Johns Hopkins Med. J. 136:109–131.

Mountcastle, V. B. 1976. The world around us: Neural command functions for selective attention. Neurosci. Res. Program Bull. [Suppl.] 14.

Mountcastle, V. B. 1978. An organizing principle for cerebral function: The unit module and the distributed system. In G. M. Edelman and V. B. Mountcastle (eds.), The Mindful Brain. Cambridge, Mass.: MIT Press, pp. 7–50.

Mountcastle, V. B. 1980. Sensory receptors and neural encoding: Introduction to sensory processes. In V. B. Mountcastle (ed.), Medical Physiology, 14th ed., Vol. 1. St. Louis: Mosby, pp. 327–347.

Mountcastle, V. B. 1984. Central nervous mechanisms in mechanoreceptive sensibility. In I. Darian-Smith (ed.), Handbook of Physiology, Section 1: The Nervous System, Vol. III, Sensory Processes. Bethesda, Md.: American Physiological Society, pp. 789–878.

Mountcastle, V. B., and Darian-Smith, I. 1968. Neural mechanisms in somesthesia. In V. B. Mountcastle (ed.), Medical Physiology, 12th ed., Vol. II. St. Louis: Mosby, pp. 1372–1423.

Mountcastle, V. B., and Henneman, E. 1952. The representation of tactile sensibility in the thalamus of the monkey. J. Comp. Neurol. 97:409–439.

Mountcastle, V. B., Lynch, J. C., Georgopoulos, A., Sakata, H., and Acuna, C. 1975. Posterior parietal association cortex of the monkey: Command functions for operations within extrapersonal space. J. Neurophysiol. 38:871–908.

Moushon, J. A., Adelson, E. H., Gizzi, M. S., and Newsome, W. T. 1985. The analysis of moving visual patterns. In C. Chagas, R. Gattass, and C. Gross (eds.), Pattern Recognition Mechanisms. Rome: Vatican Press (in press).

Mudge, A. W., Leeman, S. E., and Fischbach, G. D. 1979. Enkephalin inhibits release of substance P from sensory neurons in culture and decreases action potential duration. Proc. Natl. Acad. Sci. U.S.A. 76:526–530.

Murphy, D. L., Campbell, I., and Costa, J. L. 1978. Current status of the indoleamine hypothesis of the affective disorders. In M. A. Lipton, A. DiMascio, and K. F. Killam (eds.), Psychopharmacology: A Generation of Progress. New York: Raven Press, pp. 1235–1247.

Murray, R. G. 1973. The ultrastructure of taste buds. In I. Friedman (ed.), The Ultrastructure of Sensory Organs. New York: American Elsevier, pp. 1–81.

Myers, R. E. 1955. Interocular transfer of pattern discrimination in cats following section of crossed optic fibers. J. Comp. Physiol. Psychol. 48:470–473.

N

Nachmansohn, D. 1959. Chemical and Molecular Basis of Nerve Activity. New York: Academic Press.

Naeser, M. A., Alexander, M. P., Helm-Estabrooks, N., Levine, H. L., Laughlin, S. A., and Geschwind, N. 1982. Aphasia with predominantly subcortical lesion sites. Arch. Neurol. 39:2–14.

Nagasaki, H., Kitahama, K., Valatx, J.-L., and Jouvet, M. 1980. Sleep-promoting effect of the sleep-promoting substance (SPS) and delta sleep-inducing peptide (DSIP) in the mouse. Brain Res. 192:276–280.

Nakanishi, S., Teranishi, Y., Watanabe, Y., Notake, M., Noda, M., Kakidani, H., Jingami, H., and Numa, S. 1981. Isolation and characterization of the bovine corticotropin/β-lipotropin precursor gene. Eur. J. Biochem. 115:429–438.

Nashner, L. M. 1976. Adapting reflexes controlling the human posture. Exp. Brain Res. 26:59–72.

Nashner, L. M. 1981. Analysis of stance posture in humans. In A. L. Towe and E. S. Luschei (eds.), Handbook of Behavioral Neurobiology, Vol. 5. New York: Plenum Press, pp. 527–565.

Nathans, J., and Hogness, D. S. 1984. Isolation and nucleotide sequence of the gene encoding human rhodopsin. Proc. Natl. Acad. Sci. U.S.A. 81:4851–4855.

Nauta, W. J. H., Smith, G. P., Faull, R. L. M., and Domesick, V. B. 1978. Efferent connections and nigral afferents of the nucleus accumbens septi in the rat. Neuroscience 3:385–401.

Neher, E. 1982. Unit conductance studies in biological membranes. In P. F. Baker (ed.), Techniques in Cellular Physiology, Vol. P1/II (P. 121). County Clare, Ireland: Elsevier/North-Holland, pp. 1–16.

Neher, E., and Marty, A. 1982. Discrete changes of cell membrane capacitance observed under conditions of enhanced secretion in bovine adrenal chromaffin cells. Proc. Natl. Acad. Sci. U.S.A. 79:6712–6716.

Neher, E., and Sakmann, B. 1976. Single-channel currents recorded from membrane of denervated frog muscle fibres. Nature 260:799–802.

Nelson, R., Famiglietti, E. V., Jr., and Kolb, H. 1978. Intracellular staining reveals different levels of stratification for on- and off-center ganglion cells in cat retina. J. Neurophysiol. 41:472–483.

Nernst, W. 1888. On the kinetics of substances in solution. Translated from Z. physik. Chemie. 2:613–622, 634–637. In G. R. Kepner (ed.), Cell Membrane Permeability and Transport. Stroudsburg, Pa.: Dowden, Hutchinson & Ross, 1979, pp. 174–183.

Nestler, E. J., and Greengard, P. 1983. Protein phosphorylation in the Nervous System. New York: Wiley.

Netter, F. H. 1983. The CIBA Collection of Medical Illustrations. Vol. 1, The Nervous System, Part I, Anatomy and Physiology. West Caldwell, N.J.: CIBA.

Newton, I. 1730. Opticks: or, A Treatise on the Reflections, Refractions, Inflections and Colours of light, 4th rev. ed. London: William Innys. Reprint, New York: Dover Publications, 1952.

Nichols, T. R., and Houk, J. C. 1973. Reflex compensation for variations in the mechanical properties of a muscle. Science 181:182–184.

Nicoll, R. A. 1982. Neurotransmitters can say more than just "yes" or "no." Trends Neurosci. 5:369–374.

Nieuwenhuys, R., Voogd, J., and van Huijzen, Chr. 1981. The Human Central Nervous System: A Synopsis and Atlas, 2nd rev. ed. Berlin: Springer.

Nishihara, H. K., and Poggio, T. 1982. Hidden cues in random-line stereograms. Nature 300:347–349.

Niven, W. D. (ed.). 1890. The Scientific Papers of James Clerk Maxwell. Cambridge: The University Press.

Noback, C. R., and Demarest, R. J. 1981. The Human Nervous System: Basic Principles of Neurobiology, 3rd ed. New York: McGraw-Hill.

Nobel, D. 1966. Applications of Hodgkin–Huxley equations to excitable tissues. Physiol. Rev. 46:1–50.

Noda, M., Furutani, Y., Takahashi, H., Toyosato, M., Tanabe, T., Shimizu, S., Kikyotani, S., Kayano, T., Hirose, T., Inayama, S., and Numa, S. 1983. Cloning and sequence analysis of calf cDNA and human genomic DNA encoding α-subunit precursor of muscle acetylcholine receptor. Nature 305:818–823.

Noda, M., Shimuzu, S., Tanabe, T., Takai, T., Kayano, T., Ikeda, T., Takahashi, H., Nakayama, H., Kanaoka, Y., Minamino N., Kangawa, K., Matsuo, H., Raftery, M., Hirose, T., Inayama, S., Hayashida, H., Miyata, T., and Numa, S. 1984. Primary structure of Electrophorus electricus sodium channel deduced from cDNA sequence. Nature 312:121–127.

Noda, M., Takahashi, H., Tanabe, T., Toyosato, M., Kikyotani, S., Furutani, Y., Hirose, T., Takashima, H., Inayama, S., Miyata, T., and Numa, S. 1983. Structural homology of Torpedo californica acetylcholine receptor subunits. Nature 302:528–532.

Noda, M., Teranishi, Y., Takahashi, H., Toyosato, M., Notake, M., Nakanishi, S., and Numa, S. 1982. Isolation and structural organization of the human preproenkephalin gene. Nature 297:431–434.

Norgren, R. 1984. Central neural mechanisms of taste. In I. Darian-Smith (ed.), Handbook of Physiology, Section 1: The Nervous System, Vol. III, Sensory Processes. Bethesda, Md.: American Physiological Society, pp. 1087–1128.

Norrsell, U. 1980. Behavioral studies of the somatosensory system. Physiol. Rev. 60:327–354.

Nottebohm, F. 1979. Origins and mechanisms in the establishment of cerebral dominance. In M. S. Gazzaniga (ed.), Handbook of Behavioral Neurobiology, Vol. 2: Neuropsychology. New York: Plenum Press, pp. 295–344.

O

Oblinger, M. M., and Lasek, R. J. 1985. Selective regulation of two axonal cytoskeletal networks in dorsal root ganglion cells. In P. O'Lague (ed.), Neurobiology: Molecular Biological Approaches to Understanding Neuronal Function and Development. The Shering Corp.: UCLA Symposium on Molecular and Cellular Biology, Vol. 24. New York: Liss.

O'Brien, D. F. 1982. The chemistry of vision. Science 218:961–966.

Ochs, S. 1972. Fast transport of materials in mammalian nerve fibers. Science 176:252–260.

Ochs, S. 1975. Waller's concept of the trophic dependence of the nerve fiber on the cell body in the light of early neuron therapy. Clio Med. 10:253–265.

Ochs, S. 1982. Axoplasmic Transport and Its Relation to Other Nerve Functions. New York: Wiley.

Ogle, K. N. 1961. Optics: An Introduction for Ophthalmologists. Springfield, Ill.: Thomas.

Ohmori, H. 1984. Mechanoelectrical transducer has discrete conductances in the chick vestibular hair cell. Proc. Natl. Acad. Sci. U.S.A. 81:1888–1891.

Oldendorf, W. H. 1980. The Quest for an Image of Brain. New York: Raven Press.

Olds, J., and Milner, P. 1954. Positive reinforcement produced by electrical stimulation of septal area and other regions of rat brain. J. Comp. Physiol. Psychol. 47:419–427.

Olsen, R. W. 1982. Drug interactions at the GABA receptor-ionophore complex. Annu. Rev. Pharmacol. Toxicol. 22:245–277.

Orkand, R. K. 1977. Glial cells. In E. R. Kandel (ed.), Handbook of Physiology, Section 1: The Nervous System, Vol. I. Cellular Biology of Neurons. Bethesda, Md.: American Physiological Society, pp. 855–875.

Orton, S. T. 1937. Reading, Writing and Speech Problems in Children. New York: Norton.

Oscarsson, O. 1973. Functional organization of spinocerebellar paths. In A. Iggo (ed.), Handbook of Sensory Physiology, Vol. 2: Somatosensory System. New York: Springer, pp. 339–380.

Otsuka, M., Kravitz, E. A., and Potter, D. D. 1967. Physiological and chemical architecture of a lobster ganglion with particular reference to gamma-aminobutyrate and glutamate. J. Neurophysiol. 30:725–752.

Ottoson, D. 1971. The electro-olfactogram. In L. M. Beidler (ed.), Handbook of Sensory Physiology, Vol. IV. Chemical Senses, Part 1, Olfaction. Berlin: Springer, pp. 95–131.

Ottoson, D. 1983. Physiology of the Nervous System. New York: Oxford University Press.

Ozeki, M., and Sato, M. 1972. Responses of gustatory cells in the tongue of rat to stimuli representing four taste qualities. Comp. Biochem. Physiol. 41A:391–407.

P

Palay, S. L. 1958. The morphology of synapses in the central nervous system. Exp. Cell Res. Suppl. 5:275–293.

Palay, S. L., and Chan-Palay, V. 1977. General morphology of neurons and neuroglia. In E. R. Kandel (ed.), Handbook of Physiology, Vol. 1: The Nervous System, Part 1. Bethesda, Md.: American Physiological Society, pp. 5–37.

Pandya, D. N., and Seltzer, B. 1982. Association areas of the cerebral cortex. Trends Neurosci. 5:386–390.

Panum, P. L. 1858. Physiologische Untersuchungen über das Sehen mit zwei Augen. Kiel: Schwerssche Bucchandlung. Cited by Boring, E. G. (1942).

Pansky, B. 1982. Review of Medical Embryology. New York: Macmillan.

Papez, J. W. 1937. A proposed mechanism of emotion. Arch. Neurol. Psychiatry 38:725–743.

Pappas, G. D., and Waxman, S. G. 1972. Synaptic fine structure—morphological correlates of chemical and electrotonic transmission. In G. D. Pappas and D. P. Purpura (eds.), Structure and Function of Synapses. New York: Raven Press, pp. 1–43.

Pappenheimer, J. R. 1976. The sleep factor. Sci. Am. 235(2):24–29.

Pappenheimer, J. R., Miller, T. B., and Goodrich, C. A. 1967. Sleep-promoting effects of cerebrospinal fluid from sleep-deprived goats. Proc. Natl. Acad. Sci. U.S.A. 58:513–517.

Parkinson, J. 1817. An Essay on the Shaking Palsy. London.

Partridge, L. D. 1966. Signal-handling characteristics of load-moving skeletal muscle. Am. J. Physiol. 210:1178–1191.

Pasternak, G. W. 1981. Opiate, enkephalin, and endorphin analgesia:

Relations to a single subpopulation of opiate receptors. Neurology 31:1311–1315.

Paton, J. A., and Nottebohm, F. N. 1984. Neurons generated in the adult brain are recruited into functional circuits. Science 225:1046–1048.

Patrick, J., and Lindstrom, J. 1973. Autoimmune response to acetylcholine receptor. Science 180:871–872.

Patten, J. 1977. Neurological Differential Diagnosis. London: Starke; New York: Springer.

Patterson, P. H. 1978. Environmental determination of autonomic neurotransmitter functions. Annu. Rev. Neurosci. 1:1–17.

Patterson, H., and Purves, D. (eds.). 1982. Readings in Developmental Neurobiology. Cold Spring Harbor, New York: Cold Spring Harbor Laboratory.

Patton, H. D. 1965. Reflex regulation of movement and posture. In T. C. Ruch and H. D. Patton (eds.), Physiology and Biophysics, 19th ed. Philadelphia: Saunders, pp. 181–206.

Patton, H. D., Sundsten, J. W., Crill, W. E., and Swanson, P. D. 1976. Introduction to Basic Neurology. Philadelphia: Saunders.

Pauling, L., Itano, H. A., Singer, S. J., and Wells, I. C. 1949. Sickle Cell Anemia: A molecular disease. Science 110:543–548.

Pavlov, I. P. 1927. Conditioned Reflexes: An Investigation of the Physiological Activity of the Cerebral Cortex. G. V. Anrep (trans.) London: Oxford University Press.

Pearse, A. G. E. 1969. The cytochemistry and ultrastructure of polypeptide hormone-producing cells of the APUD series and the embryologic, physiologic and pathologic implications of the concept. J. Histochem. Cytochem. 17:303–313.

Pearse, A. G. E., Polak, J. M., and Bloom, S. R. 1977. The newer gut hormones: Cellular sources, physiology, pathology, and clinical aspects. Gastroenterology 72:746–761.

Pearson, K. 1976. The control of walking. Sci. Am. 235(6):72–86.

Penfield, W. (ed.). 1932. Cytology & Cellular Pathology of the Nervous System, Vol. 2. New York: Hoeber.

Penfield, W. 1954. Mechanisms of voluntary movement. Brain 77:1–17.

Penfield, W. 1958. Functional localization in temporal and deep Sylvian areas. Res. Publ. Assoc. Res. Nerv. Ment. Dis. 36:210–226.

Penfield, W., and Rasmussen, T. 1950. The Cerebral Cortex of Man: A Clinical Study of Localization of Function. New York: Macmillan.

Penfield, W., and Roberts, L. 1959. Speech and Brain-Mechanisms. Princeton, N.J.: Princeton University Press.

Perl, E. R. 1958. Crossed reflex effects evoked by activity in myelinated afferent fibers of muscle. J. Neurophysiol. 21:101–102.

Perl, E. R. 1968. Myelinated afferent fibres innervating the primate skin and their response to noxious stimuli. J. Physiol. (Lond.) 197:593–615.

Perry, E. K., Perry, R. H., Blessed, G., and Tomlinson, B. E. 1977. Necropsy evidence of central cholinergic deficits in senile dementia. Lancet 1:189.

Peters, A., Palay, S. L., and Webster, H. deF. 1976. The Fine Structure of the Nervous System: The Neurons and Supporting Cells. Philadelphia: Saunders.

Pfaff, D. W. 1973. Luteinizing hormone-releasing factor potentiates lordosis behavior in hypophysectomized ovariectomized female rats. Science 182:1148–1149.

Pfaff, D. W. and McEwen, B. S. 1983. Actions of estrogens and progestins on nerve cells. Science 219:808–814.

Pfaffmann, C. 1941. Gustatory afferent impulses. J. Cell. Comp. Physiol. 17:243–258.

Pfaffmann, C. 1955. Gustatory nerve impulses in rat, cat and rabbit. J. Neurophysiol. 18:429–440.

Pfenninger, K., Sandri, C., Akert, K., and Eugster, C. H. 1969. Contribution to the problem of structural organization of the presynaptic area. Brain Res. 12:10–18.

Phelps, M. E., Mazziotta, J. C., and Huang, S.-C. 1982. Study of cerebral function with positron computed tomography. J. Cerebral Blood Flow Metab. 2:113–162.

Phelps, M. E., Schelbert, H. R., and Mazziotta, J. C. 1983. Positron computed tomography for studies of myocardial and cerebral function. Ann. Intern. Med. 98:339–359.

Phillips, C. G., and Porter, R. 1977. Corticospinal Neurones: Their Role in Movement. London: Academic Press.

Phoenix, C. H., Goy, R. W., Gerall, A. A., and Young, W. C. 1959. Organizing action of prenatally administered testosterone propionate on the tissues mediating mating behavior in the female guinea pig. Endocrinology 65:369–382.

Piccolino, M., Neyton, J. Witkowsky, P., and Gerschenfeld, H. M. 1982. γ-Aminobutyric acid antagonists decrease junctional communication between L-horizontal cells of the retina. Proc. Natl. Acad. Sci. U.S.A. 79:3671–3675.

Picton, T. W., Hillyard, S. A., Krausz, H. I., and Galambos, R. 1974. Human auditory evoked potentials. I: Evaluation of components. Electroencephalogr. Clin. Neurophysiol. 36:179–190.

Pieron, H. 1913. Le Problème Physiologique du Sommeil. Paris: Masson.

Pletscher, A., Shore, P. A., and Brodie, B. B. 1956. Serotonin as a mediator of reserpine action in brain. J. Pharmacol. Exp. Ther. 116:84–89.

Plum, F., and Posner, J. B. 1980. The Diagnosis of Stupor and Coma, 3rd ed. Philadelphia: Davis.

Poggio, G. F., and Fischer, B. 1977. Binocular interaction and depth sensitivity in striate and prestriate cortex of behaving rhesus monkey. J. Neurophysiol. 40:1392–1405.

Poggio. G. F., and Mountcastle, V. B. 1960. A study of the functional contributions of the lemniscal and spinothalamic systems to somatic sensibility. Central nervous mechanisms in pain. Bull. Johns Hopkins Hosp. 106:266–316.

Poggio, G. F., and Mountcastle, V. B. 1963. The functional properties of ventrobasal thalamic neurons studied in unanesthetized monkeys. J. Neurophysiol. 26:775–806.

Poggio, T. 1984. Vision by man and machine. Sci. Am. 250(4):106–116.

Pokorny, J., Smith, V. C., Verriest, G., and Pinckers, A. J. L. G. 1979. Congenital and Acquired Color Vision Defects. New York: Grune & Stratton.

Polit, A., and Bizzi, E. 1978. Processes controlling arm movements in monkeys. Science 201:1235–1237.

Pollock, L. J., and Davis, L. 1930. The reflex activities of a decerebrate animal. J. Comp. Neurol. 50:377–411.

Pollock, L. J., and Davis, L. 1931. Studies in decerebration. VI. The effect of deafferentation upon decerebrate rigidity. Am. J. Physiol. 98:47–49.

Premack, D. 1976. Intelligence in Ape and Man. Hillsdale, N.J.: Erlbaum.

Preston, J. B., and Whitlock, D. G. 1961. Intracellular potentials recorded from motoneurons following precentral gyrus stimulation in primate. J. Neurophysiol. 24:91–100.

Price, D. L., Whitehouse, P. J., Struble, R. G., Clark, A. W., Coyle, J. T., DeLong, M. R., and Hedreen, J. C. 1982. Basal forebrain cholinergic systems in Alzheimer's disease and related dementia. Neurosci. Comment. 1(2):84–92.

Prince, D. A. 1978. Neurophysiology of epilepsy. Annu. Rev. Neurosci. 1:395–415.

Purves, D., and Lichtman, J. W. 1980. Principles of Neural Development. Sunderland Mass.: Sinauer.

Puszkin, S., Berl, S., Puszkin, E., and Clarke, D. D. 1968. Actomyosin-like protein isolated from mammalian brain. Science 161:170–171.

Pykett, I. L. 1982. NMR imaging in medicine. Sci. Am. 246(5):78–88.

Q

Quinn, W. G. 1984. Work in invertebrates on the mechanisms underlying learning. In P. Marler and H. S. Terrace (eds.), The Biology of Learning. Dahlem Konferenzen. Berlin: Springer, pp. 197–246.

R

Raftery, M. A., Hunkapiller, M. W., Strader, C. D., and Hood, L. E. 1980. Acetylcholine receptor: Complex of homologous subunits. Science 208:1454–1457.

Raisman, G. 1974. Evidence for a sex difference on the neuropil of the rat preoptic area and its importance for the study of sexually dimorphic functions. Res. Publ. Assoc. Res. Nerv. Ment. Dis. 52:42–49.

Raisman, G., and Field, P. M. 1971. Sexual dimorphism in the preoptic area of the rat. Science 173:731–733.

Rakic, P. 1971. Neuron-glia relationship during granule cell migration in developing cerebellar cortex. A Golgi and electron-microscopic study in Macacus rhesus. J. Comp. Neurol. 141:283–312.

Rakic, P. 1973. Kinetics of proliferation and latency between final cell division and onset of differentiation of cerebellar stellate and basket neurons. J. Comp. Neurol. 147:523–546.

Rakic, P. 1975. Local circuit neurons. Neurosci. Res. Program Bull. 13:289–446.

Rakic, P. 1976. Prenatal genesis of connections subserving ocular dominance in the rhesus monkey. Nature 261:467–471.

Rakic, P. 1977. Prenatal development of the visual system in rhesus monkey. Philos. Trans. R. Soc. Lond. [Biol. Sci.] 278:245–260.

Rakic, P. 1981. Development of visual centers in the primate brain depends on binocular competition before birth. Science 214:928–931.

Rakic, P., and Sidman, R. L. 1973. Weaver mutant mouse cerebellum: Defective neuronal migration secondary to abnormality of Bergmann glia. Proc. Natl. Acad. Sci. U.S.A. 70:240–244.

Rall, W. 1977. Core conductor theory and cable properties of neurons. In E. R. Kandel (ed.), Handbook of Physiology, Vol. 1: The Nervous System, Part 1. Bethesda, Md.: American Physiological Society, pp. 39–97.

Randolph, M., and Semmes, J. 1974. Behavioral consequences of selective subtotal ablations in the postcentral gyrus of Macaca mulatta. Brain Res. 70:55–70.

Ranson, S. W. 1934. The hypothalamus: Its significance for visceral innervation and emotional expression. Trans. Coll. Physicians Phila. [Ser. 4] 2:222–242.

Ranson, S. W., and Clark, S. L. 1953. The Anatomy of the Nervous System: Its Development and Function, 9th ed. Philadelphia: Saunders.

Raphan, T., and Cohen, B. 1978. Brainstem mechanisms for rapid and slow eye movements. Annu. Rev. Physiol. 40:527–552.

Rapoport, S. I. 1976. Blood–Brain Barrier in Physiology and Medicine. New York: Raven Press.

Rasmussen, T., and Milner, B. 1977. The role of early left-brain injury in determining lateralization of cerebral speech functions. Ann. N.Y. Acad. Sci. 299:355–369.

Redman, S. 1979. Junctional mechanisms at group Ia synapses. Prog. Neurobiol. 12:33–83.

Reh, T. A., and Constantine-Paton, M. 1984. Retinal ganglion cell terminals change their projection sites during larval development of Rana pipiens. J. Neurosci. 4:442–457.

Reichart, L. F. 1984. Immunological approaches to the nervous system. Science 225:1294–1299.

Reichardt, L. F., and Kelly, R. B. 1983. A molecular description of nerve terminal function. Annu. Rev. Biochem. 52:871–926.

Reichlin, S. 1978. Introduction. In S. Reichlin, R. J. Baldessarini, and J. B. Martin (eds.), The Hypothalamus. Res. Publ. Assoc. Res. Nerv. Ment. Dis. 56:1–14.

Reiman, E. M., Raichle, M. E., Butler, F. K., Herscovitch, P., and Robins, E. 1984. A focal brain abnormality in panic disorder, a severe form of anxiety. Nature 310:683–685.

Reivich, M. 1982. The use of cerebral blood flow and metabolic studies in cerebral localization. In R. A. Thompson and J. R. Green (eds.), New Perspectives in Cerebral Localization. New York: Raven Press, pp. 115–144.

Reivich, M., Kuhl, D., Wolf, A., Greenberg, J., Phelps, M., Ido, T., Casella, V., Fowler, J., Hoffman, E., Alavi, A., Som, P., and Sokoloff, L. 1979. The (^{18}F) fluorodeoxyglucose method for the measurement of local cerebral glucose utilization in man. Circ. Res. 44:127–137.

Renaud, L. P. 1981. A neurophysiological approach to the identification, connections and pharmacology of the hypothalamic tuberoinfundibular system. Neuroendocrinology 33:186–191.

Rescorla, R. A. 1978. Some implications of a cognitive perspective on Pavlovian conditioning. In S. H. Hulse, H. Fowler, and W. K. Honig (eds.), Cognitive Processes in Animal Behavior. Hillsdale, N.J.: Erlbaum, pp. 15–50.

Rescorla, R. A., and Wagner, A. R. 1972. A theory of Pavlovian conditioning: Variations in the effectiveness of reinforcement and nonreinforcement. In A. H. Black and W. F. Prokasy (eds.), Classical Conditioning II: Current Research and Theory. New York: Appleton-Century-Crofts, pp. 64–99.

Reveley, A. M., Reveley, M. A., Clifford, C. A., and Murray, R. M. 1982. Cerebral ventricular size in twins discordant for schizophrenia. Lancet 1:540–541.

Rexed, B. 1952. The cytoarchitectonic organization of the spinal cord in the cat. J. Comp. Neurol. 96:415–495.

Reznik, M. 1983. Neuropathology in seven cases of locked-in syndrome. J. Neurol. Sci. 60:67–78.

Rhode, W. S. 1971. Observations of the vibration of the basilar membrane in squirrel monkeys using the Mossbauer technique. J. Acoust. Soc. Am. 49:1218–1231.

Richter, C. P. 1942. Total self regulatory functions in animals and human beings. Harvey Lect. 38:63–103.

Riesen, A. H. 1958. Plasticity of behavior: Psychological aspects. In H. F. Harlow and C. N. Woolsey (eds.), Biological and Biochemical Bases of Behavior. Madison: University of Wisconsin Press, pp. 425–450.

Ritchie, J. M., and Rogart, R. B. 1977. The binding of saxitoxin and tetrodotoxin to excitable tissue. Rev. Physiol. Biochem. Pharmacol. 79:1–50.

Roberts, P. J., Woodruff, G. N., and Iversen, L. L. (eds.). 1978. Advances in Biochemical Psychopharmacology, Vol. 19: Dopamine. New York: Raven Press.

Robinson, D. A. 1968. Eye movement control in primates. Science 161:1219–1224.

Robinson, D. A. 1976. Adaptive gain control of vestibuloocular reflex by the cerebellum. J. Neurophysiol. 39:954–969.

Robinson, D. A. 1981. The use of control systems analysis in the neurophysiology of eye movements. Annu. Rev. Neurosci. 4:463–503.

Robinson, D. L., Goldberg, M. E., and Stanton, G. B. 1978. Parietal association cortex in the primate: Sensory mechanisms and behavioral modulations. J. Neurophysiol. 41:910–932.

Robinson, T. E., Becker, J. B., Camp, D. M and Mansour, A. 1985. Variation in the pattern of behavioral and brain asymmetries due to sex differences. In S. D. Glick (ed.), Cerebral Lateralization in Non-Human Species. Orlando, Fla.: Academic Press.

Rodieck, R. W. 1973. The Vertebrate Retina—Principles of Structure and Function. San Francisco: Freeman.

Roffwarg, H. P., Muzio, J. N., and Dement, W. C. 1966. Ontogenetic development of the human sleep–dream cycle. Science 152:604–619.

Roland, P. E., Larsen, B., Lassen, N. A., and Skinhøj, E. 1980. Supplementary motor area and other cortical areas in organization of voluntary movements in man. J. Neurophysiol. 43:118–136.

Rolls, B. J., and Rolls, E. T. 1982. Thirst. Cambridge, England: Cambridge University Press.

Rolls, E. T. 1981. Central nervous mechanism related to feeding and appetite. Br. Med. Bull. 37:131–134.

Rolls, E. T., Sanghera, M. K., and Roper-Hall, A. 1979. The latency of activation of neurones in the lateral hypothalamus and substantia innominata during feeding in the monkey. Brain Res. 164:121–135.

Roper, S. 1983. Regenerative impulses in taste cells. Science 220:1311–1312.

Rosenberg, R. L., Tomiko, S. A., and Agnew, W. S. 1984. Single-channel properties of the reconstituted voltage-regulated Na channel isolated from the electroplax of Electrophorus electricus. Proc. Natl. Acad. Sci. U.S.A. 81:5594–5598.

Rosenkilde, C. E. 1979. Functional heterogeneity of the prefrontal cortex in the monkey: A review. Behav. Neural Biol. 25:301–345.

Ross, E. D. 1981. The aprosodias: Functional–anatomical organization of the affective components of language in the right hemisphere. Arch. Neurol. 38:561–569.

Ross, E. D. 1984. Right hemisphere's role in language, affective behavior and emotion. Trends Neurosci. 7:342–346.

Roth, G. 1984. Fasciculations and their F-responses: Localisation of their axonal origin. J. Neurol. Sci. 63:299–306.

Roth, M. 1978. Diagnosis of senile and related forms of dementia. In R. Katzman, R. D. Terry, and K. L. Bick (eds.), Aging, Vol. 7: Alzheimer's Disease: Senile Dementia and Related Disorders. New York: Raven Press, pp. 71–85.

Rowland, L. P. 1977. Myasthenia gravis. In E. S. Goldensohn and S. H. Appel (eds.), Scientific Approaches to Clinical Neurology, Vol. 2. Philadelphia: Lea & Febiger, pp. 1518–1554.

Rowland, L. P. 1980. Controversies about the treatment of myasthenia gravis. J. Neurol. Neurosurg. Psychiatry 43:644–659.

Rowland, L. P. 1985. Diseases of muscle and neuromuscular junction. In J. B. Wyngaarden and L. H. Smith, Jr. (eds.), Cecil Textbook of Medicine, 17th ed. Philadelphia: Saunders, pp. 2198–2216.

Rowland, L. P. (ed.). 1982. Human Motor Neuron Diseases. New York: Raven Press.

Rowland, L. P., Hoefer, P. F. A., and Aranow, H., Jr. 1960. Myasthenic syndromes. Res. Publ. Assoc. Res. Nerv. Ment. Dis. 38:548–600.

Rowland, L. P., and Layzer, R. B. 1977. Muscular dystrophies, atrophies, and related diseases. In A. B. Baker (ed.), Clinical Neurology, Vol. 3. New York: Harper & Row, pp. 1–109.

Rozin, P., Poritsky, S., and Sotsky, R. 1971. American children with reading problems can easily learn to read English represented by Chinese characters. Science 171:1264–1267.

S

Sachar, E. J., Asnis, G., Halbreich, U., Nathan. R. S., and Halpern, F. 1980. Recent studies in the neuroendocrinology of major depressive disorders. Psychiatr. Clin. North Am. 3:313–326.

Sackett, G. P. 1966. Monkeys reared in isolation with pictures as visual input: Evidence for an innate releasing mechanism. Science 154:1468–1473.

Sacks, O. 1983. The man who mistook his wife for his hat. London Review of Books, May 19, pp. 3–5.

Saffran, E. M. 1982. Neuropsychological approaches to the study of language. Br. J. Psychol. 73:317–337.

Sakmann, B., and Neher, E. (eds.). 1983. Single-Channel Recording. New York: Plenum Press.

Salkoff, L., and Wyman, R. 1983. Ion channels in Drosophila muscle. Trends Neurosci. 6:128–133.

Salmons, S., and Sréter, F. A. 1976. Significance of impulse activity in skeletal muscle type. Nature 263:30–34.

Samorajski, T., and Ordy, J. M. 1972. Neurochemistry of aging. In C. M. Gaitz (ed.), Advances in Behavioral Biology, Vol. 3: Aging and the Brain. New York: Plenum Press, pp. 41–61.

Sanes, J. 1983. The role of extracellular matrix in neural development. Annu. Rev. Physiol. 45:581–600.

Sanger, F., and Coulson, A. R. 1975. A rapid method for determining sequences in DNA by primed synthesis with DNA polymerase. J. Mol. Biol. 94:441–448.

Sastre, J.-P., and Jouvet, M. 1979. Le comportement onirique du chat. Physiol. Behav. 22:979–989.

Satinoff, E. 1964. Behavioral thermoregulation in response to local cooling of the rat brain. Am. J. Physiol. 206:1389–1394.

Sauer, F. C. 1935. Mitosis in the neural tube. J. Comp. Neurol. 62:377–405.

Saunders, J. W., Jr. 1970. Patterns and Principles of Animal Development. New York: Macmillan.

Sawchenko, P. E., and Swanson, L. W. 1985. Localization, colocalization, and plasticity of corticotropin-releasing factor immunoreactivity in rat brain. Fed. Proc. 44:221–227.

Scatton, B., Javoy-Agid, F., Rouquier, L., Dubois, B., and Agid, Y. 1983. Reduction of cortical dopamine, noradrenaline, serotonin and their metabolites in Parkinson's disease. Brain Res. 275:321–328.

Schachter, S. 1971. Some extraordinary facts about obese humans and rats. Am. Psychol. 26:129–144.

Schally, A. V. 1978. Aspects of hypothalamic regulation of the pituitary gland. Its implications for the control of reproductive processes. Science 202:18–28.

Scharrer, E., and Scharrer, B. 1954. Hormones produced by neurosecretory cells. Recent Prog. Horm. Res. 10:183–232.

Scheibel, M. E., and Scheibel, A. B. 1958. Structural substrates for integrative patterns in the brain stem reticular core. In H. H. Jasper, L. D. Proctor, et al. (eds.), Reticular Formation of the Brain (Henry Ford Hospital International Symposium). Boston: Little, Brown, pp. 31–55.

Scheibel, M. E., and Scheibel, A. B. 1975. Structural changes in the aging brain. In H. Brody, D. Harman, and J. M. Ordy (eds.), Aging, Vol. 1: Clinical, Morphologic, and Neurochemical Aspects in the Aging Central Nervous System. New York: Raven Press, pp. 11–37.

Schell, G. R., and Strick, P. L. 1984. The origin of thalamic inputs to the arcuate premotor and supplementary motor areas. J. Neurosci. 4:539–560.

Scheller, R. H., Jackson, J. F., McAllister, L. B., Schwartz, J. H., Kandel, E. R., and Axel, R. 1982. A family of genes that codes for ELH, a neuropeptide eliciting a stereotyped pattern of behavior in Aplysia. Cell 28:707–719.

Schiffman, S. S. 1983. Taste and smell in disease. N. Engl. J. Med. 308:1337–1343.

Schildkraut, J. J. 1978. Current status of the catecholamine hypothesis of affective disorders. In M. A. Lipton, A. DiMascio, and K. F. Killam (eds.), Psychopharmacology: A Generation of Progress. New York: Raven Press, pp. 1223–1234.

Schiller, P. H. 1982. Central connections of the retinal ON and OFF pathways. Nature 297:580–583.

Schiller, P. H. 1983. Parallel channels in vision and visually guided eye movements. Invest. Ophthalmol. Vis. Sci. (ARVO Abstr.).

Schiller, P. H., True, S. D., and Conway, J. L. 1979. Effects of frontal eye field and superior colliculus ablations on eye movements. Science 206:590–592.

Schiller, P. H., True, S. D., and Conway, J. L. 1980. Deficits in eye movements following frontal eye-field and superior colliculus ablations. J. Neurophysiol. 44:1175–1189.

Schmidt, R. F., and Thews, G. (eds.). 1983. Human Physiology. M. A. Biederman-Thorson (trans.). Berlin: Springer.

Schmidt, R. H., Björklund, A., and Stenevi, U. 1981. Intracerebral grafting of dissociated CNS tissue suspensions: A new approach for neuronal transplantation to deep brain sites. Brain Res. 218:347–356.

Schmitt, F. O., Worden, F. G., Adelman, G., and Dennis, S. G. (eds.). 1981. The organization of the cerebral cortex. In: Proceedings of a Neurosciences Research Program Colloquium. Cambridge, Mass.: MIT Press.

Schnapp, B. J., and Reese, T. S. 1982. Cytoplasmic structure in rapid-frozen axons. J. Cell Biol. 94:667–679.

Schoenenberger, G. A., and Monnier, M. 1977. Characterization of a delta-electroencephalogram(-sleep)-inducing peptide. Proc. Natl. Acad. Sci. U.S.A. 74:1282–1286.

Schoener, T. W. 1971. Theory of feeding strategies. Annu. Rev. Ecol. Syst. 2:369–404.

Scott, T. R., Jr., and Erickson, R. P. 1971. Synaptic processing of taste-quality information in thalamus of the rat. J. Neurophysiol. 34:868–884.

Schramm, M., Korner, M., Neufeld, G., and Nedivi, E. 1983. The molecular mechanism of action of the β-adrenergic receptor. Cold Spring Harbor Symp. Quant. Biol. 48:187–191.

Schuetze, S. M. 1983. The discovery of the action potential. Trends Neurosci. 6:164–168.

Schultze, M. 1866. Zur Anatomie und Physiologie der Retina. Arch. Mikrouk. Anat. 2:175–286.

Schwartz, J. H. 1979. Axonal transport: Components, mechanisms, and specificity. Annu. Rev. Neurosci. 2:467–504.

Schwartz, J. H. 1980. The transport of substances in nerve cells. Sci. Am. 242(4):152–171.

Schwartz, M. F. 1985. Classification of language disorders from a psycholinguistic viewpoint. In J. Oxbury, R. Whurr, M. Coltheart, and M. Wyke (eds.), Aphasia. London: Butterworth.

Schwartz, W. J., and Gainer, H. 1977. Suprachiasmatic nucleus: Use of ^{14}C-labeled deoxyglucose uptake as a functional marker. Science 197:1089–1091.

Schwartzkroin, P. A., and Wyler, A. R. 1980. Mechanisms underlying epileptiform burst discharge. Ann. Neurol. 7:95–107.

Schworer, C. M., and Soderling, T. R. 1983. Substrate specificity of liver and calmodulin-dependent glycogen synthase kinase. Biochem. Biophys. Res. Comm. 116:412–416.

Sclafani, A. 1976. Appetite and hunger in experimental obesity syndromes. In D. Novin, W. Wyrwicka, and G. A. Bray (eds.), Hunger: Basic Mechanisms and Clinical Implications. New York: Raven Press, pp. 281–295.

Seales, D. M., Torkelson, R. D., Shuman, R. M., Rossiter, V. S., and Spencer, J. D. 1981. Abnormal brainstem auditory evoked potentials and neuropathology in "locked-in" syndrome. Neurology 31:893–896.

Sears, E. S., and Franklin, G. M. 1980. Diseases of the cranial nerves. In R. N. Rosenberg (ed.), The Science and Practice of Clinical Medicine, Vol. 5: Neurology. New York: Grune & Stratton, pp. 471–494.

Seeman, P., and Lee, T. 1975. Antipsychotic drugs: Direct correlation between clinical potency and presynaptic action on dopamine neurons. Science 188:1217–1219.

Seeman, P., Lee, T., Chau-Wong, M., and Wong, K. 1976. Antipsychotic drug doses and neuroleptic/dopamine receptors. Nature 261:717–719.

Seligman, M. E. P., and Hager, J. L. 1972. Biological Boundaries of Learning. Englewood Cliffs, N.J.: Prentice–Hall.

Serratrice, G., Cros, D., Desnuelle, C., Gastaut, J.-L., Pellissier, J.-F., Pouget, J., and Schiano, A. 1984. Neuromuscular Diseases. New York: Raven Press.

Shambes, G. M., Gibson, J. M., and Welker, W. 1978. Fractured somatotopy in granule cell tactile areas of rat cerebellar hemispheres revealed by micromapping. Brain Behav. Evol. 15:94–140.

Shepherd, G. M. 1972. Synaptic organization of the mammalian olfactory bulb. Physiol. Rev. 52:864–917.

Shepherd, G. M. 1978. Microcircuits in the nervous system. Sci. Am. 238(2):92–103.

Shepherd, G. M. 1979. The Synaptic Organization of the Brain, 2nd ed. New York: Oxford University Press.

Shepherd, G. M. 1983. Neurobiology. New York: Oxford University Press, chap. 12.

Sherk, H., and Levay, S. 1983. Contribution of the cortico-claustral loop to the receptive field properties in area 17 of the cat. J. Neurosci. 11:2121–2127.

Sherrington, C. S. 1897. The Central Nervous System. Part III of M. Foster, A Text Book of Physiology, 7th ed. London: Macmillan.

Sherrington, C. S. 1898. Decerebrate rigidity, and reflex coordination of movements. J. Physiol. (Lond.) 22:319–332.

Sherrington, C. S. 1900. The muscular sense. In E. A. Schafer (ed.), Textbook of Physiology, Vol. 2. Edinburgh: Pentland, pp. 1002–1025.

Sherrington, C. 1906. The Integrative Action of the Nervous System. Reprint, New Haven: Yale University Press, 1947.

Shkolnik, L. J., and Schwartz, J. H. 1980. Genesis and maturation of serotonin vesicles in identified giant cerebral neuron of Aplysia. J. Neurophysiol. 43:945–967.

Shik, M. L., Severin, F. V., and Orlovsky, G. N. 1966. Control of walking and running by means of electrical stimulation of the mid-brain. Biophysics 11:756–765.

Shine, J., Mason, A. J., Evans, B. A., and Richards, R. I. 1983. The kallikrein multigene family: Specific processing of biologically active peptides. Cold Spring Harbor Symp. Quant. Biol. 48:419–426.

Shurrager, P. S., and Culler, E. 1940. Conditioning in the spinal dog. J. Exp. Psychol. 26:133–159.

Shuster, M. J., Camardo, J. S., Siegelbaum, S. A., and Kandel, E. R. 1984. Cyclic AMP-dependent protein kinase closes the serotonin-sensitive K${}^+$ channels of Aplysia sensory neurones in cell-free membrane patches. Nature 313:392–395.

Siegel, G. J., Albers, R. W., Agranoff, B. W., and Katzman, R. (eds.). 1981. Basic Neurochemistry, 3rd ed. Boston: Little, Brown.

Siegel, J. M., and McGinty, D. J. 1977. Pontine reticular formation neurons: Relationship of discharge to motor activity. Science 196:678–680.

Siegelbaum, S. A., Camardo, J. S., and Kandel, E. R. 1982. Serotonin and cyclic AMP close single K${}^+$ channels in Aplysia sensory neurones. Nature 299:413–417.

Sigel, E., Stephenson, F. A., Mamalaki, C., and Barnard, E. A. 1983. A γ-aminobutyric acid/benzodiazepine receptor complex of bovine cerebral cortex. J. Biol. Chem. 258:6965–6971.

Signoret, J. L., Whiteley, A., and Lhermitte, F. 1978. Influence of choline on amnesia in early Alzheimer's disease. Lancet 2:837.

Sigworth, F. J., and Neher, E. 1980. Single Na${}^+$ channel currents observed in cultured rat muscle cells. Nature 287:447–449.

Silverman, A.-J., and Zimmerman, E. A. 1983. Magnocellular neurosecretory system. Annu. Rev. Neurosci. 6:357–380.

Simon, E. J., Hiller, J. M., and Edelman, I. 1973. Stereospecific binding of the potent narcotic analgesia [^{3}H]etorphine to rat-brain homogenate. Proc. Natl. Acad. Sci. U.S.A. 70:1947–1949.

Simpson, J. A. 1960. Myasthenia gravis: A new hypothesis. Scott. Med. J. 5:419–436.

Simpson, J. F., and Magee, K. R. 1973. Clinical Evaluation of the Nervous System, 1st ed. Boston: Little, Brown.

Sjöqvist, O. 1938. Studies on pain conduction in the trigeminal nerve. Acta Psychiatr. Neurol. [Suppl.] 17:1–139.

Skinner, B. F. 1957. Verbal Behavior. New York: Appleton–Century–Crofts.

Slaughter, M. M., and Miller, R. F. 1981. 2-Amino-4-phosphonobutyric acid: A new pharmacological tool for retina research. Science 211:182–185.

Sloan, H. E., Hughes, S. E., and Oakley, B. 1983. Chronic impairment of axonal transport eliminates taste responses and taste buds. J. Neurosci. 3:117–123.

Smit, L. M. E., Jennekens, F. G. I., Veldman, H., and Barth, P. G. 1984. Paucity of secondary synaptic clefts in a case of congenital myasthenia with multiple contractures: Ultrastructural morphology of a developmental disorder. J. Neurol. Neurosurg. Psychiatry 47:1091–1097.

Smith, A. M., Hepp-Reymond, M.-C., and Wyss, U. R. 1975. Relation of activity in precentral cortical neurons to force and rate of force change during isometric contractions of finger muscles. Exp. Brain Res. 23:321–332.

Smith, D. V., Van Buskirk, R. L., Travers, J. B., and Bieber, S. L. 1983. Coding of taste stimuli by hamster brain stem neurons. J. Neurophysiol. 50:541–558.

Smith, S. J., Augustine, G. J., and Charlton, M. P. 1985. Transmission at voltage-clamped giant synapse of the squid: Evidence for cooperativity of presynaptic calcium action. Proc. Natl. Acad. Sci. U.S.A. 82:622–625.

Smith, V. C., and Pokorny, J. 1975. Spectral sensitivity of the foveal cone photopigments between 400 and 500 nm. Vision Res. 15:161–171.

Snider, R. S., and Stowell, A. 1944. Receiving areas of the tactile, auditory, and visual systems in the cerebellum. J. Neurophysiol. 7:331–357.

Snyder, S. H. 1980. Brain peptides as neurotransmitters. Science 209:976–983.

Snyder, S. H. 1982. Neurotransmitters and CNS disease: Schizophrenia. Lancet 2:970–974.

Snyder, S. H. 1984. Drug and neurotransmitter receptors in the brain. Science 224:22–31.

Soechting, J. F., Ranish, N. A., Palminteri, R., and Terzuolo, C. A. 1976. Changes in a motor pattern following cerebellar and olivary lesions in the squirrel monkey. Brain Res. 105:21–44.

Sokoloff, L. 1984. Modeling metabolic processes in the brain in vivo. Ann. Neurol. [Suppl.] 15:S1–S11.

Solomon, F., White, C. C., Parron, D. L., and Mendelson, W. B. 1979. Sleeping pills, insomnia and medical practice (summary of report of the Institute of Medicine, National Academy of Sciences). N. Engl. J. Med. 300:803–808.

Spemann, H. 1939. Embryonic Development and Induction. New Haven: Yale University Press.

Spencer, W. A. 1977. The physiology of supraspinal neurons in mammals. In E. R. Kandel (ed.), Handbook of Physiology, Section 1: The Nervous System, Vol. I, Cellular Biology of Neurons. Bethesda, Md.: American Physiological Society, pp. 969–1021.

Spencer, W. A., and Kandel, E. R. 1961. Electrophysiology of hippocampal neurons. IV. Fast prepotentials. J. Neurophysiol. 24:272–285.

Spencer, W. A., and Kandel, E. R. 1968. Cellular and integrative properties of the hippocampal pyramidal cell and the comparative electrophysiology of cortical neurons. Int. J. Neurol. 6:266–296.

Spencer, W. A., Thompson, R. F., and Neilson, D. R., Jr. 1966. Response decrement of the flexion reflex in the acute spinal cat and transient restoration by strong stimuli. J. Neurophysiol. 29:221–239.

Sperry, R. W. 1951. Mechanisms of neural maturation. In S. S. Stevens (ed.), Handbook of Experimental Psychology. New York: Wiley, pp. 236–280.

Sperry, R. W. 1964. The great cerebral commissure. Sci. Am. 210(1):42–52.

Sperry, R. W. 1968. Mental unity following surgical disconnection of the cerebral hemispheres. Harvey Lect. 62:293–323.

Spitz, R. A. 1945. Hospitalism: An inquiry into the genesis of psychiatric conditions in early childhood. Psychoanal. Study Child 1:53–74.

Spitz, R. A. 1946. Hospitalism: A follow-up report on investigation described in Volume 1, 1945. Psychoanal. Study Child 2:113–117.

Spitz, R. A., and Wolf, K. M. 1946. Anaclitic depression: An inquiry into the genesis of psychiatric conditions in early childhood, II. Psychoanal. Study Child 2:313–342.

Spoendlin, H. 1966. Ultrastructure of the vestibular sense organ. In R. J. Wolfson (ed.), The Vestibular System and Its Diseases. Philadelphia: University of Pennsylvania Press, pp. 39–68.

Spurzheim, J. G. 1825. Phrenology, or the Doctrine of the Mind, 3rd ed. London: Knight.

Squire, L. R., Cohen, N. J., and Nadel, L. 1982. The medial temporal region and memory consolidation: A new hypothesis. In H. Weingartner and E. S. Parker (eds.), Memory Consolidation: Psychobiology of Cognition. Hillsdale, N.J.: Erlbaum, pp. 185–210.

Squire, L. R., Slater, P. C., and Chace, P. M. 1975. Retrograde amnesia: Temporal gradient in very long term memory following electroconvulsive therapy. Science 187:77–79.

Stamm, J. S. 1969. Electrical stimulation of monkey's prefrontal cortex during delayed-response performance. J. Comp. Physiol. Psychol. 67:535–546.

Starr, A. 1978. Sensory evoked potentials in clinical disorders of the nervous system. Annu. Rev. Neurosci. 1:103–127.

Stein, R. B. 1974. Peripheral control of movement. Physiol. Rev. 54:215–243.

Stein, S. C., and Langfitt, T. W. 1974. Normal-pressure hydrocephalus: Predicting the results of cerebrospinal fluid shunting. J. Neurosurg. 41:463–470.

Stellar, J. R., and Stellar, E. 1985. The Neurobiology of Motivation and Reward. New York: Springer.

Stent, G. S. (ed.). 1977. Function and Formation of Neural Systems. Dahlem Konferenzen. Berlin: Springer.

Stephan, F. K. and Zucker, I. 1972. Circadian rhythms in drinking behavior and locomotor activity of rats are eliminated by hypothalamic lesions. Proc. Natl. Acad. Sci. U.S.A. 69:1583–1586.

Steriade, M., and Hobson, J. A. 1976. Neuronal activity during the sleep-waking cycle. Prog. Neurobiol. 6:155–376.

Sternberger, L. A. 1974. Immunocytochemistry. Englewood Cliffs, N.J.: Prentice–Hall.

Stevens, C. F. 1979. The neuron. Sci. Am. 241(3):54–65.

Stevens, S. S. 1953. On the brightness of lights and the loudness of sounds. Science 118:576.

Stevens, S. S. 1961. The psychophysics of sensory function. In W. A. Rosenblith (ed.), Sensory Communication. Cambridge, Mass.: MIT Press, pp. 1–33.

Stevens, S. S. 1975. Psychophysics: Introduction to Its Perceptual, Neural, and Social Prospects. New York: Wiley.

Stewart, W. B., Kauer, J. S., and Shepherd, G. M. 1979. Functional organization of rat olfactory bulb analysed by the 2-deoxyglucose method. J. Comp. Neurol. 185:715–734.

Stiles, W. S. 1978. Mechanisms of Colour Vision. New York: Academic Press.

Stockard, J. J., and Rossiter, V. S. 1977. Clinical and pathologic correlates of brain stem auditory response abnormalities. Neurology 27:316–325.

Stone, J., Dreher, B., and Leventhal, A. 1979. Hierarchical and parallel mechanisms in the organization of visual cortex. Brain Res. Rev. 1:345–394.

Stotler, W. A. 1953. An experimental study of the cells and connections of the superior olivary complex of the cat. J. Comp. Neurol. 98:401–432.

Strauss, A. J. L., Seegal, B. C., Hsu, K. C., Burkholder, P. M., Nastuk, W. L., and Osserman, K. E. 1960. Immunofluorescence demonstration of a muscle binding, complement-fixing serum globulin fraction in myasthenia gravis. Proc. Soc. Exp. Biol. Med. 105:184–191.

Strehler, B., Hirsch, G., Gusseck, D., Johnson, R., and Bick, M. 1971. Codon-restriction theory of aging and development. J. Theor. Biol. 33:429–474.

Strehler, B. L. 1975. Implications of aging research for society. Fed. Proc. 34:5–8.

Stryer, L. 1983. Transducin and the cyclic GMP phosphodiesterase—Amplifier proteins in vision. Cold Spring Harbor Symp. Quant. Biol. 48:841–852.

Stryker, M. P., and Strickland, S. L. 1984. Physiological segregation of ocular dominance columns depends on the pattern of afferent electrical activity. Invest. Ophthalmol. Vis. Sci. [Suppl.] 25:278. (ARVO Abstr.).

Sumner, A. J. (ed.). 1980. The Physiology of Peripheral Nerve Disease. Philadelphia: Saunders.

Sundsten, J. W., and Sawyer, C. H. 1961. Osmotic activation of neurohypophyseal hormone release in rabbits with hypothalamic islands. Exp. Neurol. 4:548–561.

Suomi, S. J., and Harlow, H. F. 1975. The role and reason of peer relationships in rhesus monkeys. In M. Lewis and L. A. Rosenblum (eds.), Friendship and Peer Relations. New York: Wiley, pp. 153–185.

Sur, M., and Sherman, S. M. 1982. Retinogeniculate terminations in cats: Morphological differences between X and Y cell axons. Science 218:389–391.

Svaetichin, G., and MacNichol, E. F., Jr. 1958. Retinal mechanisms for chromatic and achromatic vision. Ann. N. Y. Acad. Sci. 74:385–404.

Swanson, L. W., and Sawchenko, P. E. 1983. Hypothalamic integration: Organization of the paraventricular and supraoptic nuclei. Annu. Rev. Neurosci. 6:269–324.

Swift, T. R. 1981. Disorders of neuromuscular transmission other than myasthenia gravis. Muscle Nerve 4:334–353.

Szentágothai, J. 1950. The elementary vestibulo-ocular reflex arc. J. Neurophysiol. 13:395–407.

Szentágothai, J. 1969. Architecture of the cerebral cortex. In H. H. Jasper, A. A. Ward, Jr., and A. Pope (eds.), Basic Mechanisms of the Epilepsies. Boston: Little, Brown, pp. 13–28.

T

Takahashi, J. S., and Zatz, M. 1982. Regulation of circadian rhythmicity. Science 217:1104–1111.

Takeuchi, A. 1977. Junctional transmission. I. Postsynaptic mechanisms. In E. R. Kandel (ed.), Handbook of Physiology, Vol. 1: The Nervous System, Part 1. Bethesda, Md.: American Physiological Society, pp. 295–327.

Talbot, S. A., and Marshall, W. H. 1941. Physiological studies on neural mechanisms of visual localization and discrimination. Am. J. Ophthalmol. 24:1255–1264.

Tanner, W. P., Jr., and Swets, J. A. 1954. A decision-making theory of visual detection. Psychol. Rev. 61:401–409.

Teitelman, G., Joh, T. H., and Reis, D. J. 1981. Linkage of the brain–skin–gut axis: Islet cells originate from dopaminergic precursors. Peptides [Suppl.] 2:157–168.

Teranishi, T., Negishi, K., and Kato, S. 1983. Dopamine modulates S potential amplitude and dye-coupling between external horizontal cells in carp retina. Nature 301:243–246.

Terenius, L. 1973. Characteristics of the "receptor" for narcotic analgesics in synaptic plasma membrane fraction from rat brain. Acta Pharmacol. Toxicol. 33:377–384.

Terman, G. W., Shavit, Y., Lewis, J. W., Cannon, J. T., and Liebeskind, J. C. 1984. Intrinsic mechanisms of pain inhibition: Activation by stress. Science 226:1270–1277.

Thach, W. T. 1978. Correlation of neural discharge with pattern and force of muscular activity, joint position, and direction of intended next movement in motor cortex and cerebellum. J. Neurophysiol. 41:654–676.

Thesleff, S., and Molgo, J. 1983. Commentary. A new type of transmitter release at the neuromuscular junction. Neuroscience 9:1–8.

Thoenen, H., Otten, U., and Schwab, M. 1979. Orthograde and retrograde signals for the regulation of neuronal gene expression: The peripheral sympathetic nervous system as a model. In F. O. Schmitt and F. G. Worden (eds.), The Neurosciences: Fourth Study Program. Cambridge, Mass.: MIT Press, pp. 911–928.

Thompson, R. F. 1975. Introduction to Physiological Psychology. New York: Harper & Row.

Thompson, R. F., Berger, T. W., and Madden, J., IV. 1983. Cellular processes of learning and memory in the mammalian CNS. Annu. Rev. Neurosci. 6:447–491.

Thompson, R. F., McCormick, D. A., Lavond, D. G., Clark, G. A., Kettner, R. E., and Mauk, M. D. 1983. The engram found? Initial localization of the memory trace for a basic form of associative learning. Prog. Psychobiol. Physiol. Psychol. 10:167–196.

Thorndike, E. L. 1911. Animal Intelligence: Experimental Studies. New York: Macmillan.

Thorpe, W. H. 1956. Learning and Instinct in Animals. Cambridge, Mass.: Harvard University Press.

Tinbergen, N. 1951. The Study of Instinct. Oxford: Clarendon Press.

Toivonen, S., Tarin, D., and Saxen, L. 1976. The transmission of morphogenetic signals from amphibian mesoderm to ectoderm in primary induction. Differentiation 5:49–55.

Tomita, T. 1976. Electrophysiological studies of retinal cell function. Invest. Ophthalmol. 15:171–187.

Tomlinson, B. E., and Henderson, G. 1976. Some quantitative cerebral findings in normal and demented old people. In R. D. Terry and S. Gershon (eds.), Aging, Vol. 3: Neurobiology of Aging. New York: Raven Press, pp. 183–204.

Toran-Allerand, C. D. 1978. Gonadal hormones and brain development: Cellular aspects of sexual differentiation. Am. Zool. 18:553–565.

Toran-Allerand, C. D. 1984. On the genesis of sexual differentiation of the central nervous system: Morphogenetic consequences of steroidal exposure and possible role of α-fetoprotein. In G. J. De Vries, J. P. De Bruin, H. B. M. Uylings, and M. A. Corner (eds.), Sex Differences in the Brain: The Relation Between Structure and Function. Prog. Brain Res. 61:63–98.

Toyka, K. V., Drachman, D. B., Pestronk, A., and Kao, I. 1975. Myasthenia gravis: Passive transfer from man to mouse. Science 190:397–399.

Tower, S. S. 1940. Pyramidal lesion in the monkey. Brain 63:36–90.

Tremblay, J. P., Laurie, R. E., and Colonnier, M. 1983. Is the MEPP due to the release of one vesicle or to the simultaneous release of several vesicles at one active zone? Brain Res. Rev. 6:299–314.

Trescher, J. H., and Ford, F. R. 1937. Colloid cysts of the third ventricle: Arch. Neurol. Psychiatry 37:959–973.

Trisler, G. D., Schneider, M. D. and Nirenberg, M. 1981. A topographic gradient of molecules in retina can be used to identify neuron position. Proc. Natl. Acad. Sci. U.S.A. 78:2145–2149.

Trotier, D., and MacLeod, P. 1983. Intracellular recordings from salamander olfactory receptor cells. Brain Res. 268:225–237.

Tucek, S. 1978. Acetycholine Synthesis in Neurons. London: Chapman & Hall.

Tucker, D. M., Watson, R. T., and Heilman, K. M. 1977. Discrimination and evocation of affectively intoned speech in patients with right parietal disease. Neurology 27:947–950.

Tulving, E. 1984. Precis of elements of episodic memory. Behav. Brain Sci. 7:223–268.

Tzartos, S. J. 1984. Monoclonal antibodies as probes of the acetylcholine receptor and myasthenia gravis. Trends Neurosci. 9:63–67.

U

Ulfhake, B. and Kellerth, J.-O. 1981. A quantitative light microscopic study of the dendrites of cat spinal α-motoneurons after intracellular staining with horseradish peroxidase. J. Comp. Neurol. 202:571–583.

Ullrich, A., Gray, A., Berman, C., Coussens, L., and Dull, T. J. 1983. Sequence homology of human and mouse β-NGF subunit genes. Cold Spring Harbor Symp. Quant. Biol. 48:435–442.

Ungerleider, L. G., and Mishkin, M. 1982. Two cortical visual systems. In D. J. Ingle, M. A. Goodale, and R. J. W. Mansfield (eds.), Analysis of Visual Behavior. Cambridge, Mass.: MIT Press, pp. 549–586.

Ungerstedt, U., Ljungberg, T., Hoffer, B., and Siggins, G. 1975. Dopaminergic supersensitivity in the striatum. In D. Calne, T. N. Chase, and A. Barbeau (eds.), Advances in Neurology, Vol. 9: Dopaminergic Mechanisms. New York: Raven Press, pp. 57–65.

Usdin, E., Kopin, I. J., and Barchas, J. (eds.). 1979. Catecholamines: Basic and Clinical Frontiers. New York: Pergamon Press.

Uttal, W. R. 1978. The Psychobiology of Mind. Hillsdale, N.J.: Erlbaum.

V

Vale, W., Spiess, J., Rivier, C., and Rivier, J. 1981. Characterization of a 41-residue ovine hypothalamic peptide that stimulates secretion of corticotropin and β-endorphin. Science 213:1394–1397.

Vallbo, A. B. 1970. Discharge patterns in human muscle spindle afferents during isometric voluntary contractions. Acta Physiol. Scand. 80:552–566.

Vallbo, Å. B. 1971. Muscle spindle response at the onset of isometric voluntary contractions in man. Time difference between fusimotor and skeletomotor effects. J. Physiol. (Lond.) 218:405–431.

Vallbo, Å. B., Hagbarth, K.-E., Torebjork, H. E., and Wallin, B. G. 1979. Somatosensory, proprioceptive, and sympathetic activity in human peripheral nerves. Physiol. Rev. 59:919–957.

Vallbo, Å. B., Olson, K. Å., Westberg, K.-G., and Clark, F. J. 1984. Microstimulation of single tactile afferents from the human hand: Sensory attributes related to unit type and properties of receptive field. Brain 107:727–749.

Van Essen, D. C. 1979. Visual areas of the mammalian cerebral cortex. Annu. Rev. Neurosci. 2:227–263.

Van Essen, D. C., and Maunsell, J. H. R. 1983. Hierarchical organization and functional streams in the visual cortex. Trends Neurosci. 6:370–375.

Van Praag, H. M. 1982. Neurotransmitters in CNS disease: Depression. Lancet 2:1259–1264.

Vaughn, J. E., Hinds, P. L., and Skoff, R. P. 1970. Electron microscopic studies of Wallerian degeneration in rat optic nerves. 1. The multipotential glia. J. Comp. Neurol. 140:175–205.

Verney, E. B. 1947. The antidiuretic hormone and the factors which determine its release. Proc. R. Soc. Lond. [Biol.] 135:25–106.

Vicario, D. S., Martin, J. H., and Ghez, C. 1983. Specialized subregions in the cat motor cortex: A single unit analysis in the behaving animal. Exp. Brain. Res. 51:351–367.

Vincent, A. 1980. Immunology of acetylcholine receptors in relation to myasthenia gravis. Physiol. Rev. 60:756–824.

Vincent, A., Newsom-Davis, J., Newton, P., and Beck, N. 1983. Acetylcholine receptor antibody and clinical response to thymectomy in myasthenia gravis. Neurology 33:1276–1281.

vom Saal, F. S., and Bronson, F. H. 1980. Sexual characteristics of adult female mice are correlated with their blood testosterone levels during prenatal development. Science 208:597–599.

von Békésy, G. 1960. Experiments in Hearing. New York: McGraw-Hill.

von Senden, M. 1932. Space and Sight. P. Heath (trans.). Glencoe, Ill.: Free Press, 1960.

Vrensen, G., Nunes Cardozo, J., Müller, L., and Van Der Want, J. 1980. The presynaptic grid: A new approach. Brain Res. 184:23–40.

W

Wagner, H. N., Jr., Burns, H. D., Dannals, R. F., Wong, D. F., Langstrom, B., Duelfer, T., Frost, J. J., Ravert, H. T., Links, J. M., Rosenbloom, S. B., Lukas, S. E., Kramer, A. V., and Kuhar, M. J. 1984. Assessment of dopamine receptor densities in the human brain with carbon-11-labeled N-methylspiperone. Ann. Neurol. [Suppl.] 15:S79–S84.

Wald, G. 1964. The receptors of human color vision. Science 145:1007–1016.

Wald, G. 1968. Molecular basis of visual excitation. Science 162:230–239.

Walford, R. L. 1974. Immunologic theory of aging: Current status. Fed. Proc. 33:2020–2027.

Walker, M. B. 1934. Treatment of myasthenia gravis with physostigmine. Lancet 1:1200–1201.

Walker, M. B. 1935. Case showing the effect of prostigmin on myasthenia gravis. Proc. R. Soc. Med. 28:759–761.

Wall, P. D., and Egger, M. D. 1971. Formation of new connexions in adult rat brains after partial deafferentation. Nature 232:542–545.

Wall, P. D., and Taub, A. 1962. Four aspects of trigeminal nucleus and a paradox. J. Neurophysiol. 25:110–126.

Walters, E. T., and Byrne, J. H. 1983. Associative conditioning of single sensory neurons suggests a cellular mechanism for learning. Science 219:405–408.

Walton, J. (ed.). 1981. Disorders of Voluntary Muscle, 4th ed. Edinburgh: Churchill Livingstone.

Warren J. M., and Akert, K. (eds.). 1964. The Frontal Granular Cortex and Behavior. New York: McGraw–Hill.

Warrington, E. K., and Weiskrantz, L. 1982. Amnesia: A disconnection syndrome? Neuropsychologia 20:233–248.

Wässle, H., Reichl, L., and Boycott, B. B. 1981. Dendritic territories of cat retinal ganglion cells. Nature 292:344–345.

Watkins, L. R., and Mayer, D. J. 1982. Organization of endogenous opiate and nonopiate pain control systems. Science 216:1185–1192.

Watson, J. B. 1930. Behaviorism, rev. ed. New York: Norton.

Watson, J. D., Tooze, J., and Kurtz, D. T. (eds.). 1983. Recombinant DNA: A Short Course. San Francisco: Freeman.

Waxman, S. G. 1982. Membranes, myelin, and the pathophysiology of multiple sclerosis. N. Engl. J. Med. 306:1529–1533.

Weber, E. H. 1846. Der Tastsinn und das Gemeingefühl. In: R. Wagner (ed.), Handworterbuch der Physiologie, Vol. III, Abt. 2. Braunschweig: Viewig, pp. 481–588.

Weeds, A. G., Trentham, D. R., Kean, C. J. C., and Buller, A. J. 1974. Myosin from cross-reinnervated cat muscles. Nature 247:135–139.

Weinberger, D. R., Wagner, R. L., and Wyatt, R. J. 1983. Neuropathological studies of schizophrenia: A selective review. Schizophr. Bull. 9:193–212.

Weinrich, M., and Wise, S. P. 1982. The pre-motor cortex of the monkey. J. Neurosci. 2:1329–1345.

Weisblat, D. A., Harper, G., Stent, G. S., and Sawyer, R. T. 1980. Embryonic cell lineages in the nervous system of the glossiphoniid leech, Helobdella triserialis. Dev. Biol. 76:58–78.

Weiss, K. R., Koch, U. T., Koester, J., Rosen, S. C., and Kupfermann, I. 1982. The role of arousal in modulating feeding behavior of Aplysia: Neural and behavioral studies. In B. G. Hoebel and D. Novin (eds.), The Neural Basis of Feeding and Reward. Brunswick, Me.: Haer Institute, pp. 25–57.

Weiss, P., and Hiscoe, H. B. 1948. Experiments on the mechanism of nerve growth. J. Exp. Zool. 107:315–395.

Werblin, F. S., and Dowling, J. E. 1969. Organization of the retina of the mudpuppy, Necturus maculosus. II. Intracellular recording. J. Neurophysiol. 32:339–355.

Werner, G., and Whitsel, B. L. 1973. Functional organization of the somatosensory cortex. In A. Iggo (ed.), Handbook of Sensory Physiology, Vol. 2: Somatosensory System. New York: Springer, pp. 621–700.

Wernicke, C. 1908. The symptom-complex of aphasia. In A. Church (ed.), Diseases of the Nervous System. New York: Appleton, pp. 265–324.

Wersäll, J., and Flock, Å. 1965. Functional anatomy of the vestibular and lateral line organs. In W. D. Neff (ed.), Contributions to Sensory Physiology Vol. 1. New York: Academic Press, pp. 39–61.

Wersäll, J., Flock, Å., and Lundquist, P.-G. 1965. Structural basis for directional sensitivity in cochlear and vestibular sensory receptors. Cold Spring Harbor Symp. Quant. Biol. 30:115–132.

Westheimer, G. 1954. Mechanism of saccadic eye movements. A.M.A. Arch. Ophthalmol. 52:710–724.

Westheimer, G. 1972. Visual acuity and spatial modulation thresholds. In D. Jameson and L. M. Hurvich (eds.), Handbook of Sensory Physiology, Vol. 7, Part 4: Visual Psychophysics. Berlin: Springer, pp. 170–187.

Westheimer, G. 1980. The eye. In V. B. Mountcastle (ed.), Medical Physiology, 14th ed., Vol. 1. St. Louis: Mosby, pp. 481–503.

Westrum, L. E., Canfield, R. C., and Black, R. G. 1976. Transganglionic degeneration in the spinal trigeminal nucleus following removal of tooth pulps in adult cats. Brain Res. 101:137–140.

Whalen, R. E., and Edwards, D. A. 1967. Hormonal determinants of the development of masculine and feminine behavior in male and female rats. Anat. Rec. 157:173–180.

Whalen, R. E., and Massicci, J. 1975. Subcellular analysis of the accumulation of estrogen by the brain of male and female rats. Brain Res. 89:255–264.

White, P., Hiley, C. R., Goodhardt, M. J., Carrasco, L. H., Keet, J. P., Williams, I. E. I., and Bowen, D. M. 1977. Neocortical cholinergic neurons in elderly people. Lancet 1:668–671.

Whitehorn, D., and Burgess, P. R. 1973. Changes in polarization of central branches of myelinated mechanoreceptor and nociceptor fibers during noxious and innocuous stimulation of the skin. J. Neurophysiol. 36:226–237.

Whitehouse, P. J., Price, D. L., Struble, R. G., Clark, A. W., Coyle, J. T., and DeLong, M. R. 1982. Alzheimer's disease and senile dementia: Loss of neurons in the basal forebrain. Science 215:1237–1239.

Whittaker, E. 1951. A History of the Theories of Aether and Electricity, Vol. I: The Classical Theories, rev. & enl. ed. London: T. Nelson and Sons.

Whittaker, V. P., Michaelson, I. A., and Kirkland, R. J. A. 1964. The separation of synaptic vesicles from nerve-ending particles ('synaptosomes'). Biochem. J. 90:293–303.

Wiersma, C. A. G. 1938. Function of the giant fibers of the central nervous system of the crayfish. Proc. Soc. Exp. Biol. Med. 38:661–662.

Wiesel, T. N., and Hubel, D. H. 1963. Single-cell responses in striate cortex of kittens deprived of vision in one eye. J. Neurophysiol. 26:1003–1017.

Wiesel, T. N., Hubel, D. H., and Lam, D. M. K. 1974. Autoradiographic demonstration of ocular-dominance columns in the monkey striate cortex by means of transneuronal transport. Brain Res. 79:273–279.

Wilks, S. 1883. Lectures on Diseases of the Nervous System Delivered at Guy's Hospital, 2nd ed. Philadelphia: P. Blakiston, Son & Co.

Willis, W. D., and Coggeshall, R. E. 1978. Sensory Mechanisms of the Spinal Cord. New York: Plenum Press.

Wilson, V. J., and Melvill Jones, G. 1979. Mammalian Vestibular Physiology. New York: Plenum Press.

Winokur, G. 1978. Mania and depression: Family studies and genetics in relation to treatment. In M. A. Lipton, A. DiMascio, and K. F. Killam (eds.), Psychopharmacology: A Generation of Progress. New York: Raven Press, pp. 1213–1221.

Wísniewski, H. M., and Terry, R. D. 1973. Morphology of the aging brain, human and animal. Neurological Aspects of Maturation and Aging. Prog. Brain Res. 40:167–186.

Witelson, S. F. 1976. Sex and the single hemisphere: Specialization of the right hemisphere for spatial processing. Science 193:425–427.

Witt, P. L., Hamm, H. E., and Bownds, M. D. 1984. Preparation and characterization of monoclonal antibodies to several frog outer segment proteins. J. Gen. Physiol. 84:251–263.

Wolpe, J. 1958. Psychotherapy by Reciprocal Inhibition. Stanford, Calif.: Stanford University Press.

Woodworth, R. S., and Sherrington, C. S. 1904. A pseudaffective reflex and its spinal path. J. Physiol. (Lond.) 31:234–243.

Woody, C. D. (ed.) 1982. Conditioning: Representation of Involved Neural Functions: New York: Plenum Press.

Woody, C. D., Swartz, B. E., and Gruen, E. 1978. Effects of acetylcholine and cyclic GMP on input resistance of cortical neurons in awake cats. Brain Res. 158:373–395.

Woolacott, M. H., and Hoyle, G. 1976. Membrane resistance changes associated with single, identified neuron learning. Soc. Neurosci. [Abstr.] 2:339.

Woolsey, C. N. 1958. Organization of somatic sensory and motor areas of the cerebral cortex. In H. F. Harlow and C. N. Woolsey (eds.), Biological and Biochemical Bases of Behavior. Madison: University of Wisconsin Press, pp. 63–81.

Woolsey, T. A., and Van der Loos, H. 1970. The structural organization of layer IV in the somatosensory region (S I) of mouse cerebral cortex. The description of a cortical field composed of discrete cytoarchitectonic units. Brain Res. 17:205–242.

Wurtz, R. H., and Albano, J. E. 1980. Visual-motor function of the primate superior colliculus. Annu. Rev. Neurosci. 3:189–226.

Wyatt, R. J., and Gillin, J. C. 1976. Biochemistry and human sleep. In R. L. Williams and I. Karacan (eds.), Pharmacology of Sleep. New York: Wiley, pp. 239–274.

Y

Yaksh, T. L., and Hammond, D. L. 1982. Peripheral and central substrates involved in the rostrad transmission of nociceptive information. Pain 13:1–85.

Yarbus, A. L. 1967. Eye Movements and Vision. B. Haigh (trans.). New York: Plenum Press.

Yates, A. J. 1970. Behavior Therapy. New York: Wiley.

Yau, K. W., and Nakatani, K. 1985. Light-induced reduction of cytoplasmic free Ca^{++} in retinal rod outer segment. Nature 313:579–582.

Yoon, M. G. 1976. Topographic polarity of the optic tectum studied by reimplantation of the tectal tissue in adult goldfish. Cold Spring Harbor Symp. Quant. Biol. 40:503–519.

Yoss, R. E., and Daly, D. D. 1957. Criteria for the diagnosis of the narcoleptic syndrome. Proc. Staff Meet. Mayo Clin. 32:320–328.

Youdim, M. B. H., Banerjee, D. K., and Pollard, H. B. 1984. Isolated chromaffin cells from adrenal medulla contain primarily monoamine oxidase B. Science 224:619–621.

Young, R. M. 1970. Mind, Brain and Adaptation in the Nineteenth Century. Oxford: Clarendon Press.

Young, R. W. 1970. Visual cells. Sci. Am. 223(4):80–91.

Young, T. 1802. The Bakerian Lecture. On the theory of light and colours. Phil. Trans. R. Soc. Lond., pp. 12–48.

Z

Zeki, S. M. 1976. The functional organization of projections from striate to prestriate visual cortex in the rhesus monkey. Cold Spring Harbor Symp. Quant. Biol. 40:591–600.

Zeki, S. 1980. The representation of colours in the cerebral cortex. Nature 284:412–418.

Zigmond, R. E. 1980. The long-term regulation of ganglionic tyrosine hydroxylase by preganglionic nerve activity. Fed. Proc. 19:3003–3008.

Zigmond, R. E., and Bowers, C. W. 1981. Influence of nerve activity on the macromolecular content of neurons and their effector organs. Annu. Rev. Physiol. 43:673–687.

Zimmerman, E. A., Carmel, P. W., Husain, M. K., Ferin, M., Tannenbaum, M., Frantz, A. G., and Robinson, A. G. 1973. Vasopressin and neurophysin: High concentrations in monkey hypophyseal portal blood. Science 182:925–927.

Illustration and Table Credits

We wish to thank all the authors who have kindly supplied us with published and unpublished materials, photographs, and information, and have given us permission to reproduce, incorporate, or quote these in the text. In addition, the following have given us permission to reproduce published textual, pictorial, or tabular materials in the book.

Academic Press: Figure 25–5 adapted from Bard, Harvey Lect. 33:143–169 (1938); Figure 30–1 adapted from Dartnall, Bowmaker, and Mollon, Colour Vision (1983); Figure 51–5 based on data from Rosenkilde, Behav. Neural Biol. 25:301–345 (1979); Figure 51–8 adapted from Sperry, Harvey Lect. 62:293–323 (1968); Figure 51–9 adapted from Levy, Trevarthen, and Sperry, Brain 95:61–78 (1972); Table 53–1 adapted from Kety, Harvey Lect. 71:1–22 (1978); Figure 56–2 adapted from Attardi and Sperry, Exp. Neurol. 7:46–64 (1963).

Acta Physiol. Scand.: Figure 54–4 adapted from Andén et al., 67:313–326.

Aerospace Medicine: Figure 49–1 adapted from Aschoff, 40:844–849 (1969).

American Elsevier (New York): Figures 32–2 and 32–3 adapted from Murray, The Ultrastructure of Sensory Organs (1973).

American Fertility Society: Figure 46–6 (part) adapted from Gay, Fertil. Steril. 23:50–63 (1972).

American Medical Association: Table 50–2 adapted from A Collaborative Study of Cerebral Death, J. Am. Med. Assoc. 237:982–986 (1977). Copyright © 1977, American Medical Associaton.

American Physiological Society: Figure 3–2C adapted from Burke and Rudomin in Kandel, Handbook of Physiology (1977); Figure 3–4B adapted from Bunge, Physiol. Rev. 48:197–251; Figure 5–4 adapted from Orkand in Kandel, Handbook of Physiology (1977); Figures 25–5 and 25–6B adapted from Marshall, Woolsey, and Bard, J. Neurophysiol. 4:1–24 (1941); Figure 25–13 adapted from Costanzo and Gardner, J. Neurophysiol. 43:1319–1341 (1980); Figure 30–7A adapted from Michael, J. Neurophysiol. 41:572–588 (1978); Figure 30–7B adapted from Michael, J. Neurophysiol. 41:1233–1249 (1978); Figure 32–6 adapted from Smith et al., J. Neurophysiol. 50:541–558 (1983); Figure 32–16 adapted from Shepherd, Physiol. Rev. 52:864–917 (1972); Figure 34–4 adapted from Partridge, Am. J. Physiol. 210:1178–1191 (1966); Figure 34–10 adapted from Matthews, Physiol. Rev. 44:219–228 (1964); Figure 38–3 adapted from Evarts, J. Neurophysiol. 31:14–27 (1968); Figure 38–5 adapted from Asanuma, Physiologist 13:143–166 (1973); Figure 38–9 adapted from Roland et al., J. Neurophysiol. 43:118–136 (1980); Figure 39–14 adapted from Allen and Tsukuhara, Physiol. Rev. 54:957–1006 (1974); Figure 43–11 adapted from Fuchs and Luschei, J. Neurophysiol. 33:382–392 (1970); Figure 47–3 (part) adapted from Satinoff, Am. J. Physiol. 206:1389–1394 (1964); Figure 48–3 adapted from Llinás and Nicholson, J. Neurophysiol. 34:532–551 (1971); Figure 60–3 adapted from Doty and Bosma, J. Neurophysiol. 19:44–60 (1956).

American Psychological Association: Figure 32–7 adapted by permission of Erickson, Psychol. Rev. 75:447–465. Copyright © 1968 by the American Psychological Association; Figure 47–3 (part) adapted from Corbit, J. Comp. Physiol. Psychol. 83:394–411 (1973); Figure 58–5 adapted from Beach, Noble, and Orndoff, J. Comp. Physiol. Psychol. 68:490–497 (1969).

American Zoologist: Figure 58–7 adapted from Toran-Allerand, 18:553–565.

Annals of Internal Medicine: Figure I–II adapted from Phelps, Schelbert, and Mazziotta, 98:339–359 (1983).

Annual Reviews, Inc.: Figure 14–4B adapted from Lefkowitz, Stadel, and Caron, Annual Review of Biochemistry, Vol. 52 (1983); Figure 25–11B adapted from Kaas, Merzenich, and Killackey, Annual Review of Neuroscience, Vol. 6 (1983); Figure 26–3 adapted from Akil et al., Annual Review of Neuroscience, Vol. 7 (1984); Figure 29–1 adapted from Van Essen, Annual Review of Neuroscience, Vol. 2 (1979); Figure 43–14 adapted from Robinson, Annual Review of Neuroscience, Vol. 4 (1981). All reproduced by copyright permission of Annual Reviews, Inc.

Archivio di Scienze Biologiche: Figure 50–5 adapted from Magni et al., 97:33–46 (1959).

Brain: Figure I–10 adapted from Ingvar and Schwartz, 97:273–288 (1974).

Brunner/Mazel: Figures 50–1 and 50–2 adapted from Kales and Kales in Usdin, Sleep Research and Clinical Practice (1973).

Cambridge University Press: Figure 55–8 adapted from Horvitz in Garrod and Feldman, Development in the Nervous System (1981).

CBS College Publishing: Figure 55–5 adapted from Bodemer, Modern Embryology. © 1968 by Holt, Rinehart and Winston, Inc. Reprinted by permission of CBS College Publishing.

Cold Spring Harbor Laboratory: Figure 13–1 adapted from Herbert et al., Symp. Quant. Biol. 48:375–384 (1983); Figure 14–4A adapted from Schramm et al., Symp. Quant. Biol. 48:187–191 (1983); Figure 29–5 adapted from Kuffler, Symp. Quant. Biol. 17:281–292 (1952); Figure 31–3 adapted from Wersäll, Flock, and Lundquist, Symp. Quant. Biol. 30:115–132 (1965); Figure 44–6 adapted from Flock, Symp. Quant. Biol. 30:133–145; Figure 62–10 adapted from Kandel et al., Symp. Quant. Biol. 48:821–830 (1983). All copyright © by The Cold Spring Harbor Laboratory.

F. A. Davis: Figure 45–7 adapted from Gatz, Manter's Essentials of Clinical Neuroanatomy and Neurophysiology, 3rd ed. (1966); Table 50–1 adapted from Plum and Posner, The Diagnosis of Stupor and Coma, 3rd ed. (1980); Figures 59–2, 59–3, 59–4, and 59–5 adapted from Duffy, Neuropathology: An Illustrated Course (1974).

Elsevier Biomedical Press, B. V. (Amsterdam): Figure 4–7 adapted from Divac et al., Brain Res. 123:197–207 (1977); Figure 9–1B adapted from Bennett, Sandri, and Akert, Brain Res. 143:43–60 (1978); Figure 32–12 adapted from Trotier and MacLeod, Brain Res. 268:225–237 (1983); Figure 38–6 adapted from Conrad et al., Brain Res. 71:507–514 (1974); Figure 42–8 adapted from Woolsey and Van der Loos, Brain Res. 17:205–242 (1970); Figure 48–12 adapted from Ayala et al., Brain Res. 52:1–17 (1973); Figure 58–6 adapted from Gorski et al., Brain Res. 148:333–346 (1978).

Elsevier Ireland (County Clare): Figure 48–10 adapted from Picton et al., Electroencephalography and Clinical Neurophysiology 36:179–190.

Elsevier/North-Holland Biomedical Press (Cambridge): Figure 9–14 adapted from Colquhoun, Trends Pharmacol. Sci. 2:212–217 (1981); Figure 16–6 adapted from Drachman, Trends Neurosci. 6:446–451 (1983); Figure 23–11 adapted from Johansson and Vallbo, Trends Neurosci. 6:27–32 (1983); Figures 62–11 and 62–12 adapted from Merzenich and Kaas, Trends Neurosci. 5:434–436 (1982).

Federal Proceedings: Figure 59–1 adapted from Strehler, 34:5–8 (1975).

Fischer (Jena): Figure 3–2A adapted from Dogiel, Der Bau der Spinalganglien des Menschen und der Säugetiere (1908).

Freeman: Figure 40–6 adapted from Watson, Tooze, and Kurtz, Recombinant DNA: A Short Course (1983). Copyright © 1983.

Garland Publishing: Figures 9–10, 9–11, and 9–12 adapted from Alberts et al., Molecular Biology of the Cell (1983).

Grune & Stratton: Figure 45–3 adapted from Sears and Franklin in Rosenberg, The Science and Practice of Clinical Medicine, Vol. 5 (1980).

Heinemann Medical Books Ltd.: Figure 9–6B adapted from Miles, Excitable Cells (1969).

Paul B. Hoeber: Figure 2–3A adapted from Penfield (ed.), Cytology & Cellular Pathology of the Nervous System, Vol. 2 (1932).

Holt, Rinehart and Winston, Inc.: Figure 49–5 adapted from Dement, in New Directions in Psychology II (1965); Figure 55–5 adapted from Bodemer, Modern Embryology. Copyright © 1968 by Holt, Rinehart and Winston, Inc. Reprinted by permission of CBS College Publishing.

International Journal of Neurology: Figure 48–2 adapted from Spencer and Kandel, 6:266–296 (1968).

Johns Hopkins University Press: Figure 16–2 adapted from Harvey, Lilienthal, and Talbot, Bull. Johns Hopkins Hosp. 69:547–577 (1941); Figure 53–1 adapted from Kety et al. in Fieve, Rosenthal, and Brill, Genetic Research in Psychiatry (1975); Figure 58–2 adapted from Money and Ehrhardt, Man and Woman, Boy and Girl (1972).

Johnson and Johnson Baby Products Co.: Figure 62–14 adapted from Merzenich in Brown, The Many Facets of Touch (1985).

Journal of Applied Physiology: Figure 34–4 adapted from Partridge, 20:150–156.

Journal of Experimental Zoology: Figure 56–5 adapted from Hamburger, 68:449–494 (1934).

Journal of Physiology (London): Figure 10–5C based on data from Finkel and Redman, 342:615–632 (1983); Figures 11–1 and 11–2 adapted from Katz and Miledi, 192:407–436 (1967); Figure 11–4 adapted from Katz and Miledi, 189:535–544 (1967); Figure 11–6A adapted from Liley, 133:571–587 (1956); Figure 11–6B adapted from Boyd and Martin, 132:74–91 (1956); Figure 18–8 adapted from Adrian and Bryant, 240:505–515 (1974); Figure 23–5 adapted from Lowenstein and Mendelson, 177:377–397 (1965); Figure 23–7 adapted from Perl, 197: 593–615 (1968); Figures 29–7, 29–8, 29–9B, 29–12, and 29–13 (part) adapted from Hubel and Wiesel, 160: 106–154; Figure 29–9A adapted from Hubel and Wiesel, 148:574–591 (1959); Figure 34–1 adapted from Henneman, 69:377–385 (1930); Figure 34–13 adapted from Crowe and Matthews, 174:109–131 (1964); Figure 34–14 adapted from Hunt and Kuffler, 113:298–315 (1951); Figure 34–2 adapted from Burke et al., 238:503–514; Figures 43–6, 43–8, and Table 43–2 adapted from Fuchs, 191:609–631 (1967); Figure 46–8 adapted from Lincoln and Wakerley, 242:533–554 (1974); Figure 48–4 adapted from Kelly and Van Essen, 238:515–547 (1974); Figure 56–8 adapted from Axelsson and Thesleff, 147:178–193 (1959).

S. Karger A. G. (Basel): Figure 39–11 adapted from Shambes, Gibson, and Welker, Brain Behav. Evol. 15:94–140 (1978).

The Lancet: Figure I–13 adapted from Cady et al., 1:1059–1062.

Lawrence Erlbaum Associates: Figure 1–8 adapted from Uttal, The Psychobiology of Mind (1978).

Lea & Febiger: Figure 48–11 adapted from Merritt, A Textbook of Neurology, 6th ed. (1979).

Life Science Associates: Figure 3–2B from Coggeshall and Mandriota, Basic Principles of Neuroscience, A Slide Set. Copyright © 1979 by Life Science Associates.

Lippincott/Harper and Row: Figure 21–8 adapted from Keibel and Mall, Manual of Human Embryology, Vol. 2 (1912); Figures 36–2 and 36–4 adapted from Collins, Illustrated Manual of Neurologic Diagnosis (1962); Figure 49–3A adapted from Feinberg in Kales, Sleep Physiology and Pathology (1969); Figure 51–1 adapted from Thompson, Introduction to Physiological Psychology (1975).

Alan R. Liss: Figure 4–9 adapted from Oblinger and Lasek in O'Lague, Neurobiology: Molecular Biological Approaches to Understanding Neuronal Function and Development. Copyright © 1985 by Alan R. Liss, Inc.; Figure 32–5 adapted from Kimura and Beidler, J. Cell. Comp. Physiol. 58:131–139 (1961); Figure 32–13 adapted from Stewart, Kauer, and Shepherd, J. Comp. Neurol. 185:715–734 (1979); Figure 55–6 adapted from Sauer, J. Comp. Neurol. 62:377–405 (1935); Figure 55–13 adapted from Rakic, J. Comp. Neurol. 141:283–312 (1971); Figure 55–14 adapted from Rakic, J. Comp. Neurol. 147:523–546 (1973); Figure 57–4 adapted from LeVay, Strycker, and Shatz, J. Comp. Neurol. 179:223–244 (1978).

Little, Brown: Figure 29–6 adapted from Brown and Herrstein, Psychology (1975); Figure 41–17 adapted from Scheibel and Scheibel in Jasper et al., Reticular Formation of the Brain (1958); Figure 48–1 adapted from Szentágothai in Jasper, Wardt, and Pope, Basic Mechanisms of the Epilepsies (1969).

Livingstone Ltd.: Figure 23–6 adapted from Boyd and Davey, Composition of Peripheral Nerves (1968).

Macmillan Journals Limited: Figure 8–9B adapted from Sigworth and Neher, 287:447–449; Reprinted by permission from Nature. Copyright © 1980 by Macmillan Journals Limited; Figure 12–7 adapted from Fernandez, Neher, and Gomperts 312:454. Reprinted by permission from Nature. Copyright © 1984 Macmillan Journals Limited; Figure 53–2B adapted from Seeman et al., 261:717–719. Reprinted by permission from Nature. Copyright © 1976 by Macmillan Journals Limited.

Macmillan Publishing Co., Inc.: Figures 1–7, 25–7, and 38–1B adapted from Penfield and Rasmussen, The Cerebral Cortex of Man (1950); Figure 21–5 adapted with permission of Macmillan Publishing Co., a Division of Macmillan, Inc., from Review of Medical Embryology by Ben Pansky, Ph.D., M.D. Copyright © 1982 by Ben Pansky; Figures 55–3 and 55–4 adapted from Saunders, Patterns and Principles of Animal Development. Copyright © 1970 by John W. Saunders, Jr.

Masson, S. A. (Paris): Figure 38–4 (part) adapted from Ghez and Vicario, J. Physiol. (Paris) 74:283–285 (1978).

McGraw–Hill Book Co.: Figure 16–8 adapted from Lindstrom in Engel and Banker, Clinical Myology (1981); Figure 17–4 adapted from Weiss and Greep, Histology (1977); Figure 19–4 adapted from Noback and Demarest, The Human Nervous System: Basic Principles of Neurology, 3rd ed. (1981); Figure 21–6 adapted from House, Pansky, and Siegel, A Systematic Approach to Neuroscience (1979); Figure 31–7 adapted from von Békésy, Experiments in Hearing (1960); Figure 45–6 adapted from Adams and Victor, Principles of Neurology (1977); Figure 51–4 adapted from Warren and Akert, The Frontal Granular Cortex and Behavior (1964); Figure I–15 adapted from Mohr, Fisher, and Adams in Isselbacher et al., Harrison's Principles of Internal Medicine, 9th ed. (1980). All reproduced by copyright permission of McGraw–Hill Book Co.

The MIT Press: Figures 11–3 and 12–6 adapted from Llinás and Heuser, Neurosci. Res. Progr. Bull. 15:555–687 (1977); Figure 12–16B adapted from Rakic, Neurosci. Res. Progr. Bull. 13:289–446 (1975); Figure 25–12B adapted from Kaas et al., Organization of the Cerebral Cortex (1981); Figure 27–6B adapted from Dowling, The Neurosciences, Fourth Study Program, pp. 163–181 (1979); Figure 31–11 adapted from Kiang, Discharge Patterns of Single Fibers in the Cat's Auditory Nerve (1965); Figure 40–3 adapted from DeLong, The Neurosciences, Third Study Program, pp. 319–325 (1974); Figure 57–8 adapted from Constantine-Paton in Schmitt et al., The Organization of the Cerebral Cortex (1981).

C. V. Mosby Co.: Figure 25–10 adapted from Mountcastle and Darian-Smith in Mountcastle, Medical Physiology, 12th ed. (1968); Figures 29–4, 29–8, and 29–11 adapted from Berne and Levy, Physiology (1983); Table II–1 adapted from Westheimer in Mountcastle, Medical Physiology, 14th ed. (1980).

New England Journal of Medicine: Figures 18–6 and 18–7 adapted from Waxman, Reprinted by permission of N. Engl. J. Med. 306:1529–1533 (1982).

New York Academy of Sciences: Table 51–1, data from Rasmussen and Milner, Ann. N.Y. Acad. Sci. 299:355–369 (1977).

W. W. Norton: Table 52–1 based in part on data from Gleitman in Gleitman and Gleitman, Psychology (1981).

Oxford Clarendon Press (London): Figure 60–1 adapted from Tinbergen, The Study of Instinct (1951).

Oxford University Press (New York): Figure 12–16A adapted from Shepherd, The Synaptic Organization of the Brain, 2nd ed. (1979); Figures 25–1A, 28–11, 31–14, and 42–1 adapted from Brodal, Neurological Anatomy in Relation to Clinical Medicine, 3rd ed. (1981); Figure 32–1C adapted from Shepherd, Neurobiology (1983); Figure 32–14 adapted from Ottoson, Physiology of the Nervous System (1983); Figure 41–16 adapted from DeArmand, Fusco, and Dewey, Structure of the Human Brain: A Photographic Atlas, 2nd ed. (1976); Figures 41–18, 41–20, 53–3, and 54–5 adapted from Cooper, Bloom, and Roth, The Biochemical Basis of Neuropharmacology, 4th ed. (1982); Figure 56–3 adapted from Lund, Development and Plasticity of the Brain (1978).

Pergamon Press: Figure 30–2 adapted from Smith and Pokorny, Vision Res. 15:161–171 (1975); Figures 44–1 and 44–9 adapted from Iurato, Submicroscopic Structure of the Inner Ear (1967); Figure 58–1 adapted from Bermant and Davidson; Biological Bases of Sexual Behavior (1974); Figure 62–13 adapted from Merzenich et al., Neuroscience 10:639–665 (1983).

Plenum Press: Figure 43–7 adapted from Yarbus, Eye Movements and Vision (1967); Figures 55–7, 55–11, and 55–12 adapted from Jacobson, Developmental Neurobiology, 2nd ed. (1978).

Princeton University Press: Figure 1–6 adapted from Penfield and Roberts, Speech and Brain Mechanisms (1959).

Proceedings of the National Academy of Sciences: Figure 10–10 adapted from Jan, Jan, and Kuffler, 76:1501–1505 (1979); Figure 14–2 adapted from Fertuck and Salpeter, 71:1376–1378 (1974); Figures 55–9 and 55–10 adapted from Le Douarin et al., 72: 728–732 (1975); Figure 56–7B adapted from Angeletti and Bradshaw, 68:2417–2420 (1971); Figures 62–4 and 62–6 adapted from Klein and Kandel, 75:3512–3516 (1978).

Proceedings of the Royal Society of London (Biological Sciences): Figure 17–5 adapted from Le Gros Clark and Penman, 114:291–313 (1981); Figure 28–13 adapted from Hubel and Wiesel, 198:1–59 (1977).

Raven Press: Figure 22–4 adapted from Oldendorf, The Quest for an Image of Brain (1980); Figure 35–8 adapted from Houk, Posture and Movement (1979); Figure 40–7 adapted from Houseman and Gusella, Molecular Genetic Neuroscience (1982); Figures 46–5 and 46–6 (part) adapted from Reichlin in Reichlin, Baldessarini, and Martin, Research Publications, Association for Research in Nervous and Mental Disease, Vol. 52, pp. 1–14 (1978); Figures 47–4 and 47–6 adapted from Keesey et al. in Novin, Wyrwicka, and Bray, Hunger: Basic Mechanisms and Clinical Implications (1976); Figure 50–4 adapted from Dement, Guilleminault, and Zarcone in Tower, The Nervous System, Vol. 2 (1975); Figures 59–6, 59–7, and 59–8 adapted from Scheibel and Scheibel in Brody, Harman, and Ordy, Aging, Vol. I (1975).

The Rockefeller University Press: Figure 4–10 adapted from Schnapp and Reese, J. Cell Biol. 94:673 (1982); Figure 9–1A adapted from Makowski et al., J. Cell Biol. 74:643 (1977); Figure 9–9 adapted from Dwyer, Adams, and Hille, J. Gen. Physiol. 75:245 (1980); Figure 12–5 adapted from Miller and Heuser, J. Cell Biol. 98:697 (1984); Figure 16–4 adapted from Berman and Patrick, J. Exp. Med. 151:204–223 (1980); Figure 34–11 adapted from Hunt, J. Gen. Physiol. 38:117–131 (1954); Figure 44–4A adapted from Flock, J. Cell Biol. 22:413–431 (1964); Figure 56–4 adapted from Barondes in Schmitt, The Neurosciences: Second Study Program (1970). All reproduced by copyright permission of the Rockefeller University Press.

The Royal Society (London): Figure 57–2C and 57–5 adapted from Hubel and Wiesel, Philos. Trans. R. Soc. Lond. [Biol. Sci.] 198:1–59 (1977); Figure 57–3 adapted from Hubel, Wiesel, and LeVay, Philos. Trans. R. Soc. Lond. [Biol. Sci.] 278:377–409 (1977).

Saunders: Figures 2–3B and 45–5B adapted from Martinez Martinez, Neuroanatomy: Development and Structure of the Central Nervous System (1982); Figures 3–1, 3–4A, 3–5, and 4–3A adapted from Peters, Palay, and Webster, The Fine Structure of the Nervous System (1976); Figure 12–3A adapted from Fawcett, The Cell, 2nd ed. (1981); Figure 16–5 adapted from Lisak and Barchi, Myasthenia Gravis (1982); Figures 31–4 and 31–5 adapted from Miller and Towe, Physiology and Biophysics, 20th ed. (1979); Figures 31–12, 41–7 through 41–13, 42–4, and 42–6 adapted from Ranson and Clark, The Anatomy of the Nervous System, 9th ed. (1953); Figure 34–12 adapted from Patton, Physiology and Biophysics, 19th ed. (1965); Figure 52–2 adapted from Patton, Crill, and Swanson, Introduction to Basic Neurology (1976); Figures I–2 (part), I–5, I–12, and Table I–1 adapted from Fishman, Cerebrospinal Fluid in Diseases of the Nervous System (1980); Figure I–14 adapted from Barnett in Wyngaarden and Smith, Textbook of Medicine, 16th ed. (1982).

Science: Figure 4–6 adapted from Ochs, 176:252–260 (1972); Table 13–2 adapted from Krieger, 222:975–985 (1983); Figure 16–3 adapted from Fambrough, Drachman, and Satyamurti, 182:293–295 (1983); Figure 25–11A adapted from Kaas et al., 204:521–523 (1979); Figure 27–2A and 27–4 adapted from O'Brien, 218:961–966 (1982); Figure 28–7 adapted from Sur and Sherman, 218:389–

391 (1982); Figure 43–15 adapted from Robinson, 161:1219–1224 (1968); Figure 49–4 adapted from Schwartz and Gainer, 197:1089–1091 (1977); Figure 50–3 adapted from Jacobson et al., 148:975–977 (1965); Figure 51–7 adapted from Geschwind and Levitsky, 161:186–187 (1968); Figure 53–2A adapted from Seeman and Lee, 188: 1217–1219 (1975); Figure 61–2 adapted from Squire, Slater, and Chace, 187:77–79 (1975); Figure 62–2 adapted from Castellucci, Carew, and Kandel, 202:1306–1308 (1978); Figure 62–7 adapted from Bailey and Chen, 220: 91–93 (1983); Figure 62–8 adapted from Carew, Hawkins, and Kandel, 219:397–400 (1983). All copyright © by the American Association for the Advancement of Science.

Scientific American (published by W. H. Freeman and Co.): Figure 1–5 adapted from Geschwind, 241(3):180–199 (1979); Figures 2–1A and 14–3 adapted from Stevens, 241(3):54–65 (1979); Figure 11–5 adapted from Llinás, 247(4):56–65 (1982); Figures 21–1, 55–1, and 55–2 adapted from Cowan, 241(3):112–133 (1979); Figure 27–2B adapted from Young, 223(4):80–91 (1970); Figure 28–2 adapted from Wald, 183(2):32–41 (1950); Figure 32–8 adapted from Amoore, Johnston, and Rubin, 210(2):42–48 (1964); Figure 35–3 adapted from Merton, 226(5):30–37 (1972); Figure 37–3 adapted from Pearson, 235(6):72–86 (1976); Figure 54–1 adapted from Kety, 241(3):202–214 (1979); Figures 58–3 and 58–4 adapted from McEwen, 235(1):48–59 (1976); Figure II–14 adapted from Poggio, 250(4):106–116 (1984). All reproduced by copyright permission of Scientific American, Inc. All rights reserved.

Scribner's: Table 49–1 adapted from Foulkes, The Psychology of Sleep (1966).

Sinauer Associates: Figures 2–3C, 29–13 (part), I–1 (part), and I–4 adapted from Kuffler and Nicholls, From Neuron to Brain (1976); Figures 9–4, 12–2, and 12–3B adapted from Kuffler, Nicholls, and Martin, From Neuron to Brain, 2nd ed. (1984); Figure 28–5 adapted from Hurvich, Color Vision (1981); Figure 56–9C adapted from Purves and Lichtman, Principles of Neural Development (1985).

Society for Neuroscience: Figure 14–1 adapted from Karlin, Neurosci. Comment. 1:111–123 (1983); Figure 30–8 adapted from Livingstone and Hubel, J. Neurosci. 4:309–356 (1984); Figure 57–6 adapted from Gilbert and Wiesel, J. Neurosci. 3:1116–1133 (1983); Figure 62–10 based on Abrams et al., Soc. Neurosci. (Abstr.) 9:168 (1983). All copyright © Society for Neuroscience.

Springer-Verlag: Figures 1–3, 21–13, 21–14, 32–15, 39–1, 40–1, 46–1, 46–3, and 47–2 adapted from Nieuwenhuys, Voogd, and van Huijzen, The Human Nervous System, 2nd rev. ed. (1981); Figures 19–7 and 29–3 adapted from Schmidt and Thews (eds.), Human Physiology (1983); Figure 31–8 adapted from Lewis and Hudspeth, Hearing—Physiological Bases and Psychophysics (1983); Figure 32–4 adapted from Burton and Benjamin, Handbook of Sensory Physiology (1971); Figure 32–10 adapted from Andres, Z. Zellforsch. 69:140–154 (1966); Figure 32–11 adapted from Ottoson, Handbook of Sensory Physiology (1971); Figure 37–2 adapted from Nashner, Exp. Brain Res. 26:59–72 (1976); Figure 38–4 (part) adapted from Vicario, Martin, and Ghez, Exp. Brain Res. 51:351–367 (1983); Figure 39–5 adapted from Eccles, Ito, and Szentágothai, The Cerebellum as a Neuronal Machine (1967); Figures 45–2, 45–4, and 45–5 adapted from Patten, Neurological Differential Diagnosis (1977); Figures II–5 and II–16 adapted from Bishop in Jung, Handbook of Sensory Physiology (1973).

Stroke: Figure I–12 adapted from Baron, Bousser, Rey, Guillard, Comar, and Castaigne, 12:454–459 (1981).

Charles C. Thomas: Figure 8–7 adapted from Hodgkin, The Conduction of the Nervous Impulse (1964); Figures II–2, II–3, II–4, II–5, II–6, and II–7 adapted from Ogle, Optics: An Introduction for Ophthalmologists (1961). All courtesy of Charles C. Thomas, Publisher, Springfield, Illinois.

University of Pennsylvania Press: Figure 44–11 adapted from Spoendlin in Wolfson, The Vestibular System and Its Diseases (1966).

University of Wisconsin Press: Figure 51–6 adapted from Harlow in Harlow and Woolsey, Biological and Biochemical Bases of Behavior (1958).

John Wiley and Sons: Table 52–1 based in part from data in Lenneberg, Biological Foundation of Language (1967); Figure 56–6 adapted from Cowan and O'Leary in Isselbacher, Medicine, Science and Society (1984).

The Williams & Wilkins Co.: Figure 16–1 adapted from Rowland, Hoefer, and Aranow, Res. Publ. Assoc. Res. Nerv. Ment. Dis. 28 (1958). Copyright © 1958 The Williams & Wilkins Co., Baltimore; Figures 24–7, 24–10, and 28–9 adapted from Carpenter, Human Neuroanatomy, 7th ed. Copyright © 1976 The Williams & Wilkins Co., Baltimore; Figure 38–10 adapted from Brinkman, J. Neurosci. 4:918–929 (1984); Figures 43–4 and I–3 adapted from Carpenter, Core Text of Neuroanatomy, 2nd ed. (1978); Figure 47–1 adapted from Di Girolamo and Rudman, Endocrinology 82:1133–1141 (1968); Table 53–2 adapted from Klein and Davis, Diagnosis and Drug Treatment of Psychiatric Disorders (1969).

The Wistar Institute: Figure 42–7 adapted from Mountcastle and Henneman, J. Comp. Neurol. 97:409–439 (1952); Figure 43–9 adapted from Hardy, Anat. Rec. 59:403–418 (1934).

William Wood: Figure 2–2B–F adapted from Cajal, Histology, 10th ed. (1933).

Yale University Press: Figure 38–1A adapted from Sherrington, The Integrative Action of the Nervous System, 2nd ed. (1947).

Zeitschrift für experimentelle angewandte Psychologie: Figure 60–5 adapted from Ahrens, 2:412–454, 599–633 (1954).

Name Index

Unless otherwise indicated, twentieth century

Subject Index

Following page numbers:
d = definition, f = figure, t = table

Declarative memory, 810d
Decomposition of movement, 520
Decortication
    effect of on emotional behavior, 623
    results of, 481
Decussation, 220d. *See also* Commissures; Corpus callosum;
        Optic chiasm
Deep nuclei, cerebellar, 503. *See also* Dentate nucleus; Fastigial
        nucleus; Interposed nucleus
Defensive conditioning, 806d
Defensive response, fixed action pattern for, 799
Degeneration
    after axotomy, 188
    spinal cord, characteristics of, 476
    terminal, 188–189d
    transneuronal, 193d
Deiters' nucleus, 480. *See also* Lateral vestibular nucleus.
    excited by fastigial nucleus, 480
Déjà vu, 10d
Delta receptor for enkephalin, 340
Delta sleep, night terrors during, 663
Delta sleep-inducing peptide, 634d
Delta waves, 643d
Delusions, in schizophrenia, 706
Dementia, 705d
    and aging of the brain, 784–792
    characteristics of, 786. *See also* Alzheimer's disease, virally
        caused, 791
Dementia praecox, 705d
Demyelination
    effect of on normal synchrony of conduction, 205
    and evoked potentials in cortex, 321–322
    multiple sclerosis, 322
    shown in patient by MRI, 281f, 282
Dendrite, 14d
    growth rate of affected by sex steroids, 779–780
    loss of with age, 789
Dendritic arbor, as receptive pole of neuron, 146
Dendritic trees, in motor neurons, 30
Dendrodendritic connections
    and olfactory bulb, 144–145
    lateral geniculate nucleus, 373
Dendrodendritic interactions, and local information processing,
        144–146
Dendrodendritic synapses, in olfactory bulb, 145
Denervating diseases, chronic, muscle fibers in, 201
Dentate nucleus, 503
    projections of, 518
Depolarization, 21d, 51f
    artificial, 50
    Ca^{++} must be released during to produce transmitter release,
        123
    commanded, 76d, 78
    effect of on action potential propagation, 72f
    effect of on Ca^{++} influx, 127
    and increased Na^+ influx, 76
    initiates action potential, 76
    paroxysmal, origin of, 646
    passive conduction of, 71–72
    role of K^+ and Na^+ in, 56
    time of, 72
Depression, 717d
    biogenic amine hypothesis of, 720–723
    genetic predisposition for, 718–719
    and loss of delta sleep, 660
    neuroendocrine functions disordered in, 724–725
    somatic treatment for, 719–720
Depressive disorders
    and defect in hypothalamus, 718
    types of, 718
Deprivation, sensory, effect of on perceptual development, 759
Deprivation, social, and effect of on early childhood
        development, 758

Depth perception
    mediation of, 759
    role of binocular vision in, 872–874
Dermatome
    as area of skin innervated by single dorsal root, 301–304, 302f
    and areas innervated by peripheral nerves, 304f
    map, as diagnostic tool, 302
    mapping of, 302, 303f
    segmental arrangement of, 473
Dermatomyositis, 206
Descending control
    muscle set point, 465–466
    spinal cord motor neurons, 435–436
    of spinal pain transmission neurons, 340
Descending influences
    controlling posture, 481. *See also* Reflex mechanisms
    modulate central motor program, 484
    and postural control, 478–481
Descending message, tonic, and locomotor output, 482–485
Descending motor commands
    mediated by corticobulbar system, 433
    mediated by corticospinal system, 433
Descending pathways, brain stem, 436–437. *See also*
        Dorsolateral pathways; Ventromedial pathways
Descending systems
    and activation of alpha and gamma neurons, 454–455
    medial and lateral, controlled by efferent spinocerebellar
        projections, 513–516
Descending tracts, spinal cord, 469, 470f. *See also* Corticospinal
        tracts; Rubrospinal tract
Determination, 731d
Deutan, 394d
Development
    brain, critical periods in, 757–770
    effects of castration on, 774
    fine tuning of brain architecture, 757–770
    nervous system, 727–792
        androgen required for emergence of male pattern, 774–775
        bipotentiality of, 774–775
        normal, and requirement for social interaction, 758
        perceptual affected by early sensory deprivation, 759
        social, critical period in, 757–759
Developmental host specificity, 773
Developmental programs
    loose vs. strict constructionists, 744
Dexamethasone
    effect of on cortisol secretion, 724
    suppression test as diagnostic assay of depression, 725
Diabetes insipidus, 23
Diabetic neuropathy, 205
Diazoacholesterol, as inducer of myotonia, 207–208
Dichotic auditory test, 682d
Diencephalon, 231d
    development of, 246, 252–257
    dorsal, CT scan through, 263f
    hypothalamus in, 5f, 6
    lesions to affect memory, 813
    as major region of CNS, 213. *See also* Hypothalamus;
        Thalamus
    MRI of, 277f
    thalamus in, 5f, 6
    tumors in may cause coma, 66f
Differentiation, 731d
    nervous system, phases of, 734
Diffraction
    causes blurs in vision, 871
    and limit of spatial resolution, 871
Diffuse reticular formation, 6d
L-Dihydroxyphenylalanine (L-DOPA), 151
    as dopaminergic agonist, 712
    and locomotion, 484
    therapy for Parkinson's disease, 531
Dimorphism, 772d

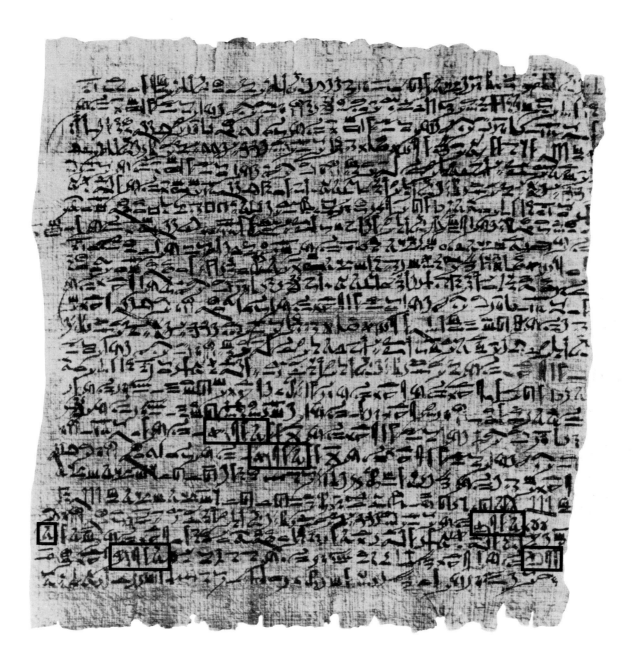

Columns II (left) and IV (right) of the Edwin Smith Surgical Papyrus

This papryus, written in the Seventeenth Century B.C., contains the earliest reference to the brain anywhere in human records. According to James Breasted, who translated and published the document in 1930, the word brain 𓄿𓇋𓇋𓊌 (*'yś*) occurs only 8 times in ancient Egyptian, 6 of them on these pages of the Smith Papyrus describing the symptoms, diagnosis and prognosis of two patients, wounded in the head, who had compound fractures of the skull. The entire treatise is now in the Rare Book Room of the New York Academy of Medicine.

Reference: Breasted, James Henry. The Edwin Smith Surgical Papyrus, 2 volumes. The University of Chicago Press, Chicago. 1930.

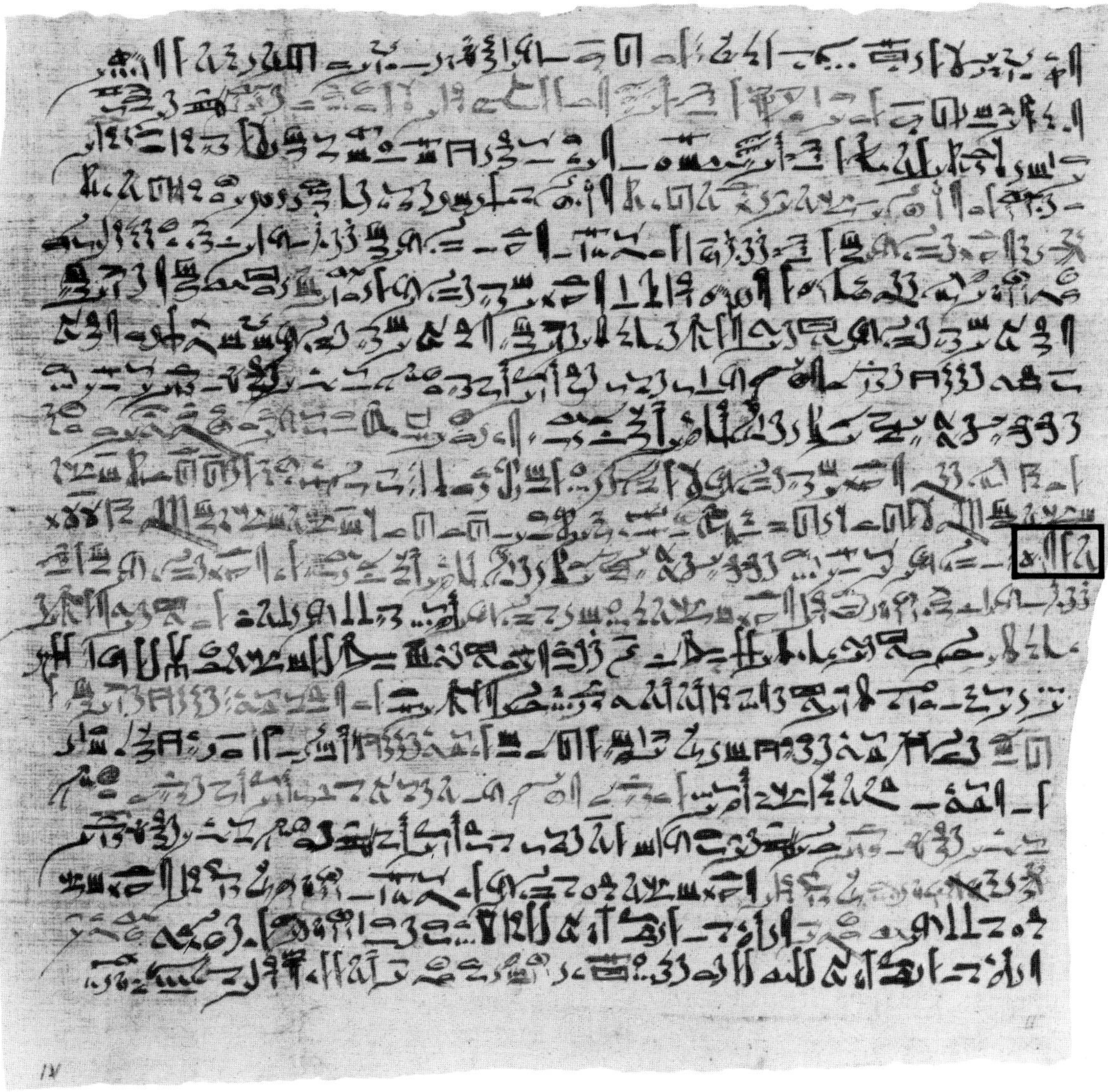